Sequelae and Long-Term Consequences of Infectious Diseases

Sequelae and Long-Term Consequences of Infectious Diseases

Edited by

Pina M. Fratamico
Eastern Regional Research Center
Agricultural Research Service
United States Department of Agriculture
Wyndmoor, Pennsylvania

James L. Smith
Eastern Regional Research Center
Agricultural Research Service
United States Department of Agriculture
Wyndmoor, Pennsylvania

Kim A. Brogden
Department of Periodontics and Dows Institute for Dental Research
College of Dentistry
University of Iowa
Iowa City, Iowa

ASM PRESS *Washington, D.C.*

American Society for Microbiology
1752 N St., N.W.
Washington, DC 20036-2904

Library of Congress Cataloging-in-Publication Data

Sequelae and long-term consequences of infectious diseases / edited by Pina M. Fratamico, James L. Smith, Kim A. Brogden.
p. ; cm.
Includes bibliographical references and index.
ISBN-13: 978-1-55581-430-4 (alk. paper)
ISBN-10: 1-55581-430-1 (alk. paper)
1. Communicable diseases—Complications. I. Fratamico, Pina M. II. Smith J. L. (James L.) III. Brogden, Kim A. IV. American Society for Microbiology.
[DNLM: 1. Communicable Diseases—complications. 2. Chronic Disease. WC 100 S479 2009]

RC112.S47 2009
616.9—dc22

2009008150

10 9 8 7 6 5 4 3 2 1

Address editorial correspondence to ASM Press, 1752 N St., N.W., Washington, DC 20036-2904, U.S.A.

Send orders to: ASM Press, P.O. Box 605, Herndon, VA 20172, U.S.A.
Phone: 800-546-2416; 703-661-1593
Fax: 703-661-1501
E-mail: books@asmusa.org
Online: http://estore.asm.org

Cover images (Top, from left.) Polymicrobial biofilm in the oral cavity (see Chapter 25); human coronary artery endothelial cells infected with *P. gingivalis* 381 (see Chapter 25); *B. burgdorferi* B31 visualized by fluorescence microscopy (Color Plate 1) (see Chapter 2); human lung tissue stained with an antibody to adenovirus E1A (Color Plate 17) (see Chapter 19); perivascular inflammatory infiltrate of the aortic wall (see Chapter 10). (Bottom, from left.) Polarized human intestinal epithelial cells infected with enteropathogenic *E. coli* (see Chapter 5); electron microscopic view of *T. whipplei* (see Chapter 11); periodic acid-Schiff–positive macrophages in lamina propria (Color Plate 7) (see Chapter 11); *Wuchereria bancrofti* (see Chapter 17); acute poststreptococcal glomerulonephritis (Color Plate 4) (see Chapter 6).

CONTENTS

CONTRIBUTORS

Fabio Albano
Department of Pediatrics, University Federico II of Naples, Via Sergio Pansini, 5, 80131 Naples, Italy

Roberto Arenas
Mycology Section, Dr. Manuel Gea González General Hospital, Tlalpan 4800, México DF 14000, Mexico

John C. Atherton
Wolfson Digestive Diseases Centre, University of Nottingham, Queen's Medical Centre, Nottingham NG7 2UH, United Kingdom

Giorgio Barbarini
Division of Infectious and Tropical Disease, Foundation IRCCS San Matteo Hospital, University of Pavia, Via Taramelli 5, 27100 Pavia, Italy

Giuseppe Barbaro
Department of Medical Pathophysiology, University La Sapienza, Rome, Italy

Myriam Bélanger
Center for Molecular Microbiology and Department of Oral Biology, College of Dentistry, University of Florida, Gainesville, FL 32610

Robert L. Bettiker
Section of Infectious Diseases, Temple University School of Medicine, Philadelphia, PA 19140

Kim A. Brogden
Dows Institute for Dental Research and Department of Periodontics, College of Dentistry, The University of Iowa, Iowa City, IA 52242

Sheldon T. Brown
Veterans Affairs Medical Center, Department of Medicine, Bronx, NY 10468

Raffaele Bruno
Division of Infectious and Tropical Disease, Foundation IRCCS San Matteo Hospital, University of Pavia, Via Taramelli 5, 27100 Pavia, Italy

Amaya L. Bustinduy
Department of Pediatrics, University Hospitals of Cleveland, Cleveland, OH 44106

Simone M. Cacciò
Department of Infectious, Parasitic and Immunomediated Diseases, Istituto Superiore di Sanità, Viale Regina Elena, 299, 00161 Rome, Italy

Kathryn M. Carbone
National Institutes of Health, MSC 4326, 8800 Rockville Pike, Bethesda, MD 20892

Teresa Corona
Instituto Nacional de Neurología y Neurocirugía, Manuel Velasco Suarez SSA, México City, Mexico

Toni Darville
Division of Infectious Diseases, Children's Hospital of Pittsburgh of University of Pittsburgh Medical Center, Pittsburgh, PA 15213

Jean-Pierre Dedet
Université Montpellier 1, CHU de Montpellier, Laboratoire de Parasitologie-Mycologie, CNRS, UMR 2724 (CNRS, IRD, and Université Montpellier 1), Montpellier, France

Gjorgi Deriban
Clinic of Gastroenterohepatology, Medical Faculty Skopje, ul. Vodnjanska 17, 1000 Skopje, Macedonia

Michael S. Donnenberg
Department of Medicine, Division of Infectious Diseases, Department of Microbiology and Immunology, University of Maryland School of Medicine, Baltimore, MD 21201

Brandy Ferguson
Duke University School of Medicine, Durham, NC 27705

Erol Fikrig
Yale University School of Medicine, Department of Internal Medicine, Infectious Diseases, 300 Cedar Street, New Haven, CT 06520-8031

Agnes Fleury
Instituto Nacional de Neurología y Neurocirugía, Manuel Velasco Suarez SSA, México City, Mexico

Ana Flisser
Facultad de Medicina, Universidad Nacional Autónoma de México (UNAM), México City, Mexico

José Flores-Rivera
Instituto Nacional de Neurología y Neurocirugía, Manuel Velasco Suarez SSA, México City, Mexico

Pina M. Fratamico
Microbial Food Safety Research Unit, Eastern Regional Research Center, Agricultural Research Service, United States Department of Agriculture, 600 East Mermaid Lane, Wyndmoor, PA 19038-6520

Alexandra H. Freeman
STD Prevention and Control Services, San Francisco Department of Public Health, San Francisco, CA 94103

Nishiena Gandhi
Department of Neurology/Neurosurgery, Johns Hopkins University School of Medicine, Baltimore, MD 21205

Thomas P. Gillis
Laboratory Research Branch at Louisiana State University, National Hansen's Disease Programs, Baton Rouge, LA 70803

Robert J. Greenstein
Veterans Affairs Medical Center, Department of Surgery, Bronx, NY 10468

Alfredo Guarino
Department of Pediatrics, University Federico II of Naples, Via Sergio Pansini, 5, 80131 Naples, Italy

Margaret R. Hammerschlag
Division of Infectious Diseases, Department of Pediatrics, SUNY Downstate Medical Center, Brooklyn, NY 11203-2098

Shizu Hayashi
James Hogg iCAPTURE Centre for Cardiovascular and Pulmonary Research, University of British Columbia, Vancouver, BC V6Z 1Y6, Canada

Richard G. Hegele
James Hogg iCAPTURE Centre for Cardiovascular and Pulmonary Research, University of British Columbia, Vancouver, BC V6Z 1Y6, Canada

James C. Hogg
James Hogg iCAPTURE Centre for Cardiovascular and Pulmonary Research, University of British Columbia, Vancouver, BC V6Z 1Y6, Canada

Joppe W. R. Hovius
Academic Medical Center, University of Amsterdam, Department of Internal Medicine, Center for Experimental and Molecular Medicine, 1105 AZ Amsterdam, The Netherlands, and Center for Infection and Immunity Amsterdam (CINIMA), Academic Medical Center, University of Amsterdam, Amsterdam, The Netherlands.

Georgia K. Johnson
Department of Periodontics, College of Dentistry, The University of Iowa, Iowa City, IA 52242

Sophie Joly
Dows Institute for Dental Research, College of Dentistry, The University of Iowa, Iowa City, IA 52242

Charles H. King
Center for Global Health and Diseases, Case Western Reserve University School of Medicine, Cleveland, OH 44106

Jeffrey D. Klausner
STD Prevention and Control Services, San Francisco Department of Public Health, San Francisco, CA 94103, and Divisions of AIDS and Infectious Diseases, Department of Medicine, University of California, School of Medicine, San Francisco, CA

Stephan A. Kohlhoff
Division of Infectious Diseases, Department of Pediatrics, SUNY Downstate Medical Center, Brooklyn, NY 11203-2098

Jeffrey D. Kravetz
Veterans Affairs Healthcare System, West Haven, CT 06516, and Yale University School of Medicine, New Haven, CT 06520

Benjamin D. Lorenz
Department of Medicine, Division of Infectious Diseases, University of Maryland School of Medicine, Baltimore, MD 21201

Per-Anders Mårdh
Department of Obstetrics and Gynaecology, Lund University, Lund, Sweden

Thomas Marth
Abteilung Innere Medizin, Krankenhaus Maria Hilf, Maria Hilf Str. 2, D-54550 Daun, Germany

E. David McIntosh
Imperial College, Faculty of Medicine, London SW7 2AZ, United Kingdom

Kåre Mølbak
Statens Serum Institut, 5 Artillerivej, 2300 Copenhagen S, Denmark

Gabriela Moreno
Mycology Section, Dr. Manuel Gea González General Hospital, Tlalpan 4800, México DF 14000, Mexico

Edoardo Pozio
Department of Infectious, Parasitic and Immunomediated Diseases, Istituto Superiore di Sanità, Viale Regina Elena, 299, 00161 Rome, Italy

Ann Progulske-Fox
Center for Molecular Microbiology and Department of Oral Biology, College of Dentistry, University of Florida, Gainesville, FL 32610

Judy R. Rees
Department of Community and Family Medicine, Dartmouth Hitchcock Medical Center, Lebanon, NH 03756

Adam Reich
Department of Dermatology, Venereology, and Allergology, Wroclaw Medical University, 50-368 Wroclaw, Poland

Karen Robinson
Centre for Biomolecular Sciences, University of Nottingham, University Park, Nottingham NG7 2RD, United Kingdom

Paolo Sacchi
Division of Infectious and Tropical Disease, Foundation IRCCS San Matteo Hospital, University of Pavia, Via Taramelli 5, 27100 Pavia, Italy

Rafik Samuel
Section of Infectious Diseases, Temple University School of Medicine, Philadelphia, PA 19140

Robert A. Schwartz
Department of Dermatology, New Jersey Medical School, Newark, NJ 07103

David S. Scollard
Laboratory Research Branch at Louisiana State University, National Hansen's Disease Programs, Baton Rouge, LA 70803

Christopher J. Silva
Foodborne Contaminants Research Unit, Agricultural Research Service, Western Regional Research Center, USDA, Albany, CA 94710

James L. Smith
Microbial Food Safety Research Unit, Eastern Regional Research Center, Agricultural Research Service, United States Department of Agriculture, 600 East Mermaid Lane, Wyndmoor, PA 19038-6520

David J. Sullivan, Jr.
Malaria Research Institute, Department of Molecular Microbiology and Immunology, Johns Hopkins University Bloomberg School of Public Health, Baltimore, MD 21205

Jacek C. Szepietowski
Department of Dermatology, Venereology, and Allergology, Wroclaw Medical University, 50-368 Wroclaw, Poland

Alje P. van Dam
Department of Medical Microbiology, Leiden University Medical Center, PO Box 9600, 2300 RC Leiden, The Netherlands

Elsa Vásquez-del-Mercado
Mycology Section, Dr. Manuel Gea González General Hospital, Tlalpan 4800, México DF 14000, Mexico

Christopher W. Woods
Duke University School of Medicine, Durham, NC 27705

PREFACE

Acute and chronic infections caused by viral, bacterial, fungal, and parasitic pathogens are still prevalent and continue to impose a large economic burden on local, national, and international economies. While acute diseases are of short duration, economic losses include those associated with treatment, recovery, and diminished worker productivity. Chronic diseases have a longer duration and result in greater economic losses related to treatment, associated disability, or death. In the United States alone, almost half of all Americans lived with at least one chronic condition (2005, 133 million people), chronic diseases accounted for 70% of all deaths, and the medical care costs of people with chronic diseases accounted for more than 75% of the nation's $2 trillion medical care costs (CDC, Chronic Disease Prevention and Health Promotion, 2008). Contributing to the costs of acute and chronic diseases are the sequelae and long-term consequences that have possible linkages to particular infections.

In *Sequelae and Long-Term Consequences of Infectious Diseases*, investigators relate many chronic illnesses, including specific types of cancers, paralysis, arthritis, peptic ulcer disease, cirrhosis, and neurological disorders, to prior infection with pathogenic microorganisms. Some associations of sequelae and infection are putative or strongly suspected, and these microbe-disease links must be unequivocally proved or disproved by rigorous studies to establish proof of causality. Certain pathogens are more likely to cause life-threatening disease and long-term sequelae in individuals with an impaired immune status, including the elderly, pregnant women, young children, organ transplant recipients, cancer patients, and individuals infected with human immunodeficiency virus. An individual's immune status, a genetic predisposition towards certain disorders, and other host and microbial factors come into play in influencing the outcome of infections with pathogens that can trigger chronic illnesses.

It is difficult to identify specific pathogens as the triggers of chronic illnesses because the effects may not be manifested until weeks or months after the acute infection has subsided. Much of the relevant literature may be scattered in numerous reports and publications that are not readily available. Medical professionals and researchers find themselves performing time-consuming and arduous searches of the scientific literature in libraries and "on-line" to find the association of specific symptoms with an underlying infectious agent. The purpose of *Sequelae and Long-Term Consequences of Infectious Diseases* is to provide a single source covering various aspects of long-term sequelae of infectious diseases. In addition to covering the diseases and their sequelae, the genetic and immunological statuses of the afflicted individuals are discussed in terms of the infection, disease progression, and symptoms as well as treatment options. The first chapter calls attention to the impediments and technical hurdles that need to be overcome to draw critical linkages between an infectious etiology and a chronic illness. Diseases caused by bacteria (*Borrelia burgdorferi*, *Chlamydia*, enteric bacteria, *Escherichia coli*, *Streptococcus*, *Staphylococcus*, *Helicobacter pylori*, *Neisseria gonorrhoeae*, *Treponema pallidum*, *Tropheryma whipplei*, and *Porphyromonas gingivalis*), parasites (*Toxoplasma gondii*, *Taenia solium*, *Cryptosporidium parvum*, *Plasmodium*, Trypanosomatidae, and helminths), various viruses, fungi, and prions are covered in subsequent chapters. In addition, there is a chapter on diseases suspected of having an infectious etiology and finally a chapter devoted to discussing the importance of epidemiological methods for confirming, refuting, or modifying links between specific microorganisms and the complications and long-term consequences. For example, epidemiological studies were critical in associating *Campylobacter* infection with Guillian-Barré syndrome; *Helicobacter pylori* infection with peptic ulcers; Epstein Barr virus with malignant disease, including Burkitt's lymphoma and Hodgkin's disease; hepatitis B virus and liver cancer; human herpesvirus 8 and Kaposi's sarcoma; and human papilloma virus with cervical cancer. The final chapter presents a brief overview of the sequelae of infectious agents and the economic burden associated with these infections and also suggests future directions towards progress on this concept.

The chapters in this text emphasize the transmissible agents that play important roles in diseases that were not originally known to be infectious in origin. The book should prove of interest to microbiologists, virologists, parasitologists, mycologists, academicians, medical students, and students in the life sciences and allied health sciences, and individuals in the pharmacological and vaccine industries and government agencies. We hope that this book will fill a critical void in the scientific literature, contributing to providing evidence of the causal links between infectious agents and chronic disorders, and most importantly, stimulating research in this area. A multidisciplinary research approach to seek answers on the causes of chronic illnesses will lead to the development of new treatments and preventive strategies that will affect the lives of a large segment of the population.

We gratefully acknowledge the assistance of James Nataro in the preparation of the book proposal, and we also extend heartfelt thanks to all of the authors of the various chapters for contributing their time, knowledge, and expertise to this endeavor. It has been a privilege and a pleasure working with such an exceptional group of professionals.

Pina M. Fratamico, James L. Smith, and Kim A. Brogden

Sequelae and Long-Term Consequences of Infectious Diseases
Edited by Pina M. Fratamico, James L. Smith, and Kim A. Brogden
© 2009 ASM Press, Washington, DC

Chapter 1

Infectious Causes of Chronic Disease: from Hypothesis to Proof

KATHRYN M. CARBONE

Infectious diseases kill more children and young adults than any other diseases, taking a huge personal and economic toll on individual households (e.g., lost wages) and across nations (e.g., slowing economies and increasing medical costs) (57, 74). Chronic diseases caused by infectious organisms vary widely, e.g., liver cancer and hepatitis B/C virus infection, cervical cancer and human papilloma virus infection, arthritis and *Borrelia burgdorferi*, lymphoma and Epstein-Barr virus infection, and ulcer/gastric cancer and *Helicobacter pylori* (17, 28, 34, 40, 50), yet they are connected by the vastness of the economic and personal costs associated with chronic disease and the psychological, technical, and medical hurdles that need to be overcome to provide causal linkages between an infectious etiology and a chronic disease. The total economic burden from infectious diseases is likely even larger than suspected, since few, if any, cost figures include chronic illnesses suspected of having a link to infectious disease, e.g., dilated myocardiopathies, multiple sclerosis, inflammatory bowel disease, diabetes, atherosclerosis, and dementia (Table 1).

Why focus on infectious diseases as etiologies of chronic disease? Unlike many incurable chronic medical diseases, diseases caused by infectious etiologies may be prevented or cured through medical treatments (e.g., vaccines or antimicrobials, respectively) that are a fraction of the cost of lifetime chronic medical care. Thus, the desire to find an infectious cause for major chronic medical illnesses stems, in part, from the hope of curing or preventing these illnesses.

TURNING THE TIDE OF MEDICAL PRACTICE: FROM HYPOTHESIS TO PROOF TO PATIENT CARE

> . . .submit your work to peer review or even better to a committee of experts. If the work receives acclaim then it means that it is part of the conventional wisdom, and is not original. If rejected it might be original; if dismissed out of hand, it probably is. (49)

Medical dogma changes slowly and with a significant degree of retrograde amnesia about the sometimes arduous process to find the "truth" about chronic disease etiologies and lodge it firmly into conventional medical wisdom. For example, it is likely that someday the fact that *Borrelia burgdorferi* is an infectious cause of a childhood arthritic syndrome that used to be diagnosed as juvenile rheumatoid arthritis will fade from clinical medical memory (10, 53, 59). Historically, many chronic, idiopathic diseases that "looked like" infections have indeed been demonstrated to be caused by infectious pathogens, and many of them are described in the chapters that follow. However, since there persist many disease syndromes that appear to be consistent with an infectious etiology for which no infection has convincingly and causally been linked, such as Crohn's disease and multiple sclerosis, research into infectious causes of chronic diseases is still an active area.

The initial proof of an infectious organism's causal link to a chronic disease often meets resistance to acceptance and requires several years of research by various teams of researchers to isolate the organism, develop a reliable clinical test, and document the association of the organism with human disease through clinical studies. Thus, identifying the "best practices" behind successful medical documentation of infectious etiologies of chronic disease will help streamline and, it is hoped, expedite the success of the process. Failure to recognize the patterns and effective pathways of this type of research forces medical scientists to "reinvent the wheel" each time it is necessary to turn prevailing medical opinion that may resist accepting these novel hypotheses and data. Further, inadvertent mistakes or poor scientific rigor/

Kathryn M. Carbone • National Institutes of Health, MSC 4326, 8800 Rockville Pike, Bethesda, MD 20892.

Table 1. Studies of economic burdens of chronic diseases in the United States[a]

Chronic illness (reference)	Estimated cost/yr (US$)[b]
Dementia (2)	148 Billion
Diabetes (69)	132 Billion
Chronic prostatitis (19)	84 Million
Cancer (49a)	72.1 Billion
End-stage kidney disease (33)	20.1 Billion
Heart failure (41)	3.2 Billion
IBD (46)	1.8 Billion

[a] The methods vary widely among studies. The citations are selected for illustrative purposes, and the cost figures cited are generally estimates—but the message is clear—chronic diseases cost a great deal. IBD, inflammatory bowel disease.
[b] May include direct medical costs, loss of productivity, or both.

methodology may produce data that *inaccurately* link an infection to a chronic disease. For this, there is a substantial price to pay; in addition to the waste of time and research resources expended and loss of patient trust, the resistance of medical dogma to the *next* novel etiological hypothesis that comes along (which may be the correct one) increases. The question is, then, how best to efficiently support high-quality, original, and creative hypothesis development and proof linking infectious pathogens to chronic diseases while avoiding erroneous associations as much as humanly possible?

An example of a "close but no cigar" association of an infectious agent with disease occurred in the late 1880s when the microbiologist Richard Pfeiffer isolated a bacillus, later named *Haemophilus influenzae*, from patients with influenza (67, 68). The general medical community accepted that this bacterium was the etiology of influenza, and the failure to identify *H. influenzae* in some patients with influenza was attributed to poor culture techniques and the fastidious nature of the agent. In 1920, when Olitzky and Gates demonstrated that the etiology of influenza was a "non-filterable" infectious agent (i.e., the early definition of a virus and therefore not a bacterium), the medical community was resistant to this shift in etiological paradigm (51). It wasn't until the next decade that influenza virus was identified in pigs and humans, and finally the acceptance of the viral etiology of influenza replaced the medical dogma of a bacterial causative agent (21, 22, 44). It bears underscoring that it took decades of scientific investigation and the development of new scientific technology/methods to identify, *and for the medical community to accept*, the correct infectious etiology of this common and serious infectious disease.

The good news is that the modern medical community is getting better at identifying and linking new infectious agents to disease syndromes. In recent history, the most infamous and most devastating new infectious pathogen to be identified as the cause of a chronic illness was, of course, human immunodeficiency virus (HIV), the etiology of AIDS (5, 9). In the early 1980s, clinicians and medical researchers noted that homosexual men were experiencing a pattern of unusual illnesses, some minor (e.g., odd mouth lesions and swollen lymph glands) and some serious (e.g., pneumocystis pneumonia, Kaposi's sarcoma, and lymphoma) (13). This new syndrome, labeled "gay compromise syndrome," "gay related immunodeficiency syndrome," or AIDS (8, 14, 70), stimulated a host of hypothesized etiologies, including abuse of chemical substances and infection with well-known viruses, such as cytomegalovirus (CMV) (26, 30, 43).

Clinicians treating the exponentially increasing numbers of disfigured, disabled, and dying patients and other medical scientists noted that both these groups, substance abusers and homosexual men, were at high risk for infectious agents transmitted through both blood and sexual contact, such as hepatitis B virus, and that this fact strongly suggested an infectious etiology of AIDS (3, 15).

In contrast to what occurred with influenza, thanks to the worldwide groundbreaking efforts of teams of clinical researchers, epidemiologists, immunologists, and virologists specializing in animal and human retroviruses, only approximately 3 years elapsed between the publication of the first patient series and the identification of the infectious etiology of AIDS. Because AIDS was demonstrated to be the result of infection with HIV, the door was opened for development of effective drugs to suppress viral replication, and treated HIV infection has gone from medical mystery and deadly epidemic in the 1980s to potentially controllable chronic disease in the 21st century (27, 47). Further progress has been made in etiologic "microbe hunting" since the 1980s. Early in the 21st century it took only a few months to identify and confirm the human coronavirus as the cause of severe acute respiratory syndrome or SARS (58, 64). Clearly, the epidemiological, medical diagnostic, and molecular biological advances and "lessons learned" in the wake of the AIDS epidemic contributed to the speed with which the agent of SARS was identified and, thankfully, contained.

Today it all seems somewhat obvious and straightforward. A postmortem on the features that contributed to the successful solving of these medical mysteries would indicate that the acute, life-threatening, and novel natures of the HIV and SARS coronavirus epidemics were critical features that stimulated an intense scientific focus on and the allocation of resources for the successful identification and linking of an infectious agent to a disease syndrome. In other words, modern medical science appears to do a good job of identifying infectious etiologies of new disease syndromes, if the disease is novel and serious. In contrast, for many well-known "idiopathic" chronic diseases that have been with us for centuries, the efforts to discover an infectious etiology, even when ultimately successful, have been less expeditious. Perhaps because these "idiopathic" illnesses have been part of the medical practice fabric for so long, there appears to be less of a sense of urgency, and, as a result, less of a coordinated, multidisciplinary research effort.

In fact, there is more than passive resistance to studies of possible infectious causes of chronic disease. In part, the skepticism is founded on experience, because many etiologic pathogens have been proposed for some of these diseases without success. When this skepticism is unfounded, it extracts a personal and professional cost for the investigators who toil to identify and study these hypotheses and for the patients who are inflicted with what might be medically curable or treatable infectious diseases. On the other hand, such resistance to change may also serve a valuable purpose, i.e., to set a high bar for scientific methods and evidence that is of the quality and robustness needed to ensure that the new hypotheses of specific etiologies of chronic idiopathic diseases are accurate and thus worthy enough to alter standard medical care.

IMPEDIMENTS TO DEMONSTRATING CAUSAL ASSOCIATIONS BETWEEN AN INFECTIOUS AGENT AND A CHRONIC DISEASE

Infectious diseases are often clinically identified based on characteristic signs of acute infection (e.g., fever and hypotension), although clearly noninfectious diseases can closely mimic the signs of infectious diseases (e.g., allergic drug reactions). Classically, infections are confirmed either by identification of the presence of the infectious agent (e.g., through culture or antigen/nucleic acid detection) or through evidence of a specific immune response, typically antibody seroconversion response. In acute infections the tight temporal association of a suspected etiologic organism with signs/symptoms/immune responses makes demonstration of the causal linkage relatively straightforward. For example, a common infectious disease such as acute measles can be easily diagnosed from clinical signs, such as Koplik's spots in the mouth, and connected with a measles virus infection by evidence of seroconversion from measles antibody-negative status prior to or early in the infection to seropositivity with high measles antibody titers following recovery and clearance of the virus (31).

The linkage of a specific organism with a specific infectious disease may be straightforward *if* the disease has classic signs and symptoms of acute infection, the disease is clinically apparent soon after infection with the organism and occurs in most or all infected individuals, the organism is a known microbe, *and* a test exists for demonstrating either the organism or the immune response to it. However, for chronic diseases caused by infectious agents, the unequivocal demonstration of a causal infectious etiology and acceptance as medical dogma are rarely so straightforward. It may instead be an arduous process, requiring (i) an astute clinical suspicion of infection in a not-classically acute infectious disease syndrome, (ii) development and validation of a suitable diagnostic test to confirm the presence of an organism (current or past infection), (iii) demonstration of a causal association of disease with the microbe through a well-designed clinical study, and (iv) a persistent group of basic scientists and clinicians to shepherd those findings into the standard medical knowledge base.

Medical advances often start with astute clinicians recognizing unexpected new patterns in their daily medical practice. This clinical acumen is hard to define, quantify, and standardize but is most worthy of mention. For example, a clinical pediatrician was one of the first who raised the alarm that viral meningitis seemed to be associated with mumps vaccination with the Urabe vaccine strain, a vaccine used in Europe, Canada, and Japan, but not the United States (45; Earl Brown, personal communications); later, numerous studies supported this theory, resulting in the large-scale removal of this vaccine from clinical use in many countries (7). As discussed above, clinicians identified the AIDS epidemic through recognition of unusual patterns of Kaposi's sarcoma, lymphoma, CMV, and pneumocystis infections in previously healthy homosexual men. It is worth highlighting this important step in medical discovery in order to encourage those clinicians on the "front lines" of medical care that their creative applications of clinical acumen count and, indeed, can jump-start new lines of medical scientific research.

Epidemiology provides a more defined and rigorous approach to recognizing and demonstrating that new patterns of disease are new infectious diseases. Epidemiology can help provide evidence supporting that a specific pattern suggests or refutes an infectious etiology of a chronic disease (see Chapter 27). Excellent examples of the usefulness of the epidemiological scientific approach and public health impact are the studies which have failed to demonstrate association between measles vaccines and autism (16a).

Some infectious diseases have life cycles and/or disease mechanisms that further complicate the ability of modern science to draw critical linkages. Increasing layers of difficulty in proving causal associations between infectious agents and chronic disease may arise from those situations in which a serious chronic disease may afflict only a small proportion of infected individuals (e.g., measles-associated subacute sclerosing panencephalitis) (55) or only after a prolonged, asymptomatic latent or persistent infection (e.g., HIV, JC virus infection and progressive multifocal leukoencephalopathy, or Epstein-Barr virus and lymphoma) (6, 12). Further, differences in host-specific genetic makeups also impact disease outcomes, as seen in the variability in risk of contracting leprosy and the variability in disease manifestations (1). In other words, matrixes of studies may need to be performed to *first* identify that a chronic disease is associated with a specific genetic marker and *then* attempt to document that there is a specific infection causing the chronic disease of interest in people with this specific genetic makeup. But there is hope, as shown by the headway made in the connections between infection and host genetic makeup in rheumatic diseases, particularly arthritis (25). Acquired host characteristics, such as malnutrition, can be variable risk factors (16). Linking specific pathogens to a chronic disease is also difficult when multiple pathogens in combination appear to be "cooperative" etiologic agents of chronic disease, as seen in periodontal disease (38). Clinical presentations of infection with the same microbe may also vary, depending upon the route of infection, the developmental age of the host at the time of infection, and the natural history of infection (e.g., whether the agent is in the acute or latent/persistent stage of infection). For example, the expressions of chronic diseases of the psychiatric, neurologic, endocrine, ophthalmologic, cardiovascular, and immune systems may vary due to all those situational factors in chronic rubella virus, CMV, and congenital and perinatal HIV infections (42). Many of the generic signs and symptoms of infectious disease, such as fever, disseminated intravascular coagulation, and shock, result from the responses of the host's immune system associated with infection, such as the often-fatal Ebola virus infection (75). Accordingly, chronic disease outcomes may be a product of the immune, fibrotic, or other maladaptive or protective host responses that are by-products of an infection, such as fibrosing mediastinitis seen in histoplasmosis infection and rheumatic syndromes following persistent hepatitis virus infections (4, 63).

TECHNICAL BARRIERS AND BRIDGES TO IDENTIFYING INFECTIOUS CAUSES OF CHRONIC DISEASE

The question remains, then, how to prevent researchers from traveling unproductive and expensive pathways to look for infectious agents when the etiology is truly not an infectious pathogen, without stifling the creative scientific process to make connections that do exist. On the path to new discoveries, scientific false starts or erroneous hypotheses/conclusions are seen even under the most rigorous experimental design and execution; however, studies that are poorly designed or executed without rigor unnecessarily divert resources and time and damage the public's trust of the scientific community.

Once a theory has been developed from clinical medicine or epidemiological study, a critical step in the search for infectious etiologies of chronic diseases is the creation and testing of a reliable, sensitive, and specific test and standards with which to confirm the presence, current or past, of a specific etiological agent. The lack of such a diagnostic test and standards significantly hinders etiological discovery and clinical practice, as seen with both Whipple's disease and Lyme disease (60, 73). In the most straightforward approach to diagnostic testing, patient samples are taken to culture for living organisms—sounds simple and works well for many standard infectious agents, but the risk with a search for unknown organisms is that the possibility of a requirement for special additives, handling, or cell substrates means that a negative result is often not meaningful (55).

Fortunately, other techniques have provided good options for the identification of infectious agents (24). For many infections, it is easier, faster, and more reproducible to demonstrate the organism's "footprint" than to recover the infectious agent itself, e.g., to identify the presence of pathogen-specific antibody or antigens using easily quantifiable methods, such as enzyme-linked immunosorbent assay. For many other infections known or suspected to be associated with chronic diseases, such as Lyme disease and hepatitis C virus-induced cirrhosis, developing reliably predictive serological assays has been difficult and not fully successful or, at the very least, controversial (32, 65, 66). Over the last decade, nucleic acid-based testing has evolved from a bench laboratory research method to a standard clinical practice, and DNA microarray, in situ hybridization, and nucleic acid sequencing are slowly but surely wending their way into clinical diagnostic laboratories (29, 36, 48). The nucleic acid amplification methods, like PCR or reverse transcriptase PCR, have sensitivity and specificity levels that are advantageous for clinical diagnosis but also carry a risk of false positive results due to contamination (71). For that reason the use of these nucleic acid amplification methods and research reports associating specific infections with chronic diseases that used these techniques were typically viewed with some skepticism; internal controls and careful handling to avoid contamination have increased the trustworthy reputation of these methods. Nonetheless, regardless of the assays used in initial demonstrations of a novel infectious agent, questions of technical artifact always arise, necessitating cooperative studies, meta-analysis of the literature, a weighing in of expert opinions, and international consensus meetings in response to the controversy generated (e.g., SV40 virus and mesothelioma) (62, 72).

Even well-intended, well-designed scientific studies and techniques and their conclusions can be subverted by sampling and sample-processing procedures that go awry. Sampling the wrong clinical site or unintentional postsampling mishandling can lead to false negative or false positive results. Further, across the board, all positive tests for the presence of organisms, even from the ill host, are susceptible to the clinical dilemma of interpreting if the host is merely colonized by an innocent microbial agent, i.e., the organism is present but not responsible for the clinical disease. Recently, increasing attention has been paid to the active symbiotic relationship of humans with their microbial flora in the mouth, gut, vagina, skin, etc., possibly complicating the situation by making the formerly distinct line between "colonizer" and "pathogen" a continuum of "microbiome" (23, 35).

If the offending pathogen is physically present or has come and gone, reliably documenting the organism or its "footprints," respectively, is a necessary (but not sufficient) step for connecting pathogens to chronic disease. A diagnostic test is needed with the robustness to be successfully utilized in the clinical and not just the research laboratory setting, as well as used by multiple laboratories with various degrees of technical expertise (39, 61). *Formal* evaluations (e.g., validations) of the sensitivity and specificity of the diagnostic test, including the use of standardized positive/negative control reagents, are an absolute necessity. Note that these developmental evaluations and validations must be carried out on "known" positive/negative control samples; although it seems obvious that a test method cannot be evaluated using unknown samples, the temptation to attempt to "test the test" and use these data to correlate an infection with a disease presentation should not occur at the same time. Only after an appropriate diagnostic test has been designed and formally evaluated in a single laboratory and validated by multiple laboratories using standardized positive and negative samples can the general scientific and medical community be assured of the durability and reliability of this diagnostic test in a variety of settings. Further, results of diagnostic tests may be less variable when these tests are designed with quantitative, automated, high-throughput numeric outputs to indicate positive or negative outcomes; by definition, any test readout that requires reader judgment or specialized reader expertise injects a significant measure of subjectivity and thus variability, making a consensus on the test's value and widespread clinical utility more difficult.

Initial clinical studies designed to test for pathogens that might be responsible for chronic diseases are often initially performed in a post hoc manner as a means of hypothesis development; medical scientists are reasonably reluctant to accept such exploratory testing results as proof of a causal association of the infection with the disease of interest. In other words, going to a laboratory freezer and performing unblinded testing on samples from poorly characterized subjects with a specific disease and then comparing the results to tests results from a set of unmatched healthy control subjects (e.g., laboratory workers who have not been age-sex-socioeconomic status-matched to the subjects) is an inadequately designed clinical study that cannot be used as evidence for proving a causal connection of a pathogen with a specific disease entity. Convincing and rigorous demonstration of a causal etiological association between an organism and a specific disease needs a high-quality "translational" type of science that connects bench research (e.g., organism identification, test development) to clinical research (e.g., well-controlled and -designed human studies). This cross-discipline research necessitates either an outstanding medical scientist with formal training in bench and clinical research or a cooperative team of scientists with complementary expertise. Application of a validated diagnostic test in prospectively designed, blinded, and well-controlled clinical studies, with sufficient numbers of carefully characterized and matched subjects with and without disease, is needed to provide a meaningful statistical analysis of the results and a reliable conclusion of causal etiological associations between infections and chronic diseases. Moreover, results from such studies performed by several independent research groups are reasonably required to provide sufficient evidence to impact medical thinking significantly.

PSYCHOLOGICAL, SOCIOLOGICAL, AND PERSONAL BARRIERS TO CHANGING MEDICAL DOGMA

Careful attention to the quality of the experimental approaches (both laboratory and clinical research), diagnostic test development, and appropriate analysis of the studies are needed to create new pathogen-disease associations that can advance current medical science. However, it is impossible to ignore the downstream psychological and sociological reaction to novel medical scientific hypotheses and data, since both accurate and inaccurate conclusions can strongly impact clinical medicine performance and even the fabric of society. If studies that have less-than-rigorous study design and execution (or have unanticipated artifacts) incorrectly suggest an association between an organism and a disease, other scientists may be inhibited from taking new (and more accurate) pathways in their research, and resources are wasted by leading others to pursue scientific inquiry down the same disingenuous pathways. When wrong conclusions or inaccurate data come to light, they can weaken public trust in medical science. Imagine the possible societal repercussions of concluding that serious psychiatric disease was caused by an infectious agent (52). Medical science discovery is a fluid and ever-moving (and oft repetitive) process, and 100% accuracy is hard if not possible to obtain; nonetheless, the responsibility to develop sound, high-quality hypotheses, testing techniques, and clinical study design should weigh heavily on all researchers and those who rely on them.

One might assume that since research is a novel and creative venture, it would follow that the novel discoveries arising from the creative scientific process would be rapidly embraced and invested into medical practice; often, however, that is not the case. In fact, the sociology of the research community seems to exhibit more of a "show me" culture, requiring multiple confirmatory studies before leaps beyond current knowledge are accepted (56). This seemingly oxymoronic response of slow acceptance of novel scientific reports has the protective effect of preventing inaccurate scientific conclusions from too rapidly becoming medical science dogma—a novel scientific finding must show robustness and stand the test of time; however, it also can make for a slow process and is sometimes personally taxing for the scientists. Some researchers who have proposed connecting a new infectious agent to a chronic disease have taken the drastic step of testing the final proof of Koch's postulates on themselves, including inducing ulcers by swallowing *Helicobacter pylori* or self-inducing (fatal) yellow fever through exposure to infected mosquitoes to test a vector hypothesis (37, 54). Another contributor to the lag time between medical discovery and medical application is the increasing pace of basic scientific discoveries in settings that lack the infrastructure needed to rapidly translate these scientific gains into medical reality (49b).

CONCLUSIONS

The combination of creative, novel thinking and essential but-not-very-glamorous rigorous diagnostic test development (e.g., assay validation and standards) makes the pursuit of infectious etiologies for chronic diseases an exciting yet challenging pursuit. This book illustrates the value of working collaboratively to seek answers that may provide more hope to those with currently incurable chronic diseases. As described in the chapters that follow, there is much we know, yet much we need to discover.

REFERENCES

1. **Alter, A., A. Alcaïs, L. Abel, and E. Schurr.** 2008. Leprosy as a genetic model for susceptibility to common infectious diseases. *Hum. Genet.* **123:**227–235.
2. **Alzheimer's Association.** 2008. 2008 Alzheimer's disease facts and figures. *Alzheimers Dement.* **4:**110–133.
3. **Ammann, A. J., M. J. Cowan, D. W. Wara, P. Weintrub, S. Dritz, H. Goldman, and H. A. Perkins.** 1983. Acquired immunodeficiency in an infant: possible transmission by means of blood products. *Lancet* **i:**956–958.
4. **Antonelli, A., C. Ferri, M. Galeazzi, C. Giannitti, D. Mmanno, G. Mieli-Vergani, E. Menegatti, T. Olivieri, M. Puoti, C. Palazzi, D. Roccatello, D. Vergani, P. Sarzi-Puttini, and F. Atzeni.** 2008. HCV infection: pathogenesis, clinical manifestations and therapy. *Clin. Exp. Rheumatol.* **26**(Suppl. 48):S39–S47.
5. **Barré-Sinoussi, F., J. C. Chermann, F. Rey, M. T. Nugeyre, S. Chamaret, J. Gruest, C. Dauguet, C. Axler-Blin, F. Vézinet-Brun, C. Rouzioux, W. Rozenbaum, and L. Montagnier.** 1983. Isolation of a T-lymphotropic retrovirus from a patient at risk for acquired immune deficiency syndrome (AIDS). *Science* **220:**868–871.
6. **Berger, J. R.** 2007. Progressive multifocal encephalopathy. *Curr. Neurol. Neurosci. Rep.* **7:**461–469.
7. **Bonnet, M. C., A. Dutta, C. Weinberger, and S. A. Plotkin.** 2006. Mumps vaccine virus strains and aseptic meningitis. *Vaccine* **24:**7037–7045.
8. **Brennan, R. O., and D. T. Durack.** 1981. Gay compromise syndrome. *Lancet* **ii:**1338–1339.
9. **Broder, S., and R. C. Gallo.** 1984. A pathogenic retrovirus (HTLV-III) linked to AIDS. *N. Engl. J. Med.* **311:**1292–1297.
10. **Burgdorfer, W.** 1994. Discovery of the Lyme disease spirochete and its relation to tick vectors. *Yale J. Biol. Med.* **57:** 515–520.
11. Reference deleted.
12. **Carbone, A., A. Gloghini, and G. Dotti.** 2008. EBV-associated lymphoproliferative disorders: classification and treatment. *Oncologist* **13:**577–585.

13. **CDC.** 1981. Kaposi's sarcoma and *Pneumocystis* pneumonia among homosexual men—New York City and California. *MMWR Morb. Mortal. Wkly. Rep.* **30:**305–308.
14. **CDC.** 1982. Update on acquired immune deficiency syndrome (AIDS)–United States. *MMWR Morb. Mortal. Wkly. Rep.* **31:**507–508, 513–514.
15. **Curran, J. W., D. N. Lawrence, H. Jaffe, J. E. Kaplan, L. D. Zyla, M. Chamberland, R. Weinstein, K. J. Lui, L. B. Schonberger, T. J. Spira, W. J. Alexander, G. Swinger, A. Ammann, S. Solomon, D. Auerbach, D. Mildvan, R. Stoneburner, J. M. Jason, H. W. Haverkos, and B. L. Evatt.** 1984. Acquired immunodeficiency syndrome (AIDS) associated with transfusions. *N. Engl. J. Med.* **310:**69–75.
16. **Curtis, L. T.** 2008. Prevention of hospital-acquired infections: review of non-pharmacological interventions. *J. Hosp. Infect.* **69:**204–219.
16a. **DeStefano, F.** 2007. Vaccines and autism: evidence does not support a causal association. *Clin. Pharmacol. Ther.* **86:**756–759.
17. **de The, G.** 1995. Viruses and human cancers: challenges for preventative strategies. *Environ. Health Perspect.* **103**(Suppl. 8):269–273.
18. Reference deleted.
19. **Duloy, A. M., E. A. Calhoun, and J. Q. Clemens.** 2007. Economic impact of chronic prostatitis. *Curr. Urol. Rep.* **8:** 336–339.
20. Reference deleted.
21. **Francis, T., Jr.** 1934. Transmission of influenza by a filterable virus. *Science* **80:**457–459.
22. **Francis, T., Jr., and T. P. Magill.** 1935. Cultivation of human influenza virus in an artificial medium. *Science* **82:**353–354.
23. **Frank, D. N., and N. R. Pace.** 2008. Gastrointestinal microbiology enters the metagenomics era. *Curr. Opin. Gastroenterol.* **24:**4–10.
24. **Gao, S. J., and P. S. Moore.** 1996. Molecular approaches to the identification of unculturable infectious agents. *Emerg. Infec. Dis.* **2:**159–167.
25. **Girschick, H. J., L. Guilherme, R. D. Inman, K. Latsch, M. Rihl, Y. Sherer, Y. Shoenfeld, H. Zeidler, S. Arienti, and A. Doria.** 2008. Bacterial triggers and autoimmune rheumatic diseases. *Clin. Exp. Rheumatol.* **26**(Suppl. 48):S12–S17.
26. **Gottlieb, M. S., R. Schroff, H. M. Schanker, J. D. Weisman, P. T. Fan, R. A. Wolf, and A. Saxon.** 1981. *Pneumocystis carinii* pneumonia and mucosal candidiasis in previously healthy homosexual men: evidence of a new acquired cellular immunodeficiency. *N. Engl. J. Med.* **305:**1425–1431.
27. **Hammer, S. M., J. J. Eron, Jr., P. Reiss, R. T. Schooley, M. A. Thompson, S. Walmsley, P. Cahn, M. A. Fischl, J. M. Gatell, M. S. Hirsch, D. M. Jacobsen, J. S. Monaer, D. D. Richman, P. G. Yeni, P. A. Volberding, and International AIDS Society–USA.** 2008. Antiretroviral treatment of adult HIV infection: 2008 recommendations of the International AIDS Society–USA panel. *JAMA* **300:**555–570.
28. **Hutton, D. W., D. Tan, S. K. So, and M. L. Brandeau.** 2007. Cost-effectiveness of screening and vaccinating Asian and Pacific Islander adults for hepatitis B. *Ann. Intern. Med.* **147:**460–469.
29. **Ieven, M.** 2007. Currently used nucleic acid amplification tests for the detection of viruses and atypicals in acute respiratory infections. *J. Clin. Virol.* **40:**259–276.
30. **Jaffe, H. W., K. Choi, P. A. Thomas, H. W. Haverkos, D. M. Auerbach, M. E. Guinan, M. F. Rogers, T. J. Spira, W. W. Darrow, M. A. Kramer, S. M. Friedman, J. M. Monroe, A. E. Friedman-Kien, L. J. Laubenstein, M. Marmor, B. Safai, S. K. Dritz, S. J. Crispi, S. L. Fannin, J. P. Orkwis, A. Kelter, W. R. Rushing, S. B. Thacker, and J. W. Curran.** 1983. National case-control study of Kaposi's sarcoma and *Pneumocystis carinii* pneumonia in homosexual men: part 1. Epidemiological results. *Ann. Intern. Med.* **99:**145–151.
31. **Jahan, S., A. M. Al Saigul, M. A. Abu Baker, A. O. Altaya, and S. A. Hamed.** 2008. Measles outbreak in Qassim, Saudi Arabia 2007: epidemiology and evaluation of the outbreak response. *J. Public Health* [Epub ahead of print.] doi:10.1093/pubmed/fdn070.
32. **Johnson, L., and R. B. Stricker.** 2004. Treatment of Lyme disease: a medicolegal assessment. *Expert Rev. Anti Infect. Ther.* **2:**533–557.
33. **Khan, S., and C. A. Amedia, Jr.** 2008. Economic burden of chronic kidney disease. *J. Eval. Clin. Pract.* **14:**422–434.
34. **Kim, J. J., and S. J. Goldie.** 2008. Health and economic implications of HPV vaccination in the United States. *N. Engl. J. Med.* **359:**821–831.
35. **Kinross, J. M., A. C. von Roon, E. Holmes, A. Darzi, and J. K. Nicholson.** 2008. The human gut microbiome: implications for future health care. *Curr. Gastroenterol. Rep.* **10:**396–403.
36. **Klouche, M., and U. Schröder.** 2008. Rapid methods for diagnosis of bloodstream infections. *Clin. Chem. Lab. Med.* **46:**888–908.
37. **Konturek, J. W.** 2003. Discovery by Jaworski of *Helicobacter pylori* and its pathogenetic role in peptic ulcer, gastritis and gastric cancer. *J. Physiol. Pharmacol.* **54**(Suppl. 3):23–41.
38. **Kuramitsu, H. K., X. He, R. Lux, M. H. Anderson, and W. Shi.** 2007. Interspecies interactions within oral microbial communities. *Microbiol. Mol. Biol. Rev.* **71:**653–670.
39. **Lalvani, A., P. L. Meroni, K. A. Millington, M. L. Modolo, M. Plebani, A. Ticani, D. Villalta, A. Doria, and A. Chiradello.** 2008. Recent advances in diagnostic technology: applications in autoimmune and infectious diseases. *Clin. Exp. Rheumatol.* **26**(Suppl. 48):S62–S66.
40. **Lee, Y.C., J. T. Lin, H. M. Wu, T. Y. Liu, M. F. Yen, H. M. Chiu, H. P. Wang, M. S. Wu, and T. Hsiu-His Chen.** 2007. Cost-effectiveness analysis between primary and secondary preventative strategies for gastric cancer. *Cancer Epidemiol. Biomarkers Prev.* **16:**875–885.
41. **Liao, L., L. A. Allen, and D. J. Whellan.** 2008. Economic burden of heart failure in the elderly. *Pharmacoeconomics* **26:**447–462.
42. **Maldonado, Y. A.** 2008. Impact of fetal and neonatal viral (and parasitic) infections on later development and disease outcome. *Nestle Nutr. Workshop Ser. Pediatr. Program* **61:**225–242.
43. **Masur, H., M. A. Michelis, J. B. Greene, I. Onorato, R. A. Stouwe, R. S. Holzman, G. Wormser, L. Brettman, M. Lange, H. W. Murray, and S. Cunningham-Rundles.** 1981. An outbreak of community-acquired *Pneumocystis carinii* pneumonia: initial manifestation of cellular immune dysfunction. *N. Engl. J. Med.* **305:**1431–1438.
44. **Maxwell, E. S., T. G. Ward, and T. E. Van Metre.** 1949. The relation of influenza virus and bacteria in the etiology of pneumonia. *J. Clin. Investig.* **28:**307–318.
45. **McDonald, J. C., D. L. Moore, and P. Quennec.** 1989. Clinical and epidemiological features of mumps meningoencephalitis and possible vaccine-related disease. *Pediatr. Infect. Dis. J.* **8:**751–755.
46. **McFarland, L. V.** 2008. State-of-the-art of irritable bowel syndrome and inflammatory bowel disease research in 2008. *World J. Gastroenterol.* **14:**2625–2629.
47. **McKellar, M. S., S. F. Callens, and R. Colebunders.** 2008. Pediatric HIV infection: the state of antiretroviral therapy. *Expert. Rev. Anti Infect. Ther.* **6:**167–180.

48. **Mikhailovich, V., D. Gryadunov, A. Kolchinsky, A. A. Makarov, and A. Zasedatelev.** 2008. DNA microarrays in the clinic: infectious diseases. *Bioessays* **30:**637–682.
49. **Morris, J.** 1993. Originality: who is to judge? *Lancet* **342:**930.
49a. **National Cancer Institute.** December 2007, posting date. Cancer trends progress report–2007 update. National Cancer Institute, NIH, DHHS, Bethesda, MD. http://progressreport.cancer.gov.
49b. **Nature Publishing Group.** 2008. To thwart disease, apply now. *Nature* **453:**823.
50. **Nichol, G., D. T. Dennis, A. C. Steere, R. Lightfoot, G. Wells, B. Shea, and P. Tugwell.** 1998. Test-treatment strategies for patients suspected of having Lyme disease: a cost effectiveness analysis. *Ann. Intern. Med.* **128:**37–48.
51. **Olitsky, P. K., and F. L. Gates.** 1920. Experimental study of the nasopharyngeal secretions from influenza patients. *JAMA* **74:**1497–1499.
52. **Planz, O., K. A. Bechter, and M. Schwemmle.** 2002. Human Borna disease virus infection, p. 179–227. *In* K. M. Carbone (ed.), *Borna Disease Virus and Its Role in Neurobehavioral Disease.* ASM Press, Washington, DC.
53. **Puius, Y. A., and R. A. Kalish.** 2008. Lyme arthritis: pathogenesis, clinical presentation and management. *Infect. Dis. Clin. North Am.* **22:**289–300.
54. **Reed, W., J. Carroll, and A. Agramonte.** 1901. The etiology of yellow fever: an additional note. *JAMA* **36:**431–440.
55. **Rima, B. K., and W. P. Duprex.** 2005. Molecular mechanisms of measles virus persistence. *Virus Res.* **111:**132–147.
56. **Rogowski, W. H., S. C. Hartz, and J. H. John.** 2008. Clearing up the hazy road from bench to bedside: a framework for integrating the fourth hurdle into translational medicine. *BMC Health Serv. Res.* **8:**194.
57. **Russel, S.** 2004. The economic burden of illness for households in developing countries: a review of studies focusing on malaria, tuberculosis and human immunodeficiency virus/acquired immunodeficiency syndrome. *Am. J. Trop. Med. Hyg.* **71**(2 Suppl.)**:**147–155.
58. **Satija, N., and S. K. Lal.** 2007. The molecular biology of SARS coronavirus. *Ann. N. Y. Acad. Sci.* **1102:**26–38.
59. **Saulsbury, F.T., and J. A. Katzmann.** 1990. Prevalence of antibody to *Borrelia burgdorferi* in children with juvenile rheumatoid arthritis. *J. Rheumatol.* **17:**1193–1194.
60. **Schneider, T., V. Moos, C. Loddenkemper, T. Marth, F. Fenollar, and D. Raoult.** 2008. Whipple's disease: new aspects of pathogenesis and treatment. *Lancet Infect. Dis.* **8:**179–190.
61. **Schrenzel, J.** 2007. Clinical relevance of new diagnostic methods for bloodstream infections. *Int. J. Antimicrob. Agents* **30**(Suppl. 1)**:**S2–S6.
62. **Shah, K. V.** 2007. SV40 and human cancer: a review of recent data. *Int. J. Cancer* **120:**215–223.
63. **Sherrick, A. D., L. R. Brown, G. F. Harms, and J. L. Myers.** 1994. The radiographic findings of fibrosing mediastinitis. *Chest* **106:**484–489.
64. **Skowronski, D. M., C. Astell, R. C. Brunham, D. E. Low, M. Petric, R. L. Roper, P. J. Talbot, T. Tam, and L. Babiuk.** 2005. Severe acute respiratory syndrome (SARS): a year in review. *Ann. Rev. Med.* **56:**357–381.
65. **Steere, A. C.** 2008. Reply to Stricker and Johnson. *Clin. Infect. Dis.* **47:**1112–1113.
66. **Stricker, R. B., and L. Johnson.** 2008. Serological tests for Lyme disease: more smoke and mirrors. *Clin. Infect. Dis.* **47:**1111–1112.
67. **Tabenberger, J.D., J. V. Hultin, and D. M. Morens.** 2007. Discovery and characterizations of the 1918 pandemic influenza virus in historical context. *Antivir. Ther.* **12:**581–591.
68. **Tognotti, E.** 2003. Scientific triumphalism and learning from facts: bacteriology and the "Spanish flu" challenge of 1918. *Soc. Hist. Med.* **16:**97–110.
69. **Urbanski, P., A. Wolf, and W. H. Herman.** 2008. Cost-effectiveness of diabetes education. *J. Am. Diet. Assoc.* **108**(4 Suppl. 1)**:**S6–S11.
70. **Vogt, M., R. Lüthy, and W. Siegenthaler.** 1982. GRID syndrome. *Dtsch. Med. Wochenschr.* **107:**1539–1542.
71. **Voisset, C., R. A. Weiss, and D. J. Griffiths.** 2008. Human RNA "rumor" viruses: the search for novel human retroviruses in chronic disease. *Microbiol. Mol. Biol. Rev.* **72:**157–196.
72. **Weiner, S. J., and S. Neragi-Miandoab.** 2008. Pathogenesis of malignant pleural mesothelioma and the role of environmental and genetic factors. *J. Cancer. Res. Clin. Oncol.* [Epub ahead of print.] doi: 10.1007/s00432-008-0444-9.
73. **Wilske, B., V. Fingerle, and U. Schulte-Spechtel.** 2007. Microbiological and serological diagnosis of Lyme borreliosis. *FEMS Immunol. Med. Microbiol.* **49:**12–21.
74. **World Health Organization.** 1999. WHO report on infectious diseases: removing obstacles to healthy development. http://www.who.int/infectious-disease-report/index-rpt99.html.
75. **Zampieri, C. A., N. J. Sullivan, and G. J. Nabel.** 2007. Immunopathology of highly virulent pathogens: insights from Ebola virus. *Nat. Immunol.* **8:**1159–1164.

Sequelae and Long-Term Consequences of Infectious Diseases
Edited by Pina M. Fratamico, James L. Smith, and Kim A. Brogden

Chapter 2

Late Manifestations of Lyme Borreliosis

Joppe W. R. Hovius, Alje P. van Dam, and Erol Fikrig

Lyme disease, also known as Lyme borreliosis, was first recognized as a distinct clinical entity in 1975 in Old Lyme, CT, in the United States, in children that were initially thought to have juvenile rheumatoid arthritis (164, 173a, 177). In retrospect, other symptoms of the disease had already been described previously in Europe, such as a cutaneous lesion named erythema chronicum migrans by Afzelius (5) and tick-borne meningoradicultis (Bannworth syndrome) (21). Lyme borreliosis has since then proven to be a common tick-borne disease in the United States, Europe, and Asia. In the United States, *Borrelia burgdorferi* sensu stricto (34), from here on referred to as *B. burgdorferi*, is the causative agent of Lyme borreliosis (172), whereas in Europe at least three major pathogenic *Borrelia* species, i.e., *B. burgdorferi*, *Borrelia garinii*, and *Borrelia afzelii*, are able to cause Lyme borreliosis (35, 189, 190). In addition, a novel *Borrelia* species, *B. spielmanii*, has been isolated from erythema migrans in Europe (150, 193).

B. burgdorferi, *B. garinii*, and *B. afzelii* can cause an expanding erythematous cutaneous lesion, designated erythema migrans, which is a sign of early infection. In later stages of infection these *Borrelia* species can disseminate and cause long-lasting disease that affects various organs, including the joints, central nervous system (CNS), skin, and heart (30, 165).

These symptoms, especially early symptoms (44, 202), usually respond well to conventional antibiotic therapy; however, if unrecognized or untreated they may become chronic and treatment may become more cumbersome (201). Recently, the Infectious Diseases Society of America has published a consensus guideline with detailed information on the diagnosis and treatment of Lyme borreliosis and related tick-borne diseases (201).

ETIOLOGY, ECOLOGY, AND EPIDEMIOLOGY

In the early 1980s, W. Burgdorfer and colleagues were the first to culture the causative agent of the disease, at that time designated Lyme disease, from ticks in an area where it was endemic (34), and this spirochete was later cultured from patients with Lyme disease (172). More than 30 years after the identification, it has become clear that the causative agent of Lyme borreliosis belongs to a broader group of spirochetes, referred to as the *Borrelia burgdorferi* sensu lato group (Table 1), encompassing the pathogenic species *B. burgdorferi* (sensu stricto), *B. garinii*, and *B. afzelii*, but also including the minimally or uncertain pathogenic and relatively infrequently found *Borrelia valaisiana*, *Borrelia bissettii*, *Borrelia lusitaniae*, and *B. spielmanii* (147, 185, 193, 195, 196, 204). These corkscrew-shaped spirochetes are distinguished from other bacteria by the location of their flagella, which run lengthwise between the inner and outer cell membrane and cause a twisting motion which allows the spirochete to move through tick and host tissues (Color Plate 1A).

The *B. burgdorferi* sensu lato genome is relatively small; e.g., the genome of *B. burgdorferi* strain B31 is approximately 1.5×10^6 base pairs, consisting of a linear chromosome and 12 linear and 9 circular plasmids (41, 57). A striking aspect of the genome is the large number of sequences that code for lipoproteins (41, 57). Some of these lipoproteins, like outer surface proteins (Osp) A and C, are differentially expressed and allow the spirochete to survive

Joppe W. R. Hovius • Academic Medical Center, University of Amsterdam, Department of Internal Medicine, Center for Experimental and Molecular Medicine, 1105 AZ Amsterdam, The Netherlands, and Center for Infection and Immunity Amsterdam (CINIMA), Academic Medical Center, University of Amsterdam, Amsterdam, The Netherlands. **Alje P. van Dam** • Department of Medical Microbiology, Leiden University Medical Center, PO Box 9600, 2300 RC Leiden, The Netherlands. **Erol Fikrig** • Yale University School of Medicine, Department of Internal Medicine, Infectious Diseases, 300 Cedar Street, New Haven, CT 06520-8031.

Table 1. The different *Borrelia burgdorferi* sensu lato species in the United States, Asia, and Europe

Borrelia species	Pathogenic (manifestation)	Geographic region
B. burgdorferi	Yes (arthritis)	United States, Europe, possibly Asia
B. garinii	Yes (neuroborreliosis)	Europe, Asia
B. afzelii	Yes (acrodermatitis chronica atrophicans)	Europe, Asia
B. japonica	No	Asia (Japan)
B. valaisiana	Uncertain	Europe, Asia
B. lusitaniae	Minimally	Europe (south)
B. spielmanii	Minimally (erythema migrans)	Europe (central)
B. andersonii	No	United States
B. bissettii	Minimally	United States
B. tanukii	No	Asia (Japan)
B. turdi	No	Asia (Japan)
B. sinica	No	Asia (China)
B. californiensis	No	United States (west)

in the different environments that the bacteria encounter during their enzootic life cycles (82). Other proteins are upregulated or downregulated during persistent infection (32, 61, 82, 107, 108, 155). Once a disseminated infection has been established, *B. burgdorferi* needs to evade adaptive host immune responses. A phenomenon that might also be important in immune evasion is recombination at the variable major protein-like sequence (*vls*) locus (10, 205), which has also been described for other *Borrelia* genospecies (194).The *vls* locus consists of a *vls* expression site (*vlsE*) and 15 unexpressed upstream silent cassettes (206). Segments of the silent *vls* cassettes randomly recombine into the *vlsE* expression site, resulting in multiple VlsE variants during the course of infection (109, 120, 206). Mutant strains lacking the *vlsE* locus and the upstream silent cassettes—or having only the *vlsE* locus, but not the silent cassettes—are able to infect immunocompetent mice but do not persist (29). The ability of wild-type *B. burgdorferi* to persist in the presence of robust anti-VlsE antibody response indicates that *vls* antigenic variation, resulting in changes of the variable regions and thereby altered antigenicity (120) of the VlsE protein, protects the spirochete from destruction by anti-VlsE antibodies. Finally, *B. burgdorferi* has been shown to survive in the extracellular matrix, hiding from host immune responses and allowing for long-lasting infection (36, 64, 106).

The obligate enzootic life cycle of the spirochetes involves ticks, mainly ticks belonging to the *Ixodes ricinus* complex, and a variety of vertebrate hosts, including small rodents, large mammals, and birds (8, 9, 82). In general, uninfected tick larvae acquire the bacterium by feeding on infected animals. Ticks remain infected during the molting period and become nymphs that can transmit spirochetes to other mammals, including humans, while taking a blood meal. Nymphs molt to become adults that can also transmit the spirochetes during feeding. After the final blood meal, adult female ticks (Color Plate 1B), which have already mated, lay (uninfected) eggs (vertical transmission rarely occurs). The hosts involved in this approximately 2-year life cycle differ for the different *Borrelia* species (Fig. 1).

Lyme borreliosis has become the most common vector-borne disease in the United States and Central Europe (171), where a large percentage of the tick population can be infected (47, 83, 85, 145). From 2002 on, the Centers for Disease Control and Prevention (CDC) reported around 20,000 confirmed cases of Lyme diseases annually (Fig. 2) however, the actual number may be between 60,000 and 100,000 cases (167). In 2005, in the 10 states where Lyme disease is most common, this came down to an average of 31.6 cases for every 100,000 persons. In 2006, Connecticut and Delaware reported over 50 cases/100,000 persons. The highest reported frequencies of the disease in Europe are in Central Europe, particularly The Netherlands, Germany, Austria, Slovenia, and Sweden (56, 80, 167). In 2006, Austria, Slovenia, and The Netherlands reported an estimated yearly incidence of over 100 cases per 100,000 residents (80). Interestingly, in the United States in only about 10% of the infected individuals does asymptomatic infection with *B. burgdorferi* seem to occur, whereas in Europe this percentage is much higher (51, 104, 175, 177, 192).

DATA ON PERSISTENCE OF *BORRELIA BURGDORFERI* INFECTION

To answer the question whether *B. burgdorferi* is capable of causing a persistent infection in mammals, animal models have been very helpful. *B. burgdorferi* has also been isolated from patient material by culture, mostly in combination with PCR, but it is

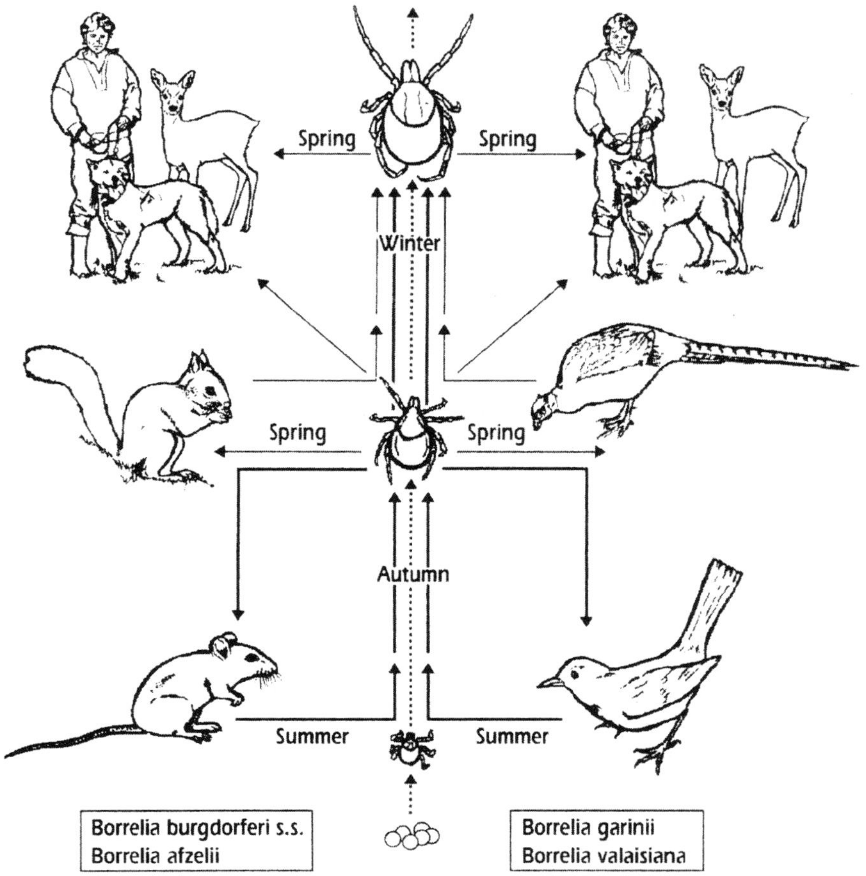

Figure 1. The obligate enzootic life cycle of *B. burgdorferi* sensu lato. (We thank K. E. Hovius for the donation of the figure.)

notoriously difficult (22, 125, 144, 156); however, culture is considered the "gold standard." In contrast, animal models allow for harvesting of multiple tissues during the course of infection and postmortem. This drastically enhances the chances of obtaining positive *Borrelia* cultures. In addition, models allow for investigating the disease in a controlled fashion with known genetic information of both host and pathogen. Models also circumvent other problems associated with culturing *B. burgdorferi* in humans; patients often live in areas where Lyme borreliosis is endemic and have a considerable risk for reinfection (127). Coinfections with other tick-borne pathogens can occur; culture could be hampered by antibiotic treatment, and inhomogeneous distribution of the bacterium through infected tissues could affect the chance to obtain positive cultures. Human Lyme borreliosis has been investigated with a variety of animal models, i.e., hamsters (89, 154), rats (27), rabbits (34, 55, 101, 132), mice (23–25, 28, 29), dogs (12, 179–182), and nonhuman primates (49, 131, 133–136, 140–142, 151, 152). The vast majority of these studies have been performed with *B. burgdorferi* (sensu stricto) isolates; therefore, the relevance of these studies for European Lyme borreliosis might be only partially applicable. We will focus on studies using the murine, canine, and nonhuman primate

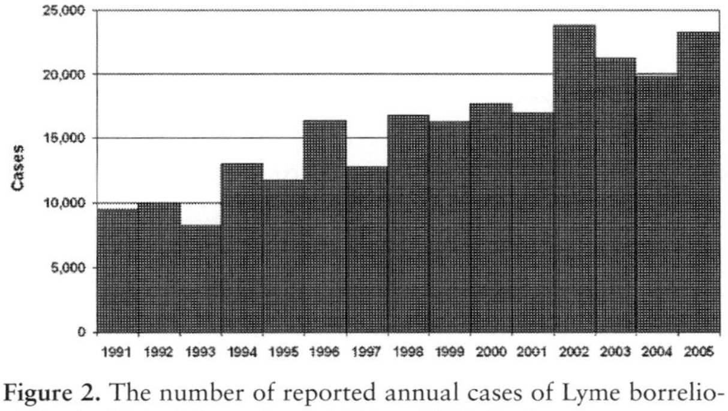

Figure 2. The number of reported annual cases of Lyme borreliosis in the United States from 1991 to 2006. Patients were reported to the Centers for Disease Control and Prevention from 1991 to 2006, and cases were defined using stringent case definitions (11). Numbers are likely to be an underestimation (167). (The figure is published courtesy of the CDC.)

model for human late Lyme borreliosis, which are the most widely used, and discuss the relevance of these findings for human disease.

The Murine Model

This model has been well established and is used by most Lyme researchers (197). In this model, mice develop acute carditis and (sub)acute arthritis (23–26, 28, 29, 197). However, mice can also be persistently infected with *B. burgdorferi* (26). Barthold and collaborators showed that in C3H/HeJ mice, an immunocompetent mouse strain susceptible to *B. burgdorferi* infection, that were intradermally inoculated with *B. burgdorferi*, viable spirochetes could be detected by culture up to 1 year postinfection in the majority of mice (26). In addition, during later stages of the disease these mice showed mild recurrent and intermittent episodes of both carditis and arthritis (26). After adequate antibiotic treatment of infected mice with ceftriaxone (16 or 50 mg/kg of body weight twice daily subcutaneously for 5 days), symptoms resolved and cultures became negative (121). In accordance, in another study, tissue samples from most, but not all, mice that were treated with ceftriaxone in a similar fashion for 5 days became negative in the PCR (115). Recently, it was shown that treatment of all (10/10) *B. burgdorferi*-infected C3H/HeJ mice with ceftriaxone (50 mg/kg once daily for 5 days administered intraperitoneally) resulted in negative tissue cultures, but that transient treatment thereafter with the immunosuppressant anti-tumor necrosis factor alpha (TNF-α) resulted in 20 to 30% (2 or 3/10) of the mice being culture positive (203). According to the authors, this proves that *B. burgdorferi* can persist after antibiotic treatment in mice. However, there were a few major shortcomings in the experimental design of this study, making it difficult to draw conclusions from this study (200). Firstly, despite the fact that 50 mg/kg ceftriaxone seems rather high, 5 days of treatment is rather short compared to the month that is usually curative in humans. Obviously, the route of administration, i.e., once daily intraperitoneally, has never been investigated in humans. Due to the short half-life of plasma levels of ceftriaxone administered through this route, compared to intravenous administration, this route of injection is likely to result in extended periods of time with insufficient antibiotic levels (200). Data on the pharmacokinetics in the individual mice would have been much appreciated. Moreover, anti-TNF-α was administered simultaneously with or shortly after the end of ceftriaxone treatment. This could have enabled weakened, but viable, spirochetes that would have normally been cleared by the immune system, to evade immune responses and cause persistent infection. Lastly, in contrast to these murine data, Steere and Angelis have recently described how they successfully used a TNF inhibitor, infliximab, to treat four patients with a late manifestation of Lyme borreliosis, i.e., antibiotic-refractory Lyme arthritis, discussed in more detail elsewhere in this chapter, without any signs of a flare-up of *B. burgdorferi* infection during the follow-up period (168). These studies illustrate that (i) *B. burgdorferi* as well as clinical symptoms of Lyme borreliosis can persist in mice, (ii) adequate antibiotic treatment leads to the disappearance of both cultivable spirochetes and clinical symptoms, (iii) some spirochetal DNA can infrequently persist, and (iv) after short-term, and potentially insufficient, treatment with ceftriaxone for 5 days, spirochetes may still reappear after severe immune suppression. The relevance of these last findings for human Lyme borreliosis remains unclear.

The Canine Model

The course of Lyme borreliosis in experimentally infected dogs was first described by Appel and colleagues (12). The authors showed that young dogs infected with *B. burgdorferi* through tick bites developed acute lameness with fibrinopurulent arthritis 2 to 5 months post-tick attachment. *B. burgdorferi*, as detected by PCR and culture, could be recovered up to 1 year after tick attachment. At this stage, dogs were asymptomatic (12). Straubinger demonstrated that the bacterium could also be isolated by culture up to 500 days after infection (179). Thus, in the canine model for Lyme borreliosis there is evidence for persistent *B. burgdorferi* infection. In addition, Straubinger et al. also showed that *B. burgdorferi* can persist after antibiotic treatment (182). Importantly, plasma levels of antibiotics were documented throughout the treatment period for some dogs in this study. Straubinger and colleagues showed that a small portion, i.e. 17% (2/12), of dogs treated with either 30 days of orally administered doxycycline (twice daily) or amoxicillin (two or three times daily), remained culture positive in only one of the many postmortem samples tested 6 months posttreatment (182). Notably, one of these dogs received amoxicillin twice daily, and although plasma levels of amoxicillin are not shown for this dog, plasma/tissue levels of antibiotic are likely to have been below the minimum inhibitory or bactericidal concentrations for considerable periods of time throughout the treatment period. This could have been the cause for the treatment failure in this particular dog. The same study also showed that in 25% (2/8) of asymptomatic dogs that were PCR positive 6 months posttreatment, antibody levels, after an initial steep decline, started rising gradually from 3 months posttreatment on, which would indicate persistent infection (182). However, these treated dogs remained culture negative and asymptomatic throughout this posttreatment period, suggesting that the bacterium is kept in control by the host immune system (182).

In a similar study, in which they studied the course of Lyme borreliosis over a period of almost 1 and a half years, Straubinger and collaborators showed that 75% (9/12) of antibiotic-treated dogs (120 days postinfection) remained positive in several tissues, as detected by PCR; however, none of these animals was culture positive (181). In addition, when these animals were treated orally with corticosteroids, i.e. prednisone, 2 mg/kg, twice a day for 14 days, all dogs previously treated with antibiotics remained asymptomatic and culture negative (181). By contrast, in control dogs, i.e., dogs that had not been treated with antibiotics, this transient immunosuppression resulted in painful and swollen joints in all four limbs. Whether or not these untreated control dogs were transiently immunosuppressed, they were culture positive in multiple tissues during the course of infection and postmortem (181). These studies by Straubinger et al. (179–182) and Appel and colleagues (12) stress that (i) dogs can be persistently infected with *B. burgdorferi*, (ii) antibiotic failure, as detected by isolation of viable spirochetes by culture, is rare (despite treatment late in the course of the disease in these studies), (iii) in the unlikely event of antibiotic failure, these data suggest that there should be at least serological evidence of ongoing infection, and (iv) in this model, the significance of merely a positive PCR—and no positive culture—after antibiotic treatment remains unclear, since, even after immunosuppression, this does not result in the detection of viable spirochetes by culture or clinical disease.

The Nonhuman Primate Model

The course of infection in macaques has been studied mostly by Pachner and colleagues and Philipp and collaborators (49, 135, 151). Besides developing arthritis and carditis, macaques develop erythema migrans when infected intradermally with *B. burgdorferi* (49, 134). Only when macaques are immunosuppressed will *Borrelia* subsequently disseminate to the CNS, where it can cause acute and chronic inflammation of the CNS, i.e., neuroborreliosis. Spirochetes can be detected in the CNS by culture and PCR in the initial stages of neuroborreliosis, before the development of intrathecal antibodies (135). Months to years postinfection, *B. burgdorferi* can be detected only by PCR, suggesting that very low pathogen loads persist. Importantly, in all organs that are infected in this model, there is no inflammation without infection; however, infection without inflammation has been observed (135). In this model, carditis is usually mild in immunocompetent macaques but can persist for years, despite low levels of spirochetes, as detected by quantitative PCR (38). In a study in which confirmed skin culture *Borrelia*-positive macaques were treated 3 months postinfection with 2 mg/kg doxycycline, twice a day for 60 days, levels of anti-C_6 antibodies waned rapidly (141). In this study, peak and trough serum levels of doxycycline were documented to ensure the minimum inhibitory concentration had been reached. C6 is a peptide that is used to detect antibodies against the most conserved invariable region, 6, of the *B. burgdorferi* protein VlsE by enzyme-linked immunosorbent assay and is thought to be a marker for persistent infection (33, 110, 116, 198). Although the authors did not perform culture or PCR in this study, these results suggest that in the nonhuman primate model for Lyme borreliosis, *Borrelia* is eradicated after antibiotic treatment (142).

Relevance of Data from Animal Studies for Human Lyme Borreliosis

Taken together, these data from the various animal models clearly demonstrate that *B. burgdorferi* can cause persistent infection. Indeed, with human studies, *B. burgdorferi* has been isolated, but only sporadically, by culture months to years after infection (16, 144, 162, 172).

The data on the persistence of *B. burgdorferi* in the various animal models after antibiotic treatment are somewhat contradictory. Nonetheless, and very importantly, in line with the canine (182) and nonhuman primate models (141), the long-term clinical outcomes of patients treated for Lyme borreliosis are generally excellent (157, 158). However, despite resolution of objective manifestations of infection after appropriate treatment regimes, a minority of patients has residual nonspecific complaints, such as fatigue, musculoskeletal pain, and loss of short-term memory and concentration, referred to as post-Lyme disease symptoms or post-Lyme disease syndrome (54, 188). These symptoms are not thought to be due to persistent and active *Borrelia* infection, since, although one group found positive *Borrelia* tissue cultures in patients even after antibiotic treatment using a new culture medium (143), other carefully conducted laboratory studies using the same medium failed to reproduce this result (117, 187). In addition, in multiple placebo-controlled treatment trials (52, 94, 99, 100, 102) patients—who had residual complaints despite antibiotic treatment for well-documented *Borrelia* infection—did not clinically respond to additional antibiotic regimes. Interestingly, children treated for Lyme borreliosis have less residual complaints than adults (59, 60). Obviously, with individual patients, physicians should be alert for recurrent signs indicating persistent infection or reinfection, such as joint swelling, skin rash, weakness of facial and other muscles, or severe headache (54). This could justify additional diagnostic tests, also aimed at excluding other causes than Lyme borreliosis, and possibly, in a minority of patients, additional or prolonged antibiotic treatment.

Regarding in vitro data that are frequently cited (by believers in long-term and repetitive treatment regimens) to explain how *B. burgdorferi* could persist after adequate treatment, it should be mentioned that, although *B. burgdorferi* may persist as cyst-like forms in vitro (7), this has never been shown to play a role in clinical practice. Furthermore, the fact that *B. burgdorferi*, although extracellular in nature (139), was shown to be able to persist intracellularly (111) does not mean that it can escape intracellular antibiotic-mediated killing, as also recently discussed by Feder and the Ad Hoc International Lyme Disease Group (54). Finally, to date, there is no scientific evidence of acquired antibiotic resistance in *B. burgdorferi* (54, 86).

Although an interesting topic, we will not discuss the different types and lengths of antibiotic therapy (166) and refer to the recently published guidelines by the Infectious Diseases Society of America (IDSA) (201).

HUMAN LATE CLINICAL MANIFESTATIONS OF LYME BORRELIOSIS

The objective clinical manifestations of Lyme borreliosis are similar worldwide, but there are regional variations, especially between the symptoms found in the United States, where Lyme borreliosis is exclusively caused by *B. burgdorferi*, and those found in Europe, where Lyme borreliosis is primarily caused by *B. afzelii* and *B. garinii*, but also *B. burgdorferi*. The disease can be divided into an acute phase, encompassing early or localized disease (days to weeks), and a late or chronic phase, representing both early disseminated (weeks to months) and late or persistent disease (months to years) (Table 2) (165, 167).

Table 2. Predominant clinical manifestations of human Lyme borreliosis in the United States and Europe[a]

Site or condition	Clinical manifestation in:	
	United States	Europe
Joints		
Acute	Severe pauciarticular arthritis[b]	Less intense and less frequent joint inflammation
Late	Antibiotic-refractory Lyme arthritis	Persistent arthritis rare
Nervous system		
Acute	Lymphocytic meningitis, radiculitis not frequently observed	Painful radiculitis[c]
Late	Encephalopathy	Chronic progressive encephalomyelitis with intrathecal antibody production[c]
	Sensory polyneuropathy	Sensory polyneuropathy (associated with ACA)
Skin		
Acute	Erythema migrans (intense inflammation, relative brief duration)	Erythema migrans (less intense inflammation, relatively longer duration)
Late	Acrodermatitis rare	Acrodermatitis chronica atrophicans relatively common[d]
Heart		
Acute	Subtle (myo)carditis with (partial) atrioventricular block	Subtle (myo)carditis with (partial) atrioventricular block
Late	Not reported	Dilated cardiomyopathy (rare)
Post-Lyme disease syndrome	Residual aspecific symptoms (fatigue, musculoskeletal and/or subtle [subjective] cognitive symptoms) with evidence for prior but not persistent *B. burgdorferi* infection[e]	Residual aspecific symptoms (fatigue, musculoskeletal and/or subtle [subjective] cognitive symptoms) with evidence for prior but not persistent *B. burgdorferi* infection[e]
Asymptomatic infection	In approximately 10% of infected individuals	Asymptomatic infection occurs much more frequently

[a]This table is modified from references 165 and 167.
[b]Almost always involving the knee.
[c]Associated with *B. garinii* infection.
[d]Associated with *B. afzelii* infection.
[e]After adequate antibiotic treatment.

For all *Borrelia* species, infection usually begins with erythema migrans, but in Europe, the skin lesion often persists for a longer period of time (183); however, 50% of patients with neuroborreliosis do not recall erythema migrans (78). Each of the *Borrelia* species may also cause longer-lasting infection of the (large) joints, heart, nervous system, or skin. However, *B. burgdorferi* is more frequently found among patients with arthritis and can cause chronic, antibiotic-refractory arthritis (173); *B. garinii* has been shown to be predominantly neurotropic and is often found to cause chronic neuroborreliosis (35, 189, 190); and *B. afzelii* often infects only the skin, where it can cause a chronic infection, acrodermatitis chronica atrophicans (165, 189, 190). All three species have been found to cause Lyme carditis; however, this seldom runs a chronic course, with the exception of the rarely observed Lyme cardiomyopathy. Although, the word "chronic" is de facto correct for these Lyme borreliosis manifestations, we prefer to refer to these manifestations as "late Lyme borreliosis" rather than "chronic Lyme borreliosis" because of the association with the post-Lyme disease syndrome, which is not associated with persistent *B. burgdorferi* infection. Another possibility to circumvent confusion of tongues would be to address these symptoms as due to persistent infection with *B. burgdorferi*.

Chronic Antibiotic-Refractory Lyme Arthritis

Although early Lyme disease may manifest itself with migratory arthralgias, Lyme arthritis is a manifestation of late disease (30, 84, 164). Months to years after exposure, intermittent recurrent attacks occur that persist for days, weeks, or months and are typically asymmetrical and pauciarticular in nature and involve one or two larger joints and almost always the knee (174) (Color Plate 2A). In a cohort of untreated patients, more than 60% of patients developed Lyme arthritis in the United Sates (165). Joint fluid white blood cell counts range from 500 to 110,000 cells/mm^3, of which most are polymorphonuclear leukocytes. The synovial lesion is similar to what has been observed in other forms of chronic inflammatory arthritis and shows synovial cell hyperplasia, vascular proliferation, and infiltration of mononuclear cells (165). From both patient (63) and experimental murine studies (118), we know that a high concentration of *B. burgdorferi*-reactive T cells is present in joint fluid from Lyme arthritis cases and that they mainly secrete Th1 cytokines, such as gamma interferon. Culture of the organism has proven to be difficult; however, *B. burgdorferi* DNA can be readily detected in synovial tissue or joint fluid from most untreated patients, even months to years after initial infection (128).

Most Lyme arthritis patients respond well to conventional antibiotic treatment strategies, such as doxycycline; however, a small percentage of patients develop chronic arthritis, defined as 1 year or more of continuous joint inflammation (174). Usually, these patients respond well to conventional therapy; however, some have chronic joint inflammation despite appropriate therapy and eradication of the spirochete as determined by PCR (40, 159). Additional antibiotics are not indicated at this stage (53, 168). Antibiotic-refractory Lyme arthritis occurs more often in the United States than in Europe (165) and has been associated with a genetic predisposition, i.e., the presence of several HLA-DR rheumatoid arthritis alleles, among which is the DRB1*0401 molecule (62). In this subset of patients, it is thought that molecular mimicry of the dominant epitope of *B. burgdorferi* OspA, $OspA_{161\text{-}175}$, and the human lymphocyte function-associated antigen (hLFA-1) is the cause for ongoing T-cell responses and joint inflammation in the absence of the causative agent. However, a recent study suggested that the majority of patients with Lyme arthritis initially do have $OspA_{161\text{-}175}$-specific T cells, but that these cells rapidly declined soon after the start of antibiotic treatment and thus are unlikely to be associated with the perpetuation of joint inflammation (91, 92). Notably, this dominant immunogenic OspA epitope is not conserved between the various *Borrelia* species, with *B. garinii* having at least five and *B. afzelii* at least eight different residues in this particular amino acid sequence, which could be an explanation for the more frequent occurrence of antibody-refractory Lyme arthritis in the United States compared to Europe (48). In addition, Shin and collaborators showed that in a comparison of synovial fluids from antibiotic-responsive and antibiotic-refractory Lyme arthritis patients, high proinflammatory chemokines and cytokines—among them CXCL 8, 9, and 10, gamma interferon, and TNF-α—persisted in the latter group (159). Thus, even when antibiotic treatment reduced or completely cleared the infection in these patients, the inflammatory response in the synovium persisted, which was associated with ongoing joint inflammation. In search of an explanation for the observed ongoing inflammation observed with antibiotic-refractory Lyme arthritis, two European studies have detected *B. burgdorferi* DNA in synovium from patients with antibiotic-refractory Lyme arthritis and assigned this as the cause for antibiotic-refractory Lyme arthritis (88, 148). However, synovium was examined only 2 or 3 months after cessation of antibiotic treatment. Indeed, other studies, in which the mean duration from the completion of antibiotic treatment to the PCR was 7 months, there was no detection of *B. burgdorferi* DNA in synovial samples from patients with antibiotic treatment-resistant Lyme arthritis (40, 159). Lastly, another major reason for the inadequate response of Lyme arthritis to antibiotic therapy is initial misdiagnosis (149, 160, 176).

Late Neurological Manifestations

Lyme neuroborreliosis implies involvement of the nervous system during systemic infection with *B. burgdorferi*. Most patients with neuroborreliosis present to a neurologist within a few weeks to months of the initial bite (137, 178). Neuroborreliosis has been classified as "early" and "chronic," and in this chapter we will refer to this classification as "early" and "late" (112, 138). Early neuroborreliosis is inflammatory in nature, with subacute lymphocytic meningitis (mostly in the United States), cranial neuritis (Bell's palsy) (Color Plate 2B), and (painful) radiculitis (mostly in Europe), giving a triad of symptoms referred to as Bannwarth's syndrome (5, 78, 90, 130, 165). In two cohorts of untreated patients in the United States and Europe, 10 to 15% developed acute neuroborreliosis (19, 164). Typically, in most patients, in both the United States and Europe, acute neurological symptoms improved or resolved in several weeks to months, even without antibiotic treatment, although a few patients had residual peripheral nervous system anomalies (3, 165).

A minority of patients will develop late neuroborreliosis with the duration of symptoms exceeding 6 months (77, 130). Months to years after the initial infection with *B. burgdorferi*, patients with late neuroborreliosis can present with a subtle encephalopathy, mainly consisting of mild cognitive disturbances (68, 73, 74, 93, 112, 164, 165). This manifestation has mostly been described in American literature (68, 93, 112, 165), and approximately 5% of untreated patients will develop such symptoms (112). In most of these patients, there is no evidence of inflammation due to *B. burgdorferi* in the CNS, and therefore, the encephalopathy might actually be an indirect effect of systemic (non-CNS) infection accompanying typical clinical findings of disseminated Lyme borreliosis (68, 71, 72, 79, 103). Similarly, in up to 30% of patients with typical manifestations of disseminated Lyme borreliosis, monoarticular large joint arthritis or a chronic or late (radiculo)-neuropathy may occur (67, 114).

In some patients suffering from encephalopathy, however, there is evidence of *B. burgdorferi* involvement in the CNS (PCR positivity in 10/11 cases [96]) or mild signs of CNS inflammation, such as mild intrathecal antibody production or pleiocytosis, in some (5/12) patients (170), and in those patients, a mild encephalomyelitis may be responsible for the observed symptoms (69, 72, 75, 96, 165, 170). Late neuroborreliosis can be treated with intravenous antibiotics (113), and neurologic abnormalities usually improve with antibiotic therapy (70); however, approximately 40% of treated patients either have no change in condition or relapse (112). In retrospect, this might be due to the fact that part of these patients actually had residual symptoms after *Borrelia* infection (post-Lyme disease syndrome) instead of symptoms due to persistent *B. burgdorferi* infection. Importantly, in patients with cognitive impairment after adequate treatment for neuroborreliosis, additional antibiotics do not have beneficial effects compared to a placebo (52, 70, 94, 99, 100, 102).

More often in Europe than in the United States, a more aggressive form of encephalomyelitis has been described, i.e., chronic progressive encephalomyelitis that is accompanied by relatively severe cerebrospinal fluid (CSF) pleiocytosis or evident intrathecal anti-*B. burgdorferi* antibody production (4, 74, 78, 130). In two studies by Hansen and colleagues and Oschmann and collaborators, 6% of these patients—patients suspected of Lyme borreliosis with either CSF pleiocytosis or specific intrathecal anti-*B. burgdorferi* antibodies—presented with a slowly progressive myelopathy beginning with an ataxic gait and gradually worsening spastic para- or tetraparesis (78, 130). Importantly, CSF abnormalities are more common with *B. garinii* infection that with *B. afzelii* infection (186). In one study, progressive sensorineural hearing loss occurred in 75% (6/8) patients with chronic progressive encephalomyelitis (78). The reaction to antibiotic treatment in these patients might be slower than the reaction to antibiotic treatment in patients with acute neuroborreliosis, but was nonetheless marked (78, 161). Finally, although unlikely, early neurological signs, such as Bannwarth's syndrome, may persist for months to years and thus become chronic (138).

Direct demonstration of *B. burgdorferi*, by PCR or culture in CSF, is not practical in clinical settings because of its low yield (198, 199). Thus, the diagnosis relies on the medical history, neurological examination, routine analysis of CSF, and antibody studies of serum and CSF (73, 77, 178). Nonetheless, the diagnosis of late neuroborreliosis is difficult, especially if cases with neurologic symptoms, but without objective CSF abnormalities, are also included in this category. These patients often present with aspecific symptoms: fatigue, malaise, myalgia, and arthralgia that can accompany any chronic infection, chronic fatigue syndrome, or fibromyalgia.

In addition, although Lyme borreliosis rarely presents with focal CNS damage on imaging studies (1, 6), the diagnosis has been considered with patients with multiple sclerosis (95). However, it was shown that reactive Lyme serology of multiple sclerosis patients, without suggestive features of Lyme disease, is unlikely to indicate neuroborreliosis (42, 43).

The only useful experimental model for neuroborreliosis is the rhesus macaque model (49, 135, 136, 140, 152).When mild immunosuppression is induced in *B. burgdorferi*-infected rhesus macaques, the spirochete establishes persistent infection in many organs, among which are the central and peripheral nervous systems (20, 37, 39, 131, 138). Inflammation in the nervous system in rhesus macaques is primarily localized to nerve roots, dorsal root ganglia, and leptomeninges, where spirochetes can also be visualized (39). T lymphocytes and plasma cells are the principal immune cells involved, and increased amounts of immunoglobulins (G and M) and C1q are found in CSF (138). These findings in the macaque model for neuroborreliosis relate to the clinical spectrum of human neuroborreliosis, with meningitis and radiculitis as the predominating symptoms, whereas parenchymal involvement is observed less frequently.

Late Cutaneous Manifestations

Erythema migrans is the most frequent clinical sign several days to weeks after *B. burgdorferi* infection and can be clinically diagnosed (124, 126, 184). Erythema migrans can be readily treated with antibiotics but, when untreated, can persist for weeks to months (123, 165). Another, spontaneously resolving early sign of *B. burgdorferi* infection is borrelial lymphocytoma, most often localized at the earlobe or nipple, consisting of lymphocytic infiltration of both the cutis as well as the subcutis (123, 165). In Europe, a chronic, slowly progressive cutaneous manifestation of late Lyme borreliosis, designated acrodermatitis chronica atrophicans (ACA), has been described as approximately 1 to 7% of European Lyme borreliosis cases (14, 18, 30, 46, 87) (Color Plate 2C). The lesion is characterized by bluish-red atrophic skin, initially in combination with edema (14, 18). Due to clinical resemblance, this late manifestation of borreliosis can be easily misdiagnosed as vascular insufficiency, especially when the lower legs are affected (18, 50). It is usually, in up to 40% of patients, associated with sensory peripheral polyneuropathy (81, 97), and although less frequently, periarticular nodules or sclerotic lesions can be observed (31). ACA is most often localized on the plantar sites of hands and feet or distal parts of the legs in female patients over 40 years of age (14, 18, 165), although ACA has been described incidentally in children (122). The onset is hardly noticeable, and the lesion slowly progresses in months to years, with edema disappearing and irreversible atrophy becoming more apparent (18). The initial presentation is usually unilateral, although in 30% of the patients, two or more extremities are affected at the time of presentation (18, 31). Similar to borrelial lymphocytoma, in Europe, ACA is usually caused by *B. afzelii*, and the causative organism has been cultured from the lesion as long as 10 years after the onset of the disease (16), indicating that the presence of the spirochete is the cause for ongoing disease. Therefore, it is not surprising that almost all patients with ACA are seropositive (17, 76) and should be treated with (oral) antibiotics (123). Serology posttreatment of patients that responded well to antibiotic treatment is not recommended, since antibodies against *B. burgdorferi* can remain detectable for months to years posttreatment (129). Notably, only 30% of ACA patients remember a tick bite or erythema migrans (15), and ACA can, therefore, be the first presenting symptom of Lyme borreliosis (18). On histological examination, pronounced lymphocyte and plasma cell infiltration of the dermis and sometimes the subcutis, with or without atrophy, can be observed (2, 45). Although suggestive for ACA, these findings are not pathognomic. Unfortunately, there is no animal model to study ACA.

Late Cardiac Involvement

Cardiac involvement in Lyme borreliosis is a rare phenomenon and is more a manifestation of early disseminated disease than a manifestation of chronic disease. This might be due to the fact that, now that Lyme borreliosis has become a well-known clinical entity, it is recognized more rapidly and patients are treated with antibiotics at an earlier stage, preventing early extracutaneous symptoms (65). Early studies showed that approximately 5% of untreated patients—most of whom acquired *B. burgdorferi* in New England, the United States—developed acute Lyme carditis (164, 169), although a later prospective study demonstrated that with only 1 of the 61 patients with early Lyme disease, also contracted in the United States, signs of Lyme carditis were observed (Color Plate 2D) (153). In Europe this percentage is estimated to be somewhat lower, i.e., 0.4 to 4% (30, 119). If Lyme carditis becomes symptomatic, symptoms are related to atrioventricular conduction abnormalities that can occur, but the overall prognosis of Lyme carditis is good, possibly even without antibiotics (191), explaining why late cardiac involvement in Lyme borreliosis is seldom observed. A rare chronic cardiac manifestation, however, is dilated cardiomyopathy and has been found in patients in Europe based on isolation of the spirochete from heart tissue (66, 105, 162) and serological studies (98, 163). Since spirochetes have rarely been isolated by culture, this might indicate that symptoms could be due to past infection and myocardial scarring rather than ongoing inflammation due to the presence of the spirochete (58). Routine therapy and screening of patients with idiopathic dilated cardiomyopathy are of limited utility and should be reserved for patients with a clear history of antecedent Lyme borreliosis symptoms or a tick bite (146).

In the murine model for Lyme carditis, different strains of laboratory mice infected with *B. burgdorferi* develop inflammation of the heart approximately 10 to 14 days after infection. The main immune cell involved is the macrophage. These mice also develop abnormalities on the electrocardiogram; however, serum markers for cardiac damage were not elevated (13). Similarly to mice, nonhuman primates develop signs of carditis after infection with *B. burgdorferi*, with T cells, plasma cells, and macrophages being the predominant immune cells. The histological abnormalities are mild, unless the macaques were transiently immunosuppressed, but can persist for years (38). However, immunocompetent nonhuman primates readily clear the spirochetes to nearly undetectable levels (as determined by quantitative PCR) (38).

CONCLUSION

Lyme borreliosis has become the most common vector-borne disease in the United States and Central Europe. However, large-scale government campaigns and active patients groups have increased awareness, which could be helpful in preventing primary cases and thereby late manifestations of Lyme borreliosis. Nonetheless, the incidence of Lyme borreliosis in the United States and Europe is still rising, and early recognition of infection remains an important issue, since early treatment regimes are generally more successful than later ones.

In this chapter, we have provided an overview of the literature on the persistence of *B. burgdorferi* infection in the various animal models for Lyme borreliosis and discussed the relevance for human disease. Comparison of data obtained from animal studies with data from human studies suggests that, in selected groups of patients with late manifestations of Lyme borreliosis, persistent *B. burgdorferi* infection is causative of the ongoing symptoms, i.e., in patients suffering from acrodermatitis chronica atrophicans or chronic neuroborreliosis and especially in patients with encephalomyelitis. In contrast, in patients presenting with other symptoms, i.e., patients with antibiotic-refractory Lyme arthritis and post-Lyme disease syndrome and possibly some of the few patients with dilated cardiomyopathy, other mechanisms than persistent *B. burgdorferi* infection seem to be involved. In addition, we have discussed the present literature on the importance of the supposed persistence of *B. burgdorferi* after antibiotic therapy. In the canine and murine, but not the nonhuman primate, models for Lyme borreliosis, there is some evidence that with animals treated for Lyme borreliosis, *B. burgdorferi* DNA can be detected in the posttreatment period. However, there are several limitations to these studies, as discussed in detail in the specific sections. Importantly, all placebo-controlled treatment trials performed to date, in patients with residual symptoms after treatment for Lyme borreliosis, show no beneficial effects of antibiotics over placebo, further questioning the relevance of the findings in the animal models. Lastly, we describe the diverse clinical and (immuno)pathogenetic aspects of the four major late manifestations of *B. burgdorferi* sensu lato infection, antibiotic-refractory Lyme arthritis, acrodermatitis chronica atrophicans, late neuroborreliosis, and dilated cardiomyopathy, combining relevant data from clinical studies as well as laboratory studies using the various animal models. The content of this chapter should provide clarity to physicians regarding the genesis of symptoms in patients with late Lyme borreliosis and could contribute to a theoretical framework for determining strategies to manage these patients and those with post-Lyme disease syndrome.

Acknowledgments. We thank K. E. Hovius for his useful suggestions regarding the section on the various animal models of Lyme borreliosis and the permission to use the figure on the life cycle of *B. burgdorferi* sensu lato, P. Speelman for the kind gift of the picture from a patient with acrodermatitis chronica atrophicans, the CDC for permission to use the figure on incidences of Lyme borreliosis in the Unites States, J. Verbunt for the Holter registration of a patient with a total atrioventricular block due to Lyme carditis, and A.C. Steere for the picture of a patient with antibiotic-refractory Lyme arthritis. The picture of the semi-engorged *I. scapularis* tick (Color Plate 1B) was taken by K. A. de Groot. Joppe W. R. Hovius is supported by ZonMw, The Netherlands organization for health research and development.

REFERENCES

1. **Aalto, A., J. Sjowall, L. Davidsson, P. Forsberg, and O. Smedby.** 2007. Brain magnetic resonance imaging does not contribute to the diagnosis of chronic neuroborreliosis. *Acta Radiol.* **48:**755–762.

2. **Aberer, E., H. Klade, and G. Hobisch**. 1991. A clinical, histological, and immunohistochemical comparison of acrodermatitis chronica atrophicans and morphea. *Am. J. Dermatopathol.* **13**:334–341.
3. **Ackermann, R., P. Horstrup, and R. Schmidt**. 1984. Tick-borne meningopolyneuritis (Garin-Bujadoux, Bannwarth). *Yale J. Biol. Med.* **57**:485–490.
4. **Ackermann, R., B. Rehse-Kupper, E. Gollmer, and R. Schmidt**. 1988. Chronic neurologic manifestations of erythema migrans borreliosis. *Ann. N. Y. Acad. Sci.* **539**:16–23.
5. **Afzelius, A.** 1921. Erythema chronicum migrans. *Acta Derm. Venereol.* **2**:120–125.
6. **Agosta, F., M. A. Rocca, B. Benedetti, R. Capra, C. Cordioli, and M. Filippi**. 2006. MR imaging assessment of brain and cervical cord damage in patients with neuroborreliosis. *AJNR Am. J. Neuroradiol.* **27**:892–894.
7. **Alban, P. S., P. W. Johnson, and D. R. Nelson**. 2000. Serum-starvation-induced changes in protein synthesis and morphology of *Borrelia burgdorferi. Microbiology* **146**:119–127.
8. **Anderson, J. F., R. C. Johnson, L. A. Magnarelli, and F. W. Hyde**. 1986. Involvement of birds in the epidemiology of the Lyme disease agent *Borrelia burgdorferi. Infect. Immun.* **51**:394–396.
9. **Anderson, J. F., and L. A. Magnarelli**. 1980. Vertebrate host relationships and distribution of ixodid ticks (Acari: Ixodidae) in Connecticut, USA. *J. Med. Entomol.* **17**:314–323.
10. **Anguita, J., V. Thomas, S. Samanta, R. Persinski, C. Hernanz, S. W. Barthold, and E. Fikrig**. 2001. *Borrelia burgdorferi*-induced inflammation facilitates spirochete adaptation and variable major protein-like sequence locus recombination. *J. Immunol.* **167**:3383–3390.
11. **Anonymous**. 1997. Case definitions for infectious conditions under public health surveillance. *MMWR Recommend. Rep.* **46**:1–55.
12. **Appel, M. J., S. Allan, R. H. Jacobson, T. L. Lauderdale, Y. F. Chang, S. J. Shin, J. W. Thomford, R. J. Todhunter, and B. A. Summers**. 1993. Experimental Lyme disease in dogs produces arthritis and persistent infection. *J. Infect. Dis.* **167**:651–664.
13. **Armstrong, A. L., S. W. Barthold, D. H. Persing, and D. S. Beck**. 1992. Carditis in Lyme disease susceptible and resistant strains of laboratory mice infected with *Borrelia burgdorferi. Am. J. Trop. Med. Hyg.* **47**:249–258.
14. **Asbrink, E., E. Brehmer-Andersson, and A. Hovmark**. 1986. Acrodermatitis chronica atrophicans—a spirochetosis. Clinical and histopathological picture based on 32 patients; course and relationship to erythema chronicum migrans Afzelius. *Am. J. Dermatopathol.* **8**:209–219.
15. **Asbrink, E., B. Hederstedt, and A. Hovmark**. 1984. The spirochetal etiology of erythema chronicum migrans Afzelius. *Acta Derm. Venereol.* **64**:291–295.
16. **Asbrink, E., and A. Hovmark**. 1985. Successful cultivation of spirochetes from skin lesions of patients with erythema chronicum migrans Afzelius and acrodermatitis chronica atrophicans. *Acta Pathol. Microbiol. Immunol. Scand. Sect. B* **93**:161–163.
17. **Asbrink, E., A. Hovmark, and B. Hederstedt**. 1985. Serologic studies of erythema chronicum migrans Afzelius and acrodermatitis chronica atrophicans with indirect immunofluorescence and enzyme-linked immunosorbent assays. *Acta Derm. Venereol.* **65**:509–514.
18. **Asbrink, E., A. Hovmark, and I. Olsson**. 1986. Clinical manifestations of acrodermatitis chronica atrophicans in 50 Swedish patients. *Zentralbl. Bakteriol. Mikrobiol. Hyg. A* **263**:253–261.
19. **Asbrink, E., I. Olsson, and A. Hovmark**. 1986. Erythema chronicum migrans Afzelius in Sweden. A study on 231 patients. *Zentralbl. Bakteriol. Mikrobiol. Hyg. A* **263**:229–236.
20. **Bai, Y., K. Narayan, D. Dail, M. Sondey, E. Hodzic, S. W. Barthold, A. R. Pachner, and D. Cadavid**. 2004. Spinal cord involvement in the nonhuman primate model of Lyme disease. *Lab. Invest.* **84**:160–172.
21. **Bannwarth A.** 1941. Chronische lymphocytare meningitis, entzundliche polyneuritis un 'Rheumatismus': ein betrag zum problem 'allergie und nervensystem'. *Arch. Psych. Nervenkrank.* **113**:284–376.
22. **Barbour, A. G.** 1984. Isolation and cultivation of Lyme disease spirochetes. *Yale J. Biol. Med.* **57**:521–525.
23. **Barthold, S. W.** 1991. Infectivity of *Borrelia burgdorferi* relative to route of inoculation and genotype in laboratory mice. *J. Infect. Dis.* **163**:419–420.
24. **Barthold, S. W., D. S. Beck, G. M. Hansen, G. A. Terwilliger, and K. D. Moody**. 1990. Lyme borreliosis in selected strains and ages of laboratory mice. *J. Infect. Dis.* **162**:133–138.
25. **Barthold, S. W., and M. de Souza**. 1995. Exacerbation of Lyme arthritis in beige mice. *J. Infect. Dis.* **172**:778–784.
26. **Barthold, S. W., M. S. de Souza, J. L. Janotka, A. L. Smith, and D. H. Persing**. 1993. Chronic Lyme borreliosis in the laboratory mouse. *Am. J. Pathol.* **143**:959–971.
27. **Barthold, S. W., K. D. Moody, G. A. Terwilliger, P. H. Duray, R. O. Jacoby, and A. C. Steere**. 1988. Experimental Lyme arthritis in rats infected with *Borrelia burgdorferi. J. Infect. Dis.* **157**:842–846.
28. **Barthold, S. W., D. H. Persing, A. L. Armstrong, and R. A. Peeples**. 1991. Kinetics of *Borrelia burgdorferi* dissemination and evolution of disease after intradermal inoculation of mice. *Am. J. Pathol.* **139**:263–273.
29. **Barthold, S. W., C. L. Sidman, and A. L. Smith**. 1992. Lyme borreliosis in genetically resistant and susceptible mice with severe combined immunodeficiency. *Am. J. Trop. Med. Hyg.* **47**:605–613.
30. **Berglund, J., R. Eitrem, K. Ornstein, A. Lindberg, A. Ringer, H. Elmrud, M. Carlsson, A. Runehagen, C. Svanborg, and R. Norrby**. 1995. An epidemiologic study of Lyme disease in southern Sweden. *N. Engl. J. Med.* **333**:1319–1327.
31. **Brehmer-Andersson, E., A. Hovmark, and E. Asbrink**. 1998. Acrodermatitis chronica atrophicans: histopathologic findings and clinical correlations in 111 cases. *Acta Derm. Venereol.* **78**:207–213.
32. **Brooks, C. S., P. S. Hefty, S. E. Jolliff, and D. R. Akins**. 2003. Global analysis of *Borrelia burgdorferi* genes regulated by mammalian host-specific signals. *Infect. Immun.* **71**:3371–3383.
33. **Bunikis, J., and A. G. Barbour**. 2002. Laboratory testing for suspected Lyme disease. *Med. Clin. North Am.* **86**:311–340.
34. **Burgdorfer, W., A. G. Barbour, S. F. Hayes, J. L. Benach, E. Grunwaldt, and J. P. Davis**. 1982. Lyme disease—a tick-borne spirochetosis? *Science* **216**:1317–1319.
35. **Busch, U., C. Hizo-Teufel, R. Boehmer, V. Fingerle, H. Nitschko, B. Wilske, and V. Preac-Mursic**. 1996. Three species of *Borrelia burgdorferi* sensu lato (*B. burgdorferi* sensu stricto, *B afzelii*, and *B. garinii*) identified from cerebrospinal fluid isolates by pulsed-field gel electrophoresis and PCR. *J. Clin. Microbiol.* **34**:1072–1078.
36. **Cabello, F. C., H. P. Godfrey, and S. A. Newman**. 2007. Hidden in plain sight: *Borrelia burgdorferi* and the extracellular matrix. *Trends Microbiol.* **15**:350–354.
37. **Cadavid, D., Y. Bai, D. Dail, M. Hurd, K. Narayan, E. Hodzic, S. W. Barthold, and A. R. Pachner**. 2003. Infection and

inflammation in skeletal muscle from nonhuman primates infected with different genospecies of the Lyme disease spirochete *Borrelia burgdorferi*. *Infect. Immun.* **71:**7087–7098.
38. **Cadavid, D., Y. Bai, E. Hodzic, K. Narayan, S. W. Barthold, and A. R. Pachner.** 2004. Cardiac involvement in non-human primates infected with the Lyme disease spirochete *Borrelia burgdorferi*. *Lab. Invest.* **84:**1439–1450.
39. **Cadavid, D., T. O'Neill, H. Schaefer, and A. R. Pachner.** 2000. Localization of *Borrelia burgdorferi* in the nervous system and other organs in a nonhuman primate model of lyme disease. *Lab. Invest.* **80:**1043–1054.
40. **Carlson, D., J. Hernandez, B. J. Bloom, J. Coburn, J. M. Aversa, and A. C. Steere.** 1999. Lack of *Borrelia burgdorferi* DNA in synovial samples from patients with antibiotic treatment-resistant Lyme arthritis. *Arthritis Rheum.* **42:**2705–2709.
41. **Casjens, S., N. Palmer, R. van Vugt, W. M. Huang, B. Stevenson, P. Rosa, R. Lathigra, G. Sutton, J. Peterson, R. J. Dodson, D. Haft, E. Hickey, M. Gwinn, O. White, and C. M. Fraser.** 2000. A bacterial genome in flux: the twelve linear and nine circular extrachromosomal DNAs in an infectious isolate of the Lyme disease spirochete *Borrelia burgdorferi*. *Mol. Microbiol.* **35:**490–516.
42. **Coyle, P. K.** 1989. *Borrelia burgdorferi* antibodies in multiple sclerosis patients. *Neurology* **39:**760–761.
43. **Coyle, P. K., L. B. Krupp, and C. Doscher.** 1993. Significance of reactive Lyme serology in multiple sclerosis. *Ann. Neurol.* **34:**745–747.
44. **Dattwyler, R. J., B. J. Luft, M. J. Kunkel, M. F. Finkel, G. P. Wormser, T. J. Rush, E. Grunwaldt, W. A. Agger, M. Franklin, D. Oswald, L. Cockey, and D. Maladorno.** 1997. Ceftriaxone compared with doxycycline for the treatment of acute disseminated Lyme disease. *N. Engl. J. Med.* **337:**289–294.
45. **de Koning, J., D. J. Tazelaar, J. A. Hoogkamp-Korstanje, and J. D. Elema.** 1995. Acrodermatitis chronica atrophicans: a light and electron microscopic study. *J. Cutan. Pathol.* **22:**23–32.
46. **Dhote, R., A. L. Basse-Guerineau, V. Beaumesnil, B. Christoforov, and M. V. Assous.** 2000. Full spectrum of clinical, serological, and epidemiological features of complicated forms of Lyme borreliosis in the Paris, France, area. *Eur. J. Clin. Microbiol. Infect. Dis.* **19:**809–815.
47. **Dolan, M. C., G. O. Maupin, B. S. Schneider, C. Denatale, N. Hamon, C. Cole, N. S. Zeidner, and K. C. Stafford III.** 2004. Control of immature *Ixodes scapularis* (Acari: Ixodidae) on rodent reservoirs of *Borrelia burgdorferi* in a residential community of southeastern Connecticut. *J. Med. Entomol.* **41:**1043–1054.
48. **Drouin, E. E., L. J. Glickstein, and A. C. Steere.** 2004. Molecular characterization of the OspA(161-175) T cell epitope associated with treatment-resistant Lyme arthritis: differences among the three pathogenic species of *Borrelia burgdorferi* sensu lato. *J. Autoimmun.* **23:**281–292.
49. **England, J. D., R. P. Bohm, Jr., E. D. Roberts, and M. T. Philipp.** 1997. Lyme neuroborreliosis in the rhesus monkey. *Semin. Neurol.* **17:**53–56.
50. **Fagrell, B., G. Stiernstedt, and J. Ostergren.** 1986. Acrodermatitis chronica atrophicans Herxheimer can often mimic a peripheral vascular disorder. *Acta Med. Scand.* **220:**485–488.
51. **Fahrer, H., S. M. van der Linden, M. J. Sauvain, L. Gern, E. Zhioua, and A. Aeschlimann.** 1991. The prevalence and incidence of clinical and asymptomatic Lyme borreliosis in a population at risk. *J. Infect. Dis.* **163:**305–310.
52. **Fallon, B. A., J. G. Keilp, K. M. Corbera, E. Petkova, C. B. Britton, E. Dwyer, I. Slavov, J. Cheng, J. Dobkin, D. R. Nelson, and H. A. Sackeim.** 2008. A randomized, placebo-controlled trial of repeated IV antibiotic therapy for Lyme encephalopathy. *Neurology* **70:**992–1003.
53. **Feder, H. M., Jr., M. Abeles, M. Bernstein, D. Whitaker-Worth, and J. M. Grant-Kels.** 2006. Diagnosis, treatment, and prognosis of erythema migrans and Lyme arthritis. *Clin. Dermatol.* **24:**509–520.
54. **Feder, H. M., Jr., B. J. Johnson, S. O'Connell, E. D. Shapiro, A. C. Steere, and G. P. Wormser.** 2007. A critical appraisal of "chronic Lyme disease." *N. Engl. J. Med.* **357:**1422–1430.
55. **Foley, D. M., R. J. Gayek, J. T. Skare, E. A. Wagar, C. I. Champion, D. R. Blanco, M. A. Lovett, and J. N. Miller.** 1995. Rabbit model of Lyme borreliosis: erythema migrans, infection-derived immunity, and identification of *Borrelia burgdorferi* proteins associated with virulence and protective immunity. *J. Clin. Investig.* **96:**965–975.
56. **Franz, J. K., and A. Krause.** 2003. Lyme disease (Lyme borreliosis). *Best Pract. Res. Clin. Rheumatol.* **17:**241–264.
57. **Fraser, C. M., S. Casjens, W. M. Huang, G. G. Sutton, R. Clayton, R. Lathigra, O. White, K. A. Ketchum, R. Dodson, E. K. Hickey, M. Gwinn, B. Dougherty, J. F. Tomb, R. D. Fleischmann, D. Richardson, J. Peterson, A. R. Kerlavage, J. Quackenbush, S. Salzberg, M. Hanson, R. van Vugt, N. Palmer, M. D. Adams, J. Gocayne, J. Weidman, T. Utterback, L. Watthey, L. McDonald, P. Artiach, C. Bowman, S. Garland, C. Fuji, M. D. Cotton, K. Horst, K. Roberts, B. Hatch, H. O. Smith, and J. C. Venter.** 1997. Genomic sequence of a Lyme disease spirochaete, *Borrelia burgdorferi*. *Nature* **390:**580–586.
58. **Gasser, R., J. Dusleag, E. Reisinger, R. Stauber, B. Feigl, S. Pongratz, W. Klein, C. Furian, and K. Pierer.** 1992. Reversal by ceftriaxone of dilated cardiomyopathy *Borrelia burgdorferi* infection. *Lancet* **339:**1174–1175.
59. **Gerber, M. A., E. D. Shapiro, G. S. Burke, V. J. Parcells, G. L. Bell, et al.** 1996. Lyme disease in children in southeastern Connecticut.. *N. Engl. J. Med.* **335:**1270–1274.
60. **Gerber, M. A., L. S. Zemel, and E. D. Shapiro.** 1998. Lyme arthritis in children: clinical epidemiology and long-term outcomes. *Pediatrics* **102:**905–908.
61. **Gilmore, R. D., Jr., R. R. Howison, V. L. Schmit, A. J. Nowalk, D. R. Clifton, C. Nolder, J. L. Hughes, and J. A. Carroll.** 2007. Temporal expression analysis of the *Borrelia burgdorferi* paralogous gene family 54 genes BBA64, BBA65, and BBA66 during persistent infection in mice. *Infect. Immun.* **75:**2753–2764.
62. **Gross, D. M., T. Forsthuber, M. Tary-Lehmann, C. Etling, K. Ito, Z. A. Nagy, J. A. Field, A. C. Steere, and B. T. Huber.** 1998. Identification of LFA-1 as a candidate autoantigen in treatment-resistant Lyme arthritis. *Science* **281:**703–706.
63. **Gross, D. M., A. C. Steere, and B. T. Huber.** 1998. T helper 1 response is dominant and localized to the synovial fluid in patients with Lyme arthritis. *J. Immunol* **160:**1022–1028.
64. **Guo, B. P., S. J. Norris, L. C. Rosenberg, and M. Hook.** 1995. Adherence of *Borrelia burgdorferi* to the proteoglycan decorin. *Infect. Immun.* **63:**3467–3472.
65. **Haddad, F. A., and R. B. Nadelman.** 2003. Lyme disease and the heart. *Front. Biosci.* **8:**s769–s782.
66. **Hajjar, R. J., and R. L. Kradin.** 2002. Case records of the Massachusetts General Hospital. Weekly clinicopathological exercises. Case 17-2002. A 55-year-old man with second-degree atrioventricular block and chest pain. *N. Engl. J. Med.* **346:**1732–1738.
67. **Halperin, J., B. J. Luft, D. J. Volkman, and R. J. Dattwyler.** 1990. Lyme neuroborreliosis. Peripheral nervous system manifestations. *Brain* **113:**1207–1221.

68. **Halperin, J. J.** 1995. Neuroborreliosis. *Am. J. Med.* **98:**52S–56S.
69. **Halperin, J. J.** 2002. Nervous system Lyme disease. *Vector Borne Zoonotic Dis.* **2:**241–247.
70. **Halperin, J. J.** 2008. Prolonged Lyme disease treatment. *Neurology* **70:**986–987.
71. **Halperin, J. J., and M. P. Heyes.** 1992. Neuroactive kynurenines in Lyme borreliosis. *Neurology* **42:**43–50.
72. **Halperin, J. J., L. B. Krupp, M. G. Golightly, and D. J. Volkman.** 1990. Lyme borreliosis-associated encephalopathy. *Neurology* **40:**1340–1343.
73. **Halperin, J. J., E. L. Logigian, M. F. Finkel, and R. A. Pearl.** 1996. Practice parameters for the diagnosis of patients with nervous system Lyme borreliosis (Lyme disease).Quality Standards Subcommittee of the American Academy of Neurology. *Neurology* **46:**619–627.
74. **Halperin, J. J., B. J. Luft, A. K. Anand, C. T. Roque, O. Alvarez, D. J. Volkman, and R. J. Dattwyler.** 1989. Lyme neuroborreliosis: central nervous system manifestations. *Neurology* **39:**753–759.
75. **Halperin, J. J., D. J. Volkman, and P. Wu.** 1991. Central nervous system abnormalities in Lyme neuroborreliosis. *Neurology* **41:**1571–1582.
76. **Hansen, K., and E. Asbrink.** 1989. Serodiagnosis of erythema migrans and acrodermatitis chronica atrophicans by the *Borrelia burgdorferi* flagellum enzyme-linked immunosorbent assay. *J. Clin. Microbiol.* **27:**545–551.
77. **Hansen, K., and A. M. Lebech.** 1991. Lyme neuroborreliosis: a new sensitive diagnostic assay for intrathecal synthesis of *Borrelia burgdorferi*-specific immunoglobulin G, A, and M. *Ann. Neurol.* **30:**197–205.
78. **Hansen, K., and A. M. Lebech.** 1992. The clinical and epidemiological profile of Lyme neuroborreliosis in Denmark 1985-1990. A prospective study of 187 patients with *Borrelia burgdorferi* specific intrathecal antibody production. *Brain* **115:**399–423.
79. **Hemmer, B., B. Gran, Y. Zhao, A. Marques, J. Pascal, A. Tzou, T. Kondo, I. Cortese, B. Bielekova, S. E. Straus, H. F. McFarland, R. Houghten, R. Simon, C. Pinilla, and R. Martin.** 1999. Identification of candidate T-cell epitopes and molecular mimics in chronic Lyme disease. *Nat. Med.* **5:**1375–1382.
80. **Hofhuis, A., J. W. van der Giessen, F. H. Borgsteede, P. R. Wielinga, D. W. Notermans, and W. van Pelt.** 2006. Lyme borreliosis in the Netherlands: strong increase in GP consultations and hospital admissions in past 10 years. *Euro. Surveill.* **11:**E060622.
81. **Hopf, H. C.** 1975. Peripheral neuropathy in acrodermatitis chronica atrophicans (Herxheimer). *J. Neurol. Neurosurg. Psychiatry* **38:**452–458.
82. **Hovius, J. W., A. P. van Dam, and E. Fikrig.** 2007. Tick-host-pathogen interactions in Lyme borreliosis. *Trends Parasitol.* **23:**434–438.
83. **Hovius, K. E., B. Beijer, S. G. Rijpkema, N. M. Bleumink-Pluym, and D. J. Houwers.** 1998. Identification of four *Borrelia burgdorferi* sensu lato species in *Ixodes ricinus* ticks collected from Dutch dogs. *Vet. Q.* **20:**143–145.
84. **Hovmark, A., E. Asbrink, and I. Olsson.** 1986. Joint and bone involvement in Swedish patients with *Ixodes ricinus*-borne *Borrelia* infection. *Zentralbl. Bakteriol. Mikrobiol. Hyg. A* **263:**275–284.
85. **Hubalek, Z., and J. Halouzka.** 1997. Distribution of *Borrelia burgdorferi* sensu lato genomic groups in Europe, a review. *Eur. J. Epidemiol.* **13:**951–957.
86. **Hunfeld, K. P., and V. Brade.** 2006. Antimicrobial susceptibility of *Borrelia burgdorferi* sensu lato: what we know, what we don't know, and what we need to know. *Wien. Klin. Wochenschr.* **118:**659–668.
87. **Huppertz, H. I., M. Bohme, S. M. Standaert, H. Karch, and S. A. Plotkin.** 1999. Incidence of Lyme borreliosis in the Wurzburg region of Germany. *Eur. J. Clin. Microbiol. Infect. Dis.* **18:**697–703.
88. **Jaulhac, B., I. Chary-Valckenaere, J. Sibilia, R. M. Javier, Y. Piemont, J. L. Kuntz, H. Monteil, and J. Pourel.** 1996. Detection of *Borrelia burgdorferi* by DNA amplification in synovial tissue samples from patients with Lyme arthritis. *Arthritis Rheum.* **39:**736–745.
89. **Johnson, R. C., N. Marek, and C. Kodner.** 1984. Infection of Syrian hamsters with Lyme disease spirochetes. *J. Clin. Microbiol.* **20:**1099–1101.
90. **Kaiser, R.** 1998. Neuroborreliosis. *J. Neurol.* **245:**247–255.
91. **Kannian, P., E. E. Drouin, L. Glickstein, W. W. Kwok, G. T. Nepom, and A. C. Steere.** 2007. Decline in the frequencies of *Borrelia burgdorferi* OspA161 175-specific T cells after antibiotic therapy in HLA-DRB1*0401-positive patients with antibiotic-responsive or antibiotic-refractory lyme arthritis. *J. Immunol.* **179:**6336–6342.
92. **Kannian, P., G. McHugh, B. J. Johnson, R. M. Bacon, L. J. Glickstein, and A. C. Steere.** 2007. Antibody responses to *Borrelia burgdorferi* in patients with antibiotic-refractory, antibiotic-responsive, or non-antibiotic-treated Lyme arthritis. *Arthritis Rheum.* **56:**4216–4225.
93. **Kaplan, R. F., M. E. Meadows, L. C. Vincent, E. L. Logigian, and A. C. Steere.** 1992. Memory impairment and depression in patients with Lyme encephalopathy: comparison with fibromyalgia and nonpsychotically depressed patients. *Neurology* **42:**1263–1267.
94. **Kaplan, R. F., R. P. Trevino, G. M. Johnson, L. Levy, R. Dornbush, L. T. Hu, J. Evans, A. Weinstein, C. H. Schmid, and M. S. Klempner.** 2003. Cognitive function in post-treatment Lyme disease: do additional antibiotics help? *Neurology* **60:**1916–1922.
95. **Karussis, D., H. L. Weiner, and O. Abramsky.** 1999. Multiple sclerosis vs Lyme disease: a case presentation to a discussant and a review of the literature. *Mult. Scler.* **5:**395–402.
96. **Keller, T. L., J. J. Halperin, and M. Whitman.** 1992. PCR detection of *Borrelia burgdorferi* DNA in cerebrospinal fluid of Lyme neuroborreliosis patients. *Neurology* **42:**32–42.
97. **Kindstrand, E., B. Y. Nilsson, A. Hovmark, R. Pirskanen, and E. Asbrink.** 1997. Peripheral neuropathy in acrodermatitis chronica atrophicans—a late *Borrelia* manifestation. *Acta Neurol. Scand.* **95:**338–345.
98. **Klein, J., G. Stanek, R. Bittner, R. Horvat, C. Holzinger, and D. Glogar.** 1991. Lyme borreliosis as a cause of myocarditis and heart muscle disease. *Eur. Heart J.* **12**(Suppl. D):73–75.
99. **Klempner, M. S.** 2002. Controlled trials of antibiotic treatment in patients with post-treatment chronic Lyme disease. *Vector Borne Zoonotic Dis.* **2:**255–263.
100. **Klempner, M. S., L. T. Hu, J. Evans, C. H. Schmid, G. M. Johnson, R. P. Trevino, D. Norton, L. Levy, D. Wall, J. McCall, M. Kosinski, and A. Weinstein.** 2001. Two controlled trials of antibiotic treatment in patients with persistent symptoms and a history of Lyme disease. *N. Engl. J. Med.* **345:**85–92.
101. **Kornblatt, A. N., A. C. Steere, and D. G. Brownstein.** 1984. Experimental Lyme disease in rabbits: spirochetes found in erythema migrans and blood. *Infect. Immun.* **46:**220–223.
102. **Krupp, L. B., L. G. Hyman, R. Grimson, P. K. Coyle, P. Melville, S. Ahnn, R. Dattwyler, and B. Chandler.** 2003.

Study and treatment of post Lyme disease (STOP-LD): a randomized double masked clinical trial. *Neurology* **60**:1923–1930.

103. **Krupp, L. B., D. Masur, J. Schwartz, P. K. Coyle, L. J. Langenbach, S. K. Fernquist, L. Jandorf, and J. J. Halperin.** 1991. Cognitive functioning in late Lyme borreliosis. *Arch. Neurol.* **48**:1125–1129.
104. **Kuiper, H., A. P. van Dam, A. W. Moll van Charante, N. P. Nauta, and J. Dankert.** 1993. One year follow-up study to assess the prevalence and incidence of Lyme borreliosis among Dutch forestry workers. *Eur. J. Clin. Microbiol. Infect. Dis.* **12**:413–418.
105. **Lardieri, G., A. Salvi, F. Camerini, M. Cinco, and G. Trevisan.** 1993. Isolation of *Borrelia burgdorferi* from myocardium. *Lancet* **342**:490.
106. **Liang, F. T., E. L. Brown, T. Wang, R. V. Iozzo, and E. Fikrig.** 2004. Protective niche for *Borrelia burgdorferi* to evade humoral immunity. *Am. J. Pathol.* **165**:977–985.
107. **Liang, F. T., M. B. Jacobs, L. C. Bowers, and M. T. Philipp.** 2002. An immune evasion mechanism for spirochetal persistence in Lyme borreliosis. *J. Exp. Med.* **195**:415–422.
108. **Liang, F. T., F. K. Nelson, and E. Fikrig.** 2002. Molecular adaptation of *Borrelia burgdorferi* in the murine host. *J. Exp. Med.* **196**:275–280.
109. **Liang, F. T., J. M. Nowling, and M. T. Philipp.** 2000. Cryptic and exposed invariable regions of VlsE, the variable surface antigen of *Borrelia burgdorferi* sl. *J. Bacteriol.* **182**:3597–3601.
110. **Liang, F. T., A. C. Steere, A. R. Marques, B. J. Johnson, J. N. Miller, and M. T. Philipp.** 1999. Sensitive and specific serodiagnosis of Lyme disease by enzyme-linked immunosorbent assay with a peptide based on an immunodominant conserved region of *Borrelia burgdorferi* VlsE. *J. Clin. Microbiol.* **37**:3990–3996.
111. **Livengood, J. A., and R. D. Gilmore, Jr.** 2006. Invasion of human neuronal and glial cells by an infectious strain of *Borrelia burgdorferi*. *Microbes Infect.* **8**:2832–2840.
112. **Logigian, E. L., R. F. Kaplan, and A. C. Steere.** 1990. Chronic neurologic manifestations of Lyme disease. *N. Engl. J. Med.* **323**:1438–1444.
113. **Logigian, E. L., R. F. Kaplan, and A. C. Steere.** 1999. Successful treatment of Lyme encephalopathy with intravenous ceftriaxone. *J. Infect. Dis.* **180**:377–383.
114. **Logigian, E. L. and A. C. Steere.** 1992. Clinical and electrophysiologic findings in chronic neuropathy of Lyme disease. *Neurology* **42**:303–311.
115. **Malawista, S. E., S. W. Barthold, and D. H. Persing.** 1994. Fate of *Borrelia burgdorferi* DNA in tissues of infected mice after antibiotic treatment. *J. Infect. Dis.* **170**:1312–1316.
116. **Marangoni, A., A. Moroni, S. Accardo, and R. Cevenini.** 2008. *Borrelia burgdorferi* VlsE antigen for the serological diagnosis of Lyme borreliosis. *Eur. J. Clin. Microbiol. Infect. Dis.* **27**:349–354.
117. **Marques, A. R., F. Stock, and V. Gill.** 2000. Evaluation of a new culture medium for *Borrelia burgdorferi*. *J. Clin. Microbiol.* **38**:4239–4241.
118. **Matyniak, J. E., and S. L. Reiner.** 1995. T helper phenotype and genetic susceptibility in experimental Lyme disease. *J. Exp. Med.* **181**:1251–1254.
119. **Mayer, W., F. X. Kleber, B. Wilske, V. Preac-Mursic, W. Maciejewski, H. Sigl, E. Holzer, and W. Doering.** 1990. Persistent atrioventricular block in Lyme borreliosis. *Klin. Wochenschr.* **68**:431–435.
120. **McDowell, J. V., S. Y. Sung, L. T. Hu, and R. T. Marconi.** 2002. Evidence that the variable regions of the central domain of VlsE are antigenic during infection with Lyme disease spirochetes. *Infect. Immun.* **70**:4196–4203.
121. **Moody, K. D., R. L. Adams, and S. W. Barthold.** 1994. Effectiveness of antimicrobial treatment against *Borrelia burgdorferi* infection in mice. *Antimicrob. Agents Chemother.* **38**:1567–1572.
122. **Muellegger, R. R., E. M. Schluepen, M. M. Millner, H. P. Soyer, M. Volkenandt, and H. Kerl.** 1996. Acrodermatitis chronica atrophicans in an 11-year-old girl. *Br. J. Dermatol.* **135**:609–612.
123. **Mullegger, R. R.** 2004. Dermatological manifestations of Lyme borreliosis. *Eur. J. Dermatol.* **14**:296–309.
124. **Nadelman, R. B., J. Nowakowski, G. Forseter, N. S. Goldberg, S. Bittker, D. Cooper, M. Aguero-Rosenfeld, and G. P. Wormser.** 1996. The clinical spectrum of early Lyme borreliosis in patients with culture-confirmed erythema migrans. *Am. J. Med.* **100**:502–508.
125. **Nadelman, R. B., J. Nowakowski, G. P. Wormser, and I. Schwartz.** 1999. How should viability of *Borrelia burgdorferi* be demonstrated? *Am. J. Med.* **106**:491–492.
126. **Nadelman, R. B., and G. P. Wormser.** 1998. Lyme borreliosis. *Lancet* **352**:557–565.
127. **Nadelman, R. B., and G. P. Wormser.** 2007. Reinfection in patients with Lyme disease. *Clin. Infect. Dis.* **45**:1032–1038.
128. **Nocton, J. J., F. Dressler, B. J. Rutledge, P. N. Rys, D. H. Persing, and A. C. Steere.** 1994. Detection of *Borrelia burgdorferi* DNA by polymerase chain reaction in synovial fluid from patients with Lyme arthritis. *N. Engl. J. Med.* **330**:229–234.
129. **Olsson, I., E. Asbrink, M. von Stedingk, and L. V. von Stedingk.** 1994. Changes in *Borrelia burgdorferi*-specific serum IgG antibody levels in patients treated for acrodermatitis chronica atrophicans. *Acta Derm. Venereol.* **74**:424–428.
130. **Oschmann, P., W. Dorndorf, C. Hornig, C. Schafer, H. J. Wellensiek, and K. W. Pflughaupt.** 1998. Stages and syndromes of neuroborreliosis. *J. Neurol.* **245**:262–272.
131. **Pachner, A. R., K. Amemiya, M. Bartlett, H. Schaefer, K. Reddy, and W. F. Zhang.** 2001. Lyme borreliosis in rhesus macaques: effects of corticosteroids on spirochetal load and isotype switching of anti-*Borrelia burgdorferi* antibody. *Clin. Diagn. Lab. Immunol.* **8**:225–232.
132. **Pachner, A. R., S. T. Braswell, E. Delaney, K. Amemiya, and E. Major.** 1994. A rabbit model of Lyme neuroborreliosis: characterization by PCR, serology, and sequencing of the OspA gene from the brain. *Neurology* **44**:1938–1943.
133. **Pachner, A. R., D. Cadavid, G. Shu, D. Dail, S. Pachner, E. Hodzic, and S. W. Barthold.** 2001. Central and peripheral nervous system infection, immunity, and inflammation in the NHP model of Lyme borreliosis. *Ann. Neurol.* **50**:330–338.
134. **Pachner, A. R., E. Delaney, T. O'Neill, and E. Major.** 1995. Inoculation of nonhuman primates with the N40 strain of *Borrelia burgdorferi* leads to a model of Lyme neuroborreliosis faithful to the human disease. *Neurology* **45**:165–172.
135. **Pachner, A. R., H. Gelderblom, and D. Cadavid.** 2001. The rhesus model of Lyme neuroborreliosis. *Immunol. Rev.* **183**:186–204.
136. **Pachner, A. R., H. Schaefer, K. Amemiya, D. Cadavid, W. F. Zhang, K. Reddy, and T. O'Neill.** 1998. Pathogenesis of neuroborreliosis—lessons from a monkey model. *Wien. Klin. Wochenschr.* **110**:870–873.
137. **Pachner, A. R., and A. C. Steere.** 1984. Neurological findings of Lyme disease. *Yale J. Biol. Med.* **57**:481–483.

138. **Pachner, A. R., and I. Steiner.** 2007. Lyme neuroborreliosis: infection, immunity, and inflammation. *Lancet Neurol.* **6:**544–552.
139. **Pal, U., and E. Fikrig.** 2003. Adaptation of *Borrelia burgdorferi* in the vector and vertebrate host. *Microbes Infect.* **5:**659–666.
140. **Philipp, M. T., M. K. Aydintug, R. P. Bohm, Jr., F. B. Cogswell, V. A. Dennis, H. N. Lanners, R. C. Lowrie, Jr., E. D. Roberts, M. D. Conway, M. Karacorlu, G. A. Peyman, D. J. Gubler, B. J. Johnson, J. Piesman, and Y. Gu.** 1993. Early and early disseminated phases of Lyme disease in the rhesus monkey: a model for infection in humans. *Infect. Immun.* **61:**3047–3059.
141. **Philipp, M. T., L. C. Bowers, P. T. Fawcett, M. B. Jacobs, F. T. Liang, A. R. Marques, P. D. Mitchell, J. E. Purcell, M. S. Ratterree, and R. K. Straubinger.** 2001. Antibody response to IR6, a conserved immunodominant region of the VlsE lipoprotein, wanes rapidly after antibiotic treatment of *Borrelia burgdorferi* infection in experimental animals and in humans. *J. Infect. Dis.* **184:**870–878.
142. **Philipp, M. T., G. P. Wormser, A. R. Marques, S. Bittker, D. S. Martin, J. Nowakowski, and L. G. Dally.** 2005. A decline in C_6 antibody titer occurs in successfully treated patients with culture-confirmed early localized or early disseminated Lyme borreliosis. *Clin. Diagn. Lab. Immunol.* **12:**1069–1074.
143. **Phillips, S. E., L. H. Mattman, D. Hulinska, and H. Moayad.** 1998. A proposal for the reliable culture of *Borrelia burgdorferi* from patients with chronic Lyme disease, even from those previously aggressively treated. *Infection* **26:**364–367.
144. **Picken, M. M., R. N. Picken, D. Han, Y. Cheng, E. Ruzic-Sabljic, J. Cimperman, V. Maraspin, S. Lotric-Furlan, and F. Strle.** 1997. A two year prospective study to compare culture and polymerase chain reaction amplification for the detection and diagnosis of Lyme borreliosis. *Mol. Pathol.* **50:**186–193.
145. **Piesman, J., K. L. Clark, M. C. Dolan, C. M. Happ, and T. R. Burkot.** 1999. Geographic survey of vector ticks (*Ixodes scapularis* and *Ixodes pacificus*) for infection with the Lyme disease spirochete, *Borrelia burgdorferi*. *J. Vector Ecol.* **24:**91–98.
146. **Pinto, D. S.** 2002. Cardiac manifestations of Lyme disease. *Med. Clin. North Am.* **86:**285–296.
147. **Postic, D., M. Garnier, and G. Baranton.** 2007. Multilocus sequence analysis of atypical *Borrelia burgdorferi* sensu lato isolates—description of *Borrelia californiensis* sp. nov., and genomospecies 1 and 2. *Int. J. Med. Microbiol.* **297:**263–271.
148. **Priem, S., G. R. Burmester, T. Kamradt, K. Wolbart, M. G. Rittig, and A. Krause.** 1998. Detection of *Borrelia burgdorferi* by polymerase chain reaction in synovial membrane, but not in synovial fluid from patients with persisting Lyme arthritis after antibiotic therapy. *Ann. Rheum. Dis.* **57:**118–121.
149. **Reid, M. C., R. T. Schoen, J. Evans, J. C. Rosenberg, and R. I. Horwitz.** 1998. The consequences of overdiagnosis and overtreatment of Lyme disease: an observational study. *Ann. Intern. Med.* **128:**354–362.
150. **Richter, D., D. B. Schlee, R. Allgower, and F. R. Matuschka.** 2004. Relationships of a novel Lyme disease spirochete, *Borrelia spielmani* sp. nov., with its hosts in Central Europe. *Appl. Environ. Microbiol.* **70:**6414–6419.
151. **Roberts, E. D., R. P. Bohm, Jr., F. B. Cogswell, H. N. Lanners, R. C. Lowrie, Jr., L. Povinelli, J. Piesman, and M. T. Philipp.** 1995. Chronic lyme disease in the rhesus monkey. *Lab. Invest.* **72:**146–160.
152. **Roberts, E. D., R. P. Bohm, Jr., R. C. Lowrie, Jr., G. Habicht, L. Katona, J. Piesman, and M. T. Philipp.** 1998. Pathogenesis of Lyme neuroborreliosis in the rhesus monkey: the early disseminated and chronic phases of disease in the peripheral nervous system. *J. Infect. Dis.* **178:**722–732.
153. **Rubin, D. A., C. Sorbera, P. Nikitin, A. McAllister, G. P. Wormser, and R. B. Nadelman.** 1992. Prospective evaluation of heart block complicating early Lyme disease. *Pacing Clin. Electrophysiol.* **15:**252–255.
154. **Schmitz, J. L., R. F. Schell, A. Hejka, D. M. England, and L. Konick.** 1988. Induction of Lyme arthritis in LSH hamsters. *Infect. Immun.* **56:**2336–2342.
155. **Schwan, T. G., J. Piesman, W. T. Golde, M. C. Dolan, and P. A. Rosa.** 1995. Induction of an outer surface protein on *Borrelia burgdorferi* during tick feeding. *Proc. Natl. Acad. Sci. USA* **92:**2909–2913.
156. **Schwartz, I., G. P. Wormser, J. J. Schwartz, D. Cooper, P. Weissensee, A. Gazumyan, E. Zimmermann, N. S. Goldberg, S. Bittker, G. L. Campbell, and C. S. Pavia.** 1992. Diagnosis of early Lyme disease by polymerase chain reaction amplification and culture of skin biopsies from erythema migrans lesions. *J. Clin. Microbiol.* **30:**3082–3088.
157. **Seltzer, E. G., M. A. Gerber, M. L. Cartter, K. Freudigman, and E. D. Shapiro.** 2000. Long-term outcomes of persons with Lyme disease. *JAMA* **283:**609–616.
158. **Shapiro, E. D.** 2002. Long-term outcomes of persons with Lyme disease. *Vector Borne Zoonotic Dis.* **2:**279–281.
159. **Shin, J. J., L. J. Glickstein, and A. C. Steere.** 2007. High levels of inflammatory chemokines and cytokines in joint fluid and synovial tissue throughout the course of antibiotic-refractory lyme arthritis. *Arthritis Rheum.* **56:**1325–1335.
160. **Sigal, L. H.** 1990. Summary of the first 100 patients seen at a Lyme disease referral center. *Am. J. Med.* **88:**577–581.
161. **Skoldenberg, B., G. Stiernstedt, M. Karlsson, B. Wretlind, and B. Svenungsson.** 1988. Treatment of Lyme borreliosis with emphasis on neurological disease. *Ann. N. Y. Acad. Sci.* **539:**317–323.
162. **Stanek, G., J. Klein, R. Bittner, and D. Glogar.** 1990. Isolation of *Borrelia burgdorferi* from the myocardium of a patient with longstanding cardiomyopathy. *N. Engl. J. Med.* **322:**249–252.
163. **Stanek, G., J. Klein, R. Bittner, and D. Glogar.** 1991. *Borrelia burgdorferi* as an etiologic agent in chronic heart failure? *Scand. J. Infect. Dis. Suppl* **77:**85–87.
164. **Steere, A. C.** 1989. Lyme disease. *N. Engl. J. Med.* **321:**586–596.
165. **Steere, A. C.** 2001. Lyme disease. *N. Engl. J. Med.* **345:**115–125.
166. **Steere, A. C.** 2003. Duration of antibiotic therapy for Lyme disease. *Ann. Intern. Med.* **138:**761–762.
167. **Steere, A. C.** 2006. Lyme borreliosis in 2005, 30 years after initial observations in Lyme Connecticut. *Wien. Klin. Wochenschr.* **118:**625–633.
168. **Steere, A. C., and S. M. Angelis.** 2006. Therapy for Lyme arthritis: strategies for the treatment of antibiotic-refractory arthritis. *Arthritis Rheum.* **54:**3079–3086.
169. **Steere, A. C., W. P. Batsford, M. Weinberg, J. Alexander, H. J. Berger, S. Wolfson, and S. E. Malawista.** 1980. Lyme carditis: cardiac abnormalities of Lyme disease. *Ann. Intern. Med.* **93:**8–16.
170. **Steere, A. C., V. P. Berardi, K. E. Weeks, E. L. Logigian, and R. Ackermann.** 1990. Evaluation of the intrathecal antibody

response to *Borrelia burgdorferi* as a diagnostic test for Lyme neuroborreliosis. *J. Infect. Dis.* **161:**1203–1209.

171. **Steere, A. C., J. Coburn, and L. Glickstein.** 2004. The emergence of Lyme disease. *J. Clin. Investig.* **113:**1093–1101.

172. **Steere, A. C., R. L. Grodzicki, A. N. Kornblatt, J. E. Craft, A. G. Barbour, W. Burgdorfer, G. P. Schmid, E. Johnson, and S. E. Malawista.** 1983. The spirochetal etiology of Lyme disease. *N. Engl. J. Med.* **308:**733–740.

173. **Steere, A. C., R. E. Levin, P. J. Molloy, R. A. Kalish, J. H. Abraham III, N. Y. Liu, and C. H. Schmid.** 1994. Treatment of Lyme arthritis. *Arthritis Rheum.* **37:**878–888.

173a. **Steere, A. C., S. E. Malawista, D. R. Snydman, R. E. Shope, W. A. Andiman, M. R. Ross, and F. M. Steele.** 1977. Lyme arthritis: an epidemic of oligoarticular arthritis in children and adults in three Connecticut communities. *Arthritis Rheum.* **20:**7–17.

174. **Steere, A. C., R. T. Schoen, and E. Taylor.** 1987. The clinical evolution of Lyme arthritis. *Ann. Intern. Med.* **107:**725–731.

175. **Steere, A. C., V. K. Sikand, R. T. Schoen, and J. Nowakowski.** 2003. Asymptomatic infection with *Borrelia burgdorferi*. *Clin. Infect. Dis.* **37:**528–532.

176. **Steere, A. C., E. Taylor, G. L. McHugh, and E. L. Logigian.** 1993. The overdiagnosis of Lyme disease. *JAMA* **269:**1812–1816.

177. **Steere, A. C., E. Taylor, M. L. Wilson, J. F. Levine, and A. Spielman.** 1986. Longitudinal assessment of the clinical and epidemiological features of Lyme disease in a defined population. *J. Infect. Dis.* **154:**295–300.

178. **Stiernstedt, G., R. Gustafsson, M. Karlsson, B. Svenungsson, and B. Skoldenberg.** 1988. Clinical manifestations and diagnosis of neuroborreliosis. *Ann. N. Y. Acad. Sci.* **539:**46–55.

179. **Straubinger, R. K.** 2000. PCR-based quantification of *Borrelia burgdorferi* organisms in canine tissues over a 500-day postinfection period. *J. Clin. Microbiol.* **38:**2191–2199.

180. **Straubinger, R. K., A. F. Straubinger, L. Harter, R. H. Jacobson, Y. F. Chang, B. A. Summers, H. N. Erb, and M. J. Appel.** 1997. *Borrelia burgdorferi* migrates into joint capsules and causes an up-regulation of interleukin-8 in synovial membranes of dogs experimentally infected with ticks. *Infect. Immun.* **65:**1273–1285.

181. **Straubinger, R. K., A. F. Straubinger, B. A. Summers, and R. H. Jacobson.** 2000. Status of *Borrelia burgdorferi* infection after antibiotic treatment and the effects of corticosteroids: an experimental study. *J. Infect. Dis.* **181:**1069–1081.

182. **Straubinger, R. K., B. A. Summers, Y. F. Chang, and M. J. Appel.** 1997. Persistence of *Borrelia burgdorferi* in experimentally infected dogs after antibiotic treatment. *J. Clin. Microbiol.* **35:**111–116.

183. **Strle, F., R. B. Nadelman, J. Cimperman, J. Nowakowski, R. N. Picken, I. Schwartz, V. Maraspin, M. E. Aguero-Rosenfeld, S. Varde, S. Lotric-Furlan, and G. P. Wormser.** 1999. Comparison of culture-confirmed erythema migrans caused by *Borrelia burgdorferi* sensu stricto in New York State and by Borrelia afzelii in Slovenia. *Ann. Intern. Med.* **130:**32–36.

184. **Strle, F., J. A. Nelson, E. Ruzic-Sabljic, J. Cimperman, V. Maraspin, S. Lotric-Furlan, Y. Cheng, M. M. Picken, G. M. Trenholme, and R. N. Picken.** 1996. European Lyme borreliosis: 231 culture-confirmed cases involving patients with erythema migrans. *Clin. Infect. Dis.* **23:**61–65.

185. **Strle, F., R. N. Picken, Y. Cheng, J. Cimperman, V. Maraspin, S. Lotric-Furlan, E. Ruzic-Sabljic, and M. M. Picken.** 1997. Clinical findings for patients with Lyme borreliosis caused by *Borrelia burgdorferi* sensu lato with genotypic and phenotypic similarities to strain 25015. *Clin. Infect. Dis.* **25:**273–280.

186. **Strle, F., E. Ruzic-Sabljic, J. Cimperman, S. Lotric-Furlan, and V. Maraspin.** 2006. Comparison of findings for patients with *Borrelia garinii* and *Borrelia afzelii* isolated from cerebrospinal fluid. *Clin. Infect. Dis.* **43:**704–710.

187. **Tilton, R. C., D. Barden, and M. Sand.** 2001. Culture of *Borrelia burgdorferi*. *J. Clin. Microbiol.* **39:**2747.

188. **Tonks, A.** 2007. Lyme wars. *BMJ* **335:**910–912.

189. **van Dam, A. P.** 2002. Diversity of Ixodes-borne Borrelia species—clinical, pathogenetic, and diagnostic implications and impact on vaccine development. *Vector Borne Zoonotic Dis.* **2:**249–254.

190. **van Dam, A. P., H. Kuiper, K. Vos, A. Widjojokusumo, B. M. de Jongh, L. Spanjaard, A. C. Ramselaar, M. D. Kramer, and J. Dankert.** 1993. Different genospecies of *Borrelia burgdorferi* are associated with distinct clinical manifestations of Lyme borreliosis. *Clin. Infect. Dis.* **17:**708–717.

191. **van der Linde, M. R.** 1991. Lyme carditis: clinical characteristics of 105 cases. *Scand. J. Infect. Dis. Suppl.***77:**81–84.

192. **Vos, K., A. P. van Dam, H. Kuiper, H. Bruins, L. Spanjaard, and J. Dankert.** 1994. Seroconversion for Lyme borreliosis among Dutch military. *Scand. J. Infect. Dis.* **26:**427–434.

193. **Wang, G., A. P. van Dam, and J. Dankert.** 1999. Phenotypic and genetic characterization of a novel *Borrelia burgdorferi* sensu lato isolate from a patient with Lyme borreliosis. *J. Clin. Microbiol.* **37:**3025–3028.

194. **Wang, G., A. P. van Dam, and J. Dankert.** 2001. Analysis of a VMP-like sequence (vls) locus in *Borrelia garinii* and Vls homologues among four *Borrelia burgdorferi* sensu lato species. *FEMS Microbiol. Lett.* **199:**39–45.

195. **Wang, G., A. P. van Dam, A. Le Fleche, D. Postic, O. Peter, G. Baranton, R. de Boer, L. Spanjaard, and J. Dankert.** 1997. Genetic and phenotypic analysis of *Borrelia valaisiana* sp. nov. (*Borrelia* genomic groups VS116 and M19). *Int. J. Syst. Bacteriol.* **47:**926–932.

196. **Wang, G., A. P. van Dam, I. Schwartz, and J. Dankert.** 1999. Molecular typing of *Borrelia burgdorferi* sensu lato: taxonomic, epidemiological, and clinical implications. *Clin. Microbiol. Rev.* **12:**633–653.

197. **Weis, J. J.** 2002. Host-pathogen interactions and the pathogenesis of murine Lyme disease. *Curr. Opin. Rheumatol.* **14:**399–403.

198. **Wilske, B.** 2002. Microbiological diagnosis in Lyme borreliosis. *Int. J. Med. Microbiol.* **291**(Suppl 33)**:**114–119.

199. **Wilske, B., V. Fingerle, and U. Schulte-Spechtel.** 2007. Microbiological and serological diagnosis of Lyme borreliosis. *FEMS Immunol. Med. Microbiol.* **49:**13–21.

200. **Wormser, G. P., S. W. Barthold, E. D. Shapiro, R. J. Dattwyler, J. S. Bakken, A. C. Steere, L. K. Bockenstedt, and J. D. Radolf.** 2007. Anti-tumor necrosis factor-alpha activation of *Borrelia burgdorferi* spirochetes in antibiotic-treated murine Lyme borreliosis: an unproven conclusion. *J. Infect. Dis.* **196:**1865–1866.

201. **Wormser, G. P., R. J. Dattwyler, E. D. Shapiro, J. J. Halperin, A. C. Steere, M. S. Klempner, P. J. Krause, J. S. Bakken, F. Strle, G. Stanek, L. Bockenstedt, D. Fish, J. S. Dumler, and R. B. Nadelman.** 2006. The clinical assessment, treatment, and prevention of lyme disease, human granulocytic anaplasmosis, and babesiosis: clinical practice guidelines by the Infectious Diseases Society of America. *Clin. Infect. Dis.* **43:**1089–1134.

202. **Wormser, G. P., R. Ramanathan, J. Nowakowski, D. McKenna, D. Holmgren, P. Visintainer, R. Dornbush, B. Singh, and R. B. Nadelman.** 2003. Duration of antibiotic therapy

for early Lyme disease. A randomized, double-blind, placebo-controlled trial. *Ann. Intern. Med.* **138:**697–704.

203. **Yrjanainen, H., J. Hytonen, X. Y. Song, J. Oksi, K. Hartiala, and M. K. Viljanen.** 2007. Anti-tumor necrosis factor-alpha treatment activates *Borrelia burgdorferi* spirochetes 4 weeks after ceftriaxone treatment in C3H/He mice. *J. Infect. Dis.* **195:**1489–1496.

204. **Zeidner, N. S., M. S. Nuncio, B. S. Schneider, L. Gern, J. Piesman, O. Brandao, and A. R. Filipe.** 2001. A Portuguese isolate of *Borrelia lusitaniae* induces disease in C3H/HeN mice. *J. Med. Microbiol.* **50:**1055–1060.

205. **Zhang, J. R., J. M. Hardham, A. G. Barbour, and S. J. Norris.** 1997. Antigenic variation in Lyme disease borreliae by promiscuous recombination of VMP-like sequence cassettes. *Cell* **89:**275–285.

206. **Zhang, J. R., and S. J. Norris.** 1998. Genetic variation of the *Borrelia burgdorferi* gene *vlsE* involves cassette-specific, segmental gene conversion. *Infect. Immun.* **66:**3698–3704.

Sequelae and Long-Term Consequences of Infectious Diseases
Edited by Pina M. Fratamico, James L. Smith, and Kim A. Brogden

Chapter 3

Chlamydia pneumoniae and *Chlamydia trachomatis*

Margaret R. Hammerschlag, Stephan A. Kohlhoff, and Toni Darville

CHARACTERISTICS OF THE ORGANISMS

Chlamydiae are obligate intracellular bacterial pathogens whose entry into mucosal epithelial cells is required for intracellular survival and subsequent growth. Chlamydiae cause a variety of diseases in animal species at virtually all phylogenic levels, from amphibians and reptiles to birds and mammals. Originally the order contained one genus, *Chlamydia*, with four recognized species: *C. trachomatis, C. psittaci, C. pneumoniae*, and *C. pecorum,* with *C. trachomatis* and *C. pneumoniae* being the most important as human pathogens. Recent taxonomic analysis using the 16S and 23S rRNA genes have found that the order *Chlamydiales* contains at least four distinct groups at the family level and that within the order *Chlamydiaceae* are two distinct lineages (65). This analysis has suggested splitting the genus *Chlamydia* into two genera, *Chlamydia* and *Chlamydophila*. Two new species, *Chlamydia muridarum* (formerly MoPn, the agent of mouse pneumonitis) and *Chlamydia suis* (gastrointestinal infection in swine) would join *C. trachomatis*. *Chlamydophila* would contain *C. pecorum* (infection in cattle, sheep, and koalas), *C. pneumoniae*, *C. psittaci* (infects primarily avian species and causes psittacosis in humans), and three new species split off from *C. psittaci*: *C. abortus* (ovine and bovine abortion), *C. caviae* (formerly the *C. psittaci* guinea pig conjunctivitis strain), and *C. felis* (keratoconjunctivitis in cats). There is continuing controversy regarding this reclassification; for the purposes of this review, we will continue to refer to *Chlamydia*.

The ability to cause persistent infection is one of the major characteristics of all chlamydial species. From a clinical standpoint, chlamydia may be the persistent infection par excellence, capable of persisting in the host for months to years, often without causing obvious illness. From a microbiologic standpoint, persistence also refers to long-term intracellular infection that can be detected by antigen, microscopy, and/or nucleic acid-based amplification methods. Chronic, persistent infection with *C. trachomatis* is well described. Chronic, persistent infection with *C. pneumoniae* is less well defined but has been implicated in the pathogenesis of several chronic diseases, initially not thought to be infectious, including asthma, arthritis, and atherosclerosis (32, 44, 60, 110, 113, 139, 210) (Table 1). However, studies of the association of *C. pneumoniae* and these disorders have been hampered by difficulty in diagnosing chronic, persistent infection with the organism, which, in turn, makes it very difficult to determine the efficacy of interventions, especially with antibiotics.

Chlamydiae have a gram-negative envelope without detectable peptidoglycan (PGN); however, recent genomic analysis has revealed that both *C. trachomatis* and *C. pneumoniae* encode proteins forming a nearly complete pathway for synthesis of PGN, including penicillin-binding proteins (74, 143, 183). Chlamydiae also share a group-specific lipopolysaccharide (LPS) antigen and utilize host adenosine triphosphate for the synthesis of chlamydial protein (183). Although chlamydiae are auxotrophic for three of four nucleoside triphosphates, they do encode functional glucose-catabolizing enzymes, which can be used for generation of ATP (183). As for PGN synthesis, for some reason these genes are turned off. This may be related to their adaptation to the intracellular environment. All chlamydiae also encode an abundant protein called the major outer membrane protein (MOMP or OmpA) that is surface exposed in *C. trachomatis* and *C. psittaci*, but apparently not in *C. pneumoniae* (183). The MOMP is the major determinant of the serologic classification of *C. trachomatis* and *C. psittaci* isolates. Chlamydiae are susceptible to antibiotics that interfere with DNA and protein synthesis, including tetracyclines,

Margaret R. Hammerschlag and Stephan A. Kohlhoff • Division of Infectious Diseases, Department of Pediatrics, SUNY Downstate Medical Center, 450 Clarkson Ave., Brooklyn, NY 11203-2098. **Toni Darville** • Division of Infectious Diseases, Children's Hospital of Pittsburgh of University of Pittsburgh Medical Center, 3705 Fifth Ave., Pittsburgh, PA 15213.

Table 1. Association of persistent *Chlamydia* infection with chronic disease in humans

Organism	Disease	Quality of evidence[a]
Chlamydia trachomatis	Trachoma	+++
	PID	+++
	Arthritis	++
Chlamydia pneumoniae	Asthma	++
	Atherosclerosis	+
	Arthritis	+
	Macular degeneration	?
	Multiple sclerosis	?
	Alzheimer's disease	?

[a]Strength of data: +, weak; ++, moderate; +++, strongest; ?, questionable, based on limited studies from one or two groups and not independently confirmed.

macrolides, and quinolones. Under certain circumstances, beta-lactam antibiotics have been demonstrated to be effective, specifically amoxicillin for the treatment of genital *C. trachomatis* infection during pregnancy (36).

Chlamydiae have a unique developmental cycle with morphologically distinct infectious and reproductive forms: the elementary body (EB) and the reticulate body (RB) (Fig. 1). Following infection, the infectious EBs, which are 200 to 400 µm in diameter, attach to the host cell by a process of electrostatic binding and are taken into the cell by endocytosis that does not depend on the microtubule system. EBs are spore like, being metabolically inactive but stable in the extracellular environment. Within the host cell, the EB remains within a membrane-lined phagosome and there is inhibition of phagosomal-lysosomal fusion. The inclusion membrane is devoid of host cell markers, but lipid markers traffic to the inclusion, which suggests a functional interaction with the Golgi apparatus. Chlamydiae appear to circumvent the host endocytic pathway, inhabiting a nonacidic vacuole, which is dissociated from late endosomes and lysosomes. EBs then differentiate into RBs that undergo binary fission. After approximately 36 hours, the RBs differentiate back into EBs. Despite the accumulation of 500 to 1,000 infectious EBs in the inclusion, host cell function is minimally disrupted. At about 48 hours, release may occur by cytolysis or by a process of exocytosis or extrusion of the whole inclusion, leaving the host cell intact. This strategy is very successful, enabling the organism to cause essentially silent, chronic infection.

IN VITRO MODELS OF CHLAMYDIAL PERSISTENCE

A number of in vitro studies have challenged this biphasic paradigm. Chlamydiae may enter a persistent state in vitro after treatment with certain cytokines, such as gamma interferon (IFN-γ); treatment with antibiotics, specifically penicillin; restriction of certain nutrients, including iron, glucose, and amino acids; infection in monocytes; and heat shock (13, 14, 55, 57, 88, 93, 152). While in the persistent state, metabolic activity is reduced and the organism is often refractory to antibiotic treatment.

These different systems produce very similar growth characteristics, including loss of infectivity and development of small inclusions containing fewer EBs and RBs and ultrastuctural findings, specifically morphologically abnormal RBs, suggesting that they are somehow altered during their otherwise normal development. These abnormal RBs are often called aberrant bodies (ABs). Abnormal chlamydial development was first described in vitro after treating *C. psittaci*- and *C. trachomatis*-infected cells with penicillin (93), which induced the development of enlarged abnormal RBs, with the formation of small daughter RBs budding from within the parent RBs. This effect was reversed following removal of the penicillin from the media. Other antibiotics, including ampicillin, erythromycin, ciprofloxacin, and ofloxacin have also been reported to produce abnormal chlamydial development. Dreses-Werringloer et al. (57) investigated the effect of ciprofloxacin and ofloxacin on established *C. trachomatis* infection (2 or 3 days postinfection) in HEp-2 cells. They found that both drugs at minimal bactericidal concentrations not only failed to eradicate chlamydia from infected cells but also induced persistent infection, which, while still being viable and metabolically active, were morphologically altered. This infection was characterized by a small number of small aberrant inclusions present through 20 days of culture.

Restriction of certain nutrients has also been demonstrated to induce persistence in chlamydiae. Harper et al. (88) observed development of large and distorted RB with decreasing concentrations of 13 amino acids and restriction of glucose with the development of *C. trachomatis* in McCoy cells. Chlamydiae require iron in order to complete their developmental cycle (55). Depletion of iron stores with deferoxamine mesylate results in delayed development, decreased infectivity of progeny EB, and the appearance of enlarged ABs. These changes are reversible upon replacing the iron in the media. Chlamydiae were found to have an iron-dependent repressor and differential transcription and protein expression profiles (55).

The effect of IFN-γ on chlamydial growth was first described by Beatty and colleagues (13, 15). IFN-γ-induced persistence is probably the best-studied model of chlamydial persistence. Beatty and colleagues

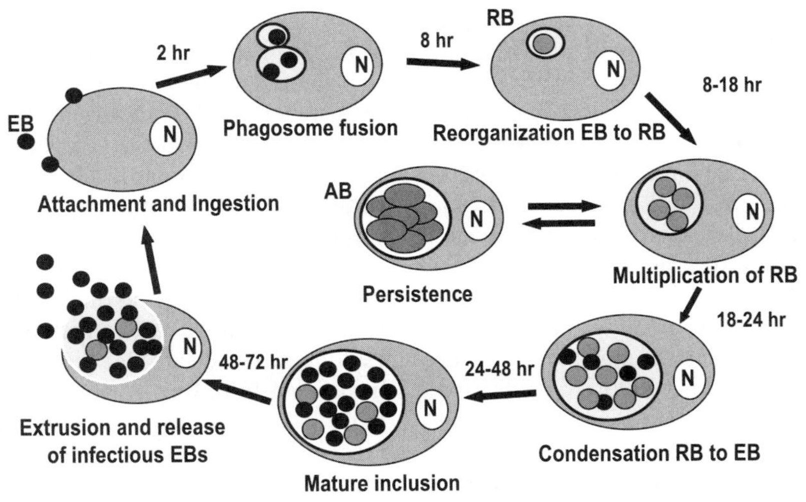

Figure 1. Life cycle of chlamydiae in epithelial cells.

demonstrated that the addition of 0.2 ng/ml of IFN-γ inhibited intracellular growth of *C. trachomatis* in HeLa cells by induction of the indoleamine 2,3-dioxygenase, leading to a persistent state. This enzyme catabolizes intracellular tryptophan, which is necessary for intracellular growth of chlamydia. Treatment with IFN-γ restricted growth and division of RBs and interrupted their differentiation to infectious EBs. The development of large aberrant RB forms combined with the absence of EBs was characteristic of persistent *C. trachomatis* infection. The aberrant chlamydial development was also concomitant with decreases in the levels of MOMP, the 60-kDa outer membrane protein, and LPS, but there was an increase in expression of heat shock protein 60 (HSP60) (13). Chlamydial growth was altered but not completely inhibited; after removal of IFN-γ from the media, infectious chlamydia could be recovered. Similar results have also been demonstrated for *C. pneumoniae* in HEp-2 cells (93). Ultrastructural analysis of IFN-γ-treated *C. pneumoniae* also reveals atypical inclusions containing large reticulate-like ABs with no evidence of redifferentiation into EBs.

Another model described by Kutlin et al. (134) is continuous infection. In contrast to the previously described models, continuous cultures become spontaneously persistent when both chlamydiae and host cells multiply freely in the absence of stress. Kutlin et al. were able to maintain *C. pneumoniae* infection in HEp-2 and A549 cells for over 4 years without centrifugation or the addition of cycloheximide or IFN-γ (134). Infection levels in these infected cells were high (70 to 80%). Ultrastructural studies revealed three types of inclusions were in these cells (133). Approximately 90% of inclusions seen were typical, large inclusions ranging from approximately 5 to 12 μm in diameter. The typical inclusions contained an average of 350 tightly packed chlamydial bodies and some extracellular material as well as membranous material. The second type of inclusions observed (altered inclusions) contained both normal EBs and RBs but in considerably lower numbers, usually approximately 70. These inclusions also contained pleomorphic ABs, which were up to 4 or 5 times the size of normal RBs (2.5 μm in diameter); their cytoplasm was very homogenous. These ABs retained an identifiable small periplasmic space and outer membrane, characteristic of the normal RBs. Altered inclusions were closely apposed to the nuclei of the HEp-2 cells. Host cell mitochondria were observed adjacent to the defined inclusion membrane.

The third type of inclusion observed was small aberrant inclusions, on average 4 μm in diameter. They contained about 60 ABs, which were similar in size to normal RBs but appeared electron dense and no longer retained a smooth spherical shape. These dense ABs retained the characteristic chlamydial outer membrane structure, with very little periplasmic space and the membranes more tightly bound to the chlamydial body, similar to normal RBs. No EBs were observed in these inclusions. These findings demonstrate that the developmental cycle of *C. pneumoniae* can combine both the typical development forms with the persistent phase in tissue culture.

Another possible mechanism of chlamydial persistence could be through a direct effect on the host cell, possibly through an effect on apoptosis, which is an important regulator of cell growth and tissue development. Apoptosis is a genetically programmed, tightly controlled process, unlike necrosis, which involves nonspecific inflammation and tissue damage as well as intracellular enzymes, condensation of the nucleus and cytoplasm, and fragmentation. Many microbial pathogens, including chlamydia, have been found to modulate cellular apoptosis in order to survive and multiply (126). *Chlamydia* species have been demonstrated to both induce and inhibit host cell apoptosis, depending on the stage of the chlamydial developmental cycle (52, 59, 67, 76, 126, 221). Chlamydiae protect infected cells against apoptosis due to external stimuli during early stages of infection and induce apoptosis of the host cell during later stages. Thus, chlamydiae may protect infected cells against cytotoxic mechanisms of the immune system, while the apoptosis observed at the end of the infection cycle may contribute to the inflammatory response, as apoptotic cells secrete proinflammatory cytokines, and facilitate the release of the organism from the infected cells. Studies using IFN-γ-treated cultures have reported that cells infected with *C. trachomatis* and *C. pneumoniae* resist apoptosis due to external ligands, via inhibition of caspace activation (52, 59). Data from studies with the long-term continuously infected cell model demonstrated marked differences in the effects of *C. pneumoniae* on apoptosis in acute and chronically infected A-549 cells (126). Acute *C. pneumoniae* infection *induced* apoptotic changes in A-549 cells within the first 24 and 48 hours postinfection. Induction of apoptosis in acute infection may facilitate release of *C. pneumoniae* from the host cell. Chronic *C. pneumoniae* infection *inhibited* apoptotic changes within the first 24 hours and up to 7 days. These results suggest that inhibition of apoptosis may help to protect the organism when it is in the persistent state.

A number of studies have examined the patterns of gene expression in various in vitro models of chlamydial persistence. The results have not been entirely consistent from study to study, even with the same model (13, 59, 91, 93, 153, 172). Initial studies of IFN-γ-treated *C. trachomatis* focused on relative levels of the MOMP and the chlamydial HSP60 (cHSP60) by immunoblotting and electron microscopy (13). Beatty and colleagues found that cHSP60 levels increased slightly and that MOMP levels decreased (13). Subsequent studies using semiquantitative reverse transcriptase PCR demonstrated selectively downregulated transcription of the *ompA* gene (91, 93). It is not clear whether the changes in expression of the MOMP and cHSP60 have any significance in chlamydial pathogenesis or are nonspecific markers of persistence. Reduced levels of the MOMP, which is an immunoprotective antigen, could enable chlamydiae, specifically *C. trachomatis*, to avoid the development of protective immunity in the host. Steady or increased levels of cHSP60 could promote immunopathology through delayed-type hypersensitivity or cross-reactivity with human HSP60 or the HSP of other bacteria (153).

Genes studied in various models of chlamydial persistence can be organized in the following categories: (i) cell division and chromosome replication and partitioning (a common characteristic of persistence in tissue culture is inhibition of cell division and continuing DNA synthesis with accumulation of chromosomes), (ii) energy metabolism, (iii) tryptophan metabolism, (iv) chlamydial protease-like activity factor, and (iv) late genes, which are genes that are generally expressed late in the chlamydial life cycle and have been found to be downregulated during persistence. It was hoped that these studies would allow identification of specific markers for persistent chlamydial infection that might have clinical application. However, as mentioned earlier the results are frequently inconsistent, some genes being upregulated in one model but downregulated in another (93).

Another novel mechanism of chlamydial persistence recently described in *C. trachomatis* is lysosome repair (14). Trachoma biovar strains are released from the host cell without concomitant host cell death. Analysis of events associated with release of chlamydia from the inclusion revealed that the host cell plasma membrane was compromised prior to rupture of the membrane of the inclusion. The disruption was accompanied by the appearance of luminal lysosomal protein LAMP-1 at the infected cell surfaces, suggesting lysosome repair of the disruptions in the host cell plasma membrane. As a result of this lysosome-mediated repair process, residual chlamydiae were retained within the host cell.

C. PNEUMONIAE AND CHRONIC DISEASE IN HUMANS

C. pneumoniae is a common human respiratory pathogen, affecting all ages with a worldwide distribution (130). The mode of transmission remains uncertain but probably involves infected respiratory tract secretions. Spread of *C. pneumoniae* within families and enclosed populations, such as military recruits, has been described. The proportion of community-acquired pneumonia in children and adults associated with *C. pneumoniae* infection has ranged from 0 to over 44%, varying with geographic location, the age group examined, and the diagnostic methods used (130). Early studies that relied on serology suggested that infection in children younger than 5 years old was rare; however, subsequent studies using culture and/or PCR have found the prevalence of infection in children beyond early infancy to be similar to that found in adults (130). Approximately

50% or more of children with culture-documented *C. pneumoniae* respiratory infection (pneumonia and asthma) are seronegative by the microimmunofluorescence (MIF) method (60, 130, 132). Prolonged respiratory infection, documented by culture, lasting from several weeks to several years after acute infection has been reported (60, 85). Hammerschlag et al. (85) first described persistent nasopharyngeal infection following acute respiratory illness in five patients for periods up to 11 months, despite treatment with multiple and prolonged courses of antibiotics. Follow-up studies of two of these patients documented persistence for 7 to 9 years (51). One patient was culture positive on 14 separate occasions over 9 years but was only intermittently symptomatic. In vitro susceptibility testing of these isolates did not demonstrate development of antibiotic resistance. Sequencing of the *omp1* gene suggested that these infections were caused by the same organism. Reliable diagnosis of respiratory infection due to *C. pneumoniae* remains difficult due to the absence of well-standardized and commercially available diagnostic tests (130). As of this writing, there are no commercially available, FDA-approved serologic or nucleic acid amplification tests for diagnosis of *C. pneumoniae* infection. Progress in the field has been hampered by inconsistent and incorrect use of the available diagnostic tests in studies, with consequent results that are often not comparable. Although the Centers for Disease Control and Prevention (CDC; United States) and the Laboratory Centre for Disease Control (Canada) published recommendations for standardizing the diagnostic approach to *C. pneumoniae* infection in 2001 (56), recent studies of in-house serologic and PCR assays for diagnosis of *C. pneumoniae* infection have suggested that there is still substantial interlaboratory variation in the performance of these tests (4a, 5, 138).

C. pneumoniae and Chronic Respiratory Disease

C. pneumoniae and asthma

Infection with *C. pneumoniae* has been linked to asthma by a large number of epidemiologic and clinical studies. Many studies reporting an association are cross-sectional studies or are limited to small case series or selected populations, such as acutely symptomatic patients. The controversy about the definition of infection and diagnostic tests contributes to the difficulty in interpreting and comparing studies. Many epidemiologic studies relied on *C. pneumoniae* serology as evidence for past or current infection, which is an approach with important limitations as described previously. Direct detection of *C. pneumoniae* by culture and/or PCR is considered more definitive evidence of current infection, but the absence of current infection does not rule out immunopathology from previous infections. The field is further complicated by differences in study populations with regard to asthma phenotype and the presence of acute symptoms. Table 2 summarizes 11 of the studies that have examined the association of *C. pneumoniae* infection and asthma, primarily with adult populations, that have been published from 1991 through 2006. There was significant heterogeneity in the methods used from study to study. Five studies relied on serology only, using different assays and criteria for determining acute or past infection. The results of only three studies utilized culture, and the prevalence ranged from 0 to 11%. Five studies used various PCR assays, including conventional and nested assays, and the positivity rate by PCR ranged from 5.4 to 21%. Identification of *C. pneumoniae* in controls ranged from 0 to 37%. In one study from the United States (141) that performed culture and nested PCR, there was significant discordance between the results from each test. This illustrates the sometimes contradictory findings regarding an association between *C. pneumoniae* and asthma, some of which may be explained by differences in populations and diagnostic methods.

C. pneumoniae infection and acute exacerbations of asthma

In 1991, Hahn et al. reported an association between serologic evidence of acute *C. pneumoniae* infection and adult onset asthma and asthmatic bronchitis in the United States (80). Studies reporting an association or lack of association between the presence of antibodies (immunoglobulin G [IgG], IgM, and IgA) or higher antibody titers (IgG) against *C. pneumoniae* and asthma have been reported since then with a variety of populations (Table 2) (2, 44, 136, 146, 198, 211). Studies that used direct detection methods (culture or PCR) were more consistent in confirming a role of *C. pneumoniae* in exacerbations of asthma (Table 2) (60, 64, 154).

Relation of *C. pneumoniae* infection to the severity and initiation of asthma

While *C. pneumoniae* appears to be clearly associated with asthma exacerbations, it has also been hypothesized to have a role in asthma pathogenesis. Infection-induced bronchiolitis, especially caused by respiratory syncytial virus, in predisposed infants has been suggested to contribute to the development of asthma (142). *C. pneumoniae*, however, does not

Table 2. Summary of clinical studies of the role of *C. pneumoniae* in asthma

Population (yr)	No. of asthma/ control	Culture-positive asthma/ control (%)	PCR-positive asthma/ control (%)	Description of (asthma/control) serology results	Comment	Reference
United States, adults (1991)	365			Positive correlation between IgG titers (MIF) and wheezing		80
Italy, adults (1994)	74/–[d]			IgG seroconversion (10%/–)[d]	Asthmatics with acute exacerbation	2
United States, children (1994)	118/41	11/4.9		No significant difference in IgG titers between groups; 58% of culture-positive asthmatics without IgG/IgM response	Asthmatics with acute exacerbation	60
Japan, adults (1998)	168/108	1.2/0	5.4/0.9	Higher prevalence of IgG and IgA in asthmatics (85%/68% and 48%/17%, respectively); mean IgG titers of 39/18	Asthmatics with acute exacerbation	154
Great Britain, adults (1998)	123/1,518			No difference in prevalence of IgG titers (≥512 and ≥64–256) between groups (5.7%/5.7% and 15%/13%, respectively)	IgG of ≥64–256 more common in subgroup of severe asthmatics (34.8%)	44
New Zealand, children, adults (2000)	96/102			No positive correlation between diagnosis of asthma and IgG titer at 11 yr and 21yr of age	Asthma-enriched birth cohort; self-reported asthma	146
Italy, children (2000)	71/80		8/2.5	Serologic response consistent with acute infection (13%/0%)	Asthmatics with acute exacerbation	64
United States, adults (2001)	55/11	0/0	12.7/0[a]	Serologic response consistent with acute infection in 42% of PCR-positive asthmatics	Stable asthmatics	141
Great Britain, adults (2004)	74/74		22/9[b]		Cases were stable atopic asthmatics, and controls were nonatopic spouses	7
Finland, adults (2005)	83/162			No difference in titers or conversion rates	Population-based cohort	169
Finland, adults (2006)	103/30		21/37[c]		Stable asthmatics	87

[a]Respiratory specimens obtained from lower airway (bronchoalveolar lavage, biopsy, or airway brushing).
[b]Positivity rate during 3-month (October to December) longitudinal study (at least one positive sample obtained on repeat sampling).
[c]Positivity rate in mild asthmatics of 20.8% and in moderate asthmatics of 22%.
[d]–, no control data.

appear to be significantly associated with respiratory infections in early infancy, including bronchiolitis (116, 131, 220). However, as infants and children do not appear to make antibody that is detectable with currently available serologic tests for *C. pneumoniae*, including the MIF test (132), serologic studies may underestimate the prevalence of infection in children. It has been noted that in children aged 2 to 14 years with lower respiratory tract infections caused by *C. pneumoniae* (as determined by PCR on nasopharyngeal aspirates and/or antibody response) wheezing was common (174). Biscardi et al. reported finding *C. pneumoniae* infection in 6% of children with new onset asthma and noted that rapid symptom recurrence occurred in all infected patients in the absence of antibiotic treatment (16).

The presence of anti-*C. pneumoniae* IgA antibodies or IgG titer has been correlated, but not consistently, with markers of asthma severity and/or wheezing (19, 20). Patients with increased antibody levels to *C. pneumoniae* have higher levels of sputum neutrophil counts and eosinophilic cationic protein (211). Evidence of infection with *C. pneumoniae* by PCR, alone or in combination with *Mycoplasma pneumoniae*, in up to 22% of patients with stable asthma symptoms may suggest chronic infection (87, 141). A greater prevalence of IgG and IgM titers (MIF) indicative of infection in the absence of direct detection of the organisms in the airway has also been reported in stable asthmatics compared to controls (128). The clinical implications of *C. pneumoniae* infection in asthmatics who have no acute symptoms are not clear; the obvious concern is that the presence of the pathogen may lead to ongoing inflammation and thus contribute to the severity and progression of asthma. The mechanisms contributing to initiation and exacerbation of asthma and those involved in chronic infection are discussed below.

Immunopathology of Infection with *C. pneumoniae* in Asthma

A number of factors precipitating asthma attacks have been identified, including allergens, exertion, and respiratory infections. Hyper-reactivity and chronic inflammation in asthma are related to and mediated by a pathogenic cytokine imbalance, including a T-helper type 2 lymphocyte (Th2)-dominant state in the airways (reviewed in reference 13) and increased IgE antibody responses in the majority of patients with allergic asthma (reviewed in reference 199). Among the candidate genes involved in Th1-Th2 differentiation status is T-bet (120). The main factors contributing to the development of the Th1-Th2 imbalance are genetic susceptibility, environmental factors, and the interaction between the innate and adaptive immune systems. The mechanisms by which *C. pneumoniae* could contribute to exacerbation or initiation of asthma are not well understood. It seems clear though that *C. pneumoniae*, as an obligate intracellular bacterium, differs in its effects on the immune systems of asthmatics from those of other bacteria and behaves in some ways similar to viral pathogens (91, 140). The role of infection in asthma and especially regulation of ongoing IgE responses in allergic asthma has received a great deal of attention. Exposure to bacterial components, especially PGNs via Toll-like receptor (TLR) 2, Nod1, and Nod2, has also been postulated to be a potential modulator of atopy (58, 74, 218). At the same time (viral) respiratory infections have been postulated to exacerbate asthma or direct predisposed individuals towards an asthma phenotype.

Immune Response to Infection with *C. pneumoniae*

Respiratory epithelial cells are usually the first cells to be infected by *C. pneumoniae* in vivo and are likely responsible for initiating the immune response by attracting antigen-presenting cells and recruiting neutrophils (62, 177). The predominant cytokines are interleukin-8 (IL-8) and to a lesser degree IL-6. IL-6 may play a role in sustaining the protective Th1-mediated immune response, while IL-10 may inhibit it (215, 208). Inflammatory responses are dependent on infection with viable bacteria (91).

It is known from animal models that cell-mediated immunity, which is regulated by differential cytokine expressions, is crucial in clearance of infections due to intracellular pathogens, including *Chlamydia* (82). Cellular memory responses to *C. pneumoniae* infection following acute infection have been described (83). Peripheral blood mononuclear cells (PBMC) may contribute not only to dissemination of the bacterium but also to immunoreactive mechanisms following infection with *C. pneumoniae* (219). *C. pneumoniae* infection induced upregulation of the CD14 molecule in Mono Mac 6 cells, a highly differentiated human monocytic cell line (90). Infection of human PBMC led to production of tumor necrosis factor alpha (TNF-α), IL-1β, IL-6, and IFN-α (112a). Stimulation with sonicated *C. pneumoniae* of human PBMC led to significant increases of the proinflammatory cytokines TNF-α and IL-1β and the anti-inflammatory cytokine IL-10, which were increased by addition of serum, but not due to complement, mannose-binding lectin or LPS-binding protein (163). Another cytokine found to be induced in human PBMC by *C. pneumoniae* is IL-12, which is important for sustaining the protective Th1 cell-mediated immune response (1). The role of professional antigen-presenting cells was addressed in a study using murine bone marrow-derived dendritic cells. While *C. pneumoniae* did not replicate to produce inclusions, stimulation was demonstrated by NF-κB activation, secretion of IL-12p40 and TNF-α, and upregulation of major histocompatibility complex (MHC) class II molecules, CD40, CD80, and CD86 (173). This was dependent on the presence of TLR2 and independent of TLR4, with the exception of IL-12p40 secretion (173). Downregulation of MHC class I antigen expression has been described (35).

Human alveolar macrophages have chlamydicidal activity, which may depend on their interaction with T cells (158). IFN-γ resulted in increased production of nitric oxide and reduction in the viability of *C. pneumoniae* in a murine macrophage cell line (34).

Host response to *C. pneumoniae* in asthmatics

Persistent infection with *C. pneumoniae* has been demonstrated in both stable asthmatics without acute respiratory symptoms and in symptomatic asthmatics for up to 6 months (17, 60). It has been hypothesized that persistence is due to an insufficient Th1 response, which may be characteristic for asthmatics (117). There are minimal data examining the immunological basis for the association between *C. pneumoniae* and asthma pathology. It is conceivable that, in analogy to the correlation of abnormal host immune response to *C. trachomatis* infection and tissue sequelae, a similar relationship exists between respiratory infection with *C. pneumoniae* and asthma pathology (89, 95, 103).

In addition to ineffective clearance of *C. pneumoniae* due to a Th2 response in asthmatics, augmentation of allergic responses is an additional concern. Enhancement of cellular proliferation after in vitro *C. pneumoniae* infection in a Th2-dominant environment was demonstrated using PBMC from *Dermatophagoides farinae*-sensitized atopic subjects; cells were cultured in the presence of Der f 2 and IL-4 (38). The antiproliferative effects of steroids were decreased by in vitro *C. pneumoniae* infection, suggesting steroid resistance (38). Two studies have shown an association between IgE-mediated wheezing and *C. pneumoniae* infection in children (61, 104). Emre et al. demonstrated the presence of specific IgE by immunoblotting in 86% of culture-positive asthmatic patients with wheezing, compared with 9% of culture-positive nonasthmatic patients with pneumonia who were not wheezing (61). Induction or augmentation of IgE responses may be mediated by generation of higher levels of Th2 and lower levels of Th1 cytokines in response to *C. pneumoniae* infection of PBMC from allergic asthmatics compared to those from nonatopic healthy controls (125).

In ovalbumin-induced allergic airway disease of newborn mice infected with *C. muridarum*, a mixed type 1 and type 2 T-cell response was observed along with mucus hypersecretion and airway hyperresponsiveness (97). In a study using *C. muridarum* infection of murine bone marrow-derived dendritic cells, which were pulsed with ovalbumin, it was demonstrated that the pathogen deviated the immune response to a Th2 response (106). Similar studies have not been reported for *C. pneumoniae*; however, a murine model of respiratory *C. pneumoniae* infection demonstrated induction of airway hyperresponsiveness (21). The above described abnormal cellular immune responses to respiratory infections like *C. pneumoniae* may in part be related to genetic variation in cytokine and immune mediator genes, such as IL-13, IL-10, transforming growth factor β, and TLR4, resulting in aberrant responses to infection and subsequent disease (92). Differences in *C. pneumoniae* IgG antibody responses were seen in asthmatic children, depending on variant mannose-binding lectin alleles (155). Human T-lymphocyte clones raised against *C. pneumoniae* EB antigens demonstrated IFN-γ production in the context of the HLA DR4 molecule, while IL-4 production was linked to antigen recognition in the context of the HLA DR15 molecule (84). An allergic asthma phenotype was related to higher prevalences of *C. pneumoniae* IgA, suggesting differences in the immune response compared to that of nonatopic asthmatics, but the correlation with direct detection of infection was not reported (156).

Inflammatory responses to infection are mediated by receptors recognizing pathogen-associated molecular patterns. These pathogen-associated molecular patterns include, among others, LPS, PGN, and muramyl dipeptide. Since *C. pneumoniae* has both intra- and extracellular developmental forms, TLR and NOD receptors are important candidate genes. Stimulation of TLR and NOD plays an important role in modulation of adaptive immune responses (74, 209). *C. pneumoniae*-induced TNF-α and IL-1β responses in human PBMC were dependent on TLR2 (163). Myd88 was critical in clearance of *C. pneumoniae* infection in mice, while TLR 2 or TLR 4 was not needed for recovery from infection (157). Recognition of chlamydial antigens by the cytosolic NOD1 receptor appeared to be of limited biological significance in a mouse study using *C. trachomatis* and *C. muridarum*, which could be explained by insufficient PGN production by *Chlamydia* (212). This may allow drawing some inferences for *C. pneumoniae*, which does not contain measurable PGN as a component of the cell wall of *Chlamydia* species, although there is a complete set of genes required for PGN biosynthesis (40, 73, 150). The degree to which *C. pneumoniae* stimulates different receptors in asthmatics and if this has a significant effect on allergic responses have not been elucidated fully.

It has been hypothesized that an inadequate or delayed clearance of the pathogen may lead to the establishment of a latent or persistent infection, which fuels a low-grade chronic immune response that causes tissue damage (210). Stimulation of tissue growth factors may contribute to structural remodeling (184). Hsp60 may play a special role, as it is the predominant chlamydial antigen during the persistent state (153). This could be analogous to the role of Hsp60 in patients with scarring trachoma (94). Chlamydial heat shock protein induced a significant inflammatory response via Myd88 in mouse macrophages, with increased and differential gene upregulation by active infection with C. *pneumoniae* in HeLa cells compared to stimulation with inactivated *C. pneumoniae* (30, 91). The role of stress and host genetics in delayed or suboptimal Th1 response to chlamydial infection and development of complications in certain individuals, as well as the role of specific *C. pneumoniae* antigens eliciting harmful immune responses in asthmatics, is unclear.

Treatment

If infection with *C. pneumoniae* contributed to inflammation in allergic asthmatics, it would be important to diagnose and treat these infections. There may also be interactions between *C. pneumoniae* infection and asthma drugs. Treatment of asthma exacerbations frequently includes systemic steroids, which have been shown to enhance the in vitro infectivity of *C. pneumoniae* (127, 207); this was reflected in significant increases of inclusions but did not affect the in vitro activities of azithromycin, erythromycin, and doxycycline against *C. pneumoniae* (207). Several studies have addressed the question of whether antibiotic treatment of *C. pneumoniae* infection in asthmatics leads to improvement in disease activity. Chlamydiae are susceptible to antibiotics that interfere with DNA and protein synthesis, including tetracyclines, macrolides, and quinolones; good correlation between in vitro susceptibility testing and eradication in patients has been demonstrated (181). However, *C. pneumoniae* is often refractory to antibiotic treatment when it is in the persistent state, which may have implications in vivo (134).

Macrolides, quinolones, and tetracyclines also have immunomodulatory activity independent of their antimicrobial activity (188, 214). The beneficial effects of azithromycin in patients with cystic fibrosis appeared to be unrelated to antibacterial activity (185, 206). A variety of mechanisms have been suggested for different classes of antibiotics. In vitro treatment of human monocytes infected with *C. pneumoniae* with levofloxacin resulted in a decrease in the number of inclusions and reduction of the cytokines TNF-α, IL-1β, IL-6, and IL-8 but did not eliminate the infection (11). One suggested mechanism for reducing the levels of inflammatory cytokines by moxifloxacin is inhibition of IκBα degradation, which may inhibit NF-κB (39). Minocycline and doxycycline have been demonstrated to suppress in vitro IgE production of asthmatic PBMC induced by IL-4 plus anti-CD40 (193).

Several studies have assessed the efficacy of antibiotics on asthmatics with proven or presumed *C. pneumoniae* infection. Emre et al. demonstrated that 75% of asthmatic children with culture-documented *C. pneumoniae* infection had long-lasting clinical and laboratory improvement of their asthma symptoms following eradication of the organism after treatment with erythromycin and clarithromycin (60). Hahn et al. reported that poorly controlled asthmatics who required daily systemic steroids had *C. pneumoniae* antibody titers (determined by MIF) of >1:256 and who were treated with clarithromycin or azithromycin demonstrated sustained improvement and good asthma control without systemic steroids (81). Subsequent placebo-controlled trials attempted to confirm the benefits suggested by these preliminary studies. A placebo-controlled 6-week trial of roxithromycin in asthmatics who were seropositive for *C. pneumoniae* demonstrated significantly higher morning peak expiratory flow in the treatment group at the end of treatment, but not at subsequent time points (20). In the absence of clear evidence that these asthmatics had persistent *C. pneumoniae* infection, one could conclude that the treatment effect was due to the anti-inflammatory action of roxithromycin, which disappeared after stopping the drug. Clarithromycin therapy of chronic, stable asthmatics improved lung function in those patients who had a positive PCR for *C. pneumoniae* or *M. pneumoniae*, suggesting an effect related to treating the infection (129). A limitation in this study was the lack of evaluation of microbiologic efficacy, in addition to the small number of patients with *C. pneumoniae* infection. A Cochrane review on this subject published in 2005 concluded that there is inconclusive evidence supporting or refuting the use of macrolides in asthmatics, indicating the need for further studies (179). Since this review, four additional randomized placebo-controlled trials were published. In 2006, Hahn et al. reported significant improvement of overall asthma symptoms, but not of Juniper Asthma Quality of Life scores, by treatment of adult asthmatics with weekly doses of azithromycin, but direct detection of *C. pneumoniae* was not performed (79). Fonseca-Aten et al. reported that when children with recurrent wheezing or asthma were treated with clarithromycin during an acute exacerbation, nasopharyngeal concentrations of TNF-α, IL-1β, and IL-10 were significantly decreased compared to those in children receiving placebo (69). Patients who had evidence of *C. pneumoniae* or *M. pneumoniae* infection (by PCR or serology by enzyme-linked immunosorbent assay) tended to show a greater reduction of mucosal cytokines, but no separate analysis for *C. pneumoniae* infection alone was provided (69). A double-blind, randomized, placebo-controlled study of telithromycin in patients with acute exacerbations of asthma found reduction of asthma symptoms among those treated with the active drug. The study could not adequately assess the effect of infection, as only one of 278 enrolled patients was positive for *C. pneumoniae* by PCR (105). A randomized controlled trial of minocycline in allergic asthmatics improved asthma symptoms and reduced total serum IgE, but not IgG, indicating a class-specific effect (47). In this study, seropositivity for *C. pneumoniae* was not significantly different between patients and controls, and no patient had positive nasopharyngeal cultures for *C. pneumoniae* (47). It appears unlikely that the beneficial effect of minocycline was due to treatment of a respiratory infection with *C. pneumoniae*.

Comparing studies of antibiotic treatment of asthmatics is complicated by the use of different criteria of *C. pneumoniae* infection status (culture, PCR, serology, or a combination of these tests), use of nonstandard methods, and the unclear definition of chronic infection. Most studies are underpowered to show the effects of infection status. The benefits of using antibiotics active against atypical bacteria in asthmatics may be due to treatment of an infection, immunomodulatory properties independent of current infection status, or a combination of these two mechanisms. Future studies therefore need to better characterize the mechanism(s) of antibiotic treatment benefits in asthmatics by documenting infection status rigorously, as well as studying immunoreactive mechanisms directed against *C. pneumoniae* before, during, and after courses of treatment. Any ongoing improvement that is maintained after stopping antibiotic therapy may be attributable to eradication of *C. pneumoniae* infection. Recurrence of symptoms and worsening of inflammatory markers would indicate a predominantly immunomodulatory effect of the antibiotic. However, such an effect may be due to suppressing immunoreactive processes in response to previous or persistent infection with *C. pneumoniae*.

C. pneumoniae and Chronic Diseases

Persistent *C. pneumoniae* infection has also been implicated in the pathogenesis of several chronic diseases, initially not thought to be infectious, including atherosclerosis, multiple sclerosis (MS), Alzheimer's disease, and macular degeneration (32, 77, 86, 99, 108, 110, 139, 196). Studies with mice have demonstrated that *C. pneumoniae* disseminates to the spleen and other organs after respiratory infection via macrophages (147, 219). However, this has not been demonstrated conclusively to occur in humans. In addition, studies of the association of *C. pneumoniae* and these disorders have been hampered by the difficulty in diagnosing chronic, persistent infection with the organism. There are no validated serologic or other surrogate markers for chronic *C. pneumoniae* infection (56). The high prevalence of chlamydial infections and transient immunity after infection makes it very difficult to even differentiate persistent infection from reinfection or even past infection. This, in turn, makes it very difficult to determine the efficacy of any therapeutic intervention.

C. pneumoniae and Atherosclerosis

Atherosclerotic heart disease is a leading cause of morbidity in developed countries and is emerging as a major health problem in many developing countries. Conventional risk factors including cigarette smoking, hypertension, and high serum lipid levels do not fully explain the incidence, prevalence, and distribution of coronary artery disease (CVD). Inflammation of the vessel wall plays an essential role in the initiation and progression of atherosclerosis, erosion, fissure, and eventual rupture of the atheromatous plaques (110). Various markers of systemic inflammation, including C-reactive protein, have been found to predict future cardiovascular events, including nonfatal and fatal myocardial infarction and stroke (110). Although inflammation is present, the exact cause is still not known. Various infectious agents have been investigated as possible etiologies for this inflammation, including cytomegalovirus, human herpesviruses, enteroviruses, *Helicobacter pylori*, bacteria involved with periodontal disease, and *C. pneumoniae*. Of these, *C. pneumoniae* has been the most extensively studied (139). The first report suggesting a possible association between *C. pneumoniae* infection and CVD came from a case-control study from Finland published in 1988, which demonstrated that patients with proven CVD were significantly more likely to have antibodies to *C. pneumoniae* than controls selected at random (184a). The presence of *C. pneumoniae* in atherosclerotic plaques of coronary arteries was demonstrated in an autopsy study from South Africa in 1992 (190). These reports were quickly followed by additional seroepidemiologic studies and studies that identified *C. pneumoniae* in atheromas by various methods, including culture, immunohistochemical staining (IHS), and PCR (24). Animal studies have demonstrated that *C. pneumoniae* can either induce or enhance the development of atherosclerosis in mice (54). In vitro studies have demonstrated that *C. pneumoniae* can infect and replicate within monocytes, macrophages, and vascular endothelial and smooth muscle cells, which are all important components of atherosclerotic plaque (32, 71, 90, 107, 110, 184). In vitro infection also results in oxidation of cellular low-density lipoprotein, the production of proinflammatory cytokines involved in atherogenesis, including TNF-α, IL-6, IL-1β, and INF-α, and the transendothelial migration of neutrophils and monocytes (32, 149). *C. pneumoniae* can induce human macrophage foam cell formation in vitro, a key event in early atheromas development (107). However, this may not be specific, as the key component appears to be the chlamydia LPS, which is conserved in all chlamydial species, including *C. trachomatis* (107).

However, no single serologic, PCR, or IHS assay has been used consistently across all studies, and these assays are not standardized. In 2002, Boman and Hammerschlag (24) reviewed 14 seroepidemiologic studies published from 1992 to 2000 and found a great deal of heterogenicity among these studies in terms of the serologic tests used and the criteria for seropositivity. In some studies, an IgG and/or IgA titer of ≥64 was used as an indicator of chronic infection; in others, the same criteria were used as indicators of *past* infection. Nine of these studies used the MIF assay; all were in-house tests. The antigen used was specified in only four of the MIF assays. The remaining studies used a variety of other methods, including genus-specific enzyme immunoassays and whole-cell immunofluorescence. However, as stated previously, MIF assays are not standardized and are subject to significant operator variation (138). As stated previously, there are no validated serologic criteria for chronic or persistent *C. pneumoniae* infection (56). Background seropositivity rates in the general population often exceed 70%, which can also make it very difficult to demonstrate an association between the presence of *C. pneumoniae* antibodies and CVD (24, 56). Earlier case-controlled studies that demonstrated an association were generally small and based on single serum samples, which does not take into account that antibody titers fluctuate over time. A meta-analysis of 12 studies found only combined odds ratios of 1.15 and 1.13 for IgG and IgA antibodies, respectively (46). Smeija et al. (192) in the Heart Outcomes Prevention and Evaluation Study (HOPE), which followed 3,168 patients for 4.5 years, found no association between *C. pneumoniae* IgG or IgA titers and subsequent cardiovascular events.

Boman and Hammerschlag (24) analyzed 43 studies published from 1992 through 2000 that examined 2,679 samples of atheromatous tissue for the presence of *C. pneumoniae* by culture, electron microscopy, PCR, and IHS. The overall rates of detection of *C. pneumoniae* ranged from 0 to 100%, with 49.7% being positive by at least one method. However, when specimens were analyzed by more than one method, the prevalence of positive specimens by at least two methods (usually IHS and PCR) was only 15.14%. As with the serological studies, there was major variation in the methods, including the antibodies and techniques for the IHS and PCR methods. IHS has also been found to have problems with interpretation and reproducibility. Hoymans et al. (98) reported that ceroid, which is an insoluble lipid present in plaque, could cause nonspecific reactions with IHS.

The extent of interlaboratory variation in performances of PCR was demonstrated by Apfalter et al. (4a), who sent a panel of 15 homogenized clinical atheroma specimens (carotid and coronary) and controls to nine laboratories in Europe and the United States for detection using PCR. The positivity rate in the clinical specimens ranged from 0 to 60%, and three laboratories identified *C. pneumoniae* in negative controls. The concordance between the assays was only 25% for one specimen. In a subsequent study, Apfalter et al. (5) demonstrated that it was practically impossible to avoid contamination with nested PCR assays. Ieven and Hoymans (102) published an analysis of studies published since 2000, many of which have used real-time PCR, that were found to be predominantly negative. Real-time PCR is much less subject to contamination from amplicon carryover. Ieven and Hoymans also noted that in studies where serology was done in addition to PCR, there was no correlation between the presence of *C. pneumoniae* in the atheroma tissue and the presence of anti-*C. pneumoniae* antibodies in individual patients (102).

Extrapolating from the observation that *C. pneumoniae* can disseminate systemically in mice after intranasal inoculation (147, 221), it has been suggested that the presence of *C. pneumoniae* in PBMCs may act as a surrogate marker for infection with *C. pneumoniae* in individuals with cardiovascular and other diseases (24). Over 20 studies examining the presence of *C. pneumoniae* DNA in PBMCs have been published, and as seen with studies of vascular tissue, the reported prevalences of *C. pneumoniae* DNA in PBMCs have also varied significantly, ranging from 0 to 59% of patients with CVD and from 0 to 46% of healthy blood donors (191). More recently, Kohlhepp et al. (124) examined PBMCs from over 300 blood donors either younger than 20 or over 60 years of age. The samples were divided and sent to two different laboratories where they were tested for *C. pneumoniae* DNA by real-time, touchdown, and nested PCR assays. Only two samples from the younger-than-20-years group were positive in one of the laboratories but were negative in the second. None of the samples for the over-60-years-old group was positive in either laboratory. This study demonstrated that two different laboratories using different extraction methods and real-time PCR targets did not detect *C. pneumoniae* DNA in both cohorts of patients, but there was evidence of interlaboratory discrepancy with two specimens.

Results of the initial seroepidemiologic and organism detection studies led to several preliminary studies which investigated the efficacy of antibiotic treatment directed at *C. pneumoniae* for the prevention of secondary cardiac events. The results of these preliminary studies suggested an effect but were underpowered and raised questions about the antibiotic regimens used, as well as how to identify patients with *C. pneumoniae* infection. The major assumption of many of the seroepidemiologic studies of the association of *C. pneumoniae* and atherosclerosis and other chronic conditions is that the presence of anti-*C. pneumoniae* antibody implies the presence of the organism somewhere in the body. However, earlier studies of patients with respiratory infection often found a poor correlation between serology and isolation of the organism from the respiratory tract (37, 100, 101).

Data on treatment of *C. pneumoniae* are also limited. *C. pneumoniae* is susceptible to antibiotics, which affect DNA and protein synthesis, including macrolides and azalides, specifically azithromycin; tetracyclines; and quinolones (189). However, in vitro activity may not always predict in vivo efficacy. Eradication rates of *C. pneumoniae* from the respiratory tract in the few studies that have assessed microbiologic efficacy rarely exceed 80% (181, 189). However, practically all pneumonia treatment studies presented or published to date have used serology alone for diagnosis, essentially limiting themselves to a clinical end point. Most studies have followed this premise: if the patient has serologic evidence of infection and clinically improves, the organism was presumed to have been eradicated. Conversely, the results of studies that have assessed microbiologic efficacy have frequently found that patients improve clinically despite persistence of the organism.

Gupta et al. (77) randomized 60 men who had prior myocardial infarction, who were seropositive by MIF (IgG ≥8) to receive either azithromycin, 500 mg/day for 3 or 6 days, or placebo. They found that the patients receiving azithromycin demonstrated a decrease in their MIF IgG titers and had a lower risk of a secondary adverse cardiac event than the patients who received the placebo. The antibiotic regimen used by Gupta et al (77) was never studied for treatment of *C. pneumoniae* infections. A study of adults with community-acquired pneumonia or bronchitis found that azithromycin at a dose of 500 mg on day 1, followed by 250 mg/day on days 2 to 5 had an 80% efficacy in eradicating *C. pneumoniae* from the respiratory tract (189). In 2005, Andraws et al. (4) performed a meta-analysis of 11 randomized trials, which enrolled a total of 19,217 patients. Seven of the trials used azithromycin, with a length of treatment ranging from 500 mg/day for 3 to 6 days to 500 to 600 mg/week for 6 weeks to 1 year. Three studies used roxithromycin for 30 days to 6 weeks; one used clarithromycin, 500 mg/day for 85 days and gatifloxacin; and one used 400 mg/day per month for 2 years. The duration of follow-up ranged from 3 months to 2 years. The results of two of six of the earlier, small studies (≤150 patients in each arm) favored antibiotic, but all of the remaining five large studies favored placebo for all end points, including total mortality and subsequent myocardial events, including infarction and unstable angina. There was also no relationship between outcome and *C. pneumoniae* serologic status. A similar analysis with similar results was published by Baker and Couch in 2007 (10). A number of possible reasons have been proposed for the failure to demonstrate a positive effect of antibiotic treatment, including the populations studied, trial design, and duration of treatment. Given the lack of a reliable marker for endovascular *C. pneumoniae* infection and the largely negative results in recent organism detection studies, it is unlikely that additional studies will demonstrate any benefit of long-term antibiotic treatment in reducing mortality or cardiovascular events in patients with CVD (99).

C. pneumoniae and Other Chronic Diseases

Chronic or persistent infection with *C. pneumoniae* has also been suggested as being related to a number of seemingly unrelated diseases and conditions, including MS, stroke, Alzheimer's disease, temporal arteritis, macular degeneration, and lung cancer. Over the past 60 years, 20 different bacteria and viruses have been proposed to be associated with MS (202). Often the results were inconsistent. The possible association of *C. pneumoniae* and MS was first described in a case study from researchers at Vanderbilt University Medical Center (VUMC), which was then followed by a series of studies from VUMC where the researchers claimed that they had identified the organism by culture and PCR (196). The hypothesis of how *C. pneumoniae* might cause MS was not clear. The results of subsequent studies from a number of other groups were conflicting; some found *C. pneumoniae* DNA in approximately 30% to over 80% of cerebrospinal fluid (CSF) samples from patients with MS and in approximately 20% of CSF samples from patients with other neurologic diseases, while others found none in CSF and brain tissue by culture and PCR (86, 202).

Several studies have also attempted to identify specific anti-*C. pneumoniae* antibodies in the oligoclonic bands in the CSF of patients with MS compared to those of patients with other neurologic diseases. As with identification of the organism, these results have also been conflicting. Much of the inconsistency of results from study to study may be due, in part, to the lack of standardized methods for *C. pneumoniae*, including serology, culture, and PCR, as has been seen with studies of respiratory infection and atherosclerosis (86). In an effort to deal with the issue of laboratory-to-laboratory differences in methods used to detect *C. pneumoniae* in studies of MS, prospectively collected CSF samples from patients with MS and other neurologic diseases were sent to laboratories at VUMC, Johns Hopkins University (JHU), University of Umea (UU) in Sweden, and subsequently also to the Centers for Disease Control and Prevention (CDC) (112). A total of 30 specimens from patients with MS and 22 controls were tested; none were positive by PCR at JHU, UU, and the CDC, but 73% of the CSF samples from patients with MS and 23% of the controls were positive by PCR at VUMC. Reasons for these discrepant results were discussed and included poor sensitivities of the assays used by JHU, UU, and the CDC or specificity problems with the assays used by VUMC. Subsequently, Tondella et al. (205) analyzed the primer sets used by VUMC in the multicenter study and sets used in previous studies from that laboratory and found high sequence similarity to human DNA, as determined by BLAST search, suggesting that these primers were not specific for just *C. pneumoniae*. This was confirmed in the laboratory using VUMC primers with commercially available human DNA.

As with the atherosclerosis, several studies examining antibiotic use and risk of MS and treatment of MS were undertaken. Woessner et al. (216) reported the results of a randomized double-blind study comparing three cycles of 6-week treatment with roxithromycin, 300 mg/day, over 12 months to a placebo group of 28 patients with MS. No significant differences were seen in expanded disability status scales or relapse rates between the two groups. Alonso et al. (3) investigated whether exposure to antibiotics active against *C. pneumoniae* might affect the risk of MS by examining data from a 1993–2000 case-control study from the United Kingdom. They identified 163 cases of MS that were followed for at least 3 years and matched them with up to 10 controls. Overall use of antibiotics or use of antibiotics with activity against *C. pneumoniae* was not associated with a decreased risk of MS.

Data on the association of *C. pneumoniae* and the other chronic conditions mentioned previously are more limited but also display the same inconsistent study-to-study results seen with CVD and MS. The possible association of *C. pneumoniae* and age-related macular degeneration (AMD) was first suggested in a seroepidemiologic study by Kalayoglu et al. in 2003 (108). AMD is the leading cause of severe visual loss in people over 60 years of age. Histopathological studies of AMD demonstrate the presence of chronic inflammation, although the role played by inflammation in this disease is not fully understood. As with atherosclerosis, *C. pneumoniae* has been proposed as a possible cause of the inflammation. Three initial reports suggested an association of AMD and exposure to *C. pneumoniae* using various serologic methods, including enzyme immunoassays and MIF assays (78). These reports were followed by two additional studies, including one from the same group that performed one of the initial studies, which did not find an association between serologic evidence of *C. pneumoniae* infection and AMD (123, 182). Subsequently, Kalayoglu et al. reported identification of *C. pneumoniae* by IHS and PCR in the choroidal neovascular membranes from four of nine patients with AMD (109). However, Kessler et al. did not identify *C. pneumoniae* DNA by PCR in the choroidal neovascular membranes from 13 consecutive patients with AMD (115). This experience is illustrative of the major problem with studies of *C. pneumoniae* and chronic diseases outside of the respiratory tract: the lack of validated, standardized methods.

C. TRACHOMATIS AND CHRONIC DISEASE IN HUMANS

Characteristically, *C. trachomatis* infections are restricted to ocular and genital tract mucosal surfaces. Infection is frequently low grade or asymptomatic and chronic in nature. Repeated infection is common, indicating that natural immunity is limited. Trachoma, due to chronic and repeated ocular infection with *C. trachomatis* serovars A, B, Ba, or C, is currently the leading cause of infectious blindness worldwide. Below the waist, three serovars of *C. trachomatis*, L_1, L_2, and L_3, are associated with lymphogranuloma venereum (LGV), a chronic sexually transmitted disease that is rare in the United States but still quite prevalent in many developing countries. LGV is characterized by spread from the genital tract to the regional nodes and rectum with chronic proctitis, sometimes leading to rectal stricture. A resurgence of this infectious syndrome has recently been noted among men who have sex with men in Western Europe and The Netherlands (165). *C. trachomatis* serovars D to K are the world's most common sexually transmitted bacterial pathogens. In men, although most infections are asymptomatic, they can cause urethritis and epididymitis. Women sustain a disproportionate share of the morbidity due to these *C. trachomatis* serovars through their well-known complications of pelvic inflammatory disease (PID), ectopic pregnancy, and tubal factor infertility. Although *C. trachomatis* infection can be treated effectively with antibiotics, infections may result in tissue damage, even with appropriate antimicrobial therapy. Thus, *C. trachomatis* causes ongoing global epidemics of infection; the associated complications of chlamydial genital infections inordinately impact women.

Unlike many other bacterial pathogens, *C. trachomatis* does not make potent toxins or tissue-damaging products; instead, it appears to induce an immune response that in the process of clearing away the bacteria results in collateral damage with inadvertent tissue destruction beyond what is needed to kill the pathogen. When *C. trachomatis* infects the eye, it causes conjunctivitis and with repeated reinfection triggers an inflammatory response that causes scarring and distortion of the eyelids. When *C. trachomatis* infects the reproductive tract, it causes inflammation in the Fallopian tubes that can lead to scars and damage that render an infected woman infertile or at elevated risk of ectopic pregnancy. Reinfection may lead to additional tissue damage via the host immune response, with each new infection reawakening the immune response and intensifying its strength.

C. trachomatis and Trachoma

It has been estimated that approximately 84 million cases of trachoma occur globally, leading to ~8 million cases of visual impairment. In developing countries, trachoma has taken the sight of some 6 million people. One hundred and fifty million people are in need of treatment, and 540 million people are at risk of getting the disease.

In areas where trachoma is endemic, infections occur early in life, with active disease persisting for several years. Poor hygiene and presence of eye-seeking flies enhance transmission of the organism. Initially, chronic follicular conjunctivitis typical of inclusion conjunctivitis develops and is followed by inflammation of the conjunctivae and involvement of the cornea. *C. trachomatis* can be isolated from conjunctival scrapings and nasopharyngeal cultures obtained from young children with active trachoma. Following severe scarring of the inner surface of the lids, trichiasis (inturning of the eyelashes) often develops. This results in further corneal ulceration, scarring, or opacification that can result in loss of visual acuity.

Treatment trials employing topical or oral antibiotics (50, 96) have been somewhat disappointing because of the short-lived impact of clinical and microbiologic effects. However, a recent study revealed that biannual mass antibiotic distribution at a high coverage level resulted in reduction of infection from 31.6% pretreatment (range, 6.1% to 48.6%) to 0.9% (range, 0.0% to 4.8%) at 24 months (144). Surgical treatments intended to repair or reduce eyelid distortion cannot restore eyesight and so far have been of limited value. The economic burden of trachoma is estimated to be approximately $2.9 billion in lost productivity per year, predominantly borne by rural populations in economically disadvantaged countries in Africa, Asia, the Middle East, and some parts of Latin America (www.trachoma.org). Ethiopia has some of the highest levels of trachoma in the world, with an active rate in children aged 1 to 10 years of 50 to 80%.

In communities where trachoma is endemic, the prevalence of active infection is inversely related to age, with the highest *C. trachomatis* bacterial loads being found in infants (194). The duration of untreated *C. trachomatis* infection is inversely related to age (10). Young preschool children who have persistent disease and chronically shed *C. trachomatis* act as an important reservoir of infection within the family unit (75, 203). Although prevalence studies have shown a predominance of children with active disease and older children and adults with healing or healed trachoma, such a progression is not observed among individuals. Rather, reversion to normal eyes and conversion to new disease were noted when cohorts of school children and families were followed longitudinally. Generally, a single serovar of *C. trachomatis* was present in all infected family members and did not vary over a 10-year observation period (75).

Patients with significant ocular scarring have significantly higher levels of antichlamydial IgG antibody compared with matched controls from areas where trachoma is endemic (49). The increased antichlamydial antibody titers likely reflect more chronic or increased numbers of repeated infections; investigations have revealed that local antichlamydial IgG is not protective against acquisition or chronicity of ocular chlamydial infection (9). Subjects recovering from human ocular chlamydial infection and that exhibit less scarring disease have enhanced lymphoproliferative responses to chlamydial antigens compared to persistently diseased controls (8, 94). Several studies have indicated that local overproduction of TNF may promote disease during human chlamydial ocular infection (24, 43, 66). Increased TNF transcripts have been observed in the inflamed conjunctiva during active trachoma (24, 66), and higher levels of TNF were found in the tear fluid of scarred individuals than in that of matched controls with normal eyes (43). By means of case-control studies, a number of genetic polymorphisms associated with increased risk of scarring sequelae have been identified, including polymorphisms of genes or promoters for TNF (162), matrix metalloproteinase 9 (MMP9) (159), IκBα (151), IFN-γ, and IL-10 (160).

A recent study carried out by Natividad et al. (161), in an African community where trachoma is endemic, revealed that susceptibility to trachomatous disease was associated with an excessive IL-10 response to *C. trachomatis* infection. This study was unique in that the investigators used the method of allele-specific quantification, which involved identifying subjects in the community who had active trachoma and were also heterozygous for the risk haplotype to overcome potential genetic and environmental confounders. They detected allelic variation in IL-10 *cis*-regulation in the conjunctival tissues of patients with active trachoma, with the risk haplotype generating relatively more IL-10 transcripts than other haplotypes in this population (average difference of 23% [95% confidence interval (CI) of 14% to 32%, $P < 0.0001$]). These findings provide a plausible functional explanation for the observed genetic association and support the hypothesis that an excessive IL-10 response to *C. trachomatis* infection is a risk factor for scarring and blindness.

C. trachomatis and Genital Tract Disease

LGV is a sexually transmitted disease caused by the L1-3 serovars of *C. trachomatis* that are endemic in tropical and subtropical areas (e.g., parts of Southeast Asia, Africa, South America, India, and the Caribbean) but rare in the United States. However, a recent resurgence of chronic proctitis due to LGV has been observed in Western Europe and the United States in men who have sex with men (68, 178). LGV is a disease of the lymphatic tissue that has acute and chronic manifestations. Unlike other anogenital *C. trachomatis* infections, where replication is confined to mucosal epithelial cells, LGV can replicate in macrophages and produce chronic invasive infection. Progression follows several defined stages similar to syphilitic infection. The primary lesion of LGV is a small, inconspicuous, asymptomatic genital papule or ulcer that heals without a scar. Days to weeks later, unilateral acute lymphadenitis with bubo formation occurs at the site of lymphatic drainage of the primary lesion; acute hemorrhagic proctitis develops following a rectal lesion. Systemic symptoms can include fever, myalgia, or headache. About one-third of inguinal buboes become fluctuant and rupture; the remainder involute slowly (204). Although most patients recover from LGV following this secondary stage, a small number develop a chronic inflammatory response with fibrosis (due to the persistence of chlamydiae in anogenital tissues) that can result in chronic genital ulcers or fistulas, rectal strictures, or genital elephantiasis. Genotyping *C. trachomatis* by nested PCR and restriction fragment length polymorphism allows a reliable diagnosis (114, 165, 166).

C. trachomatis serovars D to K are the world's most common sexually transmitted bacterial pathogens. Chlamydial genital infection primarily affects sexually active adolescents and young adults. Large-scale screening programs routinely detect infection rates of 5 to 10 percent in young adults (19 to 25 years of age) (135, 145) and 20 to 25 percent or greater in sexually active adolescents 15 to 19 years of age (23, 32, 70). Because symptoms are absent or minimal in most women and many men, a large reservoir of asymptomatic infection is present that can sustain the pathogen within a community. Presentation for diagnosis is frequently a result of screening or a contact being symptomatic. Studies in the United States have revealed that in areas where screening and treatment programs were implemented, prevalence declined (111, 187). However, other studies from Canada show increases in the number of infected individuals in areas where these programs have been implemented (27). While this increase could reflect improvements in diagnostic testing and/or changes in sexual behavior, prompt administration of antibiotics may undermine the development of natural immunity to *C. trachomatis*, leading to an increased risk of repeated infection.

Young age (less than 20 years) is the sociodemographic factor most strongly associated with chlamydial infection (relative risk among women younger than 25 years compared with older women is 2.0 to 3.5) (37, 72). Adolescents are most likely to be infected. In a recent study of 203 pregnant adolescents attending community-based public health clinics, 18 percent had chlamydial infection (164). In the United States, substantial racial/ethnic disparities are present in the prevalence of both chlamydial and gonococcal infections. One large study of U.S. female military recruits found a chlamydial prevalence of 9% that was maintained over 4 consecutive years (72). Young age, black race, home of record from the south, more than one sex partner, a new sex partner, lack of condom use, and a history of having a sexually transmitted disease were correlates of chlamydia infection.

When present, symptoms in females include mild abdominal pain, intermittent bleeding, vaginal discharge, or dysuria-pyuria syndrome. The cervix can appear normal or exhibit edema, erythema, friability, or mucopurulent discharge. The National Longitudinal Study of Adolescent Health, which collected data prospectively from 14,322 U.S adolescents and followed them into adulthood, was reported in 2004 and indicates symptoms are reported in less than 5% of infected men and women (145). Of the participants that tested positive for chlamydial infection, 95% did not report symptoms in the 24 hours preceding specimen collection. Among men with chlamydial infection, the prevalences of urethral discharge and dysuria were only 3.3% and 1.9%, respectively. Among women with chlamydial infection, the prevalences of vaginal discharge and dysuria were 0.3% and 4.2%, respectively. Among the small number of young men reporting urethral discharge ($n = 17$), the prevalence of chlamydial infection was high (38.5%). Of note, the prevalence of chlamydial infection among women reporting dysuria ($n = 232$) was 6.0%, but among those reporting vaginal discharge ($n = 98$), it was only 0.9% (145).

Some women develop ascending infection of the genital tract, resulting in endometritis and salpingitis (infection of the Fallopian tubes). The incidence of ascending infection and why ascending infection develops in some women and not others are not known. In one study, 18 of 109 (16.5%) infected asymptomatic adolescent women followed for 2 months or more became symptomatic, but only 2 (1.8%) developed clinical pelvic inflammatory disease (PID) (175). However, when women infected with both *C. trachomatis* and *Neisseria gonorrhoeae* were treated with antibiotics active only against *N. gonorrhoeae*, 6 of 20 (30 percent) developed evidence of upper genital tract infection (197). Risser et al. (180) reviewed the literature for prospective cohort studies assessing the incidence of PID following *C. trachomatis* infection. The incidence of PID varied from 0% (97.5% CI of 0 to 12%) during 1 year of follow-up of 30 women to 30% (95% CI of 12 to 54%) during 50 days of follow-up of 20 women. Studies that included asymptomatic women in other settings reported a lower incidence than those that evaluated women in sexually transmitted disease clinics. No study was of a size or quality to establish the true incidence of PID after untreated chlamydial infection.

Complications (e.g., epididymitis) affect a minority of infected men and rarely result in sequelae. Approximately 1 percent of men presenting with nongonococcal urethritis develop an acute aseptic arthritis syndrome referred to as sexually reactive arthritis. It appears to be an immune-mediated inflammatory response to an infection that occurs at a site distant from the primary infection (176). One-third of cases have the full complex of Reiter syndrome, consisting of the triad of arthritis, nonbacterial urethritis, and conjunctivitis (113). Most patients carry the histocompatibility antigen HLA-B27 (30).

The natural course of *C. trachomatis* female infection was recently described in a study of Columbian women followed for a 5-year period (148). Eighty-two women found to be positive for *C. trachomatis* at the start of the study were studied at 6-month intervals. Most of the women (70.7%) were >25 years of age, and 82.9% reported a single lifelong sex partner; thus, the potential for repeated infection from an untreated male sex partner was high. Women who had taken antibiotics effective against *C. trachomatis* while infected were excluded. Approximately 46% of the infections were persistent at 1 year, 18% at 2 years, and 6% at 4 years of follow-up, as determined by PCR of cervical scrape samples. Thus, in nearly half of this female cohort, an adaptive immune response effective in eradicating their infection or in preventing repeat infection did not develop for up to 1 year. No woman infected with chlamydiae was reported to develop PID or other chronic sequelae during the course of the study. Of those women who develop ascending infection and PID, up to 20% will become infertile; 18% will experience debilitating, chronic pelvic pain; and 9% will have a life-threatening tubal pregnancy (213). Lower abdominal pain, usually bilateral, is the most common presenting symptom. Pain may be associated with an abnormal vaginal discharge, abnormal uterine bleeding, dysuria, dyspareunia, nausea, vomiting, fever, or other constitutional symptoms. It is more commonly present in a subclinical form that lacks the typical acute symptoms but continues to lead to the associated long-term sequelae of infertility and ectopic pregnancy (63, 167). The most important causative organisms of PID are *C. trachomatis* and *N. gonorrhoeae;* well over half of cases are caused by one or both of these agents. Other microorganisms implicated in PID include organisms found in the abnormal vaginal flora of women with bacterial vaginosis, such as *Bacteroides* species, anaerobic cocci, *Mycoplasma hominis,* and *Ureaplasma urealyticum. Escherichia coli* and other enteric organisms have also been found. When women with chlamydial salpingitis are compared to women with gonococcal or with nongonococcal-nonchlamydial salpingitis, they are more likely to experience a chronic, subacute course with a longer duration of abdominal pain before seeking medical care. Yet, they have as much or more tubal inflammation at laparoscopy (201).

Most individuals with chlamydial infection spontaneously heal without a disease sequela. Individuals with severe forms of chlamydial disease often display high titers of antibody to chlamydial hsp60 antigen. Because the protein shares nearly 50% sequence identity with the human homolog, it is speculated that molecular mimicry may result in autoimmune inflammatory damage. However, high serum antibody titers to hsp60 may simply reflect increased overall exposure. In a study that controlled for level of exposure, serum antibodies to chlamydial hsp10, but not to chlamydial hsp60 or MOMP, were present at higher levels in women with tubal factor infertility (137).

Whether chlamydiae persist subclinically in the upper genital tract of women with resulting infertility remains unclear. A study by Patton et al. (170) demonstrated *C. trachomatis* DNA or antigens in 19 of 24 tubal biopsy specimens from women with postinfectious tubal infertility, 17 of whom had received anti-chlamydial antibiotics during the previous year. Serologic tests showed that all were chronically infected except one woman with IgM antibody. This is just one example of multiple studies describing the detection of chlamydial DNA or antigen in women with tubal infertility, the majority of whom are culture negative (34, 122, 195). The presence of chlamydial antigen and nucleic acids is suggestive but not proof of the presence of persistent viable organisms in the tissues. It is possible that tissue culture procedures may not be sensitive enough to detect low but potentially immunologically significant levels of replicating chlamydiae. Or, these individuals may harbor aberrant nonreplicating (and therefore nonculturable) but viable forms of chlamydiae with the capacity to stimulate immunopathologic changes. Of course, because of logistic and ethical difficulties, these studies have not examined patients over time. Thus, there is a lack of evidence for a long-term culture-negative persistent state of chlamydiae in patients with *C. trachomatis* genital tract infection.

Evidence against persistence after antimicrobial treatment comes from a study by Workowski et al. (217). Although only 20 women were studied, they were followed for up to 5 months after completion of doxycycline therapy with 384 cervical, rectal, and urethral specimens examined by culture and PCR for chlamydial DNA. All specimens were negative except for one woman with apparent reinfection with a different serotype (F) than the original infecting strain (E). Thus, this study found no evidence to indicate that doxycycline failed to eradicate lower genital tract infections and found no evidence of persistent chlamydial infection after therapy.

Thus, when patients are compliant with an active drug regimen, relapse of infection after cessation of adequate therapy is not likely a common cause of persistent or chronic infection. Rather, chronic infection may more often arise from failure to identify infections because of lack of adequate screening programs. These conclusions are supported by a study by Scholes et al. (187) in which screening and treatment of cervical chlamydial infection led to a dramatic 56 percent decrease in the incidence of PID.

In female patients with clinically suspected acute PID, pathological features that correlate both with upper genital tract infection and tubal salpingitis include presence of any neutrophils in the endometrial surface epithelium; neutrophils within gland lumens; dense subepithelial stromal lymphocytic infiltration; any stromal plasma cells; and germinal centers containing transformed lymphocytes (121). Predominant neutrophilic, lymphocytic, and plasma cell infiltrates have been described for human endocervical, endometrial, and Fallopian tube specimens from infected patients (121, 168, 171). In female patients with ectopic pregnancy who were seropositive for *C. trachomatis*, Fallopian tube biopsy specimens revealed extensive subepithelial plasma cell infiltration (26). All patients denied any history of genital tract symptoms, indicating subclinical infection of the oviduct can result in tubal disease.

TLRs are a family of surveillance proteins that recognize characteristic molecules that are expressed by bacteria, fungi, and viruses. As such, they are important components of the innate immune response which is initiated as soon as infection has been detected. These receptors are found primarily on innate immune cells, such as macrophages and dendritic cells, but are also expressed on many epithelial cells. When stimulated, these receptors drive signaling pathways that lead to activation of phagocytes and production of proinflammatory proteins called cytokines. Chlamydiae make several cell wall and outer membrane components that are recognized by TLRs. Using a mouse model of chlamydial genital infection, Darville et al. (47) revealed that TLR2 plays an essential role in the development of oviduct pathology. TLR2-deficient mice failed to develop oviduct damage when infected with *C. muridarum*, although all other aspects of their infection were similar to that seen in normal mice. Importantly, the mice were still able to mount normal anti-chlamydial antibody and cell-mediated adaptive responses, even though the signaling pathway was not operating. Thus, it seems clear that this innate immune signaling pathway is important in driving the tissue-damaging processes that result in chlamydial disease but is not needed for development of a protective response.

Genetic control of the development of genital tract disease is indicated by studies revealing genetic polymorphisms in cytokine genes, e.g., IL-10s are associated with altered risk of disease (119). There is a strong inverse relationship between age and susceptibility to chlamydial infection, even when corrected for frequency of sexual contact, suggesting effective adaptive immunity eventually develops. Lymphoproliferative responses, but not serum antibody titers, increase with age (7). Data from humans point to MHC class II-restricted $CD4^+$ T cells of the Th1 phenotype as being critical to recovery from chlamydial infection as well as having a role in protection from disease (29, 118). In a cohort of female commercial sex workers with human immunodeficiency virus, susceptibility to chlamydial PID increased as numbers of $CD4^+$ T cells decreased (118).

Debattista et al. (53) reported that PBMCs from women with chlamydial PID or a history of repeated *C. trachomatis* infection produced less IFN-γ in response to chlamydial hsp60 antigen than did women with a single episode of *C. trachomatis* infection, again suggesting an important role for host factors in protection from disease. In a prospective cohort study of commercial sex workers in Nairobi at high risk of exposure, production of IFN-γ by PBMCs stimulated with chlamydial hsp60 strongly correlated with protection against incident *C. trachomatis* infection. In contrast, levels of chlamydial EB or hsp60-specific IgA and IgG detected in endocervical mucus and plasma were not significantly associated with an altered risk of infection (42). Although antibody may not play a primary role in protection from reinfection, studies suggest it may help control the shedding of organisms and protect against upper tract disease. One study reported that the prevalence of mucosal IgA antibodies was inversely related to the quantity of *C. trachomatis* shed from the human endocervix (28), and another found the presence of serum IgA and IgG antibodies reduced the risk for ascending infection among women undergoing therapeutic abortion (30).

An effective vaccine against *C. trachomatis* will have to activate both the antibody and cellular arms of the immune system more effectively than the body's natural response does, yet somehow limit inflammation as well. A better understanding of protective host responses to chlamydiae is needed. In addition, markers for protection from upper genital tract infection and/or disease in the female will be necessary if vaccine candidates are to be tested in humans. Stimulation of long-term mucosal immunity in the genital tract is a challenge; persons are susceptible to reinfection with *C. trachomatis* after a brief period of immunity because memory cells are not retained in the genital tract. It is unclear whether all genital infections could be prevented or whether only more invasive disease, such as salpingitis, might be preventable using vaccine technology.

Although current antibiotic treatment is highly successful when administered, most persons infected with *C. trachomatis* are asymptomatic and thus go undiagnosed and untreated. Screening and treatment programs have been shown to reduce prevalence of infection and disease in the past, but recent studies indicate widespread screening and treatment may actually increase infection prevalence by blunting adaptive immunity. Therefore, a vaccine may be the only possible means whereby the morbidities associated with *C. trachomatis* infections can be prevented. More research is needed for prevention of chlamydial infections as regards effectiveness of mass screening and treatment and vaccine development.

REFERENCES

1. **Airenne, S., A. Kinnunen, M. Leinonen, P. Saikku, and H. M. Surcel.** 2002. Secretion of IL-10 and IL-12 in *Chlamydia pneumoniae* infected human monocytes, p. 77–80. Proceedings of the Tenth International Symposium on Human Chlamydial Infections. International Chlamydia Symposium, San Francisco, CA.
2. **Allegra, L., F. Blasi, S. Centanni, R. Cosentini, F. Denti, R. Raccanelli, P. Tarsia, and V. Valenti.** 1994. Acute exacerbations of asthma in adults: role of *Chlamydia pneumoniae*. *Eur. Respir. J.* 7:2165–2168.
3. **Alonso, A., S. S. Jick, H. Jick, and M. A. Hernan.** 2006. Antibiotic use and risk of multiple sclerosis. *Am. J. Epidemiol.* **163**:997–1002.
4. **Andraws, R., J. S. Berger, and D. L. Brown.** 2005. Effects of antibiotic therapy on outcomes of patients with coronary artery disease. A meta-analysis of randomized controlled trials. *JAMA* **293**:2641–2647.

4a. **Apfalter, P., F. Blasi, J. Boman, C. A. Gaydos, M. Kundi, M. Maass, A. Makristathis, A. Meijer, R. Nadrchal, K. Persson, M. L. Rotter. C. Y. W. Tong, G. Stanek, and A. M. Hirschl.** 2001. Multicenter comparison trial of DNA extraction methods and PCR assays for detection of *Chlamydia pneumoniae* in endarterectomy specimens. *J. Clin. Microbiol.* **39**:519–524.

5. **Apfalter, P., O. Assadian, F. Blasi, C. A. Gaydos, M. Kundi, M. Maass, A. Makristathis, M. Nehr, M. L. Rotter, and A. M. Hirschl.** 2002. Reliability of nested PCR for the detection of *Chlamydia pneumoniae* DNA in atheromas: results from a multicenter study applying standardized protocols. *J. Clin. Microbiol.* **40**:4428–4434.
6. **Arno, J. N., B. P. Katz, R. McBride, G. A. Carty, B. E. Batteiger, V. A. Caine, and R. B. Jones.** 1994. Age and clinical immunity to infections with *Chlamydia trachomatis*. *Sex. Transm. Dis.* **21**:47–52.
7. **Bailey, R. L., M. J. Holland, H. C. Whittle, and D. C. W. Mabey.** 1995. Subjects recovering from human ocular chlamydial infection have enhanced lymphoproliferative responses to chlamydial antigens compared with those of persistently diseased controls. *Infect. Immun.* **63**:389–392.
8. **Bailey, R. L., M. Kajbaf, H. C. Whittle, M. E. Ward, and D. C. Mabey.** 1993. The influence of local antichlamydial antibody on the acquisition and persistence of human ocular chlamydial infection: IgG antibodies are not protective. *Epidem. Infect.* **111**:315–324.

9. **Bailey, R., T. Duong, R. Carpenter, H. Whittle, and D. Mabey**. 1999. The duration of human ocular *Chlamydia trachomatis* infection is age dependent. *Epidemiol. Infect.* **123**:479–486.
10. **Baker, W. L., and K. A. Couch**. 2007. Azithromycin for secondary prevention of coronary artery disease: a meta-analysis. *Am. J. Health Syst. Pharm.* **64**:830–836.
11. **Baltch, A. L., R. P. Smioth, W. J. Ritz, A. N. Carpenter, L. H. Bopp, P. B. Michelsen, C. J. Carlyn, and J. R. Hibbs**. 2004. Effect of levofloxacin on the viability of intracellular *Chlamydia pneumoniae* and modulation of proinflammatory cytokine production by human monocytes. *Diagn. Microbiol. Infect. Dis.* **50**:205–212.
12. **Barnes, P. J.** 1994. Cytokines as mediators of chronic asthma. *Am. J. Respir. Crit. Care Med.* **150**:S42–S49.
13. **Beatty, W. L., R. P. Morrison, and G. L. Byrne**. 1994. Persistent chlamydiae: from cell culture to a paradigm form chlamydial pathogenesis. *Microbiol. Rev.* **58**:689–694.
14. **Beatty, W. L. 2007**. Lysosome repair enables host cell survival and bacterial persistence following *Chlamydia trachomatis* infection. *Cell Microbiol.* **9**:2141–2152.
15. **Beatty, W. L., R. P. Morrison, and G. L. Byrne**. 1995. Reactivation of persistent *Chlamydia trachomatis* infection in cell culture. *Infect. Immun.* **63**:199–205.
16. **Biscardi, S., M. Lorrot, E. Marc, F. Moulin, B. Boutonnat-Faucher, C. Heilbronner, J. L. Iniguez, M. Chaussain, E. Nicand, J. Raymond, and D. Gendrel**. 2004. *Mycoplasma pneumoniae* and asthma in children. *Clin. Infect. Dis.* **38**:1341–1346.
17. **Biscione, G. L., J. Corne, A. J. Chauhan, and S. L. Johnston**. 2004. Increased frequency of detection of *Chlamydophila pneumoniae* in asthma. *Eur. Resp. J.* **24**:745–749.
18. **Bjoernsson, E., E. Hjelm, C. Janson, E. Fridell, and G. Boman**. 1996. Serology of *Chlamydia* in relation to asthma and bronchial hyperresponsiveness. *Scand. J. Infect. Dis.* **28**:63–69.
19. **Black, P. N., C. R. Jenkins, R. Scicchitano, L. Allegra, F. Blasi, J. Wlodarzyck, and B. C. Cooper**. 2000. Serological evidence of infection with *Chlamydia pneumoniae* is related to the severity of asthma. *Eur. Resp. J.* **15**:254–259.
20. **Black, P. N., F. Blasi, C. R. Jenkins, R. Scicchitano, G. D. Mills, A. R. Rubinfeld, R. E. Ruffin, P. R. Mullins, J. Dangain, B. C. Cooper, D. B. David, and L. Allegra**. 2001. Trial of roxithromycin in subjects with asthma and serological evidence of infection with *Chlamydia pneumoniae*. *Am. J. Respir. Crit. Care Med.* **164**:536–541.
21. **Blasi, F., S. Aliberti, L. Allegra, G. Piatti, P. Tarsia, J. M. Ossewaarde, V. Verweij, F. P. Nijkamp, and G. Folkerts**. 2007. *Chlamydophila pneumoniae* induces a sustained airway hyperresponsiveness and inflammation in mice. *Resp. Res.* **8**:83.
22. **Blythe, M. J., B. P. Katz, D. P. Orr, V. A. Caine, and R. B. Jones**. 1988. Historical and clinical factors associated with *Chlamydia trachomatis* genitourinary infection in female adolescents. *J. Pediatr.* **112**:1000–1004.
23. **Bobo, L., N. Novak, H. Mkocha, S. Vitale, S. West, and T. C. Quinn**. 1996. Evidence for a predominant proinflammatory conjunctival cytokine response in individuals with trachoma. *Infect. Immun.* **64**:3273–3279.
24. **Boman, J., and M. R. Hammerschlag**. 2002. *Chlamydia pneumoniae* and atherosclerosis—a critical assessment of diagnostic methods and the relevance to treatment studies. *Clin. Microbiol. Rev.* **15**:1–20.
25. **Brunham, R. C., B. Binns, J. McDowell, and M. Paraskevas**. 1986. *Chlamydia trachomatis* infection in women with ectopic pregnancy. *Obstet. Gynecol.* **67**:722–726.
26. **Brunham, R. C., B. Pourbohloul, S. Mak, R. White, and M. L. Rekart**. 2005. The unexpected impact of a *Chlamydia trachomatis* infection control program on susceptibility to reinfection. *J. Infect. Dis.* **192**:1836–1844.
27. **Brunham, R. C., C. C. Kuo, L. Cles, and K. K. Holmes**. 1983. Correlation of host immune response with quantitative recovery of *Chlamydia trachomatis* from the human endocervix. *Infect. Immun.* **39**:1491–1494.
28. **Brunham, R. C., J. Kimani, J. Bwayo, G. Maitha, I. Maclean, C. Yang, C. Shen, S. Roman, N. J. Nagelkerke, M. Cheang, and F. A. Plummer**. 1996. The epidemiology of *Chlamydia trachomatis* within a sexually transmitted diseases core group. *J. Infect. Dis.* **173**:950–956.
29. **Brunham, R. C., R. Peeling, I. Maclean, J. McDowell, K. Persson, and S. Osser**. 1987. Postabortal *Chlamydia trachomatis* salpingitis: correlating risk with antigen-specific serological responses and with neutralization. *J. Infect. Dis.* **155**:749–755.
30. **Bulut, Y., E. Faure, L. Thomas, H. Karahashi, K. S. Michelsen, O. Equils, S. G. Morrison, R. P. Morrison, and M. Arditi**. 2002. Chlamydial heat shock protein 60 activates macrophages and endothelial cells through Toll-like receptor 4 and MD2 in a MyD88-dependent pathway. *J. Immunol.* **168**:1435–1440.
31. **Burstein, G. R., C. A. Gaydos, M. Diener-West, M. R. Howell, J. M. Zenilman, and T. C. Quinn**. 1998. Incident *Chlamydia trachomatis* infections among inner-city adolescent females. *JAMA* **280**:521–526.
32. **Byrne, G. I., S. I. Skarlotos, C. Grunfeld, M. V. Kalayoglu, P. Libby, P. Saikku, J. T. Summersgill, and P. Wyrick**. 2000. Collaborative multidisciplinary workshop report: interface of lipid metabolism, atherosclerosis and *Chlamydia* infection. *J. Infect. Dis.* **181**(Suppl.3):S490–S491.
33. **Campbell, L. A., D. L. Patton, D. E. Moore, A. L. Cappuccio, B. A. Mueller, and S. P. Wang**. 1993. Detection of *Chlamydia trachomatis* deoxyribonucleic acid in women with tubal infertility. *Fertil. Steril.* **59**:45–50.
34. **Carratelli, C. R., A. Rizzo, R. Paolillo, M. R. Catania, P. Catalanotti, and F. Rossano**. 2005. Effect of nitric oxide on the growth of *Chlamydophila pneumoniae*. *Can. J. Microbiol.* **51**:941–947.
35. **Caspar-Bauguil, S., B. Puissant, D. Nazzal, J. C. Lefevre, M. Thomsen, R. Salvayre, and H. Benoist.** 2000. *Chlamydia pneumoniae* induces interleukin-10 production that down-regulates major histocompatibility complex class I expression. *J. Infect. Dis.* **182**:1394–1401.
36. **Centers for Disease Control and Prevention**. 2002. Sexually transmitted disease treatment guidelines 2002. *MMWR Recommend. Rep.* **51**(RR-6):1–84.
37. **Chirgwin, K., P. M. Roblin, M. Gelling, M. R. Hammerschlag, and J. Schachter.** 1991. Infection with *Chlamydia pneumoniae* in Brooklyn. *J. Infect. Dis.* **163**:757–761.
38. **Cho, Y. S., T. B. Kim, T. H. Lee, K. A. Moon, J. Lee, Y. K. Kim, K. Y. Lee, and H. B. Moon**. 2005. *Chlamydia pneumoniae* infection enhances cellular proliferation and reduces steroid responsiveness of human peripheral blood mononuclear cells via a tumor necrosis factor-a-dependent pathway. *Clin. Exp. Allergy* **35**:1625–1631.
39. **Choi, J. H., M. J. Song, S. H. Kim, S. M. Choi, D. G. Lee, J. H. Yoo, and W. S. Shin**. 2003. Effect of moxifloxacin on production of proinflammatory cytokines from human peripheral blood mononuclear cells. *Antimicrob. Agents Chemother.* **47**:3704–3707.
40. **Chopra, I., C. Storey, T. J. Falla, and J. H. Pearce**. 1998. Antibiotics, peptidoglycan synthesis and genomics: the chlamydial anomaly revisited. *Microbiology* **144**:2673–2678.

41. **Cohen, C. R., K. M. Koochesfahani, A. S. Meier, C. Shen, K. Karunakaran, B. Ondondo, T. Kinyari, N. R. Mugo, R. Nguti, and R. C. Brunham.** 2005. Immunoepidemiologic profile of *Chlamydia trachomatis* infection: importance of heat-shock protein 60 and interferon-gamma. *J. Infect. Dis.* **192:**591–599.
42. **Conway, D. J., M. J. Holland, R. L. Bailey, A. E. Campbell, O. S. Mahdi, R. Jennings, E. Mbena, and D. C. Mabey.** 1997. Scarring trachoma is associated with polymorphism in the tumor necrosis factor alpha (TNF-α) gene promoter and with elevated TNF-α levels in tear fluid. *Infect. Immun.* **65:**1003–1006.
43. **Cook, P. J., P. Davies, W. Tunnicliffe, J. G. Ayres, D. Honeybourne, and R. Wise.** 1998. *Chlamydia pneumoniae* and asthma. *Thorax* **53:**254–259.
44. **Cunningham, A. F., S. L. Johnston, S. A. Julious, F. C. Lampe, and M. E. Ward.** 1998. Chronic *Chlamydia pneumoniae* infection and asthma exacerbations in children. *Eur. Respir. J.* **11:**345–349.
45. **Danesh, J., P. Whincup, M. Walker, L. Lennon, A. Thomson, P. Appleby, Y. Wong, M. Bernardes-Silva, and M. Ward.** 2000. *Chlamydia pneumoniae* IgG titres and coronary heart disease: prospective study and meta-analysis. *Br. Med. J.* **321:**208–213.
46. **Daoud, A., C. J. Gloria, G. Taningco, M. R. Hammerschlag, S. Weiss, M. Gelling, P. M. Roblin, and R. Joks.** 2008. Minocycline treatment results in reduced oral steroid requirements in adult asthma. *Allergy Asthma Proc.* **29:**286–294.
47. **Darville, T., J. M. O'Neill, C. W. Andrews, Jr., U. M. Nagarajan, L. Stahl, and D. M. Ojcius.** 2003. Toll-like receptor-2, but not toll-like receptor-4, is essential for development of oviduct pathology in chlamydial genital tract infection. *J. Immunol.* **171:**6187–6197.
48. **Datta, P., E. Frost, R. Peeling, S. Masinde, S. Deslandes, C. Echelu, I. Wamola, and R. C. Brunham.** 1994. Ophthalmia neonatorum in a trachoma endemic area. *Sex. Transm. Dis.* **21:**1–4.
49. **Dawson, C. R., T. Daghfous, I. Hoshiwara, K. Ramdhane, M. Kamoun, C. Yoneda, and J. Schachter.** 1982. Trachoma therapy with topical tetracycline and oral erythromycin: a comparative trial. *Bull. W. H. O.* **60:**347–355.
50. Reference deleted.
51. **Dean, D., P. Roblin, L. Mandel, J. Schachter, and M. Hammerschlag.** 1998. Molecular evaluation of serial isolates from patients with persistent *Chlamydia pneumoniae* infections, p. 219–222. *In* R. S. Stephens, G. I. Byrne, G. Christiansen, I. N. Clarke, J. T. Grayston, R. G. Rank, G. L. Ridgway, P. Saikku, J. Schachter, and W. E. Stamm (ed). *Chlamydial Infections.* Proceedings of the Ninth International Symposium on Human Chlamydia Infections. International Chlamydia Symposium, San Francisco, CA.
52. **Dean, D., and V. C. Powers.** 2001. Persistent *Chlamydia trachomatis* infections resist apoptotic stimuli. *Infect. Immun.* **69:**2442–2447.
53. **Debattista, J., P. Timms, J. Allan, and J. Allan.** 2002. Reduced levels of gamma-interferon secretion in response to chlamydial 60 kDa heat shock protein amongst women with pelvic inflammatory disease and a history of repeated *Chlamydia trachomatis* infections. *Immunol. Lett.* **81:**205–210.
54. **de Kruif, M. D., E. C. van Gorp, T. T. Keller, J. M. Ossewaarde, and H. ten Cate.** 2005. *Chlamydia pneumoniae* infections in mouse models: relevance for atherosclerosis research. *Cardiovasc. Res.* **65:**317–327.
55. **Dill, D. D., and J. E. Raulston.** 2007. Examination of an inducible expression system for limiting iron availability during *Chlamydia trachomatis* infection. *Microbes Infect.* **9:**947–953.
56. **Dowell, S. F., J. Boman, G. M. Carlone, B. S. Fields, J. Guarner, M. R. Hammerschlag, L. A. Jackson, C. C. Kuo, M. Maass, T. O. Messmer, R. W. Peeling, D. Talkington, M. L. Tondella, S. R. Zaki, and the *C. pneumoniae* workshop participants.** 2000. Standardizing *Chlamydia pneumoniae* assays: recommendations from the Centers for Disease Control and Prevention (USA), and the Laboratory Centre for Disease Control (Canada). *Clin. Infect. Dis.* **33:**492–503.
57. **Dreses-Werringloer, U., I. Padubrin, B. Jürgens-Saathoff, A. P. Hudson, H. Zeidler, and L. Köhler.** 2000. Persistence of *Chlamydia trachomatis* is induced by ciprofloxacin and ofloxacin in vitro. *Antimicrob. Agents Chemother.* **44:**3288–3297.
58. **Durkin, H. G., S. M. Chice, E. Gaetjens, H. Bazin, L. Tarcsay, and P. Dukor.** 1989. Origin and fate of IgE-bearing lymphocytes. II. Modulation of IgE isotype expression on Peyer's patch cells by feeding with certain bacteria and bacterial cell wall components or by thymectomy. *J. Immunol.* **143:**1777–1783.
59. **Eickhoff, M., J. Thalmann, S. Hess, M. Martin, T. Laue, J. Kruppa, G. Brandes, and A. Klos.** 2007. Host cell responses to *Chlamydia pneumoniae* in gamma interferon-induced persistence overlap those of productive infection and are linked to genes involved in apoptosis, cell cycle, and metabolism. *Infect. Immun.* **75:**2853–2863.
60. **Emre, U., P. M. Roblin, M. Gelling, W. Dumornay, M. Rao, M. R. Hammerschlag, and J. Schachter.** 1994. The association of *Chlamydia pneumoniae* infection and reactive airway disease in children. *Arch. Pediatr. Adolesc. Med.* **148:**727–731.
61. **Emre, U., N. Sokolovskaya, P. M. Roblin, J. Schachter, and M. R. Hammerschlag.** 1995. Detection of anti-*Chlamydia pneumoniae* IgE in children with reactive airway disease. *J. Infect. Dis.* **172:**265–267.
62. **Entrican, G., S. Wattegedera, M. Rocchi, D. C. Fleming, R. W. Kelly, G. Wathne, V. Magdalenic, and S. E. M. Howie.** 2004. Induction of inflammatory host immune responses by organisms belonging to the genera *Chlamydia/Chlamydophila. Vet. Immunol. Immunopathol.* **100:**179–186.
63. **Eschenbach, D. A., P. Wolner-Hanssen, S. E. Hawes, A. Pavletic, J. Paavonen, and K. K. Holmes.** 1997. Acute pelvic inflammatory disease: associations of clinical and laboratory findings with laparoscopic findings. *Obstet. Gynecol.* **89:**184–192.
64. **Esposito, S., F. Blasi, C. Arosio, L. Fiovavanti, L. Fagetti, R. Droghetti, P. Tarsia, N. Pincipi, and L. Allegra.** 2000. Importance of acute *Mycoplasma pneumoniae* and *Chlamydia pneumoniae* infection in children with wheezing. *Eur. Resp. J.* **16:**1142–1146.
65. **Everett, K. D. E., R. M. Bush, and A. A. Anderson.** 1999. Emended description of the order *Chlamydiales,* proposal of *Parachlamydiaceae* fam. nov. and *Simkaniaceae* fam. nov., each containing one monotypic genus, revised taxonomy of the family *Chlamydiaceae*, including a new genus and five new species, and standards for identification of organisms. *Int. J. Syst. Bacteriol.* **49:**425–440.
66. **Faal, N., R. L. Bailey, I. Sarr, H. Joof, D. C. Mabey, and M. J. Holland.** 2005. Temporal cytokine gene expression patterns in subjects with trachoma identify distinct conjunctival responses associated with infection. *Clin. Exp. Immunol.* **142:**347–353.
67. **Fan, T., H. Lu, H. Hu, L. Shi, G. A. McClarty, D. M. Nance, A. H. Greenberg, and G. Zhong.** 1998. Inhibition of apoptosis in chlamydia-infected cells: blockade of mitochondrial cytochrome c release and caspase activation. *J. Exp. Med.* **187:**487–496.

68. **Fenton, K. A., and J. Imrie.** 2005. Increasing rates of sexually transmitted diseases in homosexual men in Western Europe and the United States: why? *Infect. Dis. Clin. North Am.* **19:**311–331.
69. **Fonseca-Aten, M., P. J. Okada, K. L. Bowlware, S. Chavez-Buena, A. Mejias, A. M. Rios, K. Katz, K. Olsen, S. Ng, H. S. Jafri, G. H. McCracken, O. Ramilo, and R. D. Hardy.** 2006. Effect of clarithromycin on cytokines and chemokines in children with an acute exacerbation of recurrent wheezing: a double-blind, randomized, placebo-controlled trial. *Ann. Allergy Asthma Immunol.* **97:**457–463.
70. **Ford, C. A., B. W. Pence, W. C. Miller, M. D. Resnick, L. H. Bearinger, S. Pettingell, and M. Cohen.** 2005. Predicting adolescents' longitudinal risk for sexually transmitted infection: results from the National Longitudinal Study of Adolescent Health. *Arch. Pediatr. Adolesc. Med.* **159:**657–664.
71. **Gaydos, C. A., J. T. Summersgill, N. N. Sahney, J. A. Ramirez, and T. C. Quinn.** 1996. Replication of *Chlamydia pneumoniae* in vitro in human macrophages, endothelial cells, and aortic artery smooth muscle cells. *Infect. Immun.* **64:**1614–1620.
72. **Gaydos, C. A., M. R. Howell, T. C. Quinn, K. T. McKee, Jr., and J. C. Gaydos.** 2003. Sustained high prevalence of *Chlamydia trachomatis* infections in female army recruits. *Sex. Transm. Dis.* **30:**539–544.
73. **Ghuysen, J. M., and C. Goffin.** 1999. Lack of cell wall peptidoglycan versus penicillin sensitivity: new insights into the chlamydial anomaly. *Antimicrob. Agents Chemother.* **43:**2339–2344.
74. **Girardin, S. E., M. Jehanno, D. Mengin-Lecreulx, P. J. Sansonetti, P. M. Alzari, and D. J. Philpott.** 2005. Identification of the critical residues involved in peptidoglycan detection by Nod1. *J. Biol. Chem.* **280:**38648–38656.
75. **Grayston, J. T., S. P. Wang, L. J. Yeh, and C. C. Kuo.** 1985. Importance of reinfection in the pathogenesis of trachoma. *Rev. Infect. Dis.* **7:**717–725.
76. **Greene, W., Y. Xiao, Y. Huang, G. McClarty, and G. Zhong.** 2004. Chlamydia-infected cells continue to undergo mitosis and resist induction of apoptosis. *Infect. Immun.* **72:**451–60.
77. **Gupta, S., E. W. Leatham, D. Carrington, M. A. Mendall, J. C. Kaski, and A. J. Camm.** 1997. Elevated *Chlamydia pneumoniae* antibodies, cardiovascular events, and azithromycin in male survivors of myocardial infarction. *Circulation* **96:**404–407.
78. **Guymer, R., and L. Robman.** 2007. *Chlamydia pneumoniae* and age-related macular degeneration: a role in pathogenesis or merely a chance association? *Clin. Exper. Ophthalmol.* **35:**89–93.
79. **Hahn, D. L., M. B. Plane, O. S. Mahdi, and G. I. Byrne.** 2006. Secondary outcomes of a pilot randomized trial of azithromycin treatment for asthma. *PLOS Clin. Trials* **1:**e11.
80. **Hahn, D. L., R. W. Dodge, and R. Golubjatnikov.** 1991. Association of *Chlamydia pneumoniae* (strain TWAR) infection with wheezing, asthmatic bronchitis, and adult-onset asthma. *JAMA* **266:**225–230.
81. **Hahn, D. L., T. Anttila, P. Saikku.** 1996. Association of *Chlamydia pnuemoniae* IgA antibodies with recently symptomatic asthma. *Epidemiol. Infect.* **117:**513–517.
82. **Halme, S., and H. M. Surcel.** 1997. Cell mediated immunity to *Chlamydia pneumoniae. Scand. J. Infect. Dis.* **104**(Suppl.)**:**18–21.
83. **Halme, S., J. Latvala, R. Karttunen, I. Palatsi, P. Saikku, and H. M. Surcel.** 2000. Cell-mediated immune response during primary *Chlamydia pneumoniae* infection. *Infect. Immun.* **68:**7156–7158.
84. **Halme, S., P. Saikku, and H. M. Surcel.** 1997. Characterization of *Chlamydia pneumoniae* antigens using human T cell clones. *Scand. J. Immunol.* **45:**378–384.
85. **Hammerschlag, M. R., K. Chirgwin, P. M. Roblin, M. Gelling, W. Dumornay, L. Mandel, P. Smith, and J. Schachter.** 1992. Persistent infection with *Chlamydia pneumoniae* following acute respiratory illness. *Clin. Infect. Dis.* **14:**178–182.
86. **Hammerschlag, M. R., and G. A. Gaydos.** 2006. *Chlamydia pneumoniae* and multiple sclerosis: fact or fiction. *Lancet Neurol.* **5:**892–893.
87. **Harju, T. H., M. Leinonen, J. Nokso-Koivisto, T. Korhonen, R. Räty, Q. He, T. Hovi, J. Mertsola, A. Bloigu, P. Rytilä, and P. Saikku.** 2006. Pathogenic bacteria and viruses in induced sputum or pharyngeal secretions of adults with stable asthma. *Thorax* **61:**579–584.
88. **Harper, A., C. I. Pogson, M. L. Jones, and J. H. Pearce.** 2000. Chlamydial development is adversely affected by minor changes in amino acid supply, blood plasma amino acids levels, and glucose deprivation. *Infect. Immun.* **68:**1457–1464.
89. **Hawkins, R. A., R. G. Rank, and K. A. Kelly.** 2002. A *Chlamydia trachomatis* specific Th2 clone does not provide protection against a genital infection and displays reduced trafficking to the infected genital mucosa. *Infect. Immun.* **70:**5132–5139.
90. **Heinemann, M., M. Susa, U. Simnacher, R. Marre, and A. Essig.** 1996. Growth of *Chlamydia pneumoniae* induces cytokine production and expression of CD14 in a human monocytic cell line. *Infect. Immun.* **64:**4872–4875.
91. **Hess, S., J. Peters, G. Bartling, C. Rheinheimer, P. Hegde, M. Magid-Slav, R. Singer, and A. Klos.** 2003. More than just innate immunity: comparative analysis of *Chlamydophila pneumoniae* and *Chlamydia trachomatis* effects on host-cell gene regulation. *Cell. Microbiol.* **5:**785–795.
92. **Hoffjan, S., I. Ostrovnaja, D. Nicolae, D. L. Newman, R. Nicolae, R. Gangnon, L. Steiner, K. Walker, R. Reynolds, D. Greene, D. Mirel, J. E. Gern, R. F. Lemanske, and C. Ober.** 2004. Genetic variation in immunoregulatory pathways and atopic phenotypes in infancy. *J. Allergy Clin. Immunol.* **113:**511–518.
93. **Hogan, R. J., S. A. Mathews, S. Mukhopadhyay, J. T. Summersgill, and P. Timms.** 2004. Chlamydial persistence: beyond the biphasic paradigm. *Infect. Immun.* **72:**1843–1855.
94. **Holland, M. J., R. L. Bailey, D. J. Conway, F. Culley, G. Miranpuri, G. I. Byrne, H. C. Whittle, and D. C. Mabey.** 1996. T-helper type 1 (Th1)/Th2 profiles of peripheral blood mononuclear cells (PBMC); responses to antigens of *Chlamydia trachomatis* in subjects with severe trachomatous scarring. *Clin. Exp. Immunol.* **105:**429–435.
95. **Holland, M. J., R. L. Bailey, L. J. Hayes, H. C. Whittle, and D. C. Mabey.** 1993. Conjunctival scarring in trachoma is associated with depressed cell-mediated immune responses to chlamydial antigens. *J. Infect. Dis.* **168:**1528–1531.
96. **Holm, S. O., H. C. Jha, R. C. Bhatta, J. S. Chaudhary, B. B. Thapa, D. Davis, R. P. Pokhrel, M. Yinghui, M. Zegans, J. Schachter, K. D. Frick, L. Tapert, and T. M. Lietman.** 2001. Comparison of two azithromycin distribution strategies for controlling trachoma in Nepal. *Bull. W. H. O.* **79:**194–200.
97. **Horvat, J. C., K. W. Beagley, M. A. Wade, J. A. Preston, N. G. Hansbro, D. K. Hickey, G. E. Kaiko, P. G. Gibson, P. S. Foster, and P. M. Hansbro.** 2007. Neonatal chlamydial infection induces mixed T-cell responses that drive allergic airway disease. *Am. J. Respir. Crit. Care Med.* **176:**556–564.

98. **Hoymans, V. Y., J. M. Bosmans, D. Ursi, W. Martinet, F. L. Wuyts, E. V. Marck, M. Altwegg, C. J. Vrints, and M. M. Ieven.** 2004. Immunohistostaining assays for detection of *Chlamydia pneumoniae* in atherosclerotic arteries indicate cross-reactions with nonchlamydial plaque constituents. *J. Clin. Microbiol.* **42:**3219–3224.

99. **Hoymans, V. Y., J. M. Bosmans, M. M. Ieven, and C. J. Vrints.** 2007. *Chlamydia pneumoniae*-based atherosclerosis: a smoking gun. *Acta Cardiol.* **63:**565–571.

100. **Hyman, C. L., M. H. Augenbraun, P. Roblin, J. Schachter, and M. R. Hammerschlag.** 1991. Asymptomatic respiratory tract infection with *Chlamydia pneumoniae* TWAR. *J. Clin. Microbiol.* **29:**2082–2083.

101. **Hyman, C. L., P. M. Roblin, C. A. Gaydos, T. C. Quinn, J. Schachter, and M. R. Hammerschlag.** 1995. The prevalence of asymptomatic nasopharyngeal carriage of *Chlamydia pneumoniae* in subjectively healthy adults: assessment by polymerase chain reaction-enzyme immunoassay and culture. *Clin. Infect. Dis.* **20:**1174–1178.

102. **Ieven, M. M., and V. Y. Hoymans.** 2005. Involvement of *Chlamydia pneumoniae* in atherosclerosis: more evidence for lack of evidence. *J. Clin. Microbiol.* **43:**19–24.

103. **Igietseme, J. U., K. H. Ramsey, D. M. Magee, D. M. Williams, T. J. Kincy, and R. G. Rank.** 1993. Resolution of murine chlamydial genital infection by the adoptive transfer of a biovar-specific, TH1 lymphocyte clone. *Reg. Immunol.* **5:**317–324.

104. **Ikezawa, S.** 2001. Prevalence of *Chlamydia pneumoniae* in acute respiratory tract infection and detection of anti-*Chlamydia pneumoniae*-specific IgE in Japanese children with reactive airway disease. *Kurume Med. J.* **48:**165–170.

105. **Johnston, S. L., F. Blasi, P. N. Black, R. J. Martin, D. J. Farrell, R. B. Nieman, et al.** 2006. The effect of telithromycin in acute exacerbations of asthma. *N. Engl. J. Med.* **354:**1589–1600.

106. **Kaiko, G. E., S. Phipps, D. K. Hickey, C. E. Lam, P. M. Hansbro, P. S. Foster, and K. W. Beagley.** 2008. *Chlamydia muridarum* infection subverts dendritic cell function to promote Th2 immunity and airways hyperreactivity. *J. Immunol.* **180:**2225–2232.

107. **Kalayoglu, M. V., and G. I. Byrne.** 1998. A *Chlamydia pneumoniae* component that induces macrophage foam cell formation is chlamydial lipopolysaccharide. *Infect. Immun.* **66:**5067–5072.

108. **Kalayoglu, M. V., C. Galavan, O. S. Mahdi, G. I. Byrne, and S. Mansour.** 2003. Serological association between *Chlamydia pneumoniae* infection and age-related macular degeneration. *Arch. Ophthalmol.* **121:**478–482.

109. **Kalayoglu, M. V., D. Bula, J. Arroyo, E. S. Gragoudas, D. D'Amico, and J. W. Miller.** 2005. Identification of *Chlamydia pneumoniae* within human choroidal neovascular membranes secondary to age-related macular degeneration. *Graefes Arch. Clin. Exp. Ophthalmol.* **243:**1080–1090.

110. **Kalayoglu, M. V., P. Libby, and G. I. Byrne.** 2002. *Chlamydia pneumoniae* as an emerging risk factor in cardiovascular disease. *JAMA* **288:**2724–2731.

111. **Katz, B. P., M. J. Blythe, P. B. Van Der, and R. B. Jones.** 1996. Declining prevalence of chlamydial infection among adolescent girls. *Sex. Transm. Dis.* **23:**226–229.

112. **Kaufman, M., C. A. Gaydos, S. Sriram, J. Boman, M. L. Tondella, and H. J. Norton.** 2002. Is *Chlamydia pneumoniae* found in spinal fluid samples from multiple sclerosis patients? Conflicting results. *Mult. Scler.* **8:**289–294.

112a. **Kaukoranta-Tolvanen, S. S., A. M. Teppo, K. Laitinen, P. Saikku, K. Linnavuori, and M. Leinonen.** 1996. Growth of *Chlamydia pneumoniae* in cultured human peripheral blood mononuclear cells and induction of a cytokine response. *Microb. Pathogen.* **21:**215–221.

113. **Keat, A., B. J. Thomas, and D. Taylor Robinson.** 1983. Chlamydial infection in the aetiology of arthritis. *Br. Med. Bull.* **39:**168–174.

114. **Kellock, D. J., R. Barlow, S. K. Suvarna, S. Green, A. Eley, and K. E. Rogstad.** 1997. Lymphogranuloma venereum: biopsy, serology, and molecular biology. *Genitourin. Med.* **73:**399–401.

115. **Kessler, W., C. A. Jantos, J. Dreier, and S. Pavlovic.** 2006. *Chlamydia pneumoniae* is not detectable in subretinal neovascular membranes in the exudative stage of age-related macular degeneration. *Acta Ophthalmol. Scand.* **84:**333–337.

116. **Khan, M. A., and C. W. Potter.** 1996. The nPCR detection of *Chlamydia pneumoniae* and *Chlamydia trachomatis* in children hospitalized for bronchiolitis. *J. Infect.* **33:**173–175.

117. **Kim, C. K., S. W. Kim, C. S. Park, B. I. Kim, H. Kang, and Y. Y. Koh.** 2003. Bronchoalveolar lavage cytokine profiles in acute asthma and acute bronchiolitis. *J. Allergy Clin. Immunol.* **112:**64–71.

118. **Kimani, J., I. W. Maclean, J. J. Bwayo, K. MacDonald, J. Oyugi, G. M. Maitha, R. W. Peeling, M. Cheang, N. J. Nagelkerke, F. A. Plummer, and R. C. Brunham.** 1996. Risk factors for *Chlamydia trachomatis* pelvic inflammatory disease among sex workers in Nairobi, Kenya. *J. Infect. Dis.* **173:**1437–1444.

119. **Kinnunen, A. H., H. M. Surcel, M. Lehtinen, J. Karhukorpi, A. Tiitinen, M. Halttunen, A. Bloigu, R. P. Morrison, R. Karttunen, and J. Paavonen.** 2002. HLA DQ alleles and interleukin-10 polymorphism associated with *Chlamydia trachomatis*-related tubal factor infertility: a case-control study. *Hum. Reprod.* **17:**2073–2078.

120. **Kitamura, N., O. Kaminuma, A. Mori, T. Hashimoto, F. Kitamura, M. Miyagishi, K. Taira, and S. Miyatake.** 2005. Correlation between mRNA expression of Th1/Th2 cytokines and their specific transcription factors in human helper T-cell clones. *Immunol. Cell Biol.* **83:**536–541.

121. **Kiviat, N. B., P. Wolner-Hanssen, D. A. Eschenbach, J. N. Wasserheit, J. A. Paavonen, T. A. Bell, C. W. Critchlow, W. E. Stamm, D. E. Moore, and K. K. Holmes.** 1990. Endometrial histopathology in patients with culture-proved upper genital tract infection and laparoscopically diagnosed acute salpingitis. *Am. J. Surg. Pathol.* **14:**167–175.

122. **Kiviat, N. B., P. Wolner-Hanssen, M. Peterson, J. Wasserheit, W. E. Stamm, D. A. Eschenbach, J. Paavonen, J. Lingenfelter, T. Bell, V. Zabriskie, B. Kirby, and K. K. Holmes.** 1986. Localization of *Chlamydia trachomatis* infection by direct immunofluorescence and culture in pelvic inflammatory disease. *Am. J. Obstet. Gynecol.* **154:**865–873.

123. **Klein, R., B. E. K. Klein, M. D. Knudtson, T. Y. Wong, A. Shankar, and M. Y. Tsai.** 2005. Systemic markers of inflammation, endothelial dysfunction, and age related maculopathy. *Am. J. Ophthalmol.* **140:**35–44.

124. **Kohlhepp, S. J., J. Hardick, and C. Gaydos.** 2005. *Chlamydia pneumoniae* in peripheral blood mononuclear cells from individuals younger than 20 years and older than 60 years. *J. Clin. Microbiol.* **43:**3030.

125. **Kohlhoff, S., P. Roblin, A. Kutlin, S. Strigl, M. Nowakowski, R. Joks, and M. R. Hammerschlag.** 2005. Effect of *Chlamydia pneumoniae* infection on cytokine profiles of PBMC from asthmatics and healthy subjects. *J. Allergy Clin. Immunol.* **115:**15.

126. **Kohlhoff, S. A., A. Kutlin, P. Riska, P. M. Roblin, C. Roman, and M. R. Hammerschlag.** 2008. *In vitro* models

of acute and long term continuous infection of human respiratory epithelial cells with *Chlamydophila pneumoniae* have opposing effects on host cell apoptosis. *Microb. Pathogen.* **44**:34–42.

127. **Komura, H., H. Matsushima, K. Ouchi, M. Shirai, T. Nakazawa, and S. Furukawa.** 2003. Effect of antiasthma drugs on the growth of *Chlamydophila pneumoniae* in HEp-2 cells. *J. Infect. Chemother.* **9**:160–164.

128. **Kraft, M., G. H. Cassell, J. E. Henson, H. Watson, J. Williamson, B. P. Marmion, C. A. Gaydos, and R. J. Martin.** 1998. Detection of *Mycoplasma pneumoniae* in the airways of adults with chronic asthma. *Am. J. Resp. Crit. Care Med.* **158**:998–1001.

129. **Kraft, M., G. H. Cassell, J. Pak, and R. J. Martin.** 2002. *Mycoplasma pneumoniae* and *Chlamydia pneumoniae* in asthma: effect of clarithromycin. *Chest* **121**:1782–1788.

130. **Kumar, S., and M. R. Hammerschlag.** 2007. Acute respiratory infection due to *Chlamydia pneumoniae*: current status of diagnostic methods. *Clin. Infect. Dis.* **44**:568–576.

131. **Kumar, S., S. A. Kohlhoff, M. Gelling, P. M. Roblin, A. Kutlin, S. Kahane, M. G. Friedman, and M. R. Hammerschlag.** 2005. Infection with *Simkania negevensis* in Brooklyn, New York. *Pediatr. Infect. Dis. J.* **24**:989–992.

132. **Kutlin, A., P. M. Roblin, and M. R. Hammerschlag.** 1998. Antibody response to *Chlamydia pneumoniae* infection in children with respiratory illness. *J. Infect. Dis.* **177**:720–724.

133. **Kutlin, A., C. Flegg, D. Stenzel, T. Reznik, P. M. Roblin, S. Mathews, P. Timms, and M. R. Hammerschlag.** 2001. Ultrastructural study of *Chlamydia pneumoniae* in a continuous infection model. *J. Clin. Microbiol.* **39**:3721–3723.

134. **Kutlin, A., P. M. Roblin, and M. R. Hammerschlag.** 2002. Effect of prolonged treatment with azithromycin, clarithromycin and levofloxacin on *Chlamydia pneumoniae* in a continuous infection model. *Antimicrob. Agents Chemother.* **46**:409–412.

135. **LaMontagne, D. S., K. A. Fenton, S. Randall, S. Anderson, and P. Carter.** 2004. Establishing the National Chlamydia Screening Programme in England: results from the first full year of screening. *Sex. Transm. Infect.* **80**:335–341.

136. **Larsen, F. O., S. Norn, C. H. Mordhorst, S. P. Stahl, N. Milman, and P. Clementsen.** 1998. *Chlamydia pneumoniae* and possible relationship to asthma. *APMIS* **106**:928–934.

137. **LaVerda, D., L. N. Albanese, P. E. Ruther, S. G. Morrison, R. P. Morrison, K. A. Ault, and G. I. Byrne.** 2000. Seroreactivity to *Chlamydia trachomatis* Hsp10 correlates with severity of human genital tract disease. *Infect. Immun.* **68**:303–309.

138. **Littman, A. J., L. A. Jackson, E. White, M. D. Thornquist, C. A. Gaydos, and T. L. Vaughn.** 2004. Interlaboratory reliability of microimmunofluorescence test for measurement of *Chlamydia pneumoniae*-specific immunoglobulin A and G antibody titers. *J. Clin. Microbiol.* **11**:615–617.

139. **Liu, C., and D. D. Waters.** 2005. *Chlamydia pneumoniae* and atherosclerosis: from Koch's postulates to clinical trials. *Prog. Cardiovasc. Dis.* **47**:230–239.

140. **MacDowell, A. L., and L. B. Bacharier.** 2005. Infectious triggers of asthma. Immunol. *Allergy Clin. N. Am.* **25**:45–66.

141. **Martin, R. J., M. Kraft, H. W. Chu, E. A. Berns, and G. H. Cassell.** 2001. A link between chronic asthma and chronic infection. *J. Allergy Clin. Immunol.* **107**:595–601.

142. **Martinez, F. D.** 2003. Respiratory syncytial virus bronchiolitis and the pathogenesis of childhood asthma. *Pediatr. Infect. Dis. J.* **22**:S76–S82.

143. **McCoy, A. J., and A. T. Maurelli.** 2006. Building the invisible wall: updating the chlamydial peptidoglycan anomaly. *Trends Microbiol.* **14**:70–77.

144. **Melese, M., W. Alemayehu, T. Lakew, E. Yi, J. House, J. D. Chidambaram, Z. Zhou, V. Cevallos, K. Ray, K. C. Hong, T. C. Porco, I. Phan, A. Zaidi, B. D. Gaynor, J. P. Whitcher, and T. M. Lietman.** 2008. Comparison of annual and biannual mass antibiotic administration for elimination of infectious trachoma. *JAMA* **299**:778–784.

145. **Miller, W. C., C. A. Ford, M. Morris, M. S. Handcock, J. L. Schmitz, M. M. Hobbs, M. S. Cohen, K. M. Harris, and J. R. Udry.** 2004. Prevalence of chlamydial and gonococcal infections among young adults in the United States. *JAMA* **291**:2229–2236.

146. **Mills, G. D., J. A. Lindeman, J. P Fawcett, G. P. Herbison, and M. R. Sears.** 2000. *Chlamydia pneumoniae* serological status is not associated with asthma in children or young adults. *Int. J. Epidemiol.* **29**:280–284.

147. **Moazed, T. C., C. C. Kuo, J. T. Grayston, and L. A. Campbell.** 1998. Evidence of systemic dissemination of *Chlamydia pneumoniae* via macrophages in the mouse. *J. Infect. Dis.* **177**:1322–1325.

148. **Molano, M., C. J. Meijer, E. Weiderpass, A. Arslan, H. Posso, S. Franceschi, M. Ronderos, N. Munoz, and A. J. van den Brule.** 2005. The natural course of *Chlamydia trachomatis* infection in asymptomatic Colombian women: a 5-year follow-up study. *J. Infect. Dis.* **191**:907–916.

149. **Molestina, R. E., R. D. Miller, J. A. Ramirez, and J. T. Summersgill.** 1999. Infection of human endothelial cells with *Chlamydia pneumoniae* stimulates transendotehlial migration of neutrophils and monocytes. *Infect. Immun.* **67**:1323–1330.

150. **Moulder, J. W.** 1993. Why is Chlamydia sensitive to penicillin in the absence of peptidoglycan? *Infect. Agents Dis.* **2**:87–99.

151. **Mozzato-Chamay, N., O. S. Mahdi, O. Jallow, D. C. Mabey, R. L. Bailey, and D. J. Conway.** 2000. Polymorphisms in candidate genes and risk of scarring trachoma in a *Chlamydia trachomatis*-endemic population. *J. Infect. Dis.* **182**:1545–1548.

152. **Mpiga, P., and M. Ravaoarinoro.** 2006. *Chlamydia trachomatis* persistence: an update. *Microbiol. Res.* **161**:9–19.

153. **Mukhopadhyay, S., R. D. Miller, E. D. Sullivan, C. Theodoropoulos, S. A. Mathews, P. Timms, and J. T. Summersgill.** 2006. Protein expression profiles of *Chlamydia pneumoniae* in models of persistence versus those of heat shock stress response. *Infect. Immun.* **74**:3853–3863.

154. **Myashita, N., Y. Kubota, M. Nakajima, Y. Niki, H. Kawane, and T. Matushima.** 1998. *Chlamydia pneumoniae* and exacerbations of asthma in adults. *Ann. Allergy Asthma Immunol.* **80**:405–409.

155. **Nagy, A., G. T. Kozma, M. Keszei, A. Treszl, A. Falus, and C. Szalai.** 2003. The development of asthma in children with *Chlamydia pneumoniae* is dependent on the modifying effect of mannose-binding lectin. *J. Allergy Clin. Immunol.* **112**:729–734.

156. **Nagy, A., M. Keszei, Z. Kis, I. Budai, G. Tolgyesi, I. Ungvari, A. Falus, and C. Szalai.** 2007. *Chlamydophila pneumoniae* infection status is dependent on the subtypes of asthma and allergy. *Allergy Asthma Proc.* **28**:58–63.

157. **Naiki, Y., K. S. Michelsen, N. W. J. Schröder, R. Alsabeh, A. Slepenkin, W. Zhang, S. Chen, B. Wei, Y. Bulut, M. H. Wong, E. M. Peterson, and M. Arditi.** 2005. Myd88 is pivotal for the early inflammatory response and subsequent bacterial clearance and survival in a mouse model of *Chlamydia pneumoniae* pneumonia. *J. Biol. Chem.* **280**:29242–29249.

158. **Nakajo, M. N., P. M. Roblin, M. R. Hammerschlag, P. Smith, and M. Nowakowski**. 1990. Chlamydicidal activity of human alveolar macrophages. *Infect. Immun.* **58**:3640–3644.
159. **Natividad, A., G. Cooke, M. J. Holland, M. J. Burton, H. M. Joof, K. Rockett, D. P. Kwiatkowski, D. C. Mabey, and R. L. Bailey**. 2006. A coding polymorphism in matrix metalloproteinase 9 reduces risk of scarring sequelae of ocular *Chlamydia trachomatis* infection. *BMC Med. Genet.* **7**:40.
160. **Natividad, A., J. Wilson, O. Koch, M. J. Holland, K. Rockett, N. Faal, O. Jallow, H. M. Joof, M. J. Burton, N. D. Alexander, D. P. Kwiatkowski, D. C. Mabey, and R. L. Bailey**. 2005. Risk of trachomatous scarring and trichiasis in Gambians varies with SNP haplotypes at the interferon-gamma and interleukin-10 loci. *Genes Immun.* **6**:332–340.
161. **Natividad, A., M. J. Holland, K. A. Rockett, J. Forton, N. Faal, H. M. Joof, D. C. Mabey, R. L. Bailey, and D. P. Kwiatkowski**. 2008. Susceptibility to sequelae of human ocular chlamydial infection associated with allelic variation in IL10 *cis*-regulation. *Hum. Mol. Genet.* **17**:323–329.
162. **Natividad, A., N. Hanchard, M. J. Holland, O. S. Mahdi, M. Diakite, K. Rockett, O. Jallow, H. M. Joof, D. P. Kwiatkowski, D. C. Mabey, and R. L. Bailey**. 2007. Genetic variation at the TNF locus and the risk of severe sequelae of ocular *Chlamydia trachomatis* infection in Gambians. *Genes Immun.* **8**:288–295.
163. **Netea, M. G., B. J. Kullberg, J. M. Galama, A. F. Stalenhoef, C. A. Dinarello, and J. W. Van der Meer**. 2002. Non-LPS components of *Chlamydia pneumoniae* stimulate cytokine production through Toll-like receptor 2-dependent pathways. *Eur. J. Immunol.* **32**:1188–1195.
164. **Niccolai, L. M., K. A. Ethier, T. S. Kershaw, J. B. Lewis, and J. R. Ickovics**. 2003. Pregnant adolescents at risk: sexual behaviors and sexually transmitted disease prevalence. *Am. J. Obstet. Gynecol.* **188**:63–70.
165. **Nieuwenhuis, R. F., J. M. Ossewaarde, H. M. Gotz, J. Dees, H. B. Thio, M. G. Thomeer, J. C. den Hollander, M. H. Neumann, and W. I. van der Meijden**. 2004. Resurgence of lymphogranuloma venereum in Western Europe: an outbreak of *Chlamydia trachomatis* serovar L2 proctitis in The Netherlands among men who have sex with men. *Clin. Infect. Dis.* **39**:996–1003.
166. **Ossewaarde, J. M., M. Rieffe, G. J. van Doornum, C. J. Henquet, and A. M. van Loon**. 1994. Detection of amplified *Chlamydia trachomatis* DNA using a microtiter plate-based enzyme immunoassay. *Eur. J. Clin. Microbiol. Infect. Dis.* **13**:732–740.
167. **Paavonen, J., and M. Lehtinen**. 1996. Chlamydial pelvic inflammatory disease. *Hum. Reprod. Update* **2**:519–529.
168. **Paavonen, J., K. Teisala, P. K. Heinonen, R. Aine, S. Laine, M. Lehtinen, A. Miettinen, R. Punnonen, and P. Gronroos**. 1987. Microbiological and histopathological findings in acute pelvic inflammatory disease. *Br. J. Obstet. Gynaecol.* **94**:454–460.
169. **Pasternack, R., H. Huhtala, and J. Karjalainen**. 2005. *Chlamydophila (Chlamydia) pneumoniae* serology and asthma in adults: a longitudinal analysis. *J. Allergy Clin. Immunol.* **116**:1123–1128.
170. **Patton, D. L., M. Askienazy-Elbhar, J. Henry-Suchet, L. A. Campbell, A. Cappuccio, W. Tannous, S. P. Wang, and C. C. Kuo**. 1994. Detection of *Chlamydia trachomatis* in fallopian tube tissue in women with postinfectious tubal infertility. *Am. J. Obstet. Gynecol.* **171**:95–101.
171. **Paukku, M., M. Puolakkainen, T. Paavonen, and J. Paavonen**. 1999. Plasma cell endometritis is associated with *Chlamydia trachomatis* infection. *Am. J. Clin. Pathol.* **112**:211–215.
172. **Polkinghorne, A., R. J. Hogan, L. Vaughn, J. T. Summersgill, and P. Timms**. 2006. Differential expression of chlamydial signal transduction genes in normal and interferon gamma-induced persistent *Chlamydophila pneumoniae* infections. *Microb. Infect.* **8**:61–72.
173. **Prebeck, S., C. Kirschning, S. Durr, C. da Costa, B. Donath, K. Brand, V. Redecke, H. Wagner, and T. Miethke**. 2001. Predominant role of toll-like receptor 2 versus 4 in *Chlamydia pneumoniae*-induced activation of dendritic cells. *J. Immunol.* **167**:3316–3323.
174. **Principi, N., S. Esposito, F. Blasi, L. Allegra, and the Mowgli Study Group**. 2001. Role of *Mycoplasma pneumoniae* and *Chlamydia pneumoniae* in children with community-aquired lower respiratory tract infection. *Clin. Infect. Dis.* **32**:1281–1289.
175. **Rahm, V.-A., H. Gnarpe, and V. Odlind**. 1988. *Chlamydia trachomatis* among sexually active teenage girls. Lack of correlation between chlamydial infection, history of the patient and clinical signs of infection. *Br. J. Obstet. Gynaecol.* **95**:916–919.
176. **Rahman, M. U., R. Cantwell, C. C. Johnson, R. L. Hodinka, H. R. Schumacher, and A. P. Hudson**. 1992. Inapparent genital infection with *Chlamydia trachomatis* and its potential role in the genesis of Reiters syndrome. *DNA Cell Biol.* **11**:215–219.
177. **Rasmussen, S. J., L. Eckmann, A. J. Quayle, L. Shen, Y. X. Zhang, D. J. Anderson, J. Flerer, R. S. Stephens, and M. F. Kagnoff**. 1997. Secretion of proinflammatory cytokines by epithelial cells in response to Chlamydia infection suggests a central role for epithelial cells in chlamydial pathogenesis. *J. Clin. Investig.* **99**:77–87.
178. **Richardson, D., and D. Goldmeier**. 2007. Lymphogranuloma venereum: an emerging cause of proctitis in men who have sex with men. *Int. J. STD AIDS* **18**:11–14.
179. **Richeldi, L., G. Ferrara, T. Lasserson, and P. Gibson**. 2005. Macrolides for chronic asthma (Cochrane Review). *Cochrane Database Syst. Rev.* CD002997. doi: 10.1002/14651858.CD002997.pub3.
180. **Risser, W. L., and J. M. Risser**. 2007. The incidence of pelvic inflammatory disease in untreated women infected with *Chlamydia trachomatis*: a structured review. *Int. J. STD AIDS* **18**:727–731.
181. **Roblin, P. M., and M. R. Hammerschlag**. 1998. Microbiologic efficacy of azithromycin and susceptibility to azithromycin of isolates of *Chlamydia pneumoniae* from adults and children with community acquired pneumonia. *Antimicrob. Agents Chemother.* **42**:194–196.
182. **Robman, L., O. S. Mahdi , J. J. Wang, G. Burlutsky, P. Mitchell, G. Byrne, R. Guymer, and H. Taylor**, 2007. Exposure to *Chlamydia pneumoniae* infection and age-related macular degeneration: the Blue Mountain Eye Study. *Invest. Ophthalmol. Vis. Sci.* **48**:4007–4011.
183. **Rockey, D. D., J. Lenart, and R. S. Stephens**. 2000. Genome sequencing and our understanding of chlamydiae. *Infect. Immun.* **68**:5473–5479.
184. **Rodel, J., M. Woytas, A. Groh, K. H. Schmidt, M. Hartmann, M. Lehmann, and E. Straube**. 2000. Production of basic fibroblast growth factor and interleukin 6 by human smooth muscle cells following infection with *Chlamydia pneumoniae*. *Infect. Immun.* **68**:3635–3641.

184a. **Saikku, P., M. Leinonen, K. Mattila, M. R. Ekman, M. S. Nieminen, P. H. Makela, J. K. Huttunen, and V. Valtonen**. 1988. Serological evidence of an association of a novel

Chlamydia, TWAR, with chronic coronary heart disease and acute myocardial infarction. *Lancet* ii:983–986.

185. **Saiman, L., B. C. Marshall, N. Mayer-Hamblett, J. L. Burns, A. L. Quittner, D. A. Cibene, S. Coquilette, A. Y. Fieberg, F. J. Accurso, P. W. Campbell III, and the Macrolide Study Group.** 2003. Azithromycin in patients with cystic fibrosis chronically infected with *Pseudomonas aeruginosa*: a randomized controlled trial. *JAMA* **290:**1749–1756.
186. Reference deleted.
187. **Scholes, D., A. Stergachis, F. E. Heidrich, H. Andrilla, K. K. Holmes, and W. E. Stamm.** 1996. Prevention of pelvic inflammatory disease by screening for cervical chlamydial infection. *N. Engl. J. Med.* **334:**1362–1366.
188. **Schultz, M. J.** 2004. Macrolide activities beyond their antimicrobial effects: macrolides in diffuse panbronchiolitis and cystic fibrosis. *J. Antimicrob. Chemother.* **54:**21–28.
189. **Senn, L., M. R. Hammerschlag, and G. Greub.** 2005 Therapeutic approaches to *Chlamydia* infections. *Expert Opin. Pharmacother.* **6:**1–10.
190. **Shor, A., C. C. Kuo, and D. L. Patton.** 1992. Detection of *Chlamydia pneumoniae* in coronary arterial fatty streaks and atheromatous plaques. *S. Afr. Med. J.* **82:**158–161.
191. **Smieja, M., J. Mahoney, A. Petrich, J. Boman, and M. Chernesky.** 2002. Association of circulating *Chlamydia pneumoniae* DNA with cardiovascular disease: a systematic review. *BMC Infect. Dis.* **2:**21.
192. **Smieja, M., J. Gnarpe, E. Lonn, H. Gnarpe, G. Olsson, Q. Yi, V. Dzavik, M. Mcqueen, S. Yusuf, and Heart Outcomes Prevention and Evaluation Study (HOPE) Investigators.** 2003. Multiple infections and subsequent cardiovascular events in the Heart Outcomes Prevention and Evaluation Study (HOPE) study. *Circulation* **107:**251–257.
193. **Smith-Norowitz, T. A., M. H. Bluth, H. Drew, K. B. Norowitz, S. Chice, V. N. Shah, M. Nowakowski, A. S. Josephson, H. G. Durkin, and R. Joks.** 2002. Effect of minocycline and doxycycline on IgE responses. *Ann. Allergy Asthma Immunol.* **89:**172–179.
194. **Solomon, A. W., M. J. Holland, M. J. Burton, S. K. West, N. D. Alexander, A. Aguirre, P. A. Massae, H. Mkocha, B. Munoz, G. J. Johnson, R. W. Peeling, R. L. Bailey, A. Foster, and D. C. Mabey.** 2003. Strategies for control of trachoma: observational study with quantitative PCR. *Lancet* **362:**198–204.
195. **Soong, Y. K., S.-M. Kao, C.-H. Lee, P. S. Lee, and C. C. Pao.** 1990. Endocervical chlamydial deoxyribonucleic acid in infertile women. *Fertil. Steril.* **54:**815–818.
196. **Sriram, S., W. Mitchell, and C. Stratton.** 1998. Multiple sclerosis associated with *Chlamydia pneumoniae* infection of the CNS. *Neurology* **50:**571–572.
197. **Stamm, W. E., M. E. Guinan, C. Johnson, T. Starcher, K. K. Holmes, and W. M. McCormack.** 1984. Effect of treatment regimens for *Neisseria gonorrhoeae* on simultaneous infection with *Chlamydia trachomatis*. *N. Engl. J. Med.* **310:**545–549.
198. **Strachan, D., P. D. Carrington, M. Mendall, B. K. Butland, J. W. Yarnell, and P. Elwood.** 2000. *Chlamydia pneumoniae* serology, lung function decline, and treatment for respiratory disease. *Am. J. Respir. Crit. Care Med.* **161:**493–497.
199. **Sutton, B. J., and H. J. Gould. 1993**. The human IgE network. *Nature* **366:**421–428.
200. Reference deleted.
201. **Svensson, L., L. Westrom, K. T. Ripa, and P. A. Mardh.** 1980. Differences in some clinical and laboratory parameters in acute salpingitis related to culture and serologic findings. *Am. J. Obstet. Gynecol.* **138:**1017–1021.
202. **Swanborg, R. H., J. A. Whittum-Hudson, and A. P. Hudson.** 2003. Infectious agents and multiple sclerosis—are *Chlamydia pneumoniae* and human herpes virus 6 involved? *J. Neuroimmunol.* **135:**1–8.
203. **Taylor, H. R., J. A. Siler, H. A. Mkocha, B. Munoz, and S. West.** 1992. The natural history of endemic trachoma: a longitudinal study. *Am. J. Trop. Med. Hyg.* **46:**552–559.
204. **Thorsteinsson, S. B.** 1982. Lymphogranuloma venereum: review of clinical manifestations, epidemiology, diagnosis, and treatment. *Scand. J. Infect. Dis.* **32**(Suppl.)**:**127–131.
205. **Tondella, M. L. C., G. Galagoda, C. A. Gaydos, and J. Boman.** 2003. Is *Chlamydia pneumoniae* present in cerebrospinal fluid samples of multiple sclerosis patients? *Clin. Diag. Lab. Immunol.* **10:**977–978.
206. **Tramper-Stranders, G. A., T. F. Wolfs, A. Fleer, J. L. Kimpen, and C. K. van der Ent.** 2007. Maintenance azithromycin treatment in pediatric patients with cystic fibrosis: long-term outcomes related to macrolide resistance and pulmonary function. *Pediatr. Infect. Dis. J.* **26:**8–12.
207. **Tsumura, N., U. Emre, P. Roblin, and M. R. Hammerschlag.** 1996. The effect of hydrocortisone succinate on the growth of *Chlamydia pneumoniae* in vitro. *J. Clin. Microbiol.* **34:**2379–2381.
208. **Van Strien, R. T., R. Engel, O. Holst, A. Bufe, W. Eder, M. Waser, C. Braun-Fahrlaender, J. Riedler, D. Nowak, E. von Mutius, and the LAEX Study Team.** 2004. Microbial exposure of rural school children, as assessed by levels on N-acetyl-muramic acid in mattress dust, and its association with respiratory health. *J. Allergy Clin. Immunol.* **113:**860–867.
209. **Velasco, G., M. Campo, O. J. Manrique, A. Bellou, R. S. Arestides, B. Schaub, D. L. Perkins, and P. W. Finn.** 2005. Toll-like receptor 4 or 2 agonists decrease allergic inflammation. *Am. J. Respir. Cell. Mol. Biol.* **32:**218–224.
210. **Von Hertzen, L. C.** 2002. Role of persistent infection in the control and severity of asthma: focus on *Chlamydia pneumoniae*. *Eur. Respir. J.* **19:**546–556.
211. **Wark, P. A. B., S. L. Johnston, J. L. Simpson, M. J. Hensley, and P. G. Gibson.** 2002. *Chlamydia pneumoniae* immunoglobulin A reactivation and airway inflammation in acute asthma. *Eur. Respir. J.* **20:**834–840.
212. **Welter-Stahl, L., D. M. Ojcius, J. Viala, S. Girardin, W. Liu, C. Delarbre , D. Philpott, K. A. Kelly, and T. Darville.** 2006. Stimulation of the cytosolic receptor, Nod1, by infection with *Chlamydia trachomatis* or *Chlamydia muridarum*. *Cell. Microbiol.* **8:**1047–1057.
213. **Westrom, L., R. Joesoef, G. Reynolds, A. Hagdu, and S. E. Thompson.** 1992. Pelvic inflammatory disease and fertility. A cohort study of 1,844 women with laparoscopically verified disease and 657 control women with normal laparoscopic results. *Sex. Transm. Dis.* **19:**185–192.
214. **Williams, A. C., H. F. Galley, A. M. Watt, and N. R. Webster.** 2005. Differential effects of three antibiotics on T helper cell cytokine expression. *J. Antimicrob. Chemother.* **56:**502–506.
215. **Williams, D. M., B. G. Grubbs, T. Darville, K. Kelly, and R. R. Rank.** 1998. A role for interleukin-6 in host defense against murine *Chlamydia trachomatis* infection. *Infect. Immun.* **66:**4564–4567.
216. **Woessner, R., T. Grauer, A. Frese, F. Bethke, T. Ginger, A. Hans, and J. Treib.** 2006. Long-term antibiotic treatment with roxithromycin in patients with multiple sclerosis. *Infection* **34:**342–344.
217. **Workowski, K. A., M. F. Lampe, K. G. Wong, M. B. Watts, and W. E. Stamm.** 1993. Long-term eradication of *Chlamydia trachomatis* genital infection after antimicro-

bial therapy. Evidence against persistent infection. *JAMA* **270**:2071–2075.

218. **Yang, X., K. T. HayGlass, and R. Brunham.** 1996. Genetically determined differences in IL-10 and IFN-gamma responses correlate with clearance of *Chlamydia trachomatis* mouse pneumonitis infection. *J. Immunol.* **156:** 4338–4344.

219. **Yang, Z. P., C. C. Kuo, and J. T. Grayston.** 1995. Systemic dissemination of *Chlamydia pneumoniae* following intranasal inoculation in mice. *J. Infect. Dis.* **171**:736–738.

220. **Yeung, S. M., K. McLeod, S. P. Wang, J. T. Grayston, and E. E. Wang.** 1993. Lack of evidence of *Chlamydia pneumoniae* infection in infants with acute lower respiratory tract disease. *Eur. J. Clin. Microbiol. Infect. Dis.***12:** 850–853.

221. **Ying, S., S. F. Fischer, M. Pettengill, D. Conte, S. A. Paschen, D. M. Ojcius, and G. Häcker.** 2006. Characterization of host cell death induced by *Chlamydia trachomatis. Infect. Immun.***74**:6057–6066.

Sequelae and Long-Term Consequences of Infectious Diseases
Edited by Pina M. Fratamico, James L. Smith, and Kim A. Brogden

Chapter 4

Enteric Pathogens

Judy R. Rees

Each year in the United States, an estimated 5.2 million cases of acute bacterial gastroenteritis lead to 48,826 hospitalizations and 1,458 deaths (81). The most common agents causing acute bacterial gastroenteritis are *Campylobacter* species (2.5 million cases annually), nontyphoidal *Salmonella* species (1.4 million), *Shigella* species (0.45 million), *Escherichia coli* species (0.27 million), *Clostridium perfringens* (0.25 million), staphylococcal food poisoning (0.19 million), and *Yersinia enterocolitica* (0.1 million). While substantially less common, infections caused by *Listeria monocytogenes* and *Vibrio vulnificus* carry the greatest short-term morbidity and mortality for the infected individual. During the period 1996 through 2006, the incidence of several infections changed significantly. For example, laboratory-confirmed infections with *Campylobacter, Shigella*, and *Listeria* declined by about one-third and with *Yersinia* by about one-half. In contrast, infections with *Vibrio* species, associated most commonly with ingestion of raw seafood, increased by 78% (19). Bacterial infections caused by these organisms may occur as part of an outbreak, often associated with a single source of exposure, such as food contamination. Other, sporadic cases seem to occur in isolation, either because the diagnosed individual was the only one affected or because an outbreak was not recognized. Changing rates of bacterial gastrointestinal (GI) infections are likely to affect the incidence of their chronic complications, and this should be noted when interpreting the data presented in this chapter.

The acute symptoms of most bacterial GI infections typically include diarrhea, nausea, vomiting, abdominal pain and cramps, and dehydration. Other acute symptoms may result from hematogenous spread of the infecting organisms from the GI tract to other systems, leading to syndromes such as osteomyelitis, septic arthritis, meningitis, intracranial abscess, mycotic aneurysm, endocarditis, orchitis, and keratitis. In addition to the immediate symptoms and complications of bacterial gastroenteritis, these infections are becoming increasingly recognized for their etiologic role in chronic complications in the population. Factors affecting the symptoms, frequency, and severity of these postinfectious syndromes are not well understood. Among the complications of bacterial gastroenteritis are persistent diarrhea, inflammatory bowel disease (IBD), irritable bowel syndrome (IBS), chronic bacterial carriage, gall bladder carcinoma, hemolytic uremic syndrome, Guillain-Barré syndrome (GBS), autoimmune thyroid disease, reactive arthritides (including Reiter's syndrome and ankylosing spondylitis [AS]), atrophic rhinitis, and rhinoscleroma.

It has been estimated that chronic illness results from 2 to 3% of foodborne infections (4). In a study based on laboratory surveillance of bacterial GI infections, 3.5% of participants surveyed (8.0% of respondents) reported either persistent GI or rheumatologic symptoms between 3 and 15 months after a diagnosis of bacterial GI infections (101). However, studies of the long-term complications of GI infectious illness are hindered by logistical problems, perhaps the most substantial of which is underrecognition of the initial infection and a delay before the onset of new symptoms which, to the affected individual, may appear to be unrelated. The incidence estimates cited previously for bacterial GI infections are based on the rates of laboratory-confirmed infections, adjusted as far as possible for various factors associated with underdiagnosis of each organism. A bacterial GI infection may be subclinical or cause only mild symptoms for which patients do not seek medical advice. Of cases that come to medical attention, laboratory tests may not be ordered or patients may not provide a stool sample. Samples sent for testing may be incorrectly collected or stored, rendering them unsatisfactory for testing or giving false negative results. Thus, the majority of GI infections are never confirmed by a laboratory test, and

Judy R. Rees • Department of Community and Family Medicine, Dartmouth Hitchcock Medical Center, Lebanon, NH 03756.

the extent of underdiagnosis varies between pathogens, probably because differences in the levels of severity of symptoms determine whether medical care is sought. For example, organisms causing nonbloody diarrhea, such as *Salmonella*, are underdiagnosed and therefore underreported in the United States to such an extent that only 1 case in 38.6 will be confirmed in the laboratory (139), and it has been estimated that diarrheal illnesses in the United Kingdom may be underreported by a factor of 20 (33).

In considering the burden of GI infections in a population, it is possible to some extent to estimate the effects of underreporting and adjust for them, but the effects of underreporting on studies of the long-term sequelae of these infections are more problematic. Studies of diarrheal diseases without laboratory confirmation are likely to include syndromes caused by viral and parasitic as well as bacterial infections and by organisms or toxins that may not be identified by routine laboratory investigation. Such lack of specificity in the case definition will result in smaller measures of effect and lower incidence estimates describing the rate of complications after infection. Studies of chronic complications based on laboratory-confirmed bacterial infections probably represent the most severe clinical infections and overlook the complications that arise from all bacterial GI infections. Prospective studies based on gastroenteritis outbreaks may be highly specific, including infections with only a single bacterial strain, but these studies do not represent all GI infections. Retrospective studies in which cases are selected on the basis of the complication itself are subject to recall bias, which calls into question the initial diagnosis of a GI infection and may influence the reported severity of symptoms that an individual attributes to the GI infection. Selection bias may also hinder such studies if individuals with perceived complications of a GI infection are more likely to participate. Difficulties in the appropriateness of control selection for studies of chronic complications may also introduce bias in the assessment of risk relative to uninfected individuals. These factors make it difficult to perform reliable studies of the association between the infection and its chronic complication.

Data from small case series and other anecdotal evidence provided some of the first descriptions of a variety of long-term complications following bacterial GI infections. These earlier observations were followed later by larger case series and population-based studies that provided a better idea of the true incidence of the complications of bacterial GI infections, such as reactive arthritis and chronic bowel dysfunction.

SUSCEPTIBILITY TO BACTERIAL GI INFECTIONS

Many factors influence an individual's susceptibility to infection with the bacterial pathogens discussed in this chapter. It is less clear whether these same susceptibility factors also influence the subsequent development of chronic complications. A notable exception is the well-described predisposition of young children to symptomatic *E. coli* infection and its complication, hemolytic uremic syndrome. It is also unclear whether antibiotic use during the acute infection has any effect on the risk of subsequent complications.

The precise mechanisms underlying an individual's susceptibility to a bacterial GI infection itself may involve differences in gastric acidity, gut mucus, enteric microflora, intestinal immune factors, intestinal motility, the presence of specific receptors for microbial adhesins or toxins, and in the case of breastfed children, the presence of other factors in breast milk (75). Recent reports suggest that the use of proton pump inhibitors (PPI) to suppress gastric acid production is associated with an increased risk of bacterial gastroenteritis (relative risk 2.9; 95% confidence interval [CI] 2.5 to 3.5) in a dose-dependent manner, such that doubling the PPI dose further increases the relative risk to 5.0 (95% CI 2.7, 9.3) (37). Separate analysis of the most common pathogens identified, *Campylobacter* and *Salmonella*, suggested that PPI use increases the risk of both. Because the use of PPI in the community is increasing, this association and increased risk are potentially important, both in terms of short-term morbidity and mortality from gastroenteritis and long-term morbidity from its complications (129).

CAUSES AND SYMPTOMS OF BACTERIAL ENTERIC DISEASE

A variety of acute syndromes result from bacterial GI infections, depending on the pathologic mechanism involved. Bacterial GI infections cause symptoms in several ways (75). (i) One is a noninflammatory process mediated by toxins which alter the balance of fluid exchange across the intestine, e.g., watery diarrhea caused by *Vibrio cholerae, E. coli, Bacillus cereus, Staphylococcus aureus,* and *C. perfringens*. The toxins produced by GI pathogens may be classified as neurotoxins, enterotoxins, and cytotoxins (75). Neurotoxins usually produce enteric symptoms within 1 to 6 hours of ingestion. Examples include *S. aureus* and *B. cereus*, both of which commonly lead to nausea and vomiting and, less commonly, to diarrhea and abdominal cramps also. Although commonly regarded as enterotoxin mediated, staphylococcal food poisoning is caused by a toxin effect on the central autonomic nervous system. *Clostridium botulinum* causes a syndrome of nausea, vomiting, diarrhea, and descending weakness or paralysis, mediated by a neurotoxin. True enterotoxins have a direct effect on the intestinal mucosa that causes fluid secretion. Enterotoxins are produced by *Vibrio* species, *E. coli, Salmonella, Shigella, Klebsiella, C. perfringens*, and *B. cereus*. Cytotoxins injure the mucosa, which can result in colitis; examples include *Shigella dysenteriae, C. perfringens* and *Clostridium difficile, Vibrio* species, *S. aureus, E. coli*, and *Campylobacter jejuni*. Cytotoxins released during *E. coli* infection can cause a hemorrhagic colitis. (ii) Other infections cause an inflammatory process in which the ileal or colonic mucosa is damaged. For example, *Campylobacter* can cause a colitis resembling acute ulcerative colitis with inflammatory infiltrates and in extreme cases, bloody, exudative colitis. Other examples include dysentery caused by *Shigella, Salmonella enterica* serovar Enteritidis, and *Vibrio parahaemolyticus*. (iii) Third, enteric fever may result from penetration of the mucosa and involve the reticulo-endothelial system, e.g., infections with *Salmonella enterica* serovar Typhi (typhoid fever) and *Y. enterocolitica*.

BACTERIAL PATHOGENS CAUSING GI INFECTIOUS SYNDROMES

Salmonella

Nontyphoidal *Salmonella* species cause GI illness in the United States with an estimated incidence of 520 per 100,000 per year (19). The most commonly diagnosed species in the United States are *Salmonella enterica* serovar Typhimurium and *S.* serovar Enteritidis, which comprise 38% of *Salmonella* species laboratory isolates. Infection commonly follows ingestion of poultry, milk, and eggs. Symptoms most likely result from a combination of mucosal invasion by the pathogen and the production of enterotoxins, resulting in diarrhea, fever, cramping, and abdominal pain. Enteric fever caused by *S.* serovar Typhi and *S.* serovar Paratyphi are less common in the United States but endemic in many developing countries. Enteric fever is characterized by severe constitutional symptoms, including fever, headache, abdominal pain, and sometimes skin rash, and a chronic carrier state is recognized in a small proportion after the acute infection.

Campylobacter

An estimated 1,020 cases of *Campylobacter* infection occur per 100,000 per year in the United States. *C. jejuni is* the main causes of GI illness due to *Campylobacter*, with symptoms occurring 2 to 5 days after exposure to contaminated food or water, often raw milk or poultry. Symptoms usually consist of diarrhea, which may be bloody, abdominal pain and cramping, fever, nausea, and vomiting. *C. jejuni* can produce symptoms both by invasion and by the production of enterotoxins. Fewer than 1% of campylobacter infections are caused by other species, including *C. coli*.

Shigella

Shigella species are both waterborne and foodborne pathogens. Approximately 6 cases of *Shigella* infection occur per 100,000 per year in the United States. The majority of these are due to *S. sonnei;* the remaining 15% are caused by *S. boydii, S. dysenteriae*, and *S. flexneri*. Symptoms are usually watery or bloody diarrhea, abdominal pain, fever, and malaise.

Escherichia

The incidence of infections with *Escherichia* species is 1.77 per 100,000 per year, including both O157 and non-O157 Shiga toxin-producing *E. coli. E. coli* O157:H7 is an important cause of foodborne illness, causing a hemorrhagic colitis and infrequently, hemolytic uremic syndrome. Pathogenic *E. coli* causes disease through at least five different mechanisms; these varieties of bacteria are described as enterotoxigenic *E. coli*, enteropathogenic, enteroinvasive, enterohemorrhagic, and enteroadherent. Consumption of contaminated, undercooked meat products is the most commonly identified source of infection, but outbreaks have also been attributed to consumption of contaminated sprouts, lettuce, spinach, and unpasteurized apple juice or milk.

Yersinia

Infections with *Yersinia* occur at a rate of 0.35 per 100,000 per year in the United States. Most are caused by strains of *Y. enterocolitica* and cause fever, abdominal pain, and diarrhea, which is often bloody. Pain and fever in the absence of diarrhea may sometimes occur, and this syndrome may be mistaken for acute appendicitis. *Y. enterocolitica* can grow at temperatures used for refrigeration and is commonly acquired by consumption of undercooked pork products. In addition to reactive arthritis, infected individuals, particularly women, may develop erythema nodosum, an autoimmune skin rash commonly found on the legs and trunk.

Vibrio

Infections with several *Vibrio* species are identified in the United States, with an incidence of approximately 0.34 per 100,000 per year. *V. cholerae* is an infrequent cause of severe travelers' diarrhea in the United States, but an important one in developing countries. Outbreaks of cholera may result from contamination of drinking water with feces from an infected person, for example where there is cross-contamination of the drinking water supply by raw sewage. Two species of *Vibrio* found in salt or brackish water are *V. parahaemolyticus* and *V. vulnificans*, which may cause infection after consumption of contaminated seafood or exposure of an open wound to contaminated water. *V. vulnificans* is particularly dangerous to immunocompromised hosts and those with chronic liver disease, including alcoholics, among whom a bloodstream infection is fatal about half the time.

Listeria

Listeriosis is an important cause of serious illness in the United States, in particular because of its severity in immunocompromised hosts, including pregnant women. Approximately 0.31 cases of listeriosis are reported in the United States per 100,000 per year, and a third of cases occur among pregnant women. *Listeria* infection causes fever and muscle aches, and sometimes nausea and diarrhea. Infection may spread to the central nervous system, causing meningitis. Infection of pregnant women may lead to miscarriage, stillbirth, preterm delivery, and infection of the baby. Listeriosis is fatal in 20% of cases (81). Consumption of various raw foods is associated with *Listeria* infection, in particular unpasteurized soft cheeses and other dairy products and delicatessen foods, such as cold meats.

Clostridium

Clostridium species are responsible for several different syndromes. *C. perfringens* causes food poisoning. *C. perfringens* type C causes enteritis necroticans, a necrotic syndrome of the small intestine. *C. difficile* causes diarrhea, colitis, enterocolitis, and a pseudomembranous colitis induced by antibiotic use. Neonatal necrotizing enterocolitis may be associated with infection by *C. butyricum* and *C. perfringens*. Botulism is a rare neurological syndrome that results from the effects of a neurotoxin produced by *C. botulinum* in contaminated food products. The initial symptoms may include nausea, dry mouth, and diarrhea, but no fever, and the neurotoxin causes symmetrical cranial neuropathies and descending weakness. Treatment is based on supportive therapy, and mechanical ventilation may be required. Muscle strength improves substantially during the first 3 months, and improvement is usually complete within a year from diagnosis.

Bacillus

B. cereus typically causes one of two forms of GI disease, depending on which of two different toxins is produced. The emetic disease has an incubation period of 1 to 6 hours, and the diarrheal form has an incubation period of up to 12 hours. A typical source of *B. cereus* is contaminated fried rice, made using previously cooked rice. Typically, the spores of *B. cereus* survive cooking and germinate upon cooling, producing the toxins that cause disease.

Staphylococcus

S. aureus is a very common bacterium carried on skin and nasally, and it causes GI illness by forming heat-resistant toxins in food, which cause nausea and vomiting with a short incubation period of a half hour to 6 hours after ingestion. The illness usually resolves quickly, within 3 days.

Klebsiella

Like *E. coli, Klebsiella* species colonize the GI tract and can cause various syndromes, including pneumonia, urinary tract infection, and bacteremia. *K. rhinoscleromatis* and *K. ozaenae* cause upper respiratory tract infections and chronic nasopharyngeal complications discussed later in this chapter.

Aeromonas

Aeromonas species, commonly isolated from fresh and brackish water, are a relatively recent addition to the list of potential GI pathogens; however, there is evidence both for and against the hypothesis that *Aeromonas* causes symptomatic GI disease. *Aeromonas* has been isolated from healthy and symptomatic individuals, raising questions about its pathogenicity (4, 53). *Aeromonas hydrophila* causes diarrhea that is usually watery but can be bloody and associated with fever and abdominal pain; infection may also cause chronic colitis (144) and rarely, hemolytic uremic syndrome (11).

Plesiomonas

Plesiomonas shigelloides is also found in brackish and fresh water and has been associated with GI infectious illness acquired through foreign travel, ingestion of raw shellfish, or untreated water (54, 60). As with *Aeromonas*, chronic colitis has been documented after infection (67).

Brucella

Brucellosis is a relatively uncommon cause of GI infection in the United States, often caused by consumption of contaminated, unpasteurized milk products, including cheeses and ice cream.

LONG-TERM CONSEQUENCES AND COMPLICATIONS OF BACTERIAL ENTERIC INFECTIONS

A variety of long-term consequences have been described for bacterial enteric infections. In many cases, the relative risk posed by the various enteric pathogens and the mechanism through which these syndromes arise require further elucidation.

Chronic Diarrhea

Generally, the symptoms of an acute bacterial GI infection are self limiting. Chronic diarrhea is relatively common in some parasitic infections but may occasionally result from bacterial infections in an otherwise healthy individual. For example, persistent infection has been documented with *Salmonella, Aeromonas, Plesiomonas, Campylobacter, C. difficile,* and *Mycobacterium tuberculosis* (67). Under some circumstances, chronic symptoms may arise in immunocompromised individuals who have difficulty clearing the infectious pathogens, such as *Salmonella and Campylobacter*, from the bowel.

There is evidence that specific conditions such as IBS and Crohn's disease may be triggered by infections. However, a returning traveler with chronic diarrhea should certainly be investigated for parasitic infections (or coinfections), such as *Giardia, Cryptosporidium*, or *Cyclospora,* as well as persistent bacterial infection, before entertaining a diagnosis of postinfectious IBS or IBD.

Functional GI Disorders and Irritable Bowel Syndrome

The functional GI disorders (FGID) are diverse disorders in which chronic GI symptoms occur in the absence of a currently recognized biochemical or structural explanation. These syndromes include functional dyspepsia, functional constipation, noncardiac chest pain, and chronic abdominal pain (72, 134). However, the most common FGID is IBS, whose main characteristics are abdominal pain and a change in bowel habit. Prevalence estimates for IBS indicate that it is an important cause of morbidity and accounts for 2% of general practice consultations (132) and up to 40% of outpatient gastroenterology consultations (141).

IBS is a heterogeneous syndrome whose pathophysiology is unclear, and which has multifactorial etiologies. Much evidence now supports the existence of a disease entity termed postinfectious IBS (PI-IBS), which accounts for a small proportion of cases (47, 57, 80, 87). Psychological factors, such as anxiety and depression, also appear to play a role in the etiology and/or diagnosis of IBS. It is unclear whether psychological factors increase an individual's likelihood of diagnosis through differences in care-seeking behaviors, or whether the psychological symptoms are physiologically related to changes in the intestinal tract. A variety of stressors are known to affect intestinal motility (126), and laboratory studies have shown in animal models that stress leads to faster induction of inflammatory colitis (83).

The study of infections as a cause of IBS has one extra difficulty in addition to those general issues discussed previously. Several criteria have been described to define IBS (59, 61, 76, 82, 127, 128, 131, 133). These different criteria, when applied to different populations, can result in substantial differences in prevalence and incidence estimates (82), which hinders comparison and interpretation of studies of the chronic sequelae of GI infections. In addition, postinfectious changes in bowel habit that do not fulfill any criteria for IBS cannot easily be classified or studied. For example, a study in England identified a persistent change in bowel habit 6 months after laboratory-confirmed GI infection in 25% of participants, but only 7% of these fulfilled the Rome I criteria for IBS (87).

In 1962, Chaudhury and Truelove reported an increased incidence of symptoms now recognized as comprising part of the IBS spectrum following gastroenteritis (21). Subsequent studies reported similar findings after bacterial GI infections (47, 80, 87, 102), with a frequency of 4 to 31% (87, 92, 102,140). Some studies have identified an increased incidence of IBS following infection with specific pathogens such as *Salmonella* (80) as long as 1 year after infection. Other implicated pathogens include *Campylobacter* (92) and *Shigella* (58), and IBS may also follow infection with assorted bacterial GI pathogens (87, 92, 102). Because many GI infections are either mildly symptomatic or asymptomatic, it seems likely that unrecognized infections may cause some cases of IBS; serological studies would be necessary to investigate this further. However, few studies of IBS after bacterial gastroenteritis have included control groups.

Parry et al. (92) conducted a community-based study of patients with confirmed bacterial gastroenteritis (predominantly caused by *Campylobacter* species), and after 6 months they identified IBS according to the Rome II criteria in 16.7% of cases and 1.9% of controls (odds ratio [OR] 10.1; 95% confidence interval [CI] 3.32 to 30.69). IBS was found both in patients who sought and did not seek care for their original infectious syndrome. FGIDs were identified in 25% of cases and 2.9% of controls. Another general practice-based study estimated that the incidence of IBS after an episode of bacterial gastroenteritis was 98.2 per 10,000 person years compared with 45.3 per 10,000 person years in the control cohort (106).

In China, Wang et al. followed 295 respondents from a cohort of individuals with laboratory- or clinically confirmed bacillary dysentery (in this study most were caused by *Shigella* species) but no history of FGID (140). The incidences of IBS and FGID defined by the Rome II criteria (133) over 1 to 2 years were 8.1% and 22.4% respectively, compared with rates of 0.8% and 7.4%, respectively, in uninfected sibling or spouse controls. FGID was more likely following an episode of bacillary dysentery lasting longer than a week (OR 3.49; 95% CI 1.71 to 7.13), and even more so after an episode longer than 2 weeks (OR 4.61; 95% CI 2.14 to 9.91).

The finding that duration of symptoms predicts PI-IBS is supported by other studies (43). In the United Kingdom, individuals with laboratory-confirmed bacterial gastroenteritis (caused predominantly by *Campylobacter* or *Salmonella*) were followed for 6 months: 25% of respondents reported persistent alteration of bowel habit 6 months after the initial infection (87). However, no control group was used in this study; rather, participants were asked to compare their symptoms before and after infection, a process that may have led to recall bias. This study also found a higher risk of IBS symptoms in a dose-dependent manner among individuals with a longer duration of diarrhea during the initial infection, as well as among younger participants and women. Vomiting during the initial infection appeared to be protective against the development of IBS (OR 0.47; 95% CI 0.3 to 0.9), and it has been postulated that vomiting may reduce the infectious dose. Based on the evidence, it is tempting to suggest that early treatment of bacterial GI infections may reduce the risk of subsequent IBS; however, there is little evidence to support this hypothesis. From observational studies, in identifying risk factors for the development of IBS, it is difficult to untangle the effects of antibiotic treatment from the severity of illness being treated.

Other studies have investigated factors that may also affect an individual's risk of PI-IBS. McKendrick and Read found that patients who developed IBS after being admitted to the hospital for the initial infectious episode had a tendency to be anxious and depressed (80), but no control group was available for comparison. The nature of the association between psychological features and the development of IBS is not clear, but a common predisposition to both is possible (46, 47). Dunlop et al. found that the prevalence of psychological symptoms among individuals with PI-IBS was somewhat lower than among those with non-PI-IBS, but this did not reach statistical significance ($P = 0.3$) (30). Smoking, depression, life events, and the duration of the infectious illness may also affect risk of PI-IBS (30, 91). It is possible that psychological factors are somehow related to an intrinsic predisposition to IBS, or that they are associated with a greater likelihood of seeking medical care and subsequently being diagnosed (43, 44, 47).

Several possible mechanisms have been proposed to explain IBS after GI infection. Much evidence supports an inflammatory mechanism (45, 52, 123, 140), for example, the persistence of elevated levels of T lymphocytes in the gut (27), increased numbers of serotonin-containing enterochromaffin cells (30, 123) and chronic inflammatory cell counts in rectal mucosa (47), and increased expression of interleukin 1beta mRNA (45), as well as greater gut permeability (123). In Wang et al.'s study, 56 individuals with acute symptoms of IBS showed an increased inflammatory response in postinfectious IBS, with clustering of nerves and mast cells in the intestinal mucosa (140). Most likely, multiple factors predispose to development of IBS or FGID after bacterial enteritis, including host factors and the characteristics of the infecting organism. Future studies should be directed towards elucidating the mechanism of pathogenesis in IBS and PI-IBS and towards a determination of the possibility that antibiotic treatment of the original infection is associated with long-term outcome.

Inflammatory Bowel Disease

Crohn's disease (28) and ulcerative colitis constitute the IBDs, both of which are characterized by chronic, relapsing symptoms of diarrhea, abdominal pain, fever, and weight loss. Important differences exist in pathologic mechanisms, natural histories of the diseases, and areas of the digestive tract affected. There are several lines of evidence for a genetic predisposition in IBD (5), in particular the gene NOD2 (CARD15) (56, 89), which is thought to be involved in cytosolic receptors for pathogenic bacteria and related to resistance to infection.

Some authors have proposed that an infectious trigger may also be involved in the development of

Crohn's disease. Since *Mycobacterium avium* subsp. *paratuberculosis* was first isolated from three patients with Crohn's disease (24–26), a possible etiologic role for mycobacterial species has been the subject of an ongoing debate summarized in detail elsewhere (109). The debate intensified with a report in 1992 that the specific DNA insertion sequence IS*900* of *M. avium* subsp. *paratuberculosis* was identified in 65% of the Crohn's disease tissues tested, compared with identification in 4.3% of ulcerative colitis tissues tested (108). More recently, a larger study based on PCR gave similar results, with IS*900* identifiable in 52% of Crohn's tissue samples compared to 2% of ulcerative colitis samples and 5% of other controls (6). A meta-analysis of 28 case-control studies of this kind has since given a pooled OR of 7.01 (95% CI of 3.95 to 12.4) relative to controls without Crohn's disease (34).

While these data confirm a greater prevalence of *M. avium* subsp. *paratuberculosis* DNA in the Crohn's disease tissues tested, these observations do not identify the reason for the association. The hypothesis that Crohn's disease has an infectious etiology remains unproven, because it is unclear if the observed associations are a cause or effect of the disease. In other words, it is possible that a bacterial infection precedes and causes Crohn's disease, or it may be that the bacteria have an affinity for gut tissue already affected by Crohn's disease. The latter could reflect colonization by live bacteria, or simply deposition of dead bacteria in affected tissue. The hypothesis that Crohn's disease may be triggered by an infectious process does not seem consistent with the observation that the disease improves as a result of suppression of the immune system either through drugs or associated with low CD4 counts in HIV infection. In addition, other mycobacterial infections (*Mycobacterium avium-M. intracellulare* and *M. tuberculosis*) flourish during treatment with steroids and other immune-suppressive drugs, suggesting that active *M. avium* subsp. *paratuberculosis* infection is unlikely to account for the ongoing disease process. Trials of antimicrobial therapy have given mixed results. Variable positive effects of antimycobacterial treatment have been reported among some patients in small, uncontrolled studies (13, 14, 114), one of which included 12 patients with positive serologic tests for the p35 and p36 antigens (recombinant proteins of *M. avium* subsp. *paratuberculosis*), of whom 6 responded positively (114). More recently, a large placebo-controlled trial found evidence of a short-term improvement but no sustained benefit among Crohn's disease patients with unknown *M. avium* subsp. *paratuberculosis* status (113).

Other infectious causes have been or are being investigated in relation to Crohn's disease, including *Klebsiella* species, *Chlamydia* species, *Eubacterium* species, *Peptostreptococcus* species, *Bacteroides fragilis, Enterococcus faecalis, E. coli, C. jejuni, Campylobacter faecalis, L. monocytogenes, Brucella abortus, Yersenia pseudotuberculosis,* and *Yersenia enterocolitica* (142). Differences in colonic microflora have been reported between patients with active and inactive IBD (32), with a reduction in anaerobes and *Lactobacilli* seen when the disease is active (32). It has been hypothesized that the products of some of these normal intestinal bacteria may promote inflammation in the intestinal mucosa (10, 39, 110, 115). Surgical diversion of feces leads to improvement distal to the diversion, and this improvement is lost when continuity is restored. Lesions can be induced by instillation of fecal material into unaffected loops of bowel from susceptible individuals. The causative organism or substance has not been identified (5).

Chronic Carriage of Enteric Pathogens and Gallbladder Carcinoma

Mary Mallon ("Typhoid Mary") was a cook who, in the early 1900s, repeatedly infected her customers with *S.* serovar Typhi, killing at least three. Typhoid Mary's notoriety resulted from her persistence in her profession as a cook despite repeated warnings from New York's health department (122). Chronic carriers of foodborne illness do not experience continued symptoms of an acute infection, yet they harbor the organism persistently and may transmit the disease to others via the fecal-oral route. Chronic *Salmonella* carriers are defined as those with persistent *Salmonella* in stool or urine for at least a year. After the acute infection, approximately 0.2 to 0.6% of nontyphoidal *Salmonella* patients (85) and 5% of *S.* serovar Typhi patients (http://www.cdc.gov/ncidod/dbmd/diseaseinfo/typhoidfever_t.htm) become chronic carriers. Chronic carriers may shed the bacteria intermittently, and the gallbladder (with or without gallstones) is frequently the focus of infection. Foodhandlers infected with *Salmonella* should not return to work without evidence of clearance of the bacteria from their stool, which may be achieved with antibiotic treatment and confirmed with multiple stool cultures performed at intervals.

Several chronic infections have been shown to lead to malignant disease; for example, in immunocompetent individuals, chronic hepatitis B can lead to hepatic carcinoma; *Helicobacter pylori* is associated with gastric carcinoma; and untreated schistosomiasis causes bladder cancer. Gallbladder carcinoma is a rare cancer whose incidence varies substantially throughout the world. For example, the incidence in India is 11 times higher than that in the United States. Symptoms tend to appear late, and as a result, the prognosis is usually poor. Associated risk factors include a history of gallstones (OR 3.9; 95% CI 1.3 to 11.7) (120) and the related factors of multiparity and obesity (96). Gallstones may promote carcinogenesis through a chronic irritant effect, or via chronic stasis, they may promote chronic infection. There is evidence that bile acids may act as tumor promoters and initiators and that their composition is affected by the presence of bacteria in the bile, with an increased concentration of secondary bile acids in the bile of patients with gallbladder carcinoma, especially when the bile contains *Salmonella* (90, 121, 145). Chronic carriage of *S.* serovar Typhi, *S.* serovar Paratyphi, and *Helicobacter* in the gallbladder may predispose to carcinoma either via gallstone formation or on its own. For example, *S.* serovar Typhi Vi polysaccharide antibodies indicative of a chronic carrier state were associated with a substantially elevated risk of gallbladder carcinoma (OR 3.6; 95% CI 1.8 to 7.2) compared to controls (116). A review of 11 studies together gave combined risk ratios of 4.8 (95% CI 1.4 to 17.3) for *S.* serovar Typhi and *S.* serovar Paratyphi and 4.3 (95% CI 2.1 to 8.8) for *Helicobacter bilis* and *H. pylori* (96). The evidence supporting an association between gallbladder carcinoma and chronic carriage of these bacteria appears to present an opportunity for cancer prevention, particularly in areas in which enteric fever is endemic.

Reactive Arthritis

Reiter's syndrome, classically described as a triad of asymmetric, aseptic arthritis, urethritis, and ocular inflammation, was originally recognized as a complication of infection with a sexually transmitted disease (9). However, Reiter's syndrome or a similar arthritis without urethral or ocular symptoms may also follow enteric infection with organisms known or unknown. Several bacteria have been implicated in the development of aseptic ("reactive") arthritis. In the majority of cases, the arthritis begins within 30 days of the infection and resolves within 6 to 12 months. Some estimates of the frequency of reactive arthritis following most bacterial enteritis suggest a rate of 2 to 3% (15, 71). Data based on outbreaks of bacterial GI infection suggest a higher frequency of reactive arthritis; this may reflect differences in the severity of the infection and the pathogen causing it.

Outbreak studies typically include individuals infected with the same strain of pathogen, whereas studies of endemic disease most likely include a variety of pathogens, some of which may be more or less likely to cause a reactive arthritis. For example, 12% of individuals infected during outbreaks of *Yersinia* developed a reactive arthritis (49, 94). Based on an outbreak of *S.* serovar Enteritidis among physicians, 16% of those with symptoms developed a reactive arthritis (70). *S.* serovar Typhimurium led to reactive arthritis in 6 to14.6% of cases. The occurrence of reactive arthritis in children appears much lower. A prospective study following an outbreak of *S.* serovar Enteritidis among 286 children identified no cases of reactive arthritis at 4 months after infection (105). Two studies of separate *Salmonella* outbreaks reported that antibiotic treatment of the acute infection did not confer any benefit in reducing subsequent reactive arthritis (70, 78). Following an outbreak of *S.* serovar Typhimurium, 6.4% (n = 27) of those with GI symptoms developed reactive arthritis, which resolved within 4 months in one-third. Of patients with reactive arthritis, 37% had objective evidence of joint damage after 5 years (135). *Campylobacter* infection during a large outbreak resulted in a self-report of new arthritic symptoms among 16% of respondents, compared to 6% of controls who had an *E. coli* infection (71). *Campylobacter* patients who reported joint symptoms also reported significantly longer duration of symptoms (P = 0.0005), and 59% of those with joint symptoms reported having been treated with antibiotics for the original infection, compared to 26% of those without joint symptoms (P = 0.03). Joint symptoms occurred a median of 14 days after onset of diarrhea, and the median duration of joint symptoms was 60 days.

The pathologic mechanism underlying reactive arthritis after bacterial infection remains unclear. There may be an element of molecular mimicry involved. For example, cross-reactivity has been reported between host HLA-B27 antigens and a *Y. pseudotuberculosis* surface protein (22), and *Yersinia* species have been shown to have superantigenic properties (16, 119, 125, 136, 137). It has been suggested that *Yersinia* organisms do not proliferate within the synovium of infected animals (88, 138), but there is also some evidence to the contrary (38). PCR technology has identified fragments of DNA from a variety of gram-negative bacteria in synovial tissue or fluid of reactive arthritis patients, some but not all of which have been linked epidemiologically to reactive arthritis (17). It is not clear how these observations can be explained in terms of a pathogenic mechanism for the reactive arthritis.

Experimental data suggest that some reactive arthritides may be prevented by early treatment with antibiotics, but that treatment started after the arthritis is established is unlikely to succeed. Animal models have been used to investigate the utility of early antibiotic treatment to prevent the development of reactive arthritis caused by inoculation of infectious agents, including *Chlamydia trachomatis* and *Y. enterocolitica* (148). *C. trachomatis* causes a reactive arthritis which can be prevented by antibiotic treatment during the initial infection and also during the arthritic phase. In contrast to *Yersinia*, *Chlamydia* organisms seem to proliferate and persist for longer periods of time within host tissues, including synovial tissue, from which viable *Chlamydia* has been recovered (17, 148). In contrast, early ciprofloxacin treatment of mice artificially infected with *Y. enterocolitica* prevented the development of reactive arthritis, but treatment after the arthritis was established was not successful (148). These observations might be explained by differences in the behavior of bacteria within the joint.

Reactive arthritis, sacroiliitis, and spondylitis occur in about 20% of patients with IBDs (15). Another unusual arthritis may hold some clues to the association between the gut and reactive arthritis. From the 1950s to 1980s, intestinal bypass procedures, including jejunoileal bypass, were performed to treat morbid obesity. Between 6 and 35% of patients undergoing jejunoileal bypass reported joint symptoms, usually within 3 years after the procedure (104). Several other inflammatory processes were also seen after this kind of surgery, including tenosynovitis, myalgias, myositis, erythema nodosum, and various skin rashes. These symptoms appeared to be related to the blind loop of intestine created in the surgical procedure, which developed nonspecific changes in the mucosa and became colonized with fecal bacteria. For example, a case report described a woman with inflammatory joint and skin symptoms after jejunoileal bypass, which were refractory to medical treatment but resolved completely within 48 hours of surgical removal of the blind loop (29). Laboratory studies of HLA-B27 transgenic rats raised in a germ-free environment showed that they develop arthritis only after reintroduction of commensal gut flora (130). These intriguing relations between the intestine and the occurrence of rheumatic symptoms may eventually point to a unifying explanation underlying the association between reactive arthritis and inflammatory GI disorders, such as IBD.

A strong association has been identified with HLA-B27 among more than two-thirds of patients with Reiter's syndrome and only 10% of healthy controls (62). Several theories describe possible pathogenic mechanisms; these are described in detail elsewhere (64). One mechanism through which the HLA-B27 antigen may be involved is through molecular mimicry; cross-reactivity has been reported between it and a surface protein of *Y. pseudotuberculosis* (22). Similarity has also been found between peptides from HLA-B27 and peptides from enterobacteria (112) and other organisms (64). Another hypothesis is the arthritogenic peptide theory, in which HLA-B27 binds peptides originating either from bacteria or host and presents them to $CD8^+$ T cells (95). There is now evidence that several genes other than B27 may be involved in the pathogenesis of the spondyloarthropathies (64).

Ankylosing Spondylitis

AS is a chronic, degenerative, inflammatory arthritis that affects the spine and sacroiliac joints that typically develops in young people. It is one of the spondyloarthropathies (SpA) which is a family of conditions including reactive arthritis, psoriatic arthritis, and arthritis related to IBD and sharing a common association with the HLA-B27 antigen. AS is characterized by fusion (ankylosis) of the vertebral bodies, resulting in a rigid spine known as "bamboo spine."

The prevalence of the disease is unclear because early diagnosis is difficult and phenotypes are highly variable. Worldwide, the prevalence of AS co-varies with the prevalence of HLA B27 antigen, which is recognized as an important risk factor (63). In North America, approximately 0.3 to 1.3% of the population have evidence of AS (51). Previously, it was thought that the incidence in men was many times greater than in women, but more recent estimates suggest a narrower discrepancy (male:female, 2–3:1), perhaps because in women the condition is phenotypically different and perhaps more difficult to diagnose (68). Women report less-favorable functional outcomes than men for any given amount of damage identified radiographically, but men have more severe radiographic changes (68). Monozygotic twin concordance for AS varies in different series from 35 to 75% (97).

A pathogenic role for enteric infectious agents in AS is less clear than for reactive arthritis. Summarized elsewhere, there is evidence of increased carriage of *Klebsiella* in the intestine of AS patients with active disease and increases in antibodies to *Klebsiella* in AS patients compared to controls, and laboratory evidence linking *Klebsiella* infection and AS (77). However, there is also serologic evidence from a small case-control study supporting a lack of association between *Klebsiella* and AS (124). Further studies are needed to determine whether *Klebsiella* infection is causally associated with AS or whether the findings of studies reporting a link represent a common predisposition to both.

Guillain-Barré Syndrome

In 1859, a case series was published describing a syndrome of acute flaccid paralysis (66). In 1916, Guillain, Barré, and Strohl described in greater detail a syndrome of symmetrical flaccid paralysis, areflexia, and increased protein in the spinal fluid in the absence of cells (42). GBS is an acute inflammatory polyradiculoneuropathy in which an immune attack on peripheral nerves leads to a variety of symptoms, including muscular weakness, flaccid paralysis, and distal sensory loss. In some cases, swallowing and respiration are affected, and intensive supportive therapy, including mechanical ventilation, may be necessary. Although full recovery occurs in the majority, GBS can be fatal in 2 to 12% (40, 103) and approximately 15 to17% have a persistent long-term disability (57a, 36). In a follow-up study of patients with GBS, only 62% of the original cohort had normal or near normal health at 1 year (99). Premorbid indicators of a poorer prognosis included older age, antecedent gastroenteritis, and disability (57a).

GBS is a heterogeneous disorder now recognized as having demyelinating and axonal forms, as well as a variant known as the Fisher syndrome. Acute inflammatory demyelinating polyneuropathy is the most common form in North America and Europe. The axonal forms consist of acute motor axonal neuropathy and acute motor and sensory axonal neuropathy (55), and these forms appear to predominate in developing countries, such as China. Fisher syndrome, described in 1956, is characterized by ophthalmoplegia, ataxia, and areflexia and may progress to GBS (35).

GBS occurs at an estimated rate of 1 to 2 cases per 100,000 population per year (40, 99). Depending on the geographic area studied, 13 to 39% of cases of GBS are preceded by infection with *Campylobacter* (98, 147). A Swedish prospective study using the national laboratory reporting system estimated the incidence of GBS as 30.4 per 100,000 during the 2 months after infection, compared with 0.3 per 100,000 in the general population (79). Specific strains of *C. jejuni*, such as O serotype O:19, are disproportionately represented among those with GBS (65, 107). Other infectious agents that appear to trigger GBS include cytomegalovirus, Epstein-Barr virus and *Mycoplasma pneumoniae* (48, 111). Case reports have identified rarer triggers, such as immunization (57a), infection with herpes zoster (57a) and *Haemophilus influenzae* (84); bacterial endocarditis (7), and infection with *Coxiella burnetii* (12) or *S. aureus* (8). However, coincidental coinfection cannot be ruled out when single cases associated with unusual organisms are reported. Commonly, neurological symptoms begin 1 to 3 weeks after an infectious illness. Studies in the United Kingdom have demonstrated more severe cases of GBS following diarrheal disease, and a poorer prognosis has been seen among older individuals and among those whose GBS was preceded by diarrhea (99).

The pathogenic autoimmune process that causes GBS is thought to result from cross-reactivity between antibodies to lipopolysaccharides on the surface of the infecting organisms, such as *Campylobacter* species, and similar molecules within the host's neuronal tissue. Depending on the clinical variant of GBS, the targeted molecules may be those in the myelin sheath, Schwann cells of sensory and motor nerves, or the gangliosides of the neuronal membrane. Immune attack against different gangliosides seems to be associated with different clinical variants of GBS; for example, Fisher syndrome is associated with the presence of anti-GQ1b antibodies (23, 143). Laboratory studies have also shown that multiple ganglioside epitopes may occur in a single *Campylobacter* strain. This could be expected to give rise to mixed forms of the neuropathy; for example, a case is described in which electrophysiological and pathological investigation suggested an autoimmune response to both the myelin and axon (73).

There is evidence that the virulence of the infecting organism depends on a variety of pathogen and host factors. The former includes the chemical structure of the lipopolysaccharides on the pathogen, and the latter includes major histocompatibility complex class II genes. Different HLA alleles are known to be associated with predisposition to the different GBS subtypes (100). A comparison of sera collected from individuals infected with *Campylobacter* has shown differences in antibody responses among those with GBS and *Campylobacter*-infected controls, suggesting that factors affecting host susceptibility require further elucidation (118). Severity of the neuropathy and prognosis may be associated with the presence of anti-GM1 antibodies, although some studies did not corroborate this finding (117).

Renal Disease

Untreated dehydration associated with gastroenteritis may cause acute tubular necrosis, but the rarer complications of bacterial gastroenteritis also include renal syndromes that are not attributable to dehydration, and have substantial long-term implications. Hemolytic uremic syndrome may follow infection with *E. coli* and other pathogens, including *Campylobacter* species. Following *Campylobacter* infection, cases have also been reported of glomerulonephritis (3), immunoglobulin A nephropathy, Henoch-Schonlein purpura renal disease, tubulointerstitial nephritis, non-immunoglobulin A/Henoch-Schonlein purpura glomerulonephritis, and focal segmental glomerulosclerosis with GBS (69).

Autoimmune Thyroid Disease (AITD)

In 1835, a syndrome of goiter with exophthalmos was described by Robert Graves, after whom the disease was subsequently named (41). Graves' disease is thought to be due to an autoimmune process in which autoantibodies bind to the thyrotropin receptor. It is characterized by hyperthyroidism and its attendant symptoms, such as fatigue, weight loss with increased appetite, and nonpitting edema. AITD typically occurs between the ages of 30 and 50. As with other autoimmune diseases, it is six to eight times more common in females than males. A genetic component seems likely to affect susceptibility, and it has been suspected that an environmental trigger plays a role. Seasonal and geographic differences in the occurrence of AITD have led some to speculate an infectious trigger.

A variety of laboratory studies summarized elsewhere have demonstrated clues to an infectious etiology for AITD, in particular, a possible role for *Y. enterocolitica* triggering autoantibody formation via molecular mimicry. For example, laboratory studies have shown homology and cross-reactivity between the thyrotropin receptor and envelope proteins of *Yersinia* (74, 146). However, it is also possible that the association between *Yersinia* infection and AITD simply reflects a common susceptibility rather than a causal association. A recent Danish twin study found no statistically significant association between the presence of antibodies to *Yersinia* and thyroid autoantibodies, and in a smaller substudy, there was no serological evidence that prior *Yersinia* infection differed significantly among twins discordant for thyroid autoantibody status (50). The conflicting evidence requires further clarification.

Rhinoscleroma and Ozena

The intestinal tract of humans and animals are colonized by a variety of bacteria known collectively as the coliforms, which include *Klebsiella* species. *Klebsiella pneumoniae* most frequently causes acute respiratory or urinary tract infections and is a frequent nosocomial pathogen. Rhinoscleroma is a chronic granulomatous disease caused by *Klebsiella rhinoscleromatis*, which affects the respiratory tract, usually beginning in the nose and spreading to the pharynx in about half of cases. Further spread to adjacent areas is also described, as well as to the orbit, maxillary antrum, eustachian tube, and lower respiratory tract (2), causing significant disfiguration. Its geographic distribution is uneven, with it being endemic in areas in Eastern Europe and many developing countries (86).

Ozena, or atrophic rhinitis, is an atrophic disease of the nasal mucosa caused predominantly but not exclusively by *Klebsiella ozaenae*. It is also a chronic debilitating disease causing atrophy of the nasal mucosa and adjacent structures, including bone; widening of the nasal cavities (it is paradoxically associated with nasal congestion); and the formation of foul smelling nasal secretions and crusty discharge caused by the accumulation of bacteria. Ozena is common in tropical countries and poor populations. Many predisposing factors have been identified and are summarized elsewhere, including evidence of a genetic predisposition, chronic bacterial infection, and poor nutrition (31).

CONCLUSIONS

In summary, several important complications of bacterial GI disease have been described, and the links between the infections and their complications have only recently been recognized. Laboratory-based surveillance programs monitoring bacterial enteric infections have recently identified substantial changes in the incidences of infections caused by the major pathogens (18, 81). These programs provide an ideal platform for research to track chronic sequelae of these infections. Such studies could inform us more accurately about the burden of chronic diseases associated with these infections, the effects on susceptibility of the now widely used PPI, and whether antibiotic use for acute enteritis influences the risk and severity of these long-term complications.

REFERENCES

1. Reference deleted.
2. **Abalkhail, A., M. B. Satti, M. A. Uthman, F. Al Hilli, A. Darwish, and A. Satir.** 2007. Rhinoscleroma: a clinicopathological study from the Gulf region. *Singapore Med. J.* **48:**148–151.
3. **Andrews, P. I., G. Kainer, L. C. Yong, V. H. Tobias, and A. R. Rosenberg.** 1989. Glomerulonephritis, pulmonary hemorrhage and anemia associated with *Campylobacter jejuni* infection. *Aust. N. Z. J. Med.* **19:**721–723.
4. **Archer, D. L., and F. E. Young.** 1988. Contemporary issues: diseases with a food vector. *Clin. Microbiol. Rev.* **1:**377–398.
5. **Ardizzone, S., and G. Bianchi Porro.** 2002. Inflammatory bowel disease: new insights into pathogenesis and treatment. *J. Intern. Med.* **252:**475–496.

6. **Autschbach, F., S. Eisold, U. Hinz, S. Zinser, M. Linnebacher, T. Giese, T. Loffler, M. W. Buchler, and J. Schmidt. 2005.** High prevalence of *Mycobacterium avium* subspecies *paratuberculosis* IS900 DNA in gut tissues from individuals with Crohn's disease. *Gut* **54:**944–949.
7. **Baravelli, M., C. Fantoni, A. Rossi, P. Cattaneo, and C. Anza.** 2008. Guillain-Barre syndrome as a neurological complication of infective endocarditis. Is it really so rare and how often do we recognise it? *Int. J. Cardiol.* [Epub ahead of print.] doi:10.1016/j.ijcard.2007.11.033.
8. **Baravelli, M., A. Rossi, A. Picozzi, A. Gavazzi, D. Imperiale, P. Dario, C. Fantoni, S. Borghi, and C. Anza.** 2007. A case of Guillain-Barre syndrome following *Staphylococcus aureus* endocarditis. *Int. J. Cardiol.* **114:**E53–E55.
9. **Bauer, W., and E. P. Engeleman.** 1942. A syndrome of unknown etiology characterized by urethritis, conjunctivitis, and arthritis (so-called Reiter's disease). *Trans. Assoc. Am. Physicians* **57:**307–513.
10. **Berg, R. D.** 1996. The indigenous gastrointestinal microflora. *Trends Microbiol.* **4:**430–435.
11. **Bogdanovic, R., M. Cobeljic, M. Markovic, V. Nikolic, M. Ognjanovic, L. Sarjanovic, and D. Makic.** 1991. Haemolytic-uraemic syndrome associated with *Aeromonas hydrophila* enterocolitis. *Pediatr. Nephrol.* **5:**293–295.
12. **Bonetti, B., S. Monaco, S. Ferrari, F. Tezzon, and N. Rizzuto.** 1991. Demyelinating polyradiculoneuritis following *Coxiella burnetti* infection (Q fever). *Ital. J. Neurol. Sci.* **12:**415–417.
13. **Borody, T. J., S. Bilkey, A. R. Wettstein, S. Leis, G. Pang, and S. Tye.** 2007. Anti-mycobacterial therapy in Crohn's disease heals mucosa with longitudinal scars. *Dig. Liver Dis.* **39:**438–444.
14. **Borody, T. J., S. Leis, E. F. Warren, and R. Surace.** 2002. Treatment of severe Crohn's disease using antimycobacterial triple therapy—approaching a cure? *Dig. Liver Dis.* **34:**29–38.
15. **Braun, J., and J. Sieper.** 1999. Rheumatologic manifestations of gastrointestinal disorders. *Curr. Opin. Rheumatol.* **11:**68–74.
16. **Carnoy, C., H. Muller-Alouf, P. Desreumaux, C. Mullet, C. Grangette, and M. Simonet.** 2000. The superantigenic toxin of *Yersinia pseudotuberculosis*: a novel virulence factor? *Int. J. Med. Microbiol.* **290:**477–482.
17. **Carter, J. D.** 2006. Reactive arthritis: defined etiologies, emerging pathophysiology, and unresolved treatment. *Infect. Dis. Clin. North Am.* **20:**827–847.
18. **CDC.** 1998. Incidence of foodborne illnesses—FoodNet, 1997. *MMWR Morb. Mortal. Wkly. Rep.* **47:**782–786.
19. **CDC.** 2007. Preliminary FoodNet data on the incidence of infection with pathogens transmitted commonly through food—10 states, 2006. *MMWR Morb. Mortal. Wkly. Rep.* **56:**336–339.
20. Reference deleted.
21. **Chaudhury, N. A., and S. C. Truelove.** 1962. The irritable colon syndrome. A study of the clinical features, predisposing causes, and prognosis in 130 cases. *Q. J. Med.* **31:**307–322.
22. **Chen, J. H., D. H. Kono, Z. Yong, M. S. Park, M. M. Oldstone, and D. T. Yu.** 1987. A *Yersinia pseudotuberculosis* protein which cross-reacts with HLA-B27. *J. Immunol.* **139:**3003–3011.
23. **Chiba, A., S. Kusunoki, T. Shimizu, and I. Kanazawa.** 1992. Serum IgG antibody to ganglioside GQ1b is a possible marker of Miller Fisher syndrome. *Ann. Neurol.* **31:**677–679.
24. **Chiodini, R. J., H. J. Van Kruiningen, R. S. Merkal, W. R. Thayer, Jr., and J. A. Coutu.** 1984. Characteristics of an unclassified *Mycobacterium* species isolated from patients with Crohn's disease. *J. Clin. Microbiol.* **20:**966–971.
25. **Chiodini, R. J., H. J. Van Kruiningen, W. R. Thayer, J. A. Coutu, and R. S. Merkal.** 1984. In vitro antimicrobial susceptibility of a *Mycobacterium* sp. isolated from patients with Crohn's disease. *Antimicrob. Agents Chemother.* **26:**930–932.
26. **Chiodini, R. J., H. J. Van Kruiningen, W. R. Thayer, R. S. Merkal, and J. A. Coutu.** 1984. Possible role of mycobacteria in inflammatory bowel disease. I. An unclassified *Mycobacterium* species isolated from patients with Crohn's disease. *Dig. Dis. Sci.* **29:**1073–1079.
27. **Collins, S. M.** 1992. Is the irritable gut an inflamed gut? *Scand. J. Gastroenterol. Suppl.* **192:**102–105.
28. **Crohn, B. B., L. Ginzburg, and G. D. Oppenheimer.** 1932. Regional ileitis: a pathologic and clinical entity. *JAMA* **99:**1323–1329.
29. **Drenick, E. J., and J. J. Roslyn.** 1990. Cure of arthritis-dermatitis syndrome due to intestinal bypass by resection of nonfunctional segment of blind loop. *Dig. Dis. Sci.* **35:**656–660.
30. **Dunlop, S. P., D. Jenkins, and R. C. Spiller.** 2003. Distinctive clinical, psychological, and histological features of postinfective irritable bowel syndrome. *Am. J. Gastroenterol.* **98:**1578–1583.
31. **Dutt, S. N., and M. Kameswaran.** 2005. The aetiology and management of atrophic rhinitis. *J. Laryngol. Otol.* **119:**843–852.
32. **Fabia, R., A. Ar'Rajab, M. L. Johansson, R. Andersson, R. Willen, B. Jeppsson, G. Molin, and S. Bengmark.** 1993. Impairment of bacterial flora in human ulcerative colitis and experimental colitis in the rat. *Digestion* **54:**248–255.
33. **Feldman, R. A., and N. Banatvala.** 1994. The frequency of culturing stools from adults with diarrhoea in Great Britain. *Epidemiol. Infect.* **113:**41–44.
34. **Feller, M., K. Huwiler, R. Stephan, E. Altpeter, A. Shang, H. Furrer, G. E. Pfyffer, T. Jemmi, A. Baumgartner, and M. Egger.** 2007. *Mycobacterium avium* subspecies *paratuberculosis* and Crohn's disease: a systematic review and meta-analysis. *Lancet Infect. Dis.* **7:**607–613.
35. **Fisher, M.** 1956. An unusual variant of acute idiopathic polyneuritis (syndrome of ophthalmoplegia, ataxia and areflexia). *N. Engl. J. Med.* **255:**57–65.
36. **Forsberg, A., R. Press, U. Einarsson, J. de Pedro-Cuesta, and L. W. Holmqvist.** 2005. Disability and health-related quality of life in Guillain-Barre syndrome during the first two years after onset: a prospective study. *Clin. Rehábil.* **19:**900–909.
37. **Garcia Rodriguez, L. A., A. Ruigomez, and J. Panes.** 2007. Use of acid-suppressing drugs and the risk of bacterial gastroenteritis. *Clin. Gastroenterol. Hepatol.* **5:**1418–1423.
38. **Gaston, J. S., C. Cox, and K. Granfors.** 1999. Clinical and experimental evidence for persistent *Yersinia* infection in reactive arthritis. *Arthritis Rheum.* **42:**2239–2242.
39. **Gordon, J. I., L. V. Hooper, M. S. McNevin, M. Wong, and L. Bry.** 1997. Epithelial cell growth and differentiation. III. Promoting diversity in the intestine: conversations between the microflora, epithelium, and diffuse GALT. *Am. J. Physiol.* **273:**G565–G570.
40. **Govoni, V., and E. Granieri.** 2001. Epidemiology of the Guillain-Barre syndrome. *Curr. Opin. Neurol.* **14:**605–613.
41. **Graves, R. J.** 1835. New observed affection of the thyroid gland in females. (Clinical lectures) *London Med. Surg. J.* **7:**516–517.
42. **Guillain, G., J. A. Barré, and A. Strohl.** 1916. Sur un syndrome de radiculonebrite avec hyperalbuminose du liquide

cephalo-rachidien sans reaction cellulaire. Remarques sur les caracteres cliniques et graphiques des reflexes tendineux. *Bull. Soc. Med. Hop. Paris* **40**:1462.

43. **Gwee, K. A.** 1996. Irritable bowel syndrome: psychology, biology, and warfare between false dichotomies. *Lancet* **347**:1267.
44. **Gwee, K. A.** 1999. The many faces of irritable bowel syndrome. *Singapore Med. J.* **40**:441–442.
45. **Gwee, K. A., S. M. Collins, N. W. Read, A. Rajnakova, Y. Deng, J. C. Graham, M. W. McKendrick, and S. M. Moochhala.** 2003. Increased rectal mucosal expression of interleukin 1beta in recently acquired post-infectious irritable bowel syndrome. *Gut* **52**:523–526.
46. **Gwee, K. A., J. C. Graham, M. W. McKendrick, S. M. Collins, J. S. Marshall, S. J. Walters, and N. W. Read.** 1996. Psychometric scores and persistence of irritable bowel after infectious diarrhoea. *Lancet* **347**:150–153.
47. **Gwee, K. A., Y. L. Leong, C. Graham, M. W. McKendrick, S. M. Collins, S. J. Walters, J. E. Underwood, and N. W. Read.** 1999. The role of psychological and biological factors in postinfective gut dysfunction. *Gut* **44**:400–406.
48. **Hadden, R. D., H. Karch, H. P. Hartung, J. Zielasek, B. Weissbrich, J. Schubert, A. Weishaupt, D. R. Cornblath, A. V. Swan, R. A. Hughes, and K. V. Toyka.** 2001. Preceding infections, immune factors, and outcome in Guillain-Barre syndrome. *Neurology* **56**:758–765.
49. **Hannu, T., L. Mattila, J. P. Nuorti, P. Ruutu, J. Mikkola, A. Siitonen, and M. Leirisalo-Repo.** 2003. Reactive arthritis after an outbreak of *Yersinia pseudotuberculosis* serotype O:3 infection. *Ann. Rheum. Dis.* **62**:866–869.
50. **Hansen, P. S., B. E. Wenzel, T. H. Brix, and L. Hegedus.** 2006. *Yersinia enterocolitica* infection does not confer an increased risk of thyroid antibodies: evidence from a Danish twin study. Clin. Exp. Immunol. **146**:32–38.
51. **Helmick, C. G., D. T. Felson, R. C. Lawrence, S. Gabriel, R. Hirsch, C. K. Kwoh, M. H. Liang, H. M. Kremers, M. D. Mayes, P. A. Merkel, S. R. Pillemer, J. D. Reveille, and J. H. Stone.** 2008. Estimates of the prevalence of arthritis and other rheumatic conditions in the United States. Part I. *Arthritis Rheum.* **58**:15–25.
52. **Hiatt, R. B., and L. Katz.** 1962. Mast cells in inflammatory conditions of the gastrointestinal tract. *Am. J. Gastroenterol.* **37**:541–545.
53. **Holmberg, S. D., and J. J. Farmer, 3rd.** 1984. *Aeromonas hydrophila* and *Plesiomonas shigelloides* as causes of intestinal infections. *Rev. Infect. Dis.* **6**:633–639.
54. **Holmberg, S. D., I. K. Wachsmuth, F. W. Hickman-Brenner, P. A. Blake, and J. J. Farmer III.** 1986. *Plesiomonas* enteric infections in the United States. *Ann. Intern. Med.* **105**:690–694.
55. **Hughes, R. A., and D. R. Cornblath.** 2005. Guillain-Barre syndrome. *Lancet* **366**:1653–1666.
56. **Hugot, J. P., M. Chamaillard, H. Zouali, S. Lesage, J. P. Cezard, J. Belaiche, S. Almer, C. Tysk, C. A. O'Morain, M. Gassull, V. Binder, Y. Finkel, A. Cortot, R. Modigliani, P. Laurent-Puig, C. Gower-Rousseau, J. Macry, J. F. Colombel, M. Sahbatou, and G. Thomas.** 2001. Association of NOD2 leucine-rich repeat variants with susceptibility to Crohn's disease. *Nature* **411**:599–603.
57. **Ilnyckyj, A., B. Balachandra, L. Elliott, S. Choudhri, and D. R. Duerksen.** 2003. Post-traveler's diarrhea irritable bowel syndrome: a prospective study. *Am. J. Gastroenterol.* **98**:596–599.

57a. **The Italian Guillain-Barre Study Group.** 1996. The prognosis and main prognostic indicators of Guillain-Barre syndrome. A multicentre prospective study of 297 patients. *Brain* **119**:2053–2061.

58. **Ji, S., H. Park, D. Lee, Y. K. Song, J. P. Choi, and S. I. Lee.** 2005. Post-infectious irritable bowel syndrome in patients with *Shigella* infection. *J. Gastroenterol. Hepatol.* **20**:381–386.
59. **Jones, R., and S. Lydeard.** 1992. Irritable bowel syndrome in the general population. *Br. Med. J.* **304**:87–90.
60. **Kain, K. C., and M. T. Kelly.** 1989. Clinical features, epidemiology, and treatment of *Plesiomonas shigelloides* diarrhea. *J. Clin. Microbiol.* **27**:998–1001.
61. **Kay, L., and T. Jorgensen.** 1996. Redefining abdominal syndromes. Results of a population-based study. *Scand. J. Gastroenterol.* **31**:469–475.
62. **Keat, A.** 1983. Reiter's syndrome and reactive arthritis in perspective. *N. Engl. J. Med.* **309**:1606–1615.
63. **Khan, M. A.** 1995. HLA-B27 and its subtypes in world populations. *Curr. Opin. Rheumatol.* **7**:263–269.
64. **Kim, T. H., W. S. Uhm, and R. D. Inman.** 2005. Pathogenesis of ankylosing spondylitis and reactive arthritis. *Curr. Opin. Rheumatol.* **17**:400–405.
65. **Kuroki, S., T. Saida, M. Nukina, T. Haruta, M. Yoshioka, Y. Kobayashi, and H. Nakanishi.** 1993. *Campylobacter jejuni* strains from patients with Guillain-Barre syndrome belong mostly to Penner serogroup 19 and contain beta-*N*-acetylglucosamine residues. *Ann. Neurol.* **33**:243-247.
66. **Landry, O.** 1855. Memoire sur la paralysie du sentiment d'activite musculaire. *Gaz. Hop. Civ. Mil.* **28**:269–271.
67. **Lee, S. D., and C. M. Surawicz.** 2001. Infectious causes of chronic diarrhea. *Gastroenterol. Clin. North Am.* **30**:679–692.
68. **Lee, W., J. D. Reveille, J. C. Davis, Jr., T. J. Learch, M. M. Ward, and M. H. Weisman.** 2007. Are there gender differences in severity of ankylosing spondylitis? Results from the PSOAS cohort. *Ann. Rheum. Dis.* **66**:633–638.
69. **Lim, A., A. Lydia, H. Rim, J. Dowling, and P. Kerr.** 2007. Focal segmental glomerulosclerosis and Guillain-Barre syndrome associated with *Campylobacter* enteritis. *Intern. Med. J.* **37**:724–728.
70. **Locht, H., E. Kihlstrom, and F. D. Lindstrom.** 1993. Reactive arthritis after *Salmonella* among medical doctors—study of an outbreak. *J. Rheumatol.* **20**:845–848.
71. **Locht, H., and K. A. Krogfelt.** 2002. Comparison of rheumatological and gastrointestinal symptoms after infection with *Campylobacter jejuni/coli* and enterotoxigenic *Escherichia coli*. *Ann. Rheum. Dis.* **61**:448–452.
72. **Longstreth, G. F., W. G. Thompson, W. D. Chey, L. A. Houghton, F. Mearin, and R. C. Spiller.** 2006. Functional bowel disorders. *Gastroenterology* **130**:1480–1491.
73. **Lu, J. L., K. A. Sheikh, H. S. Wu, J. Zhang, Z. F. Jiang, D. R. Cornblath, G. M. McKhann, A. K. Asbury, J. W. Griffin, and T. W. Ho.** 2000. Physiologic-pathologic correlation in Guillain-Barre syndrome in children. *Neurology* **54**:33–39.
74. **Luo, G., G. S. Seetharamaiah, D. W. Niesel, H. Zhang, J. W. Peterson, B. S. Prabhakar, and G. R. Klimpel.** 1994. Purification and characterization of *Yersinia enterocolitica* envelope proteins which induce antibodies that react with human thyrotropin receptor. *J. Immunol.* **152**:2555–2561.
75. **Mandell, G. L., J. E. Bennett, and R. Dolin (ed.).** 2005. *Principles and Practice of Infectious Diseases*, 6th ed., vol. 1. Churchill Livingstone, Philadelphia, PA.
76. **Manning, A. P., W. G. Thompson, K. W. Heaton, and A. F. Morris.** 1978. Towards positive diagnosis of the irritable bowel. *Br. Med. J.* **2**:653–654.
77. **Martinez, A., C. Pacheco-Tena, J. Vazquez-Mellado, and R. Burgos-Vargas.** 2004. Relationship between disease activity and infection in patients with spondyloarthropathies. *Ann. Rheum. Dis.* **63**:1338–1340.

78. **Mattila, L., M. Leirisalo-Repo, P. Pelkonen, S. Koskimies, K. Granfors, and A. Siitonen.** 1998. Reactive arthritis following an outbreak of *Salmonella* Bovismorbificans infection. *J. Infect.* **36:**289–295.
79. **McCarthy, N., and J. Giesecke.** 2001. Incidence of Guillain-Barre syndrome following infection with *Campylobacter jejuni. Am. J. Epidemiol.* **153:**610–614.
80. **McKendrick, M. W., and N. W. Read.** 1994. Irritable bowel syndrome—post salmonella infection. *J. Infect.* **29:**1–3.
81. **Mead, P. S., L. Slutsker, V. Dietz, L. F. McCaig, J. S. Bresee, C. Shapiro, P. M. Griffin, and R. V. Tauxe.** 1999. Food-related illness and death in the United States. *Emerg. Infect. Dis.* **5:**607–625.
82. **Mearin, F., X. Badia, A. Balboa, E. Baro, E. Caldwell, M. Cucala, M. Diaz-Rubio, A. Fueyo, J. Ponce, M. Roset, and N. J. Talley.** 2001. Irritable bowel syndrome prevalence varies enormously depending on the employed diagnostic criteria: comparison of Rome II versus previous criteria in a general population. *Scand. J. Gastroenterol.* **36:**1155–1161.
83. **Milde, A. M., and R. Murison.** 2002. A study of the effects of restraint stress on colitis induced by dextran sulphate sodium in singly housed rats. *Integr. Physiol. Behav. Sci.* **37:**140–150.
84. **Mori, M., S. Kuwabara, M. Miyake, M. Noda, H. Kuroki, H. Kanno, K. Ogawara, and T. Hattori.** 2000. *Haemophilus influenzae* infection and Guillain-Barre syndrome. *Brain* **123:**2171–2178.
85. **Musher, D. M., and A. D. Rubenstein.** 1973. Permanent carriers of nontyphosa salmonellae. *Arch. Intern. Med.* **132:**869–872.
86. **Muzyka, M. M., and K. M. Gubina.** 1971. Problems of the epidemiology of scleroma. I. Geographical distribution of scleroma. *J. Hyg. Epidemiol. Microbiol. Immunol.* **15:**233–242.
87. **Neal, K. R., J. Hebden, and R. Spiller.** 1997. Prevalence of gastrointestinal symptoms six months after bacterial gastroenteritis and risk factors for development of the irritable bowel syndrome: postal survey of patients. *Br. Med. J.* **314:**779–782.
88. **Nikkari, S., R. Merilahti-Palo, R. Saario, K. O. Soderstrom, K. Granfors, M. Skurnik, and P. Toivanen.** 1992. *Yersinia*-triggered reactive arthritis. Use of polymerase chain reaction and immunocytochemical staining in the detection of bacterial components from synovial specimens. *Arthritis Rheum.* **35:**682–687.
89. **Ogura, Y., D. K. Bonen, N. Inohara, D. L. Nicolae, F. F. Chen, R. Ramos, H. Britton, T. Moran, R. Karaliuskas, R. H. Duerr, J. P. Achkar, S. R. Brant, T. M. Bayless, B. S. Kirschner, S. B. Hanauer, G. Nunez, and J. H. Cho.** 2001. A frameshift mutation in NOD2 associated with susceptibility to Crohn's disease. *Nature* **411:**603–606.
90. **Pandey, M., R. A. Vishwakarma, A. K. Khatri, S. K. Roy, and V. K. Shukla.** 1995. Bile, bacteria, and gallbladder carcinogenesis. *J. Surg. Oncol.* **58:**282–283.
91. **Parry, S. D., J. R. Barton, and M. R. Welfare.** 2005. Factors associated with the development of post-infectious functional gastrointestinal diseases: does smoking play a role? *Eur. J. Gastroenterol. Hepatol.* **17:**1071–1075.
92. **Parry, S. D., R. Stansfield, D. Jelley, W. Gregory, E. Phillips, J. R. Barton, and M. R. Welfare.** 2003. Does bacterial gastroenteritis predispose people to functional gastrointestinal disorders? A prospective, community-based, case-control study. 2003. Current perspective on the pathogenesis of Graves' disease and ophthalmopathy. *Endocr. Rev.* **24:**802–835.
93. Reference deleted.
94. **Press, N., M. Fyfe, W. Bowie, and M. Kelly.** 2001. Clinical and microbiological follow-up of an outbreak of *Yersinia pseudotuberculosis* serotype Ib. *Scand. J. Infect. Dis.* **33:**523–526.
95. **Ramos, M., and J. A. Lopez de Castro.** 2002. HLA-B27 and the pathogenesis of spondyloarthritis. *Tissue Antigens* **60:**191–205.
96. **Randi, G., S. Franceschi, and C. La Vecchia.** 2006. Gallbladder cancer worldwide: geographical distribution and risk factors. *Int. J. Cancer* **118:**1591–1602.
97. **Rashid, T., and A. Ebringer.** 2007. Ankylosing spondylitis is linked to *Klebsiella*—the evidence. *Clin. Rheumatol.* **26:**858–864.
98. **Rees, J. H., S. E. Soudain, N. A. Gregson, and R. A. Hughes.** 1995. *Campylobacter jejuni* infection and Guillain-Barre syndrome. *N. Engl. J. Med.* **333:**1374–1379.
99. **Rees, J. H., R. D. Thompson, N. C. Smeeton, and R. A. Hughes.** 1998. Epidemiological study of Guillain-Barre syndrome in south east England. *J. Neurol. Neurosurg. Psychiatry* **64:**74–77.
100. **Rees, J. H., R. W. Vaughan, E. Kondeatis, and R. A. Hughes.** 1995. HLA-class II alleles in Guillain-Barre syndrome and Miller Fisher syndrome and their association with preceding *Campylobacter jejuni* infection. *J. Neuroimmunol.* **62:**53–57.
101. **Rees, J. R., M. A. Pannier, A. McNees, S. Shallow, F. J. Angulo, and D. J. Vugia.** 2004. Persistent diarrhea, arthritis, and other complications of enteric infections: a pilot survey based on California FoodNet surveillance, 1998-1999. *Clin. Infect. Dis.* **38**(Suppl. 3)**:**S311–S317.
102. **Rodriguez, L. A., and A. Ruigomez.** 1999. Increased risk of irritable bowel syndrome after bacterial gastroenteritis: cohort study. *Br. Med. J.* **318:**565–566.
103. **Ropper, A. H.** 1992. The Guillain-Barre syndrome. *N. Engl. J. Med.* **326:**1130–1136.
104. **Ross, C. B., H. W. Scott, and T. Pincus.** 1989. Jejunoileal bypass arthritis. *Baillières Clin. Rheumatol.* **3:**339–355.
105. **Rudwaleit, M., S. Richter, J. Braun, and J. Sieper.** 2001. Low incidence of reactive arthritis in children following a salmonella outbreak. *Ann. Rheum. Dis.* **60:**1055–1057.
106. **Ruigomez, A., L. A. Garcia Rodriguez, and J. Panes.** 2007. Risk of irritable bowel syndrome after an episode of bacterial gastroenteritis in general practice: influence of comorbidities. *Clin. Gastroenterol. Hepatol.* **5:**465–469.
107. **Saida, T., S. Kuroki, Q. Hao, M. Nishimura, M. Nukina, and H. Obayashi.** 1997. *Campylobacter jejuni* isolates from Japanese patients with Guillain-Barre syndrome. *J. Infect. Dis.* **176**(Suppl. 2)**:**S129–S134.
108. **Sanderson, J. D., M. T. Moss, M. L. Tizard, and J. Hermon-Taylor.** 1992. *Mycobacterium paratuberculosis* DNA in Crohn's disease tissue. *Gut* **33:**890–896.
109. **Sartor, R. B.** 2005. Does *Mycobacterium avium* subspecies *paratuberculosis* cause Crohn's disease? *Gut* **54:**896–898.
110. **Sartor, R. B.** 2006. Microbial and dietary factors in the pathogenesis of chronic, immune-mediated intestinal inflammation. *Adv. Exp. Med. Biol.* **579:**35–54.
111. **Schwerer, B.** 2002. Antibodies against gangliosides: a link between preceding infection and immunopathogenesis of Guillain-Barre syndrome. *Microbes Infect.* **4:**373–384.
112. **Scofield, R. H., B. Kurien, T. Gross, W. L. Warren, and J. B. Harley.** 1995. HLA-B27 binding of peptide from its own sequence and similar peptides from bacteria: implications for spondyloarthropathies. *Lancet* **345:**1542–1544.
113. **Selby, W., P. Pavli, B. Crotty, T. Florin, G. Radford-Smith, P. Gibson, B. Mitchell, W. Connell, R. Read, M. Merrett, H. Ee, and D. Hetzel.** 2007. Two-year combination antibi-

otic therapy with clarithromycin, rifabutin, and clofazimine for Crohn's disease. *Gastroenterology* **132:**2313–2319.

114. **Shafran, I., L. Kugler, F. A. El-Zaatari, S. A. Naser, and J. Sandoval.** 2002. Open clinical trial of rifabutin and clarithromycin therapy in Crohn's disease. *Dig. Liver Dis.* **34:**22–28.
115. **Shanahan, F.** 2000. Probiotics and inflammatory bowel disease: is there a scientific rationale? *Inflamm. Bowel Dis.* **6:**107–115.
116. **Sharma, V., V. S. Chauhan, G. Nath, A. Kumar, and V. K. Shukla.** 2007. Role of bile bacteria in gallbladder carcinoma. *Hepatogastroenterology* **54:**1622–1625.
117. **Sheikh, K. A., T. W. Ho, I. Nachamkin, C. Y. Li, D. R. Cornblath, A. K. Asbury, J. W. Griffin, and G. M. McKhann.** 1998. Molecular mimicry in Guillain-Barre syndrome. *Ann. N. Y. Acad. Sci.* **845:**307–221.
118. **Sheikh, K. A., I. Nachamkin, T. W. Ho, H. J. Willison, J. Veitch, H. Ung, M. Nicholson, C. Y. Li, H. S. Wu, B. Q. Shen, D. R. Cornblath, A. K. Asbury, G. M. McKhann, and J. W. Griffin.** 1998. *Campylobacter jejuni* lipopolysaccharides in Guillain-Barre syndrome: molecular mimicry and host susceptibility. *Neurology* **51:**371–378.
119. **Sheldon, P.** 1985. Specific cell-mediated responses to bacterial antigens and clinical correlations in reactive arthritis, Reiter's syndrome and ankylosing spondylitis. *Immunol. Rev.* **86:**5–25.
120. **Shukla, V. K., H. Singh, M. Pandey, S. K. Upadhyay, and G. Nath.** 2000. Carcinoma of the gallbladder—is it a sequel of typhoid? *Dig. Dis. Sci.* **45:**900–903.
121. **Shukla, V. K., S. C. Tiwari, and S. K. Roy.** 1993. Biliary bile acids in cholelithiasis and carcinoma of the gall bladder. *Eur. J. Cancer Prev.* **2:**155–160.
122. **Soper, G.** 1939. The curious career of Typhoid Mary. *Bull. N. Y. Acad. Med.* **15:**698–712.
123. **Spiller, R. C., D. Jenkins, J. P. Thornley, J. M. Hebden, T. Wright, M. Skinner, and K. R. Neal.** 2000. Increased rectal mucosal enteroendocrine cells, T lymphocytes, and increased gut permeability following acute *Campylobacter* enteritis and in post-dysenteric irritable bowel syndrome. *Gut* **47:**804–811.
124. **Stone, M. A., U. Payne, C. Schentag, P. Rahman, C. Pacheco-Tena, and R. D. Inman.** 2004. Comparative immune responses to candidate arthritogenic bacteria do not confirm a dominant role for *Klebsiella pneumoniae* in the pathogenesis of familial ankylosing spondylitis. *Rheumatology* (Oxford) **43:**148–155.
125. **Stuart, P. M., and J. G. Woodward.** 1992. *Yersinia enterocolitica* produces superantigenic activity. *J. Immunol.* **148:**225–233.
126. **Tache, Y., V. Martinez, M. Million, and L. Wang.** 2001. Stress and the gastrointestinal tract III. Stress-related alterations of gut motor function: role of brain corticotropin-releasing factor receptors. *Am. J. Physiol. Gastrointest. Liver Physiol.* **280:**G173–G177.
127. **Talley, N. J., S. E. Gabriel, W. S. Harmsen, A. R. Zinsmeister, and R. W. Evans.** 1995. Medical costs in community subjects with irritable bowel syndrome. *Gastroenterology* **109:**1736–1741.
128. **Talley, N. J., A. R. Zinsmeister, C. Van Dyke, and L. J. Melton, 3rd.** 1991. Epidemiology of colonic symptoms and the irritable bowel syndrome. *Gastroenterology* **101:**927–934.
129. **Targownik, L. E., C. Metge, L. Roos, and S. Leung.** 2007. The prevalence of and the clinical and demographic characteristics associated with high-intensity proton pump inhibitor use. *Am. J. Gastroenterol.* **102:**942–950.
130. **Taurog, J. D., J. A. Richardson, J. T. Croft, W. A. Simmons, M. Zhou, J. L. Fernandez-Sueiro, E. Balish, and R. E. Hammer.** 1994. The germfree state prevents development of gut and joint inflammatory disease in HLA-B27 transgenic rats. *J. Exp. Med.* **180:**2359–2364.
131. **Thompson, W. G., G. Dotevall, D. A. Drossman, K. W. Heaton, and W. Kruis.** 1989. Irritable bowel syndrome: guidelines for the diagnosis. *Gastroenterol. Int.* **2:**92–95.
132. **Thompson, W. G., K. W. Heaton, G. T. Smyth, and C. Smyth.** 2000. Irritable bowel syndrome in general practice: prevalence, characteristics, and referral. *Gut* **46:**78–82.
133. **Thompson, W. G., G. F. Longstreth, D. A. Drossman, K. W. Heaton, E. J. Irvine, and S. A. Muller-Lissner.** 1999. Functional bowel disorders and functional abdominal pain. *Gut* **45**(Suppl. 2):II43–II47.
134. **Thompson, W. G., G. L. Longstreth, D. A. Drossman, K. W. Heaton, E. J. Irvin, and S. A. Muller-Lissner.** 2000. Functional bowel disorders and functional abdominal pain. *In* D. A. Drossman, E. Corazziari, N. J. Talley, W. C. Thomson, and W. E. Whitehead (ed.), *Rome II: the Functional Gastrointestinal Disorders. Diagnosis, Pathophysiology and Treatment. A Multinational Consensus,* 2nd ed. Degnon Associates, McLean, VA.
135. **Thomson, G. T., D. A. DeRubeis, M. A. Hodge, C. Rajanayagam, and R. D. Inman.** 1995. Post-*Salmonella* reactive arthritis: late clinical sequelae in a point source cohort. *Am. J. Med.* **98:**13–21.
136. **Uchiyama, T.** 1995. A novel superantigenic exotoxin from *Yersinia pseudotuberculosis* and its position in the classification of the entire bacterial toxins. *Contrib. Microbiol. Immunol.* **13:**191–194.
137. **Uchiyama, T., T. Miyoshi-Akiyama, H. Kato, W. Fujimaki, K. Imanishi, and X. J. Yan.** 1993. Superantigenic properties of a novel mitogenic substance produced by *Yersinia pseudotuberculosis* isolated from patients manifesting acute and systemic symptoms. *J. Immunol.* **151:**4407–4413.
138. **Viitanen, A. M., T. P. Arstila, R. Lahesmaa, K. Granfors, M. Skurnik, and P. Toivanen.** 1991. Application of the polymerase chain reaction and immunofluorescence techniques to the detection of bacteria in *Yersinia*-triggered reactive arthritis. *Arthritis Rheum.* **34:**89–96.
139. **Voetsch, A. C., T. J. Van Gilder, F. J. Angulo, M. M. Farley, S. Shallow, R. Marcus, P. R. Cieslak, V. C. Deneen, and R. V. Tauxe.** 2004. FoodNet estimate of the burden of illness caused by nontyphoidal *Salmonella* infections in the United States. *Clin. Infect. Dis.* **38**(Suppl. 3): S127–S134.
140. **Wang, L. H., X. C. Fang, and G. Z. Pan.** 2004. Bacillary dysentery as a causative factor of irritable bowel syndrome and its pathogenesis. *Gut* **53:**1096–1101.
141. **Wells, N. E., B. A. Hahn, and P. J. Whorwell.** 1997. Clinical economics review: irritable bowel syndrome. *Aliment. Pharmacol. Ther.* **11:**1019–1030.
142. **Welsh, K., P. Hunter, J. Colston, J. Rhodes, J. Sanderson, and J. Bower.** 2003. The Report of the NACC Expert Review Group into the evidence linking Mycobacterium paratuberculosis (MAP) and Crohn's disease. National Association for Colitis and Crohn's Disease, Hertfordshire, United Kingdom.
143. **Willison, H. J., J. Veitch, G. Paterson, and P. G. Kennedy.** 1993. Miller Fisher syndrome is associated with serum antibodies to GQ1b ganglioside. *J. Neurol. Neurosurg. Psychiatry* **56:**204–206.
144. **Willoughby, J. M., A. F. Rahman, and M. M. Gregory.** 1989. Chronic colitis after *Aeromonas* infection. *Gut* **30:**686–690.

145. **Wilpart, M.** 1991. Co-mutagenicity of bile acids: structure-activity relations. *Eur. J. Cancer Prev.* **1**(Suppl. 2):45–48.
146. **Wolf, M. W., T. Misaki, K. Bech, M. Tvede, J. E. Silva, and S. H. Ingbar.** 1991. Immunoglobulins of patients recovering from *Yersinia enterocolitica* infections exhibit Graves' disease-like activity in human thyroid membranes. *Thyroid* **1**:315–320.
147. **Yu, R. K., S. Usuki, and T. Ariga.** 2006. Ganglioside molecular mimicry and its pathological roles in Guillain-Barre syndrome and related diseases. *Infect. Immun.* **74**:6517–6527.
148. **Zhang, Y., A. Toivanen, and P. Toivanen.** 1997. Experimental *Yersinia*-triggered reactive arthritis: effect of a 3-week course of ciprofloxacin. *Br. J. Rheumatol.* **36**:541–546.

Sequelae and Long-Term Consequences of Infectious Diseases
Edited by Pina M. Fratamico, James L. Smith, and Kim A. Brogden

Chapter 5

Escherichia coli: Enteric and Extraintestinal Infections

BENJAMIN D. LORENZ AND MICHAEL S. DONNENBERG

Among the microbial flora that naturally inhabit the human gastrointestinal tract, *Escherichia coli* is the most abundant facultative anaerobe. Similarly, *E. coli* is also the most common gram-negative human pathogen. The genus *Escherichia* was named for the German-Austrian pediatrician, Theodore Escherich, who studied the enteric flora of neonates and first described the organism in 1885, applying the name *Bacillus coli commune* (39). Within the genus *Escherichia*, *E. coli* is by far the most significant; however, infections have rarely been attributed to others, such as *E. albertii* (68) and *E. fergusonii* (44). *Shigella* species, although for historic reasons classified in a distinct genus, are phylogenetically encompassed within *E. coli* (129), but in keeping with convention are discussed elsewhere (Chapter 4).

CHARACTERISTICS OF THE ORGANISM

As with other members of the family *Enterobacteriaceae*, *E. coli* is a gram-negative, facultatively anaerobic bacillus. All *Enterobacteriaceae* members are nonspore-forming, and most are motile by virtue of peritrichous flagella. With the exception of a few, *E. coli* strains are motile and grow well on nonselective media. When grown on MacConkey agar, the colonies appear pink, indicating their ability to ferment lactose, a characteristic that can be used to distinguish them from most *Salmonella* and *Shigella* species. Some diarrheagenic strains, such as most enteroinvasive *E. coli* (EIEC), are lactose negative. Accordingly, the indole test, which is positive in 99% of strains, is also critical to identification (117). *E. coli* can also be distinguished from other gram-negative bacilli by its lack of oxidase or urease activity. Other biochemical and metabolic characteristics include fermentation of glucose, xylose, and other sugars; reduction of nitrate to nitrite; and production of catalase (115).

The existence of a number of *E. coli* pathotypes capable of causing serious disease not withstanding, the vast majority of strains are poorly equipped with the genetic material of their pathogenic counterparts and lack the virulence factors that cause disease. Although many of these features are unique to specific pathotypes, common themes include the abilities to produce toxins and adhere to host cells.

Understanding the properties that facilitate pathogenicity begins by examining the anatomy of the cell. *E. coli* is surrounded by two bilayered phospholipid membranes, which sandwich the periplasmic space and peptidoglycan cell wall. The outer leaflet of the outer membrane is comprised of lipopolysaccharide (LPS), which serves as a barrier against the entry of hydrophobic molecules. Also, integrated across the outer membrane are proteins called porins, which regulate the passage of hydrophilic molecules in and out of the cell. LPS is an important virulence factor and Toll-like receptor ligand. The oligosaccharide chain attached to the LPS core, known as the O antigen, is the basis for serogroup classification, and at least 173 types have been catalogued (149). Flagella are anchored to the cell envelope through a biogenesis and export machine that crosses both membranes. Flagellin, the protein that composes most of the extracellular and filamentous portion of the flagella, comes in at least 53 antigenic varieties representing the H antigen in the serotyping scheme. Forty-three of these antigens have been mapped to a single gene locus (*fliC*), which follows the structural basis for antigenic variation: while the central region of the flagellin proteins accounts for the diverse polymorphisms, it is flanked by highly conserved terminal regions buried within the filament core (194). This antigenic diversity may provide

Benjamin D. Lorenz • Center for Drug Evaluation Research, Division of Anti-Infective and Ophthalmology Products, U.S. Food and Drug Administration, Silver Spring, MD 20933. **Michael S. Donnenberg** • Department of Medicine, Division of Infectious Diseases, and Department of Microbiology and Immunology, University of Maryland School of Medicine, Baltimore, MD 21201.

different clones a competitive advantage, since both O and H antigens are conspicuous targets of the immune system. Many virulent *E. coli* strains also produce a capsular polysaccharide (classified as K antigens). Although there are more than 80 capsular types, it is not as routinely used in serotyping (123).

Both normal hosts as well as those with compromising conditions may acquire *E. coli* infections. While members of the family *Enterobacteriaceae* are natural inhabitants of the gastrointestinal tract and are abundant in the environment, there are particular predisposing factors and circumstances that allow both intestinal and extraintestinal infections to occur in community and nosocomial settings. Of note, certain individuals, such as alcoholics, diabetics (100), and hospitalized patients (77), have higher rates of oropharyngeal colonization, while postmenopausal women have higher rates of vaginal colonization (136). Aside from the enteric pathotypes that cause diarrhea, *E. coli* is one of the most frequent causes of urinary tract infections (UTIs), neonatal meningitis, and intra-abdominal infections (30). It is a combination of such symbiotic dynamics, host susceptibilities, and various pathogenic features of these infective strains that generates the range of syndromes associated with *E. coli* and predispose the host to the complications and long-term sequelae of infection.

SPECIFIC PATHOTYPES AND SPECTRUM OF DISEASES

Humans are affected by no less than six different *E. coli* pathotypes (additional less well-characterized pathotypes will not be discussed here), each with its distinct epidemiologic patterns, virulence factors, and clinical presentation. At least five of these pathotypes cause diarrhea.

ExPEC

Although *E. coli* can cause a vast array of infections, including peritonitis, cholecystitis, cholangitis, osteomyelitis, infectious arthritis, pneumonia, and cellulitis, the most epidemiologically significant infections are those involving the urinary tract, including pyelonephritis and neonatal sepsis, including meningitis. *E. coli* strains that cause UTIs and those that cause neonatal meningitis share many features. Indeed, the same clones have been responsible for a significant proportion of both diseases, and those that cause meningitis can be considered a subset of those that cause UTIs. Many of the former express the K1 capsule. Thus, the term ExPEC has been coined to represent *E. coli* strains capable of causing diverse extraintestinal infections.

Almost half of all women will experience a UTI during their lifetime (46). On an annual basis, it is estimated that over $2.4 billion is spent in the United States on health care costs for UTIs (96). *E. coli* is by far the leading cause of UTI. In fact, a limited number of *E. coli* serotypes is responsible for approximately 80% of cases of pyelonephritis, 60% of cystitis, and 30% of asymptomatic bacteriuria (78). Significant long-term sequelae are rare but more likely to be associated with complicated infections or specific patient populations that have risk factors, such as indwelling urinary catheters, obstruction, or bladder dysfunction (46).

The pathogenesis of UTIs in otherwise healthy hosts is based first and foremost on the ability of bacteria to adhere to and colonize the urethra and bladder. Type 1 fimbriae, also called type 1 pili, are especially instrumental in colonization of the bladder. The FimH adhesin on the fimbrial tip recognizes specific mannose oligosaccharide sequences on epithelial cell surfaces. While type 1 fimbriae are critical to UTI pathogenesis, they are produced by almost all *E. coli* strains and therefore do not distinguish ExPEC from other *E. coli* strains. There are three major adherence systems specifically associated with UTIs: P fimbriae, members of the S/F1C fimbrial family, and members of the Afa afimbrial adhesin family. P fimbriae, encoded by the *pap* (pyelonephritis-associated pili) operon, for example, are expressed by a majority of *E. coli* strains isolated from otherwise healthy women with pyelonephritis, but the prevalence of these pili is lower in strains from patients with cystitis or complicated infections (32). The PapG adhesin present at the tip of P fimbriae binds to P blood group disaccharides with variable avidity, depending on the moiety (99). In addition to the ability to adhere to the urothelial cells, other factors such as flagella that are necessary for motility, contribute to virulence. Urine is an iron-poor medium, so uropathogenic *E. coli* employs the production of an array of systems, including hemolysins and siderophores, to scavenge the essential iron (4).

Similar strategies of adhesion and pathogenicity in UTIs are involved in neonatal sepsis and meningitis as well. ExPEC strains implicated in neonatal meningitis are more likely to express type 1 fimbriae, which target oligosaccharides intrinsic to brain microvascular endothelial cells (176). The K1 capsule is a major determinant that allows many strains of ExPEC associated with meningitis to produce high-grade bacteremia. Interestingly, a chemically similar capsule composed of sialic acid is produced by *Neisseria meningitidis* group B (91, 160). K1 strains have been found in more than 60% of infections associated with adverse neurological sequelae (107). These strains, however, are a heterogeneous group of *E. coli*, and no stereotypical pattern of virulence factors has been correlated with any of these outcomes (90). Cytotoxic necrotizing factor 1 toxin and an iron-regulated outer membrane protein, IbeA, are other crucial factors that contribute to the ability of ExPEC strains to cross the blood-brain barrier (66, 87). Outer membrane protein A (OmpA) also facilitates ExPEC invasion and survival within human brain microvascular endothelial cells and macrophages (158, 173). LPS activates a specific receptor, Toll-like receptor 4, and, in response, microglial cells release proinflammatory cytokines and free radicals that injure oligodendrocytes and neuronal axons (94).

E. coli is second only to *Streptococcus agalactiae* as a cause of neonatal meningitis in infants. However, with the widespread use of intrapartum antibiotic prophylaxis, the rates of group B streptococcal infections have declined (152). This has inevitably been followed by fluctuations in the incidence of ampicillin-resistant *E. coli* infections (6).

EPEC

In developing countries of Asia, Latin America, and Africa, where diarrhea is one of the most lethal threats to children under the age of five (203), enteropathogenic *E. coli* (EPEC) is a major cause of infantile diarrhea (142). The populations affected by EPEC tend to live in urban poverty with unsanitary conditions, and most infants with EPEC are malnourished or bottle-fed at baseline (41). Transmission is principally by person-to-person spread (199). The associated secretory diarrhea can be copious enough to require intravenous hydration, and food intolerance is an important complication. Children under the age of 12 months are the most at risk for EPEC infection (42), and food intolerance is significantly more frequent in infants under 6 months (40, 53). In studies that were based in Brazil, approximately one-third of the cases of diarrhea requiring hospitalization were associated with EPEC (compared to 10% of episodes in general) (43).

EPEC was the first pathotype linked to diarrhea (142). Symptoms typically include watery diarrhea and sometimes fever and vomiting. The clinical course may be persistent and can result in severe malnutrition from food intolerance and failure to meet growth curve benchmarks. The salient features of pathogenesis that define EPEC infection are the intimate attachment to the surface of intestinal epithelial cells and characteristic effacement of microvilli (Fig. 1), which occur through binding of the outer membrane protein intimin to the translocated intimin receptor (Tir) (85). Tir is injected into host cells via the bacterial type III secretion system (T3SS) and subsequently manipulates cytoskeletal proteins to alter host cell architecture (31). In addition to Tir, the T3SS injects other effector proteins into the cell that interfere with various host cell pathways, inducing microtubule dysfunction, loss of tight junction integrity, and apoptosis (23, 180). Typical strains of EPEC, which are more abundant in developing countries and may be more pathogenic, produce a bundle-forming pilus that mediates bacterial autoaggregation and initial adherence to enterocytes (54, 182). The pathogenesis of diarrhea induced by EPEC appears to be quite complex, involving loss of the microvillous absorptive surface, changes in the abundance of water channels and ion channels, and increased permeability of intestinal tight junctions.

EHEC

Shiga toxin-producing *E. coli* (STEC) strains can cause severe intestinal infections with systemic effects. Enterohemorrhagic *E. coli* (EHEC) strains are a subset of STEC that possess similar genetic elements as EPEC that encode attaching and effacing ability. Shiga toxins, also known as verotoxins, are encoded by bacteriophages (120). They are composed

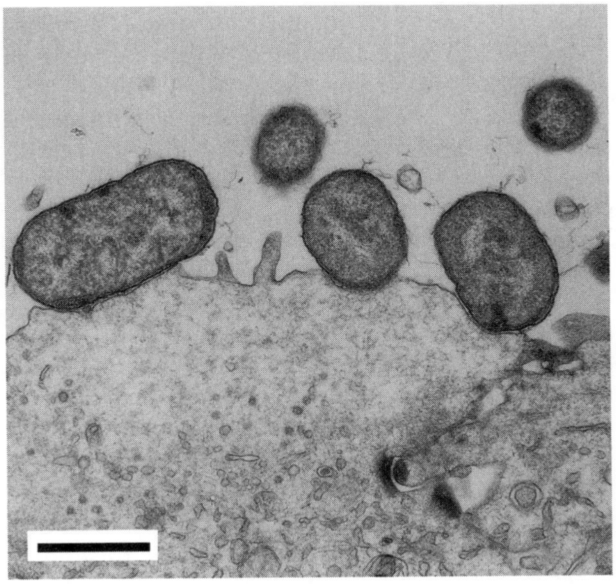

Figure 1. A transmission electron micrograph demonstrating the typical attaching and effacing effect on polarized human intestinal epithelial cells infected with EPEC. Bar, 1 μm. (Reprinted from the *Journal of Clinical Investigation* [111] with permission from the publisher.)

of a pentamer of receptor-binding B subunits and a catalytic A subunit that depurinates rRNA, causing cessation of protein synthesis, activation of the ribosome stress response, and apoptosis. Intoxication of endothelial cells leads to microvascular damage, hemorrhagic colitis, and the systemic manifestations of infection known as hemolytic-uremic syndrome (HUS). The most common serotype of EHEC is O157:H7, which can be detected by most microbiology laboratories as colorless, opaque-appearing colonies on sorbitol-MacConkey agar. However, non-O157 strains may cause 30 to 50 percent of STEC infections (112). To detect these strains and to confirm O157:H7 infections, specific assays must be performed to detect Shiga toxin.

The reservoir of EHEC strains is the gastrointestinal tract of young cattle and other large ungulates. Vegetation and food products contaminated with the feces of these animals can harbor EHEC for long periods of time: in one study, *E. coli* O157:H7 was detectable on lettuce and parsley for up to 77 and 177 days, respectively (70). Outbreaks of EHEC have been associated with consumption of undercooked beef, contaminated produce and drinking and recreational water, and petting zoos (17, 133). The infectious dose of EHEC is estimated to be less than 100 organisms (179), which also facilitates environmental and person-to-person transmission (133).

ETEC

Enterotoxogenic *E. coli* (ETEC) strains acquired by ingestion of fecally contaminated food and water are a significant cause of diarrhea in infants in developing regions (132). According to the World Health Organization, ETEC is the most commonly encountered enteropathogen in the developing world among children less than 5 years of age (198). It is also the most common cause of traveler's diarrhea (198). In the United States, ETEC is only sporadically implicated in food-borne outbreaks of gastroenteritis (27).

Certain characteristics of infection with ETEC parallel those with *Vibrio cholerae*. Like cholera, symptoms of ETEC infections include diarrhea usually without fever but often accompanied by nausea and cramps. It is not typical for stool to contain blood or leukocytes, but it can be watery and voluminous. Symptoms usually last less than 5 days, and the course is typically self limited; however, the young and malnourished are more likely to be susceptible to severe disease (132). The infectious dose in adults ranges from 10^6 to 10^8, and the incubation period ranges from 24 to 48 hours (95).

ETEC was the first pathotype for which the pathogenesis of *E. coli* as a cause of diarrhea was described. The disease requires colonization of the lumen of the small intestine and elaboration of one or more enterotoxins. The bacteria colonize the gastrointestinal tract by using fimbrial or afimbrial adhesins known as colonization factor antigens. ETEC strains produce either a heat-labile enterotoxin (LT) or a heat-stable enterotoxin (ST), or both LT and ST. LT closely resembles cholera toxin in both structure and enzymatic function and is composed of an A subunit and a pentamer of the B subunit (164). The B subunit binds to the same receptors (GM_1) as the cholera toxin in the apical membrane of enterocytes, while the A subunit proceeds into the cell via endocytosis and catalyzes the ADP ribosylation of the α subunit of the stimulatory G protein ($G\alpha_s$) in the basolateral membrane. $G\alpha_s$, in turn, constitutively activates adenylyl cyclase, resulting in elevation of cyclic AMP, which activates protein kinase A to phosphorylate and open the cystic fibrosis transmembrane conductance regulator to secrete chloride into the small bowel lumen. Sodium and free water follow the chloride by means of passive diffusion. ST binds to the guanylin receptor, a GTPase in the apical membrane, which elevates levels of cyclic GMP and also leads to chloride secretion associated with the clinical manifestation of secretory diarrhea.

EIEC

Although it has been studied to a relatively lesser degree than other pathotypes, EIEC is a sporadically reported etiology of dysentery in community-based studies worldwide (188). A major foodborne outbreak attributed to EIEC occurred in the United States in 1971 and was linked to the consumption of imported cheese (150, 184). Another outbreak in 1981 occurred in a home for people with developmental disabilities where subsequent person-to-person transmission occurred (58). EIEC, however, is transmitted primarily through food contamination.

The pathogeneses of infections with EIEC and *Shigella* seems to be highly similar. Although EIEC can generally be distinguished phenotypically by the fermentation of glucose and xylose, the differentiation between the two by microbiologic analysis can be challenging because of their genetic similarity (28). EIEC is nonmotile, lysine decarboxylase negative, and can be either lactose positive or lactose negative, which are unusual characteristics among *E. coli* strains and suggest possible convergent evolution of phenotypes with *Shigella* (130). The archetypal assay for *Shigella* and EIEC identification is the Serény test (causing keratoconjunctivitis in animal models), which demonstrates the ability of the pathogen to invade epithelial cells and spread from cell to cell (154). Both share a plasmid-encoded T3SS that confers the ability to penetrate enterocytes and then break free from the phagosome (130). Once in the cytoplasm, the bacterial invaders multiply and, by hijacking the cell's actin filament machinery, migrate through the cytoplasm and between neighboring enterocytes (30).

The clinical features of *Shigella* and EIEC are also remarkably similar. Both can produce a syndrome that typically lasts about 7 days and may progress to dysentery. Dysentery is characterized by severe abdominal cramps, fever, tenesmus, and frequent passage of small-volume stools that may contain mucus and blood (30). One important distinction, however, is the infective inoculum: for EIEC approximately 10^8 organisms are required to cause symptoms, whereas the dose for *Shigella* is on the order of 10 to 100 (36). This may account for the relatively lower propensity of person-to-person transmission with EIEC.

EAEC

Enteroaggregative *E. coli* (EAEC) strains were only appreciated as a distinct pathotype in 1987 (118), but these strains are increasingly recognized as an important cause of acute (65) and persistent diarrhea (11). EAEC affects travelers to developing countries (104), as well as children (105) and human immunodeficiency virus-infected persons (106) residing in both developing and developed regions of the world (67). Attributing symptoms to infection with EAEC in an individual with diarrhea, however, can be difficult, since EAEC has been recovered in asymptomatic individuals as well (81).

The pathogenesis of EAEC is unique because of its cascading pattern of adherence and associated mucosal damage. It can be distinguished from EPEC by identifying the aggregative phenotype exhibited with the HEp-2 cell adherence assay (118). The adherence pattern is dependent on several types of aggregative adherence fimbriae, some of which are encoded by a plasmid that confers the phenotype when transformed into laboratory *E. coli* strains (116). However, many EAEC strains produce none of the aggregative adherence fimbriae described thus far. When viewed microscopically, clusters of bacteria can be seen adhering to epithelial cells of the colonic mucosa, as well as lymphoid and absorptive surfaces of the ileum and jejunum (201). Apart from the adherence to the intestinal mucosa, two other major factors appear to contribute to the virulence of EAEC: elaboration of enterotoxins and induction of mucosal inflammation. One such toxin is aenterotoxin ST called EAST which has been found in some strains of EPEC (202) and shares some homology to the ST of ETEC (148). Another toxin that has been identified is the plasmid-encoded toxin (Pet), which induces cell rounding and dilation of crypt openings (61). Dispersin is a cell surface protein, which, as the name implies, regulates aggregation so that the bacteria spread evenly on the cell surface (156). As more information emerges about EAEC pathogenesis, attention has been focused towards host susceptibility and immune response. EAEC induces proinflammatory effects on intestinal cells mediated by interleukin 8 (IL-8), which the flagellin of EAEC strains appears to induce (167, 168). Certain polymorphisms in the promoter regions of the IL-8 gene are associated with symptomatic EAEC infection (76).

LONG-TERM CONSEQUENCES ASSOCIATED WITH THE ORGANISM

Complications of ExPEC Infections

Meningitis

Although bacterial meningitis is not a very common disease, the global burden, represented largely by the developing world, is substantial, and neurological sequelae affect a significant proportion of the survivors. Cerebrovascular complications, including focal neurologic deficits and cognitive impairment, are the most profound cause of morbidity and mortality. The prospect of recovery can be bleak despite advances in antibiotic therapy. Infants, especially in the first week of life, are the most susceptible (60). In a recent longitudinal case-control study (170), 37% of children who survived meningitis within the first month of life continued to demonstrate some neurologic or cognitive impairment when followed over a period of 9 to 10 years. A severe outcome (defined by significant functional impairment, cerebral palsy, learning deficits, an intelligence quotient less than 55, global delay, or the need for special education) was reported in 10.8% of patients. Not surprisingly, infants of lower birth weight had a higher incidence of severe, long-term outcomes: up to 44% in infants weighing less than 1,500 grams. Meningitis attributed to *E. coli* represented 38% of the cases, and the outcomes of this group did not differ significantly from the outcomes following bacterial meningitis of all types. When combined, however, all cases of gram-negative bacillary meningitis fared much more poorly, as nearly 60% had at least moderate disability (sensorineural hearing loss, mild cerebral palsy, or developmental impairment). These results were also compared to those of previous studies completed in the last two decades (107, 185), and while the mortality rates have improved (88), the trends in morbidity have remained essentially the same (18, 59). Although data that specifically distinguish cases of *E. coli* are sparse, most studies consistently show that subsequent rates of disability are comparable to (18), if not lower than (10), those after group B streptococcus infection and substantially lower than those after *Streptococcus pneumoniae*, *Haemophilus influenzae*, and other gram-negative bacilli. As with other types of bacterial meningitis, however, patients specifically with *E. coli* are also at risk for developing complications that require neurosurgical intervention, such as ventriculitis, subdural empyema, and hydrocephalus (19). Case studies of newborns following *E. coli* meningitis indicate that cerebral white matter injury due to the release of proinflammatory cytokines and free radicals from microglial cells might also be confounded by ischemia resulting from impaired cerebral autoregulation and systemic hypotension (155).

Describing early predictors of adverse outcomes following neonatal bacterial meningitis was the focus of another study (88). Term and near-term infants were followed after at least 1 year of age to evaluate for moderate or severe disability (by criteria similar to those above). Twenty-five percent of these patients had meningitis attributable to *E. coli*. Within 12 hours of admission, significant predictors included the presence of coma, the use of medication to maintain blood pressure, and leukopenia (total white blood cell count less than $5,000 \times 10^9$/liter). Seizures persisting longer than 72 hours also portended a grave prognosis. In addition, this study found that elevated total protein in the initial cerebrospinal fluid (CSF) analysis, as well as a CSF-to-blood glucose ratio of <0.5, corresponded with an adverse outcome. Although the results of CSF analysis did not reach statistical significance as a predictive factor, elevated total protein in a subsequent study (18) did.

Complications arising after a stable period of several years following *E. coli* neonatal meningitis have been described with manifestations emerging as late as adolescence. Chronic arachnoiditis may lead to spinal granulomatous adhesions (169) or late-onset myelopathy (29) marked by progressive neurological deterioration. Recurrent meningitis should raise suspicion of spinal dural defects (193). Although spontaneous *E. coli* meningitis in adults is rare, most cases represent a complication of bacteremia (113). Recurrent meningitis has been reported in adults following neurosurgical procedures (26) and in immunocompromised patients associated with superinfected, chronic fungal sinusitis (125).

Recurrent UTIs, chronic pyelonephritis, and renal scarring

The long-term impact of *E. coli* UTIs is a multifaceted process that can be influenced by host factors as well as characteristics of the pathogen. Pyelonephritis may result in chronic disease from renal scarring, which can eventually lead to renal insufficiency and hypertension.

Postinfectious sequelae associated with *E. coli* UTIs usually develop consequent to ascending infection in the setting of an abnormal urinary tract. The term "complicated," when referring to UTIs, indicates the presence of predisposing conditions, such as stones, bladder dysfunction, anatomic anomalies, or the presence of a foreign body (such as indwelling catheters or ureteral stents), which provide bacteria access to, or sanctuary in, a normally restricted and sterile site. In addition, patients belonging to certain high-risk populations have a higher risk of adverse complications following UTI. For instance, emphasematous cystitis and emphasematous pyelonephritis, which are severe necrotizing infections characterized by the formation of gas pockets, more frequently arise in patients with diabetes mellitus (127). Untreated asymptomatic bacteriuria can increase the risk of upper tract involvement and pyelonephritis during pregnancy, and women with a history of UTIs at an early age are at risk for pregnancy-induced hypertension (46). Premature contractions and other complications from UTIs can put the fetus at risk for cerebral palsy (128), developmental delay, and death (108).

Recurrent UTIs (RUTIs) are common among young women, even though they generally have anatomically and physiologically normal urinary tracts (161). Within 1 month of the first UTI episode, about 40% have recurrence, nearly 80% of which is caused by *E. coli* (69). As previously discussed, the utilization of adhesins and other virulence factors facilitate colonization of the urinary tract; however, these factors alone are not responsible for recurrence. In one study (151), young women who have the status of "non-secretor" (because they produce an abnormal ABH blood group antigen, to which *E. coli* binds with greater affinity) are not significantly more likely to suffer from RUTIs. Whether the initial strain persists within the urinary tract or reemerges after establishing a reservoir among colonic flora is an area of current controversy (145). Reemergence from an intestinal reservoir, however, is consistent with the fact that recurrences are less common in young males, and the difference can be explained by the perineal anatomy of women, in which a shorter distance from the urethra to the anus is a significant correlate to a history of RUTI (63). In fact, RUTIs in this population are more frequently associated with certain behaviors such as frequent intercourse with multiple partners, failing to void after intercourse (in some studies), and use of spermicide-based contraception (151), which increases periurethral colonization by *E. coli* (62). While asymptomatic bacteriuria or vaginal colonization may increase the risk of UTI in the elderly, there does not appear to be an associated risk for hypertension, renal scarring, or renal failure in the absence of structural or functional urinary tract abnormality (196). Beyond the cost and effort of evaluating and treating RUTIs, which can be vexing to both patient and provider, long-term consequences of uncomplicated UTIs in otherwise healthy adults are rare.

In contrast, children who present with UTIs at an early age are at the highest risk for chronic pyelonephritis and renal scarring. Damage from recurrent infection or dysfunctional urodynamics is a common theme among those who have been affected. The typical pathologic features of the kidney are corticomedullary scarring (usually overlying dilated and blunted calyces) and dilated ureters (usually indicative of chronic vesicoureteral reflux [VUR]) (22). About 10% of children who are evaluated by urography following a diagnosis of a febrile UTI have evidence of renal scarring (131). Several efforts have been made to confirm a link with infection and to what degree VUR or obstructive urinary tract malformations are predictors of renal scarring (72, 73). While most children with renal scarring (approximately 62%) do not demonstrate any VUR, the extent of scarring was proportional to the grade of reflux (72). Other studies have shown that enhanced adherence and virulence factors, such as P fimbriae, play an important role (71), but neither VUR or virulence factors associated with *E. coli* is absolutely required for scarring (97). Nevertheless, as children who are affected by renal scarring grow into adulthood, at least 10%, it can be estimated, will develop hypertension (186). Renal failure attributed to scarring from chronic pyelonephritis represents a significant portion, approximately 10% to 20%, of patients who require dialysis or renal transplant (22). Nephropathy is believed to occur when the remaining viable kidney cannot maintain the increased filtration requirements through adolescence (121). Hyperfiltration and hypertension of the remnant nephrons with ongoing tubulointerstitial disease exhaust the kidneys, which eventually falter due to focal glomerulosclerosis (13, 141).

Intestinal Complications of Intestinal *E. coli* Infections

Persistent diarrhea

While acute diarrhea is in itself a serious threat to children worldwide, persistent diarrhea, usually defined as an episode lasting more than 14 days, is also associated with severe complications, such as poor growth, developmental delay, chronic malnutrition, and high mortality. EPEC and EAEC have consistently been associated with persistent diarrhea in developing countries.

Using anthropometric data (Z scores of weight for age) as measures for protein calorie malnutrition, it was observed that food intolerance led to severe malnutrition in 31% of EPEC cases (42). Specific indications for intravenous replenishment are most often reported to be due to persistent vomiting, intense fluid and electrolyte losses, metabolic acidosis, or seizure (43). The localized adherence and the attaching and effacing models of pathogenesis have been described with patients with persistent diarrhea from food and lactose intolerance (41, 143). Ultrastructural analysis reveals distorted enterocytes, shortened microvilli, loss of the glycocalyx, and bacterial overgrowth, which accounts for the malabsorption of nutrients (12) and potentially broadens the risk of developing food allergy (191). With the repletion of fecal losses and appropriate nutrition, most of the survivors of the acute phase of diarrhea regain weight and can be weaned from parenteral support within a few days. While diarrhea can often last for more than 14 days, there is very little known about the long-term effects of diarrhea specifically due to EPEC beyond 30 days. However, diarrhea (of no specific etiology) that lasts longer than 7 days has been shown to produce linear growth deficits (determined by height-for-age Z scores) in children through the age of 5 (5). Like EPEC, EAEC infections have been linked consistently to persistent diarrhea. EAEC has been shown to induce production of the neutrophil chemokine IL-8 by intestinal epithelial cells in children with persistent diarrhea (168). Even in the absence of diarrhea, children colonized with EAEC also had elevated levels of fecal lactoferrin and IL-1β and significant growth deficits compared to children without EAEC, which may have long-term effects on physical and cognitive development (167).

IBS

Infectious diarrhea has widely been recognized as an important risk factor for irritable bowel syndrome (IBS), as about one in four patients carry a diagnosis of IBS 6 months after an acute episode (119). Enteritis caused by ETEC (122), EAEC (162), and *E. coli* O157 (33) has been implicated, as well as *Campylobacter* (166), *Salmonella* (109), *Shigella* (119, 195), parasites (163, 171), and viral pathogens (103). Several studies (178) have addressed the risk of IBS following an episode of traveler's diarrhea and have found that risk to be elevated up to six-fold in comparison to that of travelers who did not experience acute diarrhea. While the cause of the acute episode was not known, ETEC and EAEC often account for the majority of cases for travelers (34). The current definition of postinfectious IBS according to the Rome II criteria, which most studies follow, is the new onset of symptoms developing acutely after an illness characterized by two or more of the following: fever, vomiting, acute diarrhea, or positive stool culture (165). Although the pathogenesis of postinfectious IBS is not entirely understood, it has been distinguished by the symptoms of abdominal bloating, urgency, predominance of loose and watery stools (165), and a higher prevalence of psychiatric illness (e.g., anxiety, depression, neuroticism, somatization, and hypochondriasis) (56, 57). Several mechanisms have been proposed, such as increased gut permeability mediated by inflammatory cytokines (166) and increased sensitivity to rectal distention associated with the alteration of the bowel innervation (163) and psychological stressors (57). Enterochromaffin cells, which are neuroendocrine cells in the gastrointestinal tract, play an important role in peristalsis, pain perception, and intestinal secretions. They transmit various stimuli from the lumen to submucosal nerves by releasing their stores of serotonin and have been observed in increased numbers in patients with IBS following infectious diarrhea. After 2 weeks of infection, the numbers increase but tend to decline over the following 3 months (166). The duration of symptoms, however, often lasts much longer, as approximately half of the patients with postinfectious IBS still have symptoms after 5 years (165).

IBD

Crohn's disease and ulcerative colitis (UC) have long been hypothesized to be closely related with the commensal bowel flora and their interaction with the mucosa and immune system (147). Additionally, it has been observed that the use of antibiotics alters the gut flora and, to a limited degree, impacts the clinical course of inflammatory bowel disease (IBD) (1). Isolates of *E. coli* from patients with Crohn's and UC were found to be significantly more adherent to epithelial cells compared to isolates from controls (15, 50). Strains expressing the pathogenic features of EAEC (153) or a potentially new pathotype that exhibits both adherent and invasive properties (8) have also been isolated from patients with newly diagnosed or relapsing Crohn's disease and UC. Other properties have been suggested to have influence, such as hydrophobicity (14), production of Shiga-like toxins (190), outer membrane protein C (8), and the ability to bind to matrix proteins (157). The link between infection with *E. coli* and the pathogenesis of IBD, however, is still not clearly understood.

Extraintestinal Complications of Intestinal *E. coli* Infections

HUS and renal sequelae

HUS is the most lethal complication of STEC infection (84). Approximately 70% of cases of postdiarrheal HUS in the United States are caused by EHEC, 80% of which belong to serotype O157:H7 (7). HUS consists of the triad of acute renal failure, microangiopathic hemolytic anemia, and thrombocytopenia. Infants and young children are at the highest risk for HUS. In the elderly, who are also at high risk, the disease is often classified as thrombotic thrombocytopenic purpura, especially when there is associated neurological dysfunction. Although most children recover from the acute phase (overall mortality is about 9%), approximately 25% emerge with some degree of permanent renal dysfunction (49).

HUS is triggered by the systemic release of Shiga toxins produced in the colon. There are two main types of Shiga toxins, and STEC (O157 and non-O157 alike) that produce both Stx2 and Stx1, or Stx2 alone, are more likely to be associated with HUS than those that produce Stx1 only (79, 124). These toxins target glycolipid receptors (Gb3) on vascular endothelial cells, and after internalization by endocytosis, they act by cleaving the rRNA of the 60S subunit and arrest protein synthesis (137). Endothelial injury, apoptosis, and vasoactive cytokine release are harbingers of platelet aggregation and a prothrombotic state (134). The kidney vasculature appears to be particularly susceptible to these effects. As the disease progresses, glomerular endothelial cells swell and capillary lumens occlude from thrombosis (140). Arterial thrombotic microangiopathy and extensive cortical necrosis (involving more than 50% of glomeruli) are further pathologic features that demonstrate more extensive involvement associated with progression into chronic kidney disease (47). In addition to renal involvement, thrombosis and infarction may affect the central nervous system, myocardium, intestine, or other organs. The severity of the acute illness (particularly with the initial need for dialysis or extrarenal involvement) is strongly associated with a higher mortality or a poor long-term prognosis (49). During the acute phase of HUS, early signs of a poor prognosis also include leukocytosis (white blood cell count of $20,000 \times 10^9$/liter or more with neutrophilia) and hypertension (49).

If a patient remains anuric or oliguric 8 days after the onset of HUS or requires dialysis for longer than 4 weeks, then the chances of recovering renal function are poor. Such patients represent most of the 3% of cases of HUS that result in permanent end-stage renal disease (49). Several studies also suggest that there is a significant portion of patients who do not completely recover their renal function, even after initial recovery from the acute phase or milder forms of diarrhea-associated HUS. Long-term follow-up of patients who suffered only mild initial renal impairment without requiring dialysis showed that approximately 40% develop hypertension and proteinuria (47) and about 25% later deteriorated into chronic renal failure (181). Only after at least 1 year did the absence of proteinuria and hypertension with an estimated glomerular filtration rate of at least 80 ml/minute per $1.73m^2$ appear to be a reliable confirmation of a favorable long-term prognosis (49). It is suggested that patients who continue to deteriorate after a period of normal function experience progressive glomerulosclerosis related to hyperfunction of the remnant nephrons (138).

Reactive arthritis

Reactive arthritis and seronegative spondyloarthropathy are well-known consequences of the systemic inflammatory response following infectious diarrhea (38). *Campylobacter*, *Salmonella*, *Shigella*, and *Yersinia* species are most frequently associated with these syndromes (177). However, it does not appear that infection with EIEC, which closely resembles infection with *Shigella*, can also lead to reactive arthritis. Up to 4 years following an outbreak of *E. coli* O157:H7 and *Campylobacter*, there was a higher incidence of self-reported symptoms of arthralgias, enthesopathy, and low back pain in patients who had been symptomatic with acute gastroenteritis than that of patients who were asymptomatic during the outbreak (48). Expression of the type I major histocompatibility complex surface antigen HLA-B27 has been more frequently associated with severe symptoms and more features of reactive arthritis compared to the expression of HLA-B27-negative patients (38). Although the interaction of gram-negative bacteria with HLA-B27 is thought to be an important pathogenic feature that permits invasion (83), this interaction, which was demonstrated with EIEC, does not necessarily imply that infection triggers the development of arthritis. The role of HLA-B27 in reactive arthritis and the immune response that ensues following gastroenteritis remains enigmatic.

CONTROL AND TREATMENT

Public Health Strategies

As *E. coli* strains are acquired primarily through ingestion, efforts must be focused on increasing food and water safety. While providing sanitary living conditions, sources of potable water, and proper nutrition remain a priority in many developing regions, industrialized countries are also challenged by the risks inherent with the complexity and expansiveness of a global food supply (175). Exposure to foodborne pathogens has increased as food items are distributed from huge centers to increasing numbers of people and as more people eat in restaurants and food service establishments (82), where the risk of foodborne illness is greater than eating at home (80). Public health initiatives start by conducting risk assessments to define routes of transmission and critical intervention points. The prevention of illness caused by *E. coli* relies upon the surveillance of commercial food supplies with corresponding interventions to restrict distribution of contaminated products and establish safe food consumption patterns (3). After several outbreaks of *E. coli* O157 involving fresh spinach, for instance, an investigation found that the outbreak strain was isolated from feral swine and fecal contamination in the vicinity of spinach fields (74). While the use of new technology, including methods of decontamination, pasteurization, and food irradiation, may be beneficial in improving food safety (35), it is just as important to emphasize to the public the basic means of preventing transmission of enteric organisms at home, such as cooking all ground meat thoroughly (until the middle reaches a temperature of 160° F or until the juices run clear); washing hands, surfaces, and utensils that may have been contaminated by uncooked meat with soap and warm water; and avoiding unpasteurized milk or juice. More details can be found at the "Fight Bac!" website (http://www.fightbac.org). Person-to-person contact (58) and environmental exposure (17) are other important modes of transmission; during outbreaks of *E. coli* O157, person-to-person contact is responsible for approximately 14% of cases, waterborne transmission for approximately 9%, and transmission associated with animal contact for 3% (133). Knowledge of these patterns has informed additional recommendations. For example, infants and young children with diarrhea should not be permitted near public swimming areas, and all visitors of petting zoos should wash their hands afterwards.

Vaccines

The development of safe and effective vaccines for *E. coli* is beset by challenges of both clinical and financial feasibility. Nevertheless, vaccines are a rational secondary approach to the prevention of both enteric and extraintestinal *E. coli*. The two most important diarrheagenic pathotypes from a public health perspective are EHEC and ETEC. Given that *E. coli* is a natural constituent in the intestinal flora, targets of interest to produce vaccines are the unique antigens that distinguish virulent strains.

Directing immunity to Shiga toxins has been one strategy for EHEC vaccination (114). Candidate vaccines have included inactivated Stx2 toxoid: both the catalytic A subunit and the Gb3 ligand B subunit. The A-B complex is more immunogenic (102), but even the B subunit alone may potentially elicit some host damage (25, 101). In mice, inactivated Stx2 has provided protection from systemic complications of the toxin (86); however, antitoxin immunity does not necessarily prevent the attachment and colonization responsible for the clinical manifestation of diarrhea. Immunity toward the O157 polysaccharide unfortunately was not protective in murine models (20). Furthermore, there is a significant proportion of non-O157 EHEC that causes diarrhea and HUS, especially outside the United States. (79). To more effectively evoke an immune response, another approach is to administer the vaccine orally, which provides more localized exposure. There has been some initial work to construct live attenuated vectors, such as *V. cholerae*, which incorporates Stx2 and EHEC outer membrane proteins (16), or *Salmonella enterica* serovar *Landau*, which naturally express O157 (21).

Immune responses against ETEC fimbriae components have been shown to be at least partially effective in volunteers (174). Since immunity to ETEC LT toxin may also provide some protection (114), candidates for an ETEC vaccine have also included killed whole-cell formulations comprised of five strains with recombinant cholera toxin B subunit (75). One trial has used a live attenuated strain of *Shigella* to present ETEC fimbrial antigens with some encouraging response (9). Unfortunately, the large number of antigenically distinct ETEC fimbrial types is a daunting challenge to this approach.

The significant antigenic heterogeneity of ExPEC strains makes the development of an effective vaccine challenging. Initial promising results using a vaccine based upon the FimH adhesin from the type 1 pilus frequently associated with cystitis, and its chaperone protein FimC, have not been followed by further success (93). Whole-cell vaccines developed from heat-killed uropathogenic strains have the advantage of diversifying the immune response, which has been successful with *Bordetella pertussis*. However, despite having a sound concept, the development of several formulations has not convincingly yielded any success (144). K1 strains of ExPEC predominate in neonatal meningitis. However, the capsule composed of polysialic acid is not immunogenic in humans, due to its similarity to a self antigen (45).

Antibiotics, Probiotics, and Adjunctive Therapy

Extraintestinal infections

The combination of ampicillin and an aminoglycoside has traditionally been used for the treatment of gram-negative meningitis. However, ampicillin resistance in *E. coli* neonatal sepsis has exceeded 50% in some populations (60). Furthermore, when given intravenously, aminoglycoside concentrations may not exceed minimum inhibitory concentrations in CSF, which leads to the consideration of other strategies, such as intrathecal or intraventricular administration. Thus, in recent years third-generation cephalosporins or carbapenems have become the standard treatment. Given that there has been a limited decline in morbidity compared to mortality over the last two decades, antibiotic therapy appears to have a certain limit in the capacity to prevent neurological sequelae, especially when initiated late in the course. The adjunctive use of steroids for meningitis has been a controversial matter that has yet to be resolved.

Resistance is also frequently encountered with UTIs, especially in the nosocomial setting or in patients with prior antibiotic exposure. Intermittent, postcoital, or continuous prophylaxis for RUTIs may indeed become problematic with the development of resistance. Particularly concerning is the appearance of some strains that have acquired the ability to produce extended-spectrum beta-lactamase, which confers resistance to a broad array of antibiotics, including cephalosporins. Nevertheless, initiation of prophylactic antibiotics after the diagnosis of VUR may help to prevent renal scarring (110). For patients whose renal disease has progressed with evidence of proteinuria or microalbuminuria, an angiotensin-I-converting enzyme inhibitor or an angiotensin receptor blocker is the most effective therapy to preserve glomerular function (92, 187).

While it may not be practical to drink enough cranberry juice to be clinically effective for the prevention of RUTIs, there is some evidence that proanthocyanidins, which are tannins produced by many plants, can inhibit adherence of P-fimbriated *E. coli* to the uroepithelium (55, 64). In one trial involving women with UTIs caused by *E. coli*, the frequency of at least one RUTI within 6 months was significantly lower with cranberry-lingonberry juice than with both

Lactobacillus GG drink and the control (89). Further well-controlled trials are needed to establish whether capsules or tablets of cranberry concentrate may be more effective (135, 172).

Enteric infections

Most cases of diarrhea caused by *E. coli* tend to have a self-limited course and usually do not require antibiotics. Care is largely supportive and primarily entails replacement of lost fluids, either by the oral route, or parenterally, in the case of severe dehydration or persistent vomiting. Currently antibiotics are contraindicated for the treatment of EHEC, since they may actually stimulate the release of Shiga toxin (192) and increase the risk of HUS in children (197). One meta-analysis failed to show a significant risk of HUS associated with antibiotic therapy (146). However, this analysis has been criticized for including a large study in which virtually all patients received antibiotics (51). If antibiotic treatment is considered for the treatment of dysentery, care should be taken to exclude the diagnosis of Shiga toxin-producing *E. coli.* The empiric use of antibiotics, however, may have a role in the treatment of severe traveler's diarrhea (2), which is usually attributed to ETEC and has been shown to reduce symptoms associated with EAEC (52). Antimotility agents, such as loperimide, are helpful when used with fluoroquinolones. Rifaximin (an antibiotic that is not absorbed systemically) is another alternative to the fluoroquinolones indicated for travelers (37). There is no evidence to suggest that antibiotics have any impact on postinfectious sequelae, including the outcomes of IBS, IBD, or reactive arthritis. Furthermore, multidrug resistance is emerging in strains of EAEC (200) and EPEC (189).

Several conventional and inexpensive interventions are protective against EPEC infection, including colostrum, breast milk (24), and vitamin A supplementation (98). There are also emerging therapeutic strategies that may soon be realized for other intestinal *E. coli* infections. The concepts of receptor mimicry or ligand decoys and probiotics may have a special role for the treatment or prevention of EHEC disease. Polymers of globotriaosylceramide (Gb3, the receptor for Shiga toxin) could help to neutralize circulating toxin and reduce the systemic effects of HUS (183). Certain gram-negative bacteria may also express molecular mimics of host oligosaccharides and may also serve to bind toxins in the lumen and interfere with adherence of pathogens (126). The probiotics *Streptococcus thermophilus* and *Lactobacillus acidophilus* could potentially deter EIEC infection using this strategy (139). Prebiotic oligosaccharides may also have similar applications for EPEC (159). Clearly, new and innovative approaches will be required to reduce the burden of *E. coli* infections and their sequelae.

Acknowledgments. The views expressed in this chapter are those of the author and do not necessarily reflect the official policy of the Food and Drug Administration, the Department of Health and Human Services, or the United States Government.

REFERENCES

1. **Aberra, F. N., C. M. Brensinger, W. B. Bilker, G. R. Lichtenstein, and J. D. Lewis.** 2005. Antibiotic use and the risk of flare of inflammatory bowel disease. *Clin. Gastroenterol. Hepatol.* **3:**459–465.
2. **Adachi, J. A., L. Ostrosky-Zeichner, H. L. DuPont, and C. D. Ericsson.** 2000. Empirical antimicrobial therapy for traveler's diarrhea. *Clin. Infect. Dis.* **31:**1079–1083.
3. **Altekruse, S. F., M. L. Cohen, and D. L. Swerdlow.** 1997. Emerging foodborne diseases. *Emerg. Infect. Dis.* **3:**285–293.
4. **Alteri, C. J., and H. L. Mobley.** 2007. Quantitative profile of the uropathogenic *Escherichia coli* outer membrane proteome during growth in human urine. *Infect. Immun.* **75:**2679–2688.
5. **Assis, A. M., M. L. Barreto, L. M. Santos, R. Fiaccone, and G. S. da Silva Gomes.** 2005. Growth faltering in childhood related to diarrhea: a longitudinal community based study. *Eur. J. Clin. Nutr.* **59:**1317–1323.
6. **Baltimore, R. S., S. M. Huie, J. I. Meek, A. Schuchat, and K. L. O'Brien.** 2001. Early-onset neonatal sepsis in the era of group B streptococcal prevention. *Pediatrics* **108:**1094–1098.
7. **Banatvala, N., P. M. Griffin, K. D. Greene, T. J. Barrett, W. F. Bibb, J. H. Green, J. G. Wells, and Hemolytic Uremic Syndrome Study Collaborators.** 2001. The United States National Prospective Hemolytic Uremic Syndrome Study: microbiologic, serologic, clinical, and epidemiologic findings. *J. Infect. Dis.* **183:**1063–1070.
8. **Barnich, N., and A. Darfeuille-Michaud.** 2007. Adherent-invasive *Escherichia coli* and Crohn's disease. *Curr. Opin. Gastroenterol.* **23:**16–20.
9. **Barry, E. M., Z. Altboum, G. Losonsky, and M. M. Levine.** 2003. Immune responses elicited against multiple enterotoxigenic *Escherichia coli* fimbriae and mutant LT expressed in attenuated *Shigella* vaccine strains. *Vaccine* **21:**333–340.
10. **Bedford, H., J. de Louvois, S. Halket, C. Peckham, R. Hurley, and D. Harvey.** 2001. Meningitis in infancy in England and Wales: follow up at age 5 years. *BMJ* **323:**533–536.
11. **Bhan, M. K., N. Bhandari, S. Sazawal, J. Clemens, P. Raj, M. M. Levine, and J. B. Kaper.** 1989. Descriptive epidemiology of persistent diarrhoea among young children in rural northern India. *Bull. W. H. O.* **67:**281–288.
12. **Bhatnagar, S., M. K. Bhan, C. George, U. Gupta, R. Kumar, D. Bright, and S. Saini.** 1992. Is small bowel bacterial overgrowth of pathogenic significance in persistent diarrhea? *Acta Paediatr. Suppl.* **381:**108–113.
13. **Brenner, B. M.** 1983. Hemodynamically mediated glomerular injury and the progressive nature of kidney disease. *Kidney Int.* **23:**647–655.
14. **Burke, D. A., and A. T. Axon.** 1988. Hydrophobic adhesin of *E. coli* in ulcerative colitis. *Gut* **29:**41–43.
15. **Burke, D. A., and A. T. Axon.** 1988. Adhesive *Escherichia coli* in inflammatory bowel disease and infective diarrhoea. *BMJ* **297:**102–104.

16. **Butterton, J. R., E. T. Ryan, D. W. Acheson, and S. B. Calderwood**. 1997. Coexpression of the B subunit of Shiga toxin 1 and EaeA from enterohemorrhagic *Escherichia coli* in *Vibrio cholerae* vaccine strains. *Infect. Immun.* **65**:2127–2135.
17. **Centers for Disease Control and Prevention (CDC)**. 2005. Outbreaks of *Escherichia coli* O157:H7 associated with petting zoos—North Carolina, Florida, and Arizona, 2004 and 2005. *MMWR Morb. Mortal. Wkly. Rep.* **54**:1277–1280.
18. **Chang, C. J., W. N. Chang, L. T. Huang, S. C. Huang, Y. C. Chang, P. L. Hung, C. H. Lu, C. S. Chang, B. C. Cheng, P. Y. Lee, K. W. Wang, and H. W. Chang**. 2004. Bacterial meningitis in infants: the epidemiology, clinical features, and prognostic factors. *Brain Dev.* **26**:168–175.
19. **Chang, Y. C., C. C. Huang, S. T. Wang, and C. C. Chio**. 1997. Risk factor of complications requiring neurosurgical intervention in infants with bacterial meningitis. *Pediatr. Neurol.* **17**:144–149.
20. **Conlan, J. W., A. D. Cox, R. KuoLee, A. Webb, and M. B. Perry**. 1999. Parenteral immunization with a glycoconjugate vaccine containing the O157 antigen of *Escherichia coli* O157:H7 elicits a systemic humoral immune response in mice, but fails to prevent colonization by the pathogen. *Can. J. Microbiol.* **45**:279–286.
21. **Conlan, J. W., R. KuoLee, A. Webb, and M. B. Perry**. 1999. *Salmonella landau* as a live vaccine against *Escherichia coli* O157:H7 investigated in a mouse model of intestinal colonization. *Can. J. Microbiol.* **45**:723–731.
22. **Cotran, R. S., V. Kumar, and T. Collins**. 1999. *Robbins Pathologic Basis of Disease*, p. 930–996. W. B. Saunders Company, Philadelphia, PA.
23. **Crane, J. K., B. P. McNamara, and M. S. Donnenberg**. 2001. Role of EspF in host cell death induced by enteropathogenic *Escherichia coli*. *Cell. Microbiol.* **3**:197–211.
24. **Cravioto, A., A. Tello, H. Villafan, J. Ruiz, S. del Vedovo, and J. R. Neeser**. 1991. Inhibition of localized adhesion of enteropathogenic *Escherichia coli* to HEp-2 cells by immunoglobulin and oligosaccharide fractions of human colostrum and breast milk. *J. Infect. Dis.* **163**:1247–1255.
25. **Creydt, V. P., C. Silberstein, E. Zotta, and C. Ibarra**. 2006. Cytotoxic effect of Shiga toxin-2 holotoxin and its B subunit on human renal tubular epithelial cells. *Microbes Infect.* **8**:410–419.
26. **da Costa, L. B., H. Ahn, W. Montanera, and H. Ginsberg**. 2007. Repeated meningitis as a delayed complication of scoliosis surgery. *J. Spinal Disord. Tech.* **20**:333–336.
27. **Dalton, C. B., E. D. Mintz, J. G. Wells, C. A. Bopp, and R. V. Tauxe**. 1999. Outbreaks of enterotoxigenic *Escherichia coli* infection in American adults: a clinical and epidemiologic profile. *Epidemiol. Infect.* **123**:9–16.
28. **Day, W. A., and A. T. Maurelli**. 2002. *Shigella* and enteroinvasive *Escherichia coli*: paradigms for pathogen evolution and host-parasite interactions, p. 209–237. *In* M. S. Donnenberg (ed.), *Escherichia coli: Virulence Mechanisms of a Versatile Pathogen*. Academic Press, San Diego, CA.
29. **de Goede, C. G., P. E. Jardine, P. Eunson, S. Renowden, P. Sharples, and R. W. Newton**. 2006. Severe progressive late onset myelopathy and arachnoiditis following neonatal meningitis. *Eur. J. Paediatr. Neurol.* **10**:31–36.
30. **Donnenberg, M. S.** 2005. Enterobacteriaceae, p. 2567–2586. *In* G. L. Mandell, J. E. Bennett, and R. Dolin (ed.), *Mandell, Douglas, and Bennett's Principles and Practice of Infectious Diseases*. Elsevier, Philadelphia, PA.
31. **Donnenberg, M. S.** 1999. Interactions between enteropathogenic *Escherichia coli* and epithelial cells. *Clin. Infect. Dis.* **28**:451–455.
32. **Donnenberg, M. S., and R. A. Welch**. 1996. Virulence determinants of uropathogenic *Escherichia coli*, p. 135–174. *In* H. L. T. Mobley and J. W. Warren (ed.), *Urinary Tract Infections: Molecular Pathogenesis and Clinical Management*. ASM Press, Washington, DC.
33. **Dunlop, S. P., J. Hebden, E. Campbell, J. Naesdal, L. Olbe, A. C. Perkins, and R. C. Spiller**. 2006. Abnormal intestinal permeability in subgroups of diarrhea-predominant irritable bowel syndromes. *Am. J. Gastroenterol.* **101**:1288–1294.
34. **DuPont, H. L.** 2007. Therapy for and prevention of traveler's diarrhea. *Clin. Infect. Dis.* **45**(Suppl. 1):S78–S84.
35. **DuPont, H. L.** 2007. The growing threat of foodborne bacterial enteropathogens of animal origin. *Clin. Infect. Dis.* **45**:1353–1361.
36. **DuPont, H. L., S. B. Formal, R. B. Hornick, M. J. Snyder, J. P. Libonati, D. G. Sheahan, E. H. LaBrec, and J. P. Kalas**. 1971. Pathogenesis of *Escherichia coli* diarrhea. *N. Engl. J. Med.* **285**:1–9.
37. **DuPont, H. L., Z. D. Jiang, C. D. Ericsson, J. A. Adachi, J. J. Mathewson, M. W. DuPont, E. Palazzini, L. M. Riopel, D. Ashley, and F. Martinez-Sandoval**. 2001. Rifaximin versus ciprofloxacin for the treatment of traveler's diarrhea: a randomized, double-blind clinical trial. *Clin. Infect. Dis.* **33**:1807–1815.
38. **Eastmond, C. J.** 1983. Gram-negative bacteria and B27 disease. *Br. J. Rheumatol.* **22**:67–74.
39. **Escherich, T.** 1885. Die Darmbakterien des naugenborenen und sauglings. *Fortschr. Med.* **3**:515–547.
40. **Fagundes-Neto, U., and J. A. de Andrade**. 1999. Acute diarrhea and malnutrition: lethality risk in hospitalized infants. *J. Am. Coll. Nutr.* **18**:303–308.
41. **Fagundes-Neto, U., E. Freymüller, S. L. Gandolfi, and I. C. Scaletsky**. 1996. Nutritional impact and ultrastructural intestinal alterations in severe infections due to enteropathogenic *Escherichia coli* strains in infants. *J. Am. Coll. Nutr.* **15**:180–185.
42. **Fagundes-Neto, U., and I. C. Scaletsky**. 2000. The gut at war: the consequences of enteropathogenic *Escherichia coli* infection as a factor of diarrhea and malnutrition. *Sao Paulo Med. J.* **118**:21–29.
43. **Fagundes-Neto, U., L. G. Schmitz, and I. C. Scaletsky**. 1996. Acute diarrhea due to enteropathogenic *Escherichia coli*: epidemiological and clinical features in Brasilia, Brazil. *Int. J. Infect. Dis.* **1**:65–69.
44. **Farmer, J. J., III, G. R. Fanning, B. R. Davis, C. M. O'Hara, C. Riddle, F. W. Hickman-Brenner, M. A. Asbury, V. A. Lowery III, and D. J. Brenner**. 1985. *Escherichia fergusonii* and *Enterobacter taylorae*, two new species of Enterobacteriaceae isolated from clinical specimens. *J. Clin. Microbiol.* **21**:77–81.
45. **Finne, J., M. Leinonen, and P. H. Mäkelä**. 1983. Antigenic similarities between brain components and bacteria causing meningitis. Implications for vaccine development and pathogenesis. *Lancet* **ii**:355–357.
46. **Foxman, B.** 2002. Epidemiology of urinary tract infections: incidence, morbidity, and economic costs. *Am. J. Med.* **113**(Suppl. 1A):5S–13S.
47. **Gagnadoux, M. F., R. Habib, M. C. Gubler, J. L. Bacri, and M. Broyer**. 1996. Long-term (15–25 years) outcome of childhood hemolytic-uremic syndrome. *Clin. Nephrol.* **46**:39–41.
48. **Garg, A. X., J. E. Pope, H. Thiessen-Philbrook, W. F. Clark, and J. Ouimet**. 2008. Arthritis risk after acute bacterial gastroenteritis. *Rheumatology* (Oxford) **47**:200–204.
49. **Garg, A. X., R. S. Suri, N. Barrowman, F. Rehman, D. Matsell, M. P. Rosas-Arellano, M. Salvadori, R. B. Haynes, and W. F. Clark**. 2003. Long-term renal prognosis of diarrhea-as-

sociated hemolytic uremic syndrome: a systematic review, meta-analysis, and meta-regression. *JAMA* **290:**1360–1370.

50. **Giaffer, M. H., C. D. Holdsworth, and B. I. Duerden.** 1992. Virulence properties of *Escherichia coli* strains isolated from patients with inflammatory bowel disease. *Gut* **33:**646–650.
51. **Gill, C. J., D. H. Hamer, J. Lau, C. S. Wong, J. R. Brandt, P. I. Tarr, S. L. Watkins, M. A. Neill, D. G. Maki, and N. Safdar.** 2002. Risk of hemolytic uremic syndrome from antibiotic treatment of *Escherichia coli* O157:H7 colitis. *JAMA* **288:**3110–3112.
52. **Glandt, M., J. A. Adachi, J. J. Mathewson, Z. D. Jiang, D. DiCesare, D. Ashley, C. D. Ericsson, and H. L. DuPont.** 1999. Enteroaggregative *Escherichia coli* as a cause of traveler's diarrhea: clinical response to ciprofloxacin. *Clin. Infect. Dis.* **29:**335–338.
53. **Gomes, T. A., V. Rassi, K. L. MacDonald, S. R. Ramos, L. R. Trabulsi, M. A. Vieira, B. E. Guth, J. A. Candeias, C. Ivey, M. R. Toledo, et al.** 1991. Enteropathogens associated with acute diarrheal disease in urban infants in São Paulo, Brazil. *J. Infect. Dis.* **164:**331–337.
54. **Gomes, T. A., M. A. Vieira, I. K. Wachsmuth, P. A. Blake, and L. R. Trabulsi.** 1989. Serotype-specific prevalence of *Escherichia coli* strains with EPEC adherence factor genes in infants with and without diarrhea in São Paulo, Brazil. *J. Infect. Dis.* **160:**131–135.
55. **Gupta, K., M. Y. Chou, A. Howell, C. Wobbe, R. Grady, and A. E. Stapleton.** 2007. Cranberry products inhibit adherence of P-fimbriated *Escherichia coli* to primary cultured bladder and vaginal epithelial cells. *J. Urol.* **177:**2357–2360.
56. **Gwee, K. A., J. C. Graham, M. W. McKendrick, S. M. Collins, J. S. Marshall, S. J. Walters, and N. W. Read.** 1996. Psychometric scores and persistence of irritable bowel after infectious diarrhoea. *Lancet* **347:**150–153.
57. **Gwee, K. A., Y. L. Leong, C. Graham, M. W. McKendrick, S. M. Collins, S. J. Walters, J. E. Underwood, and N. W. Read.** 1999. The role of psychological and biological factors in postinfective gut dysfunction. *Gut* **44:**400–406.
58. **Harris, J. R., J. Mariano, J. G. Wells, B. J. Payne, H. D. Donnell, and M. L. Cohen.** 1985. Person-to-person transmission in an outbreak of enteroinvasive *Escherichia coli*. *Am. J. Epidemiol.* **122:**245–252.
59. **Harvey, D., D. E. Holt, and H. Bedford.** 1999. Bacterial meningitis in the newborn: a prospective study of mortality and morbidity. *Semin. Perinatol.* **23:**218–225.
60. **Heath, P. T., N. K. Nik Yusoff, and C. J. Baker.** 2003. Neonatal meningitis. *Arch. Dis. Child Fetal Neonatal Ed.* **88:**F173–F178.
61. **Henderson, I. R., S. Hicks, F. Navarro-Garcia, W. P. Elias, A. D. Philips, and J. P. Nataro.** 1999. Involvement of the enteroaggregative *Escherichia coli* plasmid-encoded toxin in causing human intestinal damage. *Infect. Immun.* **67:**5338–5344.
62. **Hooton, T. M., P. L. Roberts, and W. E. Stamm.** 1994. Effects of recent sexual activity and use of a diaphragm on the vaginal microflora. *Clin. Infect. Dis.* **19:**274–278.
63. **Hooton, T. M., A. E. Stapleton, P. L. Roberts, C. Winter, D. Scholes, T. Bavendam, and W. E. Stamm.** 1999. Perineal anatomy and urine-voiding characteristics of young women with and without recurrent urinary tract infections. *Clin. Infect. Dis.* **29:**1600–1601.
64. **Howell, A. B., N. Vorsa, M. A. Der, and L. Y. Foo.** 1998. Inhibition of the adherence of P-fimbriated *Escherichia coli* to uroepithelial-cell surfaces by proanthocyanidin extracts from cranberries. *N. Engl. J Med.* **339:**1085–1086.
65. **Huang, D. B., J. P. Nataro, H. L. DuPont, P. P. Kamat, A. D. Mhatre, P. C. Okhuysen, and T. Chiang.** 2006. Enteroaggregative *Escherichia coli* is a cause of acute diarrheal illness: a meta-analysis. *Clin. Infect. Dis.* **43:**556–563.
66. **Huang, S. H., C. Wass, Q. Fu, N. V. Prasadarao, M. Stins, and K. S. Kim.** 1995. *Escherichia coli* invasion of brain microvascular endothelial cells in vitro and in vivo: molecular cloning and characterization of invasion gene *ibe10*. *Infect. Immun.* **63:**4470–4475.
67. **Huppertz, H. I., S. Rutkowski, S. Aleksic, and H. Karch.** 1997. Acute and chronic diarrhoea and abdominal colic associated with enteroaggregative *Escherichia coli* in young children living in western Europe. *Lancet* **349:**1660–1662.
68. **Huys, G., M. Cnockaert, J. M. Janda, and J. Swings.** 2003. *Escherichia albertii sp. nov.*, a diarrhoeagenic species isolated from stool specimens of Bangladeshi children. *Int. J. Syst. Evol. Microbiol.* **53:**807–810.
69. **Ikäheimo, R., A. Siitonen, T. Heiskanen, U. Kärkkäinen, P. Kuosmanen, P. Lipponen, and P. H. Mäkelä.** 1996. Recurrence of urinary tract infection in a primary care setting: analysis of a 1-year follow-up of 179 women. *Clin. Infect. Dis.* **22:**91–99.
70. **Islam, M., M. P. Doyle, S. C. Phatak, P. Millner, and X. Jiang.** 2004. Persistence of enterohemorrhagic *Escherichia coli* O157:H7 in soil and on leaf lettuce and parsley grown in fields treated with contaminated manure composts or irrigation water. *J. Food Prot.* **67:**1365–1370.
71. **Jacobson, S. H.** 1986. P-fimbriated *Escherichia coli* in adults with renal scarring and pyelonephritis. *Acta Med. Scand. Suppl.* **713:**1–64.
72. **Jacobson, S. H., O. Eklöf, L. E. Lins, I. Wikstad, and J. Winberg.** 1992. Long-term prognosis of post-infectious renal scarring in relation to radiological findings in childhood—a 27-year follow-up. *Pediatr. Nephrol.* **6:**19–24.
73. **Jakobsson, B., U. Berg, and L. Svensson.** 1994. Renal scarring after acute pyelonephritis. *Arch. Dis. Child* **70:**111–115.
74. **Jay, M. T., M. Cooley, D. Carychao, G. W. Wiscomb, R. A. Sweitzer, L. Crawford-Miksza, J. A. Farrar, D. K. Lau, J. O'Connell, A. Millington, R. V. Asmundson, E. R. Atwill, and R. E. Mandrell.** 2007. *Escherichia coli* O157:H7 in feral swine near spinach fields and cattle, central California coast. *Emerg. Infect. Dis.* **13:**1908–1911.
75. **Jertborn, M., C. Ahrén, J. Holmgren, and A. M. Svennerholm.** 1998. Safety and immunogenicity of an oral inactivated enterotoxigenic *Escherichia coli* vaccine. *Vaccine* **16:**255–260.
76. **Jiang, Z. D., P. C. Okhuysen, D. C. Guo, R. He, T. M. King, H. L. DuPont, and D. M. Milewicz.** 2003. Genetic susceptibility to enteroaggregative *Escherichia coli* diarrhea: polymorphism in the interleukin-8 promotor region. *J. Infect. Dis.* **188:**506–511.
77. **Johanson, W. G., A. K. Pierce, and J. P. Sanford.** 1969. Changing pharyngeal bacterial flora of hospitalized patients. Emergence of gram-negative bacilli. *N. Engl. J. Med.* **281:**1137–1140.
78. **Johnson, J. R., P. L. Roberts, and W. E. Stamm.** 1987. P fimbriae and other virulence factors in *Escherichia coli* urosepsis: association with patients' characteristics. *J. Infect. Dis.* **156:**225–229.
79. **Johnson, K. E., C. M. Thorpe, and C. L. Sears.** 2006. The emerging clinical importance of non-O157 Shiga toxin-producing *Escherichia coli*. *Clin. Infect. Dis.* **43:**1587–1595.
80. **Jones, T. F., and F. J. Angulo.** 2006. Eating in restaurants: a risk factor for foodborne disease? *Clin. Infect. Dis.* **43:**1324–1328.

81. **Kang, G., S. Sheela, M. M. Mathan, and V. I. Mathan.** 1999. Prevalence of enteroaggregative and other HEp-2 cell adherent *Escherichia coli* in asymptomatic rural south Indians by longitudinal sampling. *Microbios* **100:**57–66.
82. **Kant, A. K., and B. I. Graubard.** 2004. Eating out in America, 1987-2000: trends and nutritional correlates. *Prev. Med.* **38:**243–249.
83. **Kapasi, K., and R. D. Inman.** 1992. HLA-B27 expression modulates gram-negative bacterial invasion into transfected L cells. *J. Immunol.* **148:**3554–3559.
84. **Karmali, M. A., M. Petric, C. Lim, P. C. Fleming, G. S. Arbus, and H. Lior.** 1985. The association between idiopathic hemolytic uremic syndrome and infection by verotoxin-producing *Escherichia coli. J. Infect. Dis.* **151:** 775–782.
85. **Kenny, B., R. DeVinney, M. Stein, D. J. Reinscheid, E. A. Frey, and B. B. Finlay.** 1997. Enteropathogenic *E. coli* (EPEC) transfers its receptor for intimate adherence into mammalian cells. *Cell* **91:**511–520.
86. **Keusch, G. T., D. W. Acheson, C. Marchant, and J. McIver.** 1998. Toxioid-based active and passive immunization to prevent and/or modulate hemolytic-uremic syndrome due to Shiga-producing *Escherichia coli*, p. 409–418. *In* J. B. Kaper and A. D. O'Brien (ed.), *Escherichia coli O157:H7 and Other Shiga Toxin-Producing E. coli Strains.* American Society for Microbiology, Washington, DC.
87. **Khan, N. A., Y. Wang, K. J. Kim, J. W. Chung, C. A. Wass, and K. S. Kim.** 2002. Cytotoxic necrotizing factor-1 contributes to *Escherichia coli* K1 invasion of the central nervous system. *J. Biol. Chem.* **277:**15607–15612.
88. **Klinger, G., C. N. Chin, J. Beyene, and M. Perlman.** 2000. Predicting the outcome of neonatal bacterial meningitis. *Pediatrics* **106:**477–482.
89. **Kontiokari, T., K. Sundqvist, M. Nuutinen, T. Pokka, M. Koskela, and M. Uhari.** 2001. Randomised trial of cranberry-lingonberry juice and *Lactobacillus* GG drink for the prevention of urinary tract infections in women. *BMJ* **322:**1571.
90. **Korczak, B., J. Frey, J. Schrenzel, G. Pluschke, R. Pfister, R. Ehricht, and P. Kuhnert.** 2005. Use of diagnostic microarrays for determination of virulence gene patterns of *Escherichia coli* K1, a major cause of neonatal meningitis. *J. Clin. Microbiol.* **43:**1024–1031.
91. **Korhonen, T. K., M. V. Valtonen, J. Parkkinen, V. Väisänen-Rhen, L. Wang, J. Finne, F. Ørskov, I. Ørskov, S. B. Svenson, and P. H. Mäkelä.** 1985. Serotypes, hemolysin production, and receptor recognition of *Escherichia coli* strains associated with neonatal sepsis and meningitis. *Infect. Immun.* **48:**486–491.
92. **Lama, G., M. E. Salsano, M. Pedulla, C. Grassia, and G. Ruocco.** 1997. Angiotensin converting enzyme inhibitors and reflux nephropathy: 2-year follow-up. *Pediatr. Nephrol.* **11:**714–718.
93. **Langermann, S., and W. R. Ballou, Jr.** 2001. Vaccination utilizing the FimCH complex as a strategy to prevent *Escherichia coli* urinary tract infections. *J. Infect. Dis.* **183**(Suppl. 1):S84–S86.
94. **Lehnardt, S., L. Massillon, P. Follett, F. E. Jensen, R. Ratan, P. A. Rosenberg, J. J. Volpe, and T. Vartanian.** 2003. Activation of innate immunity in the CNS triggers neurodegeneration through a Toll-like receptor 4-dependent pathway. *Proc. Natl. Acad. Sci. USA* **100:**8514–8519.
95. **Levine, M. M., D. R. Nalin, D. L. Hoover, E. J. Bergquist, R. B. Hornick, and C. R. Young.** 1979. Immunity to enterotoxigenic *Escherichia coli. Infect. Immun.* **23:**729–736.
96. **Litwin, M. S., C. S. Saigal, E. M. Yano, C. Avila, S. A. Geschwind, J. M. Hanley, G. F. Joyce, R. Madison, J. Pace, S. M. Polich, and M. Wang.** 2005. Urologic diseases in America Project: analytical methods and principal findings. *J. Urol.* **173:**933–937.
97. **Lomberg, H., P. de Man, and C. Svanborg Edén.** 1989. Bacterial and host determinants of renal scarring. *APMIS* **97:**193–199.
98. **Long, K. Z., J. I. Santos, J. L. Rosado, C. Lopez-Saucedo, R. Thompson-Bonilla, M. Abonce, H. L. DuPont, E. Hertzmark, and T. Estrada-Garcia.** 2006. Impact of vitamin A on selected gastrointestinal pathogen infections and associated diarrheal episodes among children in Mexico City, Mexico. *J. Infect. Dis.* **194:**1217–1225.
99. **Lund, B., F. Lindberg, and S. Normark.** 1988. Structure and antigenic properties of the tip-located P pilus proteins of uropathogenic *Escherichia coli. J. Bacteriol.* **170:** 1887–1894.
100. **Mackowiak, P. A., R. M. Martin, S. R. Jones, and J. W. Smith.** 1978. Pharyngeal colonization by gram-negative bacilli in aspiration-prone persons. *Arch. Intern. Med.* **138:** 1224–1227.
101. **Marcato, P., G. Mulvey, and G. D. Armstrong.** 2002. Cloned Shiga toxin 2 B subunit induces apoptosis in Ramos Burkitt's lymphoma B cells. *Infect. Immun.* **70:**1279–1286.
102. **Marcato, P., G. Mulvey, R. J. Read, H. K. Vander, P. N. Nation, and G. D. Armstrong.** 2001. Immunoprophylactic potential of cloned Shiga toxin 2 B subunit. *J. Infect. Dis.* **183:**435–443.
103. **Marshall, J. K., M. Thabane, M. R. Borgaonkar, and C. James.** 2007. Postinfectious irritable bowel syndrome after a food-borne outbreak of acute gastroenteritis attributed to a viral pathogen. *Clin. Gastroenterol. Hepatol.* **5:**457–460.
104. **Mathewson, J. J., P. C. Johnson, H. L. DuPont, D. R. Morgan, S. A. Thornton, L. V. Wood, and C. D. Ericsson.** 1985. A newly recognized cause of travelers' diarrhea: enteroadherent *Escherichia coli. J. Infect. Dis.* **151:**471–475.
105. **Mathewson, J. J., R. A. Oberhelman, H. L. DuPont, F. Javier de la Cabada, and E. V. Garibay.** 1987. Enteroadherent *Escherichia coli* as a cause of diarrhea among children in Mexico. *J. Clin. Microbiol.* **25:**1917–1919.
106. **Mayer, H. B., and C. A. Wanke.** 1995. Enteroaggregative *Escherichia coli* as a possible cause of diarrhea in an HIV-infected patient. *N. Engl. J. Med.* **332:**273–274.
107. **McCracken, G. H., Jr., L. D. Sarff, M. P. Glode, S. G. Mize, M. S. Schiffer, J. B. Robbins, E. C. Gotschlich, I. Ørskov, and F. Ørskov.** 1974. Relation between *Escherichia coli* K1 capsular polysaccharide antigen and clinical outcome in neonatal meningitis. *Lancet* **ii:**246–250.
108. **McDermott, S., V. Daguise, H. Mann, L. Szwejbka, and W. Callaghan.** 2001. Perinatal risk for mortality and mental retardation associated with maternal urinary-tract infections. *J. Fam. Pract.* **50:**433–437.
109. **McKendrick, M. W., and N. W. Read.** 1994. Irritable bowel syndrome-post *Salmonella* infection. *J. Infect.* **29:**1–3.
110. **McLorie, G. A., P. H. McKenna, B. M. Jumper, B. M. Churchill, R. F. Gilmour, and A. E. Khoury.** 1990. High grade vesicoureteral reflux: analysis of observational therapy. *J. Urol.* **144:**537–540.
111. **McNamara, B. P., A. Koutsouris, C. B. O'Connell, J. P. Nougayrede, M. S. Donnenberg, and G. Hecht.** 2001. Translocated EspF protein from enteropathogenic *Escherichia coli* disrupts host intestinal barrier function. *J. Clin. Investig.* **107:**621–629.

112. **Mead, P. S., L. Slutsker, V. Dietz, L. F. McCaig, J. S. Bresee, C. Shapiro, P. M. Griffin, and R. V. Tauxe.** 1999. Food-related illness and death in the United States. *Emerg. Infect. Dis.* **5:**607–625.
113. **Mofredj, A., J. M. Guerin, F. Leibinger, and R. Mamoudi.** 2000. Spontaneous *Escherichia coli* meningitis in an adult. *Scand. J. Infect. Dis.* **32:**699–700.
114. **Nataro, J. P.** 2004. Vaccines against diarrheal diseases. *Semin. Pediatr. Infect. Dis.* **15:**272–279.
115. **Nataro, J. P., C. A. Bopp, P. I. Fields, J. B. Kaper, and N. A. Strockbine.** 2007. *Escherichia, Shigella,* and *Salmonella*, p. 670–687. *In* P. R. Murray, E. J. Baron, J. H. Jorgensen, M. L. Landry, and M. A. Pfaller (ed.), *Manual of Clinical Microbiology*, 9th ed. vol. 1. ASM Press, Washington, DC.
116. **Nataro, J. P., Y. Deng, D. R. Maneval, A. L. German, W. C. Martin, and M. M. Levine.** 1992. Aggregative adherence fimbriae I of enteroaggregative *Escherichia coli* mediate adherence to HEp-2 cells and hemagglutination of human erythrocytes. *Infect. Immun.* **60:**2297–2304.
117. **Nataro, J. P., and J. B. Kaper.** 1998. Diarrheagenic *Escherichia coli. Clin. Microbiol. Rev.* **11:**142–201.
118. **Nataro, J. P., J. B. Kaper, R. Robins-Browne, V. Prado, P. Vial, and M. M. Levine.** 1987. Patterns of adherence of diarrheagenic *Escherichia coli* to HEp-2 cells. *Pediatr. Infect. Dis. J.* **6:**829–831.
119. **Neal, K. R., J. Hebden, and R. Spiller.** 1997. Prevalence of gastrointestinal symptoms six months after bacterial gastroenteritis and risk factors for development of the irritable bowel syndrome: postal survey of patients. *Br. Med. J.* **314:**779–782.
120. **O'Brien, A. D., J. W. Newland, S. F. Miller, R. K. Holmes, H. W. Smith, and S. B. Formal.** 1984. Shiga-like toxin-converting phages from *Escherichia coli* strains that cause hemorrhagic colitis or infantile diarrhea. *Science* **226:**694–696.
121. **O'Hanley, P.** 1996. Prospects for urinary tract infection vaccines, p. 405–425. *In* H. L. T. Mobley and J. W. Warren (ed.), *Urinary Tract Infections: Molecular Pathogenesis and Clinical Management*. ASM Press, Washington, DC.
122. **Okhuysen, P. C., Z. D. Jiang, L. Carlin, C. Forbes, and H. L. DuPont.** 2004. Post-diarrhea chronic intestinal symptoms and irritable bowel syndrome in North American travelers to Mexico. *Am. J. Gastroenterol.* **99:**1774–1778.
123. **Ørskov, I., F. Ørskov, B. Jann, and K. Jann.** 1977. Serology, chemistry, and genetics of O and K antigens of *Escherichia coli. Bacteriol. Rev.* **41:**667–710.
124. **Ostroff, S. M., P. I. Tarr, M. A. Neill, J. H. Lewis, N. Hargrett-Bean, and J. M. Kobayashi.** 1989. Toxin genotypes and plasmid profiles as determinants of systemic sequelae in *Escherichia coli* O157:H7 infections. *J. Infect. Dis.* **160:**994–998.
125. **Passeron, A., L. Capron, and G. Grateau.** 2004. Recurrent *Escherichia coli* meningitis associated with aspergillar sphenoidal sinusitis. *Scand. J. Infect. Dis.* **36:**492–493.
126. **Paton, A. W., R. Morona, and J. C. Paton.** 2006. Designer probiotics for prevention of enteric infections. *Nat. Rev. Microbiol.* **4:**193–200.
127. **Patterson, J. E., and V. T. Andriole.** 1997. Bacterial urinary tract infections in diabetes. *Infect. Dis. Clin. North Am.* **11:**735–750.
128. **Polivka, B. J., J. T. Nickel, and J. R. Wilkins III.** 1997. Urinary tract infection during pregnancy: a risk factor for cerebral palsy? *J. Obstet. Gynecol. Neonatal Nurs.* **26:** 405–413.
129. **Pupo, G. M., D. K. Karaolis, R. Lan, and P. R. Reeves.** 1997. Evolutionary relationships among pathogenic and nonpathogenic *Escherichia coli* strains inferred from multilocus enzyme electrophoresis and *mdh* sequence studies. *Infect. Immun.* **65:**2685–2692.
130. **Pupo, G. M., R. Lan, and P. R. Reeves.** 2000. Multiple independent origins of Shigella clones of *Escherichia coli* and convergent evolution of many of their characteristics. *Proc. Natl. Acad. Sci. USA* **97:**10567–10572.
131. **Pylkkänen, J., J. Vilska, and O. Koskimies.** 1981. The value of level diagnosis of childhood urinary tract infection in predicting renal injury. *Acta Paediatr. Scand.* **70:**879–883.
132. **Qadri, F., A. M. Svennerholm, A. S. Faruque, and R. B. Sack.** 2005. Enterotoxigenic *Escherichia coli* in developing countries: epidemiology, microbiology, clinical features, treatment, and prevention. *Clin. Microbiol. Rev.* **18:**465–483.
133. **Rangel, J. M., P. H. Sparling, C. Crowe, P. M. Griffin, and D. L. Swerdlow.** 2005. Epidemiology of *Escherichia coli* O157:H7 outbreaks, United States, 1982-2002. *Emerg. Infect. Dis.* **11:**603–609.
134. **Ray, P. E., and X. H. Liu.** 2001. Pathogenesis of Shiga toxin-induced hemolytic uremic syndrome. *Pediatr. Nephrol.* **16:**823–839.
135. **Raz, R., B. Chazan, and M. Dan.** 2004. Cranberry juice and urinary tract infection. *Clin. Infect. Dis.* **38:**1413–1419.
136. **Raz, R., and W. E. Stamm.** 1993. A controlled trial of intravaginal estriol in postmenopausal women with recurrent urinary tract infections. *N. Engl. J. Med.* **329:**753–756.
137. **Reisbig, R., S. Olsnes, and K. Eiklid.** 1981. The cytotoxic activity of *Shigella* toxin. Evidence for catalytic inactivation of the 60 S ribosomal subunit. *J. Biol. Chem.* **256:** 8739–8744.
138. **Repetto, H. A.** 2005. Long-term course and mechanisms of progression of renal disease in hemolytic uremic syndrome. *Kidney Int. Suppl.* **97:**S102–S106.
139. **Resta-Lenert, S., and K. E. Barrett.** 2003. Live probiotics protect intestinal epithelial cells from the effects of infection with enteroinvasive *Escherichia coli* (EIEC). *Gut* **52:**988–997.
140. **Richardson, S. E., M. A. Karmali, L. E. Becker, and C. R. Smith.** 1988. The histopathology of the hemolytic uremic syndrome associated with verocytotoxin-producing *Escherichia coli* infections. *Hum. Pathol.* **19:**1102–1108.
141. **Roberts, J. A.** 1991. Etiology and pathophysiology of pyelonephritis. *Am. J. Kidney Dis.* **17:**1–9.
142. **Robins-Browne, R. M.** 1987. Traditional enteropathogenic *Escherichia coli* of infantile diarrhea. *Rev. Infect. Dis.* **9:** 28–53.
143. **Rothbaum, R., A. J. McAdams, R. Giannella, and J. C. Partin.** 1982. A clinicopathologic study of enterocyte-adherent *Escherichia coli*: a cause of protracted diarrhea in infants. *Gastroenterology* **83:**441–454.
144. **Russo, T. A., and J. R. Johnson.** 2006. Extraintestinal isolates of *Escherichia coli*: identification and prospects for vaccine development. *Expert. Rev. Vaccines* **5:**45–54.
145. **Russo, T. A., A. Stapleton, S. Wenderoth, T. M. Hooton, and W. E. Stamm.** 1995. Chromosomal restriction fragment length polymorphism analysis of *Escherichia coli* strains causing recurrent urinary tract infections in young women. *J. Infect. Dis.* **172:**440–445.
146. **Safdar, N., A. Said, R. E. Gangnon, and D. G. Maki.** 2002. Risk of hemolytic uremic syndrome after antibiotic treatment of *Escherichia coli* O157:H7 enteritis: a meta-analysis. *JAMA* **288:**996–1001.
147. **Sartor, R. B.** 2008. Microbial influences in inflammatory bowel diseases. *Gastroenterology* **134:**577–594.

148. **Savarino, S. J., A. Fasano, J. Watson, B. M. Martin, M. M. Levine, S. Guandalini, and P. Guerry.** 1993. Enteroaggregative *Escherichia coli* heat-stable enterotoxin 1 represents another subfamily of *E. coli* heat-stable toxin. *Proc. Natl. Acad. Sci. USA* **90:**3093–3097.
149. **Scheutz, F., T. Cheasty, D. Woodward, and H. R. Smith.** 2004. Designation of O174 and O175 to temporary O groups OX3 and OX7, and six new *E. coli* O groups that include Verocytotoxin-producing *E. coli* (VTEC): O176, O177, O178, O179, O180 and O181. *APMIS* **112:**569–584.
150. **Schnurrenberger, L. W., R. Beck, and J. Pate.** 1971. Gastroenteritis attributed to imported French cheese. *MMWR Morb. Mortal. Wkly. Rpt.* **20:**427–428.
151. **Scholes, D., T. M. Hooton, P. L. Roberts, A. E. Stapleton, K. Gupta, and W. E. Stamm.** 2000. Risk factors for recurrent urinary tract infection in young women. *J. Infect. Dis.* **182:**1177–1182.
152. **Schrag, S. J., S. Zywicki, M. M. Farley, A. L. Reingold, L. H. Harrison, L. B. Lefkowitz, J. L. Hadler, R. Danila, P. R. Cieslak, and A. Schuchat.** 2000. Group B streptococcal disease in the era of intrapartum antibiotic prophylaxis. *N. Engl. J. Med.* **342:**15–20.
153. **Schultsz, C., M. Moussa, R. van Ketel, G. N. Tytgat, and J. Dankert.** 1997. Frequency of pathogenic and enteroadherent *Escherichia coli* in patients with inflammatory bowel disease and controls. *J. Clin. Pathol.* **50:**573–579.
154. **Serény, B.** 1955. Experimental *Shigella* keratoconjunctivitis: a preliminary report. *Acta Microbiol. Acad. Sci. Hung.* **2:**293–296.
155. **Shah, D. K., A. J. Daley, R. W. Hunt, J. J. Volpe, and T. E. Inder.** 2005. Cerebral white matter injury in the newborn following *Escherichia coli* meningitis. *Eur. J. Paediatr. Neurol.* **9:**13–17.
156. **Sheikh, J., J. R. Czeczulin, S. Harrington, S. Hicks, I. R. Henderson, B. C. Le, P. Gounon, A. Phillips, and J. P. Nataro.** 2002. A novel dispersin protein in enteroaggregative *Escherichia coli*. *J. Clin. Investig.* **110:**1329–1337.
157. **Shen, W., H. Steinrück, and Å. Ljungh.** 1995. Expression of binding of plasminogen, thrombospondin, vitronectin, and fibrinogen, and adhesive properties by *Escherichia coli* strains isolated from patients with colonic diseases. *Gut* **36:**401–406.
158. **Shin, S., G. Lu, M. Cai, and K. S. Kim.** 2005. *Escherichia coli* outer membrane protein A adheres to human brain microvascular endothelial cells. *Biochem. Biophys. Res. Commun.* **330:**1199–1204.
159. **Shoaf, K., G. L. Mulvey, G. D. Armstrong, and R. W. Hutkins.** 2006. Prebiotic galactooligosaccharides reduce adherence of enteropathogenic *Escherichia coli* to tissue culture cells. *Infect. Immun.* **74:**6920–6928.
160. **Siitonen, A., A. Takala, Y. A. Ratiner, A. Pere, and P. H. Mäkelä.** 1993. Invasive *Escherichia coli* infections in children: bacterial characteristics in different age groups and clinical entities. *Pediatr. Infect. Dis. J.* **12:**606–612.
161. **Sobel, J. D.** 1997. Pathogenesis of urinary tract infection. Role of host defenses. *Infect. Dis. Clin. North Am.* **11:** 531–549.
162. **Sobieszczanska, B. M., J. Osek, D. Wasko-Czopnik, E. Dworniczek, and K. Jermakow.** 2007. Association of enteroaggregative *Escherichia coli* with irritable bowel syndrome. *Clin. Microbiol. Infect.* **13:**404–407.
163. **Soyturk, M., H. Akpinar, O. Gurler, E. Pozio, I. Sari, S. Akar, M. Akarsu, M. Birlik, F. Onen, and N. Akkoc.** 2007. Irritable bowel syndrome in persons who acquired trichinellosis. *Am. J. Gastroenterol.* **102:**1064–1069.
164. **Spangler, B. D.** 1992. Structure and function of cholera toxin and the related *Escherichia coli* heat-labile enterotoxin. *Microbiol. Rev.* **56:**622–647.
165. **Spiller, R. C.** 2007. Role of infection in irritable bowel syndrome. *J. Gastroenterol.* **42**(Suppl. 17)**:**41–47.
166. **Spiller, R. C., D. Jenkins, J. P. Thornley, J. M. Hebden, T. Wright, M. Skinner, and K. R. Neal.** 2000. Increased rectal mucosal enteroendocrine cells, T lymphocytes, and increased gut permeability following acute *Campylobacter* enteritis and in post-dysenteric irritable bowel syndrome. *Gut* **47:**804–811.
167. **Steiner, T. S., A. A. Lima, J. P. Nataro, and R. L. Guerrant.** 1998. Enteroaggregative *Escherichia coli* produce intestinal inflammation and growth impairment and cause interleukin-8 release from intestinal epithelial cells. *J. Infect. Dis.* **177:**88–96.
168. **Steiner, T. S., J. P. Nataro, C. E. Poteet-Smith, J. A. Smith, and R. L. Guerrant.** 2000. Enteroaggregative *Escherichia coli* expresses a novel flagellin that causes IL-8 release from intestinal epithelial cells. *J. Clin. Investig.* **105:**1769–1777.
169. **Steinlin, M., B. Knecht, D. Konu, E. Martin, and E. Boltshauser.** 1999. Neonatal *Escherichia coli* meningitis: spinal adhesions as a late complication. *Eur. J. Pediatr.* **158:** 968–970.
170. **Stevens, J. P., M. Eames, A. Kent, S. Halket, D. Holt, and D. Harvey.** 2003. Long term outcome of neonatal meningitis. *Arch. Dis. Child Fetal Neonatal Ed.* **88:**F179–F184.
171. **Stewart, G. T.** 1950. Post-dysenteric colitis. *Br. Med. J.* **1:** 405–409.
172. **Stothers, L.** 2002. A randomized trial to evaluate effectiveness and cost effectiveness of naturopathic cranberry products as prophylaxis against urinary tract infection in women. *Can. J. Urol.* **9:**1558–1562.
173. **Sukumaran, S. K., H. Shimada, and N. V. Prasadarao.** 2003. Entry and intracellular replication of *Escherichia coli* K1 in macrophages require expression of outer membrane protein A. *Infect. Immun.* **71:**5951–5961.
174. **Tacket, C. O., R. H. Reid, E. C. Boedeker, G. Losonsky, J. P. Nataro, H. Bhagat, and R. Edelman.** 1994. Enteral immunization and challenge of volunteers given enterotoxigenic *E. coli* CFA/II encapsulated in biodegradable microspheres. *Vaccine* **12:**1270–1274.
175. **Tauxe, R. V.** 1997. Emerging foodborne diseases: an evolving public health challenge. *Emerg. Infect. Dis.* **3:**425–434.
176. **Teng, C. H., M. Cai, S. Shin, Y. Xie, K. J. Kim, N. A. Khan, C. F. Di, and K. S. Kim.** 2005. *Escherichia coli* K1 RS218 interacts with human brain microvascular endothelial cells via type 1 fimbria bacteria in the fimbriated state. *Infect. Immun.* **73:**2923–2931.
177. **Ternhag, A., A. Törner, A. Svensson, K. Ekdahl, and J. Giesecke.** 2008. Short- and long-term effects of bacterial gastrointestinal infections. *Emerg. Infect. Dis.* **14:**143–148.
178. **Thabane, M., D. T. Kottachchi, and J. K. Marshall.** 2007. Systematic review and meta-analysis: the incidence and prognosis of post-infectious irritable bowel syndrome. *Aliment. Pharmacol. Ther.* **26:**535–544.
179. **Tilden, J., Jr., W. Young, A. M. McNamara, C. Custer, B. Boesel, M. A. Lambert-Fair, J. Majkowski, D. Vugia, S. B. Werner, J. Hollingsworth, and J. G. Morris, Jr.** 1996. A new route of transmission for *Escherichia coli*: infection from dry fermented salami. *Am. J. Public Health* **86:** 1142–1145.
180. **Tomson, F. L., V. K. Viswanathan, K. J. Kanack, R. P. Kanteti, K. V. Straub, M. Menet, J. B. Kaper, and G. Hecht.** 2005. Enteropathogenic *Escherichia coli* EspG disrupts microtubules and in conjunction with Orf3 enhances pertur-

bation of the tight junction barrier. *Mol. Microbiol.* **56:** 447–464.

181. **Tönshoff, B., A. Sammet, I. Sanden, O. Mehls, R. Waldherr, and K. Schärer.** 1994. Outcome and prognostic determinants in the hemolytic uremic syndrome of children. *Nephron* **68:**63–70.
182. **Trabulsi, L. R., R. Keller, and T. A. Tardelli Gomes.** 2002. Typical and atypical enteropathogenic *Escherichia coli*. *Emerg. Infect. Dis.* **8:**508–513.
183. **Trachtman, H., A. Cnaan, E. Christen, K. Gibbs, S. Zhao, D. W. Acheson, R. Weiss, F. J. Kaskel, A. Spitzer, and G. H. Hirschman.** 2003. Effect of an oral Shiga toxin-binding agent on diarrhea-associated hemolytic uremic syndrome in children: a randomized controlled trial. *JAMA* **290:** 1337–1344.
184. **Tulloch, E. F., Jr., K. J. Ryan, S. B. Formal, and F. A. Franklin.** 1973. Invasive enteropathic *Escherichia coli* dysentery. An outbreak in 28 adults. *Ann. Intern. Med.* **79:**13–17.
185. **Unhanand, M., M. M. Mustafa, G. H. McCracken, Jr., and J. D. Nelson.** 1993. Gram-negative enteric bacillary meningitis: a twenty-one-year experience. *J. Pediatr.* **122:**15–21.
186. **Vachvanichsanong, P.** 2007. Urinary tract infection: one lingering effect of childhood kidney diseases—review of the literature. *J. Nephrol.* **20:**21–28.
187. **Venkat, K. K.** 2004. Proteinuria and microalbuminuria in adults: significance, evaluation, and treatment. *South. Med. J.* 97:969–979.
188. **Vieira, N., S. J. Bates, O. D. Solberg, K. Ponce, R. Howsmon, W. Cevallos, G. Trueba, L. Riley, and J. N. Eisenberg.** 2007. High prevalence of enteroinvasive *Escherichia coli* isolated in a remote region of northern coastal Ecuador. *Am. J. Trop. Med. Hyg.* **76:**528–533.
189. **Vila, J., M. Vargas, C. Casals, H. Urassa, H. Mshinda, D. Schellemberg, and J. Gascon.** 1999. Antimicrobial resistance of diarrheagenic *Escherichia coli* isolated from children under the age of 5 years from Ifakara, Tanzania. *Antimicrob. Agents Chemother.* **43:**3022–3024.
190. **von Wulffen, H., H. Rüssmann, H. Karch, T. Meyer, M. Bitzan, T. C. Kohrt, and S. Aleksic.** 1989. Verocytotoxin-producing *Escherichia coli* O2:H5 isolated from patients with ulcerative colitis. *Lancet* **i:**1449–1450.
191. **Walker-Smith, J. A.** 1984. Food allergy and bowel disease in childhood. *Midwife Health Visitor Community Nurse* **20:**308–316.
192. **Walterspiel, J. N., S. Ashkenazi, A. L. Morrow, and T. G. Cleary.** 1992. Effect of subinhibitory concentrations of antibiotics on extracellular Shiga-like toxin I. *Infection* **20:** 25–29.
193. **Wang, H. S., M. F. Kuo, and S. C. Huang.** 2005. Diagnostic approach to recurrent bacterial meningitis in children. *Chang Gung. Med. J.* **28:**441–452.
194. **Wang, L., D. Rothemund, H. Curd, and P. R. Reeves.** 2003. Species-wide variation in the *Escherichia coli* flagellin (H-antigen) gene. *J. Bacteriol.* **185:**2936–2943.
195. **Wang, L. H., X. C. Fang, and G. Z. Pan.** 2004. Bacillary dysentery as a causative factor of irritable bowel syndrome and its pathogenesis. *Gut* **53:**1096–1101.
196. **Warren, J. W.** 1996. Clinical presentations and epidemiology of urinary tract infections, p. 3–27. *In* H. L. T. Mobley and J. W. Warren (ed.), *Urinary Tract Infections: Molecular Pathogenesis and Clinical Management*. ASM Press, Washington, DC.
197. **Wong, C. S., S. Jelacic, R. L. Habeeb, S. L. Watkins, and P. I. Tarr.** 2000. The risk of the hemolytic-uremic syndrome after antibiotic treatment of *Escherichia coli* O157:H7 infections. *N. Engl. J. Med.* **342:**1930–1936.
198. **World Health Organization.** 1999. New frontiers in the development of vaccines against enterotoxinogenic (ETEC) and enterohaemorrhagic (EHEC) *E. coli* infections. Part I. *Wkly. Epidemiol. Rec.* **74:**98–101.
199. **Wu, S. X., and R. Q. Peng.** 1992. Studies on an outbreak of neonatal diarrhea caused by EPEC 0127:H6 with plasmid analysis restriction analysis and outer membrane protein determination. *Acta Paediatr.* **81:**217–221.
200. **Yamamoto, T., P. Echeverria, and T. Yokota.** 1992. Drug resistance and adherence to human intestines of enteroaggregative *Escherichia coli*. *J. Infect. Dis.* **165:**744–749.
201. **Yamamoto, T., S. Endo, T. Yokota, and P. Echeverria.** 1991. Characteristics of adherence of enteroaggregative *Escherichia coli* to human and animal mucosa. *Infect. Immun.* **59:**3722–3739.
202. **Yatsuyanagi, J., Y. Kinouchi, S. Saito, H. Sato, and M. Morita.** 1996. Enteropathogenic *Escherichia coli* strains harboring enteroaggregative *Escherichia coli* (EAggEC) heat-stable enterotoxin-1 gene isolated from a food-borne like outbreak. *Kansenshogaku Zasshi* **70:**73–79. (In Japanese.)
203. **Yoder, P. S., and R. C. Hornik.** 1994. Perceptions of severity of diarrhoea and treatment choice: a comparative study of HealthCom sites. *J. Trop. Med. Hyg.* **97:**1–12.

Sequelae and Long-Term Consequences of Infectious Diseases
Edited by Pina M. Fratamico, James L. Smith, and Kim A. Brogden

Chapter 6

Variable Capacity for Persistent Infection and Complications of Gram-Positive Cocci: Streptococci and Staphylococci

Brandy Ferguson and Christopher W. Woods

Gram-positive bacterial pathogens use highly efficient mechanisms to evade recognition and removal by the human immune system. Many of these bacteria produce sophisticated anti-inflammatory molecules and deploy several defensive tactics that protect against host cationic antimicrobial molecules. Others may engender a host-damaging autoimmune response that can lead to both acute and chronic manifestations. Microbial surface components recognizing adhesive matrix molecules (MSCRAMMs) are critical for the initial attachment of bacteria to the host. Cell wall teichoic acids, lipoteichoic acids, complex surface polymers, and modified membrane lipids are crucial aspects of virulence such as nasal colonization. Some isolates develop resistance mutations to common antimicrobials to prevent elimination. Still others hide either intracellularly or in a protective cocoon of biofilm on bioprosthetic devices to evade both immunological and antimicrobial stalkers. This chapter will focus on two clinically important gram-positive genera, *Staphylococcus* and *Streptococcus*, and the complications and persistent infections caused by these bacteria.

STREPTOCOCCUS

The genus *Streptococcus* belongs to the order *Lactobacillales* and the family *Streptococcaceae*. Many streptococci are part of the normal flora of the mouth, skin, intestine, and upper respiratory tract. However, certain pathogenic species of *Streptococcus* are responsible for causing diverse acute infections, including dental caries, skin and soft tissue infections, pharyngitis, pneumonia, meningitis, and endocarditis. Furthermore, in addition to these acute and subacute infections, a variety of persistent, suppurative, and postinfectious complications may occur.

The taxonomy of the streptococci is increasingly complicated. In the clinical laboratory, streptococci are differentiated based on their hemolytic properties on blood agar plates. Alpha-hemolytic streptococci partially break down hemoglobin, leaving a greenish color around a colony. Beta-hemolytic streptococci fully break down red blood cells, leaving a clear zone of true hemolysis around colonies. Beta-hemolytic streptococci are further divided into separate groups based on their Lancefield antigens. These antigens differ based on specific characteristics of the C carbohydrate on the cell wall. Lancefield antigens have letter names, A, B, C, and D through S. These letters also serve as the specific group names.

Beta-Hemolytic Streptococci

GAS (*Streptococcus pyogenes*)

Microbiological potential for complicated infection. *Streptococcus pyogenes* is beta hemolytic and, based on its Lancefield antigen, is referred to as group A streptococci (GAS). The cell wall of GAS includes a peptidoglycan layer, group-specific carbohydrates (a dimer of rhamnose and *n*-acetyl glucosamine), lipoteichoic acid, and proteins F and T. Pathogenic GAS also have a hyaluronic acid capsule that allows the bacteria to resist phagocytosis. The major somatic virulence factor is the M protein (17, 142). Strains elaborating large amounts of this protein are capable of initiating cell damage and avoid phagocytosis. Strains that do not express this protein are avirulent (86).

Variations of the N terminus on the M protein are the biochemical basis for typing GAS. Typing may be performed either serologically, based on antigenic differences, or by genotyping (*emm* typing). There are more than 120 *emm* types for GAS (39). Alternative means of strain typing GAS exist. Vir

Brandy Ferguson and Christopher W. Woods • Duke University School of Medicine, Durham, NC 27705.

typing measures restriction fragment length polymorphisms within the *emm* chromosomal region. Pulsed-field gel electrophoresis, multilocus sequence typing, and multilocus enzyme electrophoresis are new genotypic methods used today (108).

The major adherence factors for GAS are lipoteichoic acid and fibronectin binding protein (protein F), which binds to fibronectin on the human cell surface. M protein can also bind to epithelial cells and block adherence. However, some researchers have found no difference in the binding of M^+ and M^- strains of GAS to buccal epithelial cells, suggesting that the M protein is not required for attachment (15, 131).

Penicillin remains the drug of choice for treatment of GAS infections, as all isolates are quite susceptible. Erythromycin may be used to treat patients who are allergic to penicillin, but resistance to macrolides has emerged as a substantial problem in areas of high use (17, 55, 131).

Clinical presentation. *Acute GAS disease.* GAS cause acute disease by local invasion, exotoxin elaboration, or both. The two most common acute manifestations are pharyngitis and impetigo, but other acute skin and soft tissue infections include cellulitis, erysipelas, necrotizing fasciitis, myositis, myonecrosis, and the streptococcal toxic shock syndrome. Invasive sterile site infections, such as bacteremia, are less common and usually secondary to primary skin or soft tissue infections. Population-based studies in the United States estimate approximately 11,000 cases of invasive GAS (3.8 per 100,000) each year. The rate of death from invasive GAS remains 10 to 20 percent, despite improved supportive care and antibiotics (39, 142).

Complications of pharyngitis. The human pharynx is the natural reservoir for GAS. Pharyngeal carriage rates among school children are estimated to be 15 to 20%, but rates are much lower among adults. Peak incidence occurs during winter/spring and in areas of crowding (e.g., school and military barracks). Pharyngitis is the classic clinical presentation of GAS disease. Common signs and symptoms associated with streptococcal pharyngitis include purulent tonsillar exudates, fever, headache, and swollen cervical lymph nodes.

In the absence of suppurative complications, symptoms should resolve within a week of onset, even without therapy. However, if untreated, carriage may persist for several weeks, even after resolution of symptoms. Antimicrobial therapy is the standard of care to reduce duration of acute symptoms and for prevention of suppurative (e.g., peritonsillar abscesses, otitis media, and sinusitis) and postinfectious complications. Treatment also shortens transmissibility. Therapeutic options for pharyngitis include penicillin and erythromycin. GAS is completely susceptible to penicillin, amoxicillin, or ampicillin. Erythromycin-resistant strains have been reported, but the number of resistant strains in the United States remains low.

Chronic tonsillitis or recurrent disease is uncommon but can occur with inadequate response to macrolide treatment (143). Reinfection may also occur in areas of heavy carriage when type-specific antibody development has been inadequate or with the introduction of new strains. In these situations, treatment has been needed for eradication and potential persistence in households (161).

Complicated skin and soft tissue infections. Impetigo, cellulitis, and erysipelas are common GAS skin and soft tissue infections. Necrotizing fasciitis is an uncommon but severe form of skin infection. Impetigo is a superficial bacterial skin infection and frequently occurs in children. Risk factors for impetigo include poverty, poor hygiene, previous scabies infection, and residing in overcrowded areas (7, 11, 12). Over the course of a week, impetigo begins as papules (on the face or extremities), which then progress to erythematous vesicles that break to form thick, golden crusts. Cellulitis and erysipelas are infections that result from bacterial invasion into the skin. Erysipelas involves the upper dermis of the skin layer and the superficial lymphatics. In contrast, cellulitis occurs deeper into the dermis as well as subcutaneous fat. Erysipelas lesions are "raised" in appearance, with a clear line of demarcation. Cellulitis is characterized by redness, swelling, warmth, and pain or tenderness of the affected area. Systemic symptoms of both cellulitis and erysipelas may include fever, headache, and nausea. Common risk factors are immunodeficiency diabetes, skin ulceration, fungal infections, and recent surgery (7, 11, 12).

When deep infection of the subcutaneous tissue occurs, destruction of the fascia and surrounding fat can result. This infection is known as necrotizing fasciitis and is often referred to as the "flesh-eating bacteria." The bacteria actually destroy the tissue (skin and muscle) by releasing exotoxins, which activate T-cell production. This activation causes an overproduction of cytokines, which in turn triggers an excess of macrophages. Macrophages release free oxygen radicals, which damage the tissue. Individuals who have a prior history of varicella infection, blunt trauma, intravenous drug use, burns, childbirth, and surgical procedures are more predisposed to necrotizing fasciitis. Initial symptoms involve pain and swelling of the affected site, fever, diarrhea, and vomiting. The skin may turn violet in color, and blisters may begin to appear. Without treatment, tissue damage can spread, and mortality rates increase. The disease may be disfiguring, and even when treatment is initiated promptly, the mortality rate for individuals affected with necrotizing fasciitis due to streptococcal infection exceeds 50 percent (7).

Toxin-mediated infections. GAS release a variety of exotoxins (e.g., pyrogenic exotoxins and superantigens) which can facilitate primary infection and result in a number of clinical syndromes.

Scarlet fever. Scarlet fever results from infection with an erythrogenic toxin-producing strain of *S. pyogenes*. In addition to an acute pharyngitis, patients may have a "strawberry" tongue (caused by inflamed red papillae of the tongue), and a fine sandpaper rash covering the body can also result. This rash starts on the trunk and neck and then spreads to the upper and lower extremities, while sparing the face. The rash is typically followed by extensive desquamation. Severe septic or toxic forms of scarlet fever are infrequent (12).

TSS. Akin to necrotizing fasciitis, streptococcal toxic shock syndrome (TSS) is mediated by the release of exotoxins (or superantigens). These superantigens activate the immune system to release inflammatory cytokines. However, in the case of TSS, this cytokine release causes leakage of capillaries as well as tissue damage leading to shock and possible multiple organ failure. Streptococcal TSS typically begins with initial colonization and infection of the skin, pharynx, or vagina. Individuals with TSS often present with one or more of the following symptoms: abrupt onset of diffuse or localized pain or pain in an extremity. This pain can mimic that of other conditions, such as peritonitis, pelvic inflammatory disease, pneumonia, acute myocardial infarction, or cholecystitis. Other patients may complain of influenza-like symptoms—fever, chills, myalgias, nausea, or vomiting. Fever is the most common presenting symptom. Complications of streptococcal TSS can include bacteremia, acute respiratory distress syndrome, disseminated intravascular coagulation, and renal failure (11, 12).

Invasive disease. GAS bacteremia is relatively uncommon in the antibiotic era. Occasional cases are seen in young adults, during the peripartum period, and associated with surgical site infections. An upsurge in cases during the 1990s was associated with intravenous drug abusers and nosocomial outbreaks in nursing homes (90, 130). More recently, children may develop invasive disease as a complication of varicella infection (36, 155). Presentation is typically abrupt and with a case fatality rate of 25 to 40%. Infective endocarditis (IE) is an exceedingly rare consequence of GAS bacteremia. In a recent review by the International Consortium on Endocarditis (ICE) of the global distribution of endocarditis, GAS accounted for less than 0.1% of definite cases (36, 130).

Nonsuppurative sequelae. Rheumatic fever. Acute rheumatic fever (ARF) is a postinfectious syndrome characterized by inflammatory lesions involving the heart, joints, subcutaneous tissues, and central nervous system. After an initial pharyngitis, susceptible individuals may begin to experience arthritis of the large joints, carditis, valvulitis, chorea (abrupt, nonrhythmic, involuntary movements), or rash (erythema marginatum). These symptoms can last for up to 3 months. Diagnosis of rheumatic fever is made using the Jones criteria (Table 1). These criteria consist of major and minor classifications. In order to be diagnosed with rheumatic fever, a patient must have a positive streptococcal antistreptolysin O (ASO) titer and exhibit two major Jones criteria or one major with two minor Jones criteria.

The global estimated incidence of ARF (470,000 annually) and prevalence of rheumatic heart disease (15 million) heavily burden developing countries (18). After reaching all-time lows in the early 1980s, reemergence of ARF and severe GAS infections around the world highlighted the potential return of epidemic disease and its severe sequelae (108).

The issue of "rheumatogenic" strains is contentious. In the mid-1980s, a resurgence of ARF was associated with a variety of strains, but particularly

Table 1. Diagnosis of acute rheumatic fever: the Jones criteria[a] (34)

Classification	Jones criterium
Major	Carditis (40–50%)
	Polyarthritis (75%)
	Chorea (15%) "St. Vitus Dance"
	Erythema marginatum (<10%)
	Subcutaneous nodules (<10%)
Minor	
Clinical	Previous rheumatic fever
	Arthralgias
	Fever
Laboratory	Acute phase reactions include elevated sedimentation rate, C-reactive protein, leukocytosis; prolonged P-R interval plus evidence of a preceding streptococcal infection

[a] Diagnosis requires two majors or one major + two minors with a positive test for recent streptococcal infection (ASO).

prominent was an association with mucoid serotype 18 (14). Ultimately, a large variety of strains have been associated with outbreaks of ARF in the United States (types 3, 5, 6, 14, 18, 19, and 29) (73, 133). These strains do appear to share common antigenic domains against which ARF patients mount a strong immunoglobulin G (IgG) response (13). However, a subsequent reduction in the prevalence of these strains was not wholly responsible for the ultimate reduction in ARF. Furthermore, different authors identified a different group of strains, including some that were untypable (76). Ultimately, a strain that can cause pharyngitis appears to have the potential for ARF. Although not well understood, the pharynx, with its surfeit of lymphoid tissue, may be important in the abnormal immunological response.

Although poorly understood, the pathogenic mechanism for ARF is assumed to be molecular mimicry. Epitopes of streptococcal M proteins share determinants with myosin, sarcolemmal membrane proteins, synovium, and articular cartilage (31, 32, 35, 53, 146).

In patients with carditis, Zabriskie found the presence of high titers of heart-reactive antibodies in the sera of patients with ARF. Antibody titers declined rapidly 3 to 6 months after initial onset and then more gradually over the next 2 to 3 years. This group also discovered that after 5 years, these patients, in the absence of recurrent disease, had little or no detectable antibody present in their bloodstreams. Most rheumatic illnesses recur within the first 2 years after initial infection (161).

Individuals with rheumatic valvulitis have been shown to develop antibodies to the carbohydrate specific to GAS, *N*-acetylglucosamine. Antibodies to this carbohydrate will persist for years, unlike those who suffer from rheumatic carditis. The persistence of high titers is believed to be related to the slow and sustained release of valvular cross-reactive glycoproteins. These cross-reactive antibodies are a major cause of valvular damage (Color Plate 3).

A number of studies of rheumatic valvulitis and carditis have focused on the cytoskeletal components, myosin and laminin. Galvin and colleagues conducted a study of a monoclonal antibody directed against myosin and *N*-acetylglucosamine isolated from a patient suffering from rheumatic carditis. Their research showed that this antibody was cytotoxic for human endothelial cell lines and reacted against the valvular endothelium. Galvin et al. concluded that this reactivity was inhibited more by myosin than laminin, and laminin may further explain reactivity against the valve surface (53).

Host genetic susceptibility provides another conundrum. Several studies have reported both major histocompatibility complex (MHC)-related and non-MHC-related associations. In particular, an increased frequency of the MHC class II alleles HLA-DR2 (blacks) or HLA-DR4 (whites) has been reported among patients with ARF (4). However, different alleles have been identified in other geographic regions. In another report a B-cell marker (D8/17) appears to identify an ARF-susceptible population (78). Most likely, susceptibility to ARF is polygenic.

Arthritis is one of the hallmark features of ARF. In several studies of rheumatic fever-associated arthritis, patients demonstrated a decrease in complement components, C1q, C3, and C4, in their synovial fluid (161). However, Zabriskie has also proposed that antibodies to streptococcal antigens bind to the smooth muscle of blood vessel walls, causing vasculitis and resulting synovitis (161).

Treatment for rheumatic fever includes use of salicylates, steroids, and supportive care. In order to prevent recurrences, patients are given monthly injections of benzathine penicillin. ASO titers can also be monitored for any signs of reinfection. Rheumatic heart disease is the most severe sequela of ARF. It generally develops 10 to 20 years after initial infection. Mitral stenosis is the most common valvular lesion in rheumatic heart disease. Patients with mitral stenosis display dyspnea (i.e., difficulty breathing), pulmonary edema, and atrial fibrillation, and the stenotic valve can also provide an ideal nidus for IE (Color Plate 3).

POSTSTREPTOCOCCAL GLOMERULONEPHRITIS. Postinfectious acute glomerulonephritis (AGN) is an acute inflammatory lesion of the renal glomerulus with worldwide importance. Although AGN can occur after many different types of infection, poststreptococcal is the classic presentation. The disease usually follows an extrarenal infection, typically GAS; however, other groups, particularly C and G, can be associated (10, 37, 150). AGN may occur at any age but usually occurs in young children, who are most likely to have primary GAS infection. The most common antecedent infection is usually a tonsillopharyngitis. However, unlike ARF, AGN is often associated with skin infections, particularly in economically depressed populations. Oddly, ARF and AGN are unlikely to coexist. Some investigators hypothesize that impetigo may protect against pharyngitis but put an individual at greater risk for contracting ARF (7).

Approximately 1 week after a streptococcal infection of the pharynx or skin, antigen-antibody complexes are deposited in the glomerular basement membrane and activate the complement cascade, resulting in the destruction of glomeruli. Symptoms of poststreptococcal glomerulonephritis include hematuria and high blood pressure (resulting from fluid retention). As with ARF, a serotype association has been described, particularly with serotype 12. However, types 4, 25, and 49 are also considered nephritogenic, but there are many other associations that have been described, and as yet, no available biomarkers distinguish nephritogenic from nonnephritogenic strains.

The precise mechanism of glomerular injury is unknown but is clearly immunologically mediated. Possibilities include direct antibody attack on renal tissues; in fact, antigenic similarities are well described (57). However, on electron microscopy, variously sized aggregates of granular electron-dense material thought to be immune complexes are irregularly arrayed in the glomerular subepithelial space (Color Plate 4 and Fig. 1). These aggregates bind fluorescein-labeled antibodies to IgG and various components of the complement cascade. These findings are supportive of circulating immune complex-mediated disease. A number of specific antigenic targets from nephritogenic strains are currently being investigated for a pathogenic role of AGN.

Treatment is supportive and variable depending on the degree of renal injury sustained. All nonallergic patients should receive penicillin to eradicate colonization. Recovery from AGN is usually complete, with more than 90 percent of children experiencing a complete recovery. However, the outlook for adults is less clear, and the fraction who may experience residual renal dysfunction and hypertension is unknown.

Pandas. Pediatric autoimmune neuropsychiatric disorders associated with streptococcal infections (PANDAS) describes an interesting subset of childhood neuropsychiatric disorders, such as obsessive-compulsive disorder (OCD) and Tourette's syndrome, for which symptoms worsen following streptococcal infections.

Shortly after GAS infection, susceptible children may exhibit sudden-onset OCD or tic behavior.

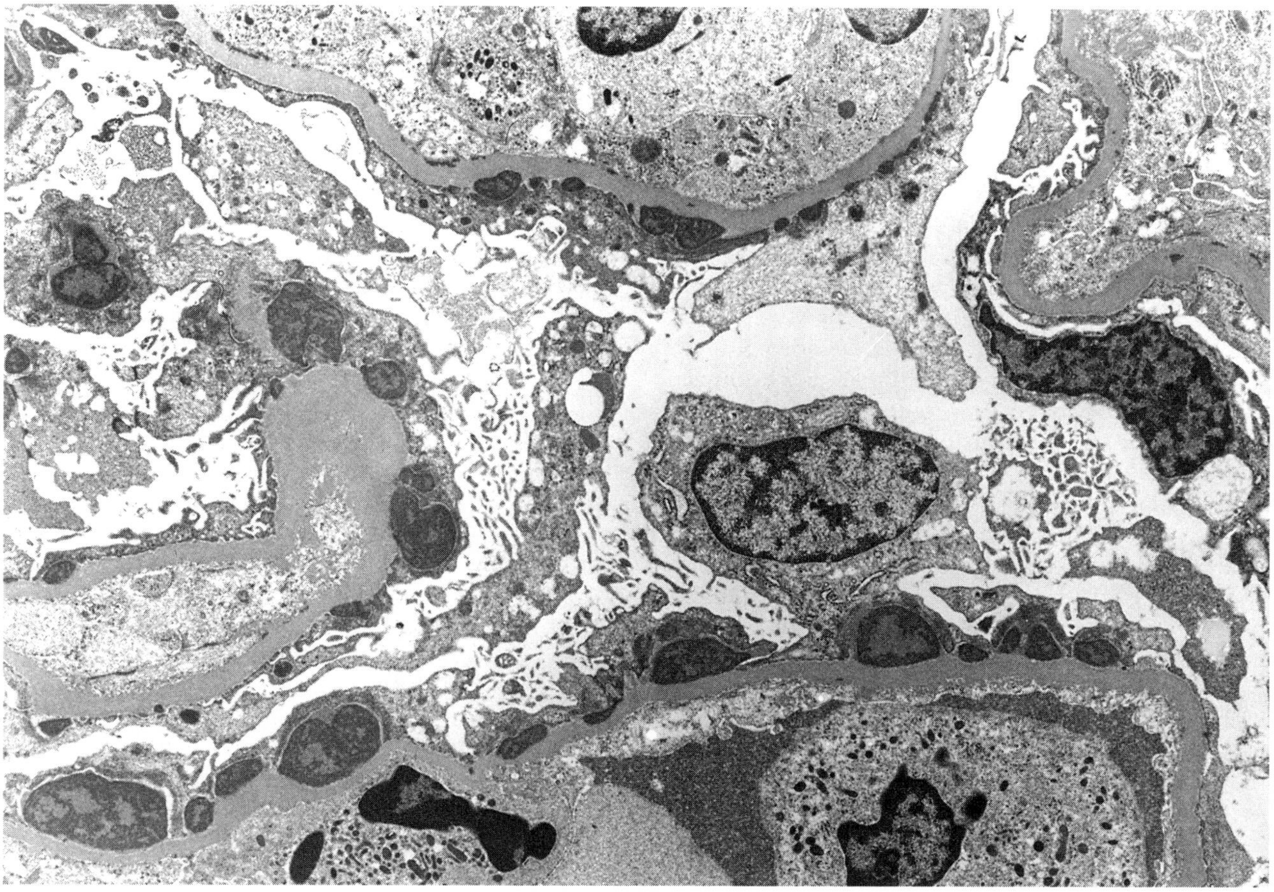

Figure 1. Electron micrograph of glomerular capillary wall in acute poststreptococcal glomerulonephritis showing hemispherical electron-dense deposit ("humps") in subepithelial space. (Courtesy of David Howell.)

Currently, there are five working criteria used to diagnose PANDAS: (i) presence of OCD and/or tic disorders, (ii) pediatric onset, (iii) abrupt onset and episodic course, (iv) association with GAS infection, and (v) association with neurological abnormalities (such as motor hyperactivity, choreoform, or tics (101). The mechanism of PANDAS is unknown, but a working hypothesis for the pathogenesis of PANDAS is that GAS infection in a susceptible host stimulates cross-reactive IgG to cellular components of the basal ganglia, most notably the putamen and caudate nucleus. When these antibodies interact with the neurons of the basal ganglia, obsessions, compulsions, and tics may manifest in children with a history of streptococcal infection (140).

Murphy and Pichichero found that even though 60 percent of patients with rheumatic fever showed significantly elevated ASO titers, those with chorea were less likely to have high ASO titers. This study also noted the absence of a strong inflammatory response in PANDAS patients (105). Veasy et al. also noted the absence of a strong inflammatory response in their study of ARF outbreaks (148). Researchers believe that symptoms of PANDAS result from a combination of local, regional, and systemic abnormalities. There is evidence that shows a genetic predisposition for tic disorders and OCD in first-degree relatives of children afflicted with PANDAS (54).

Several studies have been conducted to ascertain whether PANDAS can be mitigated with antibiotic prophylaxis. One study used a double-blind trial of azithromycin and penicillin with 23 participants. The study found that the rate of GAS infection was significantly lower during the year of antibiotic administration (0.1 per year) than during the year prior to the study (2.2 per year; $P < 0.01$), whether the subjects were treated with penicillin or azithromycin. No significant differences were found in the numbers of streptococcal infections or the numbers of neuropsychiatric exacerbations between the azithromycin or penicillin groups (54). There is suggestive evidence for the role of immunologic dysfunction in PANDAS. Snider and Swedo conducted a randomized, placebo-controlled trial of intravenous immunoglobulin and plasma exchange. They found that intravenous immunoglobulin reduced obsessions, compulsions, and tics by 45% over 1 year, while plasma exchange treatments reduced these symptoms by 58%. These results further support a potential immunologic etiology of this disease (139).

GBS (*Streptococcus agalactiae*)

Microbiological potential for complicated infection. *Streptococcus agalactiae*, referred to as group B streptococcus (GBS), is an opportunistic pathogen that colonizes the gastrointestinal and genitourinary tracts of up to 50% of healthy adults. These streptococci are facultative gram-positive diplococci that have a narrow zone of beta hemolysis on blood agar. Most isolates elaborate CAMP factor, a thermostable protein, which reacts synergistically with the β-lysin of *Staphylococcus aureus* strains to enhance their hemolysis. Capsular polysaccharide antigens allow the classification of eight distinct serotypes.

Strain-specific virulence is evident by the strain distribution of invasive isolates, with some variation by type of infection. Type IA, II, III, and V account for the vast majority of documented infections. Types IV, VI, VII, and VIII and untypable isolates are infrequently associated with invasive infection. Virulence in type III strains appears to be mediated by the elaboration of cell-associated sialic acid. Unencapsulated or sialic acid-free mutants have reduced virulence in a neonatal rat model (154).

GBS remain susceptible to beta-lactams, but the minimum inhibitory concentrations (MICs) are 4- to 10-fold higher than those for GAS. However, penicillin G remains the drug of choice in a confirmed infection, but higher doses are usually recommended. Approximately 3 to 15% of isolates are resistant to erythromycin and clindamycin. The percentages of serotype V strains that are resistant to erythromycin (34.9%) and clindamycin (22.2%) are higher than those of strains of other serotypes (93).

Clinical presentation. *Acute GBS disease.* GBS colonize the genital or lower gastrointestinal tracts of 5% to 40% of pregnant and nonpregnant women. GBS is known to cause pneumonia, septicemia, and neonatal meningitis. In pregnant women, colonization of the mammary glands with *S. agalactiae* can result in mastitis. In nonpregnant adults, GBS is also responsible for cases of sepsis and soft tissue infections. With few exceptions, persistent GBS infections are uncommon.

Neonatal disease due to GBS. Neonates develop GBS infection as a result of the birthing process. Neonatal infection is divided into early-onset and late-onset disease. Early-onset infection occurs during the first 6 days of life, and the infant is generally exposed to *S. agalactiae* before or during passage through the birth canal, but infection is believed to be caused by the ascending movement of the bacterium from the vagina through the ruptured membranes into the amniotic fluid. In the amniotic fluid, GBS multiply and later colonize the fetus' respiratory tract. As a result, the neonate can develop pneumonia. If the bacteria enter the bloodstream, septicemia can result; moreover, if the bacteria are able to penetrate the tissue, meningitis and osteomyelitis may occur. The mortality rate is 10 percent for early-onset infections (74). Serotype Ia accounts for 35 to 40% of early onset disease, while types III and V account for less (63, 94).

Late-onset neonatal GBS infection takes place approximately 7 to 90 days following birth. It is typically less common than early-onset disease. Complications of this infection include meningitis and bacteremia, and the mortality rate is lower (2 to 6 percent). Neonatal GBS sepsis is an acute disease, but morbidity due to GBS infection is high. Approximately 50% of infants who survive infection may suffer from neurological sequelae, cortical blindness, deafness, uncontrolled seizures, hydrocephalus, hearing loss, and speech and language delay (60, 128).

Skin and soft tissue infections. Nonpregnant individuals with GBS infection are likely to have skin and soft tissue infections, such as foot and decubitus ulcers, cellulitis, abscesses, and balanitis (an infection of the penis). Cellulitis is the most commonly seen GBS skin infection. In women with GBS colonization, thigh cellulitis following sexual intercourse and postcoital streptococcal sepsis can occur.

Puerperal sepsis or postpartum endometritis. Although rare, puerperal sepsis typically occurs within 12 hours of delivery. Preterm labor, internal fetal monitoring, frequent cervical examinations, and premature rupture of membranes are definite risk factors for postpartum endometritis and puerperal sepsis. Prenatal GBS screening is an important tool in preventing neonatal and puerperal sepsis (132).

IE. GBS was once a rare cause of acute mitral valve IE in the pregnant female during the preantibiotic era, but the last several decades have seen a steady increase in GBS IE. This increase is attributed to an aging population and the decline in the mortality rate of patients with underlying chronic disease. GBS IE typically affects older men and women with underlying chronic disease and involves primarily the mitral and aortic valves. GBS IE has an associated mortality rate exceeding 40% (104).

GBS IE is typically characterized by acute onset, the presence of large, friable vegetations on the heart valve, rapid valvular destruction, and frequent development of complications. Chronic complications include heart failure, emboli, septic shock, ophthalmitis, pneumonia, renal failure, and gastrointestinal bleeding. A novel insertion sequence in the hyaluronidase gene has been identified predominantly in GBS strains associated with IE (58).

Rollán and colleagues hypothesized that the acute onset, the size of vegetation, the destruction of valves, and the rate of complications are indicative of the aggressive nature of *S. agalactiae* (120). Although strains of *S. agalactiae* are generally susceptible to penicillin, an aminoglycoside is occasionally used for synergy in severe infections, e.g., meningitis or endocarditis. Surgical management of damaged valves is occasionally required (5).

Recurrent infection occurs in approximately 4% of adults surviving a bacteremic episode (62). Time to relapse with the same strain is typically much shorter (~14 weeks) than the time to a new infection with a different strain (mean of 43 weeks); many of these patients present with focal infections, such as osteomyelitis or endocarditis, at the time of relapse. Although serotype-specific antibody may be present, defects in other aspects of the host immune system may be present but are not well understood at this time. Inadequate dosage and inadequate duration of therapy are associated with relapse. Furthermore, high-dose penicillin may not eliminate mucous membrane colonization with GBS, leaving a potential source for recurrence (9).

Alpha-Hemolytic Streptococci

Streptococcus pneumoniae

Microbiological capacity for complicated infections. *Streptococcus pneumoniae* is a gram-positive, catalase-negative coccus that produces pneumolysin, which breaks down hemoglobin into a green pigment which is responsible for the zone surrounding colonies on blood agar plates. These alpha-hemolytic isolates are distinguished in the clinical laboratory from viridans group streptococci (VGS) by their susceptibility to optochin and solubility in bile salts. Most clinical isolates possess a polysaccharide capsule. Ninety serotypes have been identified on the basis of capsular antigenic differences. As with other streptococci, peptidoglycan and teichoic acid are the principal constituents of the pneumococcal cell wall.

Pneumolysin is one of the main, noncapsular virulence factors of pneumococcus. It is a thiol-activated toxin that inserts into the lipid bilayer of the cell membrane by interaction with cholesterol. Pneumolysin causes inflammation by activation complement and stimulating the release of tumor necrosis factor alpha (TNF-α) and interleukin-1 (IL-1) (121, 122). Several studies have shown that pneumolysin is cytotoxic to phagocytic cells as well as respiratory epithelial cells. Pneumolysin injection into rat lung was found to cause all the histologic findings of pneumonia (41). Immunization with pneumolysin prior to injection showed a significant decrease in virulence (1).

To cause disease, the pneumococci must adhere to human cells, replicate, and disseminate. Furthermore, they must avoid phagocytosis and damage tissue either directly or indirectly. Adherence is achieved principally through bacterial surface adhesins, such as pneumococcal surface adhesin A and choline-binding protein, and epithelial cell receptors (30). When culturing pneumococcus in vitro, transparent and opaque colonies of the organism can be found. Transparent colonies produce more adhesins, which allow for persistence in animal models. However, when opaque colonies are inoculated intraperitoneally, these colonies prove to be lethal, while transparent colonies are less likely to be deadly. It is believed that increased capsule production by opaque colonies may account for this lethal characteristic (153).

The capsule of *S. pneumoniae* plays a major role in the pathogenesis of this organism. When introduced to the host, *S. pneumoniae* evades ingestion and killing by the host's immune cells–phagocytes, polymorphonuclear leukocytes, and macrophages. Possible mechanisms for evasion of the immune system include the absence of receptors on phagocytic cells that recognize capsular polysaccharides, the presence of electrochemical forces that repel phagocytic cells, and the inactivation of the complement cascade (2).

Anticapsular antibody in humans has been found to be protective against pneumococcal infection. However, in the preantibiotic era, some individuals had the ability to recover from a pneumococcal infection without producing significant amounts of anticapsular antibody. Many adults cannot produce antibody to the pneumococcal capsule, yet they can live a life free from pneumococcus. The mechanism for decreased anticapsular antibody is not known, but many believe that IgG antibody in these individuals is less avid for the capsule (106).

It is important to note that many strains of pneumococcus are becoming increasingly resistant to penicillin and other beta-lactams due to the decreased affinity of their membrane-bound penicillin-binding proteins (48).

Factors that predispose to pneumococcal infection. Protection against infection relies heavily on components of humoral immunity, such as type-specific antibody, complement, and phagocytic cells. Several conditions can predispose individuals to infection with *S. pneumoniae*. Defective antibody formation, congenital or acquired, has the greatest impact on susceptibility to pneumococcal infection. Patients with acquired agammaglobulinemia (common variable immunodeficiency) are at a higher risk of developing infection from *S. pneumoniae*. Higher rates of pneumococcal infection have been found in those with IgG subclass deficiency and individuals with homozygous expression of the R131 allele of the FCγII receptor on polymorphonuclear leukocytes. Defective antibody production plays a major role in pneumococcus in individuals infected with human immunodeficiency virus (HIV). As CD4 lymphocytes decrease below $500/mm^3$ in HIV patients, their ability to make antibodies to pneumococcal capsular polysaccharides decreases rapidly as well. The incidence of pneumococcal bacteremia in HIV-infected individuals is approximately 10 per 1,000 per year (33, 72, 119, 125, 144, 160).

Pneumococcal infection is also more prevalent in people with multiple myeloma, lymphoma, and chronic lymphocytic leukemia. Individuals with neutropenia are prone to develop an infection from *S. pneumoniae*. Defects in the complement pathway factors, C3b, C6, C7, C8, or C9, are associated with increased susceptibility to pneumococcus. Previous hospitalization, cold exposure, stress, and infection with a prior viral illness can also predispose individuals to pneumococcal infections (42, 81, 127).

Clinical presentation. *S. pneumoniae* is a major cause of pneumonia as well as many other types of infections, such as otitis media (in children), meningitis (in adults), acute sinusitis, osteomyelitis, and sepsis. *S. pneumoniae* can also be the inciting cause of IE, pericarditis, and meningitis. It is commonly found in the nasopharynx of children and adults. Pneumonia develops if *S. pneumoniae* is aspirated into the lungs and not cleared. While in the lungs, the bacteria activate the complement complex stimulating cytokine production. White blood cells are then recruited to these areas to initiate phagocytosis of the organisms. However, the bacterium's polysaccharide capsule can protect it from macrophages, and, as a consequence, they can then enter the bloodstream. This can result in bacteremia. If the bacteria reach the meninges, joint spaces, bones, or peritoneal cavity, a patient can develop meningitis, brain abscesses, septic arthritis, or osteomyelitis. It is important to know that *S. pneumoniae* can cause suppurative infections in most areas of the body, and these can follow pneumococcal bacteremia or occur simultaneously with it. In the preantibiotic era, the pneumococcus was responsible for up to 10% of IE, but in the most recent global surveillance programs it accounts for less than 1%. When IE does occur, it is usually a fulminant presentation with high mortality.

Suppurative complications. Suppurative complications of *S. pneumoniae* infections include necrotizing pneumonia and empyema. Empyema, the most common complication of pneumococcal pneumonia in the preantibiotic era, occurred in about 5% of cases then and remains the most common at present (~2%) (92). Persistence of fever and leukocytosis after treatment is suggestive of empyema. Overall mortality for individuals with pneumococcal bacteremia is between 15 and 20 percent. These patients have the highest risk of dying within the first 72 hours after a positive pneumococcal blood culture (75).

VGS

VGS primarily reside in the respiratory and gastrointestinal tract as commensal organisms; however, on occasion they can invade and cause severe life-threatening infections that can be difficult to eradicate. Catheters, prosthetic material, and damaged valves provide hospitable conditions for VGS.

Capacity for complicated infection

VGS include primarily alpha-hemolytic and nonhemolytic bacteria and are typically not evaluated for a Lancefield designation. They consist of the normal flora of the gastrointestinal tract and are also located in the nasopharynx and gingival crevices. VGS can be differentiated from *S. pneumoniae* by resistance to optochin and lack of bile solubility. In culture, VGS can appear as spherical or ovoid cells and form chains or pairs. VGS are nonmotile and non-spore-forming organisms.

Though the taxonomic changes have been numerous, current species of VGS are typically assigned to one of the following groups: the anginosus group (*Streptococcus anginosus, S. constellatus,* and *S.* intermedius), the mitis group (*S. sanguis, S. parasanguis, S. gordonii, S. crista, S. infantis, S. mitis, S. oralis,* and *S. peroris*), the mutans group (*S. criceti, S. downei, S. macacae, S. mutans, S. rattus,* and *S. sobrinus*), and the salivarius group (*S. salivarius, S. thermophilus,* and *S. vestibularis*) (40).

VGS are bacteria of low virulence and do not possess endotoxins or elaborate exotoxins. Their pathogenicity is best exemplified by their ability to cause dental caries and IE.

S. mutans is the main causative agent of dental caries. The main virulence factors associated with the development of caries include adhesion, acidogenicity, and acid tolerance. The bacterium has the ability to bind to teeth and ferment sugar, leading to the production of acid and inducing cavities. It is believed that sucrose-independent adhesion of *S. mutans* is mainly influenced by two factors: glucosyltransferases (encoded by *gtfB, gtfC,* and *gtfD*) and antigenI/II, which is a 185-kDa surface protein (8). If *S. mutans* is introduced to the bloodstream during a dental procedure, it can travel into the bloodstream and attach itself on the endocardial surface of the heart.

VGS are now the second leading cause of IE in the developed world and remain the major cause of IE in children. Approximately 30 to 40 percent of cases of endocarditis are due to VGS, and greater than 80% of patients have underlying heart disease (80). A recent survey of endocarditis patients showed that 86% of the 607 clinical isolates were VGS, and four main species (*S. mutans, S. sanguis, S. mitis,* and *S. salivarius*) accounted for over two-thirds of isolates. However, the epidemiology of species-specific association with IE is subject to the limitations of phenotypic characterization. The ICE consortium has provided a unique opportunity to evaluate a large number of VGS isolates from patients with definite endocarditis from diverse geographic regions. Molecular characterization with sequencing of *rpoB, tuf,* and 16S sequences substantially improved identification compared with automated conventional methodology, which failed to classify the salivarius, anginosus, and gordonii groups correctly. Mitis group were the most commonly isolated VGS from patients with definite endocarditis. Interestingly, Anginosus group streptococci were infrequent (136).

A unique feature of subacute IE is the formation of the endocarditic plaque. This formation involves bacteria, platelets, coagulation factors, and leukocytes, and it is also regarded as a special kind of biofilm. The adherence of VGS to this nonbacterial thrombotic endocarditis is associated with production of an extracellular polysaccharide, dextran. The relative chance of IE among patients with bacteremia is much higher with dextran-producing organisms (113). Non-dextran-producing streptococci may produce IE in humans and adhere to artificial fibrin-platelet surfaces in vitro, which suggests that other characteristics are required.

FimA is a 36-kD protein that functions as a surface adhesin in IE when expressed by VGS. Homologues of the *fim*A gene are widely distributed among clinical strains of VGS and enterococci. Streptococcal mutants with the *fim*A gene inactivated exhibit a decrease in virulence in experimental IE.(95). Also, low fibronectin-binding mutants of *S. sanguis* have decreased ability to produce IE. Laminin-binding proteins found in *S. gordonii* have been found on the cell walls of organisms recovered from patients with IE, and the level of protein expression seemed to be regulated by the presence of dextrans. Other studies have shown the importance of platelet aggregation by *S. sanguis*, which adheres by protease-sensitive components and not extracellular matrix proteins. Platelet aggregation induced by *S. sanguis* in vivo seems to be an important virulence determinant of vegetation development and disease progression.

S. bovis strains are Lancefield group D positive, nonoral VGS that are generally found in the gastrointestinal tract of humans and many animal species. *S. bovis* has several subclasses: biotypes I and II (*S. salivarius*, *S. macedonius*, *S. galalolyticus*, and *S. infantarius*). Biotype I is more frequently associated with both bacteremia and endocarditis (67, 123). An association between *S. bovis* bacteremia and gastrointestinal malignancy is well described (82). The clinical course of *S. bovis* endocarditis is subacute and indistinguishable from VGS IE. *S. bovis* also has some unique regional distribution, including substantial increases in France and southern Europe (56). However, the epidemiology remains poorly understood.

Most strains of *VGS* and *S. bovis* are extremely sensitive to beta-lactams, and bacteremia can be treated with penicillin alone. However, because of biofilm, penicillin tolerance, and the altered metabolic state of VGS in the biofilm, endocarditis is difficult to treat and remains associated with considerable mortality, and the addition of an aminoglycoside is considered appropriate. Treatment of most VGS and *S. bovis* cases of IE with an MIC more than 0.2 ug/ml and less than 0.5ug/ml includes penicillin G with low-dose gentamicin (3mg/kg/day) (6, 118).

STAPHYLOCOCCUS

The genus *Staphylococcus* includes 32 species that belong to the order *Bacillales* and the family *Staphylococcaceae*. Ubiquitous colonizers of the skin and mucosa of most animals, the staphylococci are gram-positive cocci found singly, in pairs, or in grape-like clusters. They are nonmotile and catalase positive. Of the 16 staphylococcal species found in or on humans, only a few are pathogenic in the absence of predisposing conditions, such as immunosuppression or the presence of a foreign body. The more virulent *S. aureus* is coagulase positive, and this characteristic differentiates if in clinical microbiology laboratories.

S. aureus

S. aureus is a leading cause of bacteremia (152) and endocarditis (47) in the developed world. The increased incidence of bacteremia in the setting of prosthetic material and the rise of antibiotic resistance rates have alerted clinicians of the importance of this reemergent infection.

Capacity for complicated infection

S. aureus produces sophisticated anti-inflammatory molecules, and it employs several mechanisms protecting the bacteria against host cationic antimicrobial molecules, such as defensin-like peptides, and bacteriolytic enzymes, such as lysozymes. Cell wall teichoic acids and lipoteichoic acids, complex gram-positive surface polymers, and modified membrane lipids, such as lysylphosphatidylglycerol are crucial in defensin resistance and other important aspects of staphylococcal virulence, such as nasal colonization and biofilm formation on biomaterials.

Nasal carriage of *S. aureus* varies from 10% to 40% in both the community and the hospital environment (84). Nasal carriage is a means of spread and persistence of multidrug-resistant staphylococci, especially methicillin-resistant *S. aureus* (MRSA). Persistent carriage is associated with high risk for recurrent furunculosis and infections in susceptible populations, especially patients receiving renal replacement therapy or patients undergoing surgical procedures (19, 87, 149).

S. aureus uses highly efficient mechanisms, including surface factors and secreted proteins, to evade recognition and elimination by the innate immune system. In addition, *S. aureus* is equipped with regulatory systems that govern the microbial response to environmental stressors. Among these regulatory systems, the accessory gene regulator (*agr*) acts as a quorum-sensing control, allowing differential expression of surface adhesins (exponential) and exoproteins (stationary) during different growth phases. Inactivation of *agr* decreases pathogenicity in animal and tissue models when exoprotein expression is important but has little effect on endocarditis models in which adhesin expression is more critical for valve attachment (24, 111). There are at least four *agr* groups in *S. aureus*. Epidemiological studies have linked these groups with other markers of virulence. For example, group II is associated with vancomycin-intermediate strains, and toxic shock syndrome toxin and Panton-Valentine leukocidin are produced primarily by group III. ETA-producing strains are found to have group IV *agr*.

As with regulatory elements, *S. aureus* possesses a number of adhesins that allow adherence to a variety of host proteins. The microbial surface component reacting with MSCRAMM applies to these adhesins. More than 20 putative MSCRAMMs for *S. aureus* have been evaluated. Clumping factor A (*clf*A) and fibronectin-binding protein A (FnBPA) are associated with endocarditis, collagen-binding protein is associated with septic arthritis, protein A is an antiphagocytic factor in septic arthritis, and the extracellular adherence protein (EAP) is a T-cell immunomodulator (89, 114, 115, 117).

Persistent infection is heavily mediated by the ability to elaborate biofilm. Biofilm-producing staphylococci are described primarily as coagulase-negative staphylococci (CoNS), and they are implicated in colonization and persistence on catheters and other prosthetic materials. Polysaccharide intercellular adhesin (PIA) is elaborated by the organisms after adherence to materials. PIA is synthesized by an operon called *ica*. *S. aureus* possesses an *ica* homologue that confers the ability to produce biofilm (66). The relative importance of biofilms in comparison to MSCRAMMs in adherence and persistence is unknown at this time (28).

S. aureus strains have developed resistance mechanisms to virtually all known classes of antimicrobials. The emergence of methicillin-resistant clones, first in healthcare settings and subsequently in the community, highlights the important role of resistance in terms of public health. Methicillin resistance in *S. aureus* is conferred by a pathogenicity (or genomic) island, SCC*mec*. SCC stands for staphylococcal cassette chromosome, and *mec* is the genetic element which codes for methicillin resistance. The sizes of SCC*mec* can vary between 15 to 60kb, and SCC*mec* is virtually absent in methicillin-sensitive *S. aureus*. *mecA* mediates beta-lactam resistance and encodes the penicillin-binding protein, PBP2A. PBP2A is known to have a low affinity for methicillin and most beta-lactams, and this protein is primarily responsible for the intrinsic resistance of MRSA to beta-lactams (20, 71, 77).

Just as serious is the emergence of glycopeptide resistance at both intermediate and high levels. Intermediate resistance to glycopeptides has been reported in several developed countries. Chromosomal changes affecting the peptidoglycan wall are responsible for this reduced susceptibility, which has been associated with certain *agr* types (II), as mentioned above. Although associated with persistent MRSA bacteremia and clinical failures, glycopeptide-intermediate *S. aureus* can be hard to detect in the clinical laboratory. This is partly because of a heterogeneous phenotype. Population analysis profiles confirming heterogeneous GISA have recently associated it with persistent bacteremia in patients with MRSA endocarditis. Full vancomycin resistance (MIC, >32 mg/ml) in *S. aureus*, conferred by *vanA* acquired from vancomycin-resistant enterococci, has been achieved in the laboratory and has occurred naturally among human clinical isolates (23, 110).

Incidence of *S. aureus* bacteremia

In a review of 750 million hospitalizations in the United States from 1979 to 2000, Martin and colleagues identified 10.3 million cases of sepsis. The overall rate of sepsis increased from 82.7 to 240.4 cases per 100,000 population. Gram-positive organisms became the predominant organism in 1987 (100). A series of studies in the United States and throughout Europe supports the emergence of *S. aureus* as the leading cause of bacteremia (52, 152, 158). *S. aureus* bacteremia has typically been classified into two categories: hospital acquired (nosocomial) and community acquired. A third category of healthcare-associated bacteremia has generally been accepted now (51).

A major contributing factor to the increasing frequency of *S. aureus* bacteremia has been the progress of medical therapies and the evolution of medical interventions. This trend is due largely to increasing use of intravascular catheters and subsequent catheter-associated staphylococcal bacteremia (70). The expanding use of invasive procedures, prosthetic devices, and long-term intravascular catheters has resulted in a large population of outpatients at risk for staphylococcal bloodstream infections. The shift of acute medical care to the outpatient setting has muddled the differentiation of community-onset and hospital-acquired infection. For example, one recent analysis found that intravascular devices accounted for 22% of episodes of community-acquired *S. aureus* bacteremia (141).

Complications and risks of *S. aureus* bacteremia. In the preantibiotic era, *S. aureus* bacteremia was generally a fatal disease, with a case-fatality rate exceeding 80% (137). In the antibiotic era, *S. aureus* bacteremia remains a serious disease. One in four patients will die with or because of their *S. aureus* bacteremia (48). Furthermore, one in three *S. aureus* bacteremia patients will develop one or more acute systemic complications: septic shock, acute respiratory distress syndrome, or disseminated intravascular complications (45, 96). In addition to the acute complications that typically occur in the first 48 hours of bacteremia, localized complications may occur from hematogenous seeding or direct extension from an adjacent site of existing infection. Although endocarditis is the most important of the hematogenous complications, any organ system or prosthetic material may be involved. Complications may be evident at the time of presentation or may become apparent only during or after completion of an inadequate therapeutic regimen.

Risk factors for the development of complications of *S. aureus* bacteremia vary depending upon the route of acquisition, site of infection, presence or absence of foreign material, pathogen characteristics, and host predisposition. For instance, for patients on hemodialysis, the presence of a long-term catheter or a noncatheter device and infection with MRSA are each independently associated with complicated bacteremia (45).

Patients with community-acquired *S. aureus* bacteremia have an increased risk for metastatic complications (43, 48, 70, 88). For example, a retrospective survey of 281 cases of *S. aureus* bacteremia occurring over a 7-year period found that metastatic complications were significantly more common among patients with community-acquired rather than hospital-acquired bacteremia (43 versus 21 percent) (48). This association was confirmed in a prospective study of 113 patients with community-acquired *S. aureus* bacteremia and no history of injection drug use. Metastatic complications occurred in 90 percent of the patients (156). The explanation for this finding is not clear but could be attributed to delays in presentation and diagnosis. Importantly, these studies were performed prior to the widespread prevalence of community-acquired MRSA, and thus further investigation is needed to determine whether the propensity for metastatic complications is also seen with community-acquired MRSA strains.

Endocarditis. IE is a common and often devastating complication of *S. aureus* bacteremia. Acute IE occurs in all age groups, but it is highest in individuals more than 40 years of age. The incidence of endocarditis ranges from 10 to 13 percent in prospective, observational studies of adults and children (21, 48, 145). The risk of IE in patients with *S. aureus* bacteremia depends upon a variety of clinical factors, such as predisposing cardiac abnormalities, intravenous drug use, community-acquired bacteremia, osteomyelitis, and skin and soft tissue infections. The risk of IE is even higher in patients with a prosthetic heart valve.

For decades, IE caused by *S. aureus* has been viewed primarily as a community-acquired disease, especially with injection drug use. In contrast, patients with healthcare- or intravascular catheter-associated *S. aureus* bacteremia were considered to be at low risk for IE. *S. aureus* IE is relatively infrequent at any individual medical institution, and observations of its characteristics were previously based primarily upon relatively small samples. However, in a recent series of prospectively identified cases of *S. aureus* IE, approximately 70% of cases were healthcare associated and 39% had a presumed intravenous catheter source (49). *S. aureus* infection rates, especially bacteremia associated with healthcare contact, have increased in hospitalized patients. In fact, healthcare-associated IE has become the most common form of *S. aureus* IE. As a result, MRSA has taken prominence as a common cause of IE, and it is associated with persistent bacteremia.

Prosthetic devices. The presence of an indwelling foreign body is often both the source for staphylococcal bacteremia and an important risk factor for a complicated course. As a result, the morbidity of *S. aureus* bacteremia for patients with indwelling prostheses is significant (26). Prosthetic devices can become contaminated with staphylococci at the time of insertion or due to contiguous spread of infection or through hematogenous seeding at the time of *S. aureus* bacteremia. Once inoculated on or into a prosthetic device, *S. aureus* biofilms rapidly adapt and become highly resistant to antimicrobial therapy. Removal of the prosthesis is usually necessary for cure.

Hematogenous (metastatic) complications. Metastatic infection other than IE and prosthetic device infection via biofilms can occur in patients with *S. aureus* bacteremia. As many as 31% of these patients develop one or more metastatic infections due to *S. aureus* (70). These sites of infection are evident within the first 48 to 72 hours of hospitalization in many patients, but in some patients, metastatic seeding may not be discovered for several weeks. Demonstration of localized symptoms, such as back or joint pain should raise the suspicion of an occult site of infection in every patient with a recent history of *S. aureus* bacteremia. Common sites of metastatic disease include joints (36%), kidneys (29%), central nervous system (28%), skin (16%), the liver and spleen (13%), and bone (11%). Over half of patients with complications will have involvement of more than one site.

Hematogenous spread of *S. aureus* can result in various complications, such as vertebral osteomyelitis, septic arthritis, splenic abscesses, thrombophlebitis, meningitis, pulmonary embolism (secondary to tricuspid valve endocarditis), and bacteriuria. These diagnoses should be considered in patients with persisting fevers and/or bacteremia despite appropriate antibiotic therapy.

The most important predictors of complicated *S. aureus* infection include persistent fever or bacteremia (45, 79). Although a variety of clinical characteristics, such as skin findings, are also associated with metastatic complications among patients with *S. aureus* bacteremia, the absence of these characteristics does not ensure the absence of risk for localized disease.

Complexities of *S. aureus* bacteremia. *Prosthetic devices.* Many studies demonstrate the presence of a permanent foreign body as an independent predictor of metastatic complications following *S. aureus* bacteremia. This is true for both long-term catheters (which are potential portals of entry into the bloodstream for infecting bacteria) and noncatheter devices (which can serve as a focus for hematogenous spread). Patients with permanent pacemakers or implantable cardioverter defibrillators who develop *S. aureus* bacteremia are also at increased risk for IE or infection involving the cardiac device. In addition to device infection around the time of *S. aureus* bacteremia, the presence of prosthetic material is an important risk factor for subsequent relapsing infection (21). For example, the presence of an indwelling foreign body was the single greatest predictor of subsequent relapse among 309 prospectively identified cases of *S. aureus* bacteremia (46).

Antibiotic resistance. The steady increase of MRSA in hospitals further complicates the approach to *S. aureus* bacteremia. The past decade has seen a significant rise in rates of MRSA. Over 50% of *S. aureus* isolates from intensive-care units reported to the NNIS in 1999 were methicillin resistant, a 43% increase compared to the period of 1994 to 1998 (109). Approximately 30% of *S. aureus* bloodstream isolates in the United States are now methicillin resistant. Both widespread antibiotic use and poor adherence to infection control precautions have contributed to the rise in MRSA infection rates. The evidence regarding outcomes with MRSA bacteremia compared to those of methicillin-sensitive *S. aureus* (MSSA) bacteremia is unclear (27, 61, 107). However, some reports suggest that the genetic complement of MRSA isolates may produce a more virulent phenotype.

It is also possible that MRSA-infected patients have higher rates of complication because of treatment with vancomycin, which has been associated with high rates of clinical failure (138), prolonged bacteremia (91), and relapse (22, 46, 64). The past decade has witnessed the first clinical isolates of *S. aureus* with reduced susceptibility to vancomycin. Most of the patients were hemodialysis dependent and had deep-tissue or prosthetic device MRSA infections treated with prolonged courses of vancomycin (50).

Treatment of *S. aureus* bacteremia. The most important aspect in the treatment of *S. aureus* bacteremia is determining the extent of infection. The availability of antibiotics active against *S. aureus* raises the question of duration of treatment. A number of factors influence the duration of therapy. Of primary consideration is the presence of a removable focus of infection, such as an intravascular device. Although the prompt removal of a catheter may not prevent complications such as endocarditis (151), a number of studies have shown that only a minority of patients with catheter-associated *S. aureus* bacteremia (17% to 18%) (38, 99) can be cured with antimicrobial therapy if the catheter is not removed.

Patients with *S. aureus* bacteremia arising from a deep focus of infection, such as vertebral osteomyelitis or deep tissue abscess, are highly likely to experience a relapse of their staphylococcal infection if a short course of therapy is provided. Furthermore, the presence of a deep focus of infection is highly predictive of relapse, even with more prolonged antibiotic treatment (21, 46).

The optimal therapy for methicillin-sensitive *S. aureus* bacteremia remains the intravenous administration of a beta-lactam agent, such as nafcillin or a first-generation cephalosporin, such as cefazolin. These drugs are both bactericidal and virtually safe. For patients with MRSA infection, regardless of whether it is community acquired or not, and patients with a history of anaphylaxis to beta-lactam agents, vancomycin is the preferred therapy. However, daptomycin has recently been demonstrated to be comparable to vancomycin in a noninferiority trial for bacteremia and right-sided IE (44). Trimethroprim-sulfamethoxazole, clindamycin, minocycline, ciprofloxacin, and newer fluoroquinolones have all been used as treatment for staphylococcal infections, but all of these agents are presumed to be less effective than vancomycin and beta-lactam therapy. These alternative regimens should be used only in certain situations. Neither quinupristin-dalfopristin or linezolid are FDA approved for the treatment of *S. aureus* bacteremia.

CoNS

CoNS are generally considered to be microorganisms with low virulence for humans. However, recent evidence supports their emerging importance as true pathogens, largely as a result of medical progress at the end of the 20th century. Most infections are associated with foreign material, primarily intravenous catheters or prosthetic joints and valves. Persistent or chronic infections are common and result from the capacity to elaborate biofilm and through diverse resistance mechanisms.

Capacity for complicated infections

The group of CoNS is comprised of more than 40 species, but identification at the species level typically does not take place in the clinical laboratory

(65). However, there is growing evidence that species-level identification may alter diagnostic and therapeutic clinical decision-making. *Staphylococcus epidermidis* is the most prevalent species on human skin and mucous membranes and as a result is the most commonly retrieved specimen from clinical specimens (83).

Persistence of CoNS is primarily associated with their ability to derive and live in a biofilm on plastic surfaces. Clusters of cells elaborate and reside in an exopolysaccharide matrix. The polysaccharide (PIA) is encoded by a gene cluster, *ica*, in most CoNS species, and mutants are unable to successfully persist in animal models (66, 69). The biofilm protects embedded organisms from phagocytic cells and reduces their accessibility to antimicrobial agents. Their virulence factors are unclear, but it is believed that bacterial polysaccharide components are involved in the attachment of bacteria. While genes for toxins that are more commonly found in *S. aureus* may be found in some CoNS species, they are uncommon in *S. epidermidis* and rarely associated with disease. *S. epidermidis* has been shown to regulate its response to human antimicrobial peptides and to produce a number of factors that help protect the pathogen from the lethal effect of the peptides (102).

CoNS from healthcare-associated infections, particularly *S. epidermidis* and *Staphylococcus haemolyticus*, are highly resistant to multiple antibiotics, including methicillin. The high frequency of heterotypic resistance to methicillin confounds the detection of reduced susceptibility, which may lead to inappropriate antimicrobial regimens, but estimates approach 80% resistance (3). The methicillin resistance genes (*mecA*) are identical in *S. aureus* and *S. epidermidis*. A higher percentage of clinically significant clones contain SCC*mec* type IV (159). The emergence of vancomycin resistance and heteroresistance is increasingly important in the treatment of CoNS infections. There have been several case reports documenting CoNS with reduced susceptibility to vancomycin (126, 129, 147).

Glycopeptide resistance appears to be due to heteroresistant subpopulations of staphylococci. The mechanism of this resistance is believed to be associated with alterations in cell wall metabolism, especially cell wall thickening. Several CoNS strains have demonstrated increased cell wall thickness as well as heterogenous resistance to vancomycin (29, 59, 112, 134, 135).

Clinical presentation. CoNS are important causes of healthcare-associated infections. Community-acquired infections, such as native valve endocarditis, remain the exception. The types of infections are as variable as the medical procedures that they complicate. These include catheter and ventriculo-peritoneal shunt infections, urinary tract infections, prosthetic joint infections, and ocular infections.

Catheter-associated infections. Maki et al. concluded that all types of intravascular catheters pose differing but significant risks of developing bloodstream infections (97). Several investigations report that from 12% to 37% of all inserted catheters become infected, but most would acknowledge that all become infected eventually. *S. epidermidis* is the single most common organism infecting intravenous catheters (98). Of those infected catheters, *S. epidermidis* accounted for 50% to 75% of cultures isolated (16). Not only has there been an increase in the incidence of catheter-associated infections in hospital patients, but there has also been an increase in the incidence of catheter-associated bacteremia due to *S. epidermidis*. Patients with a catheter-associated infection due to *S. epidermidis* may have positive blood cultures but may not appear clinically ill. Infected sites may not display purulence or erythema, and bacteremia may occur with few symptoms (103, 157). Severe complications of catheter-related *S. epidermidis* bacteremia are of particular concern for immunocompromised patients, as CoNS can be a lethal pathogen in neutropenic patients.

IE. CoNS are increasingly important causes of community- and healthcare-associated IE (25, 85, 124). An international collection of isolates from patients with both prosthetic and native valve IE confirmed that *S. epidermidis* is the most common species in IE, followed by *Staphylococcus lugdunensis*, *S. hominis*, and *S. capitis* (116). A recent study investigated the relative virulence of isolates from patients with native valve endocarditis in comparison with the virulence of those from patients with prosthetic valve disease, using a *Caenorhabditis elegans* model (102). The difference in virulence levels does not appear to be associated with excess exopolysaccharide, which is the major component of CoNS biofilms. CoNS are the most common cause of bacteremia related to indwelling devices. CoNS can cause several other infections: central nervous system shunt infections, native or prosthetic valve endocarditis, urinary tract infections, and endophthalmitis. CoNS have become increasingly resistant to antibiotics.

Treatment. Methicillin and oxacillin were historically regarded as first-line treatment for CoNS infections. However, the acknowledgment of heterotypic methicillin resistance and the high prevalence of the *mec*A gene have resulted in the primary use of vancomycin for most true infections. Antimicrobials to which most CoNS remain susceptible include vancomycin, rifampin, and a number of the new gram-positive agents, including daptomycin. However, more recently, there has been an increase in the rate of vancomycin resistance in staphylococci (68, 116). Vancomycin and rifampin remain the mainstay of treatment of invasive CoNS foreign-body infections, but inducible resistance during therapy can limit the effectiveness of rifampin. Ultimately, most experts acknowledge that without removal of the offending device in prosthetic infections, the antimicrobial treatment will fail. If a device cannot be removed, then suppressive antibiotic therapy should be considered.

CONCLUSIONS

The gram-positive cocci possess a diverse variety of mechanisms for establishing and maintaining infection in the human host and for turning the host against itself. In addition to adhesins, biofilm, and resistance mutations, these organisms capitalize on immunological voids in their host and the presence of nonbiological materials to persist. Eradication of these bacteria is extremely difficult in the presence of foreign material, and its extraction is usually required.

REFERENCES

1. **Alexander, J. E., R. A. Lock, C. C. Peeters, J. T. Poolman, P. W. Andrew, T. J. Mitchell, D. Hansman and J. C. Paton.** 1994. Immunization of mice with pneumolysin toxoid confers a significant degree of protection against at least nine serotypes of *Streptococcus pneumoniae. Infect. Immun.* **62:**5683–5688.
2. **Angel, C. S., M. Ruzek, and M. K. Hostetter.** 1994. Degradation of C3 by *Streptococcus pneumoniae. J. Infect. Dis.* **170:**600–608.
3. **Archer, G. L., and M. W. Climo.** 1994. Antimicrobial susceptibility of coagulase-negative staphylococci. *Antimicrob. Agents Chemother.* **38:**2231–2237.
4. **Ayoub, E. M., D. J. Barrett, N. K. Maclaren, and J. P. Krischer.** 1986. Association of class II human histocompatibility leukocyte antigens with rheumatic fever. *J. Clin. Investig.* **77:**2019–2026.
5. **Azzam, Z. S., Y. Ron, I. Oren, W. Sbeit, D. Motlak, and N. Krivoy.** 1998. Group B streptococcal tricuspid valve endocarditis: a case report and review of literature. *Int. J. Cardiol.* **64:**259–263.
6. **Baddour, L.M., W. R. Wilson, A. S. Bayer, W. G. Fowler, Jr., A. F. Bolger, M. W. Levison, P. Ferrieri, M. A. Gerber, L. Y. Tani, M. H. Gewitz, D. C. Tong, J. M. Steckelberg, R. S. Baltimore, S. T. Shulman, J. C. Burns, D. A. Falace, J. W. Newburger, T. J. Pallasch, M. Takahashi, K. A.Taubert; Committee on Rheumatic Fever, Endocarditis, and Kawasaki Disease; Council on Cardiovascular Disease in the Young; Councils on Clinical Cardiology, Stroke, and Cardiovascular Surgery and Anesthesia; American Heart Association; and Infectious Diseases Society of America.** 2005. Infective endocarditis: diagnosis, antimicrobial therapy, and management of complications: a statement for healthcare professionals from the Committee on Rheumatic Fever, Endocarditis, and Kawasaki Disease, Council on Cardiovascular Disease in the Young, and the Councils on Clinical Cardiology, Stroke, and Cardiovascular Surgery and Anesthesia, American Heart Association: endorsed by the Infectious Diseases Society of America. *Circulation* **111:**e394–e434.
7. **Baltimore, R. S.** 1985. Treatment of impetigo: a review. *Pediatr. Infect. Dis.* **4:**597.
8. **Banas, J. A.** 2004. Virulence properties of *Streptococcus mutans. Front. Biosci.* **9:**1267–1277.
9. **Baker, C. J., and M. S. Edwards.** 2000. Group B streptococcal infections, p. 1091–1156. *In* J. S. Remington and J. O. Klein (ed.), *Infectious Diseases of the Fetus and Newborn Infant*, 5th ed. Saunders, Philadelphia, PA.
10. **Barnham, M., T. J. Thornton, and K. Lange.** 1983. Nephritis caused by *Streptococcus zooepidemicus* (Lancefield group C). *Lancet* **i:**945–948.
11. **Ben-Abraham, R., N. Keller, R. Vered, R. Harel, Z. Barzilay, and G. Paret.** 2002. Invasive group A streptococcal infections in a large tertiary center: epidemiology, characteristics and outcome. *Infection* **30:**81–85.
12. **Bernaldo de Quiros, J. C., S. Moreno, E. Cercenado, D. Diaz, J. Berenguer, P. Miralles, P. Catalán, and E. Bouza.** 1997. Group A streptococcal bacteremia. A 10-year prospective study. *Medicine* **76:**238–248.
13. **Bessen, D. E., L. G. Veasy, H. R. Hill, N. H. Augustine, and V. A. Fischetti.** 1995. Serologic evidence for a class I goup A streptococcal infection among rheumatic fever patients. *J. Infect. Dis.* **172:**1608–1611.
14. **Bisno, A. L.** 1990. The resurgence of acute rheumatic fever in the United States. *Annu. Rev. Med.* **41:**319–329.
15. **Botta, G. A.** 1981. Surface components in adhesion of group A streptococci to pharyngeal epithelial cells. *Curr. Microbiol.* **6:**101–104.
16. **Boyce, J.** 1997. Epidemiology and prevention of nosocomial infections, p. 309–329. *In* K. B. Crossley and G. L. Archer (ed.), *Staphylococci in Human Disease.* Churchill Livingstone, New York, NY.
17. **Bronze, M. S., and J. B. Dale.** 1996. The reemergence of serious group A streptococcal infections and acute rheumatic fever. *Am. J. Med. Sci.* **311:**41–54.
18. **Carapetis, J. R., A. C. Steer, E. K. Mulholland, and M. Weber.** 2005. The global burden of group A streptococcal diseases. *Lancet Infect. Dis.* **5:**685–694.
19. **Chambers, H. F.** 2001. The changing epidemiology of *Staphylococcus aureus*? *Emerg. Infect. Dis.* **7:**178–182.
20. **Chambers, H. F., B. J. Hartman, and A. Tomasz.** 1985. Increased amounts of a novel penicillin binding protein in a strain of methicillin-resistant *Staphylococcus aureus. J. Clin. Investig.* **76:**325–331.
21. **Chang, F. Y., B. B. MacDonald, J. E. Peacock. Jr., D. M. Musher, P. Triplett, J. M. Mylotte, A. O'Donnell, M. M. Wagener, and V. L. Yu.** 2003. A prospective multicenter study of *Staphylococcus aureus* bacteremia: incidence of endocarditis, risk factors for mortality, and clinical impact of methicillin resistance. *Medicine* (Baltimore). **82:**322–332.
22. **Chang, F. Y., J. E. Peacock, D. M. Musher, B. B. MacDonald, J. M. Mylotte, A. O'Donnell, M. M. Wagener, and V. L. Yu.** 2003. *Staphylococcus aureus* bacteremia: recurrence and the impact of antibiotic treatment in a prospective multicenter study. *Medicine* (Baltimore) **82:**333–339.
23. **Chang, S., D. M. Sievert, J. C. Hageman, M. L. Boulton, F. C. Tenover, F. P. Downes, S. Shah, J. T. Rudrik, G. R. Pupp,**

W. J. Brown, D. Cardo, S. K. Fridkin, and the Vancomycin-Resistant *Staphylococcus aureus* Investigative Team. 2003. Infection with vancomycin-resistant *Staphylococcus aureus* containing the *vanA* resistance gene. *N. Engl. J. Med.* **348:**1342–1347.

24. **Cheung, A. L., K. F. Eberhardt, E. Chung, M. R. Yeaman, P. M. Sullam, M. Ramos, and A. S. Bayer.** 1994. Diminished virulence of a *sar*⁻/*agr*⁻ mutant of *Staphylococcus aureus* in the rabbit model of endocarditis. *J. Clin. Investig.* **94:**1815–1822.
25. **Chu, V. H., C. H. Cabell, E. Abrutyn, G. R. Corey, B. Hoen, J. M. Miro, L. Olaison, M. E. Stryjewski, P. Pappas, K. J. Anstrom, S. Eykyn, G. Habib, N. Benito, V. J. Fowler, Jr., and International Collaboration on Endocarditis Merged Database Study Group.** 2004. Native valve endocarditis due to coagulase-negative staphylococci: report of 99 episodes from the International Collaboration on Endocarditis Merged Database. *Clin. Infect. Dis.* **39:**1527–1530.
26. **Chu, V. H., D. R. Crosslin, J. Y. Friedman, S. D. Reed, C. H. Cabell, R. I. Griffiths, L. E. Masselink, K. S. Kaye, G. R. Corey, L. B. Reller, M. E. Stryjewski, K. A. Schulman, and V. G. Fowler, Jr.** 2005. *Staphylococcus aureus* bacteremia in patients with prosthetic devices: costs and outcomes. *Am. J. Med.* **118:**1416.
27. **Cosgrove, S. E., G. Sakoulas, E. N. Perencevich, M. J. Schwaber, A. W. Karchmer, and Y. Carmeli.** 2003. Comparison of mortality associated with methicillin-resistant and methicillin-susceptible *Staphylococcus aureus* bacteremia: a meta analysis. *Clin. Infect. Dis.***36:**53–59.
28. **Cramton, S. E., C. Gerke, N. F. Schnell, W. W. Nichols, and F. Götz.** 1999. The intercellular adhesion (*ica*) locus is present in *Staphylococcus aureus* and is required for biofilm formation. *Infect. Immun.* **67:**5427–5433.
29. **Cui, L., X. Ma, K. Sato, K. Okuma, F. C. Tenover, E. M. Mamizuka, C. G. Gemmell, M. N. Kim, M. C. Ploy, N. El-Solh, V. Ferraz, and K. Hiramatsu.** 2003. Cell wall thickening is a common feature of vancomycin resistance in *Staphylococcus aureus*. *J. Clin. Microbiol.* **41:**5–14.
30. **Cundell, D. R., B. J. Pearce, J. Sandros, A. M. Naughton, and H. R. Masure.** 1995. Peptide permeases from *Streptococcus pneumoniae* affect adherence to eukaryotic cells. *Infect. Immun.* **63:**2493–2498.
31. **Cunningham, M. W., J. M. McCormack, P. G. Fenderson, M. K. Ho, E. H. Beachey, and J. B. Dale.** 1989. Human and murine antibodies cross-reactive with streptococcal M protein and myosin recognize the sequence GLN-LYS-SER-LYS-GLN in M protein. *J. Immunol.* **143:**2677–2683.
32. **Cunningham, M. W., J. M. McCormack, L. R. Talaber, J. B. Harley, E. M. Ayoub, R. S. Muneer, L. T. Chun, and D. V. Reddy.** 1988. Human monoclonal antibodies reactive with antigens of the group A *Streptococcus* and human heart. *J. Immunol.* **141:**2760.
33. **Cunningham-Rundles, C.** 1989. Clinical and immunologic analyses of 103 patients with common variable immunodeficiency. *J. Clin. Immunol.* **9:**22–33.
34. **Dajani, A. S., E. Ayoub, F. Z. Bierman, A. L. Bisno, F. W. Denny, D. T. Durack P. Ferrieri, M. Freed, M. Gerber, E. L. Kaplan, A. W. Karchme, M. Markowitz, S. H. Rahimtoola, S. T. Shulman G. Stollerman, M. Takahashi, A. Taranta, K. A. Taubert, and W. Wilson.** 1993. Guidelines for the diagnosis of rheumatic fever: Jones criteria, updated 1992. *Circulation* **87:**302–307.
35. **Dale, J. B., and E. H. Beachey.** 1985. Epitopes of streptococcal M proteins shared with cardiac myosin. *J. Exp. Med.* **162:**583–591.
36. **Davies, H. D., A. B. McGeer, B. Schwartz, K. Green, D. Cann, A. E. Simor, D. E. Low, and The Ontario Group A Streptococcal Study Group.** Invasive group A streptococcal infections in Ontario, Canada: Ontario Group A Streptococcal Study Group. *N. Engl. J. Med.* **335:**547–554.
37. **Dillon, H. C., C. W. Derrick, and M. S. Dillon.** 1974. M-antigens common to pyoderma and acute glomerulonephritis. *J. Infect. Dis.* **130:**257–267.
38. **Dugdale, D. C., and P. G. Ramsey.** 1990. *Staphylococcus aureus* bacteremia in patients with Hickman catheters. *Am. J. Med.* **89:**137–141.
39. **Enright, M. C., B. G. Spratt, A. Kalia, J. H. Cross, and D. E. Bessen.** 2001. Multilocus Sequence Typing of *Streptococcus pyogenes* and the relationships between *emm* type and clone. *Infect. Immun.***69:**2416.
40. **Facklam, R.** 2002. What happened to the streptococci: overview of the taxonomic and nonmenclature changes. *Clin. Microbiol. Rev.* **15:**613–630.
41. **Feldman, C., N. C. Munro, P. K. Jeffery, T. J. Mitchell, P. W. Andrew, G. J. Boulnois, D. Guerreiro, J. A. Rohde, H. C. Todd , P. J. Cole, and R. Wilson.** 1991. Pneumolysin induces the salient histologic features of pneumococcal infection in the rat lung in vivo. *Am. J. Respir. Cell. Mol. Biol.* **5:**416–423.
42. **Figueroa, J. E., and P. Densen.** 1991. Infectious diseases associated with complement deficiencies. *Clin. Microbiol. Rev.* **4:**359–395.
43. **Finkelstein, R., J. D. Sobel, A. Nagler, and D. Merzbach.** 1984. *Staphylococcus aureus* bacteremia and endocarditis: comparison of nosocomial and community-acquired infection. *J. Med.* **15:**193.
44. **Fowler, V. J., Jr., H. W. Boucher, G. R. Corey, E. Abrutyn, A. W. Karchmer, M. E. Rupp, D. P. Levine, H. F. Chambers, F. P. Tally, G. A. Vigliani, C. H. Cabell, A. S. Link, I. DeMeyer, S. G. Filler, M. Zervos, P. Cook, J. Parsonnet, J. M. Bernstein, C. S. Price, G. N. Forrest, G. Fätkenheuer, M. Gareca, S. J. Rehm, H. R. Brodt, A. Tice, S. E. Cosgrove and the *S. aureus* Endocarditis and Bacteremia Study Group.** 2006. Daptomycin versus standard therapy for bacteremia and endocarditis caused by *Staphylococcus aureus*. *N. Engl. J. Med.* **355:**653–665.
45. **Fowler, V. G., Jr., A. Justice, C. Moore, D. K. Benjamin, Jr., C. W. Woods, S. Campbell, L. B. Reller, G. R. Corey, N. P. J. Day, and S. J. Peacock.** 2005. Risk factors for hematogenous complications of intravascular catheter-associated *Staphylococcus aureus* bacteremia. *Clin. Infect. Dis.* **40:**695–703.
46. **Fowler, V. G., Jr., L. Kong, G. R. Corey, G. S. Gottlieb, R. S. McClelland, D. J. Sexton, D. Gesty-Palmer, and L. J. Harrell.** 1999. Recurrent *Staphylococcus aureus* bacteremia: Pulsed-field gel electrophoresis findings in 29 patients. *J. Infect. Dis.* **179:**1157–1161.
47. **Fowler, V. G., Jr., J. M. Miro, B. Hoen, C. H. Cabell, E. Abrutyn, E. Rubinstein, G. R. Corey, D. Spelman, S. F. Bradley, B. Barsic, P. A. Pappas, K. J. Anstrom, D. Wray, C. O. Fortes, I. Anguera, E. Athan, P. Jones, J. T. van der Meer, T. S. Elliott, D. P. Levine, and ICE Investigators.** 2005. *Staphylococcus aureus* endocarditis: a consequence of medical progress. *JAMA* **293:**3012–3021.
48. **Fowler, V. G., Jr., M. K. Olsen, G. R. Corey, C. W. Woods, C. H. Cabell, L. B. Reller, A. C. Cheng, T. Dudley, and E. Z. Oddone.** 2003. Clinical identifiers of complicated *Staphylococcus aureus* bacteremia. *Arch. Intern. Med.* **163:**2066–2072.
49. **Fowler, V. G., Jr., L. L. Sanders, L. K. Kong, R. S. McClelland, G. S. Gottlieb, J. Li, T. Ryan, D. J. Sexton, G. Roussakis, L. J. Harrell, and G. R. Corey.** 1999. Infective endocarditis due to *Staphylococcus aureus*: 59 prospectively identified cases with follow-up. *Clin. Infect. Dis.* **28:**106–114.

50. **Fridkin, S. K.** 2001. Vancomycin-intermediate and -resistant *Staphylococcus aureus*: what the infectious disease specialist needs to know. *Clin. Infect. Dis.* **32**:108–115.
51. **Friedman, N. D., K. S. Kaye, J. E. Stout, S. A. McGarry, S. L. Trivette, J. P. Briggs, W. Lamm, C. Clark, J. MacFarquhar, A. L. Walton, L. B. Reller, and D. J. Sexton.** 2002. Health care-associated bloodstream infections in adults: a reason to change the accepted definition of community-acquired infections. *Ann. Intern. Med.* **137**:791–797.
52. **Frimodt-Moller, N., F. Espersen, P. Skinhoj, and V. T. Rosdahl.** 1997. Epidemiology of *Staphylococcus aureus* bacteremia in Denmark from 1957 to 1990. *Clin. Microbiol. Infect.* **3**:297.
53. **Galvin, J. E., M. E. Hemric, K. Ward, and M. W. Cunningham.** 2000. Cytotoxic mAb from rheumatic carditis recognizes heart valves and laminin. *J. Clin. Investig.* **106**:217–224.
54. **Garvey, M. A., S. J. Perlmutter, A. J. Allen, S. Hamburger, L. Lougee, H. L. Leonard, M. E. Witowskiet, B. Dubbert, and S. E. Swedo.** 1999, A pilot study of penicillin prophylaxis for neuropsychiatric exacerbations triggered by streptococcal infections. *Biol. Psych.* **45**:1564–1571.
55. **Gerber, M. A.** 1995. Antibiotic resistance in group A streptococci. *Pediatr. Clin. North Am.* **42**:539–551.
56. **Giannitsioti, E., C. Chirouze, A. Bouvet, I. Béguinot, F. Delahaye, J. L. Mainardi, M. Celard, L. Mihaila-Amrouche, V. L. Moing, B. Hoen, and AEPEI Study Group.** 2007. Characteristics and regional variations of group D streptococcal endocarditis in France. *Clin. Microbiol. Infect.* **13**:770–776.
57. **Goroncy-bermes, P., J. B. Dale, E. H. Beachey, and W. Opferkuch.** 1987. Monoclonal antibody to human renal glomeruli cross-reacts with streptococcal M protein. *Infect. Immun.* **55**:2416–2419.
58. **Granlund, M., L. Oberg, M. Sellin, and M. Norgren.** 1998. Identification of a novel insertion element IS*1548*, in group B streptococci, predominantly in strains causing endocarditis. *J. Infect. Dis.* **177**:967–976.
59. **Hanaki, H., K. Kuwahara-Arai, S. Boyle-Vavra, R. S. Daum, H. Labischinski, and K. Hiramatsu.** 1998. Activated cell-wall synthesis is associated with vancomycin resistance in methicillin-resistant *Staphylococcus aureus* clinical strains Mu3 and Mu50. *J. Antimicrob. Chemother.* **42**:199–209.
60. **Hansan, S. M., N. Uldbjerg, M. Killian, and U. B. Sorensen.** 2004. Dynamics of *Streptococcus agalactiae* colonization in women during and after pregnancy and in their infants. *J. Clin. Microbiol.* **42**:83–89.
61. **Harbarth, S., O. Rutschmann, P. Sudre, and D. Pittet.** 1998. Impact of methicillin resistance on the outcome of patients with bacteremia caused by *Staphylococcus aureus*. *Arch. Intern. Med.* **158**:182–189.
62. **Harrison, L. H., A. Ali, D. M. Dwyer, J. P. Libonati, M. W. Reeves, J. A. Elliott, L. Billmann, T. Lashkerwala, and J. A. Johnson.** 1995. Relapsing invasive group B streptococcal infection in adults. *Ann. Intern. Med.* **123**:421–427.
63. **Harrison, L. H., J. A. Elliott, D. M. Dwyer, J. P. Libonati, P. Ferrieri, L. Billmann, and A. Schuchat.** 1998. Serotype distribution of invasive group B streptococcal isolates in Maryland: implications for vaccine formulation. *J. Infect. Dis.* **177**:998–1002.
64. **Hartstein, A. I., M. E. Mulligan, V. H. Morthland, and R. Y. Kwok.** 1992. Recurrent *Staphylococcus aureus* bacteremia. *J. Clin. Microbiol.* **30**:670–674.
65. **Heikens, E., A. Fleer, A. Paauw, A. Florijn, and A. C. Fluit.** 2005. Comparison of genotypic and phenotypic methods for species-level identification of clinical isolates of coagulase-negative staphylococci. *J. Clin. Microbiol.* **43**:2286–2290.
66. **Heilmann, C., O. Schweitzer, C. Gerke, N. Vanittanakom, D. Mack, and F. Götz.** 1996. Molecular basis of intercellular adhesion in the biofilm-forming *Staphylococcus epidermidis*. *Mol. Microbiol.* **20**:1083–1091.
67. **Hoen, B., C. Chirouze, C. H. Cabell, C. Selton-Suty, F. Duchêne, L. Olaison, J. M. Miro, G. Habib, E. Abrutyn, S. Eykyn, Y. Bernard, F. Marco, G. R. Corey, and International Collaboration on Endocarditis Study Group.** 2005. Emergence of endocarditis due to group D streptococci: findings derived from the merged database of the International Collaboration on Endocarditis Study Group. *Eur. J. Clin. Microbiol. Infect. Dis.* **24**:12–16.
68. **Huebner, J., and D. A. Goldman.** 1999. Coagulase-negative staphylococci: role as pathogens. *Ann. Rev. Med.* **50**:223–236.
69. **Hussain, M., A. Haggar, C. Heilmann, G. Peters, J. I. Flock, and M. Herrmann.** 2002. Insertional inactivation of Eap in *Staphylococcus aureus* strain Newman confers reduced staphylococcal binding to fibroblasts. *Infect. Immun.* **70**: 2933–2940.
70. **Ing, M. B., L. M. Baddour, and A. S. Bayer.** 1997. Bacteremia and infective endocarditis: pathogenesis, diagnosis, and complications, p. 331–354. *In* K. B. Crossley and G. L. Archer, (ed.), *The Staphylococci in Human Disease*. Churchill Livingstone, New York, NY.
71. **Ito, T., K. Okuma, X. X. Ma, H. Yuzawa, and K. Hiramatsu.** 2003. Insights on antibiotic resistance of *Staphylococcus aureus* from its whole genome: genomic island SCC. *Drug Resist. Updat.* **6**:41–52.
72. **Janoff, E. N., J. O'Brien, P. Thompson, J. Ehret, G. Meiklejohn, G. Duvall, and J. M. Douglas, Jr.** 1993. *Streptococcus pneumoniae* colonization, bacteremia, and immune response among persons with human immunodeficiency virus infection. *J. Infect. Dis.* **167**: 49–56.
73. **Johnson, D. R., D. L. Stevens, and E. L. Kaplan.** 1992. Epidemiological analysis of GAS serotypes associated with severe systemic infections, rheumatic fever or uncomplicated pharyngitis. *J. Infect. Dis.* **166**:374–382.
74. **Johri, A. K., L. C. Paoletti, P. Glaser, M. Dua, P. K. Sharma, G. Grandi, and R. Rappuoli.** 2006. Group B *Streptococcus*: global incidence and vaccine development. *Nat. Rev. Microbiol.* **4**:932–942.
75. **Kadioglu A., J. N. Weiser, J. C. Paton, and P. W. Andrew.** 2008. The role of *Streptococcus pneumoniae* virulence factors in host respiratory colonization and disease. *Nat. Rev. Microbiol.* **6**:288–301.
76. **Kaplan, E. L., D. R. Johnson, and P. P. Cleary.** 1989. GAS serotypes isolated from patients and sibling contacts during the resurgence of rheumatic fever in the US in the mid-1980s. *J. Infect. Dis.* **159**:1010–1011.
77. **Katayama, Y., T. Ito, and K. Hiramatsu.** 2000. A new class of genetic element, staphylococcus cassette chromosome *mec*, encodes methicillin resistance in *Staphylococcus aureus*. *Antimicrob. Agents Chemother.* **44**:1549–1555.
78. **Khanna, A. K., D. R. Buskirk, R. C. Williams, Jr., A. Gibofsky, M. K. Crow, A. Menon, M. Forino, H. M. Reid, T. Poon-King, P. Rubinstein, and J. B. Zabriskie.** 1989. Presence of a non-HLA B cell antigen in rheumatic fever patients and their families as defined by a monoclonal antibody. *J. Clin. Investig.* **83**:1710–1716.
79. **Khatib, R., L. B. Johnson, M. G. Fakih, K. Riederer, A. Khosrovaneh, M. Shamse Tabriz, M. Sharma, and S. Saeed.** 2006. Persistence in *Staphylococcus aureus* bacteremia: incidence, characteristics of patients and outcome. *Scand. J. Infect. Dis.* **38**:7–14.

80. **Kim, E. L., D. L. Ching, and F. D. Pien.** 1990. Bacterial endocarditis at a small community hospital. *Am. J. Med. Sci.* **299:**87–93.
81. **Kim, P., D. M. Musher, W. P. Glezen, M. C. Rodriguez-Barradas, W. K. Nahm, and C. E. Wright.** 1996. Association of invasive pneumococcal disease with season, atmospheric conditions, air pollution, and the isolation of respiratory viruses. *Clin. Infect. Dis.* **22:**100–106.
82. **Klein, R. S., R. A. Recco, M. T. Catalano, S. C. Edberg, J. I. Casey, and N. H. Steigbigel.** 1977. Association of *Streptococcus bovis* with carcinoma of the colon. *N. Engl. J. Med.* **297:**800–802.
83. **Kloos, W.** 1997. Taxonomy and systematics of staphylococci indigenous to humans, p. 113–137. *In* K. B. Crossley and G. L. Archer (ed.), *The Staphylococci in Human Disease.* Churchill Livingstone, New York, NY.
84. **Kluytmans, J., A. van Belkum, and H. Verbrugh.** 1997. Nasal carriage of *Staphylococcus aureus*: epidemiology, underlying mechanisms, and associated risks. *Clin. Microbiol. Rev.* **10:**505–520.
85. **Lalani,T., Z. Kanafani, V. H. Chu, L. L. Moore, G. R. Corey, P. Pappas, C. W. Woods, C. H. Cabell, B. Hoen, C. Selton-Suty, L. Doco-Lecompte, C. Chirouze, D. Raoult, J. M. Miro, C. A. Mestres, L. Olaison, S. Eykyn, E. Abrutyn, V. G. Fowler, Jr., and The International Collaboration on Endocarditis Merged Database Study Group.** 2006. Prosthetic valve endocarditis due to coagulase-negative staphylococci: findings from the International Collaboration on Endocarditis Merged Database. *Eur. J. Clin. Microbiol. Infect. Dis.* **25:**365–368.
86. **Lancefield, R. C.** 1962. Current knowledge of type-specific M antigens of group A streptococci. *J. Immunol.* **89:**307–313.
87. **Laupland, K. B., D. L. Church, M. Mucenski, L. R. Sutherland, and H. D. Davies.** 2003. Population-based study of the epidemiology and the risk factors for invasive *Staphylococcus aureus* infections. *J. Infect. Dis.* **187:**1452–1459.
88. **Lautenschlager, S., C. Herzog, and W. Zimmerli.** 1993. Course and outcome of bacteremia due to *Staphylococcus aureus*: evaluation of different case definitions. *Clin. Infect. Dis.* **16:**567–573.
89. **Lee, L. Y., Y. J. Miyamoto, B. W. McIntyre, M. Höök, K. W. McCrea, D. McDevitt, and E. L. Brown.** 2002. The *Staphylococcus aureus* MAP protein in an immunomodulator that interferes with T cell-mediated responses. *J. Clin. Investig.* **110:**1461–1471.
90. **Leentnek, A. L., O. Giger, and E. O'Rourke.** 1990. Group A beta-hemolytic streptococcal bacteremia and intravenous substance abuse: a growing clinical problem? *Arch. Intern. Med.* **150:**89–93.
91. **Levine, D. P., B. S. Fromm, and B. R. Reddy.** 1991. Slow response to vancomycin or vancomycin plus rifampin in methicillin-resistant *Staphylococcus aureus* endocarditis. *Ann. Intern. Med.* **115:**674–680.
92. **Light, R. W., W. M. Girard, S. G. Jenkinson, and R. B. George.** 1980. Parapneumonic effusions. *Am. J. Med.* **69:**507–512.
93. **Lin, F. Y., P. H. Azimi, L. E. Weisman, J. B. Philips III, J. Regan, P. Clark, G. G. Rhoads, J. Clemens, J. Troendle, E. Pratt, R. A. Brenner, and V. Gill.** 2000. Susceptibility profiles for group B streptococci isolated from neonates, 1995-1998. *Clin. Infect. Dis.* **31:**76–79.
94. **Lin, F. Y., J. D. Clemens, P. H. Azimi, J. A. Regan, L. E. Weisman, J. B. Philips III, G. G. Rhoads, P. Clark, R. A. Brenner, and P. Ferrieri.** 1998. Capsular polysaccharide types of group B streptococcal isolates from neonates with early-onset systemic infection. *J. Infect. Dis.* **177:**790–792.
95. **Lowrance, J. H., L. M. Baddour, and W. A. Simpson.** 1990. The role of fibronectin binding in the rat model of experimental endocarditis caused by *Streptococcus sanguis. J. Clin. Investig.* **86:**7–13.
96. **Lowy, F. D.** 1998. *Staphylococcus aureus* infections. *N. Engl. J. Med.* **339:**520–532.
97. **Maki, D. G., D. M. Kluger, and C. J. Crnich.** 2006. The risk of bloodstream infection in adults with different intravascular devices: a systematic review of 200 published prospective studies. *Mayo Clin. Proc.* **81:**1159–1171.
98. **Maki, D. G., C. E. Weise, and H. W. Sarafin.** 1977. A semi-quantitative culture method for identifying intravenous-catheter-related infection. *N. Engl. J. Med.* **296:**1305–1309.
99. **Marr, K. A., D. J. Sexton, P. J. Conlon, G. R. Corey, S. J. Schwab, and K. B. Kirkland.** 1997. Catheter-related bacteremia and outcome of attempted catheter salvage in patients undergoing hemodialysis. *Ann. Intern. Med.* **127:**275–280.
100. **Martin, G. S., D. M. Mannino, S. Eaton, and M. Moss.** 2003. The epidemiology of sepsis in the United States from 1979 through 2000. *N. Engl. J. Med.* **348:**1546–1554.
101. **Miller, D. L., and R. M. Laxe.** 2003. Pediatric autoimmune neuropsychiatric disorders associated with streptococcal infections (PANDAS). *Pediatr. Rheumatol. Online J.* **1:**140–161. http://www.pedrheumonlinejournal.org/April/review-arti.htm.
102. **Monk, A. B., S. Boundy, V. H. Chu. J. C. Bettinger, J. R. Robles, V. J. Fowler, Jr., and G. L. Archer.** 2008. Analysis of the genotype and virulence of *Staphylococcus epidermidis* isolates from patients with infective endocarditis. *Infect. Immun.* **76:**5127–5132.
103. **Moyer, M. A., L. D. Edwards, and L. Farley.** 1983. Comparative culture methods on 101 intravenous catheters. Routine, semiquantitative, and blood cultures. *Arch. Intern. Med.* **143:**66–69.
104. **Munoz, P., A. Llancaqueo, M. Rodriguez-Creixems, T. Peláez, L. Martin, and E. Bouza.** 1997. Group B streptococcus bacteremia in nonpregnant adults. *Arch. Intern. Med.* **157:**213–216.
105. **Murphy, M. L., and M. E. Pichichero.** 2002. Prospective identification and treatment of children with pediatric autoimmune neuropsychiatric disorder associated with Group A streptococcal infection (PANDAS). *Arch. Pediatr. Adolesc. Med.* **156:**356–361.
106. **Musher, D. M., J. E. Groover, D. A. Watson, J. P. Pandey, M. C. Rodriguez-Barradas, R. E. Baughn, M. S. Pollack, E. A. Graviss, M. de Andrade, and C. I. Amos.** 1997. Genetic regulation of the capacity to make immunoglobulin G to pneumococcal capsular polysaccharides. *J. Invest. Med.* **45:**57–68.
107. **Mylotte, J. M., J. R. Aeschlimann, and D. L. Rotella.** 1996. *Staphylococcus aureus* bacteremia: factors predicting hospital mortality. *Infect. Control Hosp. Epidemiol.* **17:**165–168.
108. **Nielsen, H. U., H. J. Kolmos, and N. Frimodt-Moller.** 2002. Beta-hemolytic streptococcal bacteremia: a review of 241 cases. *Scand. J. Infect. Dis.* **34:**483.
109. **NNIS.** 1999. Data summary from January 1990-May 1999. *Am. J. Infect. Control* **27:**520–532.
110. **Noble, W. C., Z. Virani, and R. G. A. Cree.** 1992. Cotransfer of vancomycin and other resistance genes from *Enterococcus faecalis* NCTC 12001 to *Staphylococcus aureus. FEMS Microbiol. Lett.* **93:**195–198.
111. **Novick, R. P.** 2003. Autoinduction and signal transduction in the regulation of staphylococcal virulence. *Mol. Microbiol.* **48:**1429–1449.
112. **Nunes, A. P., L. M. Teixeira, N. L. Iorio, C. C. Bastos, L. de Sousa Fonesca, T. Souto-Padron, and K. R. dos Santos.** 2006. Heterogenous resistance to vancomycin in *Staphylococcus epidermidis, Staphylococcus haemolyticus,*

and *Staphylococcus warneri* clinical strains: characterization of glycopeptide susceptibility profiles and cell wall thickening. *Int. J. Antimicrob. Agents* **27**:307–315.

113. **Parker, M. T., and L. C. Ball.** 1976. Streptococci and aerococci associated with systemic infection in man. *J. Med. Microbiol.* **9**:275–302.

114. **Patti, J. M., T. Bremell, D. Krajewska-Pietrasik, A. Abdelnour, A. Tarkowski, C. Rydén, and M. Höök.** 1994. The *Staphylococcus aureus* collagen adhesion is a virulence determinant in experimental septic arthritis. *Infect. Immun.* **62**:152–161.

115. **Peterson, P. K., J. Verhoef, L. D. Sabath, and P. G. Quie.** 1977. Effect of protein A on staphylococcal opsonization. *Infect. Immun.* **15**:760–764.

116. **Petti, C. A., K. E. Simmon, J. M. Miro, B. Hoen, F. Marco, V. H. Chu, E. Athan, S. Bukovski, E. Bouza, S. Bradley, V. J. Fowler, E. Giannitsioti, D. Gordon, P. Reinbott, T. Korman, S. Lang, C. Garcia de-la-Maria, A. Raglio, A. J. Morris, P. Plesiat, S. Ryan, T. Doco-Lecompte, F. Tripodi, R. Utili, D. Wray, J. J. Federspiel, K. Boisson, L. B. Reller, D. R. Murdoch, C. W. Woods, and International Collaboration on Endocarditis-Microbiology Investigators.** 2008. Genotypic diversity of coagulase-negative staphylococci causing endocarditis: a global perspective. *J. Clin. Microbiol.* **46**:1780–1784.

117. **Que, Y. A., P. Francois, J. A. Haefliger, J. M. Entenza, P. Vaudaux, and P. Moreillon.** 2001. Reassessing the role of *Staphylococcus aureus* clumping factor and fibronectin-binding protein by expression in *Lactococcus lactis*. *Infect. Immun.* **69**:6296–6302.

118. **Roberts, R. B.** 1992. Streptococcal endocarditis: the viridans and beta hemolytic streptococci, p.191. *In* D. Kaye (ed), *Infective Endocarditis*, Raven Press, Ltd, New York, NY.

119. **Rodriguez-Barradas, M. C., D. M. Musher, C. Lahart, C. Lacke, J. Groover, D. Watson, R. Baughn, T. Cate, and G. Crofoot.** 1992. Antibody to capsular polysaccharides of *Streptococcus pneumoniae* after vaccination of human immunodeficiency virus-infected subjects with 23-valent pneumococcal vaccine. *J. Infect. Dis.* **165**:553–556.

120. **Rollán, M. J., J. A. San Román, I. Vilacosta, C. Sarriá, J. López, M. Acuña, and J. L. Bratos.** 2003. Clinical profile of *Streptococcus agalactiae* native valve endocarditis. *Am. Heart J.* **146**:1095–1098.

121. **Rubins, J. B., D. Charboneau, J. C. Paton, T. J. Mitchell, P. W. Andrew, and E. N. Janoff.** 1995. Dual function of pneumolysin in the early pathogenesis of murine pneumococcal pneumonia. *J. Clin. Investig.* **95**:142–150.

122. **Rubins, J. B., and E. N. Janoff.** 1998. Pneumolysin: a multifunctional pneumococcal virulence factor. *J. Lab. Clin. Med.* **131**:21–27.

123. **Ruoff, K. L., S. I. Miller, C. V. Garner, M. J. Ferraro, and S. B. Calderwood.** 1989. Bacteremia with *Streptococcus bovis* and *Streptococcus salivarius*: clinical correlates of more accurate identification of isolates. *J. Clin. Microbiol.* **27**:305–308.

124. **Rupp, M. E., and G. L. Archer.** 1994. Coagulase-negative staphylococci: pathogens associated with medical progress. *Clin. Infect. Dis.* **19**:231–243.

125. **Sanders, L. A., G. T. Rijkers, W. Kuis, A. J. Tenbergen-Meekes, B. R. de Graeff-Meeder, I. Hiemstra, and B. J. Zegers.** 1993. Defective antipneumococcal polysaccharide antibody response in children with recurrent respiratory tract infections. *J. Allergy Clin. Immunol.* **91**:110–119.

126. **Sanyal, D., A. P. Johnson, R. C. George, B. D. Cookson, and A. J. Williams.** 1991. Peritonitis due to vancomycin-resistant *Staphylococcus epidermidis*. *Lancet* **337**:54.

127. **Savage, D. G., J. Lindenbaum, and T. J. Garrett.** 1982. Biphasic pattern of bacterial infection in multiple myeloma. *Ann. Intern. Med.* **96**:47–50.

128. **Schuchat, A.** 1998. Epidemiology of group B streptococcal disease in the United States: shifting paradigms. *Clin. Microbiol. Rev.* **11**:497–513.

129. **Schwalbe, R. S., J. T. Stapletone, and P. H. Gilligan.** 1987. Emergence of vancomycin resistance in coagulase-negative staphylococci. *N. Engl. J. Med.* **316**:927.

130. **Schwartz, B., and X. T. Ussery.** 1992. Group A streptococcal outbreaks in nursing homes. *Infect. Control Hosp. Epidemiol.* **13**:742–747.

131. **Seppälä, H., A. Nissinen, H. Järvinen, S. Huovinen, T. Henriksson, E. Herva, S. E Holm, M. Jahkola, M. L. Katila, T. Klaukka, S. Kontiainen, O. Liimatainen, S. Oinonen, L. Passi-Metsomaa, and P. Huovinen.** 1992. Resistance to erythromycin in group A streptococci. *N. Engl. J. Med.* **326**:292–297.

132. **Shet, A., and P. Ferrieri.** 2004. Neonatal and maternal group B streptococcal infections: a comprehensive review. *Indian J. Med. Res.* **120**:141–150.

133. **Shulman, S. T., G. Stollerman, B. Beall, J. B. Dale, and R. R. Tanz.** 2006. Temporal changes in streptococcal M protein types and the near-disappearance of acute rheumatic fever in the United States. *Clin. Infect. Dis.* **42**:441–447.

134. **Sieradzki, K., M. G. Pinho, and A. Tomasz.** 1999. Inactivated pbp4 in highly glycopeptide-resistant laboratory mutants of *Staphylococcus aureus*. *J. Biol. Chem.* **274**:18942–18946.

135. **Sieradzki, K., and A. Tomasz.** 1999. Gradual alterations in cell wall structure and metabolism in vancomycin-resistant mutants of *Staphylococcus aureus*. *J. Bacteriol.* **181**:7566–7570.

136. **Simmon, K. E., L. Hall, C. W. Woods, F. Marco, J. M. Miro, C. Cabell, B. Hoen, M. Marin, R. Utili, E. Giannitsioti, T. Doco-Lecompte, S. Bradley, S. Mirrett, A. Tambic, S. Ryan, D. Gordon, P. Jones, T. Korman, D. Wray, L. B. Reller, M. E. Tripodi, P. Plesiat, A. J. Morris, S. Lang, D. R. Murdoch, C. A Petti, and International Collaboration on Endocarditis Microbiology Investigators.** 2008. Phylogenetic analysis of viridans group streptococci causing endocarditis. *J. Clin. Microbiol.* **46**:3087–3090.

137. **Skinner, D., and C. S. Keefer.** 1941. Significance of bacteremia caused by *Staphylococcus aureus*. A study of 122 cases and a review of the literature concerned with experimental infection in animals. *Arch. Intern. Med.* **68**:851.

138. **Small, P. M., and H. F. Chambers.** 1990. Vancomycin for *Staphylococcus aureus* endocarditis in intravenous drug users. *Antimicrob. Agents Chemother.* **34**:1227–1231.

139. **Snider, L. A., and S. E. Swedo.** 2003. Childhood-onset obsessive disorder and tic disorders: case report and literature review. *J. Child. Adolesc. Psychopharmacol.* **13**(Supp. 1): S81–S88.

140. **Snider, L. A., and S. E. Swedo.** 2004. PANDAS: current status and directions for research. *Mol. Psych.* **9**:900–907.

141. **Steinberg, J. P., C. C. Clark, and B. O. Hackman.** 1996. Nosocomial and community-acquired *Staphylococcus aureus* bacteremias from 1980 to 1993: impact of intravascular devices and methicillin resistance. *Clin. Infect. Dis.* **23**:255–259.

142. **Stevens, D. L.** 1992. Invasive group A streptococcus infections. *Clin. Infect. Dis.* **14**:2–11.

143. **Stollerman, G. H.** 1975. *Rheumatic Fever and Streptococcal Infection*. Grune and Stratton, New York, NY.

144. **Umetsu, D. T., D. M. Ambrosino, I. Quinti, G. R. Siber, and R. S. Geha.** 1985. Recurrent sinopulmonary infection

and impaired antibody response to bacterial capsular polysaccharide antigen in children with selective IgG subclass deficiency. *N. Engl. J. Med.* **313**:1247–1251.

145. **Valente, A. M., R. Jain, M. Scheurer, V. G. Fowler, Jr., G. R. Corey, A. R. Bengur, S. Sanders, and J. S. Li.** 2005. Frequency of infective endocarditis among infants and children with *Staphylococcus aureus* bacteremia. *Pediatrics* **115**:e15–e19.

146. **Van de Rijn, I., J. B. Zabriskie, and M. McCarty.** 1977. Group A streptococcal antigens cross-reactive with myocardium: purification of heart-reactive antibody and isolation and characterization of the streptococcal antigen. *J. Exp. Med.* **146**:579.

147. **Veach, L. A., M. A. Pfaller, M. Barrett, F. P. Koontz, and R. P. Wenzel.** 1990. Vancomycin resistance in *Staphylococcus haemolyticus* causing colonization and bloodstream infection. *J. Clin. Microbiol.* **28**:2064–1068.

148. **Veasy, L. G., L. Y. Tani, and H. R. Hill.** 1994. Persistence of acute rheumatic fever in the intermountain area of the United States. *J. Pediatr.* **124**:9–16.

149. **von Eiff, C., K. Becker, K. Machka, H. Stammer, G. Peters, et al.** 2001. Nasal carriage as a source of *Staphylococcus aureus* bacteremia. *N. Engl. J. Med.* **344**:11–16.

150. **Wannamaker, L. W.** 1970. Differences between streptococcal infections of the throat and of the skin. *N. Engl. J. Med.* **282**:23–31.

151. **Watanakunakorn, C.** 1999. Increasing importance of intravascular device-associated *Staphylococcus aureus* endocarditis. *Clin. Infect. Dis.* **28**:115–116.

152. **Weinstein, M. P., M. L. Towns, S. M. Quartey, S. Mirrett, L. G. Reimer, G. Parmigiani, and L. B. Reller.** 1997. The clinical significance of positive blood cultures in the 1990s: a prospective comprehensive evaluation of the microbiology, epidemiology, and outcome of bacteremia and fungemia in adults. *Clin. Infect. Dis.* **24**:584–602.

153. **Weiser, J. N., Z. Markiewicz, E. I. Tuomanen, and J. H. Wani.** 1996. Relationship between phase variation in colony morphology, intrastrain variation in cell wall physiology, and nasopharyngeal colonization by *Streptococcus pneumoniae*. *Infect. Immun.* **64**:2240–2245.

154. **Wessels, M. R., C. E. Rubens, V. J. Benedí, and D. L. Kasper.** 1989. Definition of a bacterial virulence factor: sialylation of the group B streptococcal capsule. *Proc. Natl. Acad. Sci. USA* **86**:8983–8987.

155. **Wheeler, M. C., M. H. Roe, E. L. Kaplan, P. M. Schlievert, and J. K. Todd.** 1991. Outbreak of group A streptococcus septicemia in children: clinical, epidemiologic, and microbiological correlates. *JAMA* **266**:533–537.

156. **Willcox, P. A., B. L. Rayner, and D. A. Whitelaw.** 1998. Community-acquired *Staphylococcus aureus* bacteraemia in patients who do not abuse intravenous drugs. *Q. J. Med.* **91**:41–47.

157. **Winston, D. J., D. V. Dudnick, M. Chapin, W. G. Ho, R. P. Gale, and W. J. Martin.** 1983. Coagulase-negative staphylococcal bacteremia in patients receiving immunosuppressive therapy. *Arch. Intern. Med.* **143**:32–36.

158. **Wisplinghoff, H., T. Bischoff, S. M. Tallent, H. Seifert, R. P. Wenzel, and M. B. Edmond.** 2004. Nosocomial bloodstream infections in US hospitals: analysis of 24,179 cases from a prospective nationwide surveillance study. *Clin. Infect. Dis.* **39**:309.

159. **Wisplinghoff., H., A. E. Rosato, M. C. Enright, M. Noto, W. Craig, and G. L. Archer.** 2003. Related clones containing SCCmec type IV predominate among clinically significant *Staphylococcus epidermidis* isolates. *Antimicrob. Agents Chemother.* **47**:3574–3579.

160. **Yee, A. M., H. M. Phan, R. Zuniga, J. E. Salmon, and D. M. Musher.** 2000. Association between FcgammaRIIa-R131 allotype and bacteremic pneumonococcal pneumonia. *Clin. Infect. Dis.* **30**:25–28.

161. **Zabriskie, J. B.** 1985. Rheumatic fever: the interplay between host, genetics, and microbe. Lewis A. Conner Memorial Lecture. *Circulation* **71**:1077–1086.

Sequelae and Long-Term Consequences of Infectious Diseases
Edited by Pina M. Fratamico, James L. Smith, and Kim A. Brogden

Chapter 7

Helicobacter pylori

KAREN ROBINSON AND JOHN C. ATHERTON

CHARACTERISTICS OF THE ORGANISM

Helicobacter pylori was first described in 1983 by Barry Marshall and Robin Warren, who were awarded a Nobel prize for this work in 2005 (227, 229). This gram-negative bacterial pathogen is able to colonize and persist for life in the mucosa of the human stomach (39, 90). The bacteria are spiral bacilli which are microaerophilic, fastidious, and slow growing in vitro (165, 262). Despite not being an acidophile, *H. pylori* has several features that allow its survival in the low pH environment of the stomach. The bacteria are highly motile, with five to eight unipolar flagella (165), and can sense and respond to their environment. Rapid movement from the harsh conditions of the gastric lumen into the protective mucus layer above the epithelium appears to be essential for colonization of a new host (94, 261). In addition, the bacteria express large quantities of urease enzyme (31, 154), which catalyses the production of ammonia from urea in interstitial fluid and buffers the bacterial periplasm against gastric acid (63, 92, 358). The production of urease by *H. pylori* forms the basis of several widely used diagnostic tests (35, 168, 340).

H. pylori infections are extremely common, and approximately half the world's population have the bacteria in their stomachs (90, 337). The prevalences of infection vary in different geographical locations and are associated with socioeconomic status and living conditions, particularly in childhood (reviewed in reference 224). Based on serological testing, in developing countries, 80 to 90% of the population are thought to be infected, compared with less than 40% in developed countries (337). The acquisition of *H. pylori* occurs during childhood (125), and unless treated with antibiotics, infection persists for life (224, 344). Natural clearance of the infection is rare, if it occurs at all (103, 371). The prevalence of infection has declined over the last 30 years, particularly in developed countries. This is because fewer children are becoming infected, most likely due to improved sanitation and living conditions (303, 353). Thus, in developed countries, infection is much more common among older people (who commonly acquired the infection when children) than younger people (who acquired it more rarely as children). An epidemiological study in the United States found that less than 30% of people under 30 years old were infected compared with over 75% of those over 60 (126). Similar age-related differences have been reported in other parts of the world (197, 224, 324).

Transmission of *H. pylori* is not yet fully understood, although it is thought to be from person to person. Family studies have shown that in developed countries, the primary caregiver, usually the mother, is the most common source of her children's *H. pylori* strain, which is then likely passed between children within the family (18, 133, 361). However, *H. pylori* can be acquired from outside the family, likely from other children, and this may be the primary mode of transmission in some developing countries. The bacteria are difficult to culture from human feces, except during episodes of diarrhea, but are easily cultured from the mouth following natural gastroesophageal reflux (1, 166). Thus, it is widely thought that the oral-oral route is the most likely mode of transmission. Studies following the spread of strains between siblings and within families suggest that transmission requires close contact (19, 225). Some researchers have proposed that the infection is acquired from family members through ingestion of aerosolized vomit or diarrhea (61, 184, 206, 281). Using PCR methods, *H. pylori* has been detected at locations outside the gastrointestinal tract (e.g., atherosclerotic arterial tissue [5] and dental plaque

Karen Robinson • Centre for Biomolecular Sciences, University of Nottingham, University Park, Nottingham NG7 2RD, United Kingdom. **John C. Atherton** • Wolfson Digestive Diseases Centre, University of Nottingham, Queen's Medical Centre, Nottingham NG7 2UH, United Kingdom.

[reviewed in reference 86]), but culture of live organisms from these sites has almost always been unsuccessful (262). Several reports have described *H. pylori* isolation from domestic animals, including cats, horses, calves, pigs, and sheep (45, 81, 84.) However, most studies have shown no association between exposure to these animals and the prevalence of *H. pylori* infection, implying that they are not an important source of human infection (48). *H. pylori* DNA has also been found in water supplies, and some epidemiological evidence supports human acquisition from contaminated water. However, analysis of the *H. pylori* genome suggests that the organism does not have the necessary biochemical pathways to survive outside the human gastric niche.

DISEASES CAUSED BY THE ORGANISM

Acute Infection

Initial colonization by *H. pylori* occurs in childhood, and it is still unclear whether this is symptomatic. New infection in adults is rare: there have been isolated examples of researchers deliberately or accidentally infecting themselves (228). There have also been some deliberate human infection studies to aid vaccine research (127). Finally, acute infection by *H. pylori* is now known to be the cause of an iatrogenic illness termed "epidemic hypochlorhydria" (137). This was caused by inadequately sterilized electrodes being used to measure gastric pH in research studies; subsequent analysis of stored serum before and after showed new acquisition of *H. pylori*. The symptoms of acute *H. pylori* infection in adults are variable but usually consist of mild to moderate epigastric discomfort, anorexia, nausea, and sometimes vomiting. Physiologically, people develop acute hypochlorhydria in association with a histologically acute superficial gastritis. Symptoms usually resolve within 1 to several weeks.

Chronic Infection

Following acute infection, symptoms settle, but *H. pylori* and its associated gastric inflammation remain. The continuing histologic gastritis comprises mucosal infiltration by all classes of mononuclear immune cells, but also continuing gastric infiltration by neutrophils (300). The infection and its associated inflammation do not usually cause symptoms. However, symptoms commonly occur when an *H. pylori*-associated disease arises, such as peptic ulceration or gastric cancer.

H. pylori is the leading cause of gastric and duodenal ulceration (223), distal gastric adenocarcinoma, and gastric mucosa-associated lymphoid tissue (MALT) lymphoma (212). It has also been more controversially linked with a wide variety of medical conditions, including idiopathic thrombocytopenic purpura (ITP), atherosclerosis and stroke, hepatobiliary disease, pulmonary disease, and growth retardation in children (reviewed in reference 44). *H. pylori* infection has also been reported to have negative associations with sequelae of gastroesophageal reflux disease (GERD) (213), with allergy and asthma (58), and with autoimmune conditions, such as multiple sclerosis (208), raising the possibility that it may offer protection against some of these conditions.

One of the most remarkable features of chronic *H. pylori* infection is that it results only in overt disease in a minority of people: only 10 to 20% of *H. pylori*-infected people develop peptic ulceration in their lifetime (223), and between 0.5 and 8% develop gastric cancer, depending on the population (11, 253). Who develops disease and the great variability in disease risk between populations are influenced by several factors. These can be divided into differences in virulence between *H . pylori* strains, differences in the host immune response (some of which are genetically determined), and environmental cofactors, including smoking, diet, and possibly parasitic infection (24, 300).

Bacterial Virulence Factors and Their Association with Disease

The *cag* pathogenicity island and CagA

The virulence determinant which confers the most significant increases in the risk of peptic ulcer disease and gastric cancer is the cytotoxin-associated gene pathogenicity island (*cag* PaI) (257, 265) (Table 1). This name is misleading, as the *cag* PaI has nothing to do with the *H. pylori* toxin. It is a 40-kb segment of DNA containing 31 genes, the majority of which encode components of a type IV secretion system. This syringe-like structure penetrates gastric epithelial cells and injects CagA, the product of cytotoxin-associated gene A (*cagA*), into the cytoplasm, where it interacts with host cell signaling molecules (24) (Fig. 1). Tyrosine phosphorylation motifs (TPMs) at the C-terminal region of CagA are phosphorylated by Src kinases, permitting interaction with the protein tyrosine phosphatase SHP-2 and activation of Ras/Raf/MEK/ERK MAP kinase pathways (143). These pathways can induce signaling events associated with cellular proliferation and cell cycle arrest, and mutations in their components have been linked with cancer (55). CagA interactions within the cell may also result in cytoskeletal rearrangements, and

Table 1. *H. pylori* virulence factors and their associations with gastric disease

Virulence factor	Effect on inflammation and gastric disease	References
CagA and *cag* pathogenicity island	Activates NF-κB and proinflammatory cytokine expression. Associated with increased risk of peptic ulceration and gastric adenocarcinoma.	41, 145, 242, 275, 291, 351
VacA	Induces cytokine release from mast cells, inhibits T-cell activation and proliferation. s1/i1/m1 forms are associated with increased risk of peptic ulceration and gastric adenocarcinoma.	25, 119, 242, 298, 331, 332
DupA	Increases gastric IL-8 expression and neutrophil infiltration. Associated with increased risk of duodenal ulceration and gastric adenocarcinoma.	13, 16, 215
OipA	Increases gastric IL-8 expression and neutrophil activation. Associated with duodenal ulceration.	375
HP-NAP	Activates neutrophils and promotes Th1 immune responses. Association with disease risk unknown.	4, 192
BabA	Via adhesion, increases inflammation and epithelial proliferation. Associated with increased risk of duodenal ulceration, gastric atrophy, and gastric adenocarcinoma.	290, 380
SabA	Increases inflammation. Absence of SabA expression is associated with duodenal ulceration.	77, 285
IceA	Role in virulence unknown. Associated with duodenal ulceration and gastric adenocarcinoma.	179, 214, 276

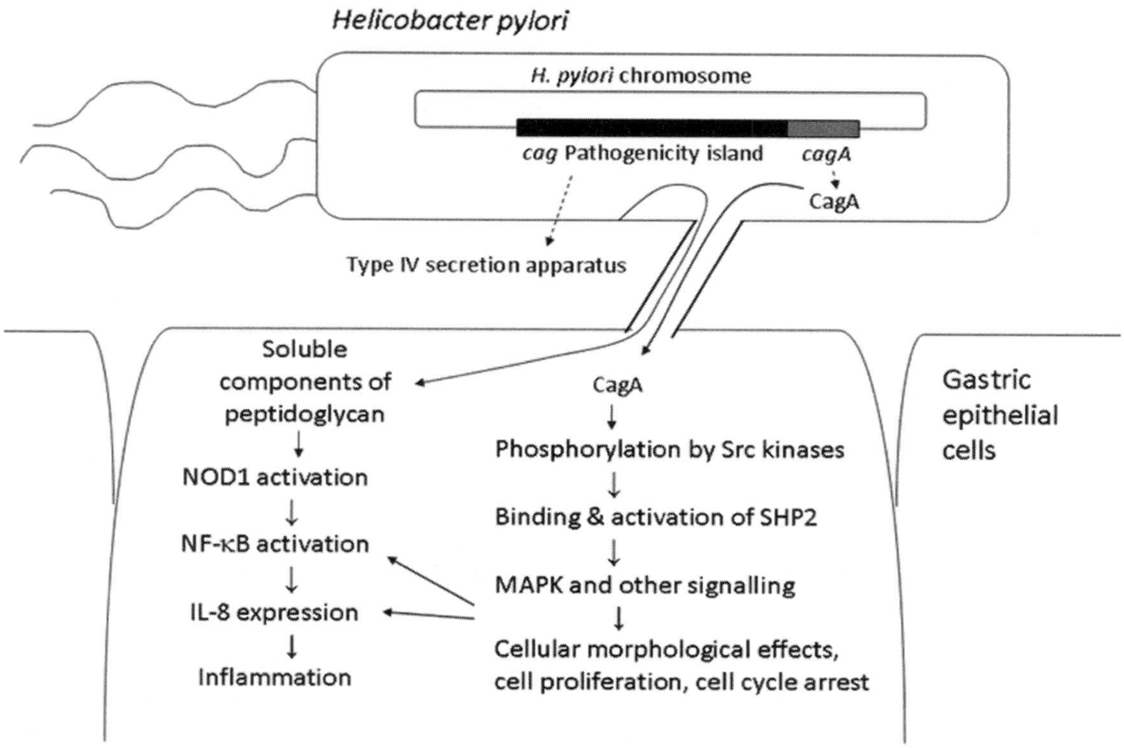

Figure 1. Host cell signalling events induced by the *cag* pathogenicity island. The *cag* PaI-encoded type IV secretion system delivers CagA into epithelial cells. CagA is phosphorylated by Scr kinases prior to its interaction with SHP-2, a protein phosphatase. Subsequent activation of MAP kinase pathways results in a number of cellular effects, including actin rearrangements, cellular proliferation and cell scattering, increased apoptosis, disruption of the cell cycle, and the expression of proinflammatory genes. In addition, when the type IV secretion system connects bacterial and epithelial cell cytoplasm, bacterial cell wall components enter the epithelial cell and activate other cell signaling pathways. Peptidoglycan components bind to and activate the intracellular pattern recognition receptor Nod1, leading to activation of NF-κB (351). This transcription factor stimulates expression of genes encoding factors which attract inflammatory cells (such as IL-8) and genes encoding antibacterial peptides (167, 175).

cultured gastric epithelial cells adopt the "hummingbird" morphology (141). Differences in the number and type of CagA TPMs are thought to control the strength of the interaction with SHP-2 and thus the magnitude of some of the effects on cell signaling (17, 142). Strains with higher numbers of CagA TPMs are associated with a greater risk of gastric adenocarcinoma, as are East Asian strains, which have a more potent CagA SHP-2 binding site. This likely contributes to the much higher incidence of gastric cancer in parts of Asia (17, 312, 384).

In addition to the effects of CagA itself, the interaction of cells with the pili of the type IV protein secretion system activates host signaling pathways which predispose to inflammation. Soluble components of the *H. pylori* peptidoglycan cell wall are translocated into epithelial cells where they activate Nod1, an intracellular innate signaling receptor (351). This in turn results in activation of the transcription factor NF-κB and expression of proinflammatory and antiapoptotic genes, such as interleukin-8 (IL-8) and cyclooxygenase-2 (COX-2) (145, 181). This is thought to be the main pathway leading to the enhanced gastric inflammation and the greatly increased risk of peptic ulceration and gastric malignancy associated with *cag*$^+$ strains.

The vacuolating cytotoxin, VacA

The vacuolating cytotoxin A (VacA) is the second important virulence factor which is linked with different disease outcomes of infection (Table 1). It is a pore-forming toxin, which allows the passage of anions and other small molecules through epithelial cell membranes (70). This underlies its most obvious in vitro effect, the induction of massive vacuoles in cultured epithelial cell lines. In addition to vacuolation, a phenomenon not usually observed in vivo, VacA affects epithelial cells in several other ways, including increasing paracellular permeability, inducing apoptosis, and interfering with cell signaling (reviewed in reference 69). VacA also has effects on the immune system, at least in vitro: it activates mast cells (332) but inhibits activation and proliferation of T cells (119).

The *vacA* gene is present in virtually all strains and encodes a preprotoxin, which is cleaved upon secretion to yield the mature 87- to 95-kDa toxin (70). This comprises a 37-kDa N terminus and 58-kDa subunits (p37 and p58, respectively) (338). The gene is polymorphic with biologically important variations in three regions (25, 298) (Fig. 2). The signal (s) region encodes the N terminus of the toxin. s1 types of VacA are active, whereas s2 types are nonvacuolating due to the presence of a hydrophilic extension on the hydrophobic N terminus of the mature toxin (204). Mid (m)-region polymorphisms influence cell specificity by affecting the binding of toxin to receptors on epithelial cells (205, 264). m1 types of VacA vacuolate a wider range of epithelial cell lines than m2 types. Finally a newly discovered intermediate region located within the p37 domain between the signal region and mid-region also determines toxicity, although the mechanism underlying this is still unknown (298). Strain genotyping studies correlating *vacA* allelic types and upper gastrointestinal disease have shown that *vacA* type s1/m1 strains are associated with duodenal and gastric ulceration and gastric adenocarcinoma (25, 109, 178, 274). However a recent study suggests that the i1 type of *vacA* may be the best marker of disease (particularly cancer) risk (298).

Other bacterial virulence factors

Several other nonconserved *H. pylori* genes and their products have been associated with disease, and for some of these there is increasing evidence of a causal pathogenic role (Table 1). Outer inflammatory protein A (OipA) is an outer membrane protein which induces IL-8 secretion from gastric epithelial cells, thereby enhancing inflammation (372). Duodenal ulcer-promoting protein A (DupA) is also thought to increase epithelial cell IL-8 expression and is variously reported to be associated with duodenal ulceration and gastric cancer (13, 16, 215). The adhesins BabA (*b*lood group *a*ntigen *b*inding adhesin A) (64) and SabA (*s*ialic *a*cid-*b*inding adhesin A) have been associated with increased inflammation (285) and may also play a role in pathogenesis by promoting colonization and inflammation.

Host and Environmental Factors Associated with Differential Disease Risk

Host genetic factors contribute to the risk of peptic ulceration and gastric adenocarcinoma, particularly polymorphisms in specific cytokine genes which lead to up- or downregulation of gastric inflammatory responses to *H. pylori.* Since chronic inflammation is a central mediator of carcinogenesis (251), it is unsurprising that cytokine polymorphisms influence the risk of gastric adenocarcinoma. Positive associations with gastric cancer have been reported with genotypes leading to high-level expression of proinflammatory IL-1β (97, 108, 294) or tumor necrosis factor alpha (TNF-α) (221), and reduced anti-inflammatory IL-10 expression (98). More recently, associations of polymorphisms in the proinflammatory genes IL-1RN, IL-8, and TNF-α with peptic ulceration have also been

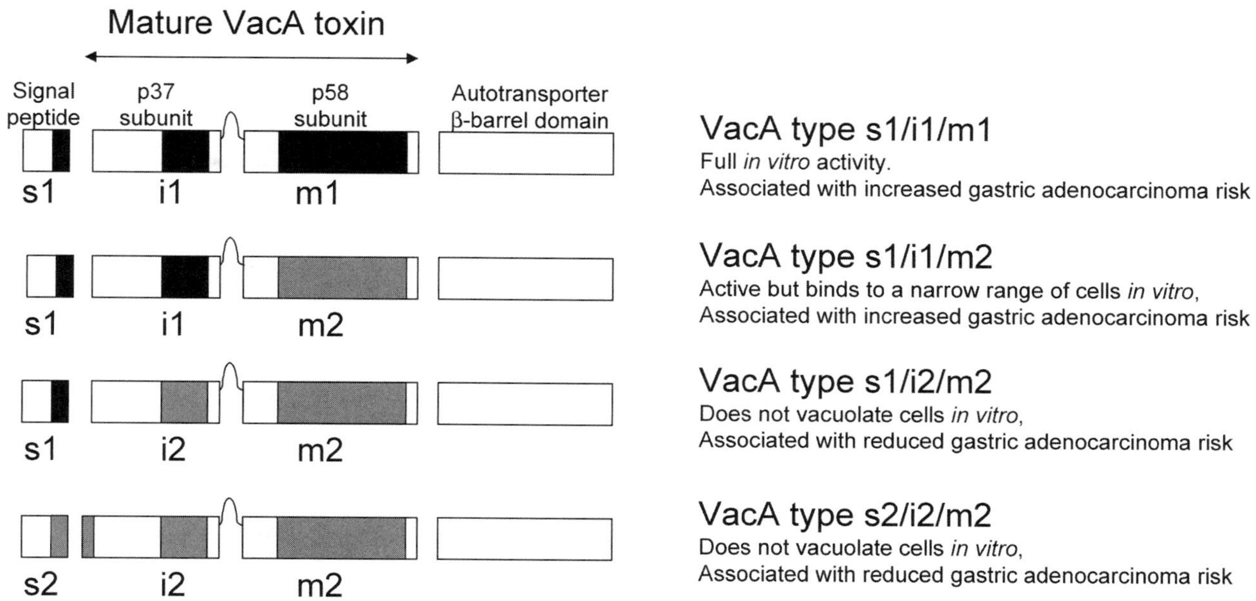

Figure 2. Effects of VacA polymorphisms on cytotoxic activity and associations with disease. The *vacA* gene varies most in the signal region (which determines cytotoxic activity and may be type s1 or s2), the intermediate region located within the p37 subunit (which determines cytotoxic activity and may be type i1 or i2), and the mid-region within the p58 subunit (which determines binding to host cells and may be type m1 or m2). Only the combinations of regions shown occur commonly.

demonstrated (130, 152, 292, 362). Experiments with transgenic mice support the central importance of these cytokines. Mice deficient in IL-10 have increased local inflammation, and this is sufficient to successfully and rapidly clear *H. pylori* infections (57). In contrast, mice deficient in the proinflammatory cytokine IL-12 are unable to clear their infections and have a reduced gastric inflammatory infiltration (2). In humans, as a further illustration of the importance of the immune response in determining disease risk, certain HLA genotypes have been found to be associated with a reduced risk of *H. pylori*-induced gastric cancer (144).

Environmental factors are also important in affecting disease risk; for example, smoking increases the risk of both peptic ulceration and gastric cancer. High-salt diets also predispose to gastric cancer, whereas diets high in antioxidants are protective (24). Recently, there has been considerable interest in whether environmentally determined differences in the acquired immune response, for example, secondary to parasite infection, may also affect disease risk (89). This could potentially help explain large variations in the worldwide gastric cancer incidence rates; these often do not correlate with the prevalence of *H. pylori* infection and cannot easily be explained by differences in smoking or diet. For example, there is at least a 10-fold higher incidence of gastric cancer in Japan compared with Nigeria, but the prevalences of *H. pylori* infection in these countries are similar (219). There is good evidence from animal models that modification of the immune response can affect the development of cancer. For example, regulatory T cells (Tregs) (Fig. 3) are able to interrupt the induction of colon cancer in mice by inhibiting the inflammatory response to *Helicobacter hepaticus* (102), and many intestinal helminths induce such Treg responses (310). Concurrent intestinal helminth infections have also been shown to modulate the proinflammatory T helper 1 (Th1) $CD4^+$ T-cell response to *Helicobacter felis* in a mouse model, and this led to reduced gastric atrophy (111). Therefore, chronic helminth infections, which are common in developing countries, could skew the human immune response to *H. pylori* in favor of anti-inflammatory Th2 or Treg resposes. It has also been shown that coinfections of mice with *H. felis* and *Toxoplasma gondii* (a potent inducer of Th1 responses) had the opposite effect of the helminth infections and enhanced gastric carcinogenesis (207). Support in humans for the modulating role of immunity comes from the detection of different immunoglobulin G (IgG) subclass responses to *H. pylori* infection in Africa compared with those in Germany and Australia (243). The serum IgG1 and IgG2 levels in African patients were suggestive of a Th2-biased cellular response, whereas Th1-biased gastric cellular responses have been demonstrated in Japan (160) and the United Kingdom (29).

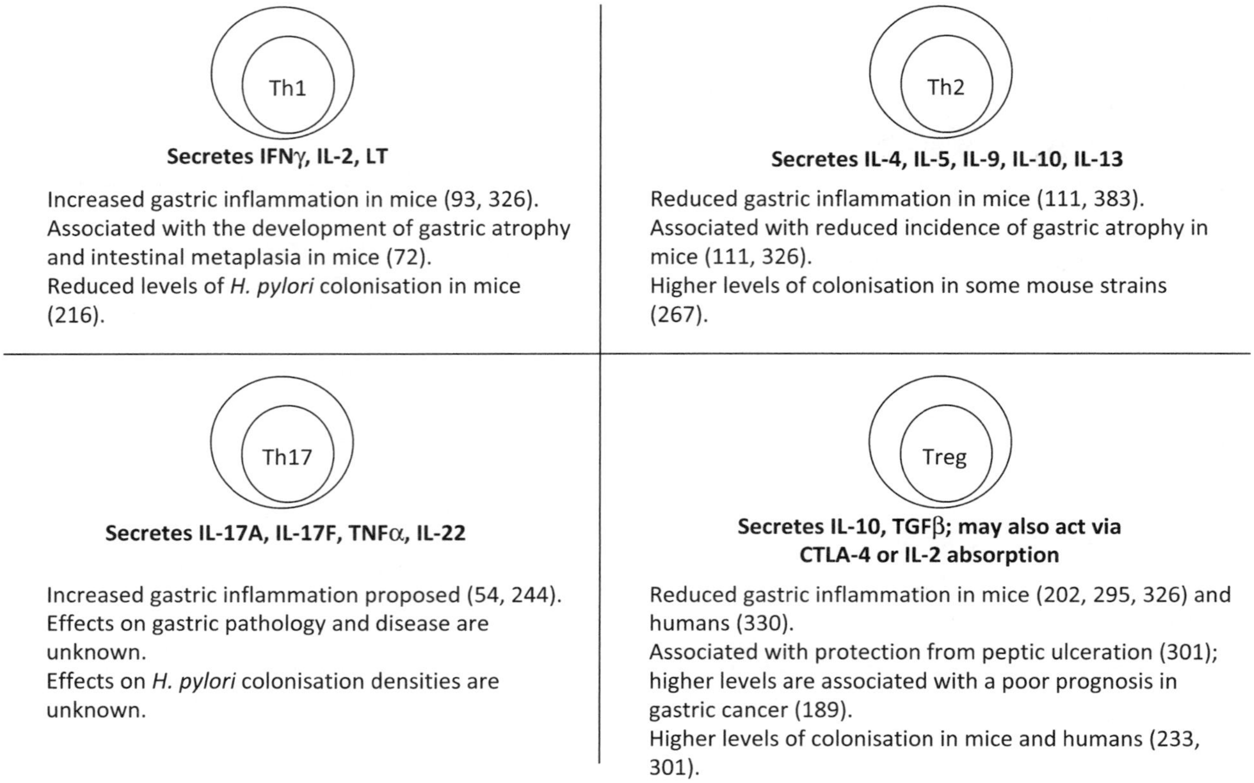
Th1
Secretes IFNγ, IL-2, LT
Increased gastric inflammation in mice (93, 326).
Associated with the development of gastric atrophy and intestinal metaplasia in mice (72).
Reduced levels of H. pylori colonisation in mice (216).
Th2
Secretes IL-4, IL-5, IL-9, IL-10, IL-13
Reduced gastric inflammation in mice (111, 383).
Associated with reduced incidence of gastric atrophy in mice (111, 326).
Higher levels of colonisation in some mouse strains (267).
Th17
Secretes IL-17A, IL-17F, TNFα, IL-22
Increased gastric inflammation proposed (54, 244).
Effects on gastric pathology and disease are unknown.
Effects on H. pylori colonisation densities are unknown.
Treg
Secretes IL-10, TGFβ; may also act via CTLA-4 or IL-2 absorption
Reduced gastric inflammation in mice (202, 295, 326) and humans (330).
Associated with protection from peptic ulceration (301); higher levels are associated with a poor prognosis in gastric cancer (189).
Higher levels of colonisation in mice and humans (233, 301).

Figure 3. $CD4^+$ T-cell subsets and their associations with *H. pylori*-induced inflammation and disease.

CHRONIC ACTIVE GASTRITIS

Colonization with *H. pylori* always results in chronic inflammation of the gastric mucosa. This is termed "active" because as well as mucosal infiltration of the whole range of mononuclear immune cells, there is continuing infiltration by neutrophils throughout the infection, which means throughout the lifetime of the host. High levels of chemokines (IL-8, GRO alpha, ENA-78, RANTES, and monocyte chemoattractant protein-1 [MCP-1]) (321, 322) are detected along with proinflammatory cytokines, such as TNF-α, IL-1β, IL-6, IL-7, IL-12, and IL-18 (30, 91, 373, 374). The gastritis itself is asymptomatic in most cases; symptoms occur if an *H. pylori*-associated disease, such as peptic ulceration, arises. Long-standing gastritis leads in some people to gastric atrophy (loss of specialized gastric glands and reduction in acid secretion), and it is on this background of "atrophic gastritis" that metaplasia, dysplasia, and adenocarcinoma can arise.

PEPTIC ULCER DISEASE

Approximately 17% of *H. pylori*-infected people develop gastric or duodenal ulceration (224), and a great deal of research has been devoted to discovering what is different in these cases. As mentioned above, host cytokine polymorphisms and expression of certain virulence factors by colonizing strains are associated with increased risk of disease. There is also increasing evidence that a subset of suppressive and anti-inflammatory $CD4^+$ lymphocytes, Tregs, may profoundly influence the development of peptic ulceration. Our recent studies have shown that peptic ulcer disease in patients was significantly associated with a lower Treg response level than that found in patients without ulcers (301). Mice with reduced numbers of $CD25^+$ Tregs develop more severe gastritis (293, 295), providing further evidence that Tregs are important for suppressing severe inflammation. Elevated levels of these cells have been found in the infected human gastric mucosa (101, 138, 293), and there is increased expression of IL-10 and TGFβ(124, 209, 301), suppressive cytokines associated with the Treg response. It has been shown in vitro that human Tregs suppress memory T-cell responses to *H. pylori* (218) and inhibit IL-8 release from gastric epithelial cells in cocultures (330). The latter effect may be through IL-10 inhibition of NF-κB activation and inflammation (301). IL-10-deficient mice have increased inflammation and, unlike wild-type mice, can clear the infection (57).

Whether ulceration occurs in the duodenal or gastric mucosa appears to be dependent upon the pattern of *H. pylori* colonization and inflammation (Fig. 4). The reasons underlying gastric inflammation patterns (antral-predominant or pan-gastric) remain unknown, but it has been suggested that *H. pylori* cannot normally colonize the gastric corpus (which contains the acid-producing parietal cells) unless individuals have a reduced capacity to produce acid (198). When the bacteria colonize the antrum of the stomach, the resulting inflammation has a profound effect on the balance of gastric acid-regulating hormones, suppressing the production of somatostatin by D cells and stimulating G cells to secrete gastrin (382, 383). Somatostatin reduces acid production by providing a negative feedback on G-cell gastrin production, so loss of somatostatin leads to hypergastrinemia and increased stimulated acid production. Somatostatin also inhibits inflammation by inhibiting dendritic cell activity and is required for IL-4-mediated resolution of *H. pylori* gastritis (171, 383). In contrast, gastrin stimulates parietal cells present in the oxyntic glands of the corpus to secrete more acid, both through direct effects on parietal cells and indirectly by stimulating histamine release from enterochromaffin-like cells. (382). Stimulated gastric hyperacidity causes damage to the duodenum, and over time this leads to gastric metaplasia there. Once epithelial cells of the gastric type are present in the duodenum, *H. pylori* can colonize it and there is a risk of duodenal ulceration.

Where distribution of the inflammation includes the proximal acid-producing part of the stomach (pan- or corpus-predominant colonization), G cells in the antrum are again stimulated to secrete increased levels of gastrin; however, in this case gastric acid output is reduced, since proinflammatory factors, such as IL-1β and TNF-α, present in the gastric corpus inhibit the secretion of acid by parietal cells. Exactly how gastric ulcers arise on this background is unknown, but they tend to occur at the vulnerable transitional zone between antral and corpus mucosa. This is thought to be due to high-level inflammation in an area of weakened gastric integrity

GASTRIC ADENOCARCINOMA

The association between *H. pylori* infection and the development of gastric cancer is now widely accepted (135, 155, 241, 270). Based on a wealth of epidemiological data, the World Health Organization and International Agency for Research on Cancer consensus group classified *H. pylori* as a biological carcinogen in 1994 (12). Gastric cancer is the fourth most common type of cancer and the second leading cause of

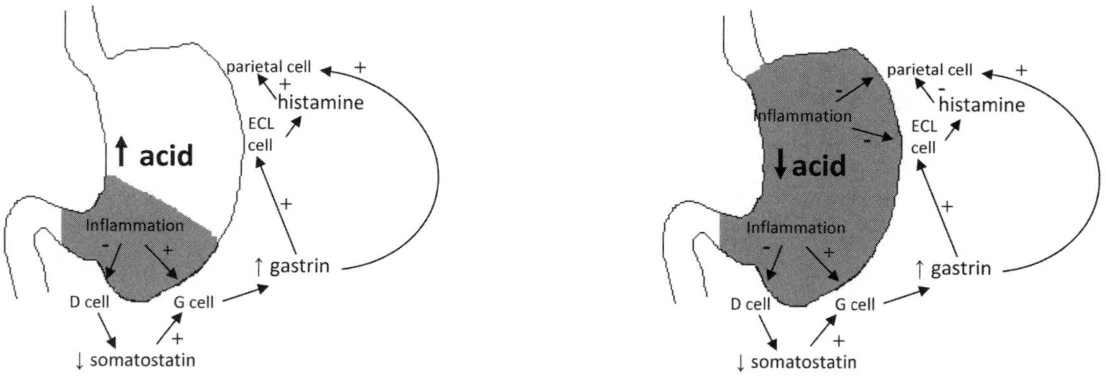

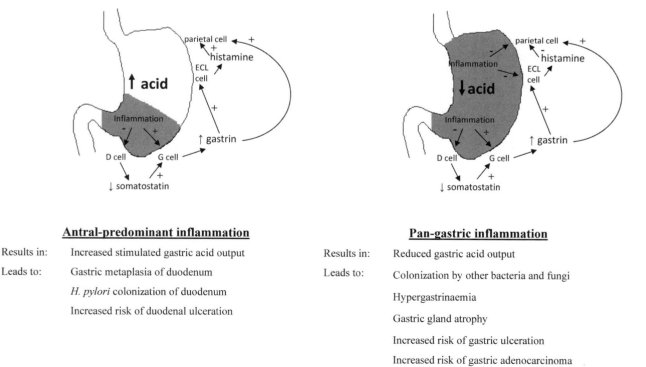

Antral-predominant inflammation

Results in: Increased stimulated gastric acid output

Leads to: Gastric metaplasia of duodenum

H. pylori colonization of duodenum

Increased risk of duodenal ulceration

Pan-gastric inflammation

Results in: Reduced gastric acid output

Leads to: Colonization by other bacteria and fungi

Hypergastrinaemia

Gastric gland atrophy

Increased risk of gastric ulceration

Increased risk of gastric adenocarcinoma

Figure 4. Colonization and gastritis patterns in the stomach: their effects on gastric acid production and their associations with duodenal and gastric ulceration.

cancer-associated death (268). Clinical manifestations usually appear late, and the prognosis is then poor, with less than a quarter of patients surviving for more than 5 years (234). *H. pylori* infection is thought to be one of several factors involved in the process of carcinogenesis, since only a small proportion of infected people go on to develop gastric cancer. The mechanisms in gastric carcinogenesis are incompletely understood, but a causal link between *H. pylori* and gastric cancer is further supported by animal models, where infection leads eventually to gastric cancer (357, 386). Several studies have reported that eradication therapy in humans and animal models leads to some regression of premalignant pathology, such as atrophy and intestinal metaplasia (52, 67, 196). However, once gastric atrophy has developed, many people will develop gastric cancer regardless of whether *H. pylori* is treated (363).

H. pylori is more closely associated with the distal (noncardia) type of gastric adenocarcinoma than the cardia type (71). There are two main forms of distal gastric cancer: the more common intestinal form occurs in the elderly, whereas the diffuse form can occur in younger adults. *H. pylori* is an important risk factor for both (22, 122, 269, 288).

Pathogenesis of Gastric Adenocarcinoma

For the intestinal type of gastric adenocarcinoma, a progressive sequence of events leading from chronic gastritis to atrophy, intestinal metaplasia, and dysplasia and culminating in the development of adenocarcinoma has been well characterized since it was first described by Correa in 1975 (68). Diffuse-type gastric cancer may arise directly from simple chronic active gastritis.

More virulent strains of *H. pylori* are more likely to cause gastric cancer. However, host genetic susceptibility is also important, and polymorphisms in many host genes have been associated with increased gastric cancer risk in infected people. These include inflammatory genes (e.g., cytokines [98, 220], Toll-like receptors [148, 369], COX-2 [211], CD14 [369, 385], and transcription factors [289]), as well as genes involved in apoptosis (153) and tissue remodeling (195). Reactive oxygen and nitrogen intermediates produced during inflammation may directly induce mutations by causing DNA damage and inhibiting DNA repair mechanisms (163, 258, 345). In addition, *H. pylori*-stimulated host signaling leads to the expression of proangiogenic and cancer-associated factors, such as IL-8, COX-2, vascular endothelial growth factor, and matrix metalloproteinases (34, 131, 183).

Elevated levels of gastrin, which regulates acid output, may also be important in gastric carcinogenesis. Gastrin is a gastrointestinal epithelial growth factor, and chronic hypergastrinemia causes increased rates of epithelial cell proliferation and eventually atrophy of gastric glands, reduced acid production and thus further hypergastrinemia in a positive feedback loop. Hypochlorydia is thought to permit colonization of the gastric mucosa by other organisms, perhaps leading to the release of oxygen and nitrogen-free radicals which might predispose to DNA damage and so to the development of gastric cancer. When transgenic INS-GAS mice (which overexpress gastrin) were infected with *Helicobacter*, gastric carcinogenesis was induced at a markedly accelerated rate compared to that seen in wild-type animals (113, 114). Gastrin also enhances the expression of several cancer-associated factors, including heparin-binding epidermal growth factor (80, 190), matrix metalloproteinases (368), trefoil factor 1 (177), and COX-2 (129, 190), and expression or activation of a range of anti-apoptotic mediators (190, 297, 342). The combination of increased epithelial cell proliferation in the presence of DNA-damaging compounds such as reactive oxygen species, together with a resistance to apoptosis, could permit the accumulation of mutations and so confer an increased risk of carcinogenesis.

The mechanisms driving the development of gastric atrophy remain poorly understood. However, several studies have demonstrated the involvement of an *H. pylori*-induced autoimmune reaction, with approximately half of infected individuals having parietal cell reactive antibodies in their serum (254). Parietal cells are rich in the H^+, K^+ proton pump ATPase, and this has been identified as a major autoantigen in patients with *H. pylori* atrophic gastritis (62). Studies of $CD4^+$ T-cell clones from the gastric mucosa of *H. pylori*-infected donors found that several bacterial components shared cross-reactive epitopes with H^+,K^+-ATPase (3, 36). Upon stimulation, the H^+,K^+-ATPase-reactive clones expressed the cytolytic molecule perforin and were able to induce apoptosis in target cells (3). Such cells therefore have the potential to cause parietal cell destruction and gastric atrophy (73).

A recent theory is that gastric adenocarcinoma arises from malignant transformation of stem cells, and in support of this, carcinogenesis is associated with disruption of stem cell signaling pathways and tissue repair mechanisms (33, 283). Many types of cancer are associated with chronic inflammatory tissue damage (251), and, since stem cells undergo continuous rounds of cell division in a chronic inflammatory environment and are long lived, they are more susceptible than other cell types to the accumulation of mutations (346). Houghton et al. (150) showed that gastric cancer in mice may be derived from bone marrow-derived stem cells (BMDCs), not from the resident gastric tissue-specific stem cells, as previously thought. In experiments using C57BL/6 mice, which had been engrafted with tagged BMDC from transgenic mice, they found that chronic *H. felis* infection resulted in a depletion of gastric mucosal stem cells and a recruitment of BMDCs into the stem cell niche. During prolonged colonization, these cells progressed to intraepithelial carcinoma. All of the neoplastic cells were derived from BMDCs, implying that in an inflammatory environment BMDCs do not differentiate properly but progress to metaplasia, dysplasia, and cancer. Identification of BMDCs as the cellular origin of *Helicobacter*-induced gastric cancer and possibly also other epithelial carcinomas associated with chronic inflammation is an important finding which, if confirmed with humans, presents opportunities for future prognostic and therapeutic strategies.

GASTRIC MALT LYMPHOMA

Gastric MALT lymphoma is an uncommon disease, with an incidence of approximately 0.8 per 100,000 per year (87). *H. pylori* is the major causative agent (reviewed in references 105, 248, and 366). Approximately 10% of cases appear to be independent of *H. pylori*, but some of these cases may be due to low-level or undiagnosed *H. pylori* infection (46, 367). MALT lymphoma has also been described in association with other gastric *Helicobacter* species which can transiently colonize humans as zoonoses.

H. pylori infection induces inflammation and the formation of lymphoid follicles in the gastric mucosa; such features are not present in the uninfected stomach (120). Gastric MALT lymphoma arises from neoplastic cells which spread from the marginal zone of lymphoid follicles to invade the epithelium (87). The tumor cells are commonly disseminated throughout the gastric mucosa, but in most cases they remain localized to the stomach for many years. Spread to regional lymph nodes occurs in at least 40% of cases (185), and migration to more distant mucosal sites in the body also commonly occurs (88). Low-grade MALT lymphomas may transform into more-aggressive diffuse large B-cell lymphomas (DLBCL) (247), although DLBCLs can also arise de novo. DLBCLs account for just over half of gastric lymphoma cases and have a much worse prognosis: 10-year survival rates for gastric MALT lymphoma and DLBCL are 90% and 45% respectively (87).

Complete regression of stomach-localized MALT lymphoma by antibiotic treatment of *H. pylori* infection is seen in the majority of cases, demonstrating both the prominent role of the infection and that it provides the ongoing stimulus to proliferation of clonal B cells (158, 246, 366). The expression of virulence factors by colonizing strains, such as *cagA* (96, 107), *iceA* (187), and *vacA* s1 (187), has been associated with increased risk of MALT lymphoma, presumably via induction of more severe mucosal inflammation. The risk factors for transformation into DLBCL, however, are unclear. High-grade lymphomas are treated with chemotherapy.

A subgroup of low-grade B-cell MALT lymphomas are associated with a chromosomal translocation between 11 and 18 [t(11;18)(q21;q21)], where chromosomal breakage results in reciprocal fusion between the activator protein-12 (*AP-12*) and *MALT-1* genes (26, 28). The product of the *AP-12–MALT-1* fusion stimulates activation of the transcription factor NF-κB, which regulates the expression of antiapoptotic genes and aids cell survival (146). Treatment for *H. pylori* in these cases is almost always ineffective (252), yet t(11;18)(q21;q21) gastric MALT lymphoma has been found to be significantly associated with *cagA*-positive *H. pylori* infections (87, 376).

IRON DEFICIENCY ANEMIA

Iron deficiency anemia (IDA), the most common form of anemia, is highly prevalent in developing countries, where *H. pylori* infection is virtually ubiquitous (328). Associations between IDA and gastritis have been reported in the literature for many years, even before the discovery of *H. pylori* (78, 159). There is now increasing evidence that *H. pylori* infection is an important causal factor in this condition (reviewed in reference 201). Annibale et al. (9) showed that the majority of patients with atrophic gastritis develop IDA, and 61% of these were infected with *H. pylori*. Apart from these epidemiological studies, several researchers have convincingly demonstrated that *H. pylori* eradication therapy alone improved erythrocyte counts and blood iron levels, in some cases leading to the complete resolution of IDA (10, 23, 226, 307, 378). Chen et al. also recently showed that treatment of the infection significantly improved the rate of recovery from IDA, when given along with ferrous succinate treatment (56). In contrast, in a study of children from rural Alaska, treatment of *H. pylori* infection did not improve iron deficiency (121).

Although the majority of reports demonstrate a role for *H. pylori* in the etiology of IDA, the mechanisms remain unclear. An obvious explanation is that ulceration caused by the infection leads to blood loss. People with ulcers often develop anemia secondary to ulcer bleeding, but most people with *H. pylori*-associated IDA do not have ulcers. A more likely explanation for the majority of *H. pylori*-associated IDA is that *H. pylori* disrupts the absorption of iron. Iron absorption is reliant upon gastric hydrochloric acid and dietary ascorbic acid (65), where gastric acid reduces ferric iron to the more readily absorbed ferrous form and ascorbic acid aids absorption further by forming soluble iron complexes. *H. pylori* infection is known to reduce both gastric acid and ascorbic acid levels (8). A further possible mechanism is that *H. pylori* sequesters iron from interstitial fluid in gastric tissue. It was recently shown that strains of *H. pylori* from patients with IDA have increased iron uptake compared with those isolated from non-IDA patients (377). *H. pylori* has several iron uptake mechanisms, but lactoferrin is thought to be the most important iron source for *H. pylori* in vivo in the human stomach, as it is secreted by neutrophils which are abundant in inflamed gastric tissue (especially in *H. pylori*-induced gastritis) (60). FeoB, a major *H. pylori* iron acquisition factor, is thought also to be important, as strains with *feoB* polymorphisms have been reported to be associated with IDA (164).

VITAMIN B_{12} DEFICIENCY

Vitamin B_{12} is another essential nutrient which requires the presence of gastric acid for its absorption. Gastric acid and pepsin release the vitamin from its protein complex in food, permitting it to bind to intrinsic factor, which is produced in the gastric corpus; this is required for B_{12} absorption (85, 182). Several researchers have reported an association between *H. pylori* infection and vitamin B_{12} deficiency and malabsorption (53, 174), even when gastric corpus atrophy is minimal (317). Gumurdulu et al. found that higher antral loads of *H. pylori* were significantly associated with vitamin B_{12} deficiency (128). In an earlier study, it was found that antibiotic treatment could improve vitamin B_{12} absorption in patients with atrophic gastritis (333), and it has now been further confirmed that *H. pylori* eradication alone restores vitamin B_{12} levels (174). The most profound form of vitamin B_{12} deficiency is pernicious anemia, which is caused by autoimmune gastritis, leading to severe inflammation and atrophy of the gastric corpus, with subsequent loss of intrinsic factor secretion by the stomach. It has been suggested that this is triggered by *H. pylori* infection (173).

EXTRAGASTRIC DISEASES

Chronic infection with *H. pylori* has been reported as a possible causal factor in several extragastric diseases, including ITP, ischemic heart disease, hepatobiliary disease, pulmonary disease, growth retardation, and Parkinson's disease.

Idiopathic Thrombocytopenic Purpura

ITP is a hematological condition in which low numbers of platelets prevent blood clotting and is characterized by extensive bruising and petechiae on the skin and mucous membranes. Children may develop an acute form of the disorder which resolves completely within a few weeks, whereas adults tend to develop chronic ITP (cITP) (162). Several studies have reported a high prevalence of *H. pylori* infection among ITP patients (reviewed in reference 117), and *H. pylori* eradication therapy has been shown to result in a significant increase in platelet counts in over 50% of cases (reviewed by reference 116). It has recently been reported that effects from this treatment are long lasting, with substantially increased platelet counts, even 4 years later (304, 309).

The relationship between *H. pylori* and cITP and the mechanisms underlying the effects of eradication of *H. pylori* infection on platelet counts remain unknown. However, more virulent strains ($cagA^+$ and *vacA* s1/m1) have been shown to be more common among patients with ITP (100), and responsiveness of ITP to *H. pylori* eradication is associated with the presence of serum CagA antibodies (186).

One proposed mechanism for *H. pylori* induction of cITP is through molecular mimicry, whereby the infection induces antibodies that cross-react with platelet membrane glycoprotein antigens (240). Cross-reactions between CagA and platelets have been demonstrated by several groups, suggesting that immunity to CagA may play a role in the pathogenesis of ITP (115, 335). A recent study examined whether platelets form immune complexes with *H. pylori* proteins (249). Immune complexes of platelets, low-molecular-weight *H. pylori* proteins, and anti-*H. pylori* antibodies were detected only when sera from patients with a positive response to *H. pylori* were used.

Host genetics appear to play a role in susceptibility to *H. pylori*-associated ITP. Patients with ITP are reported to have a lower frequency of HLA-DRB1*11 and -DQB1*03 alleles, indicating involvement of the immune system in ITP pathogenesis (350). A positive response to *H. pylori* eradication was not associated with polymorphisms in the proinflammatory genes IL-1β, IL-1RN, or TNF-α, in contrast to *H. pylori*-associated gastric cancer. Instead, certain TNF-β polymorphisms were good predictors of platelet recovery following *H. pylori* eradication (334), and it has been suggested that a +252 G/G single nucleotide polymorphism in the TNF-β gene is beneficial in controlling autoreactive B-cell responses to platelet membrane antigens (311). The association of *H. pylori* eradication and platelet count requires further investigation. There have been several unexpected findings, including the report that *H. pylori* eradication reduced platelet counts in patients with gastritis and peptic ulceration without ITP (232). *H. pylori* appears to induce platelet aggregation by several mechanisms (51), and these effects are strain dependent (66). However, in one study the administration of a proton pump inhibitor drug by itself also resulted in increased platelet counts in ITP patients, without changes in *H. pylori* antibody levels, indicating that acid suppression may be as important as *H. pylori* eradication itself in some patients (349).

Ischemic Heart Disease

Mendall et al. first reported an epidemiological association between *H. pylori* sero-prevalence and coronary heart disease in 1994 (238). Several studies have shown similar results (271, 272) and also described a higher prevalence of *H. pylori* among patients with acute myocardial infarction (278), atrial fibrillation (49), and unstable angina (279). There has been much argument over whether these associations are independent, the main potential confounder being social class. However, some studies have made strenuous efforts to correct for this, and although the size of the association is reduced (often greatly) following correction, it is rarely completely abolished. Some studies have also shown stronger associations of $CagA^+$ *H. pylori* infections with atherosclerosis (237, 287, 323), although many have not (75, 147, 188, 263). Some organisms associated with atherosclerosis, such as *Chlamydia pneumoniae,* have been cultured successfully from atherosclerotic tissue (161), but *H. pylori* has not. The presence of *H. pylori* has been detected using PCR or immunostaining in some studies (7, 20, 106), but not others (42, 359). *H. pylori* has been detected in human blood by PCR, but attempts to culture it from blood have been unsuccessful (83, 156). To test the association of *H. pylori* and atherosclerosis, several groups have investigated the effects of antibiotic therapy. Kowalski (193) reported that *H. pylori* eradication therapy significantly reduced coronary artery narrowing. Some studies have shown that *H. pylori* eradication leads to significant reductions in fibrinogen levels (raised fibrinogen being a risk factor for ischemic heart disease) (343, 381), but others have not (99, 315). This suggests that nonviable bacteria from the blood may simply be trapped within atherosclerotic plaques, rather than directly initiating atheroma development.

Nikolopoulou et al. (255) found that higher levels of the proinflammatory mediators TNF-α and sVCAM were associated with a significantly increased risk of coronary atherosclerosis, and a recent study by Danesh et al. (74) found that long-term high levels of circulating IL-6 were linked with increased risk. Since *H. pylori* induces inflammation in the gastric mucosa, it seems plausible that increased serum inflammatory mediators could explain such associations. Kowalski et al. (194) have reported that concentrations of plasma TNF-α, IL-8, and IL-1β were significantly reduced after *H. pylori* eradication, but several reports have shown comparable levels of these cytokines in patients with and without ischemic heart disease and regardless of *H. pylori* infection status (32, 79, 387). Stronger evidence suggests that *H. pylori* infection affects serum C reactive protein levels, which are an indication of systemic inflammation (49, 170, 299). Interestingly, Okada et al. (259) found that antibodies against *H. pylori* heat shock protein 60 (HSP60) which cross-reacted with the human HSP60 molecule were associated with cardiovascular disease, suggesting that autoimmune reactions may be involved in atherosclerosis.

Although there seems to be fairly broad agreement that there is no strong association between *H. pylori* and ischemic heart disease, several studies have shown that the infection modifies serum lipid levels in a way that increases the risk of atherosclerosis (147, 200). *H. pylori* eradication may reduce low-density serum lipoproteins and cholesterol (170, 222), which appears to be the most promising link between the infection and heart disease. Indeed, it has been shown in vitro that *cis*-unsaturated fatty acids, which have the capacity to prevent atherosclerosis, inhibit *H. pylori* growth (76). In addition, a cholesterol-rich diet in mice was shown to modify the T-cell response to *H. pylori* infection and alter bacterial colonization densities (370).

Hepatobiliary Disease

Serological data have shown that *H. pylori* and other *Helicobacter* species may be associated with chronic hepatobiliary diseases, such as cholesterol gallstone formation, cirrhosis, gallbladder cancer, and hepatocellular carcinoma (6, 203, 256). This association has been strengthened by studies using PCR analysis, which detected DNA from *H. pylori* and bile-resistant *Helicobacter* species, such as *H. bilis* and *H. pullorum*, in human liver and bile samples from patients with hepatic disease (112, 277, 341). However, the mere presence of bacterial DNA does not indicate that *Helicobacter* organisms are the cause of hepatobiliary disease. To address causality, Maurer et al. (235) infected mice with *H. hepaticus, H. bilis,* and *H. rodentium* and administered a lithogenic diet. Approximately 80% of these animals developed cholesterol gallstones within 8 weeks, compared to only 10% of uninfected controls. *Helicobacter* species were proposed to increase gallstone formation by releasing soluble antigens that interfere with the action of key hepatobiliary genes, and a role for *Helicobacter*-induced inflammatory cytokines was also suggested (235). Subsequently, these researchers also tested the effects of *H. pylori* infection, but this species did not induce gallstone formation (236). The data suggest that enterohepatic *Helicobacter* species play a role in gallstone formation in mice, but their effects on human disease remain unproven.

In support of a link in humans, in vitro studies have shown that *H. pylori* can survive in bile and that bile salts act as chemorepellants (134, 365). A protein present in human bile was found to react with anti-CagA antibodies, and also CagA was shown to have homology with aminopeptidase, which promotes cholesterol crystallization (110). A recent meta-analysis by Pandey (266) showed that a slightly increased risk of gallstones and benign liver disease was associated with *Helicobacter* infection (odds ratio of 1.77) but concluded that there is no evidence for a causal relationship.

Parkinson's Disease

A link between *H. pylori* infection and Parkinson's disease was first proposed in 1965 by Strang, who noted a dramatically increased frequency of peptic ulceration among Parkinson's disease patients compared to healthy controls (329). Although most Parkinson's disease patients do not have *H. pylori* infection, improvements in some aspects of Parkinsonism were seen in a trial of *H. pylori* eradication in patients (37). Unfortunately, the study was small, was terminated early, and used multiple end points, making it likely that this was a chance finding. However, if further studies confirmed the finding, a potential mechanism could be through *H. pylori*-induced chronic inflammation; systemic inflammation is associated with the worsening of chronic neurodegenerative diseases (282) and thought to exacerbate Parkinson's disease (82). *H. pylori* is known to affect drug absorption, including absorption of L-dopa, which is used to treat Parkinson's disease. Absorption is increased after eradication of the infection (286), but this does not explain the improvement in the study described above, as few of the patients involved were taking L-dopa.

Repiratory Disease

The incidence of chronic bronchitis and lung cancer is much higher in patients with peptic ulcers (21, 245), and patients with chronic bronchitis, bronchiectasis, and lung cancer have a higher sero-prevalence of *H. pylori* infection than normal controls (95, 169, 306, 348). A role for *H. pylori* virulence factors has also been proposed due to the presence of serum anti-VacA antibody among patients with lung cancer (95) and higher rates of anti-CagA antibodies in the serum of patients with chronic bronchitis (305).

Any mechanisms by which *H. pylori* might induce or exacerbate respiratory diseases remain unclear. It is thought that the risk of lung cancer could be increased via *H. pylori*-mediated upregulation of gastrin, which could stimulate tumor growth (356). Alternatively, the stimulation of increased numbers of Treg cells in response to the infection could result in suppressed tumor immunosurveillance, allowing cells to develop into cancer (354, 364). Finally, a raised level of systemic inflammatory cytokines in response to *H. pylori* could be involved (136, 149, 275).

Growth Retardation in Children

Growth retardation in children was first linked with *H. pylori* infection by Patel et al., who reported that among 7- to 11-year-old Scottish girls, height was significantly reduced in those who were *H. pylori* positive (273). Similar findings have been reported by other groups (313, 336), although growth retardation is known also to be strongly influenced by socioeconomic background and the presence of other infections and illnesses. In support of the specific association with *H. pylori,* new acquisition of *H. pylori* infection among lower-middle-class Colombian children was followed by significant retardation in growth (47, 239). There is also a higher sero-prevalence of *H. pylori* among children with delayed puberty (50, 59), and in addition, *H. pylori* infection has been proposed as a cause of low birth weight. In order to investigate this, Gobel et al. (123) mated mice following infection with *H. pylori.* No differences were found in litter size or weight between control and infected animals, and transmission of *H. pylori* from mother to pups could not be detected. They therefore suggested that low weight in babies may be due to reduced maternal milk production or impaired nutrition. Indeed, a recent study reported an increase in nutritional parameters, such as serum protein levels, following *H. pylori* eradication (118).

PROTECTIVE EFFECTS OF *H. PYLORI*

In addition to its association with gastro-duodenal and extra-gastric diseases, long-term infection with *H. pylori* has been reported to be beneficial under some circumstances. A number of researchers have reported that *H. pylori* abrogates the severity of GERD and its sequelae, and more recently there has been great interest in the possibility that the infection may help to prevent the development of allergy, asthma, and some autoimmune diseases (40, 208).

GERD and Its Complications

A relationship between *H. pylori* infection and GERD was first described by Vicari et al. in 1998 (352). These authors found the prevalence of *H. pylori* infection, particularly with *cagA*$^+$ strains, to be lower among patients with GERD, with even more marked negative associations with GERD sequelae, such as Barrett's esophagus and esophageal adenocarcinoma. This led to many studies concerning the association between *H. pylori* and GERD (reviewed in reference 318). In countries where the prevalence of *cagA*$^+$ *H. pylori* is generally high, such as in the Far East, reflux esophagitis is rare and the prevalence of *H. pylori* among patients with GERD is lower than in the general population (296). In contrast, the incidence of GERD and esophageal adenocarcinoma has increased dramatically in Western countries over the last 30 years (379), and this coincides with a reduced prevalence of *H. pylori* infection. However, as in the East, there is also a strong negative association between *H. pylori* infection (particularly *cagA*$^+$ strains) and GERD severity and complications. The overall negative association with *H. pylori* per se is weaker than in Eastern countries, possibly because strains in the West are on average less virulent.

It is thought that *H. pylori* may protect against GERD because corpus-predominant or pan-gastritis results in reduced gastric acid output (274). Although some infected people have increased gastric acid (those with antral-predominant gastritis), reduced acid is more common overall. The underlying pathological abnormality in GERD is abnormal refluxing of gastric contents into the esophagus. In people with *H. pylori* infection, this refluxate will be more acidic in people with antral-predominant gastritis and less acidic in people with pan-gastritis or corpus-predominant gastritis. Because the latter is on average more common, at a population level *H. pylori*-infected people have less-damaging gastroesophageal refluxate and so less-severe GERD symptoms, less-severe reflux esophagitis, and fewer long-term sequelae of GERD. In support of this theory, gastric atrophy associated with *cagA*$^+$ infections (where gastric acid production is particularly low) is associated with less-severe esophagitis and a reduced risk of Barrett's esophagus and esophageal adenocarcinoma (7). Infection with more virulent strains has been shown by several groups to afford a larger reduction in the risk of severe forms of GERD (15, 199, 213), although some reports refute this (180, 280). The effects of *H. pylori* eradication on development of GERD have been studied in order to confirm the association. Several groups have reported the development of GERD in patients following eradication therapy (104, 132, 308), although this is not a universal finding and individual patients may have worsening, improvement, or no change in GERD symptoms following treatment. This is to be expected, as different *H. pylori*-infected people may have hyper- or hypo-chlorhydria secondary to their infection, and treatment of the infection will at least partially reverse these conditions. Even in patients with gastric atrophy, Haruma et al. (139) showed, the intragastric pH 12 months after the eradication of *H. pylori* decreased, presumably due to some inflammation-induced reversible component accompanying the fixed reduction in acidity resulting from the atrophy.

Asthma, Atopy, and Autoimmune Diseases

Several recent reports have shown a negative association between *H. pylori* infection and the risk of atopy and asthma (58, 191, 210, 230, 284, 316). In a recent paper, Chen and Blaser (58) showed a link between *H. pylori* infection and atopic disease in early life, where people infected with CagA$^+$ strains were 37% less likely to have had childhood asthma. Several groups have also found a significantly lower prevalence of *H. pylori*-specific antibodies among people with autoimmune diseases, such as multiple sclerosis and systemic lupus erythematosus (208, 314, 360). Exacerbation of rheumatoid arthritis following the eradication of *H. pylori* has also been reported (231), suggesting that the infection may be protective against autoimmunity.

One way that *H. pylori* could protect against asthma is via prevention of GERD, since some cases of asthma may be caused or worsened by aspiration of acidic gastric juice (339). However, this cannot explain protection against allergic rhinitis and autoimmune disease. More compellingly, a role for *H. pylori* in the "hygiene hypothesis" has been proposed, in which childhood exposure to certain microorganisms (including *H. pylori*) is needed for the development of a healthy immune system (302, 319). In many developing countries, the rate of *H. pylori* infection in childhood is around 80%, but the prevalence in many developed countries has declined to below 20% (224). Concomitantly, the prevalence of atopic disease in developed countries has increased markedly over the past 50 years (27, 43). Kosunen et al. (191) reported a 3.5-fold increase in the incidence of allergy between 1973 and 1994 in Finland, which was accompanied by a 30% decrease in *H. pylori* prevalence over the same period. The proposed mechanisms behind the hygiene hypothesis include skewing of the cellular immunity from an allergy-associated Th2 response to Th1 (347) and the generation of Tregs which dampen immune responses such as those in allergy and autoimmunity (320). *H. pylori* is known to stimulate a Th1 response in the gastric mucosa and peripheral blood (327, 355), and infection with $CagA^+$ strains is reported to elicit increased human Th1 (140) and reduced Th2 responses (260). In addition, *H. pylori* infection influences the levels of gastric hormones, reducing levels of somatostatin while stimulating increased gastrin production. This is known to inhibit Th2 cytokine release and increase Th1 responses (382). However, since high levels of Th1 cytokines are not detected in the serum of those infected with *H. pylori*, it appears unlikely that the balance of T-cell immunity in general will be greatly affected.

A more plausible hypothesis is that *H. pylori*-associated Tregs are involved in suppressing the deleterious immune responses which may predispose to asthma and autoimmunity. We and others have shown that increased numbers of Tregs are present in the gastric mucosa of *H. pylori*-infected patients (217, 293, 301), and more surprisingly higher levels of these cells are found in their peripheral blood (176, 355). *H. pylori* infection is also known to induce Treg responses in the gastric mucosa, peripheral blood, and spleens of mice (172, 293). Higher levels of IL-10 mRNA have been found in *cagA*$^+$ than in *cagA* human gastric tissue samples (140, 301), perhaps explaining the stronger protective effect against asthma associated with $CagA^+$ infections (58). We have shown that there is a stronger $IL\text{-}10^+$ Treg response in individuals infected with *cagA*$^+$ strains (301). The fact that *H. pylori* stimulates a systemic Treg response supports the idea that such cells could have a more general immunoregulatory role.

The data linking *H. pylori* with protection from allergy and autoimmunity are so far mainly epidemiological. Exposure to a number of other infectious organisms has been linked with the hygiene hypothesis, including mycobacteria (347), hepatitis A (230), and parasites (14, 250). Since exposure to such organisms and *H. pylori* is similarly associated with factors such as socioeconomic status and overcrowding, we cannot be certain that any protective effects are specifically induced by *H. pylori.* To advance this field, mechanistic experiments are needed in animal models of allergy and autoimmunity, and interventional studies are needed with humans.

CONCLUSION

H. pylori is the main cause of peptic ulceration, noncardia gastric adenocarcinoma, and gastric lymphoma and has been associated with the development of several other gastric and extra-gastric diseases. In spite of this, some researchers have proposed that *H. pylori* should be regarded as a commensal organism which occasionally induces disease rather than a pathogen, since most infections are asymptomatic. Indeed, some consequences of *H. pylori* colonization on human physiology and immunity appear beneficial (38, 157). It is interesting to speculate that humans have coevolved with *H. pylori* and that our normal physiology has gradually become programmed to work in harmony with these bacteria which inhabit our stomachs throughout our lives in the absence of treatment (38). Most infections are acquired during early childhood (125), at a time when the immune system is developing (325), and this is also a common age for the development of asthma (151). From an evolutionary viewpoint, one could consider that when *H. pylori* colonization is absent, as is increasingly the case in developed countries, our immunity and gastroesophageal physiology are impaired.

REFERENCES

1. **Adams, B. L., T. C. Bates, and J. D. Oliver.** 2003. Survival of *Helicobacter pylori* in a natural freshwater environment. *Appl. Environ. Microbiol.* **69:**7462–7466.
2. **Akhiani, A. A., J. Pappo, Z. Kabok, K. Schon, W. Gao, L. E. Franzen, and N. Lycke.** 2002. Protection against *Helicobacter pylori* infection following immunization is IL-12-dependent and mediated by Th1 cells. *J. Immunol.* **169:**6977–6984.
3. **Amedei, A., M. P. Bergman, B. J. Appelmelk, A. Azzurri, M. Benagiano, C. Tamburini, R. van der Zee, J. L. Telford, C. M. Vandenbroucke-Grauls, M. M. D'Elios, and G. Del Prete.** 2003. Molecular mimicry between *Helicobacter pylori* antigens and H^+,K^+–adenosine triphosphatase in human gastric autoimmunity. *J. Exp. Med.* **198:**1147–1156.
4. **Amedei, A., A. Cappon, G. Codolo, A. Cabrelle, A. Polenghi, M. Benagiano, E. Tasca, A. Azzurri, M. M. D'Elios, G. Del Prete, and M. de Bernard.** 2006. The neutrophil-activating protein of *Helicobacter pylori* promotes Th1 immune responses. *J. Clin. Investig.* **116:**1092–1101.
5. **Ameriso, S. F., E. A. Fridman, R. C. Leiguarda, and G. E. Sevlever.** 2001. Detection of *Helicobacter pylori* in human carotid atherosclerotic plaques. *Stroke* **32:**385–391.
6. **Ananieva, O., I. Nilsson, T. Vorobjova, R. Uibo, and T. Wadstrom.** 2002. Immune responses to bile-tolerant *Helicobacter*

species in patients with chronic liver diseases, a randomized population group, and healthy blood donors. *Clin. Diagn. Lab. Immunol.* **9:**1160–1164.

7. **Anderson, L. A., S. J. Murphy, B. T. Johnston, P. Watson, H. Ferguson, K. B. Bamford, A. Ghazy, P. McCarron, J. Mc Guigan, J. V. Reynolds, H. Comber, and L. J. Murray.** 2008. Relationship between *Helicobacter pylori* infection and gastric atrophy and the stages of the oesophageal inflammation, metaplasia, adenocarcinoma sequence: results from the FINBAR case-control study. *Gut* **57:**734–9.
8. **Annibale, B., G. Capurso, E. Lahner, S. Passi, R. Ricci, F. Maggio, and G. Delle Fave.** 2003. Concomitant alterations in intragastric pH and ascorbic acid concentration in patients with *Helicobacter pylori* gastritis and associated iron deficiency anaemia. *Gut* **52:**496–501.
9. **Annibale, B., G. Capurso, G. Martino, C. Grossi, and G. Delle Fave.** 2000. Iron deficiency anaemia and *Helicobacter pylori* infection. *Int. J. Antimicrob. Agents* **16:**515–519.
10. **Annibale, B., M. Marignani, B. Monarca, G. Antonelli, A. Marcheggiano, G. Martino, F. Mandelli, R. Caprilli, and G. Delle Fave.** 1999. Reversal of iron deficiency anemia after *Helicobacter pylori* eradication in patients with asymptomatic gastritis. *Ann. Intern. Med.* **131:**668–672.
11. **Anonymous.** 2001. Gastric cancer and *Helicobacter pylori*: a combined analysis of 12 case control studies nested within prospective cohorts. *Gut* **49:**347–353.
12. **Anonymous.** 1994. Schistosomes, liver flukes and *Helicobacter pylori*. IARC Working Group on the Evaluation of Carcinogenic Risks to Humans. Lyon, 7-14 June 1994. *IARC Monogr. Eval. Carcinog. Risks Hum.* **61:**1–241.
13. **Arachchi, H. S., V. Kalra, B. Lal, V. Bhatia, C. S. Baba, S. Chakravarthy, S. Rohatgi, P. M. Sarma, V. Mishra, B. Das, and V. Ahuja.** 2007. Prevalence of duodenal ulcer-promoting gene (*dupA*) of *Helicobacter pylori* in patients with duodenal ulcer in North Indian population. *Helicobacter* **12:** 591–597.
14. **Araujo, M. I., B. S. Hoppe, M. Medeiros, Jr., and E. M. Carvalho.** 2004. *Schistosoma mansoni* infection modulates the immune response against allergic and auto-immune diseases. *Mem. Inst. Oswaldo Cruz* **99:**27–32.
15. **Arents, N. L., A. A. van Zwet, J. C. Thijs, A. M. Kooistra-Smid, K. R. van Slochteren, J. E. Degener, J. H. Kleibeuker, and L. J. van Doorn.** 2001. The importance of vacA, cagA, and iceA genotypes of *Helicobacter pylori* infection in peptic ulcer disease and gastroesophageal reflux disease. *Am. J. Gastroenterol.* **96:**2603–2608.
16. **Argent, R. H., A. Burette, V. Y. Miendje Deyi, and J. C. Atherton.** 2007. The presence of dupA in *Helicobacter pylori* is not significantly associated with duodenal ulceration in Belgium, South Africa, China, or North America. *Clin. Infect. Dis.* **45:**1204–1206.
17. **Argent, R. H., M. Kidd, R. J. Owen, R. J. Thomas, M. C. Limb, and J. C. Atherton.** 2004. Determinants and consequences of different levels of CagA phosphorylation for clinical isolates of *Helicobacter pylori*. *Gastroenterology* **127:** 514–523.
18. **Argent, R. H., R. J. Thomas, F. Aviles-Jimenez, D. P. Letley, M. C. Limb, E. M. El-Omar, and J. C. Atherton.** 2008. Toxigenic *Helicobacter pylori* infection precedes gastric hypochlorhydria in cancer relatives, and *H. pylori* virulence evolves in these families. *Clin. Cancer Res.* **14:**2227–2235.
19. **Argent, R. H., R. J. Thomas, F. Aviles-Jimenez, D. P. Letley, M. C. Limb, E. M. El-Omar, and J. C. Atherton.** 2008. Toxigenic *Helicobacter pylori* infection precedes gastric hypochlorhydria in cancer relatives, and *H. pylori* virulence evolves in these families. *Clin. Cancer Res.* **14:**2227–2235.
20. **Arias, E., H. Martinetto, M. Schultz, S. Ameriso, S. Rivera, O. Lossetti, and G. Sevlever.** 2006. Seminested polymerase chain reaction (PCR) for detecting *Helicobacter pylori* DNA in carotid atheromas. *Diagn. Mol. Pathol.* **15:**174–179.
21. **Arora, O. P., C. P. Kapoor, and P. Sobti.** 1968. Study of gastroduodenal abnormalities in chronic bronchitis and emphysema. *Am J. Gastroenterol.* **50:**289–296.
22. **Asghar, R. J., and J. Parsonnet.** 2001. *Helicobacter pylori* and risk for gastric adenocarcinoma. *Semin. Gastrointest. Dis.* **12:**203–208.
23. **Ashorn, M., T. Ruuska, and A. Makipernaa.** 2001. *Helicobacter pylori* and iron deficiency anaemia in children. *Scand. J. Gastroenterol.* **36:**701–705.
24. **Atherton, J. C.** 2006. The pathogenesis of *Helicobacter pylori*-induced gastro-duodenal diseases. *Ann. Rev. Pathol.* **1:**63–96.
25. **Atherton, J. C., P. Cao, R. M. Peek, Jr., M. K. Tummuru, M. J. Blaser, and T. L. Cover.** 1995. Mosaicism in vacuolating cytotoxin alleles of *Helicobacter pylori*. Association of specific vacA types with cytotoxin production and peptic ulceration. *J. Biol. Chem.* **270:**17771–17777.
26. **Auer, I. A., R. D. Gascoyne, J. M. Connors, F. E. Cotter, T. C. Greiner, W. G. Sanger, and D. E. Horsman.** 1997. t(11;18)(q21;q21) is the most common translocation in MALT lymphomas. *Ann. Oncol.* **8:**979–985.
27. **Austin, J. B., B. Kaur, H. R. Anderson, M. Burr, L. S. Harkins, D. P. Strachan, and J. O. Warner.** 1999. Hay fever, eczema, and wheeze: a nationwide UK study (ISAAC, international study of asthma and allergies in childhood). *Arch. Dis. Child* **81:**225–230.
28. **Baens, M., B. Maes, A. Steyls, K. Geboes, P. Marynen, and C. De Wolf-Peeters.** 2000. The product of the t(11;18), an API2-MLT fusion, marks nearly half of gastric MALT type lymphomas without large cell proliferation. *Am. J. Pathol.* **156:**1433–1439.
29. **Bamford, K. B., X. Fan, S. E. Crowe, J. F. Leary, W. K. Gourley, G. K. Luthra, E. G. Brooks, D. Y. Graham, V. E. Reyes, and P. B. Ernst.** 1998. Lymphocytes in the human gastric mucosa during *Helicobacter pylori* have a T helper cell 1 phenotype. *Gastroenterology* **114:**482–492.
30. **Bauditz, J., M. Ortner, M. Bierbaum, G. Niedobitek, H. Lochs, and S. Schreiber.** 1999. Production of IL-12 in gastritis relates to infection with *Helicobacter pylori*. *Clin. Exp. Immunol.* **117:**316–323.
31. **Bauerfeind, P., R. Garner, B. E. Dunn, and H. L. Mobley.** 1997. Synthesis and activity of *Helicobacter pylori* urease and catalase at low pH. *Gut* **40:**25–30.
32. **Bayraktaroglu, T., A. S. Aras, S. Aydemir, C. Davutoglu, Y. Ustundag, H. Atmaca, and A. Borazan.** 2004. Serum levels of tumor necrosis factor-alpha, interleukin-6 and interleukin-8 are not increased in dyspeptic patients with *Helicobacter pylori*-associated gastritis. *Mediators Inflamm.* **13:**25–28.
33. **Beachy, P. A., S. S. Karhadkar, and D. M. Berman.** 2004. Tissue repair and stem cell renewal in carcinogenesis. *Nature* **432:**324–331.
34. **Bebb, J. R., D. P. Letley, R. J. Thomas, F. Aviles, H. M. Collins, S. A. Watson, N. M. Hand, A. Zaitoun, and J. C. Atherton.** 2003. *Helicobacter pylori* upregulates matrilysin (MMP-7) in epithelial cells in vivo and in vitro in a Cag dependent manner. *Gut* **52:**1408–1413.
35. **Bell, G. D., K. Powell, J. Weil, G. Harrison, S. Brookes, and S. Prosser.** 1991. 13C-urea breath test for *Helicobacter pylori* infection. *Gut* **32:**551–552.
36. **Bergman, M. P., A. Amedei, M. M. D'Elios, A. Azzurri, M. Benagiano, C. Tamburini, R. van der Zee, C. M. Vandenbroucke-Grauls, B. J. Appelmelk, and G. Del Prete.** 2003.

Characterization of H^+,K^+-ATPase T cell epitopes in human autoimmune gastritis. *Eur. J. Immunol.* **33:**539–545.

37. **Bjarnason, I. T., A. Charlett, R. J. Dobbs, S. M. Dobbs, M. A. Ibrahim, R. W. Kerwin, R. F. Mahler, N. L. Oxlade, D. W. Peterson, J. M. Plant, A. B. Price, and C. Weller.** 2005. Role of chronic infection and inflammation in the gastrointestinal tract in the etiology and pathogenesis of idiopathic parkinsonism. Part 2: response of facets of clinical idiopathic parkinsonism to *Helicobacter pylori* eradication. A randomized, double-blind, placebo-controlled efficacy study. *Helicobacter* **10:**276–287.
38. **Blaser, M. J.** 1999. Hypothesis: the changing relationships of *Helicobacter pylori* and humans: implications for health and disease. *J. Infect. Dis.* **179:**1523–1530.
39. **Blaser, M. J., and J. C. Atherton.** 2004. *Helicobacter pylori* persistence: biology and disease. *J. Clin. Investig.* **113:** 321–333.
40. **Blaser, M. J., Y. Chen, and J. Reibman.** 2008. Does *Helicobacter pylori* protect against asthma and allergy? *Gut* **57:**561–567.
41. **Blaser, M. J., G. I. Perez-Perez, H. Kleanthous, T. L. Cover, R. M. Peek, P. H. Chyou, G. N. Stemmermann, and A. Nomura.** 1995. Infection with *Helicobacter pylori* strains possessing cagA is associated with an increased risk of developing adenocarcinoma of the stomach. *Cancer Res.* **55:**2111–2115.
42. **Blasi, F., F. Denti, M. Erba, R. Cosentini, R. Raccanelli, A. Rinaldi, L. Fagetti, G. Esposito, U. Ruberti, and L. Allegra.** 1996. Detection of *Chlamydia pneumoniae* but not *Helicobacter pylori* in atherosclerotic plaques of aortic aneurysms. *J. Clin. Microbiol.* **34:**2766–2769.
43. **Bloomfield, S. F., R. Stanwell-Smith, R. W. Crevel, and J. Pickup.** 2006. Too clean, or not too clean: the hygiene hypothesis and home hygiene. *Clin. Exp. Allergy* **36:**402–425.
44. **Bohr, U. R., B. Annibale, F. Franceschi, D. Roccarina, and A. Gasbarrini.** 2007. Extragastric manifestations of *Helicobacter pylori* infection—other *Helicobacter*s. *Helicobacter* **12**(Suppl. 1)**:**45–53.
45. **Boomkens, S. Y., J. G. Kusters, G. Hoffmann, R. G. Pot, B. Spee, L. C. Penning, H. F. Egberink, T. S. van den Ingh, and J. Rothuizen.** 2004. Detection of *Helicobacter pylori* in bile of cats. *FEMS Immunol. Med. Microbiol.* **42:**307–311.
46. **Bouzourene, H., T. Haefliger, F. Delacretaz, and E. Saraga.** 1999. The role of *Helicobacter pylori* in primary gastric MALT lymphoma. *Histopathology* **34:**118–123.
47. **Bravo, L. E., R. Mera, J. C. Reina, A. Pradilla, A. Alzate, E. Fontham, and P. Correa.** 2003. Impact of *Helicobacter pylori* infection on growth of children: a prospective cohort study. *J. Pediatr. Gastroenterol. Nutr.* **37:**614–619.
48. **Brown, L. M., T. L. Thomas, J. L. Ma, Y. S. Chang, W. C. You, W. D. Liu, L. Zhang, and M. H. Gail.** 2001. *Helicobacter pylori* infection in rural China: exposure to domestic animals during childhood and adulthood. *Scand. J. Infect. Dis.* **33:**686–691.
49. **Bunch, T. J., J. D. Day, J. L. Anderson, B. D. Horne, J. B. Muhlestein, B. G. Crandall, J. P. Weiss, D. L. Lappe, and S. J. Asirvatham.** 2008. Frequency of *Helicobacter pylori* seropositivity and C-reactive protein increase in atrial fibrillation in patients undergoing coronary angiography. *Am. J. Cardiol.* **101:**848–851.
50. **Buyukgebiz, A., B. Dundar, E. Bober, and B. Buyukgebiz.** 2001. *Helicobacter pylori* infection in children with constitutional delay of growth and puberty. *J. Pediatr. Endocrinol. Metab.* **14:**549–551.
51. **Byrne, M. F., S. W. Kerrigan, P. A. Corcoran, J. C. Atherton, F. E. Murray, D. J. Fitzgerald, and D. M. Cox.** 2003. *Helicobacter pylori* binds von Willebrand factor and interacts with GPIb to induce platelet aggregation. *Gastroenterology* **124:** 1846–1854.
52. **Cai, X., J. Carlson, C. Stoicov, H. Li, T. C. Wang, and J. Houghton.** 2005. *Helicobacter felis* eradication restores normal architecture and inhibits gastric cancer progression in C57BL/6 mice. *Gastroenterology* **128:**1937–1952.
53. **Carmel, R., G. I. Perez-Perez, and M. J. Blaser.** 1994. *Helicobacter pylori* infection and food-cobalamin malabsorption. *Dig. Dis. Sci.* **39:**309–314.
54. **Caruso, R., F. Pallone, and G. Monteleone.** 2007. Emerging role of IL-23/IL-17 axis in *H. pylori*-associated pathology. *World J. Gastroenterol.* **13:**5547–5551.
55. **Chang, F., L. S. Steelman, J. G. Shelton, J. T. Lee, P. M. Navolanic, W. L. Blalock, R. Franklin, and J. A. McCubrey.** 2003. Regulation of cell cycle progression and apoptosis by the Ras/Raf/MEK/ERK pathway. *Int. J. Oncol.* **22:** 469–480.
56. **Chen, L. H., and H. S. Luo.** 2007. Effects of *H. pylori* therapy on erythrocytic and iron parameters in iron deficiency anemia patients with *H. pylori*-positive chronic gastristis. *World J. Gastroenterol.* **13:**5380–5383.
57. **Chen, W., D. Shu, and V. S. Chadwick.** 2001. *Helicobacter pylori* infection: mechanism of colonization and functional dyspepsia. Reduced colonization of gastric mucosa by *Helicobacter pylori* in mice deficient in interleukin-10. *J. Gastroenterol. Hepatol.* **16:**377–383.
58. **Chen, Y., and M. J. Blaser.** 2007. Inverse associations of *Helicobacter pylori* with asthma and allergy. *Arch. Intern. Med.* **167:**821–827.
59. **Choe, Y. H., S. K. Kim, and Y. C. Hong.** 2000. *Helicobacter pylori* infection with iron deficiency anaemia and subnormal growth at puberty. *Arch. Dis. Child* **82:**136–140.
60. **Choe, Y. H., Y. J. Oh, N. G. Lee, I. Imoto, Y. Adachi, N. Toyoda, and E. C. Gabazza.** 2003. Lactoferrin sequestration and its contribution to iron-deficiency anemia in *Helicobacter pylori*-infected gastric mucosa. *J. Gastroenterol. Hepatol.* **18:**980–985.
61. **Chow, T. K., J. R. Lambert, M. L. Wahlqvist, and B. H. Hsu-Hage.** 1995. *Helicobacter pylori* in Melbourne Chinese immigrants: evidence for oral-oral transmission via chopsticks. *J. Gastroenterol. Hepatol.* **10:**562–569.
62. **Claeys, D., G. Faller, B. J. Appelmelk, R. Negrini, and T. Kirchner.** 1998. The gastric H^+,K^+-ATPase is a major autoantigen in chronic *Helicobacter pylori* gastritis with body mucosa atrophy. *Gastroenterology* **115:**340–347.
63. **Clyne, M., A. Labigne, and B. Drumm.** 1995. *Helicobacter pylori* requires an acidic environment to survive in the presence of urea. *Infect. Immun.* **63:**1669–1673.
64. **Colbeck, J. C., L. M. Hansen, J. M. Fong, and J. V. Solnick.** 2006. Genotypic profile of the outer membrane proteins BabA and BabB in clinical isolates of *Helicobacter pylori*. *Infect. Immun.* **74:**4375–4378.
65. **Conrad, M. E., and S. G. Schade.** 1968. Ascorbic acid chelates in iron absorption: a role for hydrochloric acid and bile. *Gastroenterology* **55:**35–45.
66. **Corcoran, P. A., J. C. Atherton, S. W. Kerrigan, T. Wadstrom, F. E. Murray, R. M. Peek, D. J. Fitzgerald, D. M. Cox, and M. F. Byrne.** 2007. The effect of different strains of *Helicobacter pylori* on platelet aggregation. *Can. J. Gastroenterol.* **21:**367–370.
67. **Correa, P., E. T. Fontham, J. C. Bravo, L. E. Bravo, B. Ruiz, G. Zarama, J. L. Realpe, G. T. Malcom, D. Li, W. D. Johnson, and R. Mera.** 2000. Chemoprevention of gastric dysplasia: randomized trial of antioxidant supplements and anti-*Helicobacter pylori* therapy. *J. Natl. Cancer Inst.* **92:** 1881–1888.

68. **Correa, P., W. Haenszel, C. Cuello, S. Tannenbaum, and M. Archer.** 1975. A model for gastric cancer epidemiology. *Lancet* **ii:**58–60.
69. **Cover, T. L., and S. R. Blanke.** 2005. *Helicobacter pylori* VacA, a paradigm for toxin multifunctionality. *Nat. Rev. Microbiol.* **3:**320–332.
70. **Cover, T. L., and M. J. Blaser.** 1992. Purification and characterization of the vacuolating toxin from *Helicobacter pylori. J. Biol. Chem.* **267:**10570–10575.
71. **Crew, K. D., and A. I. Neugut.** 2006. Epidemiology of gastric cancer. *World J. Gastroenterol.* **12:**354–362.
72. **Cui, G., J. Houghton, N. Finkel, J. Carlson, and T. Wang.** 2003. IFN-gamma infusion induces gastric atrophy, metaplasia and dysplasia in the absence of *Helicobacter pylori* infection: a role for the immune response in *Helicobacter* disease. *Gastroenterology* **124**(Suppl. 1):A19.
73. **D'Elios, M. M., M. P. Bergman, A. Amedei, B. J. Appelmelk, and G. Del Prete.** 2004. *Helicobacter pylori* and gastric autoimmunity. *Microbes Infect.* **6:**1395–1401.
74. **Danesh, J., S. Kaptoge, A. G. Mann, N. Sarwar, A. Wood, S. B. Angleman, F. Wensley, J. P. Higgins, L. Lennon, G. Eiriksdottir, A. Rumley, P. H. Whincup, G. D. Lowe, and V. Gudnason.** 2008. Long-term interleukin-6 levels and subsequent risk of coronary heart disease: two new prospective studies and a systematic review. *PLoS Med.* **5:**e78.
75. **Danesh, J., and R. Peto.** 1998. Risk factors for coronary heart disease and infection with *Helicobacter pylori*: meta-analysis of 18 studies. *BMJ* **316:**1130–1132.
76. **Das, U. N.** 1998. Hypothesis: cis-unsaturated fatty acids as potential anti-peptic ulcer drugs. *Prostaglandins Leukot. Essent. Fatty Acids* **58:**377–380.
77. **de Jonge, R., R. G. Pot, R. J. Loffeld, A. H. van Vliet, E. J. Kuipers, and J. G. Kusters.** 2004. The functional status of the *Helicobacter pylori* sabB adhesin gene as a putative marker for disease outcome. *Helicobacter* **9:**158–164.
78. **Delamore, I. W., and D. J. Shearman.** 1965. Chronic iron-deficiency anaemia and atrophic gastritis. *Lancet* **i:**889–891.
79. **Di Bonaventura, G., R. Piccolomini, A. Pompilio, R. Zappacosta, M. Piccolomini, and M. Neri.** 2007. Serum and mucosal cytokine profiles in patients with active *Helicobacter pylori* and ischemic heart disease: is there a relationship? *Int. J. Immunopathol. Pharmacol.* **20:**163–172.
80. **Dickson, J. H., A. Grabowska, M. El-Zaatari, J. Atherton, and S. A. Watson.** 2006. *Helicobacter pylori* can induce heparin-binding epidermal growth factor expression via gastrin and its receptor. *Cancer Res.* **66:**7524–7531.
81. **Dimola, S., and M. L. Caruso.** 1999. *Helicobacter pylori* in animals affecting the human habitat through the food chain. *Anticancer Res.* **19:**3889–3894.
82. **Dobbs, R. J., A. Charlett, A. G. Purkiss, S. M. Dobbs, C. Weller, and D. W. Peterson.** 1999. Association of circulating TNF-alpha and IL-6 with ageing and parkinsonism. *Acta Neurol. Scand.* **100:**34–41.
83. **Dore, M. P., G. Realdi, A. R. Sepulveda, and D. Y. Graham.** 2003. Detection of genomic *Helicobacter pylori* DNA in the blood of patients positive for the infection. *Dig. Liver Dis.* **35:**839–840.
84. **Dore, M. P., A. R. Sepulveda, H. El-Zimaity, Y. Yamaoka, M. S. Osato, K. Mototsugu, A. M. Nieddu, G. Realdi, and D. Y. Graham.** 2001. Isolation of *Helicobacter pylori* from sheep-implications for transmission to humans. *Am. J. Gastroenterol.* **96:**1396–1401.
85. **Doscherholmen, A., D. Ripley, S. Chang, and S. E. Silvis.** 1977. Influence of age and stomach function on serum vitamin B12 concentration. *Scand. J. Gastroenterol.* **12:** 313–319.
86. **Dowsett, S. A., and M. J. Kowolik.** 2003. Oral *Helicobacter pylori*: can we stomach it? *Crit. Rev. Oral Biol. Med.* **14:**226–233.
87. **Du, M. Q., and J. C. Atherton.** 2006. Molecular subtyping of gastric MALT lymphomas: implications for prognosis and management. *Gut* **55:**886–893.
88. **Du, M. Q., C. F. Xu, T. C. Diss, H. Z. Peng, A. C. Wotherspoon, P. G. Isaacson, and L. X. Pan.** 1996. Intestinal dissemination of gastric mucosa-associated lymphoid tissue lymphoma. *Blood* **88:**4445–4451.
89. **Du, Y., A. Agnew, X. P. Ye, P. A. Robinson, D. Forman, and J. E. Crabtree.** 2006. *Helicobacter pylori* and *Schistosoma japonicum* co-infection in a Chinese population: helminth infection alters humoral responses to *H. pylori* and serum pepsinogen I/II ratio. *Microbes Infect.* **8:** 52–60.
90. **Dunn, B. E., H. Cohen, and M. J. Blaser.** 1997. *Helicobacter pylori. Clin. Microbiol. Rev.* **10:**720–741.
91. **Dzierzanowska-Fangrat, K., J. Michalkiewicz, J. Cielecka-Kuszyk, M. Nowak, D. Celinska-Cedro, E. Rozynek, D. Dzierzanowska, and J. E. Crabtree.** 2008. Enhanced gastric IL-18 mRNA expression in *Helicobacter pylori*-infected children is associated with macrophage infiltration, IL-8, and IL-1 beta mRNA expression. *Eur. J. Gastroenterol. Hepatol.* **20:**314–319.
92. **Eaton, K. A., and S. Krakowka.** 1994. Effect of gastric pH on urease-dependent colonization of gnotobiotic piglets by *Helicobacter pylori. Infect. Immun.* **62:**3604–3607.
93. **Eaton, K. A., M. Mefford, and T. Thevenot.** 2001. The role of T cell subsets and cytokines in the pathogenesis of *Helicobacter pylori* gastritis in mice. *J. Immunol.* **166:** 7456–7461.
94. **Eaton, K. A., D. R. Morgan, and S. Krakowka.** 1992. Motility as a factor in the colonisation of gnotobiotic piglets by *Helicobacter pylori. J. Med. Microbiol.* **37:**123–127.
95. **Ece, F., Hataby, N. F., N. Erdal, C. Gedik, C. Guney, and F. Aksoy.** 2005. Does *Helicobacter pylori* infection play a role in lung cancer? *Respir. Med.* **99:**1258–1262.
96. **Eck, M., B. Schmausser, R. Haas, A. Greiner, S. Czub, and H. K. Muller-Hermelink.** 1997. MALT-type lymphoma of the stomach is associated with *Helicobacter pylori* strains expressing the CagA protein. *Gastroenterology* **112:**1482–1486.
97. **El-Omar, E. M., M. Carrington, W. H. Chow, K. E. McColl, J. H. Bream, H. A. Young, J. Herrera, J. Lissowska, C. C. Yuan, N. Rothman, G. Lanyon, M. Martin, J. F. Fraumeni, Jr., and C. S. Rabkin.** 2000. Interleukin-1 polymorphisms associated with increased risk of gastric cancer. *Nature* **404:**398–402.
98. **El-Omar, E. M., C. S. Rabkin, M. D. Gammon, T. L. Vaughan, H. A. Risch, J. B. Schoenberg, J. L. Stanford, S. T. Mayne, J. Goedert, W. J. Blot, J. F. Fraumeni, Jr., and W. H. Chow.** 2003. Increased risk of noncardia gastric cancer associated with proinflammatory cytokine gene polymorphisms. *Gastroenterology* **124:**1193–1201.
99. **Elizalde, J. I., J. M. Pique, V. Moreno, J. D. Morillas, I. Elizalde, L. Bujanda, C. M. De Argila, A. Cosme, A. Castiella, and E. Ros.** 2002. Influence of *Helicobacter pylori* infection and eradication on blood lipids and fibrinogen. *Aliment. Pharmacol. Ther.* **16:**577–586.
100. **Emilia, G., M. Luppi, P. Zucchini, M. Morselli, L. Potenza, F. Forghieri, F. Volzone, G. Jovic, G. Leonardi, A. Donelli, and G. Torelli.** 2007. *Helicobacter pylori* infection and chronic immune thrombocytopenic purpura: long-term results of bacterium eradication and association with bacterium virulence profiles. *Blood* **110:**3833–3841.

101. **Enarsson, K., A. Lundgren, B. Kindlund, M. Hermansson, G. Roncador, A. H. Banham, B. S. Lundin, and M. Quiding-Jarbrink.** 2006. Function and recruitment of mucosal regulatory T cells in human chronic *Helicobacter pylori* infection and gastric adenocarcinoma. *Clin. Immunol.* **121:** 358–368.
102. **Erdman, S. E., T. Poutahidis, M. Tomczak, A. B. Rogers, K. Cormier, B. Plank, B. H. Horwitz, and J. G. Fox.** 2003. CD4+ CD25+ regulatory T lymphocytes inhibit microbially induced colon cancer in Rag2-deficient mice. *Am. J. Pathol.* **162:**691–702.
103. **Everhart, J. E.** 2000. Recent developments in the epidemiology of *Helicobacter pylori*. *Gastroenterol. Clin. North. Am.* **29:**559–578.
104. **Fallone, C. A., A. N. Barkun, G. Friedman, S. Mayrand, V. Loo, R. Beech, L. Best, and L. Joseph.** 2000. Is *Helicobacter pylori* eradication associated with gastroesophageal reflux disease? *Am. J. Gastroenterol.* **95:**914–920.
105. **Farinha, P., and R. D. Gascoyne.** 2005. *Helicobacter pylori* and MALT lymphoma. *Gastroenterology* **128:**1579–1605.
106. **Farsak, B., A. Yildirir, Y. Akyon, A. Pinar, M. Oc, E. Boke, S. Kes, and L. Tokgozoglu.** 2000. Detection of *Chlamydia pneumoniae* and *Helicobacter pylori* DNA in human atherosclerotic plaques by PCR. *J. Clin. Microbiol.* **38:** 4408–4411.
107. **Ferreira-Chagas, B., G. Lasne, S. Dupouy, A. Gallois, A. Morgner, A. Menard, F. Megraud, and P. Lehours.** 2007. In vitro proinflammatory properties of *Helicobacter pylori* strains causing low-grade gastric MALT lymphoma. *Helicobacter* **12:**616–617.
108. **Figueiredo, C., J. C. Machado, P. Pharoah, R. Seruca, S. Sousa, R. Carvalho, A. F. Capelinha, W. Quint, C. Caldas, L. J. van Doorn, F. Carneiro, and M. Sobrinho-Simoes.** 2002. *Helicobacter pylori* and interleukin 1 genotyping: an opportunity to identify high-risk individuals for gastric carcinoma. *J. Natl. Cancer Inst.* **94:**1680–1687.
109. **Figueiredo, C., W. Quint, N. Nouhan, H. van den Munckhof, P. Herbrink, J. Scherpenisse, W. de Boer, P. Schneeberger, G. Perez-Perez, M. J. Blaser, and L. J. van Doorn.** 2001. Assessment of *Helicobacter pylori vacA* and *cagA* genotypes and host serological response. *J. Clin. Microbiol.* **39:**1339–1344.
110. **Figura, N., F. Cetta, M. Angelico, G. Montalto, D. Cetta, L. Pacenti, C. Vindigni, D. Vaira, F. Festuccia, A. De Santis, G. Rattan, R. Giannace, S. Campagna, and C. Gennari.** 1998. Most *Helicobacter pylori*-infected patients have specific antibodies, and some also have *H. pylori* antigens and genomic material in bile: is it a risk factor for gallstone formation? *Dig. Dis. Sci.* **43:**854–862.
111. **Fox, J. G., P. Beck, C. A. Dangler, M. T. Whary, T. C. Wang, H. N. Shi, and C. Nagler-Anderson.** 2000. Concurrent enteric helminth infection modulates inflammation and gastric immune responses and reduces *Helicobacter*-induced gastric atrophy. *Nat. Med.* **6:**536–542.
112. **Fox, J. G., F. E. Dewhirst, Z. Shen, Y. Feng, N. S. Taylor, B. J. Paster, R. L. Ericson, C. N. Lau, P. Correa, J. C. Araya, and I. Roa.** 1998. Hepatic *Helicobacter* species identified in bile and gallbladder tissue from Chileans with chronic cholecystitis. *Gastroenterology* **114:**755–763.
113. **Fox, J. G., A. B. Rogers, M. Ihrig, N. S. Taylor, M. T. Whary, G. Dockray, A. Varro, and T. C. Wang.** 2003. *Helicobacter pylori*-associated gastric cancer in INS-GAS mice is gender specific. *Cancer Res.* **63:**942-950.
114. **Fox, J. G., T. C. Wang, A. B. Rogers, T. Poutahidis, Z. Ge, N. Taylor, C. A. Dangler, D. A. Israel, U. Krishna, K. Gaus, and R. M. Peek, Jr.** 2003. Host and microbial constituents influence *Helicobacter pylori*-induced cancer in a murine model of hypergastrinemia. *Gastroenterology* **124:** 1879–1890.
115. **Franceschi, F., N. Christodoulides, M. H. Kroll, and R. M. Genta.** 2004. *Helicobacter pylori* and idiopathic thrombocytopenic purpura. *Ann. Intern. Med.* **140:**766–767.
116. **Franchini, M., M. Cruciani, C. Mengoli, G. Pizzolo, and D. Veneri.** 2007. Effect of *Helicobacter pylori* eradication on platelet count in idiopathic thrombocytopenic purpura: a systematic review and meta-analysis. *J. Antimicrob. Chemother.* **60:**237–246.
117. **Franchini, M., and D. Veneri.** 2004. *Helicobacter pylori* infection and immune thrombocytopenic purpura: an update. *Helicobacter* **9:**342–346.
118. **Furuta, T., N. Shirai, F. Xiao, M. Takashima, and H. Hanai.** 2002. Effect of *Helicobacter pylori* infection and its eradication on nutrition. *Aliment. Pharmacol. Ther.* **16:** 799–806.
119. **Gebert, B., W. Fischer, E. Weiss, R. Hoffmann, and R. Haas.** 2003. *Helicobacter pylori* vacuolating cytotoxin inhibits T lymphocyte activation. *Science* **301:**1099–1102.
120. **Genta, R. M., H. W. Hamner, and D. Y. Graham.** 1993. Gastric lymphoid follicles in *Helicobacter pylori* infection: frequency, distribution, and response to triple therapy. *Hum. Pathol.* **24:**577–583.
121. **Gessner, B. D., H. C. Baggett, P. T. Muth, E. Dunaway, B. D. Gold, Z. Feng, and A. J. Parkinson.** 2006. A controlled, household-randomized, open-label trial of the effect that treatment of *Helicobacter pylori* infection has on iron deficiency in children in rural Alaska. *J. Infect. Dis.* **193:** 537–546.
122. **Go, M. F., and D. T. Smoot.** 2000. *Helicobacter pylori*, gastric MALT lymphoma, and adenocarcinoma of the stomach. *Semin. Gastrointest. Dis.* **11:**134–141.
123. **Gobel, R., E. L. Symonds, R. N. Butler, and C. D. Tran.** 2007. Association between *Helicobacter pylori* infection in mothers and birth weight. *Dig. Dis. Sci.* **52:**3049–3053.
124. **Goll, R., F. Gruber, T. Olsen, G. Cui, G. Raschpichler, M. Buset, A. M. Asfeldt, A. Husebekk, and J. Florholmen.** 2007. *Helicobacter pylori* stimulates a mixed adaptive immune response with a strong T-regulatory component in human gastric mucosa. *Helicobacter* **12:**185–192.
125. **Goodman, K. J., and P. Correa.** 1995. The transmission of *Helicobacter pylori*. A critical review of the evidence. *Int. J. Epidemiol.* **24:**875–887.
126. **Graham, D. Y., H. M. Malaty, D. G. Evans, D. J. Evans, Jr., P. D. Klein, and E. Adam.** 1991. Epidemiology of *Helicobacter pylori* in an asymptomatic population in the United States. Effect of age, race, and socioeconomic status. *Gastroenterology* **100:**1495–1501.
127. **Graham, D. Y., A. R. Opekun, M. S. Osato, H. M. El-Zimaity, C. K. Lee, Y. Yamaoka, W. A. Qureshi, M. Cadoz, and T. P. Monath.** 2004. Challenge model for *Helicobacter pylori* infection in human volunteers. *Gut* **53:** 1235–1243.
128. **Gumurdulu, Y., E. Serin, B. Ozer, F. Kayaselcuk, K. Kul, C. Pata, M. Guclu, G. Gur, and S. Boyacioglu.** 2003. Predictors of vitamin B12 deficiency: age and *Helicobacter pylori* load of antral mucosa. *Turk. J. Gastroenterol.* **14:**44–49.
129. **Guo, Y. S., J. Z. Cheng, G. F. Jin, J. S. Gutkind, M. R. Hellmich, and C. M. Townsend, Jr.** 2002. Gastrin stimulates cyclooxygenase-2 expression in intestinal epithelial cells through multiple signaling pathways. Evidence for involvement of ERK5 kinase and transactivation of the epidermal growth factor receptor. *J. Biol. Chem.* **277:** 48755–48763.

130. **Gyulai, Z., G. Klausz, A. Tiszai, Z. Lenart, I. T. Kasa, J. Lonovics, and Y. Mandi.** 2004. Genetic polymorphism of interleukin-8 (IL-8) is associated with *Helicobacter pylori*-induced duodenal ulcer. *Eur. Cytokine Netw.* **15:**353–358.
131. **Hahm, K. B., H. Y. Lim, S. Sohn, H. J. Kwon, K. M. Lee, J. S. Lee, Y. J. Surh, Y. B. Kim, H. J. Joo, W. S. Kim, and S. W. Cho.** 2002. In vitro evidence of the role of COX-2 in attenuating gastric inflammation and promoting gastric carcinogenesis. *J. Environ. Pathol. Toxicol. Oncol.* **21:** 165–176.
132. **Hamada, H., K. Haruma, M. Mihara, T. Kamada, M. Yoshihara, K. Sumii, G. Kajiyama, and M. Kawanishi.** 2000. High incidence of reflux oesophagitis after eradication therapy for *Helicobacter pylori*: impacts of hiatal hernia and corpus gastritis. *Aliment. Pharmacol. Ther.* **14:** 729–735.
133. **Han, S. R., H. C. Zschausch, H. G. Meyer, T. Schneider, M. Loos, S. Bhakdi, and M. J. Maeurer.** 2000. *Helicobacter pylori*: clonal population structure and restricted transmission within families revealed by molecular typing. *J. Clin. Microbiol.* **38:**3646–3651.
134. **Hanninen, M. L.** 1991. Sensitivity of *Helicobacter pylori* to different bile salts. *Eur. J. Clin. Microbiol. Infect. Dis.* **10:** 515–518.
135. **Hansson, L. E., L. Engstrand, O. Nyren, D. J. Evans, Jr., A. Lindgren, R. Bergstrom, B. Andersson, L. Athlin, O. Bendtsen, and P. Tracz.** 1993. *Helicobacter pylori* infection: independent risk indicator of gastric adenocarcinoma. *Gastroenterology* **105:**1098–1103.
136. **Hardaker, E. L., A. M. Bacon, K. Carlson, A. K. Roshak, J. J. Foley, D. B. Schmidt, P. T. Buckley, M. Comegys, R. A. Panettieri, Jr., H. M. Sarau, and K. E. Belmonte.** 2004. Regulation of TNF-alpha- and IFN-gamma-induced CXCL10 expression: participation of the airway smooth muscle in the pulmonary inflammatory response in chronic obstructive pulmonary disease. *FASEB J.* **18:**191–193.
137. **Harford, W. V., C. Barnett, E. Lee, G. Perez-Perez, M. J. Blaser, and W. L. Peterson.** 2000. Acute gastritis with hypochlorhydria: report of 35 cases with long term follow up. *Gut* **47:**467–472.
138. **Harris, P. R., S. W. Wright, C. Serrano, F. Riera, I. Duarte, J. Torres, A. Pena, A. Rollan, P. Viviani, E. Guiraldes, J. M. Schmitz, R. G. Lorenz, L. Novak, L. E. Smythies, and P. D. Smith.** 2008. *Helicobacter pylori* gastritis in children is associated with a regulatory T-cell response. *Gastroenterology* **134:**491–499.
139. **Haruma, K., M. Mihara, E. Okamoto, H. Kusunoki, M. Hananoki, S. Tanaka, M. Yoshihara, K. Sumii, and G. Kajiyama.** 1999. Eradication of *Helicobacter pylori* increases gastric acidity in patients with atrophic gastritis of the corpus-evaluation of 24-h pH monitoring. *Aliment. Pharmacol. Ther.* **13:**155–162.
140. **Hida, N., T. Shimoyama, Jr., P. Neville, M. F. Dixon, A. T. Axon, T. Shimoyama, Sr., and J. E. Crabtree.** 1999. Increased expression of IL-10 and IL-12 (p40) mRNA in *Helicobacter pylori* infected gastric mucosa: relation to bacterial cag status and peptic ulceration. *J. Clin. Pathol.* **52:**658–664.
141. **Higashi, H., A. Nakaya, R. Tsutsumi, K. Yokoyama, Y. Fujii, S. Ishikawa, M. Higuchi, A. Takahashi, Y. Kurashima, Y. Teishikata, S. Tanaka, T. Azuma, and M. Hatakeyama.** 2004. *Helicobacter pylori* CagA induces Ras-independent morphogenetic response through SHP-2 recruitment and activation. *J. Biol. Chem.* **279:**17205–17216.
142. **Higashi, H., R. Tsutsumi, A. Fujita, S. Yamazaki, M. Asaka, T. Azuma, and M. Hatakeyama.** 2002. Biological activity of the *Helicobacter pylori* virulence factor CagA is determined by variation in the tyrosine phosphorylation sites. *Proc. Natl. Acad. Sci. USA* **99:**14428–14433.
143. **Higashi, H., R. Tsutsumi, S. Muto, T. Sugiyama, T. Azuma, M. Asaka, and M. Hatakeyama.** 2002. SHP-2 tyrosine phosphatase as an intracellular target of *Helicobacter pylori* CagA protein. *Science* **295:**683–686.
144. **Hirata, I., M. Murano, T. Ishiguro, K. Toshina, F. Y. Wang, and K. Katsu.** 2007. HLA genotype and development of gastric cancer in patients with *Helicobacter pylori* infection. *Hepatogastroenterology* **54:**990–994.
145. **Hirata, Y., T. Ohmae, W. Shibata, S. Maeda, K. Ogura, H. Yoshida, T. Kawabe, and M. Omata.** 2006. MyD88 and TNF receptor-associated factor 6 are critical signal transducers in *Helicobacter pylori*-infected human epithelial cells. *J. Immunol.* **176:**3796–3803.
146. **Ho, L., R. E. Davis, B. Conne, R. Chappuis, M. Berczy, P. Mhawech, L. M. Staudt, and J. Schwaller.** 2005. MALT1 and the API2-MALT1 fusion act between CD40 and IKK and confer NF-kappa B-dependent proliferative advantage and resistance against FAS-induced cell death in B cells. *Blood* **105:**2891–2899.
147. **Hoffmeister, A., D. Rothenbacher, G. Bode, K. Persson, W. Marz, M. A. Nauck, H. Brenner, V. Hombach, and W. Koenig.** 2001. Current infection with *Helicobacter pylori*, but not seropositivity to *Chlamydia pneumoniae* or cytomegalovirus, is associated with an atherogenic, modified lipid profile. *Arterioscler. Thromb. Vasc. Biol.* **21:**427–432.
148. **Hold, G. L., C. S. Rabkin, W. H. Chow, M. G. Smith, M. D. Gammon, H. A. Risch, T. L. Vaughan, K. E. McColl, J. Lissowska, W. Zatonski, J. B. Schoenberg, W. J. Blot, N. A. Mowat, J. F. Fraumeni, Jr., and E. M. El-Omar.** 2007. A functional polymorphism of toll-like receptor 4 gene increases risk of gastric carcinoma and its precursors. *Gastroenterology* **132:**905–912.
149. **Hoshi, H., I. Ohno, M. Honma, Y. Tanno, K. Yamauchi, G. Tamura, and K. Shirato.** 1995. IL-5, IL-8 and GM-CSF immunostaining of sputum cells in bronchial asthma and chronic bronchitis. *Clin. Exp. Allergy* **25:**720–728.
150. **Houghton, J., C. Stoicov, S. Nomura, A. B. Rogers, J. Carlson, H. Li, X. Cai, J. G. Fox, J. R. Goldenring, and T. C. Wang.** 2004. Gastric cancer originating from bone marrow-derived cells. *Science* **306:**1568–1571.
151. **Hsu, J. Y., S. L. King, B. I. Kuo, and C. D. Chiang.** 2004. Age of onset and the characteristics of asthma. *Respirology* **9:**369–372.
152. **Hsu, P. I., C. N. Li, H. H. Tseng, K. H. Lai, P. N. Hsu, G. H. Lo, C. C. Lo, J. J. Yeh, L. P. Ger, M. Hsiao, Y. Yamaoka, I. R. Hwang, and A. Chen.** 2004. The interleukin-1 RN polymorphism and *Helicobacter pylori* infection in the development of duodenal ulcer. *Helicobacter* **9:**605–613.
153. **Hsu, P. I., P. J. Lu, E. M. Wang, L. P. Ger, G. H. Lo, F. W. Tsay, T. A. Chen, H. B. Yang, H. C. Chen, W. S. Lin, and K. H. Lai.** 2008. Polymorphisms of death pathway genes FAS and FASL and risk of premalignant gastric lesions. *Anticancer Res.* **28:**97–103.
154. **Hu, L. T., and H. L. Mobley.** 1990. Purification and N-terminal analysis of urease from *Helicobacter pylori*. *Infect. Immun.* **58:**992–998.
155. **Hu, P. J., H. M. Mitchell, Y. Y. Li, M. H. Zhou, and S. L. Hazell.** 1994. Association of *Helicobacter pylori* with gastric cancer and observations on the detection of this bacterium in gastric cancer cases. *Am. J. Gastroenterol.* **89:** 1806–1810.
156. **Huang, Y., X. G. Fan, Z. S. Tang, L. Liu, X. F. Tian, and N. Li.** 2006. Detection of *Helicobacter pylori* DNA in

peripheral blood from patients with peptic ulcer or gastritis. *APMIS* **114:**851–856.

157. **Hunt, R. H., K. Sumanac, and J. Q. Huang.** 2001. Review article: should we kill or should we save *Helicobacter pylori*? *Aliment. Pharmacol. Ther.* **15**(Suppl. 1)**:**51–59.
158. **Hussell, T., P. G. Isaacson, J. E. Crabtree, and J. Spencer.** 1993. The response of cells from low-grade B-cell gastric lymphomas of mucosa-associated lymphoid tissue to *Helicobacter pylori*. *Lancet* **342:**571–574.
159. **Ikkala, E., H. J. Salmi, and M. Siurala.** 1970. Gastric mucosa in iron deficiency anaemia. Results of follow-up examinations. *Acta Haematol.* **43:**228–231.
160. **Itoh, T., Y. Wakatsuki, M. Yoshida, T. Usui, Y. Matsunaga, S. Kaneko, T. Chiba, and T. Kita.** 1999. The vast majority of gastric T cells are polarized to produce T helper 1 type cytokines upon antigenic stimulation despite the absence of *Helicobacter pylori* infection. *J. Gastroenterol.* **34:**560–570.
161. **Jackson, L. A., L. A. Campbell, C. C. Kuo, D. I. Rodriguez, A. Lee, and J. T. Grayston.** 1997. Isolation of *Chlamydia pneumoniae* from a carotid endarterectomy specimen. *J. Infect. Dis.* **176:**292–295.
162. **Jackson, S., P. L. Beck, G. F. Pineo, and M. C. Poon.** 2005. *Helicobacter pylori* eradication: novel therapy for immune thrombocytopenic purpura? A review of the literature. *Am. J. Hematol.* **78:**142–150.
163. **Jaiswal, M., N. F. LaRusso, and G. J. Gores.** 2001. Nitric oxide in gastrointestinal epithelial cell carcinogenesis: linking inflammation to oncogenesis. *Am. J. Physiol. Gastrointest. Liver Physiol.* **281:**G626–G634.
164. **Jeon, B. H., Y. J. Oh, N. G. Lee, and Y. H. Choe.** 2004. Polymorphism of the *Helicobacter pylori* feoB gene in Korea: a possible relation with iron-deficiency anemia? *Helicobacter* **9:**330–334.
165. **Jones, D. M., and A. Curry.** 1992. The ultrastructure of *Helicobacter pylori*, p. 29–41. *In* B. J. Rathbone and R.V. Heatley (ed.), *Helicobacter pylori and Gastroduodenal Disease*, 2nd ed. Blackwell Scientific Publications, Oxford, United Kingdom.
166. **Kabir, S.** 2001. Detection of *Helicobacter pylori* in faeces by culture, PCR and enzyme immunoassay. *J. Med. Microbiol.* **50:**1021–1029.
167. **Kaiser, V., and G. Diamond.** 2000. Expression of mammalian defensin genes. *J. Leukoc. Biol.* **68:**779–784.
168. **Kalach, N., F. Briet, J. Raymond, P. H. Benhamou, P. Barbet, M. Bergeret, L. Senouci, M. Maurel, B. Flourie, and C. Dupont.** 1998. The 13carbon urea breath test for the noninvasive detection of *Helicobacter pylori* in children: comparison with culture and determination of minimum analysis requirements. *J. Pediatr. Gastroenterol. Nutr.* **26:** 291–296.
169. **Kanbay, M., G. Gur, S. Akcay, and U. Yilmaz.** 2005. *Helicobacter pylori* seroprevalence in patients with chronic bronchitis. *Respir. Med.* **99:**1213–1216.
170. **Kanbay, M., G. Gur, M. Yucel, U. Yilmaz, and S. Boyacioglu.** 2005. Does eradication of *Helicobacter pylori* infection help normalize serum lipid and CRP levels? *Dig. Dis. Sci.* **50:**1228–1231.
171. **Kao, J. Y., A. Pierzchala, S. Rathinavelu, Y. Zavros, A. Tessier, and J. L. Merchant.** 2006. Somatostatin inhibits dendritic cell responsiveness to *Helicobacter pylori*. *Regul. Pept.* **134:**23–29.
172. **Kaparakis, M., K. L. Laurie, O. Wijburg, J. Pedersen, M. Pearse, I. R. van Driel, P. A. Gleeson, and R. A. Strugnell.** 2006. $CD4^+$ $CD25^+$ regulatory T cells modulate the T-cell and antibody responses in *Helicobacter*-infected BALB/c mice. *Infect. Immun.* **74:**3519–3529.
173. **Kaptan, K., C. Beyan, and A. Ifran.** 2006. *Helicobacter pylori* and vitamin B12 deficiency. *Haematologica* **91:**ELT10.
174. **Kaptan, K., C. Beyan, A. U. Ural, T. Cetin, F. Avcu, M. Gulsen, R. Finci, and A. Yalcin.** 2000. *Helicobacter pylori—*is it a novel causative agent in Vitamin B12 deficiency? *Arch. Intern. Med.* **160:**1349–1353.
175. **Karin, M.** 2006. Nuclear factor-kappaB in cancer development and progression. *Nature* **441:**431–436.
176. **Kenefeck, R. M. W., J. C. Atherton, and K. Robinson.** 2007. Human *Helicobacter pylori* infection induces $CD4^+$ $CD25^{hi}$ $IL\text{-}10^+$ regulatory T-cells in the peripheral blood. *Zoonoses Public Health* **54**(Suppl. 1)**:**150.
177. **Khan, Z. E., T. C. Wang, G. Cui, A. L. Chi, and R. Dimaline.** 2003. Transcriptional regulation of the human trefoil factor, TFF1, by gastrin. *Gastroenterology* **125:**510–521.
178. **Kidd, M., A. J. Lastovica, J. C. Atherton, and J. A. Louw.** 1999. Heterogeneity in the *Helicobacter pylori* vacA and cagA genes: association with gastroduodenal disease in South Africa? *Gut* **45:**499–502.
179. **Kidd, M., R. M. Peek, A. J. Lastovica, D. A. Israel, A. F. Kummer, and J. A. Louw.** 2001. Analysis of iceA genotypes in South African *Helicobacter pylori* strains and relationship to clinically significant disease. *Gut* **49:**629–635.
180. **Kiltz, U., B. Pfaffenbach, W. E. Schmidt, and R. J. Adamek.** 2002. The lack of influence of CagA positive *Helicobacter pylori* strains on gastro-oesophageal reflux disease. *Eur. J. Gastroenterol. Hepatol.* **14:**979–984.
181. **Kim, H., J. W. Lim, and K. H. Kim.** 2001. *Helicobacter pylori*-induced expression of interleukin-8 and cyclooxygenase-2 in AGS gastric epithelial cells: mediation by nuclear factor-kappaB. *Scand. J. Gastroenterol.* **36:**706–716.
182. **King, C. E., J. Leibach, and P. P. Toskes.** 1979. Clinically significant vitamin B12 deficiency secondary to malabsorption of protein-bound vitamin B12. *Dig. Dis. Sci.* **24:** 397–402.
183. **Kitadai, Y., A. Sasaki, M. Ito, S. Tanaka, N. Oue, W. Yasui, M. Aihara, K. Imagawa, K. Haruma, and K. Chayama.** 2003. *Helicobacter pylori* infection influences expression of genes related to angiogenesis and invasion in human gastric carcinoma cells. *Biochem. Biophys. Res. Commun.* **311:**809–814.
184. **Kivi, M., and Y. Tindberg.** 2006. *Helicobacter pylori* occurrence and transmission: a family affair? *Scand. J. Infect. Dis.* **38:**407–417.
185. **Ko, Y. H., J. J. Han, J. H. Noh, and H. J. Ree.** 2002. Lymph nodes in gastric B-cell lymphoma: pattern of involvement and early histological changes. *Histopathology* **40:**497–504.
186. **Kodama, M., Y. Kitadai, M. Ito, H. Kai, H. Masuda, S. Tanaka, M. Yoshihara, K. Fujimura, and K. Chayama.** 2007. Immune response to CagA protein is associated with improved platelet count after *Helicobacter pylori* eradication in patients with idiopathic thrombocytopenic purpura. *Helicobacter* **12:**36–42.
187. **Koehler, C. I., M. B. Mues, H. P. Dienes, J. Kriegsmann, P. Schirmacher, and M. Odenthal.** 2003. *Helicobacter pylori* genotyping in gastric adenocarcinoma and MALT lymphoma by multiplex PCR analyses of paraffin wax embedded tissues. *Mol. Pathol.* **56:**36–42.
188. **Koenig, W., D. Rothenbacher, A. Hoffmeister, M. Miller, G. Bode, G. Adler, V. Hombach, W. Marz, M. B. Pepys, and H. Brenner.** 1999. Infection with *Helicobacter pylori* is not a major independent risk factor for stable coronary heart disease: lack of a role of cytotoxin-associated protein A-positive strains and absence of a systemic inflammatory response. *Circulation* **100:**2326–2331.

189. **Kono, K., H. Kawaida, A. Takahashi, H. Sugai, K. Mimura, N. Miyagawa, H. Omata, and H. Fujii.** 2006. CD4(+) CD25(high) regulatory T cells increase with tumor stage in patients with gastric and esophageal cancers. *Cancer Immunol. Immunother.* **55:**1064–1071.

190. **Konturek, P. C., J. Kania, V. Kukharsky, S. Ocker, E. G. Hahn, and S. J. Konturek.** 2003. Influence of gastrin on the expression of cyclooxygenase-2, hepatocyte growth factor and apoptosis-related proteins in gastric epithelial cells. *J. Physiol. Pharmacol.* **54:**17–32.

191. **Kosunen, T. U., J. Hook-Nikanne, A. Salomaa, S. Sarna, A. Aromaa, and T. Haahtela.** 2002. Increase of allergen-specific immunoglobulin E antibodies from 1973 to 1994 in a Finnish population and a possible relationship to *Helicobacter pylori* infections. *Clin. Exp. Allergy* **32:**373–378.

192. **Kottakis, F., G. Papadopoulos, E. V. Pappa, P. Cordopatis, S. Pentas, and T. Choli-Papadopoulou.** 2008. *Helicobacter pylori* neutrophil-activating protein activates neutrophils by its C-terminal region even without dodecamer formation, which is a prerequisite for DNA protection—novel approaches against *Helicobacter pylori* inflammation. *FEBS J.* **275:**302–317.

193. **Kowalski, M.** 2001. *Helicobacter pylori* (*H. pylori*) infection in coronary artery disease: influence of *H. pylori* eradication on coronary artery lumen after percutaneous transluminal coronary angioplasty. The detection of *H. pylori* specific DNA in human coronary atherosclerotic plaque. *J. Physiol. Pharmacol.* **52:**3–31.

194. **Kowalski, M., P. C. Konturek, P. Pieniazek, E. Karczewska, A. Kluczka, R. Grove, W. Kranig, R. Nasseri, J. Thale, E. G. Hahn, and S. J. Konturek.** 2001. Prevalence of *Helicobacter pylori* infection in coronary artery disease and effect of its eradication on coronary lumen reduction after percutaneous coronary angioplasty. *Dig. Liver Dis.* **33:**222–229.

195. **Kubben, F. J., C. F. Sier, M. J. Meijer, M. van den Berg, J. J. van der Reijden, G. Griffioen, C. J. van de Velde, C. B. Lamers, and H. W. Verspaget.** 2006. Clinical impact of MMP and TIMP gene polymorphisms in gastric cancer. *Br. J. Cancer* **95:**744–751.

196. **Kuipers, E. J., G. F. Nelis, E. C. Klinkenberg-Knol, P. Snel, D. Goldfain, J. J. Kolkman, H. P. Festen, J. Dent, P. Zeitoun, N. Havu, M. Lamm, and A. Walan.** 2004. Cure of *Helicobacter pylori* infection in patients with reflux oesophagitis treated with long term omeprazole reverses gastritis without exacerbation of reflux disease: results of a randomised controlled trial. *Gut* **53:**12–20.

197. **Kumagai, T., H. M. Malaty, D. Y. Graham, S. Hosogaya, K. Misawa, K. Furihata, H. Ota, C. Sei, E. Tanaka, T. Akamatsu, T. Shimizu, K. Kiyosawa, and T. Katsuyama.** 1998. Acquisition versus loss of *Helicobacter pylori* infection in Japan: results from an 8-year birth cohort study. *J. Infect. Dis.* **178:**717–721.

198. **Kusters, J. G., A. H. van Vliet, and E. J. Kuipers.** 2006. Pathogenesis of *Helicobacter pylori* infection. *Clin. Microbiol. Rev.* **19:**449–490.

199. **Lai, C. H., S. K. Poon, Y. C. Chen, C. S. Chang, and W. C. Wang.** 2005. Lower prevalence of *Helicobacter pylori* infection with vacAs1a, cagA-positive, and babA2-positive genotype in erosive reflux esophagitis disease. *Helicobacter* **10:**577–585.

200. **Laurila, A., A. Bloigu, S. Nayha, J. Hassi, M. Leinonen, and P. Saikku.** 1999. Association of *Helicobacter pylori* infection with elevated serum lipids. *Atherosclerosis* **142:**207–210.

201. **Lee, A.** 2007. Early influences and childhood development. Does *Helicobacter* play a role? *Helicobacter* **12**(Suppl. 2): 69–74.

202. **Lee, C. W., V. P. Rao, A. B. Rogers, Z. Ge, S. E. Erdman, M. T. Whary, and J. G. Fox.** 2007. Wild-type and interleukin-10-deficient regulatory T cells reduce effector T-cell-mediated gastroduodenitis in Rag2-/- mice, but only wild-type regulatory T cells suppress *Helicobacter pylori* gastritis. *Infect. Immun.* **75:**2699–2707.

203. **Leone, N., R. Pellicano, F. Brunello, M. A. Cutufia, M. Berrutti, S. Fagoonee, M. Rizzetto, and A. Ponzetto.** 2003. *Helicobacter pylori* seroprevalence in patients with cirrhosis of the liver and hepatocellular carcinoma. *Cancer Detect. Prev.* **27:**494–497.

204. **Letley, D. P., and J. C. Atherton.** 2000. Natural diversity in the N terminus of the mature vacuolating cytotoxin of *Helicobacter pylori* determines cytotoxin activity. *J. Bacteriol.* **182:**3278–3280.

205. **Letley, D. P., J. L. Rhead, R. J. Twells, B. Dove, and J. C. Atherton.** 2003. Determinants of non-toxicity in the gastric pathogen *Helicobacter pylori*. *J. Biol. Chem.* **278:** 26734–26741.

206. **Leung, W. K., K. L. Siu, C. K. Kwok, S. Y. Chan, R. Sung, and J. J. Sung.** 1999. Isolation of *Helicobacter pylori* from vomitus in children and its implication in gastro-oral transmission. *Am. J. Gastroenterol.* **94:**2881–2884.

207. **Li, H., C. Stoicov, X. Cai, T. C. Wang, and J. Houghton.** 2003. *Helicobacter* and gastric cancer disease mechanisms: host response and disease susceptibility. *Curr. Gastroenterol. Rep.* **5:**459–467.

208. **Li, W., M. Minohara, J. J. Su, T. Matsuoka, M. Osoegawa, T. Ishizu, and J. Kira.** 2007. *Helicobacter pylori* infection is a potential protective factor against conventional multiple sclerosis in the Japanese population. *J. Neuroimmunol.* **184:**227–231.

209. **Lindholm, C., M. Quiding-Jarbrink, H. Lonroth, A. Hamlet, and A. M. Svennerholm.** 1998. Local cytokine response in *Helicobacter pylori*-infected subjects. *Infect. Immun.* **66:** 5964–5971.

210. **Linneberg, A., C. Ostergaard, M. Tvede, L. P. Andersen, N. H. Nielsen, F. Madsen, L. Frolund, A. Dirksen, and T. Jorgensen.** 2003. IgG antibodies against microorganisms and atopic disease in Danish adults: the Copenhagen Allergy Study. *J. Allergy Clin. Immunol.* **111:**847–853.

211. **Liu, F., K. Pan, X. Zhang, Y. Zhang, L. Zhang, J. Ma, C. Dong, L. Shen, J. Li, D. Deng, D. Lin, and W. You.** 2006. Genetic variants in cyclooxygenase-2: expression and risk of gastric cancer and its precursors in a Chinese population. *Gastroenterology* **130:**1975–1984.

212. **Lochhead, P., and E. M. El-Omar.** 2007. *Helicobacter pylori* infection and gastric cancer. *Best Pract. Res. Clin. Gastroenterol.* **21:**281–297.

213. **Loffeld, R. J., B. F. Werdmuller, J. G. Kuster, G. I. Perez-Perez, M. J. Blaser, and E. J. Kuipers.** 2000. Colonization with cagA-positive *Helicobacter pylori* strains inversely associated with reflux esophagitis and Barrett's esophagus. *Digestion* **62:**95–99.

214. **Louw, J. A., M. S. Kidd, A. F. Kummer, K. Taylor, U. Kotze, and D. Hanslo.** 2001. The relationship between *Helicobacter pylori* infection, the virulence genotypes of the infecting strain and gastric cancer in the African setting. *Helicobacter* **6:**268–273.

215. **Lu, H., P. I. Hsu, D. Y. Graham, and Y. Yamaoka.** 2005. Duodenal ulcer promoting gene of *Helicobacter pylori*. *Gastroenterology* **128:**833–848.

216. **Lucas, B., D. Bumann, A. Walduck, J. Koesling, L. Develioglu, T. F. Meyer, and T. Aebischer.** 2001. Adoptive transfer of $CD4^+$ T cells specific for subunit A of *Helicobacter pylori* urease reduces *H. pylori* stomach colonization in

mice in the absence of interleukin-4 (IL-4)/IL-13 receptor signaling. *Infect. Immun.* **69**:1714–1721.

217. **Lundgren, A., E. Strömberg, A. Sjöling, C. Lindholm, K. Enarsson, A. Edebo, E. Johnsson, E. Suri-Payer, P. Larsson, A. Rudin, A. M. Svennerholm, and B. S. Lundin.** 2005. Mucosal *FOXP3*-expressing CD4+ CD25high regulatory T cells in *Helicobacter pylori*-infected patients. *Infect. Immun.* **73**:523–531.

218. **Lundgren, A., E. Suri-Payer, K. Enarsson, A. M. Svennerholm, and B. S. Lundin.** 2003. *Helicobacter pylori*-specific CD4+ CD25high regulatory T cells suppress memory T-cell responses to *H. pylori* in infected individuals. *Infect. Immun.* **71**:1755–1762.

219. **Lunet, N., and H. Barros.** 2003. *Helicobacter pylori* infection and gastric cancer: facing the enigmas. *Int. J. Cancer* **106**:953–960.

220. **Macarthur, M., G. L. Hold, and E. M. El-Omar.** 2004. Inflammation and cancer II. Role of chronic inflammation and cytokine gene polymorphisms in the pathogenesis of gastrointestinal malignancy. *Am. J. Physiol. Gastrointest. Liver Physiol.* **286**:G515–G520.

221. **Machado, J. C., C. Figueiredo, P. Canedo, P. Pharoah, R. Carvalho, S. Nabais, C. Castro Alves, M. L. Campos, L. J. Van Doorn, C. Caldas, R. Seruca, F. Carneiro, and M. Sobrinho-Simoes.** 2003. A proinflammatory genetic profile increases the risk for chronic atrophic gastritis and gastric carcinoma. *Gastroenterology* **125**:364–371.

222. **Majka, J., T. Rog, P. C. Konturek, S. J. Konturek, W. Bielanski, M. Kowalsky, and A. Szczudlik.** 2002. Influence of chronic *Helicobacter pylori* infection on ischemic cerebral stroke risk factors. *Med. Sci. Monit.* **8**:CR675–CR684.

223. **Majumdar, D., J. Bebb and J. Atherton.** 2007. *Helicobacter pylori* infection and peptic ulcers. *Medicine* **35**:204–209.

224. **Malaty, H. M.** 2007. Epidemiology of *Helicobacter pylori* infection. *Best Pract. Res. Clin. Gastroenterol.* **21**:205–214.

225. **Malaty, H. M., D. Y. Graham, P. D. Klein, D. G. Evans, E. Adam, and D. J. Evans.** 1991. Transmission of *Helicobacter pylori* infection. Studies in families of healthy individuals. *Scand. J. Gastroenterol.* **26**:927–932.

226. **Marignani, M., S. Angeletti, C. Bordi, F. Malagnino, C. Mancino, G. Delle Fave, and B. Annibale.** 1997. Reversal of long-standing iron deficiency anaemia after eradication of *Helicobacter pylori* infection. *Scand. J. Gastroenterol.* **32**:617–622.

227. **Marshall, B.** 2006. *Helicobacter* connections. *ChemMedChem* **1**:783–802.

228. **Marshall, B. J., J. A. Armstrong, D. B. McGechie, and R. J. Glancy.** 1985. Attempt to fulfil Koch's postulates for pyloric Campylobacter. *Med. J. Aust.* **142**:436–439.

229. **Marshall, B. J., and J. R. Warren.** 1984. Unidentified curved bacilli in the stomach of patients with gastritis and peptic ulceration. *Lancet* **i**:1311–1315.

230. **Matricardi, P. M., F. Rosmini, S. Riondino, M. Fortini, L. Ferrigno, M. Rapicetta, and S. Bonini.** 2000. Exposure to foodborne and orofecal microbes versus airborne viruses in relation to atopy and allergic asthma: epidemiological study. *BMJ* **320**:412–417.

231. **Matsukawa, Y., Y. Asai, N. Kitamura, S. Sawada, and H. Kurosaka.** 2005. Exacerbation of rheumatoid arthritis following *Helicobacter pylori* eradication: disruption of established oral tolerance against heat shock protein? *Med. Hypotheses* **64**:41–43.

232. **Matsukawa, Y., K. Kato, Y. Hatta, M. Iwamoto, S. Mizuno, R. Kurihara, Y. Arakawa, H. Kurosaka, I. Hayashi, and S. Sawada.** 2007. *Helicobacter pylori* eradication reduces platelet count in patients without idiopathic thrombocytopenic purpura. *Platelets* **18**:52–55.

233. **Matsumoto, Y., T. G. Blanchard, M. L. Drakes, M. Basu, R. W. Redline, A. D. Levine, and S. J. Czinn.** 2005. Eradication of *Helicobacter pylori* and resolution of gastritis in the gastric mucosa of IL-10-deficient mice. *Helicobacter* **10**:407–415.

234. **Matysiak-Budnik, T., and F. Megraud.** 2006. *Helicobacter pylori* infection and gastric cancer. *Eur. J. Cancer* **42**: 708–716.

235. **Maurer, K. J., M. M. Ihrig, A. B. Rogers, V. Ng, G. Bouchard, M. R. Leonard, M. C. Carey, and J. G. Fox.** 2005. Identification of cholelithogenic enterohepatic *Helicobacter* species and their role in murine cholesterol gallstone formation. *Gastroenterology* **128**:1023–1033.

236. **Maurer, K. J., A. B. Rogers, Z. Ge, A. J. Wiese, M. C. Carey, and J. G. Fox.** 2006. *Helicobacter pylori* and cholesterol gallstone formation in C57L/J mice: a prospective study. *Am. J. Physiol. Gastrointest. Liver Physiol.* **290**: G175–G182.

237. **Mayr, M., S. Kiechl, M. A. Mendall, J. Willeit, G. Wick, and Q. Xu.** 2003. Increased risk of atherosclerosis is confined to CagA-positive *Helicobacter pylori* strains: prospective results from the Bruneck study. *Stroke* **34**:610–615.

238. **Mendall, M. A., P. M. Goggin, N. Molineaux, J. Levy, T. Toosy, D. Strachan, A. J. Camm, and T. C. Northfield.** 1994. Relation of *Helicobacter pylori* infection and coronary heart disease. *Br. Heart J.* **71**:437–439.

239. **Mera, R. M., P. Correa, E. E. Fontham, J. C. Reina, A. Pradilla, A. Alzate, and L. E. Bravo.** 2006. Effects of a new *Helicobacter pylori* infection on height and weight in Colombian children. *Ann. Epidemiol.* **16**:347–351.

240. **Michel, M., M. Khellaf, L. Desforges, K. Lee, A. Schaeffer, B. Godeau, and P. Bierling.** 2002. Autoimmune thrombocytopenic Purpura and *Helicobacter pylori* infection. *Arch. Intern. Med.* **162**:1033-1036.

241. **Miehlke, S., A. Hackelsberger, A. Meining, U. von Arnim, P. Muller, T. Ochsenkuhn, N. Lehn, P. Malfertheiner, M. Stolte, and E. Bayerdorffer.** 1997. Histological diagnosis of *Helicobacter pylori* gastritis is predictive of a high risk of gastric carcinoma. *Int. J. Cancer* **73**:837–839.

242. **Miehlke, S., C. Kirsch, K. Agha-Amiri, T. Gunther, N. Lehn, P. Malfertheiner, M. Stolte, G. Ehninger, and E. Bayerdorffer.** 2000. The *Helicobacter pylori* vacA s1, m1 genotype and cagA is associated with gastric carcinoma in Germany. *Int. J. Cancer* **87**:322–327.

243. **Mitchell, H. M., R. Ally, A. Wadee, M. Wiseman, and I. Segal.** 2002. Major differences in the IgG subclass response to *Helicobacter pylori* in the first and third worlds. *Scand. J. Gastroenterol.* **37**:517–522.

244. **Mizuno, T., T. Ando, K. Nobata, T. Tsuzuki, O. Maeda, O. Watanabe, M. Minami, K. Ina, K. Kusugami, R. M. Peek, and H. Goto.** 2005. Interleukin-17 levels in *Helicobacter pylori*-infected gastric mucosa and pathologic sequelae of colonization. *World J. Gastroenterol.* **11**:6305–6311.

245. **Møller, H., and C. Toftgaard.** 1991. Cancer occurrence in a cohort of patients surgically treated for peptic ulcer. *Gut* **32**:740–744.

246. **Montalban, C., A. Manzanal, D. Boixeda, C. Redondo, and C. Bellas.** 1995. Treatment of low-grade gastric MALT lymphoma with *Helicobacter pylori* eradication. *Lancet* **345**:798–799.

247. **Montalban, C., A. Manzanal, J. M. Castrillo, L. Escribano, and C. Bellas.** 1995. Low grade gastric B-cell MALT lymphoma progressing into high grade lymphoma. Clonal

identity of the two stages of the tumour, unusual bone involvement and leukemic dissemination. *Histopathology* **27:** 89–91.

248. **Morgner, A., E. Bayerdorffer, A. Neubauer, and M. Stolte.** 2000. Gastric MALT lymphoma and its relationship to *Helicobacter pylori* infection: management and pathogenesis of the disease. *Microsc. Res. Tech.* **48:**349–356.
249. **Morimoto, N., H. Takeuchi, T. Takahashi, T. Ueta, Y. Tanizawa, Y. Kumon, M. Kobayashi, and T. Sugiura.** 2007. *Helicobacter pylori*-associated chronic idiopathic thrombocytopenic purpura and low molecular weight *H. pylori* proteins. *Scand. J. Infect. Dis.* **39:**409–416.
250. **Mortimer, K., A. Brown, J. Feary, C. Jagger, S. Lewis, M. Antoniak, D. Pritchard, and J. Britton.** 2006. Dose-ranging study for trials of therapeutic infection with Necator americanus in humans. *Am. J. Trop. Med. Hyg.* **75:**914–920.
251. **Moss, S. F., and M. J. Blaser.** 2005. Mechanisms of disease: inflammation and the origins of cancer. *Nat. Clin. Pract. Oncol.* **2:**90–97.
252. **Nakamura, S., T. Matsumoto, S. Nakamura, Y. Jo, K. Fujisawa, H. Suekane, T. Yao, M. Tsuneyoshi, and M. Iida.** 2003. Chromosomal translocation t(11;18)(q21;q21) in gastrointestinal mucosa associated lymphoid tissue lymphoma. *J. Clin. Pathol.* **56:**36–42.
253. **Naylor, G. M., T. Gotoda, M. Dixon, T. Shimoda, L. Gatta, R. Owen, D. Tompkins, and A. Axon.** 2006. Why does Japan have a high incidence of gastric cancer? Comparison of gastritis between UK and Japanese patients. *Gut* **55:** 1545–1552.
254. **Negrini, R., L. Lisato, I. Zanella, L. Cavazzini, S. Gullini, V. Villanacci, C. Poiesi, A. Albertini, and S. Ghielmi.** 1991. *Helicobacter pylori* infection induces antibodies cross-reacting with human gastric mucosa. *Gastroenterology* **101:** 437–445.
255. **Nikolopoulou, A., D. Tousoulis, C. Antoniades, K. Petroheilou, C. Vasiliadou, N. Papageorgiou, K. Koniari, E. Stefanadi, G. Latsios, G. Siasos, and C. Stefanadis.** 11 December 2007. Common community infections and the risk for coronary artery disease and acute myocardial infarction: evidence for chronic over-expression of tumor necrosis factor alpha and vascular cells adhesion molecule-1. *Int. J. Cardiol.* [Epub ahead of print]. doi:10.1016/j.ijcard.2007.08.052.
256. **Nilsson, I., S. Lindgren, S. Eriksson, and T. Wadstrom.** 2000. Serum antibodies to *Helicobacter hepaticus* and *Helicobacter pylori* in patients with chronic liver disease. *Gut* **46:**410–414.
257. **Nomura, A. M., G. I. Perez-Perez, J. Lee, G. Stemmermann, and M. J. Blaser.** 2002. Relation between *Helicobacter pylori* cagA status and risk of peptic ulcer disease. *Am. J. Epidemiol.* **155:**1054–1059.
258. **Normark, S., C. Nilsson, B. H. Normark, and M. W. Hornef.** 2003. Persistent infection with *Helicobacter pylori* and the development of gastric cancer. *Adv. Cancer Res.* **90:**63–89.
259. **Okada, T., K. Ayada, S. Usui, K. Yokota, J. Cui, Y. Kawahara, T. Inaba, S. Hirohata, M. Mizuno, D. Yamamoto, S. Kusachi, E. Matsuura, and K. Oguma.** 2007. Antibodies against heat shock protein 60 derived from *Helicobacter pylori*: diagnostic implications in cardiovascular disease. *J. Autoimmun.* **29:**106–115.
260. **Orsini, B., B. Ottanelli, A. Amedei, E. Surrenti, M. Capanni, G. Del Prete, A. Amorosi, S. Milani, M. M. D'Elios, and C. Surrenti.** 2003. *Helicobacter pylori cag* pathogenicity island is associated with reduced expression of interleukin-4 (IL-4) mRNA and modulation of the IL-4δ2 mRNA isoform in human gastric mucosa. *Infect. Immun.* **71:**6664–6667.
261. **Ottemann, K. M., and A. C. Lowenthal.** 2002. *Helicobacter pylori* uses motility for initial colonization and to attain robust infection. *Infect. Immun.* **70:**1984–1990.
262. **Owen, R. J.** 1995. Bacteriology of *Helicobacter pylori*. *Baillieres Clin. Gastroenterol.* **9:**415–446.
263. **Ozdogru, I., N. Kalay, A. Dogan, M. T. Inanc, M. G. Kaya, R. Topsakal, I. Gul, I. Kutukoglu, H. Kilic, and N. K. Eryol.** 2007. The relationship between *Helicobacter pylori* IgG titre and coronary atherosclerosis. *Acta Cardiol.* **62:**501–505.
264. **Pagliaccia, C., M. de Bernard, P. Lupetti, X. Ji, D. Burroni, T. L. Cover, E. Papini, R. Rappuoli, J. L. Telford, and J. M. Reyrat.** 1998. The m2 form of the *Helicobacter pylori* cytotoxin has cell type-specific vacuolating activity. *Proc. Natl. Acad. Sci. USA* **95:**10212–10217.
265. **Palli, D., G. Masala, G. Del Giudice, M. Plebani, D. Basso, D. Berti, M. E. Numans, M. Ceroti, P. H. Peeters, H. B. Bueno de Mesquita, F. L. Buchner, F. Clavel-Chapelon, M. C. Boutron-Ruault, V. Krogh, C. Saieva, P. Vineis, S. Panico, R. Tumino, O. Nyren, H. Siman, G. Berglund, G. Hallmans, M. J. Sanchez, N. Larranaga, A. Barricarte, C. Navarro, J. R. Quiros, T. Key, N. Allen, S. Bingham, K. T. Khaw, H. Boeing, C. Weikert, J. Linseisen, G. Nagel, K. Overvad, R. W. Thomsen, A. Tjonneland, A. Olsen, A. Trichoupoulou, D. Trichopoulos, A. Arvaniti, G. Pera, R. Kaaks, M. Jenab, P. Ferrari, G. Nesi, F. Carneiro, E. Riboli, and C. A. Gonzalez.** 2007. $CagA^+$ *Helicobacter pylori* infection and gastric cancer risk in the EPIC-EURGAST study. *Int. J. Cancer* **120:**859–867.
266. **Pandey, M.** 2007. *Helicobacter* species are associated with possible increase in risk of biliary lithiasis and benign biliary diseases. *World J. Surg. Oncol.* **5:**94.
267. **Panthel, K., G. Faller, and R. Haas.** 2003. Colonization of C57BL/6J and BALB/c wild-type and knockout mice with *Helicobacter pylori*: effect of vaccination and implications for innate and acquired immunity. *Infect. Immun.* **71:** 794–800.
268. **Parkin, D. M., F. Bray, J. Ferlay, and P. Pisani.** 2005. Global cancer statistics, 2002. *CA Cancer J. Clin.* **55:**74–108.
269. **Parsonnet, J.** 1994. Gastric adenocarcinoma and *Helicobacter pylori* infection. *West J. Med.* **161:**60.
270. **Parsonnet, J., D. Vandersteen, J. Goates, R. K. Sibley, J. Pritikin, and Y. Chang.** 1991. *Helicobacter pylori* infection in intestinal- and diffuse-type gastric adenocarcinomas. *J. Natl. Cancer Inst.* **83:**640–643.
271. **Pasceri, V., G. Cammarota, G. Patti, L. Cuoco, A. Gasbarrini, R. L. Grillo, G. Fedeli, G. Gasbarrini, and A. Maseri.** 1998. Association of virulent *Helicobacter pylori* strains with ischemic heart disease. *Circulation* **97:**1675–1679.
272. **Pasceri, V., G. Patti, G. Cammarota, C. Pristipino, G. Richichi, and G. Di Sciascio.** 2006. Virulent strains of *Helicobacter pylori* and vascular diseases: a meta-analysis. *Am. Heart J.* **151:**1215–1222.
273. **Patel, P., M. A. Mendall, S. Khulusi, T. C. Northfield, and D. P. Strachan.** 1994. *Helicobacter pylori* infection in childhood: risk factors and effect on growth. *BMJ* **309:**1119–1123.
274. **Peek, R. M., Jr., and M. J. Blaser.** 2002. *Helicobacter pylori* and gastrointestinal tract adenocarcinomas. *Nat. Rev. Cancer* **2:**28–37.
275. **Peek, R. M., Jr., G. G. Miller, K. T. Tham, G. I. Perez-Perez, X. Zhao, J. C. Atherton, and M. J. Blaser.** 1995. Heightened inflammatory response and cytokine expression in vivo to cagA+ *Helicobacter pylori* strains. *Lab. Invest.* **73:**760–770.

276. **Peek, R. M., Jr., S. A. Thompson, J. P. Donahue, K. T. Tham, J. C. Atherton, M. J. Blaser, and G. G. Miller.** 1998. Adherence to gastric epithelial cells induces expression of a *Helicobacter pylori* gene, iceA, that is associated with clinical outcome. *Proc. Assoc. Am. Physicians* **110:**531–544.

277. **Pellicano, R., V. Mazzaferro, W. F. Grigioni, M. A. Cutufia, S. Fagoonee, L. Silengo, M. Rizzetto, and A. Ponzetto.** 2004. *Helicobacter* species sequences in liver samples from patients with and without hepatocellular carcinoma. *World J. Gastroenterol.* **10:**598–601.

278. **Pellicano, R., M. G. Mazzarello, S. Morelloni, M. Allegri, V. Arena, M. Ferrari, M. Rizzetto, and A. Ponzetto.** 1999. Acute myocardial infarction and *Helicobacter pylori* seropositivity. *Int. J. Clin. Lab. Res.* **29:**141–144.

279. **Pellicano, R., M. G. Mazzarello, S. Morelloni, M. Ferrari, P. Angelino, M. Berrutti, A. M. Torriglia, M. Rizzetto, and A. Ponzetto.** 2003. *Helicobacter pylori* seropositivity in patients with unstable angina. *J. Cardiovasc. Surg.* (Torino) **44:**605–609.

280. **Pereira-Lima, J. C., D. L. Marques, L. F. Pereira-Lima, A. P. Hornos, and C. Rota.** 2004. The role of cagA *Helicobacter pylori* strains in gastro-oesophageal reflux disease. *Eur. J. Gastroenterol. Hepatol.* **16:**643–647.

281. **Perry, S., M. de la Luz Sanchez, S. Yang, T. D. Haggerty, P. Hurst, G. Perez-Perez, and J. Parsonnet.** 2006. Gastroenteritis and transmission of *Helicobacter pylori* infection in households. *Emerg. Infect. Dis.* **12:**1701–1708.

282. **Perry, V. H., C. Cunningham, and C. Holmes.** 2007. Systemic infections and inflammation affect chronic neurodegeneration. *Nat. Rev. Immunol.* **7:**161–167.

283. **Perryman, S. V., and K. G. Sylvester.** 2006. Repair and regeneration: opportunities for carcinogenesis from tissue stem cells. *J. Cell. Mol. Med.* **10:**292–308.

284. **Pessi, T., M. Virta, K. Adjers, J. Karjalainen, H. Rautelin, T. U. Kosunen, and M. Hurme.** 2005. Genetic and environmental factors in the immunopathogenesis of atopy: interaction of *Helicobacter pylori* infection and IL4 genetics. *Int. Arch. Allergy Immunol.* **137:**282–288.

285. **Petersson, C., M. Forsberg, M. Aspholm, F. O. Olfat, T. Forslund, T. Boren, and K. E. Magnusson.** 2006. *Helicobacter pylori* SabA adhesin evokes a strong inflammatory response in human neutrophils which is down-regulated by the neutrophil-activating protein. *Med. Microbiol. Immunol.* **4:**195–206.

286. **Pierantozzi, M., A. Pietroiusti, G. Sancesario, G. Lunardi, E. Fedele, P. Giacomini, S. Frasca, A. Galante, M. G. Marciani, and P. Stanzione.** 2001. Reduced L-dopa absorption and increased clinical fluctuations in *Helicobacter pylori*-infected Parkinson's disease patients. *Neurol. Sci.* **22:**89–91.

287. **Pietroiusti, A., M. Diomedi, M. Silvestrini, L. M. Cupini, I. Luzzi, M. J. Gomez-Miguel, A. Bergamaschi, A. Magrini, T. Carrabs, M. Vellini, and A. Galante.** 2002. Cytotoxin-associated gene-A–positive *Helicobacter pylori* strains are associated with atherosclerotic stroke. *Circulation* **106:**580–584.

288. **Pinto-Santini, D., and N. R. Salama.** 2005. The biology of *Helicobacter pylori* infection, a major risk factor for gastric adenocarcinoma. *Cancer Epidemiol. Biomarkers Prev.* **14:** 1853–1858.

289. **Prasad, K. N., A. Saxena, U. C. Ghoshal, M. R. Bhagat, and N. Krishnani.** 2008. Analysis of Pro12Ala PPAR gamma polymorphism and *Helicobacter pylori* infection in gastric adenocarcinoma and peptic ulcer disease. *Ann. Oncol.* **7:** 1299–303.

290. **Prinz, C., M. Schoniger, R. Rad, I. Becker, E. Keiditsch, S. Wagenpfeil, M. Classen, T. Rosch, W. Schepp, and M. Gerhard.** 2001. Key importance of the *Helicobacter pylori* adherence factor blood group antigen binding adhesin during chronic gastric inflammation. *Cancer Res.* **61:** 1903–1909.

291. **Qiao, W., J. L. Hu, B. Xiao, K. C. Wu, D. R. Peng, J. C. Atherton, and H. Xue.** 2003. cagA and vacA genotype of *Helicobacter pylori* associated with gastric diseases in Xi'an area. *World J. Gastroenterol.* **9:**1762–1766.

292. **Queiroz, D. M., P. Bittencourt, J. B. Guerra, A. M. Rocha, G. A. Rocha, and A. S. Carvalho.** 2005. IL1RN polymorphism and cagA-positive *Helicobacter pylori* strains increase the risk of duodenal ulcer in children. *Pediatr. Res.* **58:**892–896.

293. **Rad, R., L. Brenner, S. Bauer, S. Schwendy, L. Layland, C. P. da Costa, W. Reindl, A. Dossumbekova, M. Friedrich, D. Saur, H. Wagner, R. M. Schmid, and C. Prinz.** 2006. CD25+/Foxp3+ T cells regulate gastric inflammation and *Helicobacter pylori* colonization in vivo. *Gastroenterology* **131:**525–537.

294. **Rad, R., C. Prinz, B. Neu, M. Neuhofer, M. Zeitner, P. Voland, I. Becker, W. Schepp, and M. Gerhard.** 2003. Synergistic effect of *Helicobacter pylori* virulence factors and interleukin-1 polymorphisms for the development of severe histological changes in the gastric mucosa. *J. Infect. Dis.* **188:**272–281.

295. **Raghavan, S., M. Fredriksson, A. M. Svennerholm, J. Holmgren, and E. Suri-Payer.** 2003. Absence of CD4+CD25+ regulatory T cells is associated with a loss of regulation leading to increased pathology in *Helicobacter pylori*-infected mice. *Clin. Exp. Immunol.* **132:**393–400.

296. **Raghunath, A., A. P. Hungin, D. Wooff, and S. Childs.** 2003. Prevalence of *Helicobacter pylori* in patients with gastro-oesophageal reflux disease: systematic review. *BMJ* **326:**737.

297. **Ramamoorthy, S., V. Stepan, and A. Todisco.** 2004. Intracellular mechanisms mediating the anti-apoptotic action of gastrin. *Biochem. Biophys. Res. Commun.* **323:**44–48.

298. **Rhead, J. L., D. P. Letley, M. Mohammadi, N. Hussein, M. A. Mohagheghi, M. Eshagh Hosseini, and J. C. Atherton.** 2007. A new *Helicobacter pylori* vacuolating cytotoxin determinant, the intermediate region, is associated with gastric cancer. *Gastroenterology* **133:**926–936.

299. **Rizzo, M., E. Corrado, G. Coppola, I. Muratori, and S. Novo.** 2008. Prediction of cerebrovascular and cardiovascular events in patients with subclinical carotid atherosclerosis: the role of C-reactive protein. *J. Invest. Med.* **56:** 32–40.

300. **Robinson, K., R. H. Argent, and J. C. Atherton.** 2007. The inflammatory and immune response to *Helicobacter pylori* infection. *Best Pract. Res. Clin. Gastroenterol.* **21:** 237–259.

301. **Robinson, K., R. Kenefeck, E. L. Pidgeon, S. Shakib, S. Patel, R. J. Polson, A. M. Zaitoun, and J. C. Atherton.** 2008. *Helicobacter pylori*-induced peptic ulcer disease is associated with inadequate regulatory T-cell responses. *Gut* **57:**1375–1385.

302. **Rook, G. A., and L. R. Brunet.** 2005. Microbes, immunoregulation, and the gut. *Gut* **54:**317–320.

303. **Roosendaal, R., E. J. Kuipers, J. Buitenwerf, C. van Uffelen, S. G. Meuwissen, G. J. van Kamp, and C. M. Vandenbroucke-Grauls.** 1997. *Helicobacter pylori* and the birth cohort effect: evidence of a continuous decrease of infection rates in childhood. *Am. J. Gastroenterol.* **92:**1480–1482.

304. **Rostami, N., M. Keshtkar-Jahromi, M. Rahnavardi, M. Keshtkar-Jahromi, and F. Soghra Esfahani.** 2008. Effect of eradication of *Helicobacter pylori* on platelet recovery in

patients with chronic idiopathic thrombocytopenic purpura: a controlled trial. *Am. J. Hematol.* **83:**376–381.

305. **Roussos, A., N. Philippou, V. Krietsepi, E. Anastasakou, D. Alepopoulou, P. Koursarakos, I. Iliopoulos, and K. Gourgoulianis.** 2005. *Helicobacter pylori* seroprevalence in patients with chronic obstructive pulmonary disease. *Respir. Med.* **99:**279–284.

306. **Roussos, A., F. Tsimpoukas, E. Anastasakou, D. Alepopoulou, I. Paizis, and N. Philippou.** 2002. *Helicobacter pylori* seroprevalence in patients with chronic bronchitis. *J. Gastroenterol.* **37:**332–335.

307. **Russo-Mancuso, G., F. Branciforte, M. Licciardello, and M. La Spina.** 2003. Iron deficiency anemia as the only sign of infection with *Helicobacter pylori*: a report of 9 pediatric cases. *Int. J. Hematol.* **78:**429–431.

308. **Sasaki, A., K. Haruma, N. Manabe, S. Tanaka, M. Yoshihara, and K. Chayama.** 2003. Long-term observation of reflux oesophagitis developing after *Helicobacter pylori* eradication therapy. *Aliment. Pharmacol. Ther.* **17:**1529–1534.

309. **Satake, M., J. Nishikawa, Y. Fukagawa, K. Akashi, T. Okamoto, T. Yoshida, A. Hirano, N. Maetani, Y. Iida, and I. Sakaida.** 2007. The long-term efficacy of *Helicobacter pylori* eradication therapy in patients with idiopathic thrombocytopenic purpura. *J. Gastroenterol. Hepatol.* **22:**2233–2237.

310. **Satoguina, J., M. Mempel, J. Larbi, M. Badusche, C. Loliger, O. Adjei, G. Gachelin, B. Fleischer, and A. Hoerauf.** 2002. Antigen-specific T regulatory-1 cells are associated with immunosuppression in a chronic helminth infection (onchocerciasis). *Microbes Infect.* **4:**1291–1300.

311. **Satoh, T., J. P. Pandey, Y. Okazaki, H. Yasuoka, Y. Kawakami, Y. Ikeda, and M. Kuwana.** 2004. Single nucleotide polymorphisms of the inflammatory cytokine genes in adults with chronic immune thrombocytopenic purpura. *Br. J. Haematol.* **124:**796–801.

312. **Satomi, S., A. Yamakawa, S. Matsunaga, R. Masaki, T. Inagaki, T. Okuda, H. Suto, Y. Ito, Y. Yamazaki, M. Kuriyama, Y. Keida, H. Kutsumi, and T. Azuma.** 2006. Relationship between the diversity of the cagA gene of *Helicobacter pylori* and gastric cancer in Okinawa, Japan. *J. Gastroenterol.* **41:**668–673.

313. **Sauve-Martin, H., N. Kalach, J. Raymond, L. Senouci, P. H. Benhamou, J. C. Martin, F. Briet, M. Maurel, B. Flourie, and C. Dupont.** 1999. The rate of *Helicobacter pylori* infection in children with growth retardation. *J. Pediatr. Gastroenterol. Nutr.* **28:**354–355.

314. **Sawalha, A. H., W. R. Schmid, S. R. Binder, D. K. Bacino, and J. B. Harley.** 2004. Association between systemic lupus erythematosus and *Helicobacter pylori* seronegativity. *J. Rheumatol.* **31:**1546–1550.

315. **Schweeger, I., P. Fitscha, and H. Sinzinger.** 2000. Successful eradication of *Helicobacter pylori* as determined by ^{13}C-urea breath test does not alter fibrinogen and acute phase response markers. *Thromb. Res.* **97:**411–420.

316. **Seiskari, T., A. Kondrashova, H. Viskari, M. Kaila, A. M. Haapala, J. Aittoniemi, M. Virta, M. Hurme, R. Uibo, M. Knip, and H. Hyoty.** 2007. Allergic sensitization and microbial load—a comparison between Finland and Russian Karelia. *Clin. Exp. Immunol.* **148:**47–52.

317. **Serin, E., Y. Gumurdulu, B. Ozer, F. Kayaselcuk, U. Yilmaz, and R. Kocak.** 2002. Impact of *Helicobacter pylori* on the development of vitamin B12 deficiency in the absence of gastric atrophy. *Helicobacter* **7:**337–341.

318. **Sharma, P., and N. Vakil.** 2003. Review article: *Helicobacter pylori* and reflux disease. *Aliment. Pharmacol. Ther.* **17:**297–305.

319. **Sheikh, A., and D. P. Strachan.** 2004. The hygiene theory: fact or fiction? *Curr. Opin. Otolaryngol. Head Neck Surg.* **12:**232–236.

320. **Shi, H. Z., and X. J. Qin.** 2005. CD4CD25 regulatory T lymphocytes in allergy and asthma. *Allergy* **60:**986–995.

321. **Shimoyama, T., S. M. Everett, M. F. Dixon, A. T. Axon, and J. E. Crabtree.** 1998. Chemokine mRNA expression in gastric mucosa is associated with *Helicobacter pylori* cagA positivity and severity of gastritis. *J. Clin. Pathol.* **51:**765–770.

322. **Shimoyama, T., S. M. Everett, S. Fukuda, A. T. Axon, M. F. Dixon, and J. E. Crabtree.** 2001. Influence of smoking and alcohol on gastric chemokine mRNA expression in patients with *Helicobacter pylori* infection. *J. Clin. Pathol.* **54:**332–334.

323. **Shmuely, H., D. J. Passaro, M. Vaturi, A. Sagie, S. Pitlik, Z. Samra, Y. Niv, R. Koren, D. Harell, and J. Yahav.** 2005. Association of CagA+ *Helicobacter pylori* infection with aortic atheroma. *Atherosclerosis* **179:**127–132.

324. **Sipponen, P., T. U. Kosunen, I. M. Samloff, O. P. Heinonen, and M. Siurala.** 1996. Rate of *Helicobacter pylori* acquisition among Finnish adults: a fifteen year follow-up. *Scand. J. Gastroenterol.* **31:**229–232.

325. **Smart, J. M., and A. S. Kemp.** 2001. Ontogeny of T-helper 1 and T-helper 2 cytokine production in childhood. Pediatr *Allergy Immunol.* **12:**181–187.

326. **Smythies, L. E., K. B. Waites, J. R. Lindsey, P. R. Harris, P. Ghiara, and P. D. Smith.** 2000. *Helicobacter pylori*-induced mucosal inflammation is Th1 mediated and exacerbated in IL-4, but not IFN-gamma, gene-deficient mice. *J. Immunol.* **165:**1022–1029.

327. **Sommer, F., G. Faller, P. Konturek, T. Kirchner, E. G. Hahn, J. Zeus, M. Rollinghoff, and M. Lohoff.** 1998. Antrum- and corpus mucosa-infiltrating CD4$^+$ lymphocytes in *Helicobacter pylori* gastritis display a Th1 phenotype. *Infect. Immun.* **66:**5543–5546.

328. **Stoltzfus, R. J.** 2003. Iron deficiency: global prevalence and consequences. *Food Nutr. Bull.* **24:**S99–S103.

329. **Strang, R. R.** 1965. The Association of Gastro-Duodenal Ulceration and Parkinson's Disease. *Med. J. Aust.* **1:**842–843.

330. **Stromberg, E., A. Edebo, B. S. Lundin, P. Bergin, M. Brisslert, A. M. Svennerholm, and C. Lindholm.** 2005. Down-regulation of epithelial IL-8 responses in *Helicobacter pylori*-infected duodenal ulcer patients depends on host factors, rather than bacterial factors. *Clin. Exp. Immunol.* **140:**117–125.

331. **Sundrud, M. S., V. J. Torres, D. Unutmaz, and T. L. Cover.** 2004. Inhibition of primary human T cell proliferation by *Helicobacter pylori* vacuolating toxin (VacA) is independent of VacA effects on IL-2 secretion. *Proc. Natl. Acad. Sci. USA* **101:**7727–7732.

332. **Supajatura, V., H. Ushio, A. Wada, K. Yahiro, K. Okumura, H. Ogawa, T. Hirayama, and C. Ra.** 2002. Cutting edge: VacA, a vacuolating cytotoxin of *Helicobacter pylori*, directly activates mast cells for migration and production of proinflammatory cytokines. *J. Immunol.* **168:**2603–2607.

333. **Suter, P. M., B. B. Golner, B. R. Goldin, F. D. Morrow, and R. M. Russell.** 1991. Reversal of protein-bound vitamin B12 malabsorption with antibiotics in atrophic gastritis. *Gastroenterology* **101:**1039–1045.

334. **Suzuki, T., M. Matsushima, K. Shirakura, J. Koike, A. Masui, A. Takagi, Y. Shirasugi, Y. Ogawa, T. Shirai, and T. Mine.** 2008. Association of inflammatory cytokine gene polymorphisms with platelet recovery in idiopathic thrombocytopenic purpura patients after the eradication of *Helicobacter pylori*. *Digestion* **77:**73–78.

335. **Takahashi, T., T. Yujiri, K. Shinohara, Y. Inoue, Y. Sato, Y. Fujii, M. Okubo, Y. Zaitsu, K. Ariyoshi, Y. Nakamura, R. Nawata, Y. Oka, M. Shirai, and Y. Tanizawa.** 2004. Molecular mimicry by *Helicobacter pylori* CagA protein may be involved in the pathogenesis of *H. pylori*-associated chronic idiopathic thrombocytopenic purpura. *Br. J. Haematol.* **124:**91–96.

336. **Tasar, A., E. Kibrisli, and Y. Dallar.** 2006. Seroprevalence of *Helicobacter pylori* in children with constitutional height retardation. *Turk. J. Gastroenterol.* **17:**7–12.

337. **Taylor, D. N., and M. J. Blaser.** 1991. The epidemiology of *Helicobacter pylori* infection. *Epidemiol. Rev.* **13:**42–59.

338. **Telford, J. L., P. Ghiara, M. Dell'Orco, M. Comanducci, D. Burroni, M. Bugnoli, M. F. Tecce, S. Censini, A. Covacci, Z. Xiang, et al.** 1994. Gene structure of the *Helicobacter pylori* cytotoxin and evidence of its key role in gastric disease. *J. Exp. Med.* **179:**1653–1658.

339. **Theodoropoulos, D. S., D. L. Pecoraro, and S. E. Efstratiadis.** 2002. The association of gastroesophageal reflux disease with asthma and chronic cough in the adult. *Am. J. Respir. Med.* **1:**133–146.

340. **Thijs, J. C., A. A. van Zwet, W. J. Thijs, H. B. Oey, A. Karrenbeld, F. Stellaard, D. S. Luijt, B. C. Meyer, and J. H. Kleibeuker.** 1996. Diagnostic tests for *Helicobacter pylori*: a prospective evaluation of their accuracy, without selecting a single test as the gold standard. *Am. J. Gastroenterol.* **91:**2125–2129.

341. **Tiwari, S. K., A. A. Khan, M. Ibrahim, M. A. Habeeb, and C. M. Habibullah.** 2006. *Helicobacter pylori* and other *Helicobacter* species DNA in human bile samples from patients with various hepato-biliary diseases. *World J. Gastroenterol.* **12:**2181–2186.

342. **Todisco, A., S. Ramamoorthy, T. Witham, N. Pausawasdi, S. Srinivasan, C. J. Dickinson, F. K. Askari, and D. Krametter.** 2001. Molecular mechanisms for the antiapoptotic action of gastrin. *Am. J. Physiol. Gastrointest. Liver Physiol.* **280:**G298–G307.

343. **Torgano, G., R. Cosentini, C. Mandelli, R. Perondi, F. Blasi, G. Bertinieri, T. V. Tien, G. Ceriani, P. Tarsia, C. Arosio, and M. L. Ranzi.** 1999. Treatment of *Helicobacter pylori* and *Chlamydia pneumoniae* infections decreases fibrinogen plasma level in patients with ischemic heart disease. *Circulation* **99:**1555–1559.

344. **Torres, J., G. Perez-Perez, K. J. Goodman, J. C. Atherton, B. D. Gold, P. R. Harris, A. M. la Garza, J. Guarner, and O. Munoz.** 2000. A comprehensive review of the natural history of *Helicobacter pylori* infection in children. *Arch. Med. Res.* **31:**431–469.

345. **Touati, E., V. Michel, J. M. Thiberge, N. Wuscher, M. Huerre, and A. Labigne.** 2003. Chronic *Helicobacter pylori* infections induce gastric mutations in mice. *Gastroenterology* **124:**1408–1419.

346. **Trosko, J. E., and M. H. Tai.** 2006. Adult stem cell theory of the multi-stage, multi-mechanism theory of carcinogenesis: role of inflammation on the promotion of initiated stem cells. *Contrib. Microbiol.* **13:**45–65.

347. **Trujillo, C., and K. J. Erb.** 2003. Inhibition of allergic disorders by infection with bacteria or the exposure to bacterial products. *Int. J. Med. Microbiol.* **293:**123–131.

348. **Tsang, K. W., S. K. Lam, W. K. Lam, J. Karlberg, B. C. Wong, W. H. Hu, W. W. Yew, and M. S. Ip.** 1998. High seroprevalence of *Helicobacter pylori* in active bronchiectasis. *Am. J. Respir. Crit. Care Med.* **158:**1047–1051.

349. **Tsutsumi, Y., H. Kanamori, H. Yamato, N. Ehira, T. Kawamura, S. Umehara, A. Mori, S. Obara, N. Ogura, J. Tanaka, M. Asaka, M. Imamura, and N. Masauzi.** 2005. Randomized study of *Helicobacter pylori* eradication therapy and proton pump inhibitor monotherapy for idiopathic thrombocytopenic purpura. *Ann. Hematol.* **84:**807–811.

350. **Veneri, D., G. De Matteis, P. Solero, F. Federici, C. Zanuso, E. Guizzardi, S. Arena, M. Gaio, P. Pontiero, M. M. Ricetti, and M. Franchini.** 2005. Analysis of B- and T-cell clonality and HLA class II alleles in patients with idiopathic thrombocytopenic purpura: correlation with *Helicobacter pylori* infection and response to eradication treatment. *Platelets* **16:**307–311.

351. **Viala, J., C. Chaput, I. G. Boneca, A. Cardona, S. E. Girardin, A. P. Moran, R. Athman, S. Memet, M. R. Huerre, A. J. Coyle, P. S. DiStefano, P. J. Sansonetti, A. Labigne, J. Bertin, D. J. Philpott, and R. L. Ferrero.** 2004. Nod1 responds to peptidoglycan delivered by the *Helicobacter pylori* cag pathogenicity island. *Nat. Immunol.* **5:** 1166–1174.

352. **Vicari, J. J., R. M. Peek, G. W. Falk, J. R. Goldblum, K. A. Easley, J. Schnell, G. I. Perez-Perez, S. A. Halter, T. W. Rice, M. J. Blaser, and J. E. Richter.** 1998. The seroprevalence of cagA-positive *Helicobacter pylori* strains in the spectrum of gastroesophageal reflux disease. *Gastroenterology* **115:**50-57.

353. **Vogt, T. M., and R. E. Johnson.** 1980. Recent changes in the incidence of duodenal and gastric ulcer. *Am. J. Epidemiol.* **111:**713–720.

354. **Wang, H. Y., and R. F. Wang.** 2005. Antigen-specific CD4+ regulatory T cells in cancer: implications for immunotherapy. *Microbes Infect.* **7:**1056–1062.

355. **Wang, S. K., H. F. Zhu, B. S. He, Z. Y. Zhang, Z. T. Chen, Z. Z. Wang, and G. L. Wu.** 2007. CagA+ *H. pylori* infection is associated with polarization of T helper cell immune responses in gastric carcinogenesis. *World J. Gastroenterol.* **13:**2923–2931.

356. **Wang, T. C., C. A. Dangler, D. Chen, J. R. Goldenring, T. Koh, R. Raychowdhury, R. J. Coffey, S. Ito, A. Varro, G. J. Dockray, and J. G. Fox.** 2000. Synergistic interaction between hypergastrinemia and *Helicobacter* infection in a mouse model of gastric cancer. *Gastroenterology* **118:** 36–47.

357. **Watanabe, T., M. Tada, H. Nagai, S. Sasaki, and M. Nakao.** 1998. *Helicobacter pylori* infection induces gastric cancer in mongolian gerbils. *Gastroenterology* **115:**642–648.

358. **Weeks, D. L., S. Eskandari, D. R. Scott, and G. Sachs.** 2000. A H+-gated urea channel: the link between *Helicobacter pylori* urease and gastric colonization. *Science* **287:** 482–485.

359. **Weiss, T. W., H. Kvakan, C. Kaun, M. Prager, W. S. Speidl, G. Zorn, S. Pfaffenberger, I. Huk, G. Maurer, K. Huber, and J. Wojta.** 2006. No evidence for a direct role of *Helicobacter pylori* and Mycoplasma pneumoniae in carotid artery atherosclerosis. *J. Clin. Pathol.* **59:**1186–1190.

360. **Wender, M.** 2003. Prevalence of *Helicobacter pylori* infection among patients with multiple sclerosis. *Neurol. Neurochir. Pol.* **37:**45–48. (In Polish.)

361. **Weyermann, M., G. Adler, H. Brenner, and D. Rothenbacher.** 2006. The mother as source of *Helicobacter pylori* infection. *Epidemiology* **17:**332–334.

362. **Wilschanski, M., Y. Schlesinger, J. Faber, B. Rudensky, F. S. Ohnona, S. Freier, E. Rahman, S. Refael, and D. Halle.** 2007. Combination of *Helicobacter pylori* strain and tumor necrosis factor-alpha polymorphism of the host increases the risk of peptic ulcer disease in children. *J. Pediatr. Gastroenterol. Nutr.* **45:**199–203.

363. **Wong, B. C., S. K. Lam, W. M. Wong, J. S. Chen, T. T. Zheng, R. E. Feng, K. C. Lai, W. H. Hu, S. T. Yuen, S. Y.**

Leung, D. Y. Fong, J. Ho, C. K. Ching, and J. S. Chen. 2004. *Helicobacter pylori* eradication to prevent gastric cancer in a high-risk region of China: a randomized controlled trial. *JAMA* **291:**187–194.

364. **Woo, E. Y., C. S. Chu, T. J. Goletz, K. Schlienger, H. Yeh, G. Coukos, S. C. Rubin, L. R. Kaiser, and C. H. June.** 2001. Regulatory CD4(+)CD25(+) T cells in tumors from patients with early-stage non-small cell lung cancer and late-stage ovarian cancer. *Cancer Res.* **61:**4766–4772.

365. **Worku, M. L., Q. N. Karim, J. Spencer, and R. L. Sidebotham.** 2004. Chemotactic response of *Helicobacter pylori* to human plasma and bile. *J. Med. Microbiol.* **53:** 807–811.

366. **Wotherspoon, A. C.** 2000. A critical review of the effect of *Helicobacter pylori* eradication on gastric MALT lymphoma. *Curr. Gastroenterol. Rep.* **2:**494–498.

367. **Wotherspoon, A. C., C. Ortiz-Hidalgo, M.R. Falzon and P.G. Isaacson.** 1991. *H. pylori*-associated gastritis and primary B-cell gastric lymphoma. *Lancet* **338:**175–1176.

368. **Wroblewski, L. E., D. M. Pritchard, S. Carter, and A. Varro.** 2002. Gastrin-stimulated gastric epithelial cell invasion: the role and mechanism of increased matrix metalloproteinase 9 expression. *Biochem. J.* **365:**873–879.

369. **Wu, M. S., T. Y. Cheng, C. T. Shun, M. T. Lin, L. C. Chen, and J. T. Lin.** 2006. Functional polymorphisms of CD14 and toll-like receptor 4 in Taiwanese Chinese with *Helicobacter pylori*-related gastric malignancies. *Hepatogastroenterology* **53:**807–810.

370. **Wunder, C., Y. Churin, F. Winau, D. Warnecke, M. Vieth, B. Lindner, U. Zahringer, H. J. Mollenkopf, E. Heinz, and T. F. Meyer.** 2006. Cholesterol glucosylation promotes immune evasion by *Helicobacter pylori*. *Nat. Med.* **12:** 1030–1038.

371. **Xia, H. H., and N. J. Talley.** 1997. Natural acquisition and spontaneous elimination of *Helicobacter pylori* infection: clinical implications. *Am. J. Gastroenterol.* **92:** 1780–1787.

372. **Yamaoka, Y., S. Kikuchi, H. M. el-Zimaity, O. Gutierrez, M. S. Osato, and D. Y. Graham.** 2002. Importance of *Helicobacter pylori* oipA in clinical presentation, gastric inflammation, and mucosal interleukin 8 production. *Gastroenterology* **123:**414–424.

373. **Yamaoka, Y., M. Kita, T. Kodama, N. Sawai, K. Kashima, and J. Imanishi.** 1995. Expression of cytokine mRNA in gastric mucosa with *Helicobacter pylori* infection. *Scand. J. Gastroenterol.* **30:**1153–1159.

374. **Yamaoka, Y., M. Kita, T. Kodama, N. Sawai, K. Kashima, and J. Imanishi.** 1997. Induction of various cytokines and development of severe mucosal inflammation by cagA gene positive *Helicobacter pylori* strains. *Gut* **41:**442–451.

375. **Yamaoka, Y., D. H. Kwon, and D. Y. Graham.** 2000. A M(r) 34,000 proinflammatory outer membrane protein (oipA) of *Helicobacter pylori*. *Proc. Natl. Acad. Sci. USA* **97:**7533–7538.

376. **Ye, H., H. Liu, A. Attygalle, A. C. Wotherspoon, A. G. Nicholson, F. Charlotte, V. Leblond, P. Speight, J. Goodlad, A. Lavergne-Slove, J. I. Martin-Subero, R. Siebert, A. Dogan, P. G. Isaacson, and M. Q. Du.** 2003. Variable frequencies of t(11;18)(q21;q21) in MALT lymphomas of different sites: significant association with CagA strains of *H. pylori* in gastric MALT lymphoma. *Blood* **102:**1012–1018.

377. **Yokota, S., M. Konno, E. Mino, K. Sato, M. Takahashi, and N. Fujii.** 2008. Enhanced Fe ion-uptake activity in *Helicobacter pylori* strains isolated from patients with iron-deficiency anemia. *Clin. Infect. Dis.* **46:**e31–e33.

378. **Yoshimura, M., M. Hirai, N. Tanaka, Y. Kasahara, and O. Hosokawa.** 2003. Remission of severe anemia persisting for over 20 years after eradication of *Helicobacter pylori* in cases of Menetrier's disease and atrophic gastritis: *Helicobacter pylori* as a pathogenic factor in iron-deficiency anemia. *Intern. Med.* **42:**971–977.

379. **Younes, M., D. E. Henson, A. Ertan, and C. C. Miller.** 2002. Incidence and survival trends of esophageal carcinoma in the United States: racial and gender differences by histological type. *Scand. J. Gastroenterol.* **37:**1359–1365.

380. **Yu, J., W. K. Leung, M. Y. Go, M. C. Chan, K. F. To, E. K. Ng, F. K. Chan, T. K. Ling, S. C. Chung, and J. J. Sung.** 2002. Relationship between *Helicobacter pylori* babA2 status with gastric epithelial cell turnover and premalignant gastric lesions. *Gut* **51:**480–484.

381. **Yusuf, S. W., and R. M. Mishra.** 2002. Effect of *Helicobacter pylori* infection on fibrinogen level in elderly patients with ischaemic heart disease. *Acta Cardiol.* **57:**317–322.

382. **Zavros, Y., and J. L. Merchant.** 2005. Modulating the cytokine response to treat *Helicobacter* gastritis. *Biochem. Pharmacol.* **69:**365–371.

383. **Zavros, Y., S. Rathinavelu, J. Y. Kao, A. Todisco, J. Del Valle, J. V. Weinstock, M. J. Low, and J. L. Merchant.** 2003. Treatment of *Helicobacter* gastritis with IL-4 requires somatostatin. *Proc. Natl. Acad. Sci. USA* **100:**12944–12949.

384. **Zhang, Y., R. H. Argent, D. P. Letley, R. J. Thomas, and J. C. Atherton.** 2005. Tyrosine phosphorylation of CagA from Chinese *Helicobacter pylori* isolates in AGS gastric epithelial cells. *J. Clin. Microbiol.* **43:**786–790.

385. **Zhao, D., T. Sun, X. Zhang, Y. Guo, D. Yu, M. Yang, W. Tan, G. Wang, and D. Lin.** 2007. Role of CD14 promoter polymorphisms in *Helicobacter pylori* infection—related gastric carcinoma. *Clin. Cancer Res.* **13:**2362–2368.

386. **Zheng, Q., X. Y. Chen, Y. Shi, and S. D. Xiao.** 2004. Development of gastric adenocarcinoma in Mongolian gerbils after long-term infection with *Helicobacter pylori*. *J. Gastroenterol. Hepatol.* **19:**1192–1198.

387. **Zumkeller, N., W. Koenig, M. M. Hoffmann, H. Kolb, H. Brenner, and D. Rothenbacher.** 2005. *Helicobacter pylori* seropositive subjects do not show a pronounced systemic inflammatory response even in the presence of the interleukin-1 receptor antagonist gene polymorphism. *Epidemiol. Infect.* **133:**569–572.

Sequelae and Long-Term Consequences of Infectious Diseases
Edited by Pina M. Fratamico, James L. Smith, and Kim A. Brogden

Chapter 8

Mycobacteria: Leprosy, a Battle Turned; Tuberculosis, a Battle Raging; Paratuberculosis, a Battle Ignored

R. J. Greenstein, T. Gillis, D. S. Scollard, and S. T. Brown

This chapter addresses three mycobacterial organisms that have entirely different profiles: *Mycobacterium leprae, Mycobacterium tuberculosis,* and *Mycobacterium avium* subsp. *paratuberculosis*. The disease caused by *Mycobacterium leprae* has been known since antiquity. The anti-leprosy battle has been well organized on a national as well as an international scale and is demonstrably being successfully waged. The protean diseases caused by *M. tuberculosis* are being successfully combated. But alarmingly, in concert with the rise of AIDS, the battle against *M. tuberculosis* is in danger of actually being lost. At present, one-third of humankind is infected with latent *M. tuberculosis* In complete contrast to what has occurred with *M. leprae* and *M. tuberculosis,* the vast majority of physicians are ignorant of even the existence of *M. avium* subsp. *paratuberculosis. M. avium* subsp. *paratuberculosis* causes Johne's disease in animals; however, it is not considered a cause of diseases in humans. There is increasing concern that this sanguine attitude is misplaced and that *M. avium* subsp. *paratuberculosis* may be responsible for multiple autoimmune and inflammatory diseases in humans. Because of these disparate mycobacterial profiles, this chapter is divided into three sections addressing *M. tuberculosis, M. avium* subsp. *paratuberculosis,* and *M. leprae,* separately. The interested reader who wishes to discuss specific aspects of a particular mycobacterium is encouraged to contact the author responsible for that component directly: for *M. tuberculosis,* Sheldon T. Brown (Sheldon.Brown@med.va.gov); for *M. avium* subsp. *paratuberculosis*, Robert J. Greenstein (BGAxis@aol.com); and for *M. leprae*, Tom Gillis (tgillis@lsu.edu) or David M. Scollard (dscoll1@lsu.edu).

M. TUBERCULOSIS

Tuberculosis (TB) is an ancient infection that emerged as the single most important cause of human morbidity and mortality, coinciding with the developing societal trends of increasing population concentration, commercialization, and global migration during the first and second millennia, AD. The case fatality rate had already begun to decline in developing countries by the end of the 19th century due in part to improved overall health status associated with declining poverty and crowding, vigorous public health measures, the emerging understanding of the germ theory of infection, and shifting patterns of herd immunity (86). The identification of the etiological agent led to a clearer understanding of the clinical pathogenesis of the disease, enabling the implementation of TB control programs based upon sound epidemiological principles, leading to dramatic declines in disease. These declines accelerated further in the latter half of the 20th century in technologically advanced countries following the discovery of effective antimicrobial treatment for active disease and latent infection.

"From three to five million persons die of TB every year throughout the world. Some fifty million suffer from the disease and transmit the germ of infection to their fellow man." The lead sentences from René and Jean Dubos' introduction to the first edition of *The White Plague* were written in 1952, describing the global status of the disease, which for centuries had been the leading killer of mankind (86). The time was shortly after the advent of effective combination chemotherapy capable of reliably curing the disease. New medications, programs of case finding, treatment of active disease, public

Robert J. Greenstein • Veterans Affairs Medical Center, Department of Surgery, Bronx, NY 10468. **Thomas P. Gillis and David S. Scollard** • Laboratory Research Branch at Louisiana State University, National Hansen's Disease Programs, Baton Rouge, LA 70803. **Sheldon T. Brown** • Veterans Affairs Medical Center, Department of Medicine, Bronx, NY 10468.

health measures to limit respiratory spread, prophylaxis of latent infection, and continuing *Mycobacterium bovis* BCG vaccination in high prevalence populations led to the hope for elimination of TB by the end of the 20th century (118, 151). Despite great progress in developed countries, these hopes were soon dashed by a continuing pandemic that prompted the World Health Organization to declare the worldwide epidemic of TB a global health emergency in 1993 (243). By 2000 the overall burden of TB sustained a global incidence of new disease of 8 million; its status as the leading killer of humans among infectious diseases had only recently been surpassed by AIDS. The prevalence of active TB disease was 24 million with a mean case fatality rate of 23%, and the number of people harboring latent infection was 1.86 billion, 32% of the world population (66, 87).

Several trends continue to gravely threaten progress toward further global reductions in TB. Most important is the modern plague of human immunodeficiency virus (HIV), whose central pathogenic consequence is progressive compromise of cell-mediated immune responses, the central pathway for host control of infection with TB (67). The global emergence of multidrug-resistant strains of TB diminishes the reliability of centrally important tools for TB control efforts (288). The vast reservoirs of latent infection interact with these two problems in ways that alter basic assumptions underlying conventional treatment and control programs (331).

Characteristics of the Organism

The phylum *Actinobacteria* arose relatively late in the evolution of prokaryotes, prior to emergence of eukaryotes (47, 317, 330) The genera *Corynebacterium*, *Mycobacterium*, and *Nocardia* form a subgroup of the order *Actinomycetales* that include some of the most important organisms capable of causing disease in humans and other animals (317). Members of the group have a high genomic G+C content and share similar cell wall composition.

Of the 85 species within the genus *Mycobacterium*, members of the *Mycobacterium tuberculosis* complex have evolved as one of the preeminent pathogens of man. Intimate coevolution within their mammalian hosts appears to have ancient origins, resulting in their current status as obligate intracellular parasites that occupy no known independent environmental niche (212). The complex consists of closely related species having 99.9% genetic identity. Nonetheless, they have evolved distinct characteristics through adaptation to their respective host environments, the understanding of which is beginning to reveal important details of host responses to infection and adaptive mechanisms of pathogens.

Species of the *M. tuberculosis* complex that principally cause human infection and disease are comprised of *M. tuberculosis*, *M. africanum*, and "*M. canettii*." The remaining species within the complex have a predilection for causing disease in diverse animal species, but most can cause disease in humans, particularly in the setting of deficient cell-mediated immunity. *M. microti* most commonly causes disease in voles, *M. pinnipedii* in seals, *M. caprae* in goats, and *M. bovis*, which comprises genetically distinct groups, in cows and antelope. It had long been thought that adaptation of *M. bovis* led to the emergence of *M. tuberculosis* as an outgrowth of the domestication of cattle and their resulting intimate association with humans. Recent genophenotypic analysis shows that this was not the case and that members of the *M. tuberculosis* complex with an affinity for human infection and those infecting other animal species diverged from a common ancestor (212).

Further evidence of coadaptation of subspecies of the *M. tuberculosis* complex and their hosts has become apparent through genotypic investigations of the divergent affinity of strain clusters for genetically related hosts within the same species. Just as *M. tuberculosis* has affinity for infection of humans and *M. bovis* for cattle, closely related clones of *M. tuberculosis* appear more likely to cause disease in persons with a common genetic background. Thus the Asian strain is more apt to cause disease in persons of Chinese ancestry living in the United States than are strains of European origin (113).

Clinical Disease

The clinical course of TB can be roughly divided into three phases: primary infection, latent TB, and chronic active TB (Fig. 1). The only epidemiologically important route of transmission leading to primary infection is from human to human via the inhalation of droplet nuclei from infected aerosols. The minimal infectious inoculum is calculated to be as low as one viable bacillus (287). Inhaled bacilli are phagocytosed by mechanisms that may include pathogen-directed uptake into both professional and nonprofessional phagocytes, where they are able to resist nonspecific antibacterial killing mechanisms and slowly proliferate. Once infection is established, *M. tuberculosis* primarily resides and multiplies within macrophages (MPH) and other monocytes-derived cell lines, such as dendritic cells (249, 299).

When primary infection occurs in persons with limited or absent cell-mediated immune function,

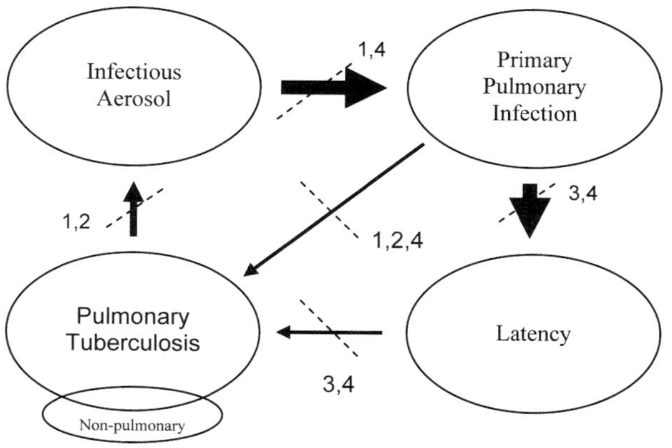

Figure 1. The cycle of TB infection and opportunities to interrupt it. Solid arrows indicate the path of various stages in the cycle of TB infection. Dashed lines indicate opportunities to interrupt the cycle of infection. Numbers refer to the most important corresponding control methods used to interrupt the cycle of infection. 1, public health and epidemiological measures; 2, multidrug treatment of active disease; 3, single-drug treatment of asymptomatic infection; 4, immunologic enhancement, including vaccination.

disease progresses from the site of inoculum and typically causes a pneumonitis that begins in the lower lung fields, becoming more widespread over many days to a few weeks. There is associated mediastinal adenopathy and increasing hematogenous spread throughout the body. Histopathology shows poorly organized epithelioid granulomas with MPH containing many acid-fast bacilli (AFB) similar to that of lepromatous leprosy and disseminated *M. avium* infection. In young children whose cell-mediated immune responses are at an intermediate stage of development, there are high rates of disseminated disease, including the devastating complication of miliary disease and tuberculous meningitis. A fulminant pneumonitis with widely disseminated disease and bacillemia can occur in patients with profound immunodeficiency, such as advanced AIDS, or those receiving intensive immune suppression to treat cancer or for organ transplantation (4, 37, 88). The rapidity of progression of disease in such patients is the opposite extreme from those who contain the initial infection with few or no sequelae other than residual granuloma and amnestic immunity reflected by hypersensitivity response to purified protein derivative (PPD) (tuberculin skin test). It also sharply contrasts with the indolent course commonly associated with active TB. Intermediate clinical syndromes therefore reflect a continuous spectrum in the balance between effective and ineffective host responses, and a preponderance of pathology appears to result from collateral damage from the ongoing inflammatory events that accompany this process (105).

The clinical fate of infection with *M. tuberculosis* follows the onset of effective antigen directed host cell-mediated immune responses and depends upon a balance between the ability of these mechanisms to successfully kill or inhibit the replication of intracellular bacilli and the opposing capacity of the bacteria to resist these mechanisms, permitting multiplication and spread. The immunological evolution of the host response has been a productive focus of research, having the ultimate aim of developing more effective vaccines. The interaction between the organism and the host is highly dynamic. The revolution in genomics has created the opportunity to study these relationships at an increasingly refined level (4, 96, 214). The pivotal role of gamma interferon (IFN-γ) for the activation of MPH was worked out in cell culture systems and has been verified through the use of gene knockout animal models and in molecular studies from human disease (104). TB successfully resists the bactericidal activity of reactive oxygen intermediates, but the succeeding amplification cascades involving tumor necrosis factor alpha (TNF-α) and reactive nitrogen intermediates are clearly of central importance for the elaboration of effective intracellular mycobactericidal activity (184). Dramatic evidence for the importance of TNF-α in maintaining persistence of immunological control in humans is provided by cases of relapsed TB in persons treated with TNF receptor antagonists (171). When immune responses are successful, bacilli may be contained in granuloma at the initial site of infection and associated regional lymph nodes, where viable bacilli may persist in semi-dormancy for many years, undergoing occasional subclinical cycles of replication. This is the stage of latent TB (52).

Chronic active clinical TB results from an incompletely effective host response. The wide individual variation in the ability to suppress infection accounts for wide diversity in time course and clinical manifestations of tuberculous disease. The most common outcome is spread to the apical lobes with subsequent inflammation, caseation necrosis and parenchymal tissue destruction leading to cavity formation and fibrosis (328). Chronic progression of apical pulmonary TB is the most common form of the disease. In the early stages, there are typically few symptoms other than a progressive cough, nonproductive at first, which is indistinguishable from a chronic smoker's cough, accompanied by increasing malaise. These symptoms do not at first interfere with normal activities of daily living. As the burden of infection gradually builds and symptoms intensify over periods of time varying from months to years, there is a parallel increased capacity for contagious aerosolization, particularly after the development of cavitary disease. With disease progression there are an increasing frequency and severity of systemic features of chronic infection, including fevers, night sweats, weight loss, and anorexia. Many of these symptoms are the consequence of an intensifying systemic chronic inflammatory state with chronic elevations of circulating proinflammatory cytokines (105). Medical attention is often not sought until after these symptoms develop. Even in an advanced stage, the symptomatic presentation of TB can be confused with other chronic illnesses. A number of other chronic intracellular infections, such as histoplasmosis, nocardiosis, and *M. avium* complex infections, as well as conditions without known infectious etiology, such as sarcoidosis, cannot be confidently distinguished from pulmonary TB on purely clinical grounds. Since dyspnea is commonly absent and chest auscultation may yield only subtle findings, clinicians not living in areas where TB is endemic may often discount the likelihood of TB in favor of more familiar diagnoses. The diagnosis of extrapulmonary TB can be even more challenging, but the public health risk of transmission is not generally as serious.

Whether spread to the lung apex is due to hematogenous spread or to auto-reinfection from the site of primary infection is controversial (328). It has been convincingly modeled in animals, and there is evidence that the immune response is initiated in lymph nodes and not at the site of inoculation in the lungs (328, 332). It is therefore likely that hematogenous dissemination does commonly occur in association with primary infection in persons who subsequently control the infection. This accounts for the higher rate of extrapulmonary disease occurring during a relapse of latent infection, particularly in the setting of acquired deficiencies of cell-mediated immunity.

Extrapulmonary TB, with rare exception, occurs as a result of hematogenous dissemination. It may present concurrently with progressive pulmonary infection or may be the dominant clinical syndrome during reactivation of latent infection. The protean clinical manifestations of TB vary widely depending upon the organ affected, the burden of infection, and the robustness of the host immune response. Reactivation within the lining of cavities of the pleura, pericardium, and peritoneum leads to diffuse granulomatous studding of the serosal surface with chronic mononuclear infiltration and progressive fibrosis that may lead to restrictive disease. Mass lesions and abscess formation can occur in single or multiple sites and tissues, often mimicking metastatic neoplasia (37, 163). Another feature shared with solid neoplastic tumors is that TB is one of the few infections that readily transgress the fascial planes between tissues, which can lead to fistulization between organs or to the skin. Vertebral osteomyelitis and discitis, the most common presentation of tuberculous osteomyelitis, is often complicated by contiguous epidural and psoas muscle abscess formation and is a common form of reactivated disease in persons with mild to moderate impairments of immune function (213). These presentations may develop gradually, with symptoms developing over weeks to months and then chronically progressing for years if untreated. Renal TB may progress asymptomatically for years.

TB can also manifest with rapid progression to fulminant disease in just a few weeks, usually in the setting of moderate to severe immunosuppression. Tuberculous meningitis is a particularly devastating form of extrapulmonary TB that occurs most commonly in young children and in patients with AIDS. The characteristic radiographic picture of miliary TB requires prompt recognition and empiric initiation of treatment if serious morbidity or death is to be avoided. Primary infection in patients with advanced AIDS or those treated with prolonged high-dose corticosteroids or chemotherapy can develop rapidly progressive, diffuse pneumonitis, leading to respiratory failure (88).

Each of these clinical stages presents particular opportunities and challenges for prevention, diagnosis, and treatment of the individual patient. When recognized early enough, individual management can usually be expected to result in a cure if the organism is susceptible to the chosen antimicrobials and the patient adheres to the regimen. The emergence of extensively drug-resistant TB may place curative outcomes beyond reach with currently available therapies (114).

The remainder of this section will address aspects of current understanding and critical gaps in knowledge that need to be filled if the global burden of disease due to infection is to be reduced. Selection will be principally from the societal perspective of interventions that can reduce the transmission and thereby diminish the disease.

Control of TB

The cycle of infection with TB provides three principal opportunities to intervene and control its spread: prevention of person-to-person transmission; stimulation of effective host responses to prevent, immunologically control, or eliminate infection; and effective antimicrobial treatment of the organism, whether for active disease or for paucibacillary latent infection (Fig. 1). It is widely recognized that successful control or elimination of TB will require an integrated convergence of strategies in all three domains. Each of these opportunities has been the subject of intense effort and remarkable advances in medical science. Existing and new obstacles to successful intervention have correspondingly been identified as priority areas for treatment, public health policy, and research (243).

Prevention of Person-to-Person Spread

If person-to-person contagion with TB were eliminated, there would be no other environmental source from which TB might be reintroduced as an infection of humans. Respiratory transmission of infection is the fundamental event that allows for persistence and propagation of TB, and TB control programs are therefore directed toward the prevention, identification, and treatment of pulmonary TB. The spread of TB within a population can decrease as long as the number of patients newly infected by a person with active disease is lower than the number of new infections that will, on average, result in a case of active disease. This is conventionally regarded as fewer than 10 to 20 persons infected per index case, although this number varies, as risk of progression to active disease varies within a population. This simple concept is the foundation for all public health measures relevant to TB control. Its application is exemplified in the World Health Organization global TB control strategy for directly observed therapy (DOTS) centered on government commitment to sustained TB control, active surveillance, standardized treatment under case management conditions, availability of effective drugs, and a system to monitor treatment outcomes (243). Impressive gains followed the implementation of DOTS in the early 1990s, with dramatic declines in pulmonary TB in some countries that had previously witnessed expanding or resurgent rates of disease (294).

There are several threats to the future success of these strategies. The expectation of a stable rate of active disease in relation to the rate of infection is often altered by local circumstance. The most dramatic example is the influence of concurrent HIV infection, which transforms the approximate 10% lifetime rate of active TB to a 10% annual risk, roughly a 10-fold increase in the rate of active disease and opportunity for transmission. This leads to a greatly increased demand on public health services, already tested by the spread of HIV within countries with limited resources and which must now contend with greatly expanded requirements for case finding, contact tracing, prophylaxis, and treatment if the spread of TB is to be contained. The effects of poverty, malnutrition and famine, population displacements due to societal upheaval, and crowding can also lead to increased proportions of active disease (86). Many countries have effectively implemented the WHO/International Union Against Tuberculosis and Lung Disease (IUALTD) program, often with creative adaptations to overcome local obstacles, and resources from a variety of governmental and nongovernmental agencies have been dedicated to the effort (294). However, other countries have been slow to adopt effective control measures, often because of political instability or inadequate appreciation of the extent of the problem. Many of these countries are those with high rates of latent endemic TB and epidemic spread of HIV (51, 231) Failure or delays in implementation of control programs in these settings will inevitably lead to increases in cases of active disease and increases in reservoirs of latent infection that may potentially lead to further active disease and spread through travel and migration. Establishing comprehensive and sustainable public health programs for TB control remains the greatest pragmatic challenge in global efforts to reverse the spread of TB.

Variation in strain virulence is well recognized, but its influence on overall epidemiological trends is less clear. There is increasing evidence that some strains of TB may be hypervirulent, which could significantly change the epidemiologic dynamic of contagious spread and attendant control measures (179, 308, 334). In contrast, there is also evidence for the diminished virulence of drug-resistant strains of TB and, while it is hoped that this will support the near-term aims of control programs, the heterogeneity of these effects makes this prospect unreliable (60, 61). New outbreaks from lingering reservoirs of latent drug-resistant infection have occurred, and some of these have been associated with strains that appear to be hypervirulent (48–50). Future reactivation of latent infection caused by resistant bacilli is certain to occur, which further underscores the need for sustained vigilance and global commitments to surveillance long after near-term successes in reducing rates of active disease. The alternative is the development of improved methods to prevent and cure infection in exposed individuals.

Diagnostic Testing

An essential requirement for the success of TB control programs, including the DOTS initiatives, is early detection of active disease and reliable identification of newly infected contacts. Initial presumptive detection of active disease is made on clinical grounds since results of culture may not be available for weeks, even with optimal technology. Clinical suspicion for TB may be strongly influenced by practitioner experience and, because of broad overlap with other clinical syndromes, is roughly proportional to the regional prevalence of disease. When clinically suspected, preliminary diagnosis is presumptively confirmed by the microscopic finding of AFB in sputum. However, there is wide variation on the technical performance of this labor-intensive examination, which is only 75% sensitive under optimal circumstances. It is commonly held that sputum smears that do not show AFB indicate that a person is minimally contagious, even if active TB is subsequently verified by culture. Recent evidence challenges this assumption and suggests that up to 17% of transmission may occur from index cases of TB that are smear negative but culture positive (19). More rapid molecular amplification-based techniques are available in resource rich countries, but they are unlikely to be widely available for many years. While highly specific, their diagnostic sensitivity is, so far, not reliably greater than conventional culture (58). Recent improvements of culture have been demonstrated for assays of cerebral spinal fluid using real-time nested PCR that reopen the question of whether sensitivity can be improved from other clinical specimens (301). Mapping of the proteome of *M. tuberculosis* reveals a significant number of previously unrecognized products, some of which may prove useful for the development of antigen capture assays (233). Improved diagnostic tests for active TB remain a priority, whether using genetic amplification or specific antigen capture assays. Their utility will ultimately depend upon speed, ease of use, and cost.

Molecular technologies are becoming increasingly accessible and may be of particular importance as heterogeneous patterns of drug resistance become more widespread. It takes a minimum of several weeks for culture-based antimicrobial susceptibility testing of TB to be reported. Uncertainty about the appropriate treatment regimen can lead to potential for disease progression, further transmission, or errors in choice of initial therapy that may lead to development of further resistance while waiting for results. One of the ways that TB differs importantly from most bacterial pathogens is that there is little or no horizontal exchange of genetic material (196). All known drug resistance is therefore a result of clonal proliferation of chromosomal mutations, and these are fairly easy to identify. Amplification assays for identification of particular resistance mutations are now available, and the development of composite assays for the full range of drug resistance mutations is certainly feasible (164). Rapid susceptibility testing using genetically modified mycobacteriophages continues to be an attractive technology (146). Such assays can theoretically be applied directly to diagnostic specimens or after a brief period of incubation, thereby hastening availability of critical data to guide antimicrobial interventions. These technologies will be of increasing importance as the problem of drug resistance evolves.

The tuberculin skin test for delayed-type hypersensitivity reactions to PPD extracts from cultures of TB, useful in increasing the index of suspicion for smear-negative and extrapulmonary disease, is reactive in the majority of immunologically healthy infected contacts of persons with active TB and remains the current clinical standard for diagnosis of latent infection. However, there are significant limitations to PPD testing that lead to the need for alternative or complementary methods. PPD test results may be compromised by improper technique in administration and interpretation of the test, leading to both false-negative and false-positive results. The test must be read from 2 to 5 days after administration and follow-up of subjects who do not return for reading is a problem (136, 152). False-negative results due to anergy, which is very common in the setting of HIV, can miss identifying those most at risk for progression to active disease following infection. False-positive results can occur due to cross reactivity from prior vaccination with BCG or to subclinical infection with ubiquitous environmental mycobacteria and may lead to unnecessary treatment with the potential for uncommon but serious toxicity. Once a person has a reactive tuberculin skin test and has received prophylaxis or been treated for active disease, the test can no longer be used to identify reinfection at a later date (262). Therefore, there is a critical need to identify reliable and inexpensive alternatives to tuberculin skin testing for both active and latent infection.

Tests for latent TB are all based upon host immune responses, whereas tests for active TB may detect products of the organism, the host immune response, or both. Measurement of IFN-γ production in response to the TB-specific early secretory antigenic target 6 (ESAT-6) and culture filtrate protein 10 (CFP-10) are both sensitive and specific, since they do not cross-react with BCG or common nontuberculous mycobacteria (99). They have been incorporated into recently commercialized assays that are undergoing widespread evaluation (203, 230). Positive results lack complete concordance with PPD testing, which may be an attribute of improved specificity. However, they require carefully handled fresh whole blood, lose sensitivity with increasing immune compromise of the host, and are relatively expensive tests that may be of limited use in resource-poor settings. There is renewed interest in serodiagnosis of both latent and active TB using antibodies to novel antigens (2). Serodiagnosis may have advantages of specificity and rapid turnaround at relatively low cost. To date, the major limitation of serological assays continues to be poor sensitivity. There is consequently a continuing need for simple, sensitive, and specific diagnostic tools for both latent and active infection with TB.

Immunological Treatment of TB

Immunological control is the rule in healthy persons who are infected with TB. Ninety-five percent of the time, this control is established within a few weeks and lasts for life in up to 90 percent of those infected. Persistence of viable bacilli contained by granuloma in a dormant state are thought to be the most common outcome after infection with TB. Eradication of initial infection by innate immunity and sterilization of latent infection probably occur but are much less common outcomes. Nonetheless, such evidence for the capacity of immune mechanisms to clear infection or to prevent active disease suggests that prophylactic vaccination should be an achievable aim and that vaccine-directed clearance of persistent infection may be achievable (285).

All antimicrobial vaccine strategies are designed to activate host immune responses capable of suppressing or eliminating a pathogen. Within the cycle of infection with *M. tuberculosis* (Fig. 1), they may act to (i) stimulate host-directed immune responses to recognize and clear organisms at the time of initial infection, (ii) stimulate host immune responses to ensure the induction of latency and prevent the development of active disease, (iii) stimulate host immune responses to restrict dissemination of the organism, or (iv) stimulate host-directed immune responses to clear latent infection.

The laboratory attenuated *M. bovis* bacillus Calmette-Guérin (BCG) is one of the earliest bacterial vaccines developed; has proven efficacy in reducing the incidence of disseminated TB, particularly in healthy children; and remains in common use in countries with high rates of endemic infection. However, BCG vaccination has not reliably reduced rates of pulmonary TB in adults; it leads to tuberculin skin test conversion, thus eliminating one of the most useful screening diagnostic tests, and its use is not without hazards, especially in immunocompromised hosts who may develop disseminated infection after vaccination (103, 116) While of great importance to TB control programs, it is clear that BCG vaccination does not reliably prevent infection or latency and thus cannot be the centerpiece of TB elimination programs, similar to those for smallpox and polio. Efforts to understand the details of host pathogen interactions, identify immune-reactive bacillary antigens, and identify methods of antigen delivery leading to effective immunity have therefore been a research priority.

The availability of powerful molecular methods coupled with the complete sequencing of the genome of TB has led to great advances in the understanding of the organism and its interaction with host responses (63, 234). There is an increasing understanding of the remarkable adaptations that have permitted TB to occupy its niche as a parasite of MPH, cells whose major role is to initiate powerful processes of antigen-directed immunity and when activated to recognize and kill pathogens. These adaptations include pathogen-influenced changes in normal host protective responses, such as alterations in the maturation of macrophage-directed bactericidal mechanisms, including inhibition of phagosome-lysosome fusion, inhibition of the acidification of phago-lysosomal vesicles, and induction of cytokine responses that result in a shift from Th1- to Th2-type immunity, among others (26, 249).

The mechanisms by which *M. tuberculosis* survives within a hostile intracellular milieu and interacts with host immune mechanisms are complex, and a comprehensive treatment is beyond the scope of this chapter. However, a number of areas of current understanding are worth highlighting for what they reveal about the pathogenesis of TB and for further work that needs to be done.

The complex mycobacterial cell wall stands at the interface of microbe-host interactions and has remarkable biological properties (16). The understanding of the synthetic pathways and structure of the cell well is nearly complete, along with an increasingly detailed understanding of its role in interacting with host cells (32). Pathways of cell wall synthesis are particularly attractive as targets for drug development for new classes of anti-TB chemotherapy. The initiation of phagocytosis is modified by components of the bacterial cell wall that redirect trafficking of host intracellular signaling so that normal processes of phagosome and lysosome fusion are interrupted (45, 85, 249). Immunoreactive cell wall antigens, including lipoarabinomannan, phenolic glycolipids (PGL), and mycolic acids, are of particular importance as targets of cell-mediated immune responses and in turn influence the pathway of immune activation that ensues. The dogma that specific immunity requires protein or polysaccharide antigenic epitopes was overturned by the finding that CD-1-restricted antigen presentation of mycobacterial glycolipids depended upon the lipid moiety of these cell wall components (36).

Host antimicrobial mechanisms are further modified by secreted proteins. The ESAT-6 and CFP-10 family of secreted proteins, used in newly developed diagnostic assays, contribute to inhibition of the acidification of lysosomal vesicles required for activation of lytic enzymes in activated MPH (302). The Ag85 family of major secreted proteins has mycolyl transferase activity, functions as fibronectin binding proteins, and is highly immunoreactive. They are of particular interest as vaccine candidates, and clinical trials are currently underway (285). Recent studies suggest that a relatively small proportion of secreted proteins and their functions have been characterized (194). More detailed understanding of these proteins is needed both to understand their function and to assess their potential as candidates for diagnostic tests or as targets for treatment interventions. A limitation of these studies is that they focus on products of culture-adapted organisms that are of uncertain relevance to in vivo phenotypes during different phases of infection.

It is now feasible to model transcriptional responses of both the organism and host cells to describe their interactive responses over time using microarray methods (299). The main limitation of these techniques is that they are currently applied in the controlled context of cell culture coinfection. The in vivo interactive milieu is far more complex, such that models developed in cell culture may not be of direct relevance. However, tools obtained from these in vitro studies may be used to probe in vivo models to more closely reveal details of host-pathogen interactions. If vaccine strategies capable of reliably sterilizing infection in the immunocompetent host are to be developed, insights from these studies will contribute importantly to their foundation. Of particular interest will be vaccination of latent TB with the aim of clearing reservoirs of viable but metabolically dormant bacilli.

Antimicrobial Treatment of TB

Development of drugs capable of curing active TB and preventing progression to disease among recently infected contacts was one of the medical triumphs of the last century (256). The predictable development of resistance in the setting of single-drug therapy was soon apparent, and the requirement for multidrug therapy, including drugs that were bactericidal, was established. Incremental improvements led to regimens with less toxicity and greater efficacy that allowed the term of treatment to be reduced from an average of 30 months to 6 months for treatment of drug-susceptible strains. However, the only meaningful additions to the armamentarium of useful agents for the treatment of TB in the last 30 years have been members of the fluoroquinolone class of DNA gyrase inhibitors. Meanwhile, strains of TB resistant to all classes have emerged. When highly immunocompromised patients are infected with such strains, there is a high likelihood of progressive, communicable disease with no meaningful treatment option. The development of new drugs with bactericidal activity against the organism and which are not cross-resistant with current classes of drugs is imperative (80).

There are two important categories of treatment that need to be addressed, latent infection and active disease. Latent infection is most commonly treated with a single bactericidal agent, usually isoniazid (INH), for a period of at least 6 months. The aim is to prevent the development of active disease in persons recently infected or who have evidence of past untreated disease. This is somewhat misleadingly referred to as prophylaxis. It is more appropriately conceptualized as treatment of infection with a bacillary burden that is below the threshold required to select for spontaneous resistance. For many years, it was unclear if the treatment of latent infection was curative and therefore protective against remote reactivation. No definitive studies of this question have been conducted in humans because of logistical difficulties and the potential confounding effect of unrecognized reinfection. There is indirect evidence for sterilization from animal models, but the time course of disease and clinical conditions differ so widely from infection in humans that their relevance remains speculative (207). However, the concurrent epidemics of TB and HIV strongly suggest that monotherapy of latent TB with INH may often be sterilizing. Reactivation of latent TB is one of the earliest opportunistic infections that occurs as immunological function declines due to HIV, and that is why TB is globally the most common AIDS-defining condition. Prior to the advent of effective antiretroviral therapy, the greatest improvements in health outcomes were achieved by using prophylactic antimicrobial medications for opportunistic infections to which patients were most susceptible. For HIV-infected persons who had a history at any time of a reactive tuberculin skin test, the standard has been a 9- to 12-month course of INH. Studies comparing treated with untreated patients before the advent of highly active antiretroviral therapy show marked reductions in active disease and no difference between immunocompetent and anergic patients (117, 331). For patients adherent to prophylaxis for tuberculin positivity or treatment for active disease, recurrence of TB is most commonly due to reinfection rather than to relapse, despite the progression of HIV to profound levels of immunosuppression (278, 289). It is not known whether prophylaxis of patients exposed to drug-resistant TB is similarly effective or how best to construct prophylactic regimens for such patients.

From an epidemiological perspective, latent reservoirs of infection constitute the greatest potential source of future transmission and perpetuation of human TB. Confident elimination of this reservoir would dramatically reduce the uncertainties and time needed for sustained TB control efforts, if they are to be effective (112). If management of active infection is successful, then knowledgeable treatment of reservoirs of latent infection, currently one-third of the world population, will be necessary to prevent recurrent outbreaks. Development of vaccines that lead to host elimination of latent infection would be the most efficient strategy for reduction of latent reservoirs. However, since an increasing proportion of reactivated TB is likely to occur in persons unable to mount an effective vaccine response, there is a need for a parallel effort to develop convenient, nontoxic antimycobacterial drugs that lead to reliable sterilization of latent TB. Carefully constructed human trials will need to be conducted to validate these treatments since animal models insufficiently reflect human infection (207).

M. AVIUM SUBSP. *PARATUBERCULOSIS*

In this section, I will introduce *M. avium* subsp. *paratuberculosis*, enumerate its salient characteristics, and briefly discuss its pervasiveness in the agricultural community, where it is freely acknowledged to cause Johne's disease (161). Next, I will show how live *M. avium* subsp. *paratuberculosis* is transmitted to humans.

Then I will deal with what are, in my opinion, the two most important reasons that *M. avium* subsp. *paratuberculosis* has not been acknowledged to be a human pathogen. The first is that, in humans, *M. avium* subsp. *paratuberculosis* exists in the cell wall-deficient form. The second is that, unknowingly, the medical profession has been treating *M. avium* subsp. *paratuberculosis* infections since 1942, when Nana Svartz introduced sulfasalazine into clinical practice.

Since prevailing medical dogma does not consider *M. avium* subsp. *paratuberculosis* to be zoonotic, there is not a single human disease that is accepted as being caused by *M. avium* subsp. *paratuberculosis*. Thus it is not possible to address the chronic effect of *M. avium* subsp. *paratuberculosis* in any particular human disease. As a consequence, this section will deal with possible diseases in man that may be caused by *M. avium* subsp. *paratuberculosis* and how that diagnosis may be established. The circumstantial evidence that accounts for including these diseases will be presented. Suggestions will be made as to how to test the hypothesis that a given disease may be caused by *M. avium* subsp. *paratuberculosis*, as will the ethical dilemmas that will need to be addressed in the performance of such studies.

Characteristics of the Organism

For the uninitiated, *M. avium* subsp. *paratuberculosis* should be considered a mycobacterium that is distinct from *M. avium* subsp. *avium* and *M. avium* subsp. *silvaticum* (309). The last two have much more in common phylogenetically with each other than with *M. avium* subsp. *paratuberculosis* (309). The importance of this *M. avium*/*M. avium* subsp. *paratuberculosis* distinction will become apparent when we discuss certain in vitro inhibition studies (vide infra).

Cell wall

M. avium subsp. *paratuberculosis* exists in cell wall-containing and cell wall-deficient forms. Characteristically, *M. avium* subsp. *paratuberculosis* in ruminants has a characteristic complex cell wall that is identified by the acid-/alcohol-fast stain described by Ziehl in 1882 (339) and Neelsen in 1883 (219). In contrast, in humans, with two exceptions (245, 284), *M. avium* subsp. *paratuberculosis* is found in the cell wall-deficient form (54, 55).

M. avium subsp. *paratuberculosis* Culture

Within the agricultural community, much attention has been given to the successful culture of *M. avium* subsp. *paratuberculosis*. It must be emphasized that culture of *M. avium* subsp. *paratuberculosis*, although difficult, is possible. This is in contrast to the culture of *M. tuberculosis*, which is relatively easy, and *M. leprae*, for which in vitro culture has never been achieved.

From the perspective of this general audience, several factors should be stressed concerning *M. avium* subsp. *paratuberculosis* culture. The cell wall-containing form is relatively easier to culture than the cell wall-deficient form. Culture requires specific medium (generally Middlebrook based [73]). Additionally, since *M. avium* subsp. *paratuberculosis* is constitutively unable to celate iron, Mycobactin J (Allied Monitor, Fayette, MO) *must* be added to the culture medium. This applies to both primary culture and passaged strains. When performing primary isolation, the addition of Herrold's egg yolk is required. Any attempt to isolate cell wall-containing or -deficient *M. avium* subsp. *paratuberculosis* without these two agents will not be successful.

Pivotal in the theses posited in this section are the ability to quantify *M. avium* subsp. *paratuberculosis* growth and the inhibition of that growth by agents being studied. *M. avium* subsp. *paratuberculosis* grows very slowly, its tardiness being exceeded only by *M. leprae*. As a consequence, an agar-based slope that contains the obligate Mycobactin J and Herrold's egg yolk is only of use for evaluating very potent bactericidal agents. Such slopes are incapable of providing sufficient sensitivity to generate the data that will be presented and discussed below.

Quantifying *M. avium* subsp. *paratuberculosis* Growth

Several commercially available methods quantify mycobacterial growth in liquid culture. They quantify the consumption of oxygen, the release of CO_2 (138), or the increasing pressure within a sealed container as the strains grow.

CO_2 release measurement requires the Bactec 460 radiometric $^{14}CO_2$ quantifying system (Becton-Dickenson, NJ). There are two major drawbacks to the Bactec system, as a consequence of which it is being phased out. The first is that it quantifies ^{14}C in the form of $^{14}CO_2$ (70, 204). Thus, its use requires compliance with onerous, obligatory, nuclear regulatory requirements and documentation. Additionally, the Bactec system is only semiautomatic. Vials have to be transferred from the incubator and hand-loaded onto the $^{14}CO_2$ detector on a daily basis. The $^{14}CO_2$ release by the growing bacteria is quantified by the integral detector and presented as arbitrary growth index units. The range is 0 to 999. Once $>$ 999, the results are no longer meaningful. By quantifying $^{14}CO_2$ release on a daily basis, a cumulative growth index unit is obtained. The undeniable advantage of the Bactec system is that it is exquisitely sensitive (326).

The oxygen consumption (MIGT; Becton-Dickerson, NJ) method relies on a fluorescent probe being activated as growing bacteria consume O_2 and the O_2 tension falls. The major advantage is that this is a completely automated system. Once inoculated and the appropriate agent added, the vial is placed in the MIGT 960 incubator and requires no further physical manipulation until the integral computer determines whether growth has occurred or not. Data are presented as the number of days required for the computer to decide that log phase growth has occurred, and at these numbers of days, a given vial is declared positive. Another advantage is that this system does not use radionucleotides, obviating the need for meticulous regulatory agent documentation. Although of use in studying potent antimycobacterial agents (253), its disadvantage is that it is not as sensitive as the Bactec 460 system.

Simply put, the subtle 5 amino-salicylic acid (5-ASA) data discussed below could only have been detected using the Bactec system. If only the MIGT system had been used (282), the insights presented below could not have been made.

Diseases Caused by *M. avium* subsp. *paratuberculosis*

In ruminants, *M. avium* subsp. *paratuberculosis* causes Johne's disease (161), a chronic wasting intestinal diarrheal affliction. *M. avium* subsp. *paratuberculosis* is endemic worldwide. In animals with Johne's disease, *M. avium* subsp. *paratuberculosis* is disseminated (11), is found in milk, and has in utero transmission to the fetus (305, 327). Animals may become infected in utero, during parturition, from infected milk, or from environmental sources, such as contaminated water and/or food. Animals with Johne's disease will have chronic diarrhea and weight loss. Since *M. avium* subsp. *paratuberculosis* grows so slowly, animals being raised for meat production may well be slaughtered before Johne's disease retards their growth. However, cattle being bred for milk production survive for longer periods ($>$5 years), permitting Johne's disease to manifest itself. In such a case, an indication to cull an infected animal is when their Johne's disease impairs their milk production. In 1913, the diagnosis of Johne's disease was predominantly made by the Ziehl (339)-Neelsen (219) stain.

Johne's disease occurs on all continents. Initially, the disease was predominately found in ruminants, including cattle (161), sheep (271), bison (38), and red deer (218), but it has now spread to other species, including wild animals, such as ferrets in Scotland (17) and guanacos in Argentina (165), that ingest animals suffering from Johne's disease. The prevalence of Johne's disease is increasing, and the financial losses attributed to it are measured in billions of dollars. *M. avium* subsp. *paratuberculosis* causes chronic intestinal inflammation in nonhuman primates, such as stumptail macaque monkeys (*Macaca arctoides*) (201).

Johne's disease is evocative of inflammatory bowel disease (IBD) in humans. The disease in humans that is most commonly implicated as being caused by *M. avium* subsp. *paratuberculosis* is Dalziel's disease (72) (most frequently referred to as Crohn's disease [69]). In 1913, when Dalziel first reported his disease, he commented on its similarity to Johne's disease (72). However, since *M. avium* subsp. *paratuberculosis* is in the cell wall-deficient form, the

Ziehl-Neelsen stain, described in 1882, was negative. As a consequence, it has been assumed that Johne's and Dalziel's/Crohn's diseases had different causes. Subsequently, *M. avium* subsp. *paratuberculosis* RNA (206), DNA (reviewed in reference 130; 260), and *M. avium* subsp. *paratuberculosis*-specific proteins (94, 95) have been identified, and culture of *M. avium* subsp. *paratuberculosis* (40, 54–56, 216, 217), including from the milk of women with Dalziel/Crohn's disease (217) and from the blood of patients with IBD (216) has been achieved. It must be emphasized that some laboratories cannot replicate these findings (reviewed in reference 130). Possible technical explanations for this lack of reproducibility have been addressed (130).

There is now an additional insight that may in part explain the lack of reproducibility in detecting *M. avium* subsp. *paratuberculosis*-associated markers from one institution to another. Recent observations show unsuspected anti-*M. avium* subsp. *paratuberculosis* antibiotic activity of routinely used immune modulator (135, 282) and anti-inflammatory (43) agents, which are used in the therapy of IBD. The use of these multiple agents in the therapy of a variety of autoimmune and inflammatory diseases has until now been considered irrelevant when addressing the possible zoonosis of *M. avium* subsp. *paratuberculosis*.

In the event that *M. avium* subsp. *paratuberculosis* is eventually accepted as being zoonotic (133), the question will need to be asked how does *M. avium* subsp. *paratuberculosis* get from infected animals to humans. *M. avium* subsp. *paratuberculosis* has been cultured from US chlorinated potable municipal water (206) and pasteurized milk in the United States (91) and Europe (14, 122). These data are of considerable importance, as they identify one of several critical elements that will need to be addressed in the control of *M. avium* subsp. *paratuberculosis*. *M. avium* subsp. *paratuberculosis* will need to be removed from, or adequately pasteurized in, the food chain (82, 119–123) and the potable, chlorinated municipal water supply of humans (323).

In my opinion, there are two critical elements that have been responsible for the failure to recognize *M. avium* subsp. *paratuberculosis* as a human pathogen. The first, addressed above, is the fact that in humans, *M. avium* subsp. *paratuberculosis* is present in the cell wall-deficient, or L, form. The second is that the medical profession has, unknowingly, been treating *M. avium* subsp. *paratuberculosis* since Svartz introduced sulfasalazine in 1942 (295).

Sulfasalazine is a conjugate of two molecules, sulfapyridine and 5-ASA. Enteric enzymes cleave the intact molecule into its two components on its passage through the intestinal lumen. Sulfasalazine or its 5-ASA moiety is now "the most widely prescribed medication in the therapy of IBD" (20), with the greatest efficacy in ulcerative colitis (126, 127, 291, 306). This is despite the fact that "the mechanism of action [of 5-ASA] in the therapy of IBD is 'uncertain'" (20).

Sulfapyridine is acknowledged to be an antibiotic (97, 325). However, prevailing medical dogma holds that "it is unlikely that [sulfasalazine's] antibacterial activity accounts for its clinical efficacy" (20). Svartz herself considered 5-ASA to be an antibiotic (295–297). However in 1977, the independent efficacies of sulfapyridine and 5-ASA were compared in a 2-week study on ulcerative proctitis (15). Inflammation was more diminished in patients treated with 5-ASA. At that time, a 5-ASA antibiotic effect had not been demonstrated in vitro. As a consequence, 5-ASA became known as an "anti-inflammatory" agent. It was presumed by medical professionals that the anti-inflammatory effect was primary and that 5-ASA was treating a primary "autoimmune" disease.

But what if 5-ASA is an anti-*M. avium* subsp. *paratuberculosis* antibiotic? Then the anti-inflammatory effect of 5-ASA would be secondary. That 5-ASA is an anti-*M. avium* subsp. *paratuberculosis* antibiotic (135) should not be surprising. Para-aminosalicylic acid (PAS) was the first mass-produced anti-TB medication (185). Structurally, 5-ASA differs minimally from PAS. The amino group is on the fifth, rather than the fourth, carbon atom of the benzene ring (see Fig. 2). It is intriguing to observe the difference associated with the minimal spatial repositioning of the amino group from C4 to C5. Even more remarkable is the specificity of 5-ASA for *M. avium* subsp. *paratuberculosis*. PAS has both anti-*M. avium* subsp. *paratuberculosis* and anti-TB activity, whereas 5-ASA has no role whatsoever in the therapy of TB.

In 1940, Bernheim noted that adding salicylates to mycobacteria doubled their oxygen consumption (23). This was followed by Lehrmann's insightful intuition that a modified salicylate molecule might have anti-TB activity. The result was the first mass-produced anti-TB molecule. PAS was introduced in 1943 in World War II-isolated neutral Sweden (255). Stunningly, and unrecognized until 2007, a year earlier a fellow Swede had introduced an almost identical molecule, 5-ASA (295) (Fig. 2), that has now been demonstrated to have anti-*M. avium* subsp. *paratuberculosis* activity (135), albeit at a far lower potency than PAS (author's unpublished data). Sixty years after Bernheim's observation, in 2000, possible molecular mechanisms accounting for the action of salicylates and the competitive inhibition of its derivatives have been identified. Salicylate-induced growth arrest is associated with inhibition of p70s6k and

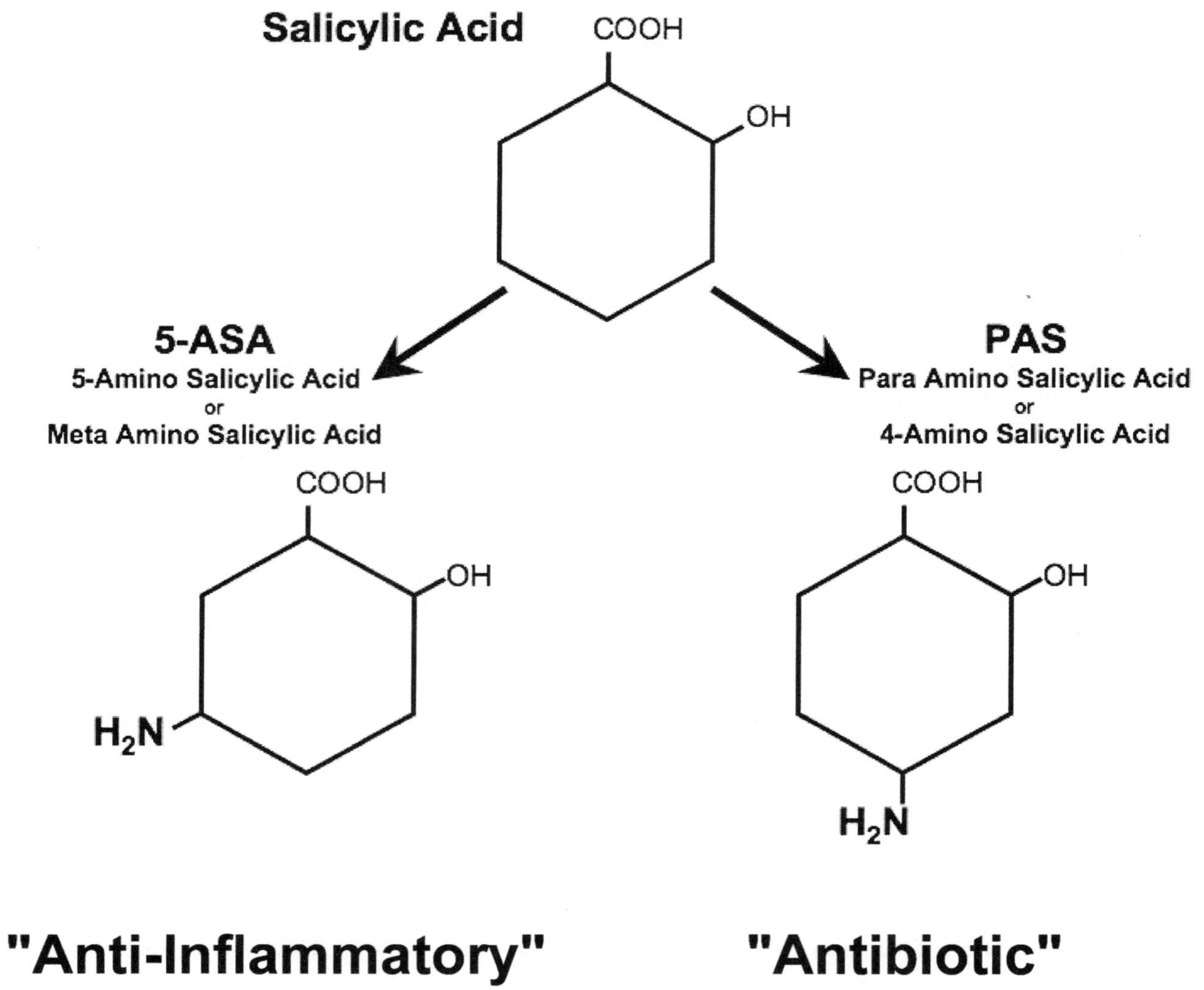

Figure 2. Salicylic acid and derivatives.

downregulation of c-myc, cyclin D1, cyclin A, and proliferating cell nuclear antigen (183).

Inhibition of *M. avium* subsp. *paratuberculosis* growth will, in my opinion, eventually establish *M. avium* subsp. *paratuberculosis* as a major human pathogen, responsible for far more than just IBD. I now posit that any disease that is treated with 5-ASA, without a known mechanism of action, but because of empirically observed efficacy, should be evaluated for the possibility that *M. avium* subsp. *paratuberculosis* is the instigating agent.

Other agents that are used because of clinical efficacy, but without a specific mechanism of action, are called "immuno-modulators" because their use is attended by a decrease in proinflammatory cytokines. This fall in cytokine levels has been presumed to be their primary mechanism of action. Recently, immuno-modulators—methotrexate (134), the thiopurine azothioprine (282), and its metabolite 6 mercaptopurine (134, 282)—have been shown to be anti-*M. avium* subsp. *paratuberculosis* antibiotics. It is therefore possible that the decrease in proinflammatory cytokines is a secondary, physiological response as an instigating *M. avium* subsp. *paratuberculosis* infection is treated. We recommend that other immuno-modulators that are used to treat "autoimmune" and "inflammatory" diseases (44), such as thalidomide (8, 43) and the "immuno-suppressives" cyclosporine

A (139, 190), tacrolimus (78, 174, 222), and rapamycin (106, 199), should now be evaluated for possible anti-*M. avium* subsp. *paratuberculosis* activity.

Most commonly, *M. avium* subsp. *paratuberculosis* is considered possibly causative of Dalziel's (Crohn's) disease. Dalziel's/Crohn's disease and ulcerative colitis (UC) are referred to under the rubric of IBD. Conventionally they are considered to be distinct and separate diseases. Since first seeing the *M. avium* subsp. *paratuberculosis* RNA data in my laboratory in 1996 (206), in presentations at professional conferences (R. J. Greenstein, presented at the Inflammatory Bowel Disease Research Drives Clinics, Genetics, Barrier Function, Immunologic and Microbial Pathways, Munster, Germany, 2 and 3 September 2005; R. J. Greenstein, presented at the Johne's Disease Integrated Program, 2nd Annual Conference, University of California-Davis, Sacramento, CA, 26-29 January 2006), and while peer-reviewing manuscripts (13, 216, 333), I have suggested that Dalziel's/Crohn's disease and UC were part of a spectrum of human intestinal *M. avium* subsp. *paratuberculosis* infection. This would make IBD analogous to the lepromatous and tuberculoid forms of leprosy—a clinically diverse spectrum of the same disease caused by a single mycobacterium (144). This "spectrum" concept has been previously presented (130).

It is now 95 years since Dalziel considered the possibility that *M. avium* subsp. *paratuberculosis* caused human intestinal disease. The possible intestinal/*M. avium* subsp. *paratuberculosis* connection is still not settled. Nevertheless, there are disquieting data that suggest that multiple other "autoimmune" and "inflammatory" diseases should be intensively investigated for the possibility that they may be caused by *M. avium* subsp. *paratuberculosis*.

Common Pathways in Prokaryotes and Eukaryotes

At the subcellular level, there is an obligate commonality in basic cellular functions that occurs in both prokaryotes and eukaryotes. For example, both may need to replicate DNA. Both utilize folic acid as an integral part of that process. A pivotal difference is that eukaryotes are able to utilize environmental folic acid, whereas prokaryotes have to generate the folic acid themselves. It should therefore come as no surprise that agents that are used to interrupt cellular processes in eukaryotes (for example, methotrexate) may also have a profound effect on prokaryotes.

High Dose versus Low Dose

A detailed dosage analysis of agents that may have an effect on both prokaryotes and eukaryotes and that are used in apparently paradoxical diseases reveals an intriguing divergence into low and high doses. For example, methotrexate is a dihydrofolate reductase inhibitor. It interferes with folic acid synthesis and therefore adenine production and consequently DNA replication. Methotrexate is used to treat both eukaryotic malignancies and a variety of "autoimmune" and "inflammatory" conditions. When used to treat human malignancies, such as multiple myeloma, the high dose that is used may be as much as 7,500 mg in a 70-kg person (102). In noteworthy contrast, the chronic dose that is used to treat "inflammatory" diseases, such as Dalziel's/Crohn's is 25 mg a week (98). Another antimetabolite used to treat both eukaryotic malignancies and inflammatory conditions is 6-mercaptopurine (6-MP). In high doses, it is used to treat reticuloendothelial malignancies (42), such as childhood acute lymphoblastic leukemia at a dose of 1 g/M^2/IV (311). In contrast, the low dose of 6-MP that is used for IBD is ~50 mg/day (24).

It is possible that the high dose of these antimetabolites is treating eukaryotic malignancies and the low dose is treating an unsuspected (possibly *M. avium* subsp. *paratuberculosis*) bacterial infection. If this hypothesis is correct, the prevailing dogma that low-dose therapy acts by immune suppression (226, 254) is wrong. The decrease in proinflammatory cytokines that attends the use of these antimetabolites would simply represent a normal secondary physiological response as an underlying (possibly *M. avium* subsp. *paratuberculosis*) infection was being treated.

In the event that the *M. avium* subsp. *paratuberculosis* "infectious" hypothesis suggested above is correct, there are multiple consequences that the medical profession will need to consider. The first is that prevailing dogma does not advocate chronic, unending antimicrobial therapy for infectious diseases. The intention of antibiotic therapy is to permit a competent immune system as rapidly as possible to be able to deal with an exogenous infection. A concern is that chronic therapy will, inevitably, result in the emergence of prokaryotic antibiotic-resistant strains. With two slowly replicating mycobacteria (*M. leprae* and *M. tuberculosis*), an effort is made to limit treatment to $\leq$ 2 years. One reason is to maximize patient compliance. Additionally, for both *M. leprae* (34) and *M. tuberculosis*, multiple-drug therapy (MDT) is usually considered obligatory, to prevent the emergence of resistant mycobacterial strains. It appears as though the medical profession has serendipitously been performing MDT in the "inflammatory" diseases that may be caused by *M. avium* subsp. *paratuberculosis*. Sulfasalazine has two agents with anti-*M. avium* subsp. *paratuberculosis* action

(135), and these are often used in concert with other agents that have (134, 282), or I hypothesize may have, anti-*M. avium* subsp. *paratuberculosis* activity (89, 106, 190, 312).

Secondly, attention will need to be paid to immunocompromised individuals, who are not able to mount an effective immune response to an invading microorganism. For example, *M. avium* infections in an HIV/AIDS immunocompromised individual require continuous anti-*M. avium* therapy. If the anti-HIV therapy is unable to maintain an adequate CD4 count and anti-Avium therapy has been stopped, the *M. avium* infection will recur.

Several genetic defects have been identified in humans that are associated with diseases (148), some of which I suggest may be caused by *M. avium* subsp. *paratuberculosis*. The NOD2/Card15 genetic region codes for the ability to detect invading microorganisms, including *M. tuberculosis* (101). The NOD2/Card15 genes are in turn regulated by signals from Toll-like receptors (TLR) (31, 221). Both NOD2 and TLR govern an appropriate response to bacterial muramyl dipeptide (177) using NF-κB (193), IL-1β (220), and IL-6 activation (220, 221) in a "tissue-specific and context-dependent NOD2 transcript isoform pattern" (252). A defect in the NOD2/Card15 gene has been identified in Dalziel's/Crohn's disease (154, 228). Subsequently, the NOD2/Card15 defect has been shown to impair IL-1β production (193) and NF-κB (193) activation.

Finally, TLR4 Asp299Gly and Thr399Ile polymorphisms are associated with specific IBD phenotypes (31). The NOD2/Card15 defect is also associated with an impaired intestinal response to bacterial muramyl dipeptide (177). This is of relevance because humans are continually exposed to viable *M. avium* subsp. *paratuberculosis* enterically (91, 122). The NOD2/Card15 defect is associated with Dalziel's/Crohn's disease, but not ulcerative colitis (141). It is therefore possible that the NOD2/Card15 defect predisposes to Dalziel's/Crohn's disease by impairing the normal physiological protective responses to *M. avium* subsp. *paratuberculosis* (18, 130).

Defects in the natural resistance-associated macrophage protein 1 (Nramp1) gene are incontrovertibly associated with an increased susceptibility to a variety of intracellular pathogens, including *Salmonella*, *Leishmania* (28, 29), and mycobacteria (41). Specific mycobacterial diseases associated with Nramp1 defects include leprosy (3, 100, 314), TB (particularly the cavitary form [1]), *Mycobacterium avium-M. intracellulare* (153), and *M. avium* complex (303). Nramp1 defects have been associated with IBD (both Dalziel's/Crohn's disease and UC) in a Japanese population (178), an observation that is compatible with *M. avium* subsp. *paratuberculosis* being the etiological agent.

As a consequence of the foregoing, I suggest that diseases of unknown etiology that are associated with defects in NOD2/Card15 or Nramp1 systems should be reevaluated as being caused by infective agents (including *M. avium* subsp. *paratuberculosis*). Defects in the NOD2/CARD15 system have been noted in multiple sclerosis, systemic lupus erythematosus (77), and psoriatic arthropathy (237). In the Nramp1 system, diseases that should be evaluated include rheumatoid arthritis (248, 276, 277, 283, 336, 337) and type 1 diabetes (176, 224, 293, 300). Sarcoidosis should be investigated as being caused by *M. avium* subsp. *paratuberculosis*, as Nramp1 defects have been found in individuals with sarcoidosis from Poland (84), but not African Americans with sarcoidosis (195) or individuals with sarcoidosis from Japan. (5).

In addition to the Nramp1/type 1 diabetes connection (176, 224, 293, 300), others have found an increase in *M. avium* subsp. *paratuberculosis*-specific antigens (273) and *M. avium* subsp. *paratuberculosis* bacteremia (272) and suggest that *M. avium* subsp. *paratuberculosis* should be considered an environmental trigger of type 1 diabetes. Yet others have commented on the parallel increases in IBD, multiple sclerosis (124) and type one diabetes (251) but do not consider *M. avium* subsp. *paratuberculosis* potentially culpable.

Interpreting serology testing in mycobacterial diseases should be approached with caution. For example, in humans there is no connection between having a NOD2 defect and the incidence of *M. avium* subsp. *paratuberculosis* serology status (25). Likewise, it is of interest that only 40 to 50% of individuals with paucibacillary leprosy will have serum antibodies to leprosy-specific PGL-1 (59, 247).

Epidemiology and "Cure"

An intensely skeptical medical profession was reluctant to consider that *Helicobacter pylori* could be the major etiological agent causing gastric ulcers (197, 198, 319, 320). The pivotal finding that convinced the doubters was that gastric ulcers were cured when the *H. pylori* infection was eradicated (319). Epidemiological data were of secondary importance.

Similarly, a dubious medical community has been reluctant to acknowledge that *M. avium* subsp. *paratuberculosis* might be zoonotic unless and until a cure is achieved (274). This desirable objective unfortunately shows a lack of understanding of the complexity of dealing with mycobacterial diseases.

The cure data are not, and never will be, as clean as those achieved with simple infections such as *H. pylori*. Lessons from both TB and leprosy are critical in developing an understanding of responses to appropriate antibiotics that are reasonable to anticipate when considering possible *M. avium* subsp. *paratuberculosis* zoonosis.

The other two components of this chapter enunciate in detail that even with the most intensive MDT regimes, neither *M. leprae* (74, 321) nor *M. tuberculosis* (182, 232) is eradicated. Although quiescent, these persistent mycobacteria will reactivate under immuno-compromising conditions, such as HIV/AIDS (68, 76, 192), nutritional depletion, or cancer chemotherapy, with pathological consequences (142, 318).

Accordingly, particularly in individuals with genetic defects that may render them immune-incompetent to fight *M. avium* subsp. *paratuberculosis*, with probable *M. avium* subsp. *paratuberculosis* latency, persistence, and continual reinfection, a "cure" cannot be expected.

In all future trials concerning the possible zoonosis of *M. avium* subsp. *paratuberculosis*, determining each individual's genetic predisposition should be an integral component of the protocol. Such patients should be, prospectively, subjected to a subset analysis that assumes individuals with the NOD2 or Nramp1 defects will be "once infected, never cured." Such individuals should be expected to have a relapse when anti-*M. avium* subsp. *paratuberculosis* therapy is withheld. Lessons from leprosy (74, 321) and TB (182, 232) indicate that, in individuals with the wild-type genome, if *M. avium* subsp. *paratuberculosis* is indeed zoonotic, symptomatic progression may occur, despite apparently adequate therapy.

Cancer as a Consequence of Chronic Inflammation

It is well established that *H. pylori*-induced chronic enteric infectious inflammation causes gastric adenocarcinoma in humans and animal models (250), and clearing *H. pylori* infection protects humans from developing gastric cancer (227). Possible adjunct mechanisms include TLR-mediated responses to chronic infections resulting in an unregulated repair process, the consequence of which may be malignancy (92, 111).

It is not surprising that IBD is associated with an increase in intestinal malignancies both in Dalziel's/Crohn's disease (129) and UC (137, 186). These include lymphoma (12, 128) and adenocarcinoma (166). However, evocative of the protective effect of eradicating *H. pylori*, there are increasingly compelling data that therapy with 5-ASA, an anti-*M. avium* subsp. *paratuberculosis* antibiotic (135), may be protective against colorectal cancer in UC (187, 315, 316).

Circumstantial evidence for the potential zoonosis of *M. avium* subsp. *paratuberculosis* may be gleaned from the dose-dependent malignant potential of several medications used to treat a variety of human diseases. There is an association of chronic IBD and intestinal malignancy, particularly lymphoma. There is a concern that the use of 6-MP (200) and azathioprine (110) may increase the incidence of malignancies. Some authors conclude that the malignancy potential outweighs the potential benefit (30). Others conclude exactly the opposite, that the benefits of using azathioprine in IBD outweigh the risks of developing an azathioprine-induced malignancy (188). However, we suggest that low-dose 6-MP and azathioprine are anti- *M. avium* subsp. *paratuberculosis* antibiotics (134, 282). Accordingly, analogous to the protective effect of eradicating *H. pylori*, suppressing *M. avium* subsp. *paratuberculosis* should prevent the chronic infections' neoplastic potential of *M. avium* subsp. *paratuberculosis*. In contrast, the high doses used to treat reticuloendothelial malignancies do predispose to subsequent malignancies (167, 215). Rational studies should now be designed to study the protective effect of treating possible *M. avium* subsp. *paratuberculosis* infections with low-dose immunosuppressant medication, whose mode of action may well be as anti-*M. avium* subsp. *paratuberculosis* agents.

Several other diseases are empirically treated with the low-dose anti-inflammatory and immunomodulatory agents that are used to treat IBD. These include irritable bowel syndrome (21, 263) and rheumatoid (22, 244, 295, 322) and psoriatic arthritis (150). Other potential *M. avium* subsp. *paratuberculosis*-associated systemic diseases include pulmonary (156, 202) and cerebral sarcoidosis (93) as well as type 1 diabetes (83, 272, 273) and possibly some neurodegenerative diseases (46, 65, 77, 124, 266).

Treatments/Control

Control of Johne's disease has several components. The first is controlling the disease within the animal community. The second is preventing the transmission of viable *M. avium* subsp. *paratuberculosis* to humans through the food chain and water supply. In terms of antibiotic therapy, in animals there is the cost of therapy compared to the monetary value of the animal. For humans, the medical profession will need to understand that many of the agents they at present employ as nonspecific immune-modulators, anti-inflammatories, and immunosuppressants are probably acting as anti-*M. avium* subsp. *paratuberculosis* antibiotics. Future antibiotic trials that are ethical (334a) will need to take these data into account. Possible studies might compare infliximab or humera alone in the placebo group, with the same agents coadministered with anti-*M. avium* subsp. *paratuberculosis* agents.

M. avium subsp. *paratuberculosis* antibiotic susceptibility studies will need to be performed if *M. avium* subsp. *paratuberculosis* zoonosis is to be accepted. However, few laboratories can successfully culture the cell wall-deficient form of *M. avium* subsp. *paratuberculosis* that exists in humans (40, 54, 216), a process that may take up to 18 months (54). Nucleic acid-based methods may need to be developed to more rapidly determine the presence of *M. avium* subsp. *paratuberculosis* RNA (indicating viability) (206), potential infectivity (157, 259), and antibiotic susceptibility (191).

An entire veterinary literature deals with control in the agricultural domain. Briefly, simple husbandry methods are recommended within infected herds (125). It is also possible that breeding animals that are innately able to combat *M. avium* subsp. *paratuberculosis* may prove a viable option (210). However, the most promising intervention may well be vaccination (53, 149, 172, 310).

Physicians are used to the concept of vaccination being a prophylactic intervention (159, 169). However, with other mycobacterial diseases, particularly leprosy (79, 168, 338) and Johne's disease (162), vaccination may actually be therapeutic. Thus, the development of vaccination against *M. avium* subsp. *paratuberculosis*-specific antigens (39, 149) may be of utility both in postexposure therapy and prophylaxis against *M. avium* subsp. *paratuberculosis.*

M. LEPRAE

M. leprae infection in humans is characterized by insidious onset and a chronic course, which, if untreated, may cause loss of sensory perception in fingers and toes, paralysis, deformity, blindness, and laryngeal involvement that, although rare today, can be fatal. Skin, oral, and pharyngeal mucosae and peripheral nerves are primarily involved, although deep infection (e.g., liver and bone marrow) and transient bacteremia are well documented. The exact mode of transmission has not been determined, but both respiratory and direct skin contact are possible. The incubation time is very long, typically 2 to 5 years, but occasionally up to 20 years. The two major complications of leprosy are neuropathy and acute inflammatory syndromes collectively termed reactions. Reactions are poorly understood phenomena and represent the greatest challenges in both clinical management of leprosy and in our understanding of the basic mechanisms of pathogenesis in this disease. Good medical treatment for *M. leprae* infection is now widely available and constitutes the primary strategy for disease control. Dapsone, the initial curative agent, was first demonstrated to be effective in leprosy in the 1940s, in studies at Carville, LA, United States. Today dapsone is combined with rifampin in 6- to 12-month regimens for the treatment of the forms of disease with few bacilli. For patients with heavy bacterial infection, an additional agent, clofazimine, is used in regimens of 12 to 24 months. Ofloxacin, clarithromycin, and minocycline are additional effective agents that can be substituted for the others when necessary (211). Vaccines designed specifically for leprosy control are in development based on documented protection observed in some populations following BCG vaccination for TB.

Host Susceptibility and Immunity

Available evidence suggests that approximately 95% of adults have native resistance to this infection, and genetic determinants of overall susceptibility are now being identified (267). A locus in the regulatory gene PACRG is the first to be associated with overall susceptibility to leprosy (205). This gene codes for an E3 ligase in the ubiquitin proteasome pathway, and this finding has opened new possibilities for the study of mechanisms of antigen processing that may be related to innate resistance to infection with *M. leprae*. Other genes associated with innate resistance/susceptibility are now also being described (6), which may implicate other mechanisms of innate resistance.

Among susceptible individuals, *M. leprae* elicits a uniquely broad spectrum of cell-mediated immunity (CMI) (Fig. 3). Based on clinical, microbiological, and histopathological appearances, the disease is classified into categories of those with a very high bacterial load and a very disorganized inflammatory response (lepromatous [LL]) at one extreme and those with rare bacilli and a well-organized granulomatous response (tuberculoid [TT]) at the other (246). However, unlike patients with many other infections which have these extreme polar manifestations, *most* leprosy patients fall within a broad borderline category, further divided into borderline lepromatous (BL), mid-borderline (BB), and borderline tuberculoid (BT). Since the mid-1960s, the basis for this diversity has been recognized as the capability of the host to develop CMI to *M. leprae* (286). This capability is severely lacking in lepromatous patients but is expressed as a high degree of CMI in the

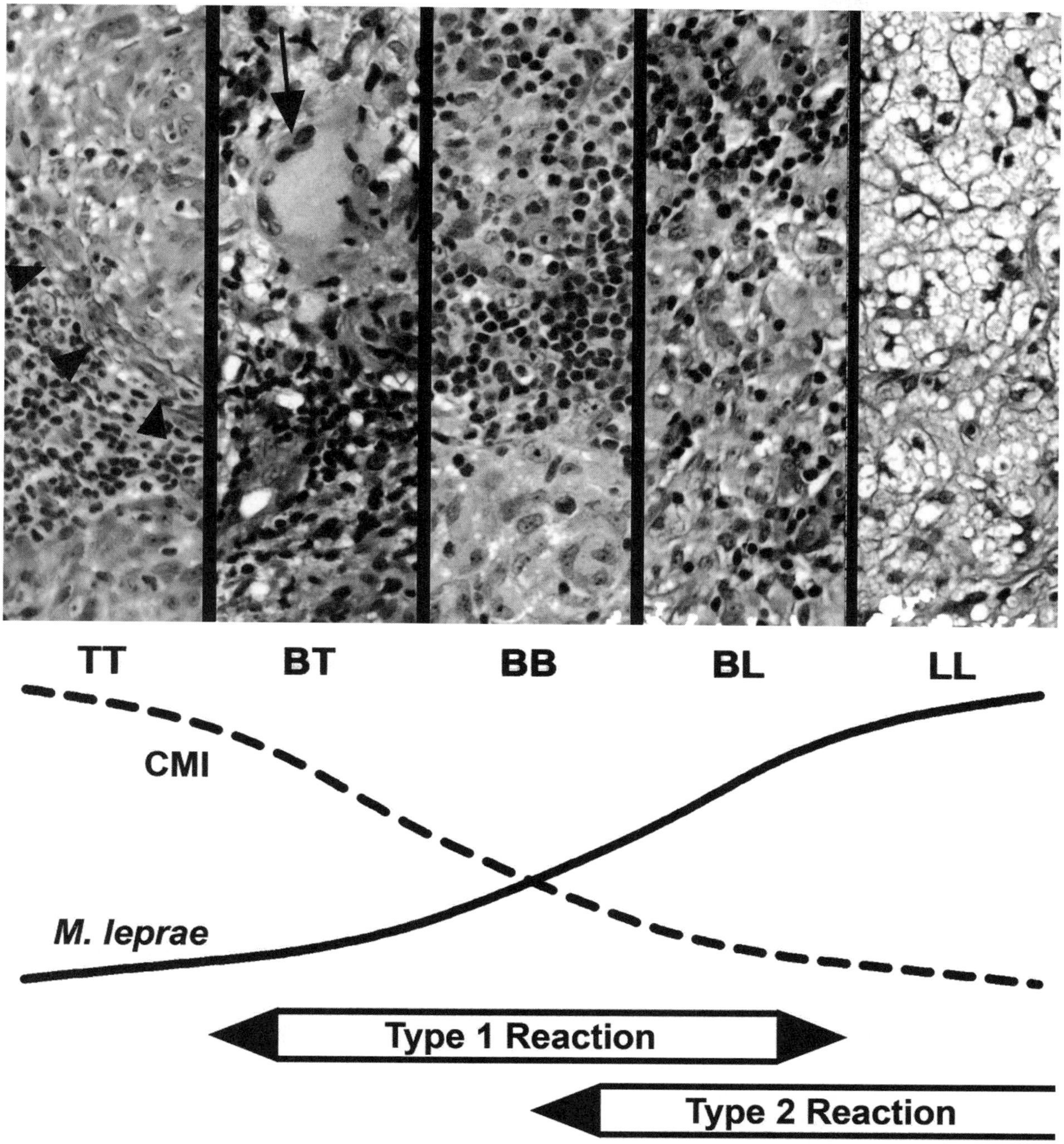

Figure 3. The immunopathologic spectrum of leprosy. Representative sections of human skin biopsy specimens illustrate the full spectrum of inflammation seen in leprosy. Well-organized granulomatous inflammation characterizes polar TT lesions; the perimeter of the epithelioid center of a granuloma is outlined by the arrowheads. In borderline tuberculoid (BT) lesions, the granulomas are less well organized but still contain typical features, such as giant multi-nucleated cells (arrow). BB lesions contain both well-formed granulomas (bottom of BB panel) and disorganized areas (top of panel). Disorganization becomes more pronounced and foamy histiocytes become more prominent in BL lesions, and polar LL lesions are composed of the completely disorganized sheets of foamy MPH. Most patients are classified in the broad borderline region. As indicated in the diagram, the number of bacilli present in lesions (solid line) varies from rare in TT lesions to abundant in LL ones. This is inversely related to the patient's degree of CMI to *M. leprae*. The open arrows indicate the portions of the spectrum in which patients are at risk for T1R or T2R, reversal or ENL leprosy reactions, respectively. [Modified from Frankel, R. I., and D. M. Scollard. Leprosy. *In* Philip Brachman and Elias Abrutyn (ed.), *Bacterial Infections of Humans*, 3rd ed. Springer, in press.]

granulomas of tuberculoid lesions, with intermediate degrees of CMI in the borderline categories.

Molecular immunological studies have provided an increasingly detailed description of the immunological status of the different types of cutaneous leprosy lesions, but the precise mechanisms by which this organism can elicit the entire range of CMI remain to be determined. MPH and dendritic cells (DC) play critical roles as antigen-presenting cells in the afferent limb of the response. Because *M. leprae* contains many lipid-rich antigenic molecules, the capability of CD1-mediated presentation of these antigens by DC is of particular interest (155, 180), and TLR1 and -2 have been observed to be expressed more strongly on monocytes and DC within tuberculoid lesions than in lepromatous lesions (180). A provocative study has reported that mycobacterial antigen activation of TLR2 on monocytes from tuberculoid leprosy patients induced differentiation into cells bearing the dendritic cell-specific intercellular adhesion molecule grabbing nonintegrin (DC-SIGN) MPH and $CD1b^+$ DC (181).

Monocytes from lepromatous patients, under the same conditions, differentiated into $DC\text{-}SIGN^+$ but not $CD1b^+$ cells, suggesting that monocytes from lepromatous patients may not be able to generate the cellular immune response seen in tuberculoid disease. Immunostaining of these molecules in skin biopsies from tuberculoid versus lepromatous lesions revealed patterns consistent with the in vitro observations, but it is not known whether cells from borderline patients would show different degrees of expression of these molecules. The number and percentage of $CD4^+$ T cells decline from the tuberculoid to the lepromatous poles of leprosy, while little change is seen in the number of $CD8^+$ cells (208). $CD8^+$ cells are found in the periphery of tuberculoid granulomas but are interspersed randomly throughout the disorganized infiltrates of lepromatous lesions. It is not clear whether T cells perform significant cytotoxic functions in leprosy lesions, although cells containing molecules such as granulysin are found in leprosy (225), and $CD4^+$ and $CD8^+$ cytotoxic cells can lyse *M. leprae*-infected MPH in vitro (57) (143). Tuberculoid lesions exhibit a TH1 cytokine pattern, while a TH2 pattern is generally observed in lepromatous lesions (335). Such studies have not yet carefully evaluated the entire spectrum of leprosy to determine which, if any, of the cytokines involved show a graduated expression across the spectrum. With current knowledge of the complexity of cytokine pathways and interactions, it is necessary to evaluate lesions with respect to a larger array of cytokines and chemokines and their associated transcription factors and receptors. A number of genes for immunologically important molecules, such as major histocompatibility complex class II, TLRs, and vitamin D receptors, have been associated with different capabilities in developing cellular immunity to *M. leprae* (310a) (reviewed in reference 268). It is likely that these and future discoveries in human genetics will guide future research into the mechanisms underlying the wide diversity of acquired immune responses to this pathogen.

Leprosy and Nerves

Unique among bacterial pathogens, *M. leprae* infects peripheral nerves and parasitizes Schwann cells (SC). Recent evidence suggests that bacilli probably enter nerves via their blood supply (270). In tissue sections, both bacilli and inflammation are typically perineurial as well as endoneurial. Focal nerve function impairment occurs very early in this disease, since anesthesia (or hypaesthesia) is the distinguishing clinical feature of the earliest cutaneous lesions of leprosy. Without treatment, neuropathy is slowly progressive. Neuritis may also occur long after cure of the infection, and it has recently been recognized that neuropathic pain may develop in some patients (147).

Immunological and inflammatory events occur in and around nerves throughout the course of this disease, and in this context three discrete neuropathic phenomena are observed: (i) infection of SC, (ii) demyelination, and (iii) axonal atrophy. The mechanisms, interrelationship, and even the sequence of these phenomena are not clearly understood. Although nerve biopsy is seldom performed, histopathological observations suggest that the immunological and inflammatory processes involving nerves are very similar to those studied more extensively with the skin (160). Similarly, minimal opportunities have been available to directly assess nerve lesions using contemporary molecular tools, but evidence to date supports the concept that the immune-inflammatory events within nerves parallel those in the skin (173). Since SC have been very accessible for in vitro experimentation, they have been studied extensively in vitro, using, until recently, only rodent cell models. SC bind *M. leprae* via a number of surface molecules (239) and ingest the bacilli without major deleterious effects to the host or the pathogen. Some studies have observed that after *M. leprae* infection, SC-SC and SC-axon interactions are normal (140), but other investigators have reported demyelination following SC exposure to *M. leprae* (240). Follow-up studies have reported that after the binding of *M. leprae* to the ErbB2 receptor on SC, demyelination is induced via a unique signaling pathway involving Erk1 and -2, bypassing the standard neuregulin-Erb signaling pathway (304). A humanized antibody to Erb2 inhibits this process, offering unique possibilities of application of these findings to the treatment or prevention of nerve injury in leprosy. Analysis of human SC gene transcription using global microarray technologies has shown the alteration of several hundreds of gene transcripts during *M. leprae* infection in vitro (Diana Williams, personal communication). SC are capable of antigen presentation, and infected SC can be targeted by *M. leprae*-specific T cells in vitro (290). TLR2 is expressed on SC, and activation via TLR2 has been postulated as another mechanism leading to nerve injury (229). Further critical evaluation of the role that infection of SC plays in leprosy neuritis remains an important priority for leprosy, since SC are essential to the maintenance of the nerve.

Segmental demyelination has been demonstrated clearly in teased fiber studies of human nerves from patients with well-established lepromatous disease (298). How early in the course of disease does demyelination occur? What are the mechanisms leading to demyelination? These are still unanswered questions in leprosy, although the latter has been the subject of recent, provocative studies in vitro and in rodent models. Rambukkana and colleagues have reported very rapid demyelination following binding of *M. leprae* to the ErbB2 receptor in SC-neuron cocultures in vitro (304).

Axonal atrophy has been implicated as another possible mechanism of neuropathy (281). In studies of biopsies of affected human nerves, ultrastructural evidence of reduction of axonal caliber was observed, with compaction of neurofilaments at the periphery of these axons (261). Biochemical evidence indicated abnormalities of phosphorylation of neurofilament proteins. Dephosphorylation of neurofilament proteins has been observed in a variety of neurological disorders but, as in leprosy, the mechanisms responsible for this are poorly understood. Axonal atrophy in leprosy is intriguing and requires much more study because it is a mechanism that is probably not SC-dependent. Elucidating the mechanism for axonal atrophy may help us understand the functional impairment that occurs in nonmyelinated nerve fibers.

Leprosy Reactions

Two types of reactions acutely complicate the otherwise indolent course of leprosy in 40 to 50% of patients. Type 1 reactions (T1R, or reversal reactions) occur in patients whose immune response is in the large borderline portion of the leprosy spectrum, between the tuberculoid and lepromatous poles. T1R develop slowly, usually as exacerbations of preexisting lesions, and appear to be consequences of spontaneous activation or upgrading of cellular immunity to *M. leprae*. Increased levels of several proinflammatory cytokines, including IL-1, IL-2, IL-12, IFN-γ, and TNF-α, or expression of mRNA for these cytokines have been reported in several studies of T1R lesions (reviewed in [268]), supporting clinical and histopathological impressions that patients' cellular immunity is enhanced during these reactions. Elevation of circulating levels of the chemokine CXCL-10 (IP10), an inducer of IFN-γ, has also been observed in some patients with T1R (D. Scollard, unpublished data). Gradual upgrading also occurs in many patients who do not have an acute reaction, and it is possible that the mechanisms are similar in both situations, but on a different time scale. Recently, T1R have been observed as immune reconstitution phenomena in patients with leprosy and AIDS after highly active antiretroviral treatment (235) and in other patients after transient inhibition of TNF-α with humanized antibody (269). These observations suggest that some degree of transient immune inhibition may be a common event preceding or precipitating T1R. No animal models are available to test these hypotheses regarding T1R, however, and such possibilities must therefore be addressed in clinical studies. Recent genetic studies have identified some candidate genes that may confer increased susceptibility to T1R (242).

Treatment with corticosteroids alleviates the symptoms of these reactions and prevents or reduces the nerve damage that often accompanies them, but this often requires moderate or high doses of prednisone for many weeks. Although the anti-inflammatory effects of corticosteroids are beneficial, available evidence suggests that the underlying mechanisms of T1R may continue in spite of corticosteroid treatment (7). In a small study, pentoxyfylline or thalidomide treatment of T1R (but not prednisone) resulted in reduced mRNA transcripts for TNF, IFN, IL-6, and IL-12p40, and IL-10 in skin lesions (209). The resolution of the reactions themselves may thus depend on immunoregulatory mechanisms that remain to be elucidated. No specific laboratory tests are available for the diagnosis of these reactions or for assessment of the severity or resolution of these reactions.

T2R (*erythema nodosum leprosum* [ENL]) occur only in patients with a high bacterial load and little or no cellular immunity to *M. leprae,* i.e., lepromatous disease. These reactions develop abruptly, as crops of red, tender nodules on various parts of the body, not correlated with the location of prior lepromatous lesions. Biopsies of these lesions reveal acute inflammation, with focal infiltrates of polymorphs, superimposed upon the chronic inflammation and high mycobacterial load of lepromatous (LL-BL) leprosy. The natural course of ENL is typically 10 to 14 days, but it is frequently recurrent, and without treatment, severe tissue damage (including acute neuritis) often results. The incidence of T2R appears to have declined after the widespread implementation of multidrug therapy which includes daily doses of clofazimine, an agent with notable anti-inflammatory effects in addition to its antimycobacterial actions. The T2R is widely regarded as an immune complex-mediated disorder, although the evidence for this is not fully convincing. T2R were observed in several lepromatous patients who received experimental treatment with intralesional injections of IFN-γ (258); exogenous IFN-γ also appeared to induce appreciable levels of circulating TNF-α in these patients. The mechanisms by which exogenous IFN-γ might induce or precipitate the acute inflammatory infiltrates in T2R has not been determined. Recent studies, however, have observed elevated levels of IFN-γ and IL-6 receptor (but not IL-6) in patients with T2R, and these fell after corticosteroid treatment (158). Corticosteroids and thalidomide reduce the inflammation in ENL, but the mechanism by which thalidomide exerts this anti-inflammatory/ immunoinhibitory effect is also unclear, partly due to conflicting evidence from clinical studies. Early reports (257) suggested that thalidomide inhibited the production of TNF-α, but a recent report has suggested that the benefit from thalidomide in T2R is a result of stimulation (rather than inhibition) of TNF-α and IL-12 (145).

Characteristics of the Pathogen

The etiologic agent of leprosy, *M. leprae*, continues to test the microbiologist's skill when studying straightforward aspects of physiology, genetics, and pathogenesis. This is due exclusively to our inability to grow the agent in vitro under axenic culture conditions, forcing investigators to rely on in vivo-grown (nude mouse and armadillo) bacteria for basic biochemical and genetic studies. *M. leprae* harvested from infected tissues appear as pleomorphic rods with an average length of 2.1 micrometers and width of 0.25 to 0.3 micrometers. The bacteria are considered gram-positive but can be differentially stained, appearing acid fast using the Ziehl-Neelsen stain on smears or the Fite stain in paraffin-embedded tissue sections.

Early cultivation studies focused on supplements needed for culturing other slow-growing mycobacterial species. These studies reached their peak with the definition of culture maintenance conditions for *M. leprae*, when techniques were developed for monitoring *M. leprae* viability by measuring cellular ATP levels (75, 81), palmitate oxidation (107), and phenolic glycolipid-1 biosynthesis (109). These procedural advancements allowed Franzblau and Harris (108) to define pH, oxygen, and temperature optima for *M. leprae* under specific axenic culture conditions. While the various readout systems for *M. leprae* metabolism are indirect measures of viability, studies have confirmed the relationship between palmitate oxidation activity levels in culture and growth of *M. leprae* in animals (307). Studies showed that *M. leprae* preferred acidic (pH 5.1 to 5.6) growth conditions under reduced oxygen concentrations (2.5 to 10%) within a temperature range of 30 to 33°C.

These culture optima seem to support our current understanding of the specialized niche in which *M. leprae* survives, indeed prospers, as an obligate intracellular parasite. For example, *M. leprae* grows best in tissues that are cooler than the core body temperature of humans (27). In humans this includes the skin, superficial nerves, mucosa of the upper respiratory tract, and the anterior portion of the eye. In mice this includes the foot pad (279, 280) and in susceptible nine-banded armadillos, whose body temperature ranges from 30 to 35°C (175), this includes almost all tissues.

At the cellular level *M. leprae* resides primarily inside phagocytic cells of the monocytes/MPH lineage and SC. Phagocytosis of nonpathogenic mycobacteria by a MPH sets in motion a series of events culminating with their death and destruction. Primary among these steps is phagosome-lysosome fusion resulting in a lowering of pH in the phagosome. Pathogenic mycobacteria have been shown to resist phaogosome-lysosome fusion and block full acidification, which, based on in vitro growth studies described above, may not be inhospitable to *M. leprae* in the early phagosome. In contrast, surviving a highly oxygenated environment that can produce reactive oxygen intermediates during the oxidative burst associated with macrophage activation may be somewhat more challenging for *M. leprae* due to its demonstrated lack of a functional catalase gene (64). However, *M. leprae's* observed resistance to killing by toxic oxygen radicals suggests that other enzymes, such as superoxide dismutases (SodA and SodC) and alkyl hydroperoxide reductase (AphC), must provide sufficient resistance to reactive oxygen intermediates and supports the observation that *M. leprae*'s preference for a microaerophilic environment in axenic culture could be maintained in vivo.

Unfortunately, viability monitoring with markers like palmitate oxidation, PGL-1 biosynthesis, or other indicators of cellular energetics has not led to a new round of investigations aimed at unlocking the mystery of *M. leprae*'s metabolism and how it informs our understanding of *M. leprae*'s unique virulence and related pathogenicity. Tools for studying the genetic makeup of *M. leprae* need expanding to determine whether in vitro cultivation is possible, and, if possible, we need to apply well-established tools for genetic manipulation of pathogens in an attempt to understand *M. leprae's* niche-adapted lifestyle in nature. New ways to study *M. leprae* genes, their expression, and their effects on physiologic and biochemical transformations leading to growth, transmission, and continued parasitism of humans and other hosts are urgently needed.

Genomic research has produced new and innovative approaches for studying massive amounts of data generated over the last few years from DNA sequencing projects. Initial comparisons of *M. leprae*'s genome with that of *M. tuberculosis* (62) and more recently with those of other mycobacterial species (292) have made it possible to assign potential gene function to many of *M. leprae*'s genes. Comparative studies suggest that *M. leprae* has undergone an extreme case of reductive evolution (64). This is most evident with *M. leprae*'s reduced genome size in comparison to those of all other mycobacteria species sequenced thus far (Table 1). The precise method by which the genome has become smaller in terms of functional open reading frames is unknown. However, downsizing is reflected in the number of inactivated genes (genes lost through mutation and pseudogenes) with the accompanying reduction in G+C content (58% for *M. leprae* versus 66% for *M. tuberculosis*), which is thought to be associated with nonsynonymous nucleotide substitutions, once a gene has become nonfunctional and is therefore no longer under selective pressure (115).

M. leprae's annotated genome contains approximately 1,800 open reading frames, compared to over 4,000 open reading frames predicted for *M. tuberculosis*. Peppered throughout *M. leprae*'s genome are approximately 1,100 inactivated genes. In comparison, *M. tuberculosis* has been reported to contain less than 10 pseudogenes (62). The result of this downsizing leaves *M. leprae* with less than 50% of its genome encoding functional genes; in comparison, 90% of the genome of *M. tuberculosis* and other fully functional mycobacterial genomes, such as *M. bovis* and *Mycobacterium marinum,* encode fully functional genes. It is interesting to note that comparisons with *Mycobacterium ulcerans*, a mycobacterial pathogen thought to be undergoing niche adaptation and associated reductive evolution of its genome, suggest that specialization in terms of endosymbiosis or host adaptation may be associated with these dramatic genome compressions stemming from lateral gene transfer (in the case of *M. ulcerans*), accumulated insertion sequences, increased numbers of pseudogenes, and multiple DNA deletions and rearrangements (292). Further comparative work in this area is important to elucidate basic mechanisms associated with selective pressure(s) leading to genome plasticity and restructuring. More specifically, for the leprosy bacillus, these kinds of studies may provide new ways of thinking about mechanisms involved in host-pathogen coevolution, which may give rise to unanticipated opportunities to configure new treatment modalities for disease management of both obligate and facultative intracellular pathogens causing chronic diseases in humans.

Early studies of *M. leprae*'s metabolic capabilities were aimed at determining whether special media could be formulated to support in vitro growth of the bacilli and to learn more about pathways that could be exploited for developing new antileprosy drugs. Genomic data have dramatically expanded our understanding of basic anabolic and catabolic pathways, but a much-anticipated explanation of *M. leprae*'s nonculturability in vitro remains elusive (35, 90, 324). *M. leprae* is not unusual when compared to other mycobacteria, in that it has the capacity to generate energy by oxidizing glucose to pyruvate

Table 1. Genome comparisons[b]

Organism	Genome size (bp)	No. of CDS[a]	No. of pseudogenes	G+C content (%)
M. leprae	3,268,203	1,806	1,133	57.8
M. ulcerans	5,632,000	4,160	771	65.7
	(174,155)	(81)	(0)	(62.8)
M. marinum	6,636,827	5,426	Unknown[c]	65.7
M. tuberculosis	4,411,532	4,267	6	65.6
M. bovis	4,345,492	4,336	31	65.6
M. avium subspecies *paratuberculosis*[d]	4,829,781	4,396	(Not stated)	69.3

[a]CDS, coding sequences (includes protein coding, and rRNA and tRNA genes; cmr.tigr.org or genolist.pasteur.fr).
[b]Values in parentheses are for the self-replicating virulence plasmid, in addition to the 5.6-Mb chromosome.
[c]Exact number unknown but estimated to be very low.
[d]See reference 189.

through the Embden-Mayerhoff-Parnas pathway. In addition to glycolysis for energy production, genome and biochemical analyses suggest that both *M. leprae* and *M. tuberculosis* rely heavily upon lipid degradation and the glyoxylate shunt for energy. *M. leprae* contains a full complement of genes for B-oxidation but, compared to *M. tuberculosis*, very few genes capable of lipolysis. Does *M. leprae*'s strict intracellular parasitism and its reliance on SC and MPH for survival tell us something about the permissive nature of these cells for *M. leprae*'s metabolic inefficiencies? Moreover, is this host-parasite relationship a reflection of the inevitable coevolution of single-cell and multicellular organisms interacting over time? Studies focused on metabolomics of intracellular symbiotic and parasitic relationships need further exploration from the standpoint of understanding biological balance and evolution. *M. leprae* may be the first recognized, but certainly not the only, organism undergoing dramatic reductive evolutionary processes. In terms of *M. leprae*'s chronic nature and long-term consequences as a human pathogen, studies directed at the metabolic capability of *M. leprae* within its host cell may uncover new ideas for treating not only the bacterial infection but also host responses triggered in response to infection and resulting in reactions (see Leprosy Reactions) that lead to significant morbidity.

Fundamental to understanding the pathogenicity of *M. leprae* is defining the composite phenotype of the bacillus and determining gene expression related to intracellular survival and virulence. Gene identification through comparative genomic studies with known functional homologues is the first step in defining some of these disease-causing capabilities. Next must come an understanding of which genes are expressed during infection and, if possible, the temporal events associated with gene expression during infection. At present this can be accomplished only at the most elementary level, using tools measuring gene transcription of *M. leprae* during infection. Williams et al. (329) successfully demonstrated this approach using reverse-transcriptase polymerase chain reaction and cross-species (*M. tuberculosis*) DNA microarrays to examine *M. leprae* gene transcription during infection. Transcripts were identified for 221 open reading frames and included genes involved in cell division, DNA replication, protein secretion, intermediary metabolism and energy production, and transport and storage of iron and a subset of genes associated with virulence in *M. tuberculosis*.

Recognizing that *M. leprae* and *M. tuberculosis* are unique pathogens causing significantly different pathology in humans should not divert our attention from commonalities that exist. For example, metabolic similarities exist regarding oxidation of lipids as a prime carbon source for energy production during certain stages of infection. In addition, shared cell wall components, some of which appear to act as adhesins, are important in establishing infection (33, 223, 236, 238, 264, 265) and subsequent pathology. Aspects of the chronic nature of the infections caused by these two pathogens may exist as well. For example, the long-recognized but little understood biological states of persistence of *M. leprae* in leprosy (321) and *M. tuberculosis* in TB (182, 232) have led to studies aimed at identifying metabolic changes in *M. tuberculosis* that render it nonreplicating, or dormant, but very much alive and potentially capable of reactivation with pathological consequences (142, 318). Most of these studies have modeled dormancy using bacteria grown in culture under defined conditions leading to stationary growth, reproducing a form of dormancy. While it is not clear whether all conditions have been met for reproducing the nonreplicative state of *M. tuberculosis* in vivo, studies like these may further our understanding of a critical physiological adaptation used by at least two major mycobacterial pathogens of man. Persistence remains a major obstacle for managing leprosy and TB and, if understood more fully, could lead to improved treatment regimens and better control of both diseases.

Vaccines

Despite significantly improved access to drugs globally, new cases of leprosy continue to be reported at around one-quarter to one-half million per year (10). Implementation of WHO-recommended multidrug therapy has raised the hope of reducing leprosy to manageable levels globally. Unfortunately, this has not been the case in resource-poor areas of the world, and global elimination of the disease does not appear imminent. It is likely that steps toward improved control will require additional intervention strategies, such as improving early diagnosis and developing and applying therapeutic and prophylactic vaccines. By far the intervention strategy with the greatest potential impact would be an effective vaccine against leprosy. Strategies for controlling infectious diseases can benefit from vaccines in that they may be applied as prophylactic (preexposure as first demonstrated against viruses in 1798 [159] and to date most effectively against leprosy using BCG [71, 340], Mycobacterium w [170, 275], and the ICRC bacillus [241]) or therapeutic (postexposure [79, 168, 169, 338]) interventions. Both may be important steps in any campaign to control leprosy. Vaccines have the added potential advantage of providing protracted protection against infection as a result of their ability to induce long-lived immunological memory in the host. Additionally, an appropriately designed potent vaccine should protect against many, if not all, drug-resistant mutants of the infectious agent, an inevitability in leprosy that cannot be minimized.

REFERENCES

1. **Abe, T., Y. Iinuma, M. Ando, T. Yokoyama, T. Yamamoto, K. Nakashima, N. Takagi, H. Baba, Y. Hasegawa, and K. Shimokata.** 2003. NRAMP1 polymorphisms, susceptibility and clinical features of tuberculosis. *J. Infect.* **46:**215–220.
2. **Abebe, F., C. Holm-Hansen, H. G. Wiker, and G. Bjune.** 2007. Progress in serodiagnosis of *Mycobacterium tuberculosis* infection. *Scand. J. Immunol.* **66:**176–191.
3. **Abel, L., F. O. Sanchez, J. Oberti, N. V. Thuc, L. V. Hoa, V. D. Lap, E. Skamene, P. H. Lagrange, and E. Schurr.** 1998. Susceptibility to leprosy is linked to the human NRAMP1 gene. *J. Infect. Dis.* **177:**133–145.
4. **Aguado, J. M., J. A. Herrero, J. Gavalda, J. Torre-Cisneros, M. Blanes, G. Rufi, A. Moreno, M. Gurgui, M. Hayek, C. Lumbreras, C. Cantarell, et al.** 1997. Clinical presentation and outcome of tuberculosis in kidney, liver, and heart transplant recipients in Spain.*Transplantation* **63:**1278–1286.
5. **Akahoshi, M., M. Ishihara, N. Remus, K. Uno, K. Miyake, T. Hirota, K. Nakashima, A. Matsuda, M. Kanda, T. Enomoto, S. Ohno, H. Nakashima, J. L. Casanova, J. M. Hopkin, M. Tamari, X. Q. Mao, and T. Shirakawa.** 2004. Association between IFNA genotype and the risk of sarcoidosis. *Hum. Genet.* **114:**503–509.
6. **Alcais, A., A. Alter, G. Antoni, M. Orlova, V. T. Nguyen, M. Singh, P. R. Vanderborght, K. Katoch, M. T. Mira, H. T. Vu, T. H. Ngyuen, N. B. Nguyen, M. Moraes, N. Mehra, E. Schurr, and L. Abel.** 2007. Stepwise replication identifies a low-producing lymphotoxin-alpha allele as a major risk factor for early-onset leprosy. *Nat. Genet.* **39:**517–522.
7. **Andersson, A. K., M. Chaduvula, S. E. Atkinson, S. Khanolkar-Young, S. Jain, L. Suneetha, S. Suneetha, and D. N. Lockwood.** 2005. Effects of prednisolone treatment on cytokine expression in patients with leprosy type 1 reactions. *Infect. Immun.* **73:**3725–3733.
8. **Anonymous.** 1998. The thalidomide comeback. *HIV Hotline* **8:**7, 9, 15.
9. Reference deleted.
10. **Anonymous.** 2006. Global strategy for further reducing the leprosy burden and sustaining leprosy control activities 2006–2010. Operational guidelines. *Lepr. Rev.* **77:**IX, X, 1–50.
11. **Antognoli, M. C., F. B. Garry, H. L. Hirst, J. E. Lombard, M. M. Dennis, D. H. Gould, and M. D. Salman.** 2008. Characterization of *Mycobacterium avium* subspecies *paratuberculosis* disseminated infection in dairy cattle and its association with antemortem test results. *Vet. Microbiol.* **127:**300–308.
12. **Askling, J., L. Brandt, A. Lapidus, P. Karlen, M. Bjorkholm, R. Lofberg, and A. Ekbom.** 2005. Risk of haematopoietic cancer in patients with inflammatory bowel disease. *Gut* **54:**617–622.
13. **Autschbach, F., S. Eisold, U. Hinz, S. Zinser, M. Linnebacher, T. Giese, T. Loffler, M. W. Buchler, and J. Schmidt.** 2005. High prevalence of *Mycobacterium avium* subspecies *paratuberculosis* IS*900* DNA in gut tissues from individuals with Crohn's disease. *Gut* **54:**944–949.
14. **Ayele, W. Y., P. Svastova, P. Roubal, M. Bartos, and I. Pavlik.** 2005. *Mycobacterium avium* subspecies *paratuberculosis* cultured from locally and commercially pasteurized cow's milk in the Czech Republic. *Appl. Environ. Microbiol.* **71:** 1210–1214.
15. **Azad Khan, A. K., J. Piris, and S. C. Truelove.** 1977. An experiment to determine the active therapeutic moiety of sulphasalazine. *Lancet* **ii:**829–831.
16. **Barksdale, L., and K. S. Kim.** 1977. Mycobacterium. *Bacteriol. Rev.* **41:**217–372.
17. **Beard, P. M., M. J. Daniels, D. Henderson, A. Pirie, K. Rudge, D. Buxton, S. Rhind, A. Greig, M. R. Hutchings, I. McKendrick, K. Stevenson, and J. M. Sharp.** 2001. Paratuberculosis infection of nonruminant wildlife in Scotland. *J. Clin. Microbiol.* **39:**1517–1521.
18. **Behr, M. A., M. Semret, A. Poon, and E. Schurr.** 2004. Crohn's disease, mycobacteria, and NOD2. *Lancet Infect. Dis.* **4:**136–137.
19. **Behr, M. A., S. A. Warren, H. Salamon, P. C. Hopewell, D. L. Ponce, C. L. Daley, and P. M. Small.** 1999. Transmission of *Mycobacterium tuberculosis* from patients smear-negative for acid-fast bacilli. *Lancet* **353:**444–449.
20. **Berardi, R. R.** 1996. Inflammatory bowel disease, p. 483–502. *In* E. T. Herfindal and D. R. Gourley (ed.), *Textbook of Therapeutics. Drugs and Disease Management*, vol. 1. Williams and Wilkins, Baltimore, MD.
21. **Bercik, P., E. F. Verdu, and S. M. Collins.** 2005. Is irritable bowel syndrome a low-grade inflammatory bowel disease? *Gastroenterol. Clin. North Am.* **34:**235–245.
22. **Bernadsky, S., A. Clarke, and S. Suissa.** 2008. Hematologic malignant neoplasms in drug exposure in rheumatoid arthritis. *Arch. Intern. Med.* **168:**378–381.
23. **Bernheim, F.** 1940. The effect of salicylate on the oxygen uptake of the tubercle bacillus. *Science* **92:**204.
24. **Bernstein, C. N., L. Artinian, P. A. Anton, and F. Shanahan.** 1994. Low-dose 6-mercaptopurine in inflammatory bowel disease is associated with minimal hematologic toxicity. *Dig. Dis. Sci.* **39:**1638–1641.
25. **Bernstein, C. N., M. H. Wang, M. Sargent, S. R. Brant, and M. T. Collins.** 2007. Testing the interaction between NOD-2 status and serological response to *Mycobacterium paratuberculosis* in cases of inflammatory bowel disease. *J. Clin. Microbiol.* **45:**968–971.
26. **Bhatt, K., and P. Salgame.** 2007. Host innate immune response to *Mycobacterium tuberculosis*. *J. Clin. Immunol.* **27:**347–362.
27. **Binford, C. H.** 1956. Comprehensive program for the inoculation of human leprosy into laboratory animals. *US Public Health Rep.* **71:**995–996.
28. **Blackwell, J. M.** 1996. Genetic susceptibility to leishmanial infections: studies in mice and man. *Parasitology* **112**(Suppl.)**:** S67–S74.
29. **Blackwell, J. M.** 1998. Genetics of host resistance and susceptibility to intramacrophage pathogens: a study of multicase families of tuberculosis, leprosy and leishmaniasis in north-eastern Brazil. *Int. J. Parasitol.* **28:**21–28.
30. **Bouhnik, Y., M. Lemann, J. Y. Mary, G. Scemama, R. Tai, C. Matuchansky, R. Modigliani, and J. C. Rambaud.** 1996. Long-term follow-up of patients with Crohn's disease treated with azathioprine or 6-mercaptopurine. *Lancet* **347:**215–219.
31. **Brand, S., T. Staudinger, F. Schnitzler, S. Pfennig, K. Hofbauer, J. Dambacher, J. Seiderer, C. Tillack, A. Konrad, A. Crispin, B. Goke, P. Lohse, and T. Ochsenkuhn.** 2005. The role of Toll-like receptor 4 Asp299Gly and Thr399Ile polymorphisms and CARD15/NOD2 mutations in the susceptibility and phenotype of Crohn's disease. *Inflamm. Bowel Dis.* **11:**645–652.

32. **Brennan, P. J.** 2003. Structure, function, and biogenesis of the cell wall of *Mycobacterium tuberculosis*. *Tuberculosis* (Edinburgh) **83:**91–97.
33. **Brennan, P. J., and V. D. Vissa.** 2001. Genomic evidence for the retention of the essential mycobacterial cell wall in the otherwise defective *Mycobacterium leprae*. *Lepr. Rev.* **72:**415–428.
34. **Britton, W. J., and D. N. Lockwood.** 2004. Leprosy. *Lancet* **363:**1209–1219.
35. **Brosch, R., S. V. Gordon, K. Eiglmeier, T. Garnier, and S. T. Cole.** 2000. Comparative genomics of the leprosy and tubercle bacilli. *Res. Microbiol.* **151:**135–142.
36. **Brosch, R., S. V. Gordon, M. Marmiesse, P. Brodin, C. Buchrieser, K. Eiglmeier, T. Garnier, C. Gutierrez, G. Hewinson, K. Kremer, L. M. Parsons, A. S. Pym, S. Samper, D. van Soolingen, and S. T. Cole.** 2002. A new evolutionary scenario for the *Mycobacterium tuberculosis* complex. *Proc. Natl. Acad. Sci. USA* **99:**3684–3689.
37. **Brown, S. T., and P. L. Almenoff.** 1992. Pulmonary mycobacterial infections associated with neoplasia. *Semin.Respir. Infect.* **7:**104–113.
38. **Buergelt, C. D., A. W. Layton, P. E. Ginn, M. Taylor, J. M. King, P. L. Habecker, E. Mauldin, R. Whitlock, C. Rossiter, and M. T. Collins.** 2000. The pathology of spontaneous paratuberculosis in the North American bison (*Bison bison*). *Vet. Pathol.* **37:** 428–438.
39. **Bull, T. J., S. C. Gilbert, S. Sridhar, R. Linedale, N. Dierkes, K. Sidi-Boumedine, and J. Hermon-Taylor.** 2007. A novel multi-antigen virally vectored vaccine against *Mycobacterium avium* subspecies *paratuberculosis*. *PLoS ONE* **2:**e1229.
40. **Bull, T. J., E. J. McMinn, K. Sidi-Boumedine, A. Skull, D. Durkin, P. Neild, G. Rhodes, R. Pickup, and J. Hermon-Taylor.** 2003. Detection and verification of *Mycobacterium avium* subsp. *paratuberculosis* in fresh ileocolonic mucosal biopsy specimens from individuals with and without Crohn's disease. *J. Clin. Microbiol.* **41:**2915–2923.
41. **Buschman, E., S. Vidal, and E. Skamene.** 1997. Nonspecific resistance to *Mycobacteria*: the role of the Nramp1 gene. *Behring Inst. Mitt.* **(99):**51–57.
42. **Calabresi, P., and B. A. Chabner.** 1990. Chemotherapy of neoplastic diseases, p. 1202–1208. *In* L. S. Goodman, A. Gilman, T. Rall, A. S. Nies, and P. Taylor (ed.), *The Pharmacological Basis of Therapeutics*, 8th ed. Pergamon Press, New York, NY.
43. **Caprilli, R., E. Angelucci, A. Cocco, A. Viscido, V. Annese, S. Ardizzone, L. Biancone, F. Castiglione, M. Cottone, G. Meucci, P. Paoluzi, C. Papi, G. C. Sturniolo, and M. Vecchi.** 2005. Appropriateness of immunosuppressive drugs in inflammatory bowel diseases assessed by RAND method: Italian Group for IBD (IG-IBD) position statement. *Dig. Liver Dis.* **37:**407–417.
44. **Caprilli, R., E. Angelucci, A. Cocco, A. Viscido, and M. Zippi.** 2004. Efficacy of conventional immunosuppressive drugs in IBD. *Dig. Liver Dis.* **36:**766–780.
45. **Casali, N., A. M. White, and L. W. Riley.** 2006. Regulation of the *Mycobacterium tuberculosis mce1* operon. *J. Bacteriol.* **188:**441–449.
46. **Casetta, I., G. Iuliano, and G. Filippini.** 2007. Azathioprine for multiple sclerosis. *Cochrane Database Syst. Rev.*: CD003982.
47. **Cavalier-Smith, T.** 2006. Origin of mitochondria by intracellular enslavement of a photosynthetic purple bacterium. *Proc. Biol. Sci.* **273:**1943–1952.
48. **CDC.** 2002. Tuberculosis outbreak on an American Indian reservation—Montana, 2000-2001. *MMWR Morb. Mortal. Wkly. Rep.* **51:**232–234.
49. **CDC.** 2005. Multidrug-resistant tuberculosis in Hmong refugees resettling from Thailand into the United States, 2004–2005. *MMWR Morb. Mortal. Wkly. Rep.* **54:**741–744.
50. **CDC.** 2007. Extensively drug-resistant tuberculosis—United States, 1993-2006. *MMWR Morb. Mortal. Wkly. Rep.* **56:**250–253.
51. **Chaisson, R. E., and N. A. Martinson.** 2008. Tuberculosis in Africa–combating an HIV-driven crisis. *N. Engl. J. Med.* **358:**1089–1092.
52. **Chan, J., and J. Flynn.** 2004. The immunological aspects of latency in tuberculosis. *Clin. Immunol.* **110:**2–12.
53. **Chen, L. H., K. Kathaperumal, C. J. Huang, S. P. McDonough, S. Stehman, B. Akey, J. Huntley, J. P. Bannantine, C. F. Chang, and Y. F. Chang.** 2008. Immune responses in mice to *Mycobacterium avium* subsp. *paratuberculosis* following vaccination with a novel 74F recombinant polyprotein. *Vaccine* **26:**1253–1262.
54. **Chiodini, R. J., H. J. Van Kruiningen, R. S. Merkal, W. R. Thayer, Jr., and J. A. Coutu.** 1984. Characteristics of an unclassified *Mycobacterium* species isolated from patients with Crohn's disease. *J. Clin. Microbiol.* **20:**966–971.
55. **Chiodini, R. J., H. J. Van Kruiningen, W. R. Thayer, Jr., and J. Coutu.** 1986. Spheroplastic phase of mycobacteria isolated from patients with Crohn's disease. *J. Clin. Microbiol.* **24:**357–363.
56. **Chiodini, R. J., H. J. Van Kruiningen, W. R. Thayer, R. S. Merkal, and J. A. Coutu.** 1984. Possible role of mycobacteria in inflammatory bowel disease. I. An unclassified *Mycobacterium* species isolated from patients with Crohn's disease. *Dig. Dis. Sci.* **29:**1073–1079.
57. **Chiplunkar, S., G. De Libero, and S. H. Kaufmann.** 1986. *Mycobacterium leprae*-specific Lyt-2^+ T lymphocytes with cytolytic activity. *Infect. Immun.* **54:**793–797.
58. **Cho, S. N., and P. J. Brennan.** 2007. Tuberculosis: diagnostics. *Tuberculosis* (Edinburgh) **87**(Suppl. 1):S14–S17.
59. **Cho, S. N., R. V. Cellona, L. G. Villahermosa, T. T. Fajardo, Jr., M. V. Balagon, R. M. Abalos, E. V. Tan, G. P. Walsh, J. D. Kim, and P. J. Brennan.** 2001. Detection of phenolic glycolipid I of *Mycobacterium leprae* in sera from leprosy patients before and after start of multidrug therapy. *Clin. Diagn. Lab. Immunol.* **8:**138–142.
60. **Cohen, T., and M. Murray.** 2004. Modeling epidemics of multidrug-resistant *M. tuberculosis* of heterogeneous fitness. *Nat. Med.* **10:**1117–1121.
61. **Cohen, T., B. Sommers, and M. Murray.** 2003. The effect of drug resistance on the fitness of *Mycobacterium tuberculosis*. *Lancet Infect. Dis.* **3:**13–21.
62. **Cole, S. T.** 1998. Comparative mycobacterial genomics. *Curr. Opin. Microbiol.* **1:**567–571.
63. **Cole, S. T., R. Brosch, J. Parkhill, T. Garnier, C. Churcher, D. Harris, S. V. Gordon, K. Eiglmeier, S. Gas, C. E. Barry, F. Tekaia, K. Badcock, D. Basham, D. Brown, T. Chillingworth, R. Connor, R. Davies, K. Devlin, T. Feltwell, S. Gentles, N. Hamlin, S. Holroyd, T. Hornsby, K. Jagels, A. Krough, J. McLean, S. Moule, L. Murphy, K. Oliver, J. Osborne, M. A. Quail, M. A. Rajandream, J. Rogers, S. Rujtter, K. Seeger, J. Skelton, R. Squares, S. Squares, J. E. Sulston, K. Taylor, S. Whitehead, and B. G. Barrell.** 1998. Deciphering the biology of *Mycobacterium tuberculosis* from the complete genome sequence. *Nature* **393:**537–544.
64. **Cole, S. T., K. Eiglmeier, J. Parkhill, K. D. James, N. R. Thomson, P. R. Wheeler, N. Honore, T. Garnier, C. Churcher, D. Harris, K. Mungall, D. Basham, D. Brown, T. Chillingworth, R. Connor, R. M. Davies, K. Devlin, S. Duthoy, T. Feltwell, A. Fraser, N. Hamlin, S. Holroyd, T. Hornsby, K. Jagels, C. Lacroix, J. Maclean, S. Moule, L. Murphy,**

K. Oliver, M. A. Quail, M. A. Rajandream, K. M. Rutherford, S. Rutter, K. Seeger, S. Simon, M. Simmonds, J. Skelton, R. Squares, S. Squares, K. Stevens, K. Taylor, S. Whitehead, J. R. Woodward, and B. G. Barrell. 2001. Massive gene decay in the leprosy bacillus. *Nature* **409:**1007–1011.

65. **Comabella, M., L. Altet, F. Peris, P. Villoslada, A. Sanchez, and X. Montalban.** 2004. Genetic analysis of SLC11A1 polymorphisms in multiple sclerosis patients. *Mult. Scler.* **10:**618–620.

66. **Corbett, E. L., T. Bandason, Y. B. Cheung, S. Munyati, P. Godfrey-Faussett, R. Hayes, G. Churchyard, A. Butterworth, and P. Mason.** 2007. Epidemiology of tuberculosis in a high HIV prevalence population provided with enhanced diagnosis of symptomatic disease. *PLoS Med.* **4:**e22.

67. **Corbett, E. L., and K. M. De Cock.** 2001. The clinical significance of interactions between HIV and TB: more questions than answers. *Int. J. Tuberc. Lung Dis.* **5:**205–207.

68. **Corbett, E. L., C. J. Watt, N. Walker, D. Maher, B. G. Williams, M. C. Raviglione, and C. Dye.** 2003. The growing burden of tuberculosis: global trends and interactions with the HIV epidemic. *Arch. Intern. Med.* **163:**1009–1021.

69. **Crohn, B. B., L. Ginzberg, and G. D. Oppenheimer.** 1932. Regional ileitis. *J. Amer. Med. Assoc.* **99:**1323–1328.

70. **Cummings, D. M., D. Ristroph, E. E. Camargo, S. M. Larson, and H. N. Wagner, Jr.** 1975. Radiometric detection of the metabolic activity of *Mycobacterium tuberculosis*. *J. Nucl. Med.* **16:**1189–1191.

71. **Cunha, S. S., N. Alexander, M. L. Barreto, E. S. Pereira, I. Dourado, M. de Fatima Maroja, Y. Ichihara, S. Brito, S. Pereira, and L. C. Rodrigues.** 2008. BCG revaccination does not protect against leprosy in the Brazilian Amazon: a cluster randomised trial. *PLoS Negl. Trop. Dis.* **2:**e167.

72. **Dalziel, T. K.** 1913. Chronic intestinal enteritis. *Br. Med. J.* **ii:**1068–1070.

73. **Damato, J. J., and M. T. Collins.** 1990. Growth of *Mycobacterium paratuberculosis* in radiometric, Middlebrook and egg-based media. *Vet. Microbiol.* **22:**31–42.

74. **Dasananjali, K., P. A. Schreuder, and C. Pirayavaraporn.** 1997. A study on the effectiveness and safety of the WHO/MDT regimen in the northeast of Thailand; a prospective study, 1984-1996. *Int. J. Lepr. Other Mycobact. Dis.* **65:**28–36.

75. **David, H. L., N. Rastogi, C. Frehel, and M. Gheorghiu.** 1982. Reduction of potassium tellurite and ATP content in *Mycobacterium leprae*. *Ann. Microbiol.* (Paris) **133:**129–139.

76. **De Francesco, M. A., D. Colombrita, G. Pinsi, F. Gargiulo, S. Caligaris, D. Bertelli, F. Martinelli, J. Gao, and A. Turano.** 1996. Detection and identification of *Mycobacterium avium* in the blood of AIDS patients by the polymerase chain reaction. *Eur. J. Clin. Microbiol. Infect. Dis.* **15:**551–555.

77. **De Jager, P. L., R. Graham, L. Farwell, S. Sawcer, A. Richardson, T. W. Behrens, A. Compston, D. A. Hafler, J. Kere, T. J. Vyse, and J. D. Rioux.** 2006. The role of inflammatory bowel disease susceptibility loci in multiple sclerosis and systemic lupus erythematosus. *Genes Immun.* **7:**327–34.

78. **de Oca, J., L. Vilar, J. Castellote, R. Sanchez Santos, D. Pares, S. Biondo, A. Osorio, C. del Rio, E. Jaurrieta, and J. Marti Rague.** 2003. Immunodulation with tacrolimus (FK506): results of a prospective, open-label, non-controlled trial in patients with inflammatory bowel disease. *Rev. Esp. Enferm. Dig.* **95:**459–464, 465–470.

79. **De Sarkar, A., I. Kaur, B. D. Radotra, and B. Kumar.** 2001. Impact of combined Mycobacterium w vaccine and 1 year of MDT on multibacillary leprosy patients. *Int. J. Lepr. Other Mycobact. Dis.* **69:**187–194.

80. **de Souza, M. V.** 2006. Promising drugs against tuberculosis. *Recent Patents Anti-Infect. Drug Disc.* **1:**33–44.

81. **Dhople, A. M., and L. C. Lamoureux.** 1991. Factors influencing the in vitro growth of *Mycobacterium leprae*: effect of sulfhydryl compounds. *Microbiol. Immunol.* **35:**209–213.

82. **Djonne, B., M. R. Jensen, I. R. Grant, and G. Holstad.** 2003. Detection by immunomagnetic PCR of *Mycobacterium avium* subsp. *paratuberculosis* in milk from dairy goats in Norway. *Vet. Microbiol.* **92:**135–43.

83. **Dow, C. T.** 2006. Paratuberculosis and type I diabetes: is this the trigger? *Med. Hypotheses* **67:**782–785.

84. **Dubaniewicz, A., S. E. Jamieson, M. Dubaniewicz-Wybieralska, M. Fakiola, E. Nancy Miller, and J. M. Blackwell.** 2005. Association between SLC11A1 (formerly NRAMP1) and the risk of sarcoidosis in Poland. *Eur. J. Hum. Genet.* **13:**829–34.

85. **Dubnau, E., P. Fontan, R. Manganelli, S. Soares-Appel, and I. Smith.** 2002. *Mycobacterium tuberculosis* genes induced during infection of human macrophages. *Infect. Immun.* **70:**2787–2795.

86. **Dubos, R. J., and J. Dubos.** 1952. *The White Plague: Tuberculosis, Man and Society*. Little, Brown and Company, Boston, MA.

87. **Dye, C., S. Scheele, P. Dolin, V. Pathania, and M. C. Raviglione.** 1999. Consensus statement. Global burden of tuberculosis: estimated incidence, prevalence, and mortality by country. WHO Global Surveillance and Monitoring Project. *JAMA* **282:**677–686.

88. **Edlin, B. R., J. I. Tokars, M. H. Grieco, J. T. Crawford, J. Williams, E. M. Sordillo, K. R. Ong, J. O. Kilburn, S. W. Dooley, K. G. Castro, W. R. Jarvis, and S. D. Holmberg.** 1992. An outbreak of multidrug-resistant tuberculosis among hospitalized patients with the acquired immunodeficiency syndrome. *N. Engl. J. Med.* **326:**1514–1521.

89. **Ehrenpreis, E. D., S. V. Kane, L. B. Cohen, R. D. Cohen, and S. B. Hanauer.** 1999. Thalidomide therapy for patients with refractory Crohn's disease: an open-label trial. *Gastroenterology* **117:**1271–1277.

90. **Eiglmeier, K., J. Parkhill, N. Honore, T. Garnier, F. Tekaia, A. Telenti, P. Klatser, K. D. James, N. R. Thomson, P. R. Wheeler, C. Churcher, D. Harris, K. Mungall, B. G. Barrell, and S. T. Cole.** 2001. The decaying genome of *Mycobacterium leprae*. *Lepr. Rev.* **72:**387–398.

91. **Ellingson, J. L., J. L. Anderson, J. J. Koziczkowski, R. P. Radcliff, S. J. Sloan, S. E. Allen, and N. M. Sullivan.** 2005. Detection of viable *Mycobacterium avium* subsp. *paratuberculosis* in retail pasteurized whole milk by two culture methods and PCR. *J. Food Prot.* **68:**966–972.

92. **El-Omar, E. M., M. T. Ng, and G. L. Hold.** 2008. Polymorphisms in Toll-like receptor genes and risk of cancer. *Oncogene* **27:**244–252.

93. **El-Zaatari, F. A., D. Y. Graham, K. Samuelsson, and L. Engstrand.** 1997. Detection of *Mycobacterium avium* complex in cerebrospinal fluid of a sarcoid patient by specific polymerase chain reaction assays. *Scand. J. Infect. Dis.* **29:**202–204.

94. **El-Zaatari, F. A., S. A. Naser, L. Engstrand, P. E. Burch, C. Y. Hachem, D. L. Whipple, and D. Y. Graham.** 1995. Nucleotide sequence analysis and seroreactivities of the 65K heat shock protein from *Mycobacterium paratuberculosis*. *Clin. Diagn. Lab. Immunol.* **2:**657–664.

95. **El-Zaatari, F. A., S. A. Naser, and D. Y. Graham.** 1997. Characterization of a specific *Mycobacterium paratuberculosis* recombinant clone expressing 35,000-molecular-weight antigen and reactivity with sera from animals with clinical and subclinical Johne's disease. *J. Clin. Microbiol.* **35:**1794–1799.

96. **Ernst, J. D., G. Trevejo-Nunez, and N. Banaiee.** 2007. Genomics and the evolution, pathogenesis, and diagnosis of tuberculosis. *J. Clin. Investig.* **117:**1738–1745.

97. **Evans, G. M., and W. F. Gaisford.** 1938. Treatment of pneumonia with 2-(p aminobenzenesulphonamido) pyridine. *Lancet* ii:14–19.
98. **Feagan, B. G., J. Rochon, R. N. Fedorak, E. J. Irvine, G. Wild, L. Sutherland, A. H. Steinhart, G. R. Greenberg, R. Gillies, M. Hopkins, et al.** 1995. Methotrexate for the treatment of Crohn's disease. *N. Engl. J. Med.* **332:**292–297.
99. **Ferrara, G., M. Losi, R. D'Amico, P. Roversi, R. Piro, M. Meacci, B. Meccugni, I. M. Dori, A. Andreani, B. M. Bergamini, C. Mussini, F. Rumpianesi, L. M. Fabbri, and L. Richeldi.** 2006. Use in routine clinical practice of two commercial blood tests for diagnosis of infection with *Mycobacterium tuberculosis*: a prospective study. *Lancet* **367:**1328–1334.
100. **Ferreira, F. R., L. R. Goulart, H. D. Silva, and I. M. Goulart.** 2004. Susceptibility to leprosy may be conditioned by an interaction between the NRAMP1 promoter polymorphisms and the lepromin response. *Int. J. Lepr. Other Mycobact. Dis.* **72:**457–467.
101. **Ferwerda, G., S. E. Girardin, B. J. Kullberg, L. Le Bourhis, D. J. de Jong, D. M. Langenberg, R. van Crevel, G. J. Adema, T. H. Ottenhoff, J. W. Van der Meer, and M. G. Netea.** 2005. NOD2 and Toll-like receptors are nonredundant recognition systems of *Mycobacterium tuberculosis*. *PLoS Pathog.* **1:**279–285.
102. **Findley, R. S., and C. L. Fortner.** 1996. Methotrexate in non-Hodgkin's lymphoma, p. 1509–1513. *In* E. T. Herfindal and D. R. Gourley (ed.), *Textbook of Therapeutics: Drugs and Disease Management*, 6th ed., vol.1. Williams & Wilkins, Baltimore, MD.
103. **Fine, P. E.** 1995. Variation in protection by BCG: implications of and for heterologous immunity. *Lancet* **346:**1339–1345.
104. **Flynn, J. L.** 2004. Immunology of tuberculosis and implications in vaccine development. *Tuberculosis* (Edinburgh) **84:**93–101.
105. **Flynn, J. L., and J. Chan.** 2001. Immunology of tuberculosis. *Annu. Rev. Immunol.* **19:**93–129.
106. **Foroncewicz, B., K. Mucha, L. Paczek, A. Chmura, and W. Rowinski.** 2005. Efficacy of rapamycin in patient with juvenile rheumatoid arthritis. *Transpl. Int.* **18:**366–368.
107. **Franzblau, S. G.** 1988. Oxidation of palmitic acid by *Mycobacterium leprae* in an axenic medium. *J. Clin. Microbiol.* **26:**18–21.
108. **Franzblau, S. G., and E. B. Harris.** 1988. Biophysical optima for metabolism of *Mycobacterium leprae*. *J. Clin. Microbiol.* **26:**1124–1129.
109. **Franzblau, S. G., E. B. Harris, and R. C. Hastings.** 1987. Axenic incorporation of [U-14C]palmitic acid into the phenolic glycolipid-1 of *Mycobacterium leprae*. *FEMS Microbiol. Lett.* **48:**407–411.
110. **Fraser, A. G., T. R. Orchard, E. M. Robinson, and D. P. Jewell.** 2002. Long-term risk of malignancy after treatment of inflammatory bowel disease with azathioprine. *Aliment. Pharmacol. Ther.* **16:**1225–1232.
111. **Fukata, M., and M. T. Abreu.** 2008. Role of Toll-like receptors in gastrointestinal malignancies. *Oncogene* **27:**234–243.
112. **Gabriela, M. G., P. Rodrigues, F. M. Hilker, N. B. Mantilla-Beniers, M. Muehlen, P. A. Cristina, and G. F. Medley.** 2007. Implications of partial immunity on the prospects for tuberculosis control by post-exposure interventions. *J. Theor. Biol.* **248:**608–617.
113. **Gagneux, S., and P. M. Small.** 2007. Global phylogeography of *Mycobacterium tuberculosis* and implications for tuberculosis product development. *Lancet Infect. Dis.* **7:**328–337.
114. **Goldman, R. C., K. V. Plumley, and B. E. Laughon.** 2007. The evolution of extensively drug resistant tuberculosis (XDR-TB): history, status and issues for global control. *Infect. Disord. Drug Targets* **7:**73–91.
115. **Gomez-Valero, L., E. P. Rocha, A. Latorre, and F. J. Silva.** 2007. Reconstructing the ancestor of *Mycobacterium leprae*: the dynamics of gene loss and genome reduction. *Genome Res.* **17:**1178–1185.
116. **Gonzalez, B., S. Moreno, R. Burdach, M. T. Valenzuela, A. Henriquez, M. I. Ramos, and R. U. Sorensen.** 1989. Clinical presentation of bacillus Calmette-Guerin infections in patients with immunodeficiency syndromes. *Pediatr. Infect. Dis. J.* **8:**201–206.
117. **Gourevitch, M. N., D. Hartel, P. A. Selwyn, E. E. Schoenbaum, and R. S. Klein.** 1999. Effectiveness of isoniazid chemoprophylaxis for HIV-infected drug users at high risk for active tuberculosis. *AIDS* **13:**2069–2074.
118. **Grange, J. M.** 1990. Drug resistance and tuberculosis elimination. *Bull. Int. Union Tuberc. Lung Dis.* **65:**57–59.
119. **Grant, I. R.** 1998. Does *Mycobacterium paratuberculosis* survive current pasteurization conditions? *Appl. Environ. Microbiol.* **64:**2760–2761.
120. **Grant, I. R., H. J. Ball, and M. T. Rowe.** 1998. Effect of high-temperature, short-time (HTST) pasteurization on milk containing low numbers of *Mycobacterium paratuberculosis*. *Lett. Appl. Microbiol.* **26:**166–170.
121. **Grant, I. R., H. J. Ball, and M. T. Rowe.** 1998. Isolation of *Mycobacterium paratuberculosis* from milk by immunomagnetic separation. *Appl. Environ. Microbiol.* **64:**3153–3158.
122. **Grant, I. R., E. I. Hitchings, A. McCartney, F. Ferguson, and M. T. Rowe.** 2002. Effect of commercial-scale high-temperature, short-time pasteurization on the viability of *Mycobacterium paratuberculosis* in naturally infected cows' milk. *Appl. Environ. Microbiol.* **68:**602–607.
123. **Grant, I. R., L. M. O'Riordan, H. J. Ball, and M. T. Rowe.** 2001. Incidence of *Mycobacterium paratuberculosis* in raw sheep and goats' milk in England, Wales and Northern Ireland. *Vet. Microbiol.* **79:**123–131.
124. **Green, C., L. Elliott, C. Beaudoin, and C. N. Bernstein.** 2006. A population-based ecologic study of inflammatory bowel disease: searching for etiologic clues. *Am. J. Epidemiol.* **164:**615–623.
125. **Green, J. P.** 2004, posting date. Guidance on control of Johne's disease in dairy herds. Department for Environment Food and Rural Affairs (DEFRA). http://www.defra.gov.uk/animalh/diseases/pdf/johnesguidance.pdf.
126. **Green, J. R., J. A. Gibson, G. D. Kerr, E. T. Swarbrick, A. J. Lobo, C. D. Holdsworth, J. P. Crowe, K. J. Schofield, M. D. Taylor, et al.** 1998. Maintenance of remission of ulcerative colitis: a comparison between balsalazide 3 g daily and mesalazine 1.2 g daily over 12 months. *Aliment. Pharmacol. Ther.* **12:**1207–1216.
127. **Green, J. R., A. J. Lobo, C. D. Holdsworth, R. J. Leicester, J. A. Gibson, G. D. Kerr, H. J. Hodgson, K. J. Parkins, M. D. Taylor, et al.** 1998. Balsalazide is more effective and better tolerated than mesalamine in the treatment of acute ulcerative colitis. *Gastroenterology* **114:**15–22.
128. **Greenstein, A. J., G. E. Mullin, J. A. Strauchen, T. Heimann, H. D. Janowitz, A. H. Aufses, Jr., and D. B. Sachar.** 1992. Lymphoma in inflammatory bowel disease. *Cancer* **69:**1119–1123.
129. **Greenstein, A. J., D. Sachar, A. Pucillo, I. Kreel, S. Geller, H. D. Janowitz, and A. Aufses, Jr.** 1978. Cancer in Crohn's disease after diversionary surgery. A report of seven carcinomas occurring in excluded bowel. *Am. J. Surg.* **135:**86–90.
130. **Greenstein, R. J.** 2003. Is Crohn's disease caused by a mycobacterium? Comparisons with leprosy, tuberculosis, and Johne's disease. *Lancet Infect. Dis.* **3:**507–514.

131. Reference deleted.
132. Reference deleted.
133. **Greenstein, R. J., and M. T. Collins.** 2004. Emerging pathogens: is *Mycobacterium avium* subspecies *paratuberculosis* zoonotic? *Lancet* **364:**396–397.
134. **Greenstein, R. J., L. Su, V. Haroutunian, A. Shahidi, and S. T. Brown.** 2007. On the action of methotrexate and 6-mercaptopurine on *M. avium* subspecies *paratuberculosis*. *PLoS ONE* **2:**e161.
135. **Greenstein, R. J., L. Su, A. Shahidi, and S. T. Brown.** 2007. On the action of 5-amino-salicylic acid and sulfapyridine on *M. avium* including subspecies *paratuberculosis*. *PLoS ONE* **2:**e516.
136. **Grzybowski, S., E. A. Allen, W. A. Black, C. W. Chao, D. A. Enarson, J. L. Isaac Renton, S. H. Peck, and H. J. Xie.** 1987. Inner-city survey for tuberculosis: evaluation of diagnostic methods. *Am. Rev. Respir. Dis.* **135:**1311–1315.
137. **Gumaste, V., D. B. Sachar, and A. J. Greenstein.** 1992. Benign and malignant colorectal strictures in ulcerative colitis. *Gut* **33:**938–941.
138. **Gumber, S., and R. J. Whittington.** 2007. Comparison of BACTEC 460 and MGIT 960 systems for the culture of *Mycobacterium avium* subsp. *paratuberculosis* S strain and observations on the effect of inclusion of ampicillin in culture media to reduce contamination. *Vet. Microbiol.* **119:**42–52.
139. **Guslandi, M., and A. Tittobello.** 1992. Cyclosporin for Crohn's disease? *Drugs* **43:**440–442.
140. **Hagge, D., S. O. Robinson, D. Scollard, G. McCormick, and D. L. Williams.** 2002. A new model for studying the effects of *Mycobacterium leprae* on Schwann cell and neuron interactions. *J. Infect. Dis.* **186:**1283–1296.
141. **Hampe, J., A. Cuthbert, P. J. Croucher, M. M. Mirza, S. Mascheretti, S. Fisher, H. Frenzel, K. King, A. Hasselmeyer, A. J. MacPherson, S. Bridger, S. van Deventer, A. Forbes, S. Nikolaus, J. E. Lennard-Jones, U. R. Foelsch, M. Krawczak, C. Lewis, S. Schreiber, and C. G. Mathew.** 2001. Association between insertion mutation in NOD2 gene and Crohn's disease in German and British populations. *Lancet* **357:** 1925–1928.
142. **Hampshire, T., S. Soneji, J. Bacon, B. W. James, J. Hinds, K. Laing, R. A. Stabler, P. D. Marsh, and P. D. Butcher.** 2004. Stationary phase gene expression of *Mycobacterium tuberculosis* following a progressive nutrient depletion: a model for persistent organisms? *Tuberculosis* (Edinburgh) **84:** 228–238.
143. **Hancock, G. E., A. Molloy, B. K. Ab, R. Kiessling, M. Becx-Bleumink, Z. A. Cohn, and G. Kaplan.** 1991. In vivo administration of low-dose human interleukin-2 induces lymphokine-activated killer cells for enhanced cytolysis in vitro. *Cell. Immunol.* **132:**277–284.
144. **Hansen, G. A.** 1874. Undersogelser angaende spedalskhedens arsager. *Norsk Magazin for Laegevidenskaben* **4:**1–88.
145. **Haslett, P. A., P. Roche, C. R. Butlin, M. Macdonald, N. Shrestha, R. Manandhar, J. Lemaster, R. Hawksworth, M. Shah, A. S. Lubinsky, M. Albert, J. Worley, and G. Kaplan.** 2005. Effective treatment of erythema nodosum leprosum with thalidomide is associated with immune stimulation. *J. Infect. Dis.* **192:**2045–2053.
146. **Hazbon, M. H., N. Guarin, B. E. Ferro, A. L. Rodriguez, L. A. Labrada, R. Tovar, P. F. Riska, and W. R. Jacobs, Jr.** 2003. Photographic and luminometric detection of luciferase reporter phages for drug susceptibility testing of clinical *Mycobacterium tuberculosis* isolates. *J. Clin. Microbiol.* **41:**4865–4869.
147. **Hietaharju, A., R. Croft, R. Alam, P. Birch, A. Mong, and M. Haanpaa.** 2000. Chronic neuropathic pain in treated leprosy. *Lancet* **356:**1080–1081.
148. **Hill, A. V.** 1998. The immunogenetics of human infectious diseases. *Annu. Rev. Immunol.* **16:**593–617.
149. **Hines, M. E., II, S. Stiver, D. Giri, L. Whittington, C. Watson, J. Johnson, J. Musgrove, M. Pence, D. Hurley, C. Baldwin, I. A. Gardner, and S. Aly.** 2007. Efficacy of spheroplastic and cell-wall competent vaccines for *Mycobacterium avium* subsp. *paratuberculosis* in experimentally-challenged baby goats. *Vet. Microbiol.* **120:**261–283.
150. **Ho, P., I. N. Bruce, A. Silman, D. Symmons, B. Newman, H. Young, C. E. Griffiths, S. John, J. Worthington, and A. Barton.** 2005. Evidence for common genetic control in pathways of inflammation for Crohn's disease and psoriatic arthritis. *Arthritis Rheum.* **52:**3596–3602.
151. **Holm, J.** 1959. How can elimination of tuberculosis as a public health problem be achieved. *Am. Rev. Tuberc.* **79:**690–694.
152. **Howard, T. P., and D. A. Solomon.** 1988. Reading the tuberculin skin test. Who, when, and how? *Arch. Intern. Med.* **148:**2457–2459.
153. **Huang, J. H., P. J. Oefner, V. Adi, K. Ratnam, S. J. Ruoss, E. Trako, and P. N. Kao.** 1998. Analyses of the *NRAMP1* and *IFN-γR1* genes in women with *Mycobacterium avium-intracellulare* pulmonary disease. *Am. J. Respir. Crit. Care Med.* **157:**377–381.
154. **Hugot, J. P., M. Chamaillard, H. Zouali, S. Lesage, J. P. Cezard, J. Belaiche, S. Almer, C. Tysk, C. A. O'Morain, M. Gassull, V. Binder, Y. Finkel, A. Cortot, R. Modigliani, P. Laurent-Puig, C. Gower-Rousseau, J. Macry, J. F. Colombel, M. Sahbatou, and G. Thomas.** 2001. Association of NOD2 leucine-rich repeat variants with susceptibility to Crohn's disease. *Nature* **411:**599–603.
155. **Hunger, R. E., P. A. Sieling, M. T. Ochoa, M. Sugaya, A. E. Burdick, T. H. Rea, P. J. Brennan, J. T. Belisle, A. Blauvelt, S. A. Porcelli, and R. L. Modlin.** 2004. Langerhans cells utilize CD1a and langerin to efficiently present nonpeptide antigens to T cells. *J. Clin. Investig.* **113:**701–708.
156. **Ikonomopoulos, J. A., V. G. Gorgoulis, N. G. Kastrinakis, A. A. Galanos, A. Karameris, and C. Kittas.** 2000. Experimental inoculation of laboratory animals with samples collected from sarcoidal patients and molecular diagnostic evaluation of the results. *In Vivo* **14:**761–765.
157. **Ivnitski, D., D. J. O'Neil, A. Gattuso, R. Schlicht, M. Calidonna, and R. Fisher.** 2003. Nucleic acid approaches for detection and identification of biological warfare and infectious disease agents. *Biotechniques* **35:**862–869.
158. **Iyer, A., M. Hatta, R. Usman, S. Luiten, L. Oskam, W. Faber, A. Geluk, and P. Das.** 2007. Serum levels of interferon-gamma, tumour necrosis factor-alpha, soluble interleukin-6R and soluble cell activation markers for monitoring response to treatment of leprosy reactions. *Clin. Exp. Immunol.* **150:**210–216.
159. **Jenner, E.** 1798. *An inquiry into the causes and effects of the Variolae Vaccinae, a disease discovered in some of the western counties of England, particularly Gloucestershire, and known by the name of the cow-pox*, 1st ed. Sampson Low Berwick St. (printed for the author), London, England.
160. **Job, C. K.** 1994. Pathology of leprosy, p. 193–224. *In* R. C. Hastings (ed.), *Leprosy*, 2nd ed. Churchill Livingstone, Edinburgh, United Kingdom.
161. **Johne, H. A., and L. Frothingham.** 1895. Ein eigenthumlicher fall von tuberculose beim rind (A particular case of tuberculosis in a cow). *Dtsch. Zeitschr. Tiermed. Vergl. Pathol.* **21:**438–454.

162. **Kalis, C. H., J. W. Hesselink, H. W. Barkema, and M. T. Collins.** 2001. Use of long-term vaccination with a killed vaccine to prevent fecal shedding of *Mycobacterium avium* subsp *paratuberculosis* in dairy herds. *Am. J. Vet. Res.* **62:** 270–274.

163. **Kaplan, M. H., D. Armstrong, and P. Rosen.** 1974. Tuberculosis complicating neoplastic disease: a review of 201 cases. *Cancer* **33:**850–858.

164. **Kapur, V., L. L. Li, M. R. Hamrick, B. B. Plikaytis, T. M. Shinnick, A. Telenti, W. R. Jacobs, Jr., A. Banerjee, S. Cole, K. Y. Yuen, J. E. Clarridge III, B. N. Kreiswirth, and J. M. Musser.** 1995. Rapid *Mycobacterium* species assignment and unambiguous identification of mutations associated with antimicrobial resistance in *Mycobacterium tuberculosis* by automated DNA sequencing. *Arch. Pathol. Lab. Med.* **119:** 131–138.

165. **Karesh, W. B., M. M. Uhart, E. S. Dierenfeld, W. E. Braselton, A. Torres, C. House, H. Puche, and R. A. Cook.** 1998. Health evaluation of free-ranging guanaco (Lama guanicoe). *J. Zoo Wildl. Med.* **29:**134–141.

166. **Karlen, P., R. Lofberg, O. Brostrom, C. E. Leijonmarck, G. Hellers, and P. G. Persson.** 1999. Increased risk of cancer in ulcerative colitis: a population-based cohort study. *Am. J. Gastroenterol.* **94:**1047–1052.

167. **Karran, P., and N. Attard.** 2008. Thiopurines in current medical practice: molecular mechanisms and contributions to therapy-related cancer. *Nat. Rev. Cancer* **8:**24–36.

168. **Katoch, K.** 1996. Immunotherapy of leprosy. *Indian J. Lepr.* **68:**349–361.

169. **Katoch, K., P. Singh, T. Adhikari, S. K. Benara, H. B. Singh, D. S. Chauhan, V. D. Sharma, M. Lavania, A. S. Sachan, and V. M. Katoch.** 2008. Potential of Mw as a prophylactic vaccine against pulmonary tuberculosis. *Vaccine* **26:**1228–1234.

170. **Katoch, V. M.** 1981. A report on the biochemical analysis of *Mycobacterium* W. *Lepr. India* **53:**385–369.

171. **Keane, J., S. Gershon, R. P. Wise, E. Mirabile-Levens, J. Kasznica, W. D. Schwieterman, J. N. Siegel, and M. M. Braun.** 2001. Tuberculosis associated with infliximab, a tumor necrosis factor alpha-neutralizing agent. *N. Engl. J. Med.* **345:**1098–1104.

172. **Kennedy, D. J., and G. Benedictus.** 2001. Control of *Mycobacterium avium* subsp. *paratuberculosis* infection in agricultural species. *Rev. Sci. Tech.* **20:**151–179.

173. **Khanolkar-Young, S., N. Rayment, P. M. Brickell, D. R. Katz, S. Vinayakumar, M. J. Colston, and D. N. Lockwood.** 1995. Tumour necrosis factor-alpha (TNF-α) synthesis is associated with the skin and peripheral nerve pathology of leprosy reversal reactions. *Clin. Exp. Immunol.* **99:**196–202.

174. **Kino, T., H. Hatanaka, M. Hashimoto, M. Nishiyama, T. Goto, M. Okuhara, M. Kohsaka, H. Aoki, and H. Imanaka.** 1987. FK-506, a novel immunosuppressant isolated from a *Streptomyces*. I. Fermentation, isolation, and physico-chemical and biological characteristics. *J. Antibiot.* (Tokyo) **40:**1249–1255.

175. **Kirchheimer, W. F., and E. E. Storrs.** 1971. Attempts to establish the armadillo (*Dasypus novemcinctus* Linn.) as a model for the study of leprosy. I. Report of lepromatoid leprosy in an experimentally infected armadillo. *Int. J. Lepr. Other Mycobact. Dis.* **39:**693–702.

176. **Kissler, S., P. Stern, K. Takahashi, K. Hunter, L. B. Peterson, and L. S. Wicker.** 2006. In vivo RNA interference demonstrates a role for Nramp1 in modifying susceptibility to type 1 diabetes. *Nat. Genet.* **38:**479–483.

177. **Kobayashi, K. S., M. Chamaillard, Y. Ogura, O. Henegariu, N. Inohara, G. Nunez, and R. A. Flavell.** 2005. Nod2-dependent regulation of innate and adaptive immunity in the intestinal tract. *Science* **307:**731–734.

178. **Kojima, Y., Y. Kinouchi, S. Takahashi, K. Negoro, N. Hiwatashi, and T. Shimosegawa.** 2001. Inflammatory bowel disease is associated with a novel promoter polymorphism of natural resistance-associated macrophage protein 1 (NRAMP1) gene. *Tissue Antigens* **58:**379–384.

179. **Kong, Y., M. D. Cave, L. Zhang, B. Foxman, C. F. Marrs, J. H. Bates, and Z. H. Yang.** 2007. Association between *Mycobacterium tuberculosis* Beijing/W lineage strain infection and extrathoracic tuberculosis: insights from epidemiologic and clinical characterization of the three principal genetic groups of *M. tuberculosis* clinical isolates. *J. Clin. Microbiol.* **45:**409–414.

180. **Krutzik, S. R., M. T. Ochoa, P. A. Sieling, S. Uematsu, Y. W. Ng, A. Legaspi, P. T. Liu, S. T. Cole, P. J. Godowski, Y. Maeda, E. N. Sarno, M. V. Norgard, P. J. Brennan, S. Akira, T. H. Rea, and R. L. Modlin.** 2003. Activation and regulation of Toll-like receptors 2 and 1 in human leprosy. *Nat. Med.* **9:**525–532.

181. **Krutzik, S. R., B. Tan, H. Li, M. T. Ochoa, P. T. Liu, S. E. Sharfstein, T. G. Graeber, P. A. Sieling, Y. J. Liu, T. H. Rea, B. R. Bloom, and R. L. Modlin.** 2005. TLR activation triggers the rapid differentiation of monocytes into macrophages and dendritic cells. *Nat. Med.* **11:**653–660.

182. **Kusner, D. J.** 2005. Mechanisms of mycobacterial persistence in tuberculosis. *Clin. Immunol.* **114:**239–247.

183. **Law, B. K., M. E. Waltner-Law, A. J. Entingh, A. Chytil, M. E. Aakre, P. Norgaard, and H. L. Moses.** 2000. Salicylate-induced growth arrest is associated with inhibition of p70s6k and down-regulation of c-myc, cyclin D1, cyclin A, and proliferating cell nuclear antigen. *J. Biol. Chem.* **275:** 38261–38267.

184. **Lazarevic, V., D. Nolt, and J. L. Flynn.** 2005. Long-term control of *Mycobacterium tuberculosis* infection is mediated by dynamic immune responses. *J. Immunol.* **175:**1107–1117.

185. **Lehmann, J.** 1946. Para-aminosalicylic acid in the treatment of tuberculosis. *Lancet* **i:**15–16.

186. **Lennard-Jones, J. E., D. M. Melville, B. C. Morson, J. K. Ritchie, and C. B. Williams.** 1990. Precancer and cancer in extensive ulcerative colitis: findings among 401 patients over 22 years. *Gut* **31:**800–806.

187. **Levine, J. S., and R. Burakoff.** 2007. Chemoprophylaxis of colorectal cancer in inflammatory bowel disease: current concepts. *Inflamm. Bowel Dis.* **13:**1293–1298.

188. **Lewis, J. D., J. S. Schwartz, and G. R. Lichtenstein.** 2000. Azathioprine for maintenance of remission in Crohn's disease: benefits outweigh the risk of lymphoma. *Gastroenterology* **118:**1018–1024.

189. **Li, L., J. P. Bannantine, Q. Zhang, A. Amonsin, B. J. May, D. Alt, N. Banerji, S. Kanjilal, and V. Kapur.** 2005. The complete genome sequence of *Mycobacterium avium* subspecies *paratuberculosis*. *Proc. Natl. Acad. Sci. USA* **102:** 12344–12349.

190. **Lichtiger, S., D. H. Present, A. Kornbluth, I. Gelernt, J. Bauer, G. Galler, F. Michelassi, and S. Hanauer.** 1994. Cyclosporine in severe ulcerative colitis refractory to steroid therapy. *N. Engl. J. Med.* **330:**1841–1845.

191. **Lindler, L. E., and W. Fan.** 2003. Development of a 5' nuclease assay to detect ciprofloxacin resistant isolates of the biowarfare agent *Yersinia pestis*. *Mol. Cell. Probes* **17:**41–47.

192. **Lucas, S.** 1993. Human immunodeficiency virus and leprosy. *Lepr. Rev.* **64:**97–103.

193. **Maeda, S., L. C. Hsu, H. Liu, L. A. Bankston, M. Iimura, M. F. Kagnoff, L. Eckmann, and M. Karin.** 2005. Nod2 mutation in Crohn's disease potentiates NF-$\kappa\beta$ activity and IL-1β processing. *Science* **307:**734–738.

194. **Malen, H., F. S. Berven, K. E. Fladmark, and H. G. Wiker.** 2007. Comprehensive analysis of exported proteins from

Mycobacterium tuberculosis H37Rv. *Proteomics* **7:**1702–1718.

195. **Maliarik, M. J., K. M. Chen, R. G. Sheffer, B. A. Rybicki, M. L. Major, J. Popovich, Jr., and M. C. Iannuzzi.** 2000. The natural resistance-associated macrophage protein gene in African Americans with sarcoidosis. *Am. J. Respir. Cell. Mol. Biol.* **22:**672–675.
196. **Marri, P. R., J. P. Bannantine, and G. B. Golding.** 2006. Comparative genomics of metabolic pathways in *Mycobacterium* species: gene duplication, gene decay and lateral gene transfer. *FEMS Microbiol. Rev.* **30:**906–925.
197. **Marshall, B. J.** 1983. Unidentified curved bacilli on gastric epithelium in active chronic gastritis. *Lancet* **i:**1273–1275.
198. **Marshall, B. J., and J. R. Warren.** 1984. Unidentified curved bacilli in the stomach of patients with gastritis and peptic ulceration. *Lancet* **i:**1311–1315.
199. **Matsuda, C., T. Ito, J. Song, T. Mizushima, H. Tamagawa, Y. Kai, Y. Hamanaka, M. Inoue, T. Nishida, H. Matsuda, and Y. Sawa.** 2007. Therapeutic effect of a new immunosuppressive agent, everolimus, on interleukin-10 gene-deficient mice with colitis. *Clin. Exp. Immunol.* **148:**348–359.
200. **Matula, S., V. Croog, S. Itzkowitz, N. Harpaz, C. Bodian, S. Hossain, and T. Ullman.** 2005. Chemoprevention of colorectal neoplasia in ulcerative colitis: the effect of 6-mercaptopurine. *Clin. Gastroenterol. Hepatol.* **3:**1015–1021.
201. **McClure, H. M., R. J. Chiodini, D. C. Anderson, R. B. Swenson, W. R. Thayer, and J. A. Coutu.** 1987. *Mycobacterium paratuberculosis* infection in a colony of stumptail macaques (*Macaca arctoides*). *J. Infect. Dis.* **155:**1011–1019.
202. **McFadden, J. J., and H. M. Fidler.** 1996. Mycobacteria as possible causes of sarcoidosis and Crohn's disease. Soc. *Appl. Bacteriol. Symp. Ser.* **25:**47S–52S.
203. **Menzies, D., M. Pai, and G. Comstock.** 2007. Meta-analysis: new tests for the diagnosis of latent tuberculosis infection: areas of uncertainty and recommendations for research. *Ann. Intern. Med.* **146:**340–354.
204. **Middlebrook, G., Z. Reggiardo, and W. D. Tigertt.** 1977. Automatable radiometric detection of growth of *Mycobacterium tuberculosis* in selective media. *Am. Rev. Respir. Dis.* **115:**1066–1069.
205. **Mira, M. T., A. Alcais, V. T. Nguyen, M. O. Moraes, C. Di Flumeri, H. T. Vu, C. P. Mai, T. H. Nguyen, N. B. Nguyen, X. K. Pham, E. N. Sarno, A. Alter, A. Montpetit, M. E. Moraes, J. R. Moraes, C. Dore, C. J. Gallant, P. Lepage, A. Verner, E. Van De Vosse, T. J. Hudson, L. Abel, and E. Schurr.** 2004. Susceptibility to leprosy is associated with PARK2 and PACRG. *Nature* **427:**636–640.
206. **Mishina, D., P. Katsel, S. T. Brown, E. C. Gilberts, and R. J. Greenstein.** 1996. On the etiology of Crohn disease. *Proc. Natl. Acad. Sci. USA* **93:**9816–9820.
207. **Miyazaki, E., R. E. Chaisson, and W. R. Bishai.** 1999. Analysis of rifapentine for preventive therapy in the Cornell mouse model of latent tuberculosis. *Antimicrob. Agents Chemother.* **43:**2126–2130.
208. **Modlin, R. L., J. Melancon-Kaplan, S. M. M. Young, C. Pirmez, H. Kino, J. Convit, T. H. Rea, and B. R. Bloom.** 1988. Learning from lesions: patterns of tissue inflammation in leprosy. *Proc. Nat. Acad. Sci. USA* **85:**1213–1217.
209. **Moraes, M. O., E. N. Sarno, R. M. Teles, A. S. Almeida, B. C. Saraiva, J. A. Nery, and E. P. Sampaio.** 2000. Anti-inflammatory drugs block cytokine mRNA accumulation in the skin and improve the clinical condition of reactional leprosy patients. *J. Invest. Dermatol.* **115:**935–941.
210. **Mortensen, H., S. S. Nielsen, and P. Berg.** 2004. Genetic variation and heritability in the antibody response to *Mycobacterium avium* subspecies *paratuberculosis* in Danish holstein cows. *J. Dairy Sci.* **87:**2108–2113.
211. **Moschella, S. L.** 2004. An update on the diagnosis and treatment of leprosy. *J. Am. Acad. Dermatol.* **51:**417–426.
212. **Mostowy, S., and M. A. Behr.** 2005. The origin and evolution of *Mycobacterium tuberculosis*. *Clin. Chest Med.* **26:**207–216.
213. **Mulleman, D., S. Mammou, I. Griffoul, A. Avimadje, P. Goupille, and J. P. Valat.** 2006. Characteristics of patients with spinal tuberculosis in a French teaching hospital. *Joint Bone Spine* **73:**424–427.
214. **Nagabhushanam, V., A. Solache, L. M. Ting, C. J. Escaron, J. Y. Zhang, and J. D. Ernst.** 2003. Innate inhibition of adaptive immunity: *Mycobacterium tuberculosis*-induced IL-6 inhibits macrophage responses to IFN-γ. *J. Immunol.* **171:**4750–4757.
215. **Nair, B., S. Sukumar, G. K. Poolari, and T. Appu.** 2007. Azathioprine-induced squamous cell carcinoma of the kidney. *Scand. J. Urol. Nephrol.* **41:**173–175.
216. **Naser, S. A., G. Ghobrial, C. Romero, and J. F. Valentine.** 2004. Culture of *Mycobacterium avium* subspecies *paratuberculosis* from the blood of patients with Crohn's disease. *Lancet* **364:**1039–1044.
217. **Naser, S. A., D. Schwartz, and I. Shafran.** 2000. Isolation of *Mycobacterium avium* subsp *paratuberculosis* from breast milk of Crohn's disease patients. *Am. J. Gastroenterol.* **95:**1094–1095.
218. **Nebbia, P., P. Robino, E. Ferroglio, L. Rossi, G. Meneguz, and S. Rosati.** 2000. Paratuberculosis in red deer (*Cervus elaphus hippelaphus*) in the western Alps. *Vet. Res. Commun.* **24:**435–443.
219. **Neelsen, F. C. A.** 1883. Ein casuistischer Bietrag zur Lehre von der Tuberkulose. *Zbl. med. Wiss.* **21:**497–501.
220. **Netea, M. G., T. Azam, G. Ferwerda, S. E. Girardin, M. Walsh, J. S. Park, E. Abraham, J. M. Kim, D. Y. Yoon, C. A. Dinarello, and S. H. Kim.** 2005. IL-32 synergizes with nucleotide oligomerization domain (NOD) 1 and NOD2 ligands for IL-1beta and IL-6 production through a caspase 1-dependent mechanism. *Proc. Natl. Acad. Sci. USA* **102:**16309–16314.
221. **Netea, M. G., G. Ferwerda, D. J. de Jong, T. Jansen, L. Jacobs, M. Kramer, T. H. Naber, J. P. Drenth, S. E. Girardin, B. J. Kullberg, G. J. Adema, and J. W. Van der Meer.** 2005. Nucleotide-binding oligomerization domain-2 modulates specific TLR pathways for the induction of cytokine release. *J. Immunol.* **174:**6518–6523.
222. **Ng, S. C., N. Arebi, and M. A. Kamm.** 2007. Medium-term results of oral tacrolimus treatment in refractory inflammatory bowel disease. *Inflamm. Bowel Dis.* **13:**129–134.
223. **Ng, V., G. Zanazzi, R. Timpl, J. Talts, J. L. Salzer, P. J. Brennan, and A. Rambukkana.** 2000. Role of the cell wall phenolic glycolipid-1 in the peripheral nerve predilection of *Mycobacterium leprae*. *Cell* **103:**511–529.
224. **Nishino, M., H. Ikegami, T. Fujisawa, Y. Kawaguchi, Y. Kawabata, M. Shintani, M. Ono, and T. Ogihara.** 2005. Functional polymorphism in Z-DNA-forming motif of promoter of SLC11A1 gene and type 1 diabetes in Japanese subjects: association study and meta-analysis. *Metabolism* **54:**628–633.
225. **Ochoa, M. T., S. Stenger, P. A. Sieling, S. Thoma-Uszynski, S. Sabet, S. Cho, A. M. Krensky, M. Rollinghoff, E. Nunes Sarno, A. E. Burdick, T. H. Rea, and R. L. Modlin.** 2001. T-cell release of granulysin contributes to host defense in leprosy. *Nat. Med.* **7:**174–179.
226. **Ogata, H., and T. Hibi.** 2003. Cytokine and anti-cytokine therapies for inflammatory bowel disease. *Curr. Pharm. Des.* **9:**1107–1113.

227. **Ogura, K., Y. Hirata, A. Yanai, W. Shibata, T. Ohmae, Y. Mitsuno, S. Maeda, H. Watabe, Y. Yamaji, M. Okamoto, H. Yoshida, T. Kawabe, and M. Omata.** 2008. The effect of *Helicobacter pylori* eradication on reducing the incidence of gastric cancer. *J. Clin. Gastroenterol.* **42:**279–283.

228. **Ogura, Y., D. K. Bonen, N. Inohara, D. L. Nicolae, F. F. Chen, R. Ramos, H. Britton, T. Moran, R. Karaliuskas, R. H. Duerr, J. P. Achkar, S. R. Brant, T. M. Bayless, B. S. Kirschner, S. B. Hanauer, G. Nunez, and J. H. Cho.** 2001. A frameshift mutation in NOD2 associated with a susceptability to Crohn's disease. *Nature* **411:**603–606.

229. **Oliveira, R. B., M. T. Ochoa, P. A. Sieling, T. H. Rea, A. Rambukkana, E. N. Sarno, and R. L. Modlin.** 2003. Expression of Toll-like receptor 2 on human Schwann cells: a mechanism of nerve damage in leprosy. *Infect. Immun.* **71:**1427–1433.

230. **Pai, M., K. Gokhale, R. Joshi, S. Dogra, S. Kalantri, D. K. Mendiratta, P. Narang, C. L. Daley, R. M. Granich, G. H. Mazurek, A. L. Reingold, L. W. Riley, and J. M. Colford, Jr.** 2005. *Mycobacterium tuberculosis* infection in health care workers in rural India: comparison of a whole-blood interferon gamma assay with tuberculin skin testing. *JAMA* **293:**2746–2755.

231. **Paralkar, V.** 2008. Worlds apart—tuberculosis in India and the United States. *N. Engl. J. Med.* **358:**1092–1095.

232. **Parrish, N. M., J. D. Dick, and W. R. Bishai.** 1998. Mechanisms of latency in *Mycobacterium tuberculosis*. *Trends Microbiol.* **6:**107–112.

233. **Pearce, M. J., P. Arora, R. A. Festa, S. M. Butler-Wu, R. S. Gokhale, and K. H. Darwin.** 2006. Identification of substrates of the *Mycobacterium tuberculosis* proteasome. *EMBO J.* **25:**5423–5432.

234. **Philipp, W. J., S. Poulet, K. Eiglmeier, L. Pascopella, V. Balasubramanian, B. Heym, S. Bergh, B. R. Bloom, W. R. Jacobs, Jr., and S. T. Cole.** 1996. An integrated map of the genome of the tubercle bacillus, *Mycobacterium tuberculosis* H37Rv, and comparison with *Mycobacterium leprae*. *Proc. Natl. Acad. Sci.USA* **93:**3132–3137.

235. **Pignataro, P., S. Rocha Ada, J. A. Nery, A. Miranda, A. M. Sales, H. Ferrreira, V. Valentim, and P. N. Suffys.** 2004. Leprosy and AIDS: two cases of increasing inflammatory reactions at the start of highly active antiretroviral therapy. *Eur. J. Clin. Microbiol. Infect. Dis.* **23:**408–411.

236. **Prigozy, T. I., P. A. Sieling, D. Clemens, P. L. Stewart, S. M. Behar, S. A. Porcelli, M. B. Brenner, R. L. Modlin, and M. Kronenberg.** 1997. The mannose receptor delivers lipoglycan antigens to endosomes for presentation to T cells by CD1b molecules. *Immunity* **6:**187–197.

237. **Rahman, P., S. Bartlett, F. Siannis, F. J. Pellett, V. T. Farewell, L. Peddle, C. T. Schentag, C. A. Alderdice, S. Hamilton, M. Khraishi, Y. Tobin, D. Hefferton, and D. D. Gladman.** 2003. CARD15: a pleiotropic autoimmune gene that confers susceptibility to psoriatic arthritis. *Am. J. Hum. Genet.* **73:** 677–681.

238. **Rambukkana, A., J. L. Salzer, P. D. Yurchenco, and E. I. Tuomanen.** 1997. Neural targeting of *Mycobacterium leprae* mediated by the G domain of the laminin alpha 2 chain. *Cell* **88:**811–821.

239. **Rambukkana, A., H. Yamada, G. Zanazzi, T. Mathus, J. L. Salzer, P. D. Yurchenco, K. P. Campbell, and V. A. Fischetti.** 1998. Role of alpha 2-dystroglycan as a Schwann cell receptor for *Mycobacterium leprae*. *Science* **282:** 2076–2079.

240. **Rambukkana, A., G. Zanazzi, N. Tapinos, and J. L. Salzer.** 2002. Contact-dependent demyelination by *Mycobacterium leprae* in the absence of immune cells. *Science* **296:**927–931.

241. **Ranadive, K. J., C. V. Bapat, and V. R. Khanolkar.** 1962. Studies of pathogenicity of the ICRC bacillus isolated from human lepromatous leprosy. *Int. J. Lepr.* **30:**442–456.

242. **Ranque, B., V. T. Nguyen, H. T. Vu, T. H. Nguyen, N. B. Nguyen, X. K. Pham, E. Schurr, L. Abel, and A. Alcais.** 2007. Age is an important risk factor for onset and sequelae of reversal reactions in Vietnamese patients with leprosy. *Clin. Infect. Dis.* **44:**33–40.

243. **Raviglione, M. C., and A. Pio.** 2002. Evolution of WHO policies for tuberculosis control, 1948–2001. *Lancet* **359:** 775–780.

244. **Rhodes, J. M., and P. Collins.** 2006. Lessons for inflammatory bowel disease from rheumatology. *Dig. Liver Dis.* **38:**157–162.

245. **Richter, E., J. Wessling, N. Lugering, W. Domschke, and S. Rusch-Gerdes.** 2002. *Mycobacterium avium* subsp. *paratuberculosis* infection in a patient with HIV, Germany. *Emerg. Infect. Dis.* **8:**729–731.

246. **Ridley, D. S., and W. H. Jopling.** 1966. Classification of leprosy according to immunity—a five-group system. *Int. J. Lepr. Other Mycobact. Dis.* **34:**255–273.

247. **Roche, P. W., W. J. Britton, S. S. Failbus, H. Ludwig, W. J. Theuvenet, and R. B. Adiga.** 1990. Heterogeneity of serological responses in paucibacillary leprosy—differential responses to protein and carbohydrate antigens and correlation with clinical parameters. *Int. J. Lepr. Other Mycobact. Dis.* **58:**319–327.

248. **Rodriguez, M. R., M. F. Gonzalez-Escribano, F. Aguilar, A. Valenzuela, A. Garcia, and A. Nunez-Roldan.** 2002. Association of NRAMP1 promoter gene polymorphism with the susceptibility and radiological severity of rheumatoid arthritis. *Tissue Antigens* **59:**311–315.

249. **Rohde, K., R. M. Yates, G. E. Purdy, and D. G. Russell.** 2007. *Mycobacterium tuberculosis* and the environment within the phagosome. *Immunol. Rev.* **219:**37–54.

250. **Romero-Gallo, J., E. J. Harris, U. Krishna, M. K. Washington, G. I. Perez-Perez, and R. M. Peek, Jr.** 2008. Effect of *Helicobacter pylori* eradication on gastric carcinogenesis. *Lab. Invest.* **88:**328–336.

251. **Rook, G. A., V. Adams, J. Hunt, R. Palmer, R. Martinelli, and L. R. Brunet.** 2004. Mycobacteria and other environmental organisms as immunomodulators for immunoregulatory disorders. *Springer Semin. Immunopathol.* **25:**237–255.

252. **Rosenstiel, P., K. Huse, A. Franke, J. Hampe, K. Reichwald, C. Platzer, R. G. Roberts, C. G. Mathew, M. Platzer, and S. Schreiber.** 2007. Functional characterization of two novel 5' untranslated exons reveals a complex regulation of NOD2 protein expression. *BMC Genomics* **8:**472.

253. **Rusch-Gerdes, S., G. E. Pfyffer, M. Casal, M. Chadwick, and S. Siddiqi.** 2006. Multicenter laboratory validation of the BACTEC MGIT 960 technique for testing susceptibilities of *Mycobacterium tuberculosis* to classical second-line drugs and newer antimicrobials. *J. Clin. Microbiol.* **44:** 688–692.

254. **Rutgeerts, P.** 2002. A critical assessment of new therapies in inflammatory bowel disease. *J. Gastroenterol. Hepatol.* **17**(Suppl.):S176–S185.

255. **Ryan, F.** 1992. *The Forgotten Plague: How the Battle against Tuberculosis Was Won—and Lost*. Little Brown & Co., Boston, MA.

256. **Ryan, F.** 1992. *Tuberculosis: the Greatest Story Never Told*. Swift Publishers, Worcestershire, England.

257. **Sampaio, E. P., M. O. Hernandez, D. S. Carvalho, and E. N. Sarno.** 2002. Management of erythema nodosum

leprosum by thalidomide: thalidomide analogues inhibit *M. leprae*-induced TNFα production in vitro. *Biomed. Pharmacother.* **56**:13–19.

258. **Sampaio, E. P., A. L. Moreira, E. N. Sarno, A. M. Malta, and G. Kaplan.** 1992. Prolonged treatment with recombinant interferon gamma induces erythema nodosum leprosum in lepromatous leprosy patients. *J. Exp. Med.* **175**:1729–1737.
259. **Sampath, R., T. A. Hall, C. Massire, F. Li, L. B. Blyn, M. W. Eshoo, S. A. Hofstadler, and D. J. Ecker.** 2007. Rapid identification of emerging infectious agents using PCR and electrospray ionization mass spectrometry. *Ann. N. Y. Acad. Sci.* **1102**:109–120.
260. **Sanderson, J. D., M. T. Moss, M. L. V. Tizard, and J. Hermon-Taylor.** 1992. *Mycobacterium paratuberculosis* DNA in Crohn's disease tissue. *Gut* **33**:890–896.
261. **Save, M. P., V. P. Shetty, K. T. Shetty, and N. H. Antia.** 2004. Alterations in neurofilament protein(s) in human leprous nerves: morphology, immunohistochemistry and Western immunoblot correlative study. *Neuropathol. Appl. Neurobiol.* **30**:635–650.
262. **Sbarbaro, J. A.** 1985. Tuberculin test. A re-emphasis on clinical judgement. *Am. Rev. Respir. Dis.* **132**:177–178.
263. **Scanu, A. M., T. J. Bull, S. Cannas, J. D. Sanderson, L. A. Sechi, G. Dettori, S. Zanetti, and J. Hermon-Taylor.** 2007. *Mycobacterium avium* subspecies *paratuberculosis* infection in cases of irritable bowel syndrome and comparison with Crohn's disease and Johne's disease: common neural and immune pathogenicities. *J. Clin. Microbiol.* **45**:3883–3890.
264. **Schlesinger, L. S.** 1993. Macrophage phagocytosis of virulent but not attenuated strains of *Mycobacterium tuberculosis* is mediated by mannose receptors in addition to complement receptors. *J. Immunol.* **150**:2920–2930.
265. **Schlesinger, L. S., and M. A. Horwitz.** 1991. Phenolic glycolipid-1 of *Mycobacterium leprae* binds complement component C3 in serum and mediates phagocytosis by human monocytes. *J. Exp. Med.* **174**:1031–1038.
266. **Schott, E., F. Paul, J. T. Wuerfel, F. Zipp, B. Rudolph, B. Wiedenmann, and D. C. Baumgart.** 2007. Development of ulcerative colitis in a patient with multiple sclerosis following treatment with interferon beta 1a. *World J. Gastroenterol.* **13**:3638–3640.
267. **Schurr, E., A. Alcais, M. Singh, N. Mehra, and L. Abel.** 2007. Mycobacterial infections: PARK2 and PACRG associations in leprosy. *Tissue Antigens* **69**(Suppl. 1):231–233.
268. **Scollard, D. M., L. B. Adams, T. P. Gillis, J. L. Krahenbuhl, R. W. Truman, and D. L. Williams.** 2006. The continuing challenges of leprosy. *Clin. Microbiol. Rev.* **19**:338–381.
269. **Scollard, D. M., M. P. Joyce, and T. P. Gillis.** 2006. Development of leprosy and type 1 leprosy reactions after treatment with infliximab: a report of 2 cases. *Clin. Infect. Dis.* **43**:e19–e22.
270. **Scollard, D. M., G. McCormick, and J. Allen.** 1999. Localization of *Mycobacterium leprae* to endothelial cells of epineural and perineural blood vessels and lymphatics. *Am. J. Pathol.* **154**:1611–1620.
271. **Scott-Orr, H.** 1998. Ovine Johne's disease. *Aust. Vet. J.* **76**:31.
272. **Sechi, L. A., D. Paccagnini, S. Salza, A. Pacifico, N. Ahmed, and S. Zanetti.** 2008. *Mycobacterium avium* subspecies *paratuberculosis* bacteremia in type 1 diabetes mellitus: an infectious trigger? *Clin. Infect. Dis.* **46**:148–149.
273. **Sechi, L. A., V. Rosu, A. Pacifico, G. Fadda, N. Ahmed, and S. Zanetti.** 2008. Humoral immune responses of type 1 diabetes patients to *Mycobacterium avium* subsp. *paratuberculosis* lend support to the infectious trigger hypothesis. *Clin. Vaccine Immunol.* **15**:320–326.
274. **Selby, W., P. Pavli, B. Crotty, T. Florin, G. Radford-Smith, P. Gibson, B. Mitchell, W. Connell, R. Read, M. Merrett, H. Ee, and D. Hetzel.** 2007. Two-year combination antibiotic therapy with clarithromycin, rifabutin, and clofazimine for Crohn's disease. *Gastroenterology* **132**:2313–2319.
275. **Sharma, P., R. Mukherjee, G. P. Talwar, K. G. Sarathchandra, R. Walia, S. K. Parida, R. M. Pandey, R. Rani, H. Kar, A. Mukherjee, K. Katoch, S. K. Benara, T. Singh, and P. Singh.** 2005. Immunoprophylactic effects of the anti-leprosy Mw vaccine in household contacts of leprosy patients: clinical field trials with a follow up of 8-10 years. *Lepr. Rev.* **76**:127–143.
276. **Shaw, M. A., D. Clayton, S. E. Atkinson, H. Williams, N. Miller, D. Sibthorpe, and J. M. Blackwell.** 1996. Linkage of rheumatoid arthritis to the candidate gene NRAMP1 on 2q35. *J. Med. Genet.* **33**:672–677.
277. **Shaw, M. A., D. Clayton, and J. M. Blackwell.** 1997. Analysis of the candidate gene NRAMP1 in the first 61 ARC National Repository families for rheumatoid arthritis. *J. Rheumatol.* **24**:212–214.
278. **Shen, G., Z. Xue, X. Shen, B. Sun, X. Gui, M. Shen, J. Mei, and Q. Gao.** 2006. The study recurrent tuberculosis and exogenous reinfection, Shanghai, China. *Emerg. Infect. Dis.* **12**:1776–1778.
279. **Shepard, C. C.** 1965. Stability of *Mycobacterium leprae* and temperature optimum for growth. *Int. J. Lepr.* **33**:541–550.
280. **Shepard, C. C., and J. A. Habas.** 1967. Relation of infection to tissue temperature in mice infected with *Mycobacterium marinum* and *Mycobacterium leprae*. *J. Bacteriol.* **93**:790–796.
281. **Shetty, V. P., N. H. Antia, and J. M. Jacobs.** 1988. The pathology of early leprous neuropathy. *J. Neurol. Sci.* **88**:115–131.
282. **Shin, S. J., and M. T. Collins.** 2008. Thiopurine drugs (azathioprine and 6-mercaptopurine) inhibit *Mycobacterium paratuberculosis* growth in vitro. *Antimicrob. Agents Chemother.* **52**:418–426.
283. **Singal, D. P., J. Li, Y. Zhu, and G. Zhang.** 2000. NRAMP1 gene polymorphisms in patients with rheumatoid arthritis. *Tissue Antigens* **55**:44–47.
284. **Singh, A. V., S. V. Singh, G. K. Makharia, P. K. Singh, and J. S. Sohal.** 2007. Presence and characterization of *Mycobacterium avium* subspecies *paratuberculosis* from clinical and suspected cases of Crohn's disease and in the healthy human population in India. *Int. J. Infect. Dis.* **12**:190–197.
285. **Skeiky, Y. A., and J. C. Sadoff.** 2006. Advances in tuberculosis vaccine strategies. *Nat. Rev. Microbiol.* **4**:469–476.
286. **Skinsnes, O. K.** 1964. The immunopathologic spectrum of leprosy, p. 152–182. *In* R. G. Cochrane (ed.), *Leprosy in Theory and Practice*. John Wright & Sons Ltd, Bristol, United Kingdom.
287. **Smith, D. W., and G. E. Harding.** 1977. Animal model of human disease. Pulmonary tuberculosis. Animal model: experimental airborne tuberculosis in the guinea pig. *Am. J. Pathol.* **89**:273–276.
288. **Snider, D. E., Jr., and K. G. Castro.** 1998. The global threat of drug-resistant tuberculosis. *N. Engl. J. Med.* **338**:1689–1690.
289. **Sonnenberg, P., J. Murray, J. R. Glynn, S. Shearer, B. Kambashi, and P. Godfrey-Faussett.** 2001. HIV-1 and recurrence, relapse, and reinfection of tuberculosis after cure: a cohort study in South African mineworkers. *Lancet* **358**:1687–1693.

290. **Spierings, E., T. De Boer, L. Zulianello, and T. H. Ottenhoff.** 2000. Novel mechanisms in the immunopathogenesis of leprosy nerve damage: the role of Schwann cells, T cells and *Mycobacterium leprae*. *Immunol. Cell. Biol.* **78:**349–355.

291. **Stenson, W. F., and J. Korznik.** 2003. Inflammatory bowel disease, p. 1727–1828. *In* T. Yamada (ed.), *Textbook of Gastroenterology*, 4th ed, vol. 2. Lippincott Williams & Wilkins, Philadelphia, PA.

292. **Stinear, T. P., T. Seemann, S. Pidot, W. Frigui, G. Reysset, T. Garnier, G. Meurice, D. Simon, C. Bouchier, L. Ma, M. Tichit, J. L. Porter, J. Ryan, P. D. Johnson, J. K. Davies, G. A. Jenkin, P. L. Small, L. M. Jones, F. Tekaia, F. Laval, M. Daffe, J. Parkhill, and S. T. Cole.** 2007. Reductive evolution and niche adaptation inferred from the genome of *Mycobacterium ulcerans*, the causative agent of Buruli ulcer. *Genome Res.* **17:**192–200.

293. **Stober, C. B., S. Brode, J. K. White, J. F. Popoff, and J. M. Blackwell.** 2007. Slc11a1, formerly Nramp1, is expressed in dendritic cells and influences major histocompatibility complex class II expression and antigen-presenting cell function. *Infect. Immun.* **75:**5059–5067.

294. **Suarez, P. G., C. J. Watt, E. Alarcon, J. Portocarrero, D. Zavala, R. Canales, F. Luelmo, M. A. Espinal, and C. Dye.** 2001. The dynamics of tuberculosis in response to 10 years of intensive control effort in Peru. *J. Infect. Dis.* **184:**473–478.

295. **Svartz, N.** 1942. Salazopyrin, a new sulfanilamide preparation. A. Therapeutic results in rheumatic polyarthritis. B. Therapeutic results in ulcerative colitis. C. Toxic manifestations in treatment with sulfanilamide preparations. *Acta Med. Scandinavica* **110:**577–598.

296. **Svartz, N.** 1948. The treatment of 124 cases of ulcerative colitis with salazoprine and attempts of desensibilization in cases of hypertsensitiveness to sulfa. *Acta Med. Scandinavica* **139**(Suppl. 206):465–472.

297. **Svartz, N.** 1988. Sulfasalazine: II. Some notes on the discovery and development of salazopyrin. *Am. J. Gastroenterol.* **83:**497–503.

298. **Swift, T. R.** 1974. Peripheral nerve involvement in leprosy: quantitative histologic aspects. *Acta Neuropathol.* (Berlin) **29:**1–8.

299. **Tailleux, L., S. J. Waddell, M. Pelizzola, A. Mortellaro, M. Withers, A. Tanne, P. R. Castagnoli, B. Gicquel, N. G. Stoker, P. D. Butcher, M. Foti, and O. Neyrolles.** 2008. Probing host pathogen cross-talk by transcriptional profiling of both Mycobacterium tuberculosis and infected human dendritic cells and macrophages. *PLoS ONE* **3:** e1403.

300. **Takahashi, K., J. Satoh, Y. Kojima, K. Negoro, M. Hirai, Y. Hinokio, Y. Kinouchi, S. Suzuki, N. Matsuura, T. Shimosegawa, and Y. Oka.** 2004. Promoter polymorphism of SLC11A1 (formerly NRAMP1) confers susceptibility to autoimmune type 1 diabetes mellitus in Japanese. *Tissue Antigens* **63:**231–236.

301. **Takahashi, T., and T. Nakayama.** 2006. Novel technique of quantitative nested real-time PCR assay for Mycobacterium tuberculosis DNA. *J. Clin. Microbiol.* **44:** 1029–1039.

302. **Tan, T., W. L. Lee, D. C. Alexander, S. Grinstein, and J. Liu.** 2006. The ESAT-6/CFP-10 secretion system of *Mycobacterium marinum* modulates phagosome maturation. *Cell.* Microbiol. **8:**1417–1429.

303. **Tanaka, E., T. Kimoto, H. Matsumoto, K. Tsuyuguchi, K. Suzuki, S. Nagai, M. Shimadzu, H. Ishibatake, T. Murayama, and R. Amitani.** 2000. Familial pulmonary *Mycobacterium avium* complex disease. *Am. J. Respir. Crit. Care Med.* **161:**1643–1647.

304. **Tapinos, N., M. Ohnishi, and A. Rambukkana.** 2006. ErbB2 receptor tyrosine kinase signaling mediates early demyelination induced by leprosy bacilli. *Nat. Med.* **12:** 961–966.

305. **Thompson, B. R., R. G. Clark, and C. G. Mackintosh.** 2007. Intra-uterine transmission of *Mycobacterium avium* subsp. *paratuberculosis* in subclinically affected red deer (*Cervus elaphus*). *N. Z. Vet. J.* **55:**308–313.

306. **Travis, S. P.** 2002. Which 5-ASA? *Gut* **51:**548–549.

307. **Truman, R. W., and J. L. Krahenbuhl.** 2001. Viable *M. leprae* as a research reagent. *Int. J. Lepr. Other Mycobact. Dis.* **69:**1–12.

308. **Tsolaki, A. G., S. Gagneux, A. S. Pym, Y.-O. L. G. de la Salmoniere, B. N. Kreiswirth, D. van Soolingen, and P. M. Small.** 2005. Genomic deletions classify the Beijing/W strains as a distinct genetic lineage of *Mycobacterium tuberculosis*. *J. Clin. Microbiol.* **43:**3185–3191.

309. **Turenne, C. Y., D. M. Collins, D. C. Alexander, and M. A. Behr.** 2008. *Mycobacterium avium* subsp. *paratuberculosis* and *Mycobacterium avium* subsp. *avium* are independently evolved pathogenic clones of a much broader group of *M. avium* organisms. *J. Bacteriol.* **190:** 2479–2487.

310. **Uzonna, J. E., P. Chilton, R. H. Whitlock, P. L. Habecker, P. Scott, and R. W. Sweeney.** 2003. Efficacy of commercial and field-strain *Mycobacterium paratuberculosis* vaccinations with recombinant IL-12 in a bovine experimental infection model. *Vaccine* **21:**3101–3109.

310a. **Vanderborght, P. R., H. J. Matos, A. M. Salles, S. E. Vasconcellos, V. F. Silva-Filho, T. W. Huizinga, T. H. Ottenhoff, E. P. Sampaio, E. N. Sarno, A. R. Santos, and M. O. Moraes.** 2004. Single nucleotide polymorphisms (SNPs) at −238 and −308 positions in the TNFα promoter: clinical and bacteriological evaluation in leprosy. *Int. J. Lepr. Other Mycobact. Dis.* **72:**143–148.

311. **van der Werff, T. B. J., S. Suciu, A. Thyss, Y. Bertrand, L. Norton, F. Mazingue, A. Uyttebroeck, P. Lutz, A. Robert, P. Boutard, A. Ferster, E. Plouvier, P. Maes, M. Munzer, D. Plantaz, M. F. Dresse, P. Philippet, N. Sirvent, C. Waterkeyn, E. Vilmer, N. Philippe, and J. Otten.** 2005. Value of intravenous 6-mercaptopurine during continuation treatment in childhood acute lymphoblastic leukemia and non-Hodgkin's lymphoma: final results of a randomized phase III trial (58881) of the EORTC CLG. *Leukemia* **19:**721–726.

312. **van Dieren, J. M., E. J. Kuipers, J. N. Samsom, E. E. Nieuwenhuis, and C. J. van der Woude.** 2006. Revisiting the immunomodulators tacrolimus, methotrexate, and mycophenolate mofetil: their mechanisms of action and role in the treatment of IBD. *Inflamm. Bowel Dis.* **12:**311–327.

313. Reference deleted.

314. **Vejbaesya, S., P. Mahaisavariya, P. Luangtrakool, and C. Sermduangprateep.** 2007. TNF alpha and NRAMP1 polymorphisms in leprosy. *J. Med. Assoc. Thai.* **90:**1188–1192.

315. **Velayos, F. S., E. V. Loftus, Jr., T. Jess, W. S. Harmsen, J. Bida, A. R. Zinsmeister, W. J. Tremaine, and W. J. Sandborn.** 2006. Predictive and protective factors associated with colorectal cancer in ulcerative colitis: a case-control study. *Gastroenterology* **130:**1941–1949.

316. **Velayos, F. S., J. P. Terdiman, and J. M. Walsh.** 2005. Effect of 5-aminosalicylate use on colorectal cancer and dysplasia risk: a systematic review and metaanalysis of observational studies. *Am. J. Gastroenterol.* **100:**1345–1353.

317. **Ventura, M., C. Canchaya, A. Tauch, G. Chandra, G. F. Fitzgerald, K. F. Chater, and D. van Sinderen.** 2007. Genomics of *Actinobacteria*: tracing the evolutionary history of an ancient phylum. *Microbiol. Mol. Biol. Rev.* **71:**495–548.

318. **Voskuil, M. I., K. C. Visconti, and G. K. Schoolnik.** 2004. *Mycobacterium* tuberculosis gene expression during adaptation to stationary phase and low-oxygen dormancy. *Tuberculosis* (Edinburgh) **84:**218–227.
319. **Warren, J., H. Rees, and T. Cox.** 1986. Remission of Crohn's disease with tuberculosis chemotherapy. *N. Engl. J. Med.* **314:**182.
320. **Warren, J. R.** 1983. Unidentified curved bacilli on gastric epithelium in active chronic gastritis. *Lancet* **i:**1273.
321. **Waters, M. F., R. J. Rees, A. C. McDougall, and A. G. Weddell.** 1974. Ten years of dapsone in lepromatous leprosy: clinical, bacteriological and histological assessment and the finding of viable leprosy bacilli. *Lepr. Rev.* **45:**288–298.
322. **Weinblatt, M. E., A. L. Maier, P. A. Fraser, and J. S. Coblyn.** 1998. Longterm prospective study of methotrexate in rheumatoid arthritis: conclusion after 132 months of therapy. *J. Rheumatol.* **25:**238–242.
323. **Whan, L. B., I. R. Grant, H. J. Ball, R. Scott, and M. T. Rowe.** 2001. Bactericidal effect of chlorine on *Mycobacterium paratuberculosis* in drinking water. *Lett. Appl. Microbiol.* **33:**227–231.
324. **Wheeler, P. R. 2001.** The microbial physiologist's guide to the leprosy genome. *Lepr. Rev.* **72:**399–407.
325. **Whitby, L. E. H.** 1938. Chemotherapy of pneumoccal and other infections with 2-(p aminobenzenesulphonamido) pyridine. *Lancet* **i:**1210–1212.
326. **Whittington, R. J., I. Marsh, S. McAllister, M. J. Turner, D. J. Marshall, and C. A. Fraser.** 1999. Evaluation of modified BACTEC 12B radiometric medium and solid media for culture of *Mycobacterium avium* subsp. *paratuberculosis* from sheep. *J. Clin. Microbiol.* **37:**1077–1083.
327. **Whittington, R. J., and P. A. Windsor.** 8 October 2007. In utero infection of cattle with *Mycobacterium avium* subsp. *paratuberculosis*: a critical review and meta-analysis. *Vet. J.* [Epub ahead of print.] DOI:10.1016/j.tvjl.2007.08.023.
328. **Wiegeshaus, E., V. Balasubramanian, and D. W. Smith.** 1989. Immunity to tuberculosis from the perspective of pathogenesis. *Infect. Immun.* **57:**3671–3676.
329. **Williams, D. L., M. Torrero, P. R. Wheeler, R. W. Truman, M. Yoder, N. Morrison, W. R. Bishai, and T. P. Gillis.** 2004. Biological implications of *Mycobacterium leprae* gene expression during infection. *J. Mol. Microbiol. Biotechnol.* **8:**58–72.
330. **Woese, C. R.** 1987. Bacterial evolution. *Microbiol. Rev.* **51:**221–271.
331. **Woldehanna, S., and J. Volmink.** 2004. Treatment of latent tuberculosis infection in HIV infected persons. *Cochrane Database Syst. Rev.* **1:**CD000171.
332. **Wolf, A. J., L. Desvignes, B. Linas, N. Banaiee, T. Tamura, K. Takatsu, and J. D. Ernst.** 2008. Initiation of the adaptive immune response to *Mycobacterium* tuberculosis depends on antigen production in the local lymph node, not the lungs. *J. Exp. Med.* **205:**105–115.
333. **Wolters, F. L., M. G. Russel, J. Sijbrandij, T. Ambergen, S. Odes, L. Riis, E. Langholz, P. Politi, A. Qasim, I. Koutroubakis, E. Tsianos, S. Vermeire, J. Freitas, G. van Zeijl, O. Hoie, T. Bernklev, M. Beltrami, D. Rodriguez, R. W. Stockbrugger, and B. Moum.** 2005. Phenotype at diagnosis predicts recurrence rates in Crohn's disease. *Gut* **55:**1124–1130.
334. **Wong, K. C., W. M. Leong, H. K. Law, K. F. Ip, J. T. Lam, K. Y. Yuen, P. L. Ho, W. S. Tse, X. H. Weng, W. H. Zhang, S. Chen, and W. C. Yam.** 2007. Molecular characterization of clinical isolates of *Mycobacterium tuberculosis* and their association with phenotypic virulence in human macrophages. *Clin. Vaccine Immunol.* **14:**1279–1284.
334a. **World Medical Association.** 1964–2004. World Medical Association declaration of Helsenki. Ethical principles for medical research involving human subjects. http://www.wma.net/e/policy/b3.htm.
335. **Yamamura, M., K. Uyemura, R. J. Deans, K. Weinberg, T. H. Rea, B. R. Bloom, and R. L. Modlin.** 1991. Defining protective responses to pathogens: cytokine profiles in leprosy lesions. *Science* **254:**277–279. (Erratum, **255:**12, 1992.)
336. **Yang, Y. S., S. J. Kim, J. W. Kim, and E. M. Koh.** 2000. NRAMP1 gene polymorphisms in patients with rheumatoid arthritis in Koreans. *J. Korean Med. Sci.* **15:**83–87.
337. **Yen, J. H., C. H. Lin, W. C. Tsai, T. T. Ou, C. C. Wu, C. J. Hu, and H. W. Liu.** 2006. Natural resistance-associated macrophage protein 1 gene polymorphisms in rheumatoid arthritis. *Immunol. Lett.* **102:**91–97.
338. **Zaheer, S. A., R. Mukherjee, B. Ramkumar, R. S. Misra, A. K. Sharma, H. K. Kar, H. Kaur, S. Nair, A. Mukherjee, and G. P. Talwar.** 1993. Combined multidrug and *Mycobacterium* w vaccine therapy in patients with multibacillary leprosy. *J. Infect. Dis.* **167:**401–410.
339. **Ziehl, F.** 1882. Zur Farbung des Tuberkelbacillus. *Dtsch. Med. Wschr.* **8:**451.
340. **Zodpey, S. P.** 2007. Protective effect of bacillus Calmette Guerin (BCG) vaccine in the prevention of leprosy: a meta-analysis. *Indian J. Dermatol. Venereol. Leprol.* **73:**86–93.

Sequelae and Long-Term Consequences of Infectious Diseases
Edited by Pina M. Fratamico, James L. Smith, and Kim A. Brogden

Chapter 9

Complications and Long-Term Sequelae of Infections by *Neisseria gonorrhoeae*

PER-ANDERS MÅRDH

THE GONOCOCCUS

The species *Neisseria gonorrhoeae* in the genus *Neisseria* belongs to the family *Neisseriaceae*, which consists mostly of gram-negative cocci that divide in two planes at right angles to each other (95). Gonococci can be detected in Gram- and methylene blue-stained smears of body secretions, in which characteristic "coffee bean" diplococci can be seen. Diplococci found phagocytized by polymorphonuclear leukocytes (PML) constitute a pathognomonic sign of gonorrhea affecting the genital tract (81). Gonococci may also be detected in the rectum in patients with gonococcal proctitis (23); in eye secretions in cases of gonococcal conjunctivitis (4), including in newborns with ophthalmia neonatorum (45); in the oropharynx of patients with gonococcal pharyngitis (55); and in skin blisters in cases of disseminated gonococcal infections (i.e., gonococcal septicemia) (57).

The gonococcus is a smart invader! Once inside PML, the gonococcus delays apoptosis of the host cell (93). Gonococci of some strains are even able to multiply inside PML (92). Both these characteristics constitute newly discovered virulence factors of *N. gonorrhoeae*. Tumor necrosis factor alpha-induced apoptosis may be inhibited by epithelial cell-associated gonococci, which is believed to contribute to the establishment of gonococcal infections (64). Gonococcal endotoxin may slow down or even eliminate mucociliary wave activity (47), which may favor the development of cervicitis and salpingitis (infection and inflammation of the fallopian tubes). Both in the cervical channel and in the fallopian tubes, there are ciliated cells, which can transport away microbes, as well as secretions and spermatozoa. The majority of genes considered virulence genes are also shared by nonpathogenic, harmless commensals of the family *Neisseria*, such as *N. lactamica* (94), and by the variants of *N. gonorrhoeae* not requiring blood in gonococcal agar media and CO_2 for growth (21).

Immunity to gonococcal infections is poor. Repeated attacks of gonorrhea are common in individuals who frequently expose themselves to the risk of contracting the infection. The prevalence of complications of gonorrhea depends not only on the number of individuals who become infected but also on the characteristics of the gonococcal strains causing the infection. For example, disseminated gonococcal infections are particularly common with strains resistant to the killing effect of serum components. Such strains often belong to serogroup WI (69). They are also more common in salpingitis cases and as causative agents of tubal factor infertility (TFI) and ectopic pregnancy.

EPIDEMIOLOGY OF GONORRHEA

Marked Variations in the Number of Detected Cases of Gonorrhea

There are obvious difficulties in fully explaining the marked variations in the reported number of cases of gonorrhea, including the associated complications and long-term sequelae observed over the past years. This difficulty became particularly obvious when comparing the epidemiology of *N. gonorrhoeae* and *Chlamydia trachomatis*, organisms which spread by the same mode but have had different epidemiological patterns. During the past century, there were three prevalence peaks of gonorrhea. In Europe, the first two peaks occurred during World Wars I and II, while the third occurred during the early 1970s. In most Western countries, there has been a dramatic decrease in gonorrhea cases. In the United States, there was a 74.3% reduction in the number of reported cases from 1975 through 1997 (42). A study

Per-Anders Mårdh • Department of Obstetrics and Gynaecology, Lund University, Lund, Sweden.

done in the Liverpool area in England reported that 47 (1%) of 4,680 women had a positive Gen-Probe Aptima Combo 2 assay for *N. gonorrhoeae,* whereas the corresponding percentage for 473 men tested was 1.7 (40). Recently, many countries have experienced an increase in the number of diagnosed and reported cases of gonorrhea. For example, the CDC (Centers for Disease Control and Prevention) reported that in the western states of the United States, there has been an increase of gonorrhea from 57.2 to 81.5 cases per 100,000 population from 2000 to 2005 (10).

Double Infections with Gonococci and Other Organisms

The use of nucleic acid-based tests has offered the possibility to test for coinfections with *C. trachomatis* and *N. gonorrhoeae*. Among persons aged 15 to 29 years in The Netherlands, 605 chlamydia-negative samples were selected for nucleic acid-based tests for *N. gonorrhoeae*. None were positive for *N. gonorrhoeae*, while 4 (2.4%) of 166 chlamydia-positive cases also had gonorrhea (102). In the total population of 21,000 persons screened, the positive rate for *C. trachomatis* was 2% (95% confidence interval of 1.7 to 2.3). These authors recommended that only chlamydia-positive cases should be tested for gonococcal infection in screening surveys. Therefore, the occurrence not only of postgonococcal urethritis but also of postchlamydia urethritis caused by *N. gonorrhoeae* and/or by mycoplasmas should be considered.

In addition to *N. gonorrhoeae* and *C. trachomatis*, *Mycoplasma* species such as *M. hominis* (2, 53, 58) and *M. genitalium* (13) may cause genital infection. The mycoplasma organisms may occur in coinfections with *N. gonorrhoeae.* In gonococcal urethritis in males, the concurrent presence of mycoplasma and/or chlamydia may require different antibiotic therapies from those required to cure gonococcal infections. Bacteria that normally cause upper respiratory tract infections, e.g., *Haemophilus influenzae* and group A streptococci, may also cause female genital infections, including pelvic inflammatory disease (PID), and they are often overlooked.

Impact of Screening Programs on the Detection of Gonorrhea Cases

An increase in the reported number of *N. gonorrhoeae* cases may be due to the start of or extension of screening programs for detection of *C. trachomatis* (46). This is due to the fact that currently used laboratory methods offer detection of both organisms, even if the primary intention was to detect *Chlamydia*. Thus, test kits for *N. gonorrhoeae* are offered free of charge by the same commercial companies from which one purchases the chlamydia tests (40). The influence of screening programs on the outcome of surveillance systems for these agents relates, among other things, to which individuals participate in the screening. If the individuals have not previously been enrolled in such a screening program, the number of detected cases is usually high in contrast to testing samples from previously screened populations. The most "rewarding" result will be obtained if partners of infected individuals are also notified and screened.

In the past, routine screening for *N. gonorrhoeae* was done in most maternal health care units, but since gonorrhea has become rather uncommon in such settings, screening is often not performed. However, the failure to screen pregnant woman may result in sequelae, such as blindness in newborns and postpartum infertility in the mother.

Value of Sentinel Studies

It has been common to trust data from sentinel studies in the analysis of changes in the epidemiology of diseases, i.e., data collected from one and the same clinics/laboratories over a number of years. However, in the case of gonorrhea, the value of sentinel studies will be hampered due to (i) frequent changes of laboratory methods used for detection of *N. gonorrhoeae*, (ii) changes in staff who perform screening for gonococcal infection, (iii) variations in economic support for the best diagnostic services for gonorrhea and for notification of partners of gonorrhea patients, and (iv) changes of therapy from "trial and error" to using drugs based on the results of antibiotic susceptibility tests of the gonococcal strain recovered from each infected individual. On the other hand, effective diagnostic services, obligatory partner notification, and treatment based on susceptibility data will favor combating a gonococcal epidemic and reduce the number of complications and long-term sequelae of gonorrhea.

Does Gonorrhea Enhance the Risk of HIV Infection?

In in vitro studies, the presence of *N. gonorrhoeae* enhances uptake of type 1 human immunodeficiency virus (HIV) into dendritic cells (109). However, it is not known if gonorrhea also enhances infection by HIV in vivo. There have been speculations that the HIV epidemic initially resulted in less sexual risk-taking in some populations, which led to a decrease in the number of gonorrhea cases. When antiviral therapy became available, AIDS may have been regarded as being less dangerous and thereby contributed to increased sexual risk behavior, leading to the increases in gonorrhea and other sexually transmitted infections (STIs).

LONG-TERM SEQUELAE OF GONORRHEA: DIAGNOSTIC CONSIDERATIONS

Potential Problems in Evaluation of the Role of *Neisseria gonorrhoeae* Infection in TFI

In epidemiological studies of long-term sequelae of gonorrhea, it is essential to remember that there is often a long lag time between the infection and the diagnosis of sequelae such as TFI. TFI is characterized by occlusion of the fallopian tubes, which prevents the implantation of the fertilized egg into the uterine mucosa. The prevalence of TFI correlates with gonococcal salpingitis that had been contracted many years before TFI was diagnosed. In many developed countries, women are becoming pregnant for the first time more than a decade after the most common period for contracting STIs, including gonorrhea. As a consequence, there are very few prospective studies of TFI with a convincingly long follow-up period.

Another problem in studies of long-term sequelae of gonorrhea is that at the time when the diagnosis was made, other infectious agents may have been involved in coinfections with *N. gonorrhoeae*, agents that were rarely diagnosed at that time, such as *C. trachomatis*. Routine diagnostic services for *C. trachomatis* were first offered in 1976 in Lund, Sweden, by employing cycloheximide-treated McCoy cell cultures (82). At that time, no less than one-fourth of all women with gonorrhea seen at the gynecological department were coinfected with *C. trachomatis* (83). Likewise, approximately one-third of all women with a genital chlamydia infection also had gonorrhea. Monitoring for possible coinfections with gonorrhea should be a natural complement in the etiological work-up of all patients presenting with genital discharge. In recent years, the introduction of nucleic acid-based technologies has made detection of coinfections an easier task, as diagnostic kits are offered which allow concomitant detection of *C. trachomatis* and *N. gonorrhoeae*. However, data collected before *C. trachomatis* was included in the microbiological diagnostic battery make the determination of the unique impact of gonococcal infections on many earlier cases of TFI impossible. Furthermore, the disappearance of detectable antibodies against *N. gonorrhoeae* and *C. trachomatis* due to the long lag time between the contraction of a gonococcal infection and the initiation of retrospective investigations of TFI complicates etiological studies of the condition. Moreover, detection of the causative agent(s) may not be possible, as the patient could have received antibiotics for upper respiratory or urinary tract infections or the gonorrhea may have spontaneously resolved.

Infections by *C. trachomatis* may develop into a low-grade chronic infection that can be detected in fallopian tubal tissue samples using in situ hybridization techniques (73) or other tests demonstrating chlamydia nucleic acid sequences. Chronic chlamydia infections may result in overrepresentation of *C. trachomatis* as an etiological agent causing long-term sequelae, such as TFI. Infections by *N. gonorrhoeae* may more commonly resolve and/or more easily be eradicated by antibiotic therapy than those by *C. trachomatis* and thereby lead to an underestimation of gonococci as the etiological agent. Antibodies against various disease agents may persist for quite different periods of time, which limits the value of follow-up testing of persons in studies of sequelae. Recently, *M. hominis* has been reconfirmed as still another infectious agent independently associated with TFI (2, 53). *M. hominis* is an agent for which diagnostic services are not widely available, and therefore, determination of the role of *M. hominis* is not often done.

Value of Different Microbiological Laboratory Tools To Establish the Impact of Gonococcal Infections in Long-Term Sequelae

The widely used PCR tests for *C. trachomatis* available from Abbott or Roche that are based on a sequence in the cryptic plasmids which are found in the vast majority of strains of *C. trachomatis* did not detect chlamydia infection in one-third to more than half of all tested persons in different counties in Sweden. A retest of these individuals by the use of other technologies, such as the 16S RNA-based chlamydia test from GenProbe, indicated that they were infected with *C. trachomatis*. Therefore, a study on acute salpingitis and TFI based on the Abbott or Roche PCR tests would have resulted in a skewed distribution of the relative importance of gonorrhea versus genital chlamydia infections in these diseases. In attempts to establish the impact of infections with *N. gonorrhoeae* on sequelae, it is essential to know not only the sensitivity and specificity but also the positive and negative predictive values for the diagnostic method(s) employed. Some tests may not work very well in populations in which the prevalence of the infection under study is low (71).

Culture

Gonococcal culture results are highly dependent on the source of the blood used to produce chocolate agar for isolation studies. As a general rule, culture techniques should be more sensitive than microscopy. If this is not the case, there are reasons to believe that the medium is not optimal. The percentage of gonorrhea cases detected by microscopy of Gram-stained genital secretion was only 70% compared to culture isolation from women seen at U.S. venereal disease clinics (43). However, in long-standing gonococcal infections, the percentage of culture-positive females is even lower than that found by microscopy. In a study of male sexually transmitted disease (STD) clinic patients in the United Kingdom, Ryder and Ivens (86) made the provocative statement that it would cost £5,700 to detect an additional case of gonorrhea by performing both microscopy and culture, and they argued for reconsideration of whether cultures should be done at all in screening for gonorrhea. One traditional method to increase the isolation frequency of bacteria has been to use enrichment broth media. Such enrichment media for *N. gonorrhoeae* has been described (50, 96). It is somewhat surprising that such media have not been used in routine diagnosis of gonorrhea. In heterosexual persons, cultures of rectal, in addition to urethral and cervical, specimens may add approximately 5% to the detection rate of gonorrhea. This percentage is considerably higher in men who have sex with men (MSM). If optimal diagnostic services that include testing each gonococcal isolate for its antibiotic susceptibility are not done, the infected persons may have increased risks for developing long-term sequelae.

Nucleic Acid-Based Tests

DNA- and RNA-based diagnostic methods for gonorrhea are valuable, particularly when used in settings where gonococcal culture techniques are not used or are of low quality. On the other hand, the use of PCR tests in screening for gonococci in low-prevalence populations may have a low positive predictive value (44). Furthermore, PCR tests may detect other *Neisseria* species, particularly in tests of pharyngeal and rectal samples (for which PCR tests are not recommended by the FDA). Mangold and coworkers (44) used a method based on 16S rRNA real-time/melt curve analyses to confirm positive tests for *N. gonorrhoeae* by Roche's COBAS Amplicor PCR test. Their method confirmed that species other than *N. gonorrhoeae* were responsible for most of the false-positive tests. The relative value of real-time PCR tests (29) compared with those of other methods that are used in screening programs for gonorrhea still requires further evaluation. Inhibitory substances present in urine may require retesting of specimens when using PCR tests for diagnosing gonorrhea (27). With the introduction of PCR, it seems to have become "old fashioned" to isolate gonococci by culture. However, culture should still have a central diagnostic role for gonorrhea.

Serology

A number of techniques have been used to study serum antibodies to *N. gonorrhoeae,* including complement fixation, immunofluorescence, passive hemolysis, and indirect hemagglutination assays (48, 87). However, serology has never been a standard means to diagnose gonococcal infections but is valuable in seroepidemiological studies of resolved gonococcal infections. A population-based study in Greenland serves as an example. Gonococcal antibody-positive women had an age span from early prepubertal to late postmenopausal age. Antibody-positive men were found in all age groups (49) (Fig.1). This indicates that when a study of the epidemiology of sequelae of gonorrhea in a population is conducted, it is essential to consider the gender ratios in that population.

Miettinen et al. (58) and Baczynska et al. (2) found serological evidence that *N. gonorrhoeae*, *C. trachomatis*, and *M. hominis* were independently associated with TFI. This stresses the importance of a multimicrobial approach in studies of sequelae of infections that are sexually transmitted.

In acute STIs, there may be no detectable immunoglobulin M (IgM) antibodies. The demonstration of IgM antibodies and then the production of IgG antibodies to the same agent have traditionally been considered a sign that a given agent has caused the infection. The lack of detectable IgM antibodies to *C. trachomatis* as the causative agent of salpingitis exemplifies this diagnostic limitation. The use of IgA antibodies to diagnose genital infections by STD agents is not feasible since there is a poor correlation of IgA to current infections. Another problem that occurs when using serology in studies of long-term sequelae is that the antibodies detected may not be an indication of the complication under study, but rather may be a response to an uncomplicated infection, such as gonococcal urethritis or cervicitis, and not a response to PID. Another way to study the impact of specific organisms on long-term sequelae is to detect antibodies to heat shock proteins, such as chlamydia heat shock protein 60 (chsp60) in studies of TFI. The presence of such antibodies indicated

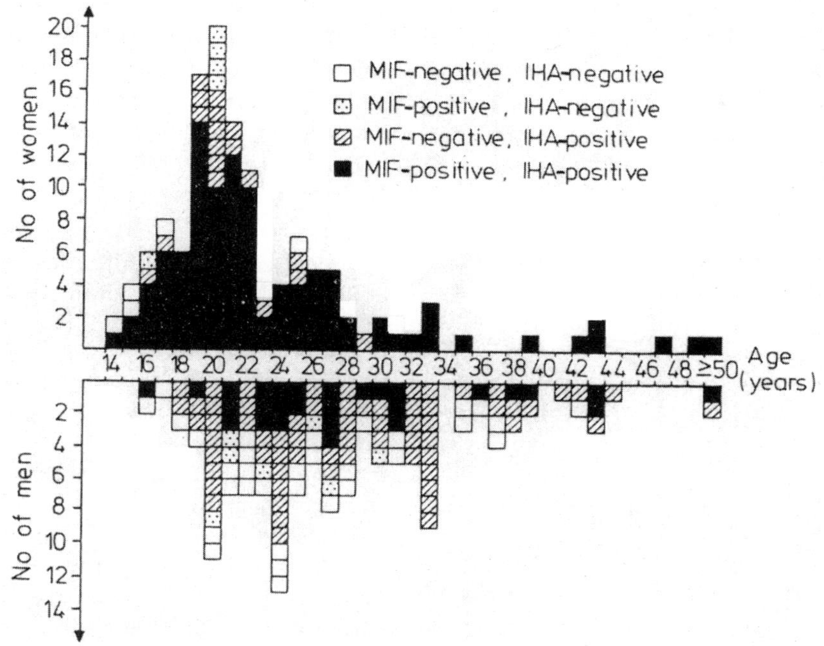

Figure 1. Microimmunofluorescent (MIF) and indirect hemagglutination (IHA) antibodies to *Neisseria gonorrhoeae* in males and females attending a venereal disease clinic in Greenland.

that there was a two- to threefold increased risk of having had one or more episodes of salpingitis associated with *C. trachomatis* (74).

Sampling: How and from Where?

Sampling, particularly from the male urethra may be so painful that the infected person may not show up again for testing after therapy. This obstacle may influence combating any infectious epidemic in which the etiological diagnosis involves urethral sampling. Rumors circulate among men about this "horrible" procedure, leading to the failure of men to show up for gonorrhea screening. Often urethral samples are collected with the patient standing up, which is painful, and may result in mucosal lesions, which may cause urethral stricture as a long-term sequela (see below). The patient may also faint when standing up and fall to the floor with risks for a serious outcome. Therefore, the patient should lie down and the penis should be lifted up, which will allow the sampling stick to be introduced into the urethra to a depth that is optimal for sampling and is pain free.

In selected groups of patients, for example, in MSM, gonococcal infections may be missed if extragenital sites, such as the rectum and the oropharynx, are not screened for *N. gonorrhoeae*. Kent and coworkers (39) found that 64% of such men, when tested by nucleic acid amplification only from the urethra, gave a negative test result for *N. gonorrhoeae* compared to men subjected to sampling at extragenital sites; therefore, urethral sampling alone would give an incorrect diagnosis. In studies of long-term sequelae of STIs in this group of patients, the impact of gonococcal infections may be underestimated if multiple sites are not sampled.

Attempts have been made to increase the detection rate of oral-pharyngeal gonorrhea by collection of samples either as a water rinse or with an oral-pharyngeal rinse solution, instead of by using swabs. Papp et al. (72) analyzed rinse solutions by a Gen-Probe PCR. The use of self-sampled vaginal swabs instead of other genital specimens for detection of gonorrhea and chlamydial infections has been evaluated. When using nucleic acid-based detection methods, such samples are preferred over earlier recommended types of samples, such as urine and cervical swabs (30).

SPECIFIED COMPLICATIONS AND LONG-TERM SEQUELAE OF GONORRHEA

PID (Endometritis and Salpingitis)

Gonococcal endometritis is usually regarded as part of an ascending infection reaching the fallopian tubes leading to salpingitis. Since it is difficult to distinguish between these entities clinically, the term pelvic inflammatory disease (PID) is used to cover both conditions. Gonococcal endometritis is characterized by an intensive plasma cell infiltration in the endometrium (Color Plate 5), a characteristic also found in chlamydial endometritis (51). Early descriptions of gonococcal endometritis may have overlooked a concomitant infection with *C. trachomatis*, an organism generally undiagnosed at the time. Thus, it is unclear to what extent gonorrhea exclusively or in combination with a chlamydia infection corresponds to the original description of gonococcal endometritis. Sequelae of endometritis include abortion or fertility problems related to the process of implantation of a fertilized ovum in the uterine mucosa.

The prevalence of salpingitis as a complication of cervical gonorrhea seems to be related to the serovars of *N. gonorrhoeae* that were circulating in the community at the time of the study period. In addition, the epidemiology of gonococcal septicemia is dependent on the dominant serovar type(s) (87). The diagnosis of gonococcal endometritis may be established by performing endometrial aspirates, and salpingitis may be established by visual inspection of the fallopian tubes (34) during laparoscopy and laparotomy or "by robot keyhole (minimally invasive) surgery." A high proportion of all gonorrhea cases present with few symptoms, and the patient does not consult a physician; therefore, clinically "silent" cases of salpingitis are not diagnosed. Many women diagnosed with TFI cannot remember if they had an episode that may have been salpingitis. The percentage of "silent" cases is not known, and it is not known if the percentage of cases has changed over time. The difficulty in diagnosing ascending genital infections has hampered studies of long-term sequelae of PID.

There are four types of infections that can lead to PID and its long-term sequelae; the infective agents may occur alone or in various combinations. In addition to *N. gonorrhoeae*, *C. trachomatis* (52), *M. hominis* (53), and *M. genitalium* (1, 13) can be involved. The last agent seems, however, to be less commonly involved in ascending genital infections in the female than the other three microorganisms. This is in contrast to nongonococcal urethritis in males in which *M. genitalium* is a common cause. The spread of gonococci to the fallopian tubes is canalicular through the uterus, while *M. hominis* may be spread to the parametrial lymphatics (59, 61).

Double or even multiple infections with *N. gonorrhoeae*, *C. trachomatis*, and *M. hominis* are common. The relative proportion of each agent as the cause of salpingitis is, of course, dependent on the local epidemic situation. Since *Mycoplasma* infections are nonreportable, their epidemiology is poorly documented. Potential coinfection with more than one organism in cervical, uterine, and tubal infections is of concern when choosing an antibiotic(s). If diagnostic services for detecting microbial organisms are poor, it will be difficult to determine an "umbrella" regimen for treatment of all of the organisms that may be involved in the infection. If the laboratory is to perform diagnostic tests for all possible agents, different sampling and transportation requirements must be followed.

Increased Risk for Infertility with an Increased Number of Salpingitis Episodes

In one study in Sweden from 1970 to 1980, when infections with both *N. gonorrhoeae* and *C. trachomatis* were common in women with acute salpingitis, the risk of future involuntary childlessness increased by 25% with each new episode of salpingitis. Women with a history of a resolved ascending genital infection should be informed about this increased risk if they become reinfected; however, this type of counseling is seldom performed. Furthermore, women with a vaginal flora change, e.g., with bacterial vaginosis or the "lactobacilli deficiency syndrome," may run a particular risk for repeated tubal infections with non-STD agents ascending from the vagina. An attempt to correct the vaginal flora to a lactobacilli-dominated flora is essential to protect the fertility of these particular women.

Postpartum PID and the "One-Child Sterility Syndrome"

Testing of pregnant women for *N. gonorrhoeae* in maternal health care units is seldom done since gonorrhea has become uncommon in pregnant women. In the long run, however, this may result in an increase in postpartum infertility as a long-term sequela in mothers, as well as blindness in the offspring. A gonococcal infection, which may have been transmitted to a primipara woman by an unfaithful husband, may result in an ascending genital infection after the delivery, when canalicular spread again becomes possible. The postpartum infection may cause infertility in the mother, a phenomenon known as "the one-child sterility syndrome."

TFI

Serological studies have demonstrated that gonococci, chlamydia, and mycoplasma organisms are independently associated with TFI (1, 58). A recent serological study did not, however, find any evidence of an association between TFI and a resolved infection with *M. genitalium* (36).

There are a number of obstacles in the evaluation of the impact of gonorrhea on TFI. Today, the mean age when women in many Western communities become pregnant for the first time has steadily increased. The time lag between a primary tubal infection and when a woman conceives may often be more than 15 years. Thus, the time span between contracting gonorrhea and when TFI is first diagnosed makes it difficult to define the relative importance of *N. gonorrheae* and other organisms in TFI. The relative impact of different organisms on TFI has also changed over the years. At present, it is believed that chlamydia infections cause more cases of TFI than gonorrhea.

Pathological Alterations of Tubal Tissue in Salpingitis Leading to Infertility as a Long-Term Sequela

Both gonococci and chlamydia organisms can cause a profound destruction of the tubal epithelium (62) (Color Plate 6). With tubal tissue cell cultures experimentally infected with either *M. hominis* or *M. genitalium*, a characteristic swelling or "ballooning" of the cilia has been observed (1, 3). Experimental infection of tissue cell cultures of tubal epithelium by *N. gonorrhoeae,* as well as treatment of such cultures with purified gonococcal endotoxin, caused a slowing down of the mucociliary wave activity of the ciliated epithelium (47) (Fig. 2). This phenomenon, occurring in vivo, may interfere with removal of microbes invading the tube. The concentration of tumor necrosis factor alpha in the mucosa of tissue cell cultures of tubal epithelium infected by gonococci correlates with sloughing of ciliated cells (56). There is an intracellular uptake of gonococci in mucosal, nonciliated tubal cells following enfolding of the bacteria by cellular pseudopods. Pseudopods are formed after mucosal cells are exposed to endotoxin excreted by the gonococci (Fig. 3). Inside mucosal cells, the gonococcus is safe from the influence of immune defense mechanisms mediated by antibodies and complement factors and from digestion by PML. Gonococcal lipid A has been considered as an important tissue-damaging component. Both an increased adhesiveness and enhanced internalization of *N. gonorrhoeae,* as well as changes in the expression of the CD66 and synecan-1 receptors, can be demonstrated in oviduct epithelium obtained from women carrying copper T intrauterine devices (IUD) and in Norplant users, compared with women not using any of these contraceptive methods (19). IUD users have a threefold greater risk of developing salpingitis if they contract STIs compared to nonusers (105).

How a concomitant tubal infection with gonococci and chlamydia organisms correlates with the development of tubal tissue damage and its long-term sequelae is not known. Chlamydial tubal infections downregulate the local immune response, and

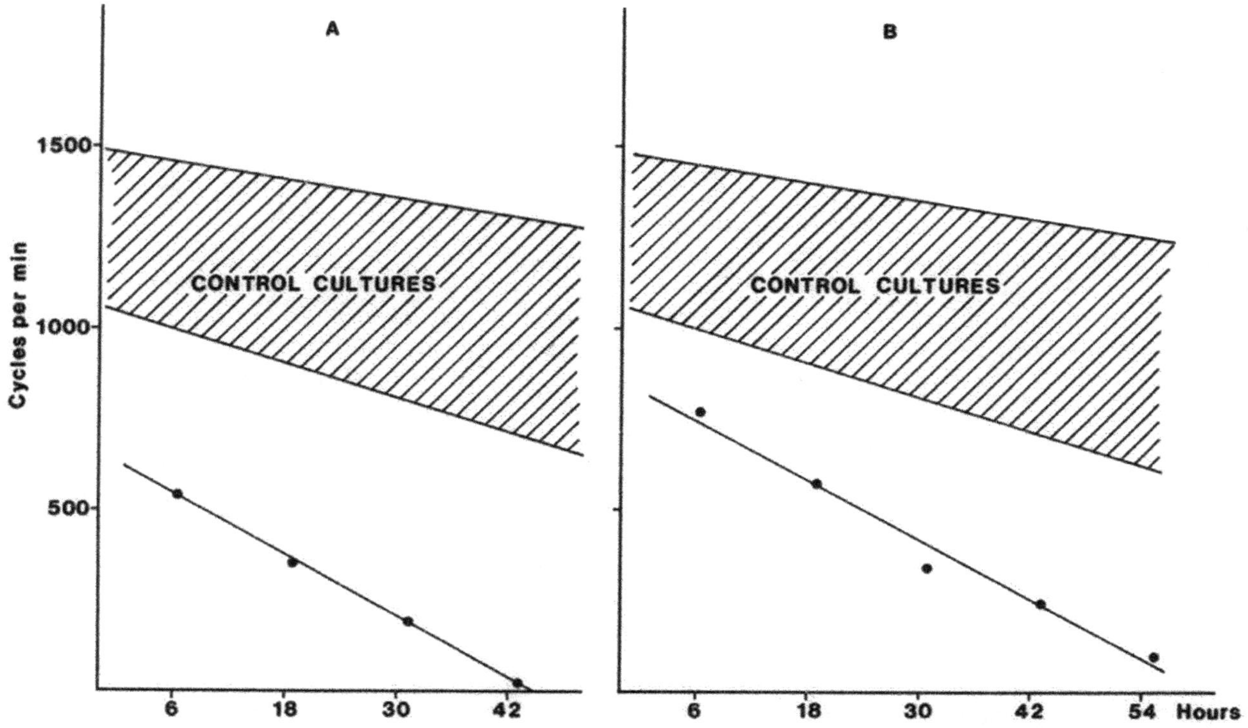

Figure 2. Influence of cell-free culture filtrates of *N. gonorrhoeae* (A) and purified gonococcal endotoxin (B) on mucociliary wave activity in tissue cell culture of human fallopian tube epithelium.

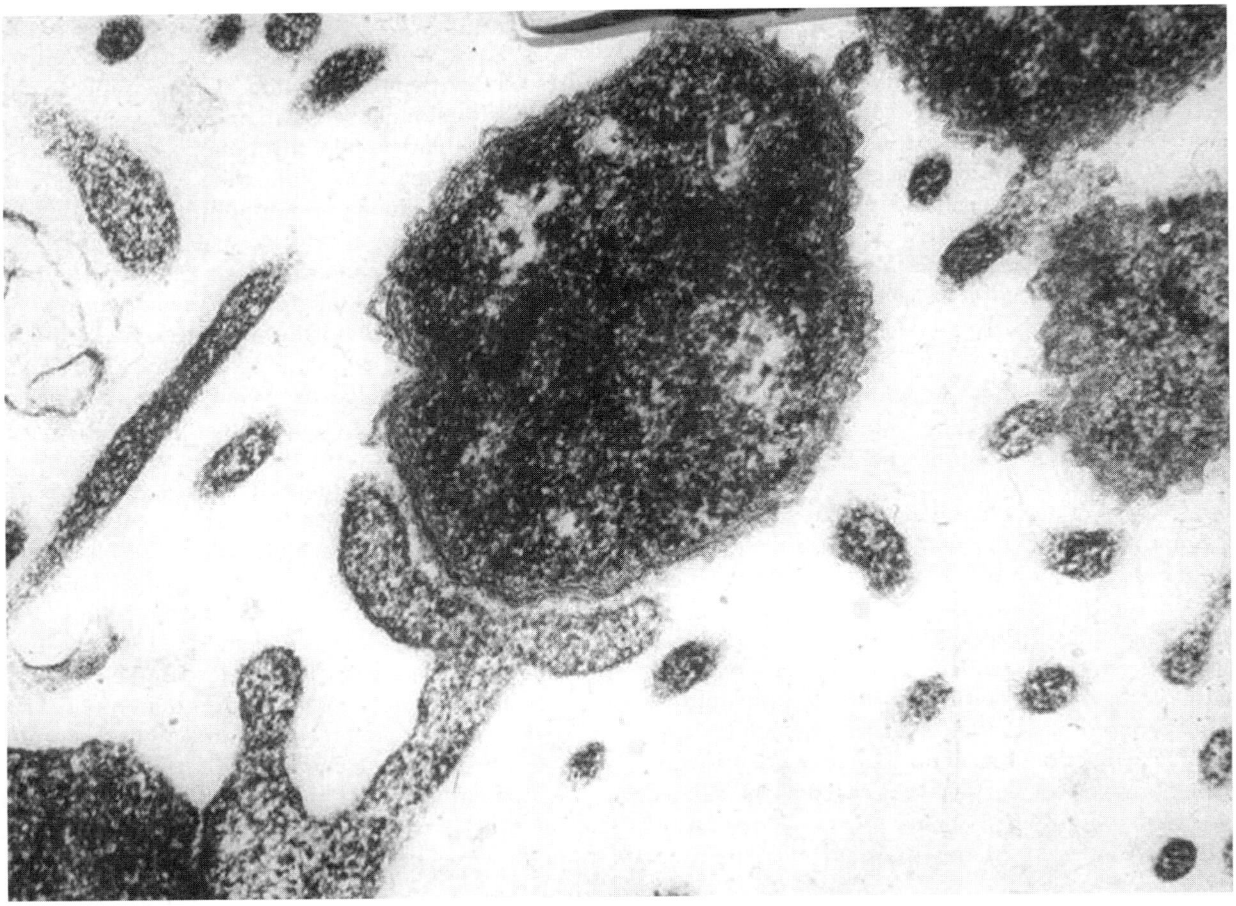

Figure 3. Electron micrograph showing gonococci and gonococcal endotoxin blebs, which can be seen as indistinct structures outside the epithelial cells. The endotoxin, in turn, influences the host cells to produce pseudopodia. There is a repelling force between gonococci and host cells, which are both negatively charged. The tip of a cell pseudopodium and the tip of a gonococcal pilus represent a minimal contact surface with a minimum of physical repelling force, which will facilitate the initial phase of an intracellular uptake of gonococci.

the reproductive rate of chlamydia organisms in the tubes is low. Both of these factors will favor the development of a chronic, low-grade tubal infection by the organisms. The process may slowly cause tubal tissue degradation, resulting in obliteration of the fallopian tubes followed by subfertility or infertility, particularly if the salpingitis affects both sides.

Ectopic Pregnancy

Ectopic or extrauterine pregnancy may be another long-term sequela of gonococcal salpingitis (58). The number of diagnosed and reported cases of ectopic pregnancy depends on the diagnostic criteria used. There has been a marked drop in the reported rate of ectopic pregnancy in many countries, including the United States and Canada. It is tempting to believe that at least part of the reduced number of ectopic pregnancies is related to the marked drop in gonococcal infections seen in most countries. However, the rate of hospital diagnoses of ectopic pregnancy has decreased, as many cases are now treated in private practices. Ectopic pregnancy often occurs many years after an episode of gonorrhea.

Women carrying an IUD run an increased risk of developing both PID and ectopic pregnancy (105, 107). The individual role of infections by *N. gonorrhoeae* and *C. trachomatis* may be difficult to establish retrospectively in a given case of ectopic pregnancy. In a study of *M. genitalium,* there was no serological evidence of an association with ectopic pregnancy (36).

Adverse Pregnancy Outcome after IVF May Indirectly Be Linked to Gonorrhea

As a consequence of TFI due to an infection by *N. gonorrhoeae,* couples who wish to have children may try to conceive by in vitro fertilization (IVF). Such a procedure involves a greater risk of adverse pregnancy outcome compared to conception by natural means. If more than one egg is transferred at IVF, there is a risk of twins or even multifetal pregnancies. Multiple pregnancies are associated with an increased rate of premature delivery, which in turn means a threat of stillbirth or severe neonatal central nervous system and pulmonary complications in the newborn. A preterm delivery may also affect the normal mental development of the child.

Perihepatitis (Fitz-Hugh-Curtis Syndrome)

The spread of gonococci from the fallopian tubes into the abdominal cavity and onto the surface of the liver was believed to be the cause of Fitz-Hugh-Curtis syndrome. The syndrome is characterized by the liver surface being covered by a layer of fibrinous mucus, which gives it a pale white color that can easily be seen through a laparoscope. There is generally only a slight increase in serum liver transamines. Liver biopsies reveal a slight congestion in the capillaries close to the liver surface. There may also be "violin string" adhesions in the abdominal cavity (see below). However, it is now obvious that *C. trachomatis*, not *N. gonorrhoeae*, is the most common cause of perihepatitis (54). It may even be questioned if gonorrhea can induce Fitz-Hugh-Curtis syndrome at all. Hormonal oral contraceptives containing estrogen may interfere with the spread of chlamydia organisms from the fallopian tubes to the abdominal cavity.

Chronic Abdominal Pain—a Sequela of Gonococcal Salpingitis?

Chronic abdominal pain following salpingitis has been associated with formation of "violin string" adhesions (108). They may hinder the free movement of the intestines and other intra-abdominal structures. There has been no consensus on whether or not the "strings" should be cut in an attempt to increase mobility of the intestines in order to reduce the risk for chronic abdominal pain. "Violin string" adhesions have been associated with both gonococcal and chlamydial abdominal infections. The spread of tubal infections to the abdominal cavity is influenced by the use of hormonal contraceptives, particularly estrogen-containing contraceptives. In a study of women with chlamydia salpingitis and who were taking contraceptive pills, only 3% developed chlamydial perihepatitis, compared to 27% of women not using such contraceptives (Mårdh et al., unpublished data). Therefore, women on such pills may be protected against spread of tubal infections to the abdominal cavity compared to nonusers. Thus, there are pros and cons for oral versus barrier contraceptive methods when focusing on the risk of developing long-term sequelae from salpingitis.

Periappendicitis

Periappendicitis is characterized by serosal inflammation of the appendix without mucosal involvement. Cases of periappendicitis have been described in the surgical literature as a complication of abdominal surgery or sepsis. One abstract of a study of periappendicitis starts as follow: "Periappendicitis has heretofore been regarded as a pathologic curiosity with little clinical significance" (20). In their series of 292 appendectomized patients, 41 actually had periappendicitis. It is notable that there were 32 females in this group, but only 9 males, with a mean age of 29 years. The authors end their abstract by concluding that identification of periappendicitis is of "definite clinical significance." Periappendicitis may also result in chronic abdominal pain as a long-term sequela. As periappendicitis may be a complication of acute salpingitis, a gynecological examination ought to be a standard procedure in young women in whom appendicitis is diagnosed. Mårdh and Wölner-Hanssen (54) indicated that periappendicitis can be caused by *C. trachomatis*. In their series of periappendicitis cases, gonorrhea was not diagnosed.

The presence of an STI should be sought in periappendicitis cases: if the person is positive, then the proper antibiotic can be prescribed and the person's partner notified. It is not known if estrogen-containing contraceptives may protect women against *Chlamydia*-induced perihepatitis and periappendicitis.

Sacroiliitis

Sacroiliitis is a painful spondylitis that may be associated with fallopian tube infections (25, 70). In a study of 57 salpingitis patients, 39 (68%) had signs of sacroiliitis, whereas this condition was seen in only 1 (3%) of 31 healthy controls (25). Sacroiliitis belongs to a group of complications that is particularly common in HLA-27-positive persons. It is also associated with uveitis. The condition is not merely due to an invasion of a microbial agent, but rather linked to an immunological process. However, Hagenfeldt and Szanto (25) found the frequencies of HLA-27 positivity to be similar in their salpingitis patients and healthy controls. Olhagen (70) reported that HLA-27-negative patients developed ankylosing spondylitis less often than those who were HLA-27 positive.

Urethral Stricture

Urethral stricture is one of the long-term sequelae of gonorrhea. However, the prevalence of urethral stricture after gonococcal urethritis in males and particularly in females is poorly documented. A frequency of 3% of urethral stricture after gonococcal urethritis has been cited in the older literature before the antibiotic era (32). It is not known if chlamydial infections are causes of urethral stricture and to what extent coinfections with *C. trachomatis* and *N. gonorrhoeae* increase the risk of stricture. Likewise, it is not known to what extent, if any, traumatic lesions from urethral sampling in urethritis cases contribute to the frequency of urethral stricture. Catherization for medical reasons or performed as a part of a sexual stimulation may also be an etiological factor. Urinary tract infections and hydronephosis may be secondary sequelae of urethral stricture, which in turn may severely interfere with kidney function. Focus on urethral stricture as a long-term sequela of gonorrhea has partly faded away and seems to have become less of a medical problem due to effective antibiotic therapy.

Epididymitis/Vasitis and Infertility

Epididymitis is a rather uncommon complication of urethritis, which only infrequently results in infertility, partly because it generally does not affect both sides. There are no recent data that are suitable for establishing the risk for infertility as a long-term sequela of gonococcal epididymitis. Epididymitis is often associated with oligoospermia, which may contribute to male subfertility. An obstacle in long-term retrospective studies performed in order to determine a possible role of gonococcal epididymitis in male infertility has been the possible involvement of double infections with *C. trachomatis*. In studies from the 1970s and 1980s, chlamydia-associated epididymitis cases were more common than those caused by *N. gonorrhoeae* (28, 31). Today most cases of male infertility following infections are due to a resolved episode of mumps involving the testicles. Gram-negative bacteria, such as *Escherichia coli*, are involved in epididymitis in elderly men, particularly in men with prostate enlargement and a history of urinary tract infections.

In ascending gonococcal infections in males, the vas deferens may be affected with swelling of the mucosal surface causing partial or total obliteration of the spermatic cord. This, in turn, may result in transient or long-term fertility problems. Chlamydial infections may cause vasitis with obliteration of the duct, as demonstrated in experimentally infected grivet monkeys (60). Genital infectious conditions, possibly including infections by *N. gonorrhoeae*, may result in thrombosis of pelvic vessels, which recently has been identified as a possible cause of ejaculation problems, with the possibility of fertility problems.

Disseminated Gonococcal Infection

Disseminated gonococcal infection (DGI) (gonococcal septicaemia) is a term covering bacteremia and the appearance of hemorrhagic pustules on a pink base, often covering interphalangeal joints. There may also be macules with pinpoint vesiculation and a vasculitis rash (35). Biopsies of such lesions show a dense neutrophilic infiltrate with leukocytoclasis and a fibrin deposit in the superficial and deep dermal vessels (57). As the gonococcus is a gram-negative bacterium, "gram-negative" shock may develop in DGI, which can be fatal, particularly if misdiagnosed and treated with vasoconstriction therapy. In DGI, there may also be arthralgia and septic arthritis, which affect large joints, particularly the knees. Endocarditis is another very rare complication of DGI (see below).

The prevalence of DGI is highly related to the characteristics of the strains of *N. gonorrhoeae* circulating in the population. Several studies have demonstrated that gonococcal strains causing DGI differ from those found in uncomplicated gonorrhea. The latter strains more frequently belong to serogroup WIG, in contrast to those not causing sepsis (69, 88). These DGI strains are often resistant to killing by serum. Others have demonstrated that DGI strains, which contain the protein IAN, are resistant to the bactericidal action of serum (65). Strains causing DGI often produce colonies of the transparent phenotype. O'Brien and coworkers (69) found 90% of strains recovered from cases with DGI to produce transparent colonies on chocolate agar. Power and coworkers (76), in contrast to earlier studies, did not find a correlation between strains recovered from patients with DGI and the *pglA* gene and its phase-variable allele. No particular gonococcal auxotype has been associated with DGI.

Gonococcal Endocarditis and Meningitis

Endocarditis may become a complication of gonococcal septicaemia (14), which may result in heart failure, a serious, although rare, long-term sequela of gonorrhea. Gonococcal meningitis is an extremely rare condition, and only a few cases, confirmed by culture studies, have been reported (6). There is an old saying "the gonococcus and the meningococcus are two brothers, but they never meet." This saying seems true as far as the central nervous system is concerned. It should be pointed out that the presence of meningococci in clinical specimens may cause a positive PCR test for *N. gonorrhoeae*, giving a false diagnosis of gonorrhea. This is one reason why gonococcal PCR tests have not been recommended for extragenital samples.

Gonococcal Arthritis and Reiter's Syndrome

The nomenclature and definitions for conditions affecting the joints have changed over the years, making it difficult to compare "older" and "newer" studies with regard to their association to gonococcal infections. Gonorrhea was a common infection in cases diagnosed as "Romanus spondarthritis" or "uroarthritis" during the 1940s and 1950s, when postgonorrhea cases constituted 35 to 50% of all such cases (70). In the past, *N. gonorrhoeae* was the most common cause of septic monoarticular and oligoarticular arthritis (80, 81). The recent marked drop in the prevalence of "uroarthritis" associated with gonorrhea is believed to relate to the use of antibiotic therapy at an early stage of infection.

Reiter's syndrome may be associated with enterically and sexually transmitted infections and often occurs after the first sexual contact with a new partner. The exact contribution of gonorrhea to Reiter's syndrome is unclear. Joint involvement in the syndrome (apart from those of the eyes and genital tract, i.e., uveitis and urethritis) is due to the triggering of immunological reactions rather than microbial invasion of the joints.

Neonatal Conjunctivitis

Neonatal gonococcal conjunctivitis (ophthalmia neonatorum) may result in blindness, therefore constituting one of the most serious sequelae of infections with *N. gonorrhoeae*. Medical textbooks state that neonatal gonococcal conjunctivitis may run an extremely rapid course, resulting in blindness within a few hours after the eyes have become infected. The diagnosis of neonatal gonococcal conjunctivitis can be rapidly established by microscopy by staining eye secretions with methylene blue and Gram stain and/or by fluorescent gonococcal antibody preparations. Gonococcal cultures and antibiotic susceptibility tests of isolated gonococcal strains should be performed. Obviously, a child with gonococcal conjunctivitis should always be given general antibiotic therapy as soon as possible. In addition, the parents should be treated.

Proper administration of silver nitrate after birth can prevent gonococcal conjunctivitis. Credé's prophylaxis is a classic example of the importance of public health recommendations. Its efficacy was early proven by the marked drop in the number children registered at blind schools (89). In areas where gonorrhea has become a rare infection in pregnant women, the Credé prophylaxis has often been excluded as a preventive measure. Nonetheless, routine follow-up inspection of the eyes of newborns should be carried out in instances where the Credé procedure is not performed.

In those cases where conjunctivitis develops in a newborn after a week or more, it is generally caused by *C. trachomatis*. Such an infection typically begins on one side and later spreads to the other eye. Chlamydial conjunctivitis is not prevented by silver nitrate and should be treated by general antibiotic therapy, not by antibiotic eye drops. Chlamydial conjunctivitis (neonatal inclusion conjunctivitis) has been reported as a long-term consequence of chlamydia infection of the neonate (66). Microscopy of eye secretion to detect chlamydia-infected cells has been used to diagnose neonatal inclusion conjunctivitis. To what extent double infections with *C. trachomatis* and *N. gonorrhoeae* contribute to the course of eye infections in newborns is not known.

Keratoconjunctivitis in Adults

Gonococcal eye infections may cause irreversible blindness not only in newborns but also in older children and adults (99). Corneal melting, corneal perforation, iris prolapse, and endophthalmitis with enucleation are known manifestations of the condition. Severe loss of vision with gonococcal eye infections may occur after leucomata (corneal opacity) and can be a sequela after healing of corneal ulcerations (90). Postgonococcal conjunctivitis also may be due to a concomitant chlamydia infection (97).

Pharyngitis

The clinical findings in pharyngeal pharyngitis may vary from slight erythema to severe ulceration with a pseudomembraneous coating. It can either be symptomatic or asymptomatic. The highest prevalence for gonococcal pharyngitis has been observed in MSM and who practice insertive oral sex. In a study of such men performed from 2001 to 2003, the prevalence of gonococcal pharyngitis was 5.5%, with an incidence of 11.2 cases per 100 person-years (67). In another study, pharyngeal colonization by *N. gonorrhoeae* was found in 9.2% of MSM cases (39). Pharyngeal colonization by gonococci may persist for months. Sequelae from gonococcal pharyngitis have not yet been documented.

Remember That Your Case May Represent a Complication of Genital Gonorrhea!

Of the papers on complications and sequelae from gonorrhea published during the past decade, most are just "case reports." Such reports often stem from countries where gonorrhea is still relatively common. These cases include corneal perforation (4), orbital cellulitis (79), septic arthritis (9), septic arthritis presenting without urethritis (41), migratory arthralgias and generalized exanthema (104), and vasculitis (35). Long-standing pharyngitis (67), septicemia in pregnant women (9, 75), and gonococcal endocarditis (14) are other conditions that may be caused by *N. gonorrhoeae*.

Infections with *Neisseria meningitidis* in Conditions Also Known To Be Associated with Gonorrhea

Some of the uncommon manifestations seen in gonococcal infections may also occur in infections with *N. meningitidis*, including pericarditis (15, 16, 33), cellulitis (38), keratitis (100), corneal perforation (4), periorbital cellulitis (12), endophthalmia (78), neonatal sepsis (17), arthritis (85), and arthritis-dermatitis syndrome (98). *N. meningitidis* has also been claimed to be a rare causative agent of urethritis in males (77, 98). It should be pointed out that it is essential to include isolation studies and not depend only on PCR tests, in order to prevent etiological errors. In culture studies, it is essential to include the conventional biomarkers used for speciation of *Neisseria* isolates.

PRIMARY AND SECONDARY INTERVENTIONS TO REDUCE COMPLICATIONS AND SEQUELAE OF GONORRHEA

Credè Prophylaxis

As described above, the use of silver nitrate eye drops to prevent blindness as a serious long-term sequela of gonorrhea is a classic example of successful primary prevention in medicine. Application of silver nitrate creates, however, an inflammatory reaction, i.e., conjunctivitis, which is believed to interfere with contact between the baby and the mother. This has been used as an argument to stop Credé prophylaxis, particularly in settings where gonorrhea has become uncommon in pregnant women.

Screening for Gonorrhea by Culture Methods

Historically, prevention of gonorrhea has included screening programs, employing isolation of *N. gonorrhoeae*. Such measures have been performed in STI clinics, but less commonly in other settings, including maternal service centers. With the introduction of PCR tests for *C. trachomatis,* the commercial kits commonly used also include tests for *N. gonorrhoeae*. This has resulted in wider screening for gonorrhea. The gonococcal tests have generally been offered free of charge to laboratories purchasing chlamydia test kits. If separate gonococcal and chlamydia tests are requested, the cost of screening increases.

Condom Use

Apart from screening for gonorrhea, campaigns for condom use have dominated the primary preventive initiatives to reduce the prevalence of gonorrhea and other STIs. Condom campaigns were intensified after the HIV epidemic began. These campaigns have had a limited effect on the spread of many STDs, in spite of exceptional allocation of economic resources to advertise the importance of condom use. There is also a behavior problem regarding condoms. The gap between purchasing condoms and their actual use in situations where gonorrhea and other STIs may be contracted has overestimated the condom as an alternative tool to prevent STDs.

Microcides

Vaginal application of nonoxynol-9 and other microcides is not an effective means of protecting women from STIs (18). In addition, resistance of the gonococcus to microcides has been demonstrated in vitro. Monlca and Hillier (63) have shown that most clinical strains (17/25) of *N. gonorrhoeae* were resistant to 20% nonoxynol-9. They suggested that a large number of clinical isolates should be tested before undertaking a clinical trial to determine the usefulness of vaginal microbiocides.

Gonococcal Vaccine—Still Far Away?

There have been a number of attempts to produce a gonococcal vaccine, but without any real success (95). The interest in producing vaccines against *N. gonorrhoeae* was quite active until the early 1990s. When the prevalence of gonorrhea started to decrease in Western industrial countries, resources for STI vaccine production were instead allocated to vaccines against human papilloma viruses (already on the market now) and HIV (now in field studies, but so far with disappointing results).

Vaccines against the gonococcal porin protein and pilus antigens have been produced (7, 101). Some protection against gonorrhea has been achieved with these vaccines but generally only against experimental rechallenge with the same strain. One problem in the development of gonococcal vaccines is the great variation in antigenicity among gonococcal strains.

Secondary Prevention by Using Effective Antibiotic Therapies

Before penicillin resistance emerged in gonococcal strains, this antibiotic was traditionally the drug of choice for therapy of gonorrhea. There are few organisms that initially had a lower MIC (minimum inhibitory concentration) to any antibiotic than gonococci to penicillin. After withdrawal of penicillin for general treatment of gonorrhea, the number of penicillin-sensitive strains decreased from 19.6% in 1991 to 6.3% in 2003 (103).

If beta-lactamase-producing strains of gonococci are exposed to penicillin, there is a drug-dose-related increase in the resistance to penicillin, since enzyme production is induced by the antibiotic. Studies from India indicate that only 4% of gonococci are penicillin resistant (5); half of the resistant strains produced beta-lactamase. Another recent study from India also indicated that half of gonococcal isolates produced beta-lactamase (91).

In analyzing the effect of any antibiotic therapy, it is essential to differentiate between microbiological and clinical cure. This became very obvious in males who developed nongonococcal urethritis or postgonococal urethritis with persistent signs of urethritis, without the presence of gonococci being demonstrated after penicillin therapy. It then became obvious that there must be one or more causative agents of urethritis besides *N. gonorrhoeae*. The causative organism was resistant to penicillin, unlike *N. gonorrhoeae*. *C. trachomatis* was later established as the main cause of nongonococcal urethritis, an agent not susceptible to standard regimens used to treat gonorrhea. Tetracyclines may cure a few cases of gonorrhea, but they do cure the majority of the cases of chlamydial infection.

Erythromycin is not effective against *M. hominis* but is active against other *Mycoplasma* species. Cephalosporins have been the first line alternatives for treatment of gonorrhea; however, they have a poor effect against *C. trachomatis*.

In secondary prevention, it is important to continuously perform antibiotic susceptibility surveys on *N. gonorrhoeae* isolates to ensure optimal therapy. Health officials must continuously update their therapy recommendations after any change in antibiotic susceptibility of circulating gonococcal strains. CDC recommendations banned the general use of fluoroquinolones for treatment of gonorrhea, since there is increasing resistance to these antibiotics (11). In 2007, the CDC also banned their routine use in therapy of endometritis and salpingitis cases, i.e., in PID. From 1999 to 2003, the percentage of strains of gonococci resistant to fluoroquinolones isolated in the United States increased from 0.4 to 4.1% (103). Resistance to ceftriaxone has, however, remained uncommon (103), and ceftriaxone has been considered the drug of choice for the cure of gonococcal infection, regardless of the prevalence of concomitant chlamydial infections or the choice of antichlamydial agent (22). Azithromycin has remained a therapeutic alternative for gonorrhea, genital chlamydial infections, and *M. genitalium* (8).

Contrary to antibiotic susceptibility problems in the treatment of gonorrhea, uncomplicated genital infections by *C. trachomatis* have remained curable with the recommended standard drug regimens, which have included tetracyclines, azithromycin, and erythromycin. The physician should, however, be cautious about prescribing tetracycline and erythromycin to pregnant women. Tetracyclines prescribed in high doses may result in bone malformation of the fetus if instituted during the second and third trimesters. There is a slight increase of heart malformation in the offspring of mothers treated with erythromycin during early pregnancy (37). Decreased susceptibility to one or more of tetracyclines, erythromycins, and azithromycin have been reported in a few strains of *C. trachomatis* (24), but it is not clear to what extent the results of in vivo susceptibility tests for *C. trachomatis* really mirror the clinical effect of the drugs. It is important to know if the recommended therapies for genital chlamydia infections will also cure a concomitant gonococcal infection. Likewise, it would be of interest to know to what extent gonorrhea may be cured by drugs commonly prescribed for respiratory tract infections.

Follow-up after Antibiotic Therapy Needed?

There is still no general consensus on if follow-up tests should be required in gonorrhea cases detected by PCR assays, such as the APTIMA Combo 2, and which have been given standard recommended therapies (68). Formerly, authorities in some countries, including Sweden, required two culture follow-up studies on all antibiotic-treated gonorrhea patients diagnosed using urethral/cervical and rectal samples. Culture and antibiotic susceptibility tests of all isolated gonococcal strains were also required.

Therapy of Sexual Partners

One important measure in secondary prevention of gonorrhea is the performance of partner notification.

There is a debate whether all partners, independent of the result of tests for *N. gonorrhoeae*, should be given antibiotic therapy. It is important to reach all consorts of the index case to avoid the possibility of reinfection of the index case. Attempts have been made to distribute sampling kits to partners via surface mail, which are to be sent back for analysis. Distribution of antibiotics to partner(s) of the index case has also been tested as a secondary prevention strategy (84).

Possible Impact of Antibiotic Therapy for Salpingitis To Prevent TFI

The effect of various antibiotic therapies of acute salpingitis on reduction of TFI and the consequent rate of involuntary childlessness is poorly documented. In fact, there are very few studies which have had a follow-up period long enough to allow such an assessment (26, 106). The lack of distinct end points for the cure of PID also constitutes an obstacle in studies concerning the effect of any therapy on salpingitis. Tubal infections may be difficult to eradicate by antibiotic therapy. Antibiotics may fail to penetrate injured tubal tissue to reach therapeutic concentrations. The effectiveness of antibiotics may be dependent on whether the patient has earlier experienced one or more episodes of salpingitis, since the penetration of antibiotics becomes less effective with each new episode of tubal infection. To be able to perform a study on the influence of different antibiotic therapies on TFI, one must consider the fact that salpingitis may have multiple microbial etiologies with organisms that have different antibiotic susceptibilities. One obstacle in retrospective analyses of TFI may be that appropriate samples were not saved for future analyses, making it impossible to test for all of the organisms that may have been involved.

CONCLUSIONS

To what extent the decrease of gonorrhea cases that has occurred will result in a decrease in severe sequelae remains to be seen. However, in most countries, the cases of gonorrhea appear to be again increasing in spite of access to microbiological diagnostic services, effective antibiotic therapy, and screening programs, and an improved insight that partner notification constitutes an important part of the management of gonococcal infections. Studies should be conducted to determine if there is a "hard core" of individuals who are responsible for maintaining gonorrhea in the population and to what extent they spread the infection.

REFERENCES

1. **Baczynska, A., P. Funch, J. Fedder, H. J. Knudsen, S. Birkelund, and G. Christiansen.** 2007. Morphology of human Fallopian tubes after infection with *Mycoplasma genitalium* and *Mycoplasma hominis*—in vitro organ culture study. *Hum. Reprod.* **22:**968–979.
2. **Baczynska, A., H. F. Svenstrup, J. Fedder, S. Birkelund, and G. Christiansen.** 2005. The use of enzyme-linked immunosorbent assay for detection of *Mycoplasma hominis* antibodies in infertile women serum samples. *Hum. Reprod.* **20:**1277–1285.
3. **Baldetorp, B., P.-A. Mårdh, and L. Weström.** 1983. Studies of ciliated epithelia of the human genital. IV. Mucocilary wave-activity on organ cultures of human fallopian tubes challenged with *Mycoplasma hominis*. *Sex. Trans. Dis.* **10:**363–365.
4. **Bastion M. L., K. Prakash, V. C. Siow, and S. S. Loh.** 2006. Bilateral corneal perforation in a sexually active adult male with gonococcal conjunctivitis. *Med. J. Malaysia* **61:**366–388.
5. **Bhatambare, G. S., and R. P. Karyayakarte.** 2001. Penicillin-resistant *Neisseria gonorrhoeae* at Aurangabad. *Indian J. Med. Microbiol.* **19:**155–156.
6. **Billings F. T., V. A. Evans, P. S. Wittinger, and H. E. Rowen.** 1991. "Primary" gonococcal meningitis. *Sex. Trans. Dis.* **18:** 129–130.
7. **Boslego, J. W., E. C. Tramont, R. C. Chung, D. G. McChesney, J. Ciak, J. C. Sadoff, M. V. Piziak, J. D. Brown, C. C. Brinton, Jr., and S. W. Wood.** 1991. Efficacy trial of a parenteral gonococcus pilus vaccine in men. *Vaccine* **9:**154–162.
8. **Brihmer, C., P.-A. Mårdh, I. Kallings, S. Osser, M. Robech, B. Sikström, and L. Wagner.** 1996. Efficiency and safety of azithromycin and lymecycline in the treatment of genital chlamydial infections in women. *Scand. J. Infect. Dis.* **28:** 451–458.
9. **Burgis J. T., and H. Nawaz III.** 2006. Disseminated gonococcal infection in pregnancy presenting as meningitis and dermatitis. *Obstet. Gynecol.* **108:**798–801.
10. **Centers for Disease Control and Prevention (CDC).** 2007. Increases in gonorrhea—eight Western states, 2000–2006. *MMWR Morb. Mortal. Wkly. Rep.* **16:**222–225.
11. **Centers for Disease Control and Prevention (CDC).** 2007. Update of CDC's sexually transmitted diseases treatment guidelines 2006; fluoroquinolones no longer recommended for treatment of gonococcal infections. *MMWR Morb. Mortal. Wkly. Res.* **56:**332–336.
12. **Chand, D. V., C. K. Hoyen, E. G. Leonard, and G. A. McComsey.** 2005. First reported case of *Neisseria meningitides* periorbital celllulitis associated with meningitis. *Pediatrics* **116:**e874–e875.
13. **Cohen C. R., N. R. Mugo, S. G. Astete, R. Odondo, L. E. Manhart, J. A. Kielbauch, W. E. Stamm, P. G. Waiyaki, and P. A. Totten.** 2005. Detection of *Mycoplasma genitalium* in women with laparoscopically diagnosed acute salpingitis. *Sex. Trans. Infect.* **81:**463–466.
14. **Cove-Smith, A., and J. L. Klein.** 2006. Gonococcal endocarditis: forgotten but not yet gone. *Scand. J. Infect. Dis.* **38:** 696–697.
15. **de Souza A. L., and A. C. Seguro.** 2007. Pericarditis secondary to *Neisseria meningitidis*. A potential cytokine network pathway. *Endocardiography* **24:**780–781.
16. **Duchateau, F. X., F. Companion, S. Rosenstingel, A. Fillion, B. Bonneton, and J. Mautz.** 2007. Serogroup C meningococcus presenting as pericarditis in a 55-year-old woman without medical history. *Ann. Fr. Anesth. Reanim.* **26:**452–454. (In French.)

17. **Falcao, M. C., S. B. Andrade, M. E. Ceccon, and F. A. Costa Vaz.** 2007. Neonatal sepsis and meningitis caused by *Neisseria meningitidis*: a case report. *Rev. Inst. Med. Trop. Sao Paulo* **49:**191–194.
18. **FDA.** 2007. Over-the-counter vaginal contraceptive and spermicide drug products containing nonoxynol-9; required labeling. Final rule. *Fed. Regist.* **72:**72769–72785.
19. **Fernandez, R., P. Nelson, J. Delgado, J. Aguilera, R. Massai, L. Velasquez, M. Imarai, H. G. Croxatto, and H. Cardenas.** 2001. Increased adhesiveness and internalization of *Neisseria gonorrhoeae* and changes in the expression of epithelial gonococcal receptors in the fallopian tube of copper T and Norplant users. *Hum. Reprod.* **16:**463–468.
20. **Fink A. S., C. A. Kosakowsky, J. R. Hiatt, and A. J. Cochran.** 1990. Periappendicitis is a significant clinical finding. *Am. J. Surg.* **159:**564–568.
21. **Garcia, C. S., R. Massa, A. Famiglietti, C. Vay, and G. Gutkind.** 2004. Unusual phenotypic characteristic of *Neisseria gonorrhoeae* from male patients who have sex with men. *Rev. Argent. Microbiol.* **36:**78–80.
22. **Genc, M., and P.-A. Mårdh.** 1997. Cost-effective treatment of uncomplicated gonorrhoea including co-infection with *Chlamydia trachomatis*. *Pharmacoeconomics* **12:**374–383.
23. **Grover, D., K. P. Prime, M. V., G. Ridgway, and R. J. Gilson.** 2006. Rectal gonorrhoea in man—is microscopy still a useful tool? *Int. J. STD AIDS* **17:**277–279.
24. **Guashino, S., and G. Ricci.** 2002. How, and how efficiently, can we treat *Chlamydia trachomatis* infections in women? *Best Pract. Res. Clin. Obstet. Gynaecol.* **16:**875–888.
25. **Hagenfeldt, K., and E. Szanto.** 1980. Sacroiliitis in women—a late sequela to acute salpingitis. *Am. J. Obstet. Gynecol.* **138:**1039–1041.
26. **Haggerty, C. L., and R. B. Ness.** 2006. Epidemiology, pathogenesis and treatment of pelvic inflammatory disease. *Expert Rev. Anti Inf. Ther.* **4:**235–237.
27. **Harwick, C., D. White, and H. Osman.** 2007. An audit of the results of the Roche Amplicor gonorroea test on female genital samples—a cheaper and more sensitive method than culture in an urban English population. *Int. J. STD AIDS* **18:**347–348.
28. **Hawkins, D. A., D. Taylor-Robinson, B. J. Thomas, and J. R. Harris.** 1986. Microbiological survey of acute epididymitis. *Genitourin. Med.* **62:**343–344.
29. **Hjelmevoll, S. O., M. E. Olsen, J. U. Sollid, H. Haaheim, M. Unemo, and V. Skogen.** 2006. A fast real-time polymerase chain reaction method for sensitive and specific detection of the *Neisseria gonorrhoeae* porA pseudogene. *J. Mol. Diagn.* **8:**574–581.
30. **Hobbs, M. M., B. van der Pol, P. Totten, C. A. Gaydos, A. Wald, T. Warren, R. L. Winer, R. L. Cook, C. D. Deal, M. E. Rogers, J. Schachter, K. K. Holmes, and D. H. Martin.** 2008. From the NIH: proceedings of a workshop on the importance of self-obtained vaginal specimens for detection of sexually transmitted infections. *Sex. Transm. Dis.* **35:**8–13.
31. **Holmes, K. K., R. E. Berger, and E. R. Alexander.** 1979. Acute epididymitis: etiology and therapy. *Arch. Androl.* **3:**309–316.
32. **Hook, E. W., and H. H. Handsfield.** 1999. Gonococcal infections in the adult, p. 451–466. *In* K. K. Holmes , P. F. Sparling, P.-A. Mårdh, S. M. Lemon, W. E. Stamm, P. Piot, and J. N. Wasserheit (ed.), *Sexually Transmitted Diseases,* 3rd ed. McGraw-Hill, New York, NY.
33. **Hussein, A., K. S. Prasad, D. Bhattacharyya, and K. El-Bouni.** 2005. C2 deficiency primary meningococcal arthritis of the elbow by *Neisseria meningitidis* in a 12-year-old girl. *Infection* **35:**287–288.
34. **Jacobson, L., and L. Weström.** 1969. Objectified diagnosis of acute pelvic inflammatory disease. *Am. J. Obstet. Gynecol.* **105:**1088–1098.
35. **Jain, S., H. N. Win, V. Chalam, and L. Yee.** 2007. Disseminated gonococcal infection presenting as vasculitic rash: a case report. *J. Clin. Pathol.* **60:**90–91.
36. **Jurstrand, M., J. S. Jensen, A. Magnusson, F. Kamvendo, and H. Fredlund.** 2007. A serological role of *Mycoplasma genitalium* in pelvic inflammatory disease and ectopic pregnancy. *Sex. Trans. Dis.* **97:**1118–1125.
37. **Källén, B. A., and P. Otterblad-Olausson.** 2003. Maternal drug use in early pregnancy and infant cardiovascular defect. *Reprod. Toxicol.* **17:**255–261.
38. **Kennedy, K. J., J. Roy, and P. Lamberth.** 2006. Invasive meningococcal disease presenting with cellulites. *Med. J. Austr.* **184:**421.
39. **Kent, C. K., J. K. Chaw, W. Wong, S. Liska, S. Gibson, G. Hubbard, and J. D. Klausner.** 2005. Prevalence of rectal, urethral, and pharyngeal chlamydia and gonorrhea detected in 2 clinical settings among men who have sex with men: San Francisco, California, 2003. *Clin. Infect. Dis.* **41:**67–74.
40. **Lavelle, S. J., K. E. Jones, H. Mallison, and A. M. Webb.** 2006. Finding, confirming, and managing gonorrhoea in a population screened for chlamydia using the Gen-Probe Aptima Combo2 assay. *Sex. Trans. Dis.* **82:**221–224.
41. **Le Berre, J. P., J. Samy, E. Garrabé, I. Imbert, J. Magnin, and D. Lechevalier.** 2007. Arthritis without urethritis: remember the gonococcus. *Rev. Med. Interne* **28:**183–185. (In French.)
42. **Little, J. W.** 2006. Gonorrhea: update. *Oral. Surg. Med. Oral Pathol. Oral Radiol. Endod.* **101:**137–143.
43. **Lossik, J. G., M. P. Smelzer, and J. W. Curran.** 1982. The value of cervical gram-staining in the diagnosis and treatment of gonorrhea in a venereal disease clinic. *Sex. Trans. Dis.* **9:**124–127.
44. **Mangold, K. A., M. Regner, M. Tajuddin, A. M. Tajuddin, L. Jennings, H. Du, and K. L. Kaul.** 2007. *Neisseria* species identification assay for the confirmation of *Neisseria gonorrhoeae*-positive results of the COBAS Amplicor PCR. *J. Clin. Microbiol.* **45:**1403–1409.
45. **Marchers, C. A., and C. R. Dawson.** 1971. Sequelae of neonatal inclusion conjunctivitis and associated disease in parents. *Am. J. Ophthalmol.* **71:**861–867.
46. **Mårdh, P.-A.** 2004. How wide spread are STIs? Need for improvements in surveillance systems and interpretation of test results, as exemplified by chlamydial infections. *Rev. Pract. Gynecol.* **4:**141–147.
47. **Mårdh, P.-A., B. Baldetorp, C. H. Håkansson, H. Fritz, and L. Weström.** 1979. Studies on ciliated epithelia of the human genital tract. III. Mucociliary wave pattern in organ cultures of human Fallopian tubes challenged with *Neisseria gonorrhoeae* and gonococcal endotoxin. *Brit. J. Vener. Dis.* **55:**256–264.
48. **Mårdh, P.-A., T. Buchanan, P. Christiansen, D. Danielsson, I. Lind, and K. Reimann.** 1978. Comparison of four serological tests for detection of gonococcal antibodies in patients with complicated infection, p. 377–381. *In* G. F. Brooks, E. C. Gotschlich, K. K. Holmes, W. D. Sawyer, and F. E. Young (ed). *Immunology of Neisseria gonorrhoeae*. American Society for Microbiology, Washington, DC.
49. **Mårdh, P.-A., I. Lind, E. From, and A-L. Andersen.** 1980. Prevalence of *Chlamydia trachomatis Neisseria gonorrhoeae* infections in Greenland. *Brit. J. Vener. Dis.* **56:**327–331.
50. **Mårdh, P.-A., D. Mårtensson, and L. V. Soltesz.** 1978. An effective, simplified culture medium for *Neisseria gonorrhoeae*. *Sex. Trans. Dis.* **5:**5–9.

51. **Mårdh, P.-A., B. R. Möller, H. J. Ingerslev, E. Nüssler, L. Weström, and P. Wölner-Hanssen.** 1981. Endometritis caused by *Chlamydia trachomatis*. *Brit. J. Vener. Dis.* **57**:191–195.
52. **Mårdh, P.-A., T. Ripa., L. Svensson, and L. Weström.** 1977. *Chlamydia trachomatis* infection in patients with acute salpingitis *N. Engl. J. Med.* **296**:1377–1379.
53. **Mårdh, P.-A., and L. Weström.** 1970. Tubal and cervical culture in acute salpingitis with special references to *Mycoplasma hominis* and T-strain mycoplasmas. *Brit. J. Vener. Dis.* **48**:179–186.
54. **Mårdh, P.-A., and P. Wölner-Hanssen.** 1985. Periappendicitis and chlamydial salpingitis. *Surg. Gynecol. Obstet.* **160**: 304–306.
55. **Matsumoto, T., T. Matsumoto, K. Takahshi, T. Ikuyama, D. Yokoo, Y. Ando, Y. Sato, M. Kurashima, H. Shimokawa, and S. Yanai.** 2006. Multiple doses of cefodizime are necessary for the treatment of *Neisseria gonorrhoeae* pharyngeal infection. *J. Infect. Chemother.* **12**:145–147.
56. **McGee, X. A., R. L. Jensen, C. M. Clemens, D. Taylor-Robinson, A. P. Johnson, and C. R. Gregg.** 1999. Gonococcal infection of human fallopian tube mucosa in organ culture. Relationship of mucosal tissue TNF-alpha concentration to sloughing of ciliated cells. *Sex. Trans. Dis.* **26**:160–165.
57. **Mehrany, K., J. M. Kist, W. J. O'Connor, and D. J. DiCaudo.** 2003. Disseminated gonococcemia. *Int. J. Dermatol.* **42**:208–209.
58. **Miettinen, A., P. K. Heinonen, K. Teisala, K. Hakkarainen, and R. Punnonen.** 1990. Serological evidence for the role of *Neisseria gonorrhoeae*, and *Mycoplasma hominis* in the etiology of tubal factor infertility and ectopic pregnancy. *Sex. Trans. Dis.* **17**:10–14.
59. **Möller, B. R., and E. A. Freundt.** 1979. Experimental infection of the genital tract of female grivit monkeys by *Mycoplasma hominis*: effect of different routes of infection. *Infect. Immun.* **26**:1123–1128.
60. **Möller, B. R., and P.-A. Mårdh.** 1980. Experimental epididymitis and urethritis in grivit monkeys provoked by *Chlamydia trachomatis*. *Fertil. Steril.* **34**:275–279.
61. **Möller, B. R., P.-A. Mårdh, S. Ahrons, and E. Nüssler.** 1981. Infection with *Chlamydia trachomatis, Mycoplasma hominis* and *Neisseria gonorrhoeae* in patients with acute pelvic inflammatory disease. *Sex Trans. Dis.* **8**:198–202.
62. **Möller, B. R., L.Weström, S.Ahrons, K. T. Ripa, L. Svensson, C. von Mecklenburg, H. Henrikson, and P.-A. Mårdh.** 1979. *Chlamydia trachomatis* infection of the Fallopian tubes. Histological finding in two patients. *Brit. J. Vener. Dis.* **55**:422–428.
63. **Monlca, B. J., and S. L. Hillier.** 2005. Why nonoxynol-9 may have failed to prevent acquisition of *Neisseria gonorrhoeae* in clinical trials. *Sex. Trans. Dis.* **32**:491–494.
64. **Morales, P., P. Reyes, M. Vargas, M. Rios, M. Imarai, H. Cardenas, H. Croxatto, P. Orihuela, R. Vargas, J. Fuhrer, J. E. Heckels, M. Christodoulides, and L. Velasquez.** 2006. Infection of human tube epithelial cells with *Neisseria gonorrhoeae* protects cells from tumor necrosis factor alpha-induced apoptosis. *Infect Immun.* **74**:3643–3650.
65. **Morello, J. A., and M. Bohnhoff.** 1989. Serovars and serum resistance of *Neisseria gonorrhoeae* from disseminated and uncomplicated infections. *J. Infect. Dis.* **160**:1012–1017.
66. **Mordhorst, C. H., and C. Dawson.** 1971 .Sequelae of neonatal inclusion conjunctivitis and associated disease in parents. *Am. J. Ophthalmol.* **71**:861–867.
67. **Morris, S. R., J. D. Klausner, S. P. Buchbinder, S. L. Wheeler, B. Koblin, T. Coates, M. Chesney, and G. N. Colfax.** 2006. Prevalence and incidence of pharyngeal gonorrhea in a longitudinal sample of men who have sex with men. The EXPLORE study. *Clin. Infect. Dis.* **43**:1284–1289.
68. **Moss, S., and H. Mallison.** 2007. The contribution of APTTIMA Combo 2 assay to the diagnosis of gonorrhoea. *Int. J. STD/AIDS* **18**:551–554.
69. **O'Brien, J. P., D. L. Goldenberg, and P. A. Rice.** 1983. Disseminated gonococcal infection: a prospective analysis of 49 patients and a review of pathophysiology and immune mechanisms. *Medicine* (Baltimore) **62**:395–406.
70. **Olhagen, B.** 1983. Urogenital syndromes and spondarthritis. *Br. J. Rheumatol.* **22**:33–40.
71. **Østergaard, L.** 2002. Microbiological aspects of the diagnosis of *Chlamydia trachomatis*. *Best Pract. Res. Clin. Obstet. Gynecol.* **16**:789–799.
72. **Papp, J. R., K. Ahrens, C. Phillips, C. K. Kent, S. Phillips, and J. D. Klausner.** 2007. The use and performance of oral rinses to detect pharyngeal *Neisseria gonorrhoeae* and *Chlamydia trachomatis* infections. *Diagn. Microbial. Infect. Dis.* **59**:259–264.
73. **Patton, D. L., M. Askienazy-Elbhar, J. Henry-Suchet, L. A. Campbell, A. Cappuccio, W., Tannous, S. P. Wang, and C. C. Kuo.** 1994. Detection of *C. trachomatis* in fallopian tube tissue in women with postinfectious tubal infertility. *Am. J. Obstet. Gynecol.* **171**:95–101.
74. **Peeling, R. W., J. Kimani, F. Plummer, I. MacLean, M. Cheang, J. Bwayo, and R. C. Brunham.** 1997. Antibody to chlamydial hsp60 predicts an increased risk for chlamydial pelvic inflammatory disease. *J. Infect. Dis.* **175**:1153–1158.
75. **Phupong, V., T. Sittisomwong, and W. Wisawasukmongchol.** 2005. Disseminated gonococcal infection during pregnancy. *Arch. Gynecol. Obstet.* **273**:185–186.
76. **Power, P. M., S. C. Ku, K. Rutter, M. J. Warren, E. A. Limnios, J. W. Tapsall, and M. P. Jennings.** 2007. The phase-variable allele of the pilus glycosylation gene *pglA* is not strongly associated with strains of *Neisseria gonorrhoeae* isolated from patients with disseminated gonococcal infection. *Infect. Immun.* **75**:3202–3204.
77. **Quarto, M, S. Barbuti, C. Germinario, G. A. Vena, and C. Foti.** 1991. Urethritis caused by *Neisseria meningitidis*: a case report. *Eur. J. Epidemiol.* **7**:699–701.
78. **Quintyn, J. C., S. Poupelin, S. Fajoles-Vasseneix, and G. Brasseur.** 2006. Meningococcal endoophthalmitis without meningitis. *J. Fr. Ophthalmol.* **29**:e 24.
79. **Raja, N. S., and N. N. Singh.** 2005. Bilateral cellulitis due to *Neisseria gonorrhoeae* and *Staphylococcus aureus*: a previously unreported case. *J. Med. Microbiol.* **54**:609–911.
80. **Rice, P. A.** 2005. Gonococcal arthritis (disseminated gonococcal infection). *Infect. Dis. Clin. North Am.* **19**:853–861.
81. **Rice, P. A., and H. H. Handsfield.** 1999. Arthritis associated with sexually transmitted diseases, p. 921–935. *In* K. K. Holmes, P. F. Sparling, P.-A. Mårdh, S. M. Lemon, W. E. Stamm, P. Piot, and J. N. Wasserheit (ed). *Sexually Transmitted Diseases,* 3rd ed. McGraw-Hill, New York, NY.
82. **Ripa, K. T., and P.-A. Mårdh.** 1977. Cultivation of *Chlamydia trachomatis* in cycloheximide-treated McCoy cells. *J. Clin. Microbiol.* **6**:328–331.
83. **Ripa, K. T., L. Svenssson, P.-A. Mårdh, and L. Weström.** 1978. *Chlamydia trachomatis* in gynecological out-patients. Obstet. Gynecol. **52**:698–702.
84. **Rogers, M. E.** 2007. Patient-delivered partner treatment and other partner management strategies for sexually transmitted diseases used by New York City healthcare providers. *Sex. Trans. Dis.* **34**:88–92.
85. **Rondier, J., J. Cayla, C. Fayeton, and B. Gallet.** 1981. Meningococcal arthritis simulating articular gonorrhea. *Rev. Rhum. Mal. Osteoartic.* **48**:249–251.

86. **Ryder, N., and D. Ivens.** 2005. Male urethral gonorrhoea—5,700 pounds per positive test? *Int. J. STD AIDS* **16:**638.
87. **Sandström, E., and D. Danielsson.** 1975. A survey of gonococcal serology, p. 253–259. *In* D. Danielsson, I. Juhlin, and P.-A. Mårdh (ed.), *Genital Infections and Their Complications.* Almquist and Wiksell International, Stockholm, Sweden.
88. **Sandström, E. G., J. S. Knapp, L. B. Reller, S. E. Thompson, E. E. Hook III, and K. K. Holmes.** 1984. Serogrouping of *Neisseria gonorrhoeae*: correlation of serogroup with disseminated gonococcal infection. *Sex. Transm. Dis.* **11:**77–80.
89. **Schaller, U. C., and V. Klauss.** 2001. Is Credé's prophylaxis for ophthalmia neonatorum still valid? *Bull. W. H. O.* **79:**262–263.
90. **Schwab, L., and T. Tizazu.** 1985. Destructive epidemic *Neisseria gonorrhoeae. Brit. J. Ophthalmol.* **69:**525–529.
91. **Sethi, B., D. Sharma, S. D. Mehta, B. Singh, M. Smriti, B. Kumar, and M. Sharma.** 2006. Emergence of ciprofloxacin resistant *Neisseria gonorrhoeae* in north India. *Indian J. Med. Res.* **123:**707–710.
92. **Simons, M. P., W. M. Nauseef, and M. A. Apicella.** 2005. Interaction of *Neisseria gonorrhoeae* with adherent polymorphonuclear leukocytes. *Infect. Immun.* **73:**1971–1977.
93. **Simons, M. P.,W. M. Nauseef, T. S. Griffith, and M. A. Apicella.** 2006. *Neisseria gonorrhoeae* delays the onset of apoptosis in polymorphonuclear leukocytes. *Cell. Microbiol.* **8:**1780–1790.
94. **Snyder, L. A., and N. J. Saunders.** 2006. The majority of genes in the pathogenic *Neisseria* species are present in non-pathogenic *Neisseria lactamica*, including those designated as "virulence genes." *BMC Genomics* **7:**128.
95. **Sparling, P. F.** 1999. Biology of *Neisseria gonorrhoeae*, p. 433–450. *In* K. K. Holmes, P. F. Sparling, P.-A. Mårdh, S. M. Lemon, W. E. Stamm, P. Piot, and J. N. Wasserheit (ed.), *Sexually Transmitted Diseases,* 3rd ed. McGraw-Hill, New York, NY.
96. **Soltèsz, L. V., and P.-A. Mårdh.** 1980. Serum-free liquid medium for *Neisseria gonorrhoeae. Cur. Microbiol.* **4:**45–49.
97. **Stenberg, K., and P.-A. Mårdh.** 1990. Chlamydial conjunctivitis in neonates and adults: history, clinic and follow-up of 133 cases. *Acta Ophthalmology* **68:**651–657.
98. **Sun, H. Y., I. C. Chang, M. J. Chen, C. C. Hung, and S. C. Chang.** 2004. Acute urethritis and arthritis-dermatitis syndrome due to *Neisseria meningitidis. J. Formos. Med. Assoc.* **103:**858–859.
99. **Symes, R. J., C. J. Catt, and J. J. Males.** 2007. Diffus lamellar keratitis associated with gonococcal keratoconjunctivitis 3 years after laser in situ keratomileusis. *J. Cataract Refract. Surg.* **33:**323–325.
100. **Tan, C. S., F. U. Krishnan, F. Y. Foo, J. C. Pan, and L. W. Voon.** 2006. *Neisseria meningitidis* keratitis in adults: a case series. *Ann. Acad. Med. Singapore.* **35:**837–839.
101. **Tramont, E. C., J. C. Sadoff, J. W. Boslego, J. Ciak, D. W. McChesney, C. C. Brinton, S. W. Wood, and E. Takufuji.** 1981. Gonococcal pilus vaccine. Studies of antigenity and inhibition of attachment. *Infect. Immun.* **68:**881–888.
102. **van Bergen, J. E., J. Spaargaren, H. M. Götz, I. K.Veldhuijzen, P. J. Bindels, T. J. Coenen, J. Broer, F. de Groot, C. J. Hoebe, J. H. Richardus, D. van Schaik, M. Verhooren, and PILOT CT study group.** 2006. Population prevalence of *Chlamydia trachomatis* and *Neisseria gonorrhoeae* in the Netherlands. Should asymptomatic persons be tested during population-based Chlamydia screening also for gonorrhoea or only if chlamydial infection is found? *BMC Infect. Dis.* **6:**42.
103. **Wang, S. A., A. B. Harvey, S. M. Conner, A. A. Zaidi, J. S. Knapp, W. L. Whittington, C. del Rio, F. N. Judson, and K. K. Holmes.** 2007. Antimicrobial resistance for *Neisseria gonorrhoeae* in the United States, 1988 to 2003: the spread of fluoroquinolone resistance. *Ann. Intern. Med.* **147:**81–88.
104. **Weber, M., and H. Gerber.** 1994. Gonorrheal arthritis. *Schweiz Rundsch. Med. Prax.* **83:**46–48. (In German.)
105. **Weström, L., L. P. Bengtsson, and P.-A. Mårdh.** 1976. The risk of pelvic inflammatory disease in women using intrauterine contraceptive devices as compared to non-users. *Lancet* **ii:**221–224.
106. **Weström, L., S. Iosif, S. Svensson, and P.-A. Mårdh.** 1979. Infertility after acute salpingitis with different antibiotics, p. 47–50. *In Sexually Transmitted Disease: Reappraisal of the Role of Vibramycin (Doxycycline).* Science and Medicine Publishing Co., New York, NY.
107. **Weström, L., L. P. Bengtsson, and P.-A. Mårdh.** 1981. Incidence, trends, and risks of ectopic pregnancy in a population of women. *Br. Med. J.* **282:**15–18.
108. **Wölner-Hansen, P., L. Weström, and P.-A. Mårdh.** 1980. Perihepatitis in chlamydial salpingitis. *Lancet* **i:**901–904.
109. **Zhang, J., G. Li, A. Bafica, M. Pantelic, P. Zhang, H. Broxmeyer, Y. Liu, L. Wetzler, J. J. He, and T. Chen.** 2005. *Neisseria gonorrhoeae* enhances infection of dendritic cells by HIV type 1. *J. Immunol.* **174:**7995–8002.

Sequelae and Long-Term Consequences of Infectious Diseases
Edited by Pina M. Fratamico, James L. Smith, and Kim A. Brogden

Chapter 10

Sequelae and Long-Term Consequences of Syphilis Infection

Jeffrey D. Klausner and Alexandra H. Freeman

While tremendous advances in the prevention, control, and treatment of syphilis have occurred in industrialized nations, syphilis remains endemic and often untreated in many less developed countries. Maternal syphilis infection remains common in those areas, and congenital syphilis may be two- or threefold more common than perinatal human immunodeficiency virus (HIV) infections (49). Chronic untreated infection can lead to significant morbidity, serious life-threatening sequelae, and premature death. Due to the relative paucity of complications of syphilis in resource-rich areas currently, clinical research of syphilis has all but ground to a halt. Few infectious disease researchers study the pathogenesis of syphilis infection, and much of the current clinical knowledge of syphilis comes from an era before the advent of antibiotics. Soon after the discovery of penicillin in 1943, the use of penicillin rapidly became the standard of care, such that penicillin eluded rigorous evaluation through controlled clinical trials. In this chapter we briefly review the biology, epidemiology, and natural history of syphilis. Further, we characterize the infectious complications and sequelae of untreated syphilis infection by organ system from natural history studies and more recent case reports.

BIOLOGY OF *TREPONEMA PALLIDUM* SUBSP. *PALLIDUM*

Syphilis is caused by infection with the spirochetal bacterium *Treponema pallidum* subspecies *pallidum* (48). *T. pallidum* is a highly motile organism with tapering ends presenting between 6 and 14 spirals. Of uniform cylindrical shape, the bacteria measure approximately 6 to 15 micrometers in length and 0.25 micrometers in width (43). Recent molecular sequencing has determined the genomic sequence of *T. pallidum* to be 1,138,006 base pairs with 1,041 open reading frames (9). *T. pallidum* is a slowly metabolizing organism with an average multiplying time of approximately 30 hours (29). Humans are the only host for the organism. Laboratory study of the pathogen is difficult, as *T. pallidum* cannot be cultivated in artificial media. Most laboratory systems perpetuate the organism in rabbits and identify a rich source of the organism in rabbit testes. Traditional Gram staining cannot render the organism visible under light microscopy, such that a specialized system using refracted light on a darkened background (dark-field microscopy) is used to identify the spirochete in clinical specimens. Silver stain (Warthin-Starry) is used in histological specimens. While PCR has been used to amplify genetic elements of *T. pallidum* in clinical specimens, there are no current FDA-cleared molecular amplification assays in use in routine clinical practice. The clinical diagnosis of syphilis is based on characteristic findings on the skin and mucous membranes and confirmed with serologic assays measuring antibodies to nontreponemal (rapid plasma reagin [RPR] or venereal disease research laboratory tests) and treponemal antigens (*Treponemal pallidum* particle agglutination, fluorescent *Treponemal* absorption, and enzyme immunoassays).

EPIDEMIOLOGY

The epidemiology of syphilis follows two distinct patterns between developed and developing countries. Syphilis incidence in developed nations declined

Jeffrey D. Klausner • STD Prevention and Control Services, San Francisco Department of Public Health, San Francisco, CA 94103, and Divisions of AIDS and Infectious Diseases, Department of Medicine, University of California, School of Medicine, San Francisco, CA. **Alexandra H. Freeman** • STD Prevention and Control Services, San Francisco Department of Public Health, San Francisco, CA 94103.

dramatically after the introduction of mass population screening programs and the advent of penicillin therapy. In 2000, infectious syphilis was at a historic low in the United States, with only 9,756 primary and secondary cases compared with about 100,000 cases in 1946 (6). Similar declines have been observed across Europe and Australia (7). Currently, syphilis has experienced a resurgence in high-risk subpopulations in developed countries, particularly among men who have sex with men (7, 25, 60). Reversal of the control of syphilis in disenfranchised heterosexual subpopulations has also been observed in major metropolitan areas in the Southeast of the United States (6).

The unmitigated persistence of syphilis in less developed countries starkly contrasts with the changing epidemiology of syphilis in developed nations. Regional data of the World Health Organization from the Western Pacific, Sub-Saharan Africa, South Asia, and South America demonstrate that on average about 5% of pregnant women seeking antenatal care services have evidence of recent syphilis infection (49). The unfortunate recent acquisition of syphilis and high rates of infection in pregnant women results in a large number of miscarriages, stillbirths, and newborns with congenital infection. Estimates of the burden of syphilis suggest that congenital syphilis may be two or three times more common globally than perinatal HIV infection (49).

The well-documented increase of syphilis in China (population 1.3 billion) has further raised global concern about syphilis (4). An aggressive venereal disease control policy of the Chinese government from the 1950s to the 1970s effectively eliminated syphilis in China. Despite those efforts, as well as recent sociopolitical and economic changes in China, recent data showed a 250- and 1,000-fold increase in adult and congenital cases, respectively, in the last decade (Fig. 1) (4).

NATURAL HISTORY

Our current understanding of the natural course of syphilitic infection among untreated individuals is largely based on historical data from the preantibiotic era. The Oslo study was a large prospective natural history study in which Boeck observed approximately 2,000 patients with primary and secondary syphilis admitted to the Oslo Clinic from 1891 to 1910. The study was later continued by Bruusgaard and further investigated by Gsetland from 1949 to 1951. Approximately one-third of untreated individuals developed clinical manifestations of tertiary disease, including late benign syphilis, neurosyphilis, and cardiovascular syphilis (13). From 1932 to 1972 in Macon County, AL, the U.S. Public Health Service conducted the Tuskegee Syphilis Study to observe untreated syphilis

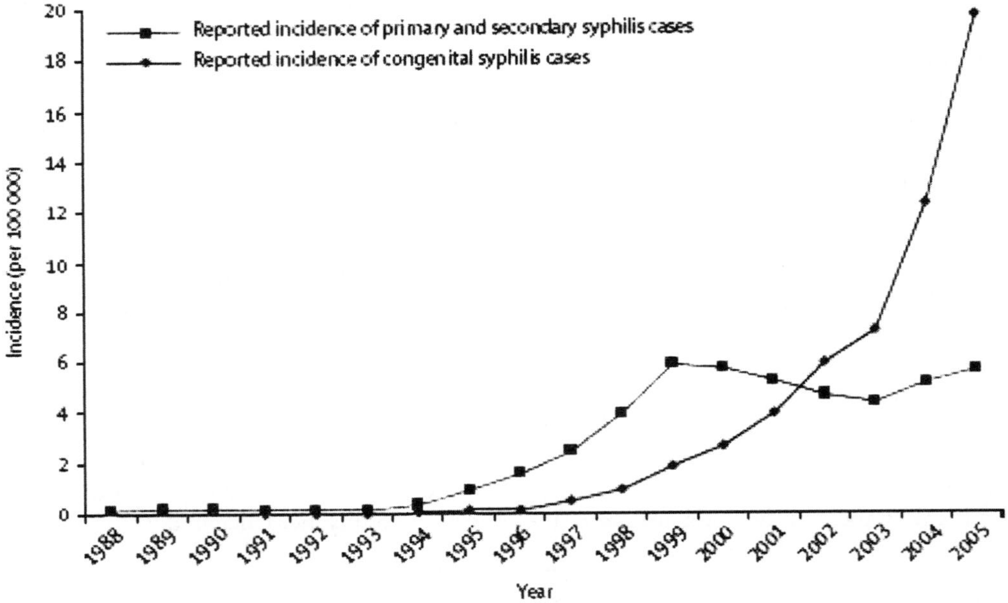

Figure 1. Reported incidence of primary and secondary syphilis and congenital syphilis, China 1988–2005. (Reprinted from the *Lancet* [4] with permission from Elsevier.)

infection among African American men. The Tuskegee Study was unethical, as informed consent from patients was not obtained, and most notably, treatment was withheld from study participants after the discovery of penicillin; no findings from the Tuskegee Study will be discussed in this chapter.

The natural course of untreated syphilis is characterized by several periods of clinical disease of primary, secondary, and tertiary stages as well as latent asymptomatic periods. Infectious syphilis includes the primary and secondary periods, and because secondary recurrences can occur in the early latent stage, some experts include early latent disease as potentially infectious. In most untreated individuals, syphilis infection will be cleared by the host's immune system. However, in about a third of patients, latent syphilis may progress into tertiary disease (13).

Syphilis is transmitted through direct contact with an infectious lesion. The primary modes of transmission are sexual contact and maternal transmission during pregnancy. Upon infection, the motile spirochete *T. pallidum* enters through subclinical areas of microtrauma of the skin or normal mucosa (30), locally multiplying, with resultant systemic dissemination in less than 24 hours (47). A primary chancre develops at the site of inoculation due to local infiltration of immune cells. The incubation period for the primary lesion is on average 3 weeks, ranging between 10 and 90 days. The chancre characterizes primary syphilis, marking the first clinical manifestation of infection.

The primary chancre of syphilis is a sharply defined lesion at the site of infection. Chancres may vary in size but are usually singular and indurated (33, 61). In men, primary lesions are most commonly found on the penis (Fig. 2), and anorectal lesions are common among men who have sex with men (36). In women, chancres most commonly occur on the labia majora and labia minora, while they may also be found on the fourchette and perineum (53). Other sites include the male prepuce, scrotum, rectum or anus, mouth, or nipple. The primary lesion is frequently accompanied by nontender regional lymphadenopathy.

In untreated syphilis, spontaneous healing of the primary chancre generally occurs within a few weeks, disappearing before manifestations of secondary syphilis. Primary symptoms may, however, persist for up to 3 months, being evident at onset of the secondary stage. That overlap in clinical manifestations of primary and secondary syphilis is more common in patients coinfected with HIV (62).

Secondary syphilis generally appears 6 weeks to several months after infection and is characterized by a widespread skin reaction. Common clinical manifestations include local or generalized cutaneous rash, fatigue, fever, mucous membrane lesions or "patches" on the tongue, and buccal mucosa, skin

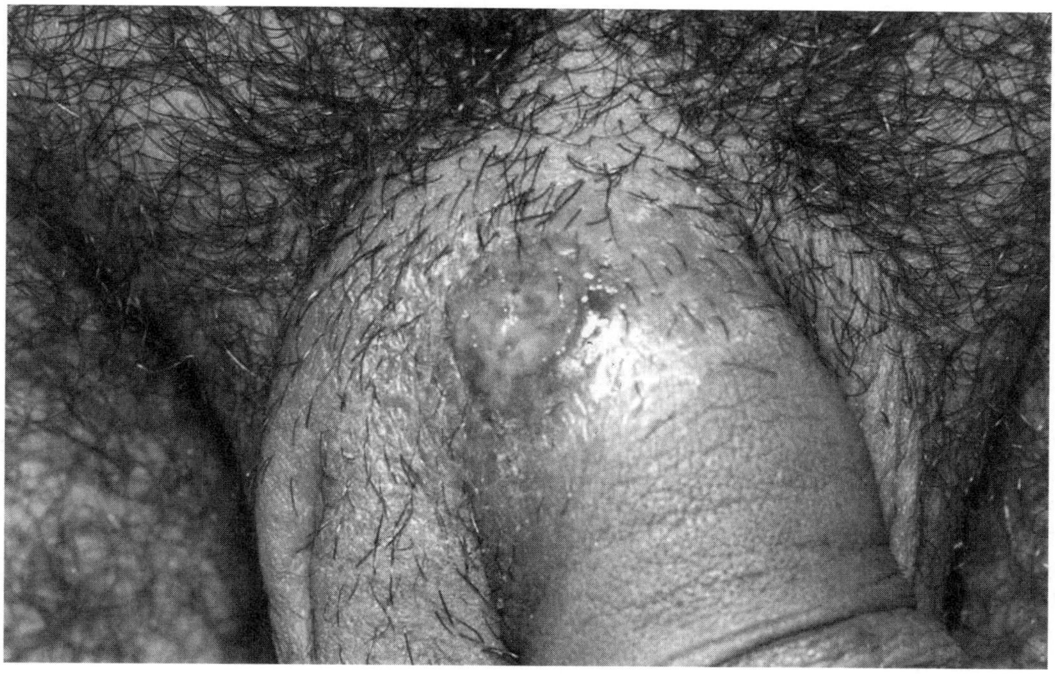

Figure 2. Primary chancre of the penis.

lesions, or maculopapular rash on the palms and soles, trunk, and extremities (53). In adults, skin lesions are usually bilateral and symmetrical. Papular lesions may also occur on the face, chin, upper trunk, or palms—essentially anywhere on the skin and mucous membranes. Those skin lesions are not, however, vesicular or bulbous, as may occur in early congenital syphilis of infants. Papular lesions of secondary syphilis are typically painless and range in size from 5 to 10 mm (51). These lesions can also coalesce to form infectious plaques called condylomata lata on warm, moist areas. Other manifestations of secondary syphilis may include uveitis, alopecia, and hepatitis (29). A symptomatic sore throat may also develop due to an inflammatory response of the tonsils and pharynx (53).

The natural course of syphilitic disease among most untreated individuals includes an asymptomatic latent stage. Latent syphilis is defined as a lack of clinical manifestations, beginning with the resolution of secondary symptoms. During this period the organism burden may be low but found throughout the host body. About one-third of persons with late latent disease may develop late symptomatic or tertiary disease (13). A reactive serologic test may be the only indication of chronic infection.

GENERAL PATHOPHYSIOLOGY OF CHRONIC INFECTION—CHRONIC INFLAMMATORY REACTION

Long-term syphilitic infection in untreated individuals occurs in patients who have not immunologically cleared infection. Ultimately, chronic inflammation in end organs results in organ damage and failure. These end-organ or tissue-specific changes include fibrosis, sclerosis, scarring, and loss of normal tissue parenchyma. Chronic inflammation is characterized by lymphocytic infiltration, a high concentration of plasma cells, and increased fibroblastic activity. In addition, treponemes reside in the lymph space around capillaries, resulting in an endarteritis with subsequent tissue degeneration due to cellular necrosis, which is due to inadequate blood supply (53).

Gumma or gummatous tissue changes are inflammatory masses of lymphocytic and plasma cells with extensive local endarteritis. Subsequent obliteration of the vascular supply leads to massive central necrosis and the appearance of giant cells. If this process occurs in the skin or in mucous membranes, superficial firm or rubbery lesions may appear often, with central softening of necrotic tissue. The central area may eventually break down into crater-like ulcers. Those ulcers will usually heal, but in untreated disease relapses or recurrences can occur. Depending on the location (e.g., skin, bone, or brain), the effects of such gumma will differ.

LATE SYPHILIS OF THE SKIN

Untreated, chronic syphilis infection may result in a myriad of skin manifestations (22, 42). Macular depigmentation can occur on the side of the neck, appearing similar to vitiligo (53). However, vitiligo is usually larger, with slightly hyperpigmented borders and a geographic contour. Historically, the skin lesions of syphilis were referred to as syphilids. Such late syphilids can be nodular, nodulo-ulcerative (ulcerative including multiple and deep lesions), nonulcerative, or gummatous (22, 52). Nodular lesions may be intact gumma. Syphilids may be scaly in appearance, similar to the lesions of psoriasis. Solitary gumma may be cutaneous or subcutaneous (Fig. 3). Lesions may be indurated with an arc-like or polcyclic configuration, forming a ring or half-ring of scalloped chains (53).

Late syphilids of the lip and mucous membranes may be nodular, nodulo-ulcerative, and ulcerative. Lesions of the tongue may appear as glossitis, which may be sclerosing or have fissures or associated leukoplakia. Solitary gumma or perforating gumma may occur in the soft palate, and lesions such as leukoplakia of the buccal mucosa or commissures may occur. Finally there may be gummatous infiltration of the lip.

The differential diagnoses of lesions of the skin and mucous membranes are broad and will depend on the local epidemiology of other infectious diseases and neoplasms. Conditions to consider in the different

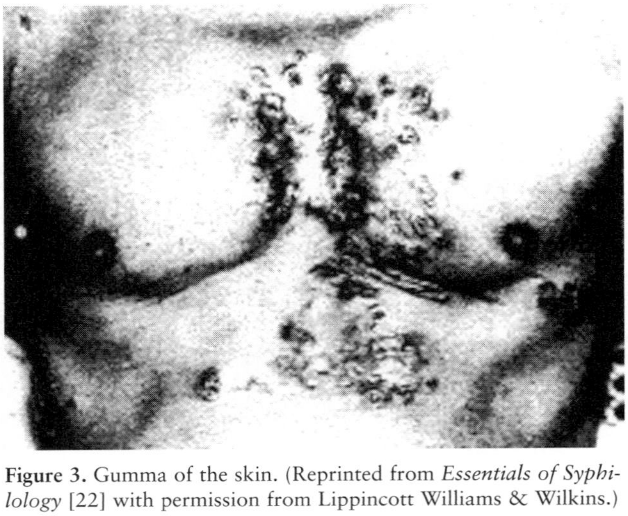

Figure 3. Gumma of the skin. (Reprinted from *Essentials of Syphilology* [22] with permission from Lippincott Williams & Wilkins.)

diagnoses of skin lesions include Hodgkins disease; mycosis fungoides; tuberculids (tuberculosis); systemic lupus erythematous; fungal infections, like sporotrichosis or blastomycosis; and malignancies (e.g., sarcomas) as well as conditions like granuloma annulare.

LATE SYPHILIS OF MUSCULOSKELETAL SYSTEM

T. pallidum disseminates early within the body and localizes within the bone marrow and the richly vascularized periosteum and dependent areas of the long bones (53). Characteristic skeletal changes result from late periostitis of the long bones and shoulder girdle. Reports of syphilis of the clavicle and clavicular swelling were common in the preantibiotic era. Radiographic findings include periosteal thickening, elevation, irregularities of the bony outer surface, and increased density along the surface below the periosteum (53). Evidence of osteitis and osteoperiostitis, as well as thickening and increased bone density may not be uniform. *T. pallidum* invasion of cavities of the long bones and flat bones of the face and skull may result in sequestra formation. In the early 20th century, Skinner reported various radiographic abnormalities, such as worm-eaten areas of destruction or necrosis, irregular contour of the periosteum, moth-eaten appearance of tissue around the abnormal periosteum, sclerosis (increased density) of bone, and bulging of the periosteum from subperiosteal infiltration (53).

Gummatous osteomyelitis—tertiary disease—may involve the entire bone marrow with proliferative and destructive changes and may be more marked in less dense bone tissue and at the end of the bones. Involvement of tissues around affected bone may occur with a reactive inflammatory process. Benign gummatous infiltrations of muscles (e.g., biceps) may occur; however, reports are rare.

Cranial osteoperiostitis and thickening and infiltration of the periosteum can occur in association with chronic inflammatory changes, which may appear normal on X-ray radiography.

In early reports, osteitis of the palate and septum were the most frequently cited locations of disease, although that may be substantially biased by ascertainment. Cases of palatal or septal disease may have been more likely to seek medical attention. In his review of data from the Mayo Clinic (239 cases), Stokes reported a high percentage of cranial and nasopalatine lesions (42%), which was followed by abnormalities of the tibia (26%), clavicle (7.5%), and the shoulder girdle, including the sternum and ribs (10%) (53). The most common lesions were periostitis (53%), osteomyelitis (20%), and arthritis (12%) (53).

As early as 1868, Charcot described tabetic arthropathy or deinnervation dystrophy of various joints (Charcot joint) (53). At that time, it was unclear whether the joint disease was due to syphilitic disease of the joint or was secondary due to the loss of nerve function at the joint. Abnormalities were reported in the joints of the foot, ankle, hip, and shoulder. Classically, involvement of the joints is usually absent (53). Occasionally, simple effusions and mild joint inflammation (syphilitic pseudo-rheumatism) have been reported as being associated with syphilis in the older literature but causality remains uncertain. Syphilitic bursitis may also occur.

In terms of the differential diagnoses of bony lesions, older reports suggested that syphilitic bony lesions were usually hyperplastic and the result of increased osteoblastic activity, while malignancy or tuberculosis were often destructive and necrotic (53). The exception was syphilitic cranial bone disease that resulted in bone loss. Bony lesions often coexisted with late cutaneous lesions. Clinically, syphilis osseous involvement was characterized by nocturnal bone pain. Such reports may have been characterized as bony involvement in tertiary disease because more recent report of syphilitic bone disease in early syphilis described lytic and destructive lesions (15, 23).

Two recent case reports described syphilitic bony lesions in patients with HIV infection (15, 23). The first case presented a patient with painful nodules on the front and vertex of his head. The patient had a serum RPR titer of 1:128. Penicillin therapy was associated with resolution of the lesions and decline in the syphilis titer. The second case was an African American male with a painful lump on his chest. A magnetic resonance image (MRI) of the chest showed a sternal lesion (Fig. 4). The diagnosis was confirmed by a PCR that amplified *T. pallidum* DNA in a biopsy sample of the lesion. The bony lesion resolved after penicillin therapy.

While these case reports raised concern about the possible increase of syphilitic bony disease in the era of AIDS, such complications of syphilis appear to be uncommon. Historically, the most comprehensive review of bony disease and syphilis was by Reynolds and Wasserman in 1942 (45). They reviewed 10,000 cases of early syphilis and found only 15 cases of osteitis. Another review of 854 patients with secondary syphilis described only 2 patients with osteitis (36). Our recent clinical experience with syphilis in San Francisco in HIV-infected patients has not identified any cases with concomitant bony disease.

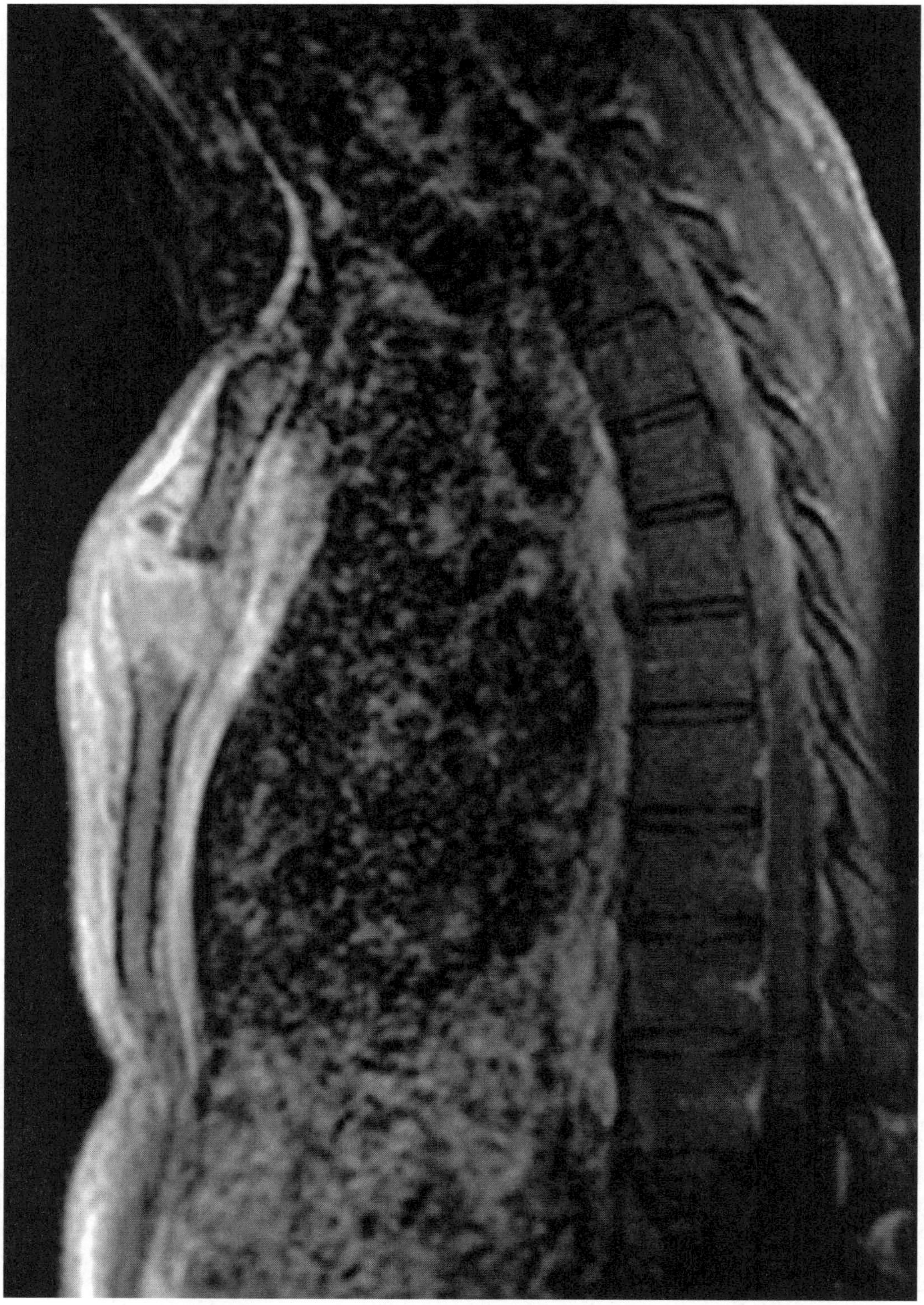

Figure 4. Sternal bony lesion shown by magnetic resonance imaging (MRI). (Reprinted from *AIDS Patient Care and STDs* [23] with permission from Mary Anne Liebert, Inc.)

LATE SYPHILIS OF THE GASTROINTESTINAL SYSTEM

Syphilis of the gastrointestinal system is generally much less common than syphilis of the skin or cardiovascular or nervous system. However, both the liver and spleen are highly vascularized organs and remain targets for the dissemination of infection. Syphilis of the liver has been described, mostly related to gummatous infiltration or the presence of gumma near critical structures (e.g, portal vein and biliary duct). Single and multiple gummas in the liver may occur and range in size from pinhead lesions to a large single gumma (53). Gummatous hepatitis may be diffuse or localized, and the clinical manifestations depend on the location of the lesions. If gumma abut a portal vein, ascites may develop. Jaundice from diffuse, interstitial disease may occur from obstruction of the bile ducts.

In chronic infection, fibrotic replacement of the liver may lead to cirrhosis and vascular damage to the portal circulation (53). The enlarged liver then becomes small, hard, and atrophic. Perihepatitis can occur from extension of a localized inflammatory process to the peritoneum, leading to adhesions and biliary tract disease, obstruction, and cholecystitis. The frequency of direct gall bladder disease appears unknown and has not been reported. Perilymphatic tissue around the liver or biliary system may become involved. Clinical manifestations of chronic syphilitic liver disease may include weight loss, jaundice, pain, fever, and ascites. Liver disease is often associated with other late manifestations, particularly syphilids in the skin or mucous membranes (53).

Syphilis of the esophagus is very rare, but cases have been described with ulcers, strictures, or mass lesions. Gastric ulceration is poorly documented, and while cases have been reported, causality is unclear (54). Gastric symptoms usually have been related to neurologic involvement of the vagus nerve, abdominal ganglia, and the sympathetic nervous system and represent neurologic rather than primary gastrointestinal disease. The differential diagnosis of esophageal or gastric disease must include malignancies and other infectious diseases (e.g., herpes simplex virus and cytomegalovirus). Syphilis of the small or large intestine appears to be very, very rare. In one case series of over 19,000 autopsies by Frankel, only three cases of intestinal disease were identified (53).

More recent reports of syphilis and gastrointestinal disease have focused on hepatic gumma presenting as mass lesions in the liver of unknown etiology (5, 31). After imaging and collection of tissue, syphilis was diagnosed on the basis of histology (Fig. 5). The authors emphasized the treatable nature of those lesions and the importance of including syphilis in the differential diagnosis and work-up of hepatic lesions (31). In addition, one case series described seven cases of hepatitis associated with early syphilis infection in HIV-infected individuals (37). While the role of HIV infection was unclear, all patients had elevations in liver enzymes that resolved with penicillin therapy. The authors concluded that syphilitic hepatitis was due to a periportal inflammatory response associated with treponemal hepatic invasion (37).

SYPHILIS OF THE GENITOURINARY SYSTEM

Syphilis of the genitourinary system appears to be even more uncommon than syphilis of the gastrointestinal tract. Most reports have cited renal disease due to immune complex formation and resultant glomerulonephritis (2). In the preantibiotic era, orchitis and testicular gumma were reported, but the relationship of syphilis to orchitis is not known (53).

A case report in 1975 described nephrosis in a 20-year old black man with a confirmed serum syphilis titer of 1:64 (10). The results of his renal biopsy demonstrated early membranous glomerulonephritis characterized by subepithelial basement-membrane deposits. Antibody elution studies confirmed the presence of antitreponemal antibodies within the immune complex deposits. The patient's nephrosis responded within days to penicillin treatment (10).

SYPHILIS OF THE CARDIOVASCULAR SYSTEM

Syphilis of the cardiovascular system is perhaps among the best-described medical conditions of the first half of the 20th century. Medical scientists performed and reported on extensive pathological work and clinical studies during that time.

Due to the vascular distribution and direct pathogenic effect of *T. pallidum* on blood vessels, there are multiple cardiovascular effects. The two pathophysiologic mechanisms resulting in clinical disease include chronic inflammation, with replacement of normal tissue with fibrous tissue and endarteritis resulting in ischemic or necrotic changes in the affected tissue and organs.

Chronic inflammation in the wall of the aorta, for example, results in normal elastic tissue being replaced by fibrous tissue and the weakening of the vessel wall, leading to the characteristic bulge of an aneurysm (53). Furthermore, chronic inflammation in the myocardium may result in fibrotic replacement

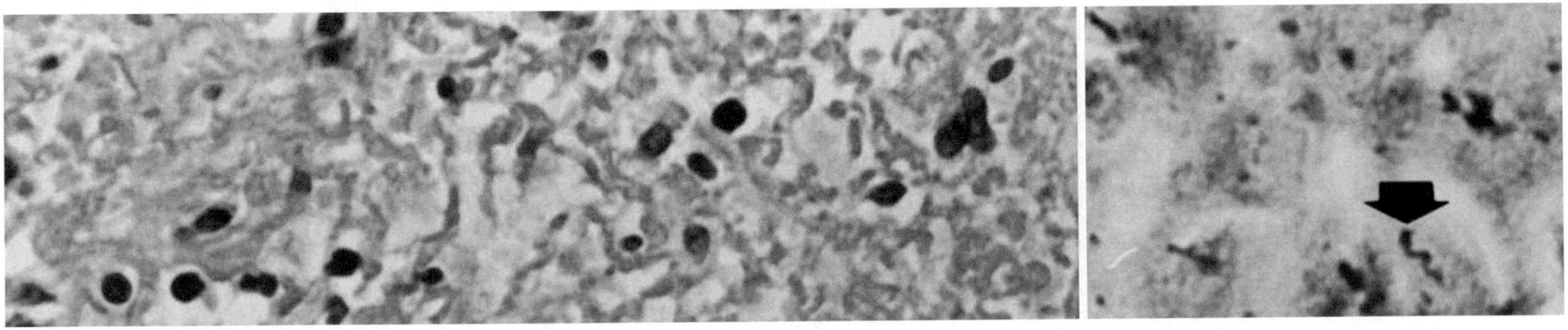

Figure 5. Fine-needle liver aspiration biopsy in hepatic tertiary disease. (Reprinted from *Digestive Diseases and Sciences* [31] with permission from Springer.)

of the myocardial tissue, leading to myocardial tissue degeneration, arrhythmias, and electrophysiologic abnormalities due to a damaged conduction system. Reported electrocardiographic abnormalities include abnormal T-wave morphology, QRS changes, inverted T waves, tachycardia, and bradycardia.

In contrast, fibrotic constriction of arteries, such as the vessels of the vasa vasorum that feed the wall of the aorta (the vasa vasorum supply nutrients to the aortic adventitia or wall of large arteries), or the narrowing of the ostia of the coronary arteries may lead to necrosis of aortic or myocardial tissue, causing aortic rupture or myocardial infarction and hemodynamic collapse (24).

The discovery of *T. pallidum* in the wall of the aorta was first accomplished by Reuter in 1906 and confirmed by Wright and Richardson in the United States in 1909 (44). An association between syphilis and aneurysm was first made by Lancisi as early as 1724 (53). In 1875, Welch reported a study of 117 cases of "fibroid aortitis" in which 46% had syphilis (53). Infiltration of the aortic wall with *T. pallidum* was associated with subsequent fibrotic replacement of the elastica, resulting in the weakening of the aortic ring and destruction of the mobility and competence of the aortic valve (53).

Based on prior natural history studies and the work of a variety of clinical investigators, it was estimated that aortitis may occur in about 75% of patients with untreated syphilis and among those about 10 to 15% may have clinical complications (21, 53). The time to clinical manifestations is at least 10 years after initial infection. Finally, cardiovascular syphilis is the predominant cause of death in those who die as a result of syphilis (21).

The symptoms of cardiovascular syphilis are myriad. Classic presentations include chest pain, dyspnea, cough, and hoarseness consistent with stretching or compression of the laryngeal nerve from a thoracic aneurysm. Aortitis does not include hoarseness. Chest pain is more diffuse but may include dyspnea, palpitations, indigestion, and angina.

Various clinical signs of aortitis and valvulitis include systolic and diastolic murmurs, hypertension, and left ventricular hypertrophy. Thoracic aneurysms may present with precordial dullness, bruits, vocal cord paralysis, diffuse loss of the radial pulse, marked differences in the blood pressure between arms, mediastinitis, a nondilating or small pupil on the affected side due to involvement of the sympathetic trunk, diastolic hypotension, and abnormalities on chest X-ray (21, 52). Further complications of a thoracic aneurysm can include spinal cord involvement, resulting in weakness or paralysis, or erosion of the vessel wall, leading to nerve compression, which results in radicular or referred pain.

Peripheral vascular disease is rarely associated with syphilis. Vasomotor spasm is inconsistent with syphilis. Peripheral vascular sclerosis leading to cool, blue, ulcerated, or gangrenous digits have an uncertain association with syphilis. Obliterative endarteritis, while seen in organ disease, is a diagnosis by exclusion in peripheral vascular disease.

Gumma of tertiary disease may involve the epicardium, visceral pericardium, or myocardium but seems to be very rare. The location of these gummatous lesions will result in a variety of clinical manifestations.

Aortitis and Aortic Valve Disease

Involvement of the aortic root is the most common manifestation of cardiovascular syphilis. Stokes reported on 200 cases of syphilis and aortic disease (53). Syphilitic aortitis was usually asymptomatic for a long period until valvular disease developed. The aortic root was the most vulnerable to aortitis, perhaps due to the rich vascularization of that segment of the aorta. Inflammation of adventitia begins near the vasa vasorum with lymphocytic infiltration. Coined "tree barking," the atherotic changes produce a characteristic pattern in the wall of the aorta (16). Intimal thickening leads to sclerosis, distortions, and abnormal architecture of the aortic ring. While the aortic valve may develop nodular infiltrations and subsequent stenosis, aortic insufficiency is more common due the weakening of the aortic ring. Additionally, lymphatic infiltration and inflammation results in peri-aortitis and mediastinitis. In another series, Stokes reported on 190 patients with cardiovascular syphilis: 104 had symptomatic aortitis, 61 had an aortic aneurysm, 38 had congestive heart failure, 4 had hypertension and renal disease, 2 had endarteritis, and 1 had phlebitis. The peak age of cases was 46 to 50 years; 54% had neurosyphilis as well (53).

Aortic insufficiency due to syphilis has a poor prognosis, with overall 10-year survival of 30 to 40% (26, 58). Chronic aortic insufficiency may lead to congestive heart failure. Data on clinical outcomes after aortic valve replacement in syphilis are limited, but clinical case series suggest valve replacement early in the course of disease was associated with benefit (14).

Aneurysm

While aortic aneurysms due to syphilis are among the less common of cardiovascular manifestations, they are the most dramatic. Aortic aneurysm and French disease (syphilis) were described in the last half of the 16th century (32). Most aneurysms occur in the ascending aortic arch and can become quite large before symptoms develop. Following the ascending aorta, the transverse aorta and then the descending arch are the next most common sites. The prognosis of patients with a syphilitic aortic aneurysm is very poor, with 80% dying at 2 years (21).

A recent case was described by Jackman and Radolf of an 82-year-old Hispanic woman who initially presented with fever, possible pneumonia, and a serum syphilis serology of 1:2, confirmed by a reactive treponemal test. Over about a 10-month period, syphilitic aortitis manifested as a thoracic aneurysm, resulting in aortic dissection and her death. Microscopic findings included an inflammatory infiltrate in the adventitia of the aorta with lymphocytes and plasma cells about the vasa vasorum (Fig. 6) (21). The media of the vessel had elastic fiber degeneration in a lamellar fashion with irregular scars. In their careful review of prior cases, Jackman and Radolf described syphilitic aneurysms as "fusiform or saccular and when saccular, the aneurysm may communicate with the aortic lumen." Notable in that report were the radiographic images by MRI which demonstrated the saccular nature of the aneurysm (Fig. 7). Those MRI images may have been more suggestive of syphilitic disease than the traditional arteriogram. While the authors hypothesized about the preferential role of MRI in the differential diagnosis of thoracic aneurysms, more research and experience are needed.

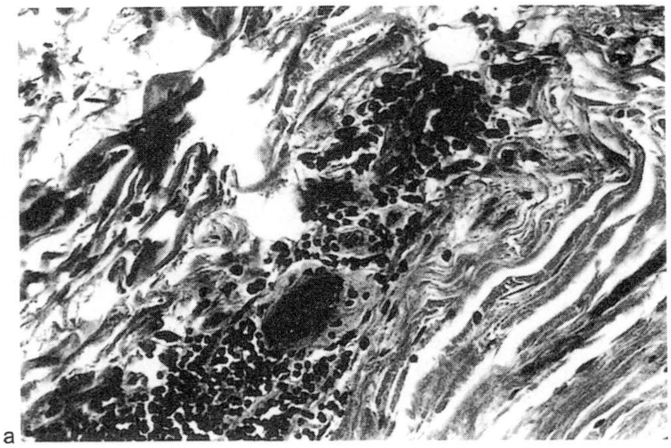

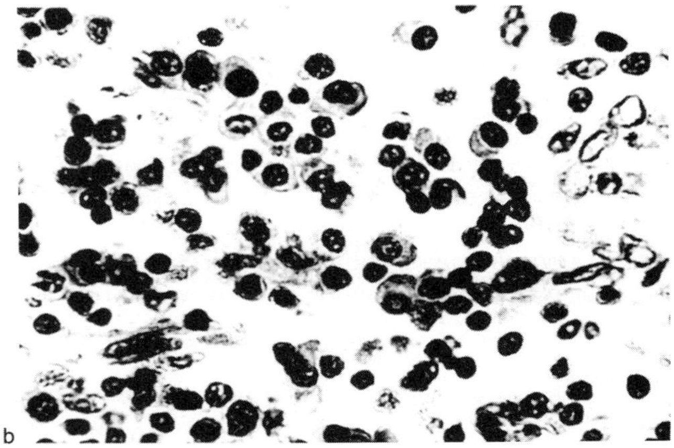

Figure 6. Postmortem microscopic findings showing perivascular inflammatory infiltrate of the aortic wall (a) and higher resolution plasma cells and lymphocytes (b). (Reprinted from *American Journal of Medicine* [21] with permission from Elsevier.)

Coronary Ostial Disease

Involvement of the cardiac sinuses of Valsalva may produce stenosis of coronary ostia, with possible extension into the coronary arteries themselves (Fig. 8). Coronary ostial stenosis is the second most common complication of syphilitic aortitis (21). Angina is the most common clinical manifestation, yet myocardial infarction is rare. The slow progression of disease along with the concomitant development of collateral vascularization of the myocardium has been suggested to protect the myocardium from ischemic disease (3).

SYPHILIS OF THE CENTRAL NERVOUS SYSTEM

Perhaps the most well-known and feared complication of syphilis infection is syphilis of the brain. Syphilitic dementia or general paresis has captured the imagination of the general population, and while today it is a rare event, in the early part of the last century it was the principal cause of acquired insanity. There are different manifestations and underlying pathophysiologic mechanisms causing syphilis of the central nervous system. Similar to cardiovascular syphilis, the main mechanisms of disease result from chronic inflammation, microvascular compromise, or gummatous infiltration. The inflammatory process can occur directly in the parenchyma of the brain, resulting in neuronal loss. Elevation of the white blood cell count in cerebrospinal fluid is the sine qua non of cerebral inflammation, and experts state that without such an increase, syphilis of the central nervous system (excluding the ocular system) can be ruled out (50).

Meningovascular Disease

Early reports described ruptured small arterioles in the brain leading to hemiplegia (53). For example, Stokes described a patient with a ruptured aneurysm

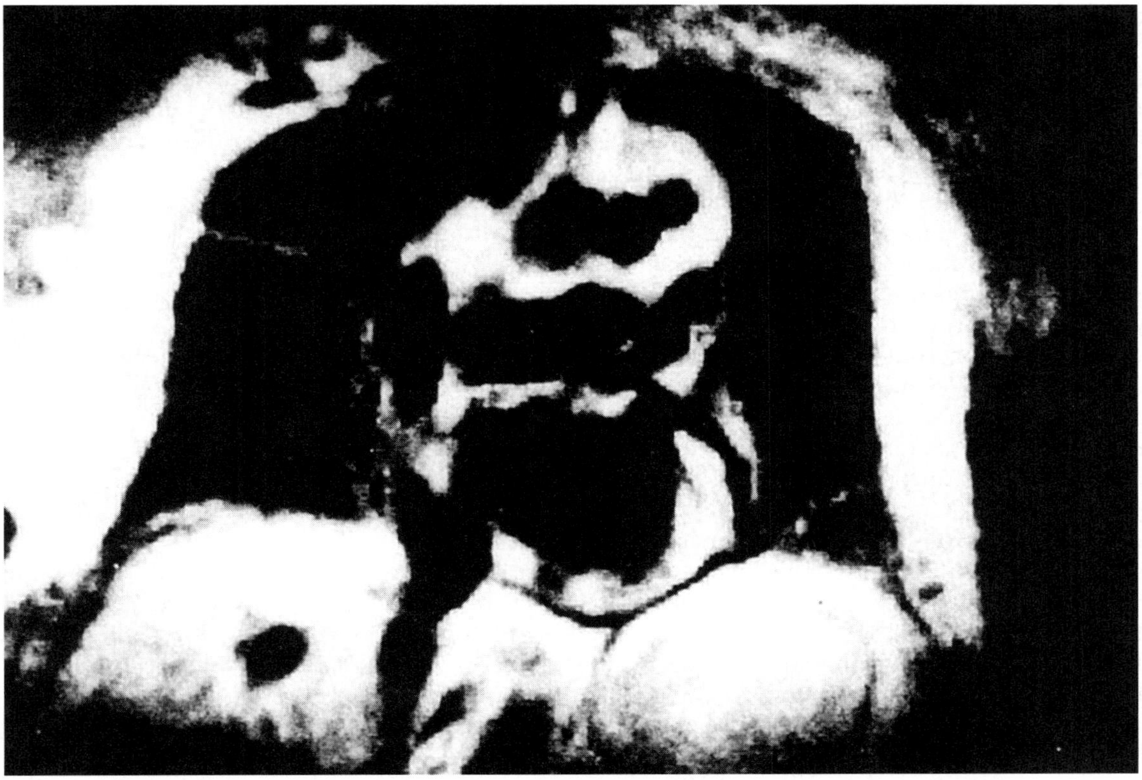

Figure 7. Magnetic resonance imaging MRI showing saccular aneurysm. (Reprinted from the *American Journal of Medicine* [21] with permission from Elsevier.)

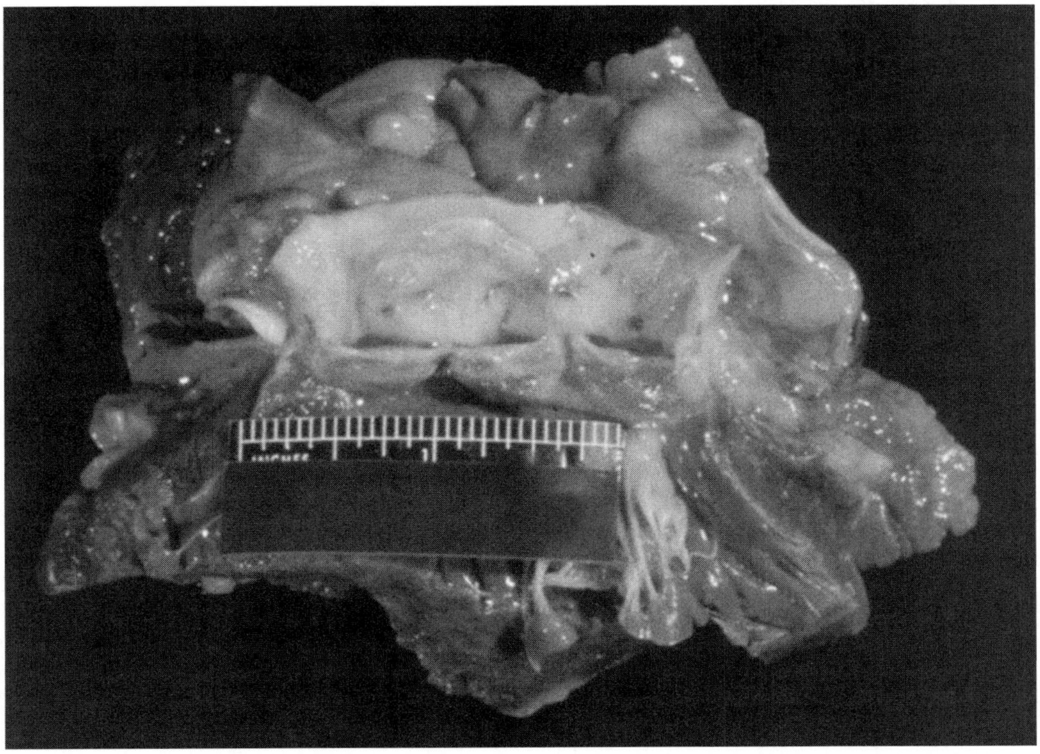

Figure 8. Gross autopsy photograph showing coronary artery ostial narrowing by syphilitic aortitis. (Republished with permission of Joseph A. Prahlow, forensic pathologist, South Bend Medical Foundation and Indiana University School of Medicine, South Bend at the University of Notre Dame, South Bend, IN.)

of the lenticulostriate artery of internal capsule resulting in severe motor dysfunction (53). Endarteritis may lead to thromboses and cerebral ischemia. Involvement of the cerebrovascular system has been called meningovascular neurosyphilis. After the advent of penicillin therapy, meningovascular syphilis was rare. In the Oslo series of 953 untreated cases, meningovascular complications usually presented 10 to 20 years after infection (13). Meningovascular involvement has been characterized by some authors as involving mesodermal tissues as opposed to the ectodermal tissues involved in progressive parenchymal disease (39). Such mesodermal disease causes meningitis, cranial nerve deficits, or cerebrovascular accidents. In Merritt's summary of the neurosyphilis of patients in New York City, published in 1938, only 80 patients out of approximately 2,000 had this form of central nervous system involvement (35). Others have stated that meningovascular syphilis may represent about 10% of cases of central nervous system disease (18).

Because in syphilitic meningitis the vascular involvement and inflammatory response occur at the base of the brain where there is a rich supply of blood vessels, clinical presentations often involve the cranial nerves, I, II, III, IV, VI , VII, and VIII. Furthermore, in vascular disease, the circle of Willis, as well as smaller capillaries, can be involved, causing strokes and hemorrhages.

The histopathology of meningovascular syphilis shows arteritis with infiltration of lymphocytes and plasma cells of the vasa vasorum, adventitia, and media in medium and large arteries (52). Occlusion of the vasa vasorum leads to destruction of the smooth muscle and elastic tissue in the media of larger vessels. Concentric proliferation of subintimal fibroblasts narrows the lumen until occlusion occurs by thrombus.

The symptoms and laboratory findings in meningovascular syphilis can include hemiparesis or hemiplegia, aphasia, and seizures (52). Ischemic territory may include the middle cerebral artery, resulting in abnormalities in language, speech, and motor function. While the symptoms may appear abruptly, about half of cases may have a prodrome with headache, dizziness, insomnia, memory loss, and mood changes.

On cerebral angiography, findings can include "beading" of the anterior or middle cerebral arteries and segmental dilatation of the pericallosal arteries (28). Cerebral vascular syphilis tends to affect the more distal portion of the internal carotid artery and the proximal portions of its branches compared with cerebroatherosclerotic disease, which tends to involve more proximal aspects of the carotid, e.g, at the carotid bifurcation (52).

Meningovascular disease can also affect the spinal cord (1). Syphilitic meningomyelitis and spinal vascular syphilis can cause acute transverse myelitis. Such spinal cord disease, however, has been rare. Spinal vascular disease can result in transection of the spinal cord at the thoracic level with abrupt onset of flaccid paraplegia, at the sensory level on the trunk, and urinary retention (52).

Parenchymal Disease

Central nervous system involvement of the cerebral parenchymal tissue may result from particular neurotropic strains of *T. pallidum* with a predilection for neuroinvasion (53, 55). In the last century it was shown that there was a high concordance of neurological involvement in conjugal cases (53). The frequency and clinical significance of neuroinvasion are areas of intense debate. In a study among about 500 patients with early syphilis who underwent cerebrospinal fluid analysis, about 25% had some evidence of neuroinvasion (46). In a historic series by Mattauschek and Pilcz reported by Stokes among 4,134 Austrian Army officers with syphilis, 4.8% had paresis, 2.7% had tabes dorsalus, and 2.3% cerebrospinal syphilis (53). Other studies have shown that men have greater central nervous system involvement than women. Looking at 70,000 first admissions to 48 hospitals in 16 states, May found 11% of patients with paresis (53).

General Paresis

General paresis is an inflammatory process of the brain (52). The pathologic findings in cerebral disease include a diffuse inflammatory reaction in the cerebrum; localizing about the blood vessels and the meninges, with "coat-sleeve" lymphocytic and plasma cell infiltration about the capillaries; and degeneration of parenchymal cells with reactive gliosis (53). The encephalitis is chronic and usually manifests in middle or late adulthood after a 15- to 25-year incubation period (52).

There is a wide range of manifestations associated with a progressive dementia. Defects in judgment, emotional lability, grandiose delusions, megalomania, and depression have been described. Further reports include paresthesias, such as fleeting attacks of numbness, tingling, prickling, feelings of constriction, and cold or warm sensations. Various forms of sexual dysfunction, including hypersexuality, have also been described. General paresis may include paralysis, focal paralysis, catatonia, senility, amnesia, clouded consciousness, irritability, violence, and tremors (53).

Neurologic findings include pupillary changes; facial changes, with flattening of the nasolabial fold; tremors of facial muscles; and impaired writing and speech. Untreated paresis may last for months to years. Further complications may include communicating hydrocephalus. With the advent of computer-assisted tomography, a computer-assisted tomography scan may show decreased attenuation of cerebral white matter in frontal regions, parietal and ventricular dilatation (11). Pathologic findings include thickening of the meninges; cerebral atrophy, particularly of the frontal lobe or temporal lobe; and demyelination of white matter.

Tabes Dorsalis

Tabes dorsalis, syphilitic involvement of the spinal cord, impacted about one-third of patients with neurosyphilis in the preantibiotic era (53). Currently, tabes dorsalis is a very rare condition. Similar to that of general paresis, the incubation period ranges from 15 to 25 years. Clinical symptoms include lightning pains, paresthesias, decreased reflexes, difficulty walking, and poor pupillary responses to light. Tabes dorsalis is a disease of the dorsal roots of the spinal nerves with ascending degeneration of the spinal cord (53). Because the arterial blood supply is dominant to the posterior aspects of the spinal cord, the sensory horns, and posterolateral columns, the anterior aspects of the spinal cord and motor areas are less affected. Lightning pains (73 to 88%), visual symptoms (44%), difficulties in urination (43 to 68%), abnormalities in peripheral sensation, difficulty in walking, and eye findings, like strabismus and diplopia, are not uncommon (53). Table 1 shows a range of clinical findings described by Merritt (35).

Early signs of tabes dorsalis include loss of vibration sense and the inability to feel passive movement in the joints. Over time there may be a loss of deep pain perception, with patchy areas of numbness or increased pain sensitivity. Decreased knee and ankle reflexes were characterized with preserved muscle strength until end-stage disease (52, 53). Neuromuscular or skeletal abnormalities included a broad-based walk, Charcot's joints resulting from a loss of nerve function serving large joints like the knee, foot ulcers, and spinal abnormalities.

For tabes dorsalis, clinicians have described "cushion feet" or the feeling of walking on cotton, a girdle sensation or tightening of the waist or lower thorax, lightning pains up and down the spine, ringing ears, dizziness, impaired vision, double vision, deafness, facial palsy, seizures, and language and speaking difficulties (53). Urinary retention may result in overflow incontinence with difficulty in initiating a urine stream and postvoid dribbling. A classic description of tabes dorsalis includes patients who walk with their heels landing hard on the floor, knees positioned outward with their feet slapping.

Table 1. Tabes dorsalis: signs and symptoms[a]

Symptom or sign	% Cases
Symptoms	
Lightning pains	75
Ataxia	42
Bladder disturbances	33
Paresthesias	24
Visceral crises	18
Visual loss (optic atrophy)	16
Rectal incontinence	14
Signs	
Pupillary abnormalities	94
Argyll Robertson pupils	48
Absent ankle jerks	94
Absent knee jerks	81
Romberg's sign	55
Impaired vibratory sense	52
Impaired position sense	45
Impaired touch and pain sense	13
Ocular palsies	10
Charcot's joints	7

[a]Adapted from Sparling (52) with permission from McGraw-Hill Companies, Inc.

Visceral crises resulting from specific spinal cord involvement was described in the early medical literature (53). Gastric crisis with intense epigastric pain, nausea, and vomiting was the most common. Intestinal crises with abdominal pain and diarrhea, rectal crises with painful tenesmus, and laryngeal crises with pain in the larynx, hoarseness, and stridor were less common.

Cerebral Gummas

Finally, more recent reports of cerebral gumma have been described in HIV-infected patients and diagnosis has been aided with the use of PCR assays (Fig. 9a, b, c, and d) (19, 54, 58). The authors reported space-occupying lesions in the brain manifesting with stroke-like syndromes and focal motor seizures. Gummatous lesions may be solitary or multiple. Overall, however, such clinical disease is rare and does not appear to be increased in the era of AIDS. The importance of microbiological diagnosis versus empirical therapy is unclear (41).

SYPHILIS OF THE VISUAL SYSTEM

Syphilis of the ocular system can occur at the level of the cerebrum, optic nerve, other cranial nerves, retina, and eye. The nerves that enervate the muscles that control eye movement and constriction or

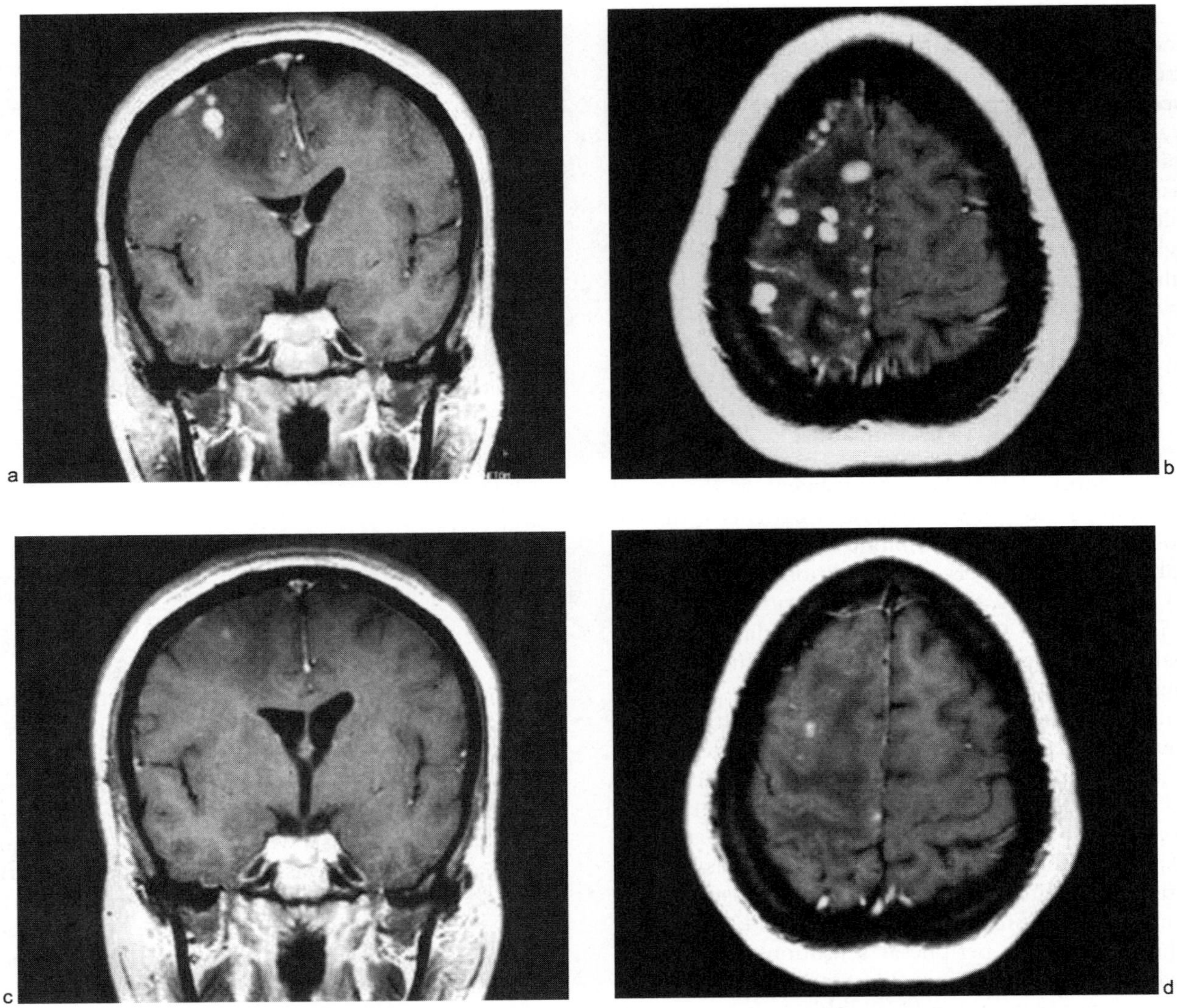

Figure 9. MRI (a and b) showing multiple cerebral syphilitic gummas in patient with HIV and RPR titer of 1:32. Significant improvement shown after treatment with penicillin (c and d). (Republished from reference 45a with permission from the *Massachusetts Medical Society.*)

dilation of the pupil can be affected resulting in abnormal, bilateral or unilateral physical findings of the eye. In one series of 126 cases of neurosyphilis, 63% had pathologic eye findings, including 35% with Argyll-Robertson pupils (a pupil that is nonreactive to light but constricts during accommodation) (53). Optic neuritis and atrophy can lead to visual loss.

Keratitis, iritis, and anterior uveitis (posterior is less common) may be associated with secondary syphilis; however, given the association of ocular disease with neurosyphilis, cerebrospinal fluid examination is warranted (27). A recent review of ocular syphilis emphasized the importance of excluding syphilis infection in all ocular inflammatory conditions (12).

PREGNANCY AND CONGENITAL SYPHILIS

Untreated syphilis infection during pregnancy may have a devastating impact on the developing fetus, even in the absence of maternal clinical manifestations. Untreated maternal infection during pregnancy may result in stillbirth, preterm labor or delivery, fetal growth retardation, or congenital infection (17, 38, 40). Severe pregnancy outcomes associated with maternal syphilis emphasize the need for women to receive antenatal syphilis screening. Prenatal diagnosis of syphilis in pregnancy as well as timely treatment is critical in the prevention of congenital syphilis. It is estimated that about 26% of stillbirths in developing countries are due to syphilis infection (34).

Newly acquired infection with *T. pallidum* invades the placenta during the first trimester of pregnancy. Further risk of transmission decreases with the duration of untreated maternal infection (59). Mothers with latent-stage infection are less likely to transmit syphilis to the fetus.

Maternal syphilitic infection can result in premature death of the developing fetus, resulting in spontaneous abortions or stillbirths. Depending on the duration of fetal infection, the stillbirth may be macerated at delivery. Historical studies estimated that approximately 30% of untreated maternal syphilis pregnancies result in second-trimester spontaneous abortion or stillbirth (20, 59). Further data have suggested that untreated early latent maternal syphilis infection may lead to congenital syphilis infection (40%), preterm birth (20%), and healthy uninfected infants (20%) (8).

Several recent reports in developing countries have highlighted the significant impact of maternal syphilis on the fetus. Studies in Tanzania and Malawi suggest that high-titer active syphilis (RPR titer

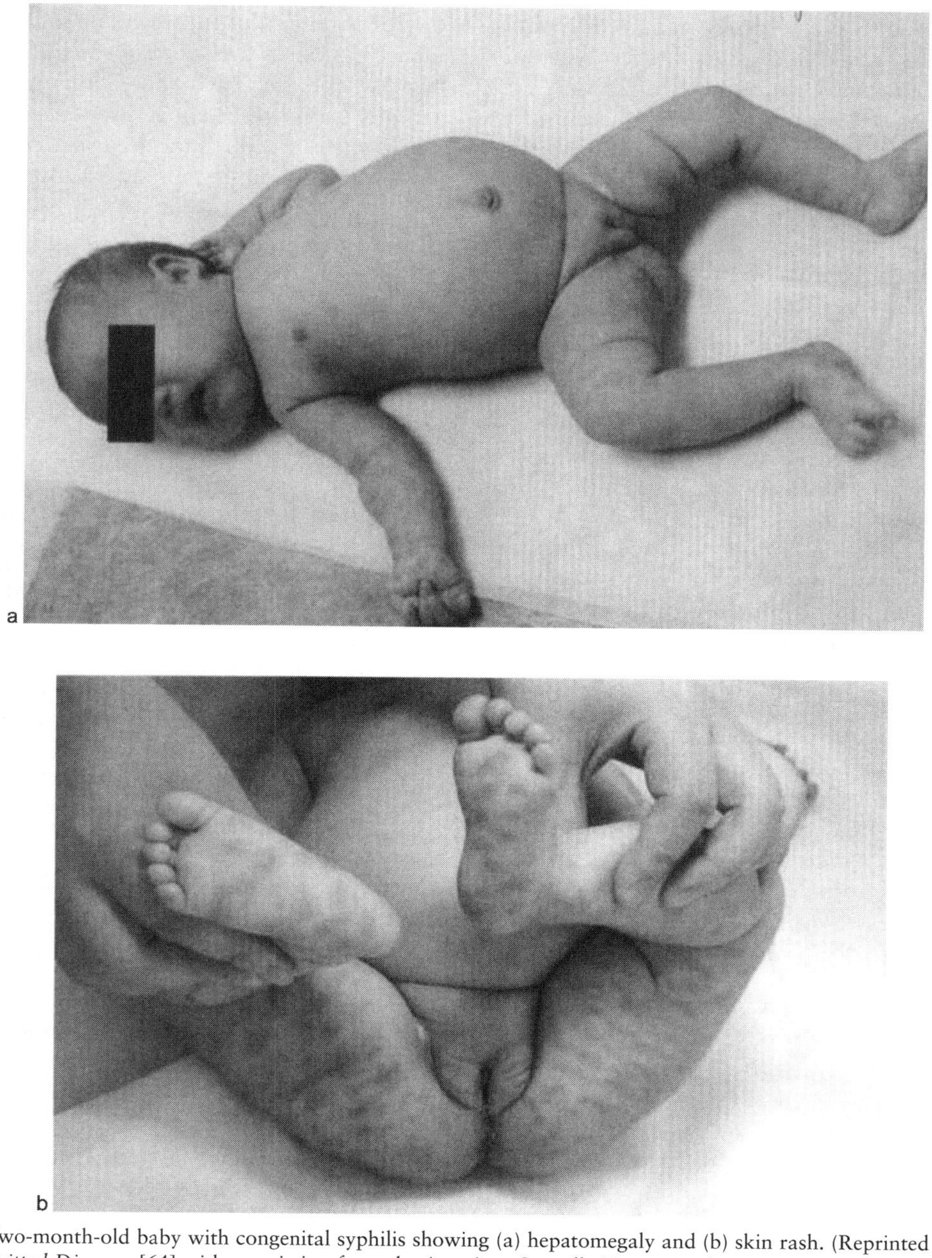

Figure 10. Two-month-old baby with congenital syphilis showing (a) hepatomegaly and (b) skin rash. (Reprinted from *Sexually Transmitted Diseases* [64] with permission from the American Sexually Transmitted Diseases Association.)

greater than or equal to 1:8) has been strongly associated with stillbirths, preterm birth, and low-birth-weight live births (34, 56). Overall, women with high-titer syphilis were at a fourfold increased risk of any adverse pregnancy outcome compared with seronegative women.

Pathologic findings in syphilis-related stillbirths include enlarged liver and spleen, chondro-epiphysitis; fibrotic changes in the lung, liver, spleen, and pancreas (with separation of the lobules and acini); and internal hemorrhage (53). Osteochondritis may also be seen. The myocardium may become involved with fatty changes and perivascular lymphocytic infiltration.

Live births with congenitally acquired syphilis may manifest by week 3 of life. Snuffles (hemorrhagic or purulent nasal discharge is often diagnostic) and cutaneous lesions on the chin and circumoral area, palms, or soles are characteristic (53). Fissuring ("hacking" of the lip), lesions at the angles of mouth (eczema-like), scarring of chin ("rhagades"), mucous patches, and anal condyloma lata may appear. An enlarged spleen and bony lesions are diagnostic of congenital syphilis (Fig. 10a and b). Increased irritability and restlessness as well as an abnormal cry (aphonic) may be typical.

Bony involvement may be seen with an epiphyseal lesion. Thickening and irregularity of the epiphyseal line may be replaced with fatty degeneration and necrosis between the epiphysis and diaphysis. Fetal cranial lesions are unusual.

Other characteristic findings include interstitial keratitis, which usually manifests at 5 to 16 years of age and may result in inflammation of the entire corneal thickness; Hutchinson incisors; mulberry molars; cranial VIII-related nerve deafness; saber shin tibia; nasal septum osteitis; and dactylitis with fusiform swelling of the proximal phalanx and abnormal facies, with a flattened bridge of the nose (53). In Stokes' series, eye lesions were most common, followed by bony changes and teeth abnormalities. The Hutchinson triad was the combined findings of interstitial keratitis, abnormal teeth, and cranial nerve VIII-related deafness.

CONCLUSIONS

The clinical manifestations of untreated syphilis infection are due to a chronic inflammatory process with resultant fibrosis that can impact almost any body system. *T. pallidum* has a predilection for highly vascularized tissue, like the brain and heart. Chronic inflammation results in a weakened architecture of the tissue and endarteritis causing vascular compromise. The lack of blood supply to tissue can cause ischemic changes and necrosis. While the consequences of untreated syphilis appear rare in the current era of widespread antibiotic use and the continued susceptibility of *T. pallidum* to penicillin in areas where syphilis control programs do not exist, endemic syphilis takes a significant toll on maternal-child health and is the most important preventable cause of spontaneous terminations of pregnancy, premature delivery, and still birth.

Because most tissue damage from chronic syphilis infection is irreversible and occasionally lethal, renewed emphasis must be placed on the primary prevention of syphilis infection through the development of an effective vaccine. Research into the basic biology of *T. pallidum* must be expanded, including the identification of a reliable means of in vitro cultivation. While the early detection and treatment of syphilis can prevent clinical sequelae, in much of the world such screening and treatment programs do not exist, causing undue pain and human suffering.

Acknowledgment. We acknowledge Joanne Carpio for her research and administrative assistance in the production of this chapter.

REFERENCES

1. **Adams, R. D., and H. H. Merritt.** 1994. Meningeal and vascular syphilis of the spinal cord. *Medicine* **23:**181–214.
2. **Baughn, R. E.** 1986. Characterization of the antigenic determinants and host components in immune complexes from patients with secondary syphilis. *J. Immunol.* **136:**1406–1414.
3. **Burch, G. E., and T. Winsor,** 1942. Syphilitic coronary stenosis, with myocardial infarction. *Am. Heart J.* **24:**740–751.
4. **Chen, Z. Q., G. C. Zhang, X. D. Gong, C. Lin, X. Gao, G. J. Liang, X. L. Yue, X. S. Chen, and M. S. Cohen.** 2007. Syphilis in China: results of a national surveillance programme. *Lancet* **369:**132–138.
5. **Chen, J. F., W. X. Chen, H. Y. Zhang, and W. Y. Zhang.** 2008. Peliosis and gummatous syphilis of the liver: a case report. *World J. Gastroenterol.* **14:**1961–1963.
6. **Centers for Disease Control and Prevention.** 2007. Sexually transmitted disease surveillance 2006. U.S. Department of Health and Human Services, Atlanta, GA.
7. **Fenton, K. A., R. Breban, R. Vardavas, J. T. Okano, T. Martin, S. Aral, and S. Blower.** 2008. Infectious syphilis in high-income settings in the 21st century. *Lancet Infect. Dis.* **8:**244–253.
8. **Fiumara, N. J., W. L. Fleming, J. G. Downing, and F. L. Good.** 1952. The incidence of prenatal syphilis at the Boston City Hospital. *N. Engl. J. Med.* **247:**48–52.
9. **Fraser, C. M., S. J. Norris, G. M. Weinstock, O. White, G. G. Sutton, R. Dodson, M. Gwinn, E. K. Hickey, R. Clayton, and K. A. Ketchum.** 1998. Complete genome sequence of *Treponema pallidum*, the syphilis spirochete. *Science* **281:**375.
10. **Gamble, C. N., and J. B. Reardan.** 1975. Immunopathogenesis of syphilitic glomerulonephritis. Elution of antitreponemal antibody from glomerular immune-complex deposits. *N. Engl. J. Med.* **292:**449–454.
11. **Ganti, S. R., M. Cohen, P. Sane, and S. K. Hilal.** 1981. Computed tomography of cerebral syphilis. *J. Comput. Assist. Tomogr.* **5:**345–347.
12. **Gaudio, P. A.** 2006. Update on ocular syphilis. *Curr. Opin. Ophthalmol.* **17:** 562.

13. **Gjestland, T.** 1955. The Oslo study of untreated syphilis; an epidemiologic investigation of the natural course of the syphilitic infection based upon a re-study of the Boeck-Bruusgaard material. *Acta Derm. Venereol. Suppl.* (Stockholm) **35**(Suppl. 34):3–368.
14. **Grabau, W., R. Emanuel, D. Ross, J. Parker, and M. Hegde.** 1976. Syphilitic aortic regurgitation. An appraisal of surgical treatment. *Br. Med. J.* **52**:366.
15. **Gurland, I. A., L. Korn, L. Edelman, and F. Wallach.** 2001. An unusual manifestation of acquired syphilis. *Clin. Infect. Dis.* **32**:667–669.
16. **Heggtveit, H. A.** 1964. Syphilitic aortitis A clinicopathologic autopsy study of 100 cases, 1950 to 1960. *Circulation* **29**:346–355.
17. **Hollier, L. M., T. W. Harstad, P. J. Sanchez, D. M. Twickler, and G. D. Wendel, Jr.** 2001. Fetal syphilis: clinical and laboratory characteristics. *Obstet. Gynecol.* **97**:947–53.
18. **Holmes, M. D.** 1984. Clinical features of meningovascular syphilis. *Neurology* **34**:553–556.
19. **Horowitz, H. W., M. P. Valsamis, V. Wicher, F. Abbruscato, S. A. Larsen, G. P. Wormser, and K. Wicher.** 1994. Cerebral syphilitic gumma confirmed by the polymerase chain reaction in a man with human immunodeficiency virus infection. *N. Engl. J. Med.* **331**:1488.
20. **Ingraham, N. R., Jr.** 1950. The value of penicillin alone in the prevention and treatment of congenital syphilis. *Acta Derm. Venereol. Suppl.* (Stockholm) **31**:60–87.
21. **Jackman, J. D., Jr., and J. D. Radolf.** 1989. Cardiovascular syphilis. *Am. J. Med.* **87**:425–33.
22. **Kampmeier, R. H.** 1943. *Essentials of Syphilology*, 3rd ed. JB Lippincott Company, Philadelphia, PA.
23. **Kandelaki, G., R. Kapila, and H. Fernandes.** 2007. Destructive osteomyelitis associated with early secondary syphilis in an HIV-positive patient diagnosed by *Treponema pallidum* DNA polymerase chain reaction. *AIDS Patient Care STDS* **21**:229–233.
24. **Kennedy, J. L. W., J. J. Barnard, and J. A. Prahlow.** 2006. Syphilitic coronary artery ostial stenosis resulting in acute myocardial infarction and death. *Cardiology* **105**:25–29.
25. **Klausner, J. D., C. K. Kent, W. Wong, J. McCright, and M. H. Katz.** 2005. The public health response to epidemic syphilis, San Francisco, 1999-2004. *Sex. Transm. Dis.* **32**(Suppl. 10):S11–S18.
26. **Leonard, J. C., and W. G. Smith.** 1957. Syphilitic aortic incompetence with special reference to prognosis and effect of treatment. *Lancet* **272**:234–240.
27. **Levy, J. H., R. A. Liss, and A. M. Maguire.** 1989. Neurosyphilis and ocular syphilis in patients with concurrent human immunodeficiency virus infection. *Retina* **9**:175–180.
28. **Liebeskind, A., S. Cohen, R. Anderson, M. M. Schechter, and L. H. Zingesser.** 1973. Unusual segmental cerebrovascular changes. *Radiology* **106**:119–122.
29. **Lukehart, S. A.** 2008. Biology of treponemes, p. 661–684. *In* K. K. Holmes, P. F. Sparling, P. A. Mardh, S. M. Lemon, W. E. Stamm, P. Piot, and J. N. Wasserheit (ed.), *Sexually Transmitted Diseases,* 4th ed. McGraw-Hill, New York, NY.
30. **Mahoney, J. F., and K. K. Bryant.** 1933. Contact infection of rabbits in experimental syphilis. *Am. J. Syphilis* **17**: 188–193.
31. **Maincent, G., H. Labadie, M. Fabre, P. Novello, K. Derghal, C. Patriarche, and H. Licht.** 1997. Case report: tertiary hepatic syphilis A treatable cause of multinodular liver. *Dig. Dis. Sci.* **42**:447–450.
32. **Major, R. H.** 1932. *Classic Descriptions of Disease*, p. 415–418. Charles C. Thomas, Springfield, IL.
33. **Mandell, G. L.** 2004. *Essential Atlas of Infectious Diseases.* Current Medicine, Philadelphia, PA.
34. **McDermott, J., R. Steketee, S. Larsen, and J. Wirima.** 1993. Syphilis-associated perinatal and infant mortality in rural Malawi. *Bull. W. H. O.* **71**:773–780.
35. **Merritt, H. H., H. Houston, R. D. Adams, and H. C. Solomon.** 1946. *Neurosyphilis.* Oxford University Press, New York, NY.
36. **Mindel, A., S. J. Tovey, D. J. Timmins, and P. Williams.** 1989. Primary and secondary syphilis, 20 years' experience. 2. Clinical features. *Br. Med. J.* **65**:1.
37. **Mullick, C. J., A. P. Liappis, D. A. Benator, A. D. Roberts, D. M. Parenti, and G. L. Simon.** 2004. Syphilitic hepatitis in HIV-infected patients: a report of 7 cases and review of the literature. *Clin. Infect. Dis.* **39**:e100–e105.
38. **Mullick, S., D. Watson-Jones, M. Beksinska, and D. Mabey.** 2005. Sexually transmitted infections in pregnancy: prevalence, impact on pregnancy outcomes, and approach to treatment in developing countries. *Br. Med. J.* **81**:294.
39. **Musher, D. M., and R. E. Baughn.** 1994. Neurosyphilis in HIV-infected persons. *N. Engl. J. Med.* **331**:1516.
40. **Navas, R. M., R. Parra, M. Pacheco, J. Gomez, I. Bermudez, and A. J. Rodriguez-Morales.** 2006. Congenital bilateral microphthalmos after gestational syphilis. *Indian J. Pediatr.* **73**:935–936.
41. **Quinn, P., L. Weisberg, L. C. Roeske, P. R. Kennedy, J. L. Suarez, D. Mlakar, and S. M. Snodgrass.** 1997. Cerebral syphilitic gumma. *N. Engl. J. Med.* **336**:1027.
42. **Rademacher, S. E., and J. D. Radolf.** 1996. Prominent osseous and unusual dermatologic manifestations of early syphilis in two patients with discordant serological statuses for human immunodeficiency virus infection. *Clin. Infect. Dis.* **23**:462–467.
43. **Radolf, J. D., K. R. O. Hazlett, and S. A. Lukehart.** 2006. Pathogenesis of syphilis, p. 197–236. *In* J. D. Radolf and S. A. Lukehart, *Pathogenic Treponema. Molecular and Cellular Biology.* Caister Academic Press, Norfolk, England.
44. **Reuter, K.** 1989. Neue befunde von Sprichaete pallida im menschlichen korper und ihre bedeutung fur die atiologie der syphilis. *Z Hyg Infectionskrankh 1906* **54**:49–62.
45. **Reynolds, F., and H. Wasserman.** 1942. Destructive osseous lesions in early syphilis. *Arch. Intern. Med.* **69**:263–276.
45a. **Roeske, L. C., and P. R. Kennedy.** 1996. Syphilitic gummas in a patient with human immunodeficiency virus infection. *New Engl. J. Med.* **335**:1123.
46. **Rolfs, R. T., M. R. Joesoef, E. F. Hendershot, A. M. Rompalo, M. H. Augenbraun, M. Chiu, G. Bolan, S. C. Johnson, P. French, E. Steen, J. D. Radolf, S. Larsen, et al.** 1997. A randomized trial of enhanced therapy for early syphilis in patients with and without human immunodeficiency virus infection. *N. Engl. J. Med.* **337**:307–314.
47. **Salazar, J. C., A. Rathi, N.L. Michael, J. D. Radolf, and L. L. Jagodzinski.** 2007. Assessment of the kinetics of *Treponema pallidum* dissemination into blood and tissues in experimental syphilis by real-time quantitative PCR. *Infect. Immun.* **75**:2954–2958.
48. **Schaudinn, F., and E. Hoffmann.** 1905. Vorläufiger Bericht über das Vorkommen von Spirochaeten in syphilitischen Krankheitsprodukten und bei Papillomen. *Arb. Kaiserl. Gesundheitsamte* **22**:527–534.
49. **Schmid, G. P., B. P. Stoner, S. Hawkes, and N. Broutet.** 2007. The need and plan for global elimination of congenital syphilis. *Sex. Transm. Dis.* **34**: S5–S10.
50. **Simon, R.** 2007. Nuerosyphilis, p. 130–137. *In* J. D. Klausner and E. W. Hook, *Current Diagnosis and Treatment of Sexually Transmitted Diseases.* McGraw-Hill, New York, NY.
51. **Singh, A. E., and B. Romanowski.** 1999. Syphilis: review with emphasis on clinical, epidemiologic, and some biologic features. *Clin. Microbiol. Rev.* **12**:187–209.

52. **Sparling P. F., M. N. Swartz, D. M. Musher, and B. P. Healy.** 2008. Clinical manifestations of syphilis, p. 661–684. *In* K. K. Holmes, P. F. Sparling, P. A. Mardh, S. M. Lemon, W. E. Stamm, P. Piot, and J. N. Wasserheit, *Sexually Transmitted Diseases,* 4th ed. McGraw-Hill, New York, NY.
53. **Stokes, J. H., H. Beerman, and N. R. Ingraham.** 1944. *Modern Clinical Syphilology: Diagnosis, Treatment, Case Study,* 3rd ed. W. B. Saunders, Philadelphia, PA.
54. **Suarez, J. I., D. Mlakar, and S. M. Snodgrass.** 1996. Cerebral syphilitic gumma in an HIV-negative patient presenting as prolonged focal motor status epilepticus. *N. Engl. J. Med.* **335:**1159.
55. **Tantalo, L. C., S. A. Lukehart, and C. M. Marra.** 2005. Treponema pallidum strain-specific differences in neuroinvasion and clinical phenotype in a rabbit model. *J. Infect. Dis.* **191:**75–80.
56. **Watson-Jones, D., J. Changalucha, B. Gumodoka, H. Weiss, M. Rusizoka, L. Ndeki, A. Whitehouse, R. Balira, J. Todd, and D. Ngeleja.** 2002. Syphilis in pregnancy in Tanzania. I. impact of maternal syphilis on outcome of pregnancy. *J. Infect. Dis.* **186:**940–947.
57. **Webster, B., C. Rich, Jr., P. M. Densen, J. E. Moore, C. S. Nicol, and P. Padget.** 1953. Studies in cardiovascular syphilis. III. The natural history of syphilitic aortic insufficiency. *Am. Heart J.* **46:**117–145.
58. **Weinert, L. S., R. S. Scheffel, G. Zoratto, V. Samios, M. W. Jeffmann, J. M. Dora, and L. Z. Goldani.** 2008. Cerebral syphilitic gumma in HIV-infected patients: case report and review. *Int. J. STD AIDS* **19:**62–64.
59. **Weiss, R. S., and H. L. Joseph. 1951.** *Syphilis.* Nelson, New York, NY.
60. **Williams, L. A., J. D. Klausner, W. L. Whittington, H. H. Handsfield, C. Celum, and K. K. Holmes.** 1999. Elimination and reintroduction of primary and secondary syphilis. *Am. J. Public Health* **89:**1093.
61. **Wong, T. Y., and M. C. Mihm, Jr.** 1994. Images in clinical medicine. Primary syphilis. *N. Engl. J. Med.* **331:**1492.
62. **Zetola, N. M. and J. D. Klausner.** 2007. Syphilis and HIV infection: an update. *Clin. Infect. Dis.* **44:**1222–1228.
63. **Zhou, P., Y. Qian, J. Xu, Z. Gu, and K. Liao.** 2007. Occurrence of congenital syphilis after maternal treatment with azithromycin during pregnancy. *Sex. Transm. Dis.* **34:**472.

Sequelae and Long-Term Consequences of Infectious Diseases
Edited by Pina M. Fratamico, James L. Smith, and Kim A. Brogden

Chapter 11

Whipple's Disease

THOMAS MARTH AND GJORGI DERIBAN

Whipple's disease (WD) is a rare multisystemic chronic infection caused by the rod-shaped bacterium *Tropheryma whipplei*. The disease may occur in people of all ages but most frequently affects middle-aged white males. Patients usually present with symptoms of weight loss, arthralgia, diarrhea, and abdominal pain. Involvement of the heart, lung, and central nervous system (CNS) is also common. A significant number of patients do not have these classic signs and symptoms. Therefore, WD should also be considered in the differential diagnoses of inflammatory rheumatic diseases, malabsorption syndromes, and endocrine disorders and in a variety of neurological disorders.

The diagnosis is established by small-bowel biopsy in which the samples show inclusions in macrophages of the lamina propria staining with periodic acid-Schiff (PAS). The inclusions present remnants of the causative organism *T. whipplei*.

The first published case was by G. H. Whipple in 1907. He described a 36-year-old physician suffering from diarrhea, polyarthritis, and bronchitis. The symptoms persisted over a 5-year period, and the patient finally died.

Untreated, WD is chronic, progressive, and fatal (89). Many studies have proven that the majority of patients when treated with antibiotics achieve rapid clinical improvement and maintain a long-lasting remission. About 20% of patients do not respond sufficiently to antibiotic therapy, and up to 40% have relapses afterwards, as reported in reviews, more frequently with CNS involvement (44, 61).

CHARACTERISTICS OF THE ORGANISM

T. whipplei is a rod-shaped bacterium measuring 0.25 by 1.5 to 2.5 μm. Morphologically, the organism uniformly possesses a trilaminar plasma membrane and a surrounding homogenous cell wall of 20-nm thickness, with two inner layers and an outer trilaminar membrane-like structure (17, 20, 27, 109) (Fig. 1). Due to the frequent intestinal symptoms, an oral route of acquisition is generally assumed. *T. whipplei* passes the stomach and enters the proximal small intestine, where the bacteria invade the mucosa. From the mucosa, bacteria are spread via the lymphatic system into the blood (27, 48).

Typically, *T. whipplei* is found in macrophages of the lamina propria of the small bowel and its lymphatic drainage. The bacillus can be observed within cells in various stages of degradation. When observed on light microscopy, the remnants of digested bacteria present as PAS-positive granular foamy inclusions in large macrophages (Color Plate 7). The PAS positivity is believed to be a reaction with bacterial capsular mucopolysaccharides located in the cell wall. In florid disease, undigested bacteria can also be seen in the extracellular space. During antibiotic treatment, there is a continuous decrease in the number of PAS-positive macrophages, and the organisms disappear, usually slowly, from the lamina propria, resulting in clinical improvement (103).

WD bacteria have also been observed in endothelial and epithelial cells, muscle cells, and in various cells of the immune system, including polymorphonuclear leukocytes, plasma cells, mast cells, and intraepithelial lymphocytes (26).

The nature of this bacterium was difficult to establish. It has an atypical morphology for a gram-positive or a gram-negative bacillus. Phylogenetic analysis of the *T. whipplei* 16S rRNA gene sequence established that this bacterium is an actinomycete (94, 108). A detailed analysis placed the organism in an intermediate position between cellulomonads and a group of actinomyces with group B peptidoglycan (72). These groups of bacteria are predominantly environmental bacteria and can be found in soil, water, and plants.

Thomas Marth • Abteilung Innere Medizin, Krankenhaus Maria Hilf, Maria Hilf Str. 2, D-54550 Daun, Germany.
Gjorgi Deriban • Clinic of Gastroenterohepatology, Medical Faculty Skopje, ul. Vodnjanska 17, 1000 Skopje, Macedonia.

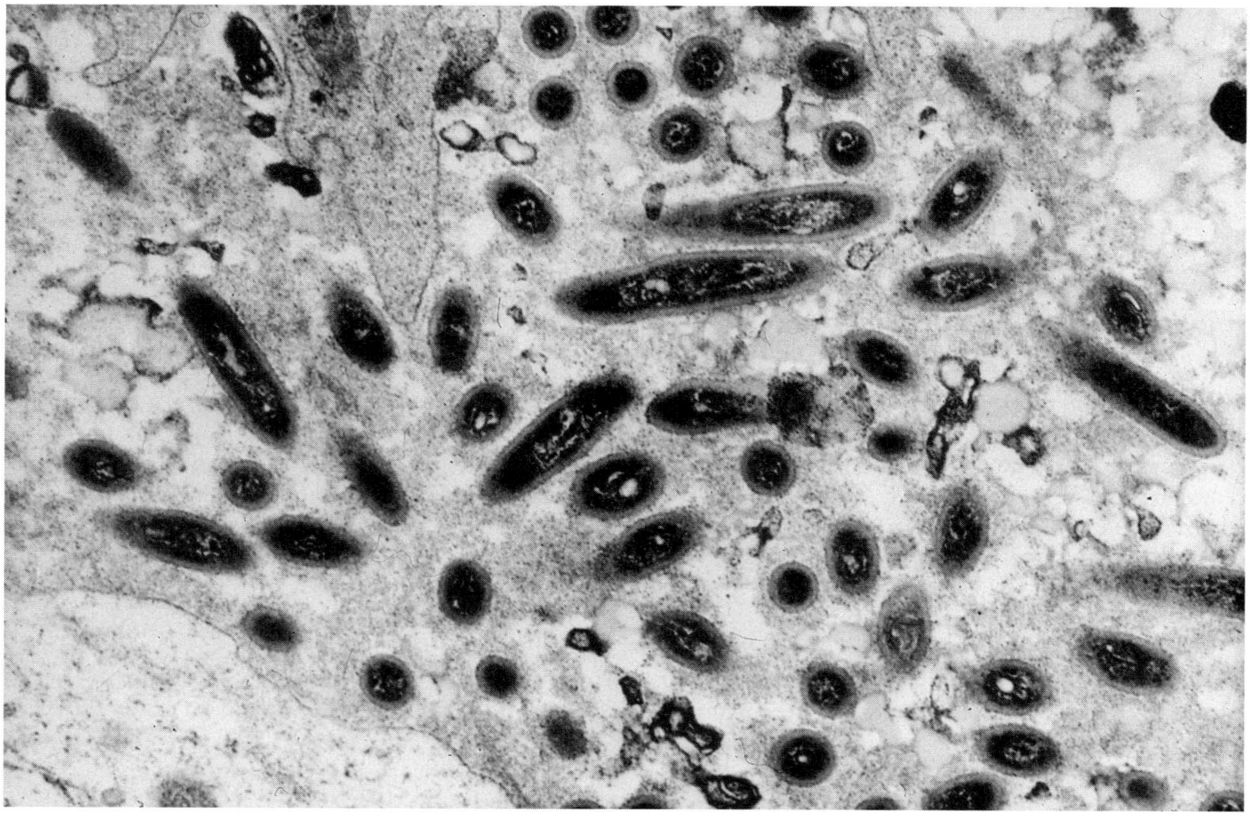

Figure 1. Electron microscopic view of *T. whipplei*.

The bacillus has been propagated in peripheral blood mononuclear cells deactivated by interleukin-4 and interleukin-10 (100). In 1999, stable growth of the bacillus was established in human fibroblast cells. Raoult et al. were able to show that *T. whipplei* is a slowly growing organism, with an estimated doubling time of 17 days; however, newer studies with axenic media show a much faster replication rate (95). The site of multiplication in vivo is still controversial. It has been suggested that this bacteria multiplies in the digestive lumen and becomes phagocytized and then degraded in macrophages. *T. whipplei* replicates also within peripheral blood mononuclear cells and within HeLa cells, where the bacillus actively multiplies in acidic vacuoles at pH 5 (52, 92). The high acidity may impair antibiotic activity, and this may be the cause for the lack of efficacy of some antibiotics.

T. whipplei shows genetic heterogeneity, and the genomic variants have been presumed to be associated with geographic distribution. There is no clear link between genotype and symptom pattern: some strains could be pathogenic, others cause atypical symptoms, and some are nonpathogenic (52, 66a).

The habitat of *T. whipplei* is unknown, but PCR studies suggest that the bacterium is ubiquitously present (73). *T. whipplei* was found by PCR in 17 of 46 (37%) influxes to sewage treatment plants. The 17 influxes testing positive came from residential and agricultural communities in the vicinity of Vienna, Austria, whereas all influxes from industrial sites remained negative (101).

Whipple's disease occurs usually in middle-aged individuals and is approximately eight times more common in men than in women (26, 79). There are several cases of familial clustering, but most of the analyzed cases do not exhibit familial components.

The disorder has been most frequently described with Caucasian populations of Europe and North America. A few cases have been reported with Hispanic, Black, Native American, and Asian populations. Most of the cases come from rural regions, and farming is a frequently documented occupation (26). There is no valid estimate of the WD prevalence; so far, more than 1,000 cases have been reported worldwide (41). The annual incidence in middle Europe may be around 1 in 10^6 (31).

There was some controversy regarding the prevalence of *T. whipplei* in healthy persons, since *T. whipplei* DNA was found in the saliva from 19 to 35% of healthy subjects. According to recent data from Relman and Raoult, *T. whipplei* DNA could not be identified in samples from duodenal biopsies from healthy persons, while 0.6% and 1.5% of healthy persons had *T. whipplei* DNA in saliva and stool, respectively (37, 41, 74). Amsler reported the occurrence of *T. whipplei* in stool samples from 13 of 208 (6%) healthy control individuals and in 5 of 196 (2.5%) diseased control patients (3). The number of positive stool samples was considerably higher from workers at sewage treatment plants. In a survey conducted by Schöniger-Hekele, 25% of the sewage plant workers tested positive for *T. whipplei* in stool by nested PCR, whereas only 7% of diseased controls (without antibiotic treatment at this point in time) tested positive for *T. whipplei* in stool (101). This confirms the observation that close contact to sewage water increases the likelihood of excreting *T. whipplei* in stool. The same study showed a high percentage of excretors of *T. whipplei* amongst patients with liver cirrhosis and hepatocellular carcinoma. Patients with various other diagnoses (with exception of one patient with chronic obstructive pulmonary disease and one with chronic cardiac disease) were negative for *T. whipplei* in stool. Immunocompromised and immunosuppressed patients were also stool-negative for *T. whipplei* (101). This finding shows that a more specific immune derangement, like the recently described *T. whipplei*-specific reduced Th1 response, is likely to play a crucial role in the pathogenesis.

PATHOGENESIS

Despite the presumed ubiquitous presence of *T. whipplei*, WD is extremely rare. The defective immune response in patients with clinically alert WD would have to be quite specific since these patients are not generally predisposed to other infections. Only a few cases have pointed to the possibility that WD also occurs in a setting of immunodeficiency, immunosuppression, or concomitantly with other infections (10, 54, 83). In patients already infected with *T. whipplei*, immunosuppression accelerates the course of the infection and especially triggers the occurrence of intestinal manifestations. Mahnel et al. found that prior to establishing the diagnosis of WD (patients usually presenting with polyarthritis), initiation of immunosuppressive therapy due to long-standing suspected rheumatoid arthritis led to diarrhea and finally to the diagnosis of WD (71). Immunodeficiency influences the progress of WD, but the question of whether WD patients have a primary immune defect or an immune defect induced by the actinomycete remains unanswered (79).

The role of a genetic susceptibility is controversial since small case series have described an overexpression of the HLA-B27 positivity in about a quarter of patients (43), whereas others have not supported this association (7). Biagi et al. found in WD patients an association with DRB1*13, DQB1*06, B*44, and Cw*05, but no HLA-B27 overexpression (81a).

PAS stain and immunohistochemistry as detection methods, using a computerized system of image analysis, allow the quantification of intestinal macrophagic infiltration and quantification of infected cells in intestinal WD. Percentages of macrophagic infiltration in intestinal biopsy specimens range from 20.3% before antibiotic therapy to 13.4% after antibiotic therapy, compared to 2.1% in controls (65).

Results of older histological studies (27, 56) have shown that despite the influx of macrophages, intestinal tissue has little lymphocytic infiltration and a few plasma cells in WD. A secondary loss of lymphocytes caused by intestinal lymphangiectasia could cause this lack of lymphocytes. Other, more profound changes in immunity have also been identified. Populations of T cells are characterized by a low CD4/CD8 T-cell ratio, increased cell activation markers, and a shift toward a mature T-cell subpopulation (80). The reduced proliferative response of peripheral T cells occurs in response to phytohemagglutinin, concanavalin A, and antibodies to CD2 (25, 56, 78, 80, 82). Serum factors may play a role in downregulating T-cell-mediated responses.

The small-bowel mucosa contains a low number of immunoglobulin A (IgA)-positive B cells but an increased number of surface IgM-positive B cells (33). A literature review by Fenollar et al. (40) reports that up to 40% of WD patients have hypereosinophilia; others report eosinophilia at a lower percentage (25, 29). The reason for this is unknown (40). Secretory IgA concentrations measured in intestinal aspirates and humoral immune responses to infectious agents in the periphery are normal. Serum concentrations of total IgG are normal in most cases, whereas IgM concentrations are low and those of IgA high in acute stages of the disease (25, 30, 71, 76).

T. whipplei multiplies in macrophages but not in monocytes from healthy subjects. Unlike in healthy subjects, in patients with WD, *T. whipplei* multiplies in both monocytes and macrophages. (24). The replication of *T. whipplei* in monocytes and macrophages correlates with interleukin-16 overexpression and thioredoxin downregulation. Untreated WD patients reveal elevated serum levels of interleukin-16 (24). The elevated levels normalize after successful antibiotic treatment. The role of interleukin-16 in the pathophysiology of WD is also confirmed by the finding that antibodies neutralizing interleukin-16 inhibit the growth of *T. whipplei* in macrophages (11, 22, 23, 24).

Several studies have shown defective macrophage function in WD patients, and this seems to be of central importance in the development of the disease. Recently, it has been shown that intestinal macrophages of WD patients display in vivo the phenotype of M2/alternatively activated macrophages that favor the development of Th2 response and inhibit protective Th1 polarization (23).

Macrophages from affected patients phagocytize bacteria normally but are unable to degrade bacterial antigens efficiently (26). The decreased ability to cope with intracellular infection could be related to a reduced CD11b expression. The CD11b molecule serves as a facilitator of microbial phagocytosis, has a role in antigen processing, and mediates intracellular killing of ingested bacteria that is induced by IFN-γ (80). Patients with inactive disease have in general a lower-than-normal number of circulating cells expressing CD11b, while during active disease intestinal macrophages do not express CD11b (22, 23, 34).

Studies have also shown low interleukin-12 production in macrophages (22, 77, 78) and in vitro replication of *T. whipplei* in macrophages deactivated by interleukin-4 and interleukin-10 (100). Moos et al. found that WD patients showed reduced or absent *T. whipplei*-specific Th1 response, whereas their capacity to react to other common antigens like tetanus toxoid, tuberculin, actinomycetes, *Giardia lamblia*, or cytomegalovirus was not reduced compared with that of controls (86). This defective immune response specific to *T. whipplei* persists independent of disease activity and treatment. Even in successfully treated WD patients, the Th1 reactivity remains repressed.

In conclusion, the subtle defects of cellular immunity that involve activation and interaction of macrophages and T cells probably contribute to an important part of a disturbed phagocytosis, disturbed intracellular degradation, and an impaired immunological clearance of *T. whipplei*. This allows an invasion from the gastrointestinal mucosa to peripheral organs and may result in a chronic infection and eventually in a fatal course of the disease.

DISEASES CAUSED BY THE ORGANISM AND LONG-TERM CONSEQUENCES

WD is characterized with many patients by two stages—a prodromal stage and a progressive stage. The prodromal stage is often characterized by protean symptoms, arthralgia, arthritis, and nonspecific findings. In the progressive stage, weight loss, diarrhea, and arthropathies can be found in up to 75% of patients. The clinical presentation in the progressive stage can vary to a great extent and even in the absence of gastrointestinal symptoms, cardiac or CNS symptoms may occur (40, 44, 45, 71, 76). The average time between the prodromal stage and the progressive stage is 6 years (41, 71).

Immunosuppressive therapy with corticosteroids, azathioprine, or other immunosuppressants accelerates the progression to a progressive-state stage and the diagnosis (71). Gastrointestinal symptoms usually lead to the diagnosis of WD. The median time to occurrence of gastrointestinal symptoms after initiation of immunosuppressive therapy is 4 months, and another 2 months are necessary to establish the diagnosis of WD (71).

Classic WD

The common presenting clinical features of WD are weight loss, arthropathy, diarrhea, abdominal pain, low-grade fever, and peripheral lymphadenopathy (Table 1). Although WD has traditionally been regarded as a gastrointestinal disease, the first symptom preceding the diagnosis by a mean of 8 years is usually arthropathy. In one large series, arthropathy as a prodromal symptom was found in 63% of patients (81). The arthropathy, often accompanied by myalgias, consists of chronic migratory nondestructive and seronegative joint disease, involving predominantly

Table 1. Percentage of individuals with Whipple's disease showing specific clinical features

Major clinical feature or frequent sign/symptom	% of individuals with feature
Major clinical features	
Weight loss	90
Arthropathy	85
Diarrhea	75
Abdominal pain	60
Frequent signs/symptoms	
Fever	45
Lymphadenopathy	45
Hyperpigmentation	35
Hypotension	35
Peripheral edema	30
Cardiac murmurs	30
Occult bleeding	25
Myalgia	25
Abdominal mass	20
CNS involvement	15
Chronic cough	15
Splenomegaly	15
Hepatomegaly	10
Ascites	10

the peripheral joints (26, 79). On rare occasions spondyloarthopathy, hypertrophic osteoarthropathy, and infection of knee prostheses have been described (47). Joint deformity, persisting destructive joint changes, or vertebral involvement (2) associated with WD are very rare (6, 98), and on radiography, the joints usually appear normal (66). Joint symptoms often diminish, for unknown reasons, with the occurrence of intestinal symptoms. Within 2 to 4 weeks after initiation of antibiotic therapy, the joint symptomatology improves (44, 76).

Weight loss is a major symptom by the time of diagnosis and is present in two-thirds of the patients more than 4 years before diagnosis (26, 76). Most patients respond well to antibiotic treatment and regain their initial weight after several months. Watery diarrhea resulting from small intestine involvement is usually episodic and accompanied by colicky abdominal pain. Steatorrhea occurs rarely, and 20 to 30% of patients have evidence of occult blood in their stools. These symptoms with concomitant anorexia lead to full malabsorption syndrome (26). Diarrhea responds well to antibiotic therapy and often resolves within 1 or several weeks of therapy initiation. Endoscopic lesions disappear 6 to 9 months after antibiotics (49). Twelve to 18 months after the onset of antibiotic therapy, most of the intestinal villi have a normal architecture (26, 58).

In about half of the patients, systemic symptoms occur (26, 44). Frequent features of WD are intermittent low-grade fever, night sweats, and a peripheral and abdominal lymphadenopathy. However, few patients experience prolonged fevers or lymphadenopathy after therapy induction.

Cardiac Involvement

Cardiac involvement associated with WD was first described by Upton in 1952 (104) and since then has been reported with a wide range (17 to 55%) of patients with classic WD (29). In contrast, autopsy studies showed in 79% of cases involvement of the pericardium, myocardium, or endocardium (26, 35). The common clinical presentations are cardiac murmurs and insufficiency of the valves, necessitating valve replacement. Clinically apparent endocarditis is less frequent, and compared to other causes of endocarditis, congestive heart failure and fever are observed less frequently in patients with Whipple's endocarditis (40, 41). Recent reports have described a syndrome of "blood culture-negative endocarditis" in patients with *T. whipplei* infection but negative duodenal biopsies and no other evidence of WD. In these cases, PCR may be useful to confirm a presumed diagnosis of *T. whipplei* endocarditis, which then should lead to an effective treatment regimen (16, 55, 61).

Geissdörfer et al. reported a 69-year-old patient suffering from severe aortic regurgitation requiring aortic valve replacement. *T. whipplei was* detected in the explanted aortic valve by broad-range PCR amplification. The histological examination of the aortic valve was compatible with Whipple's disease. Duodenal biopsy was negative, and the patient had no symptoms of WD (50). Naegeli et al. reported a very unusual presentation of culture-negative Whipple's endocarditis with transient ischemic attack followed by recurrent strokes. Transesophageal echocardiography revealed 2.5-cm gross pedunculated vegetations on both leaflets of the mitral valve. The diagnosis was established by histological examination of the explanted native mitral valve and PCR. A small-bowel biopsy and an examination of the cerebral spinal fluid, obtained after valve replacement, were negative by microscopy and PCR (87).

WD endocarditis occurs in 88% of patients with native valves without underlying disease. In endocarditis due to other causes, the percentage associated with native valves without previous diseases is significantly lower. Indeed, only 11% of patients with Q fever endocarditis, 22% of patients with *Bartonella henselae* endocarditis, and 46% of patients with blood culture-positive endocarditis, have native valves (14, 40, 107).

Pathologic valve alterations in WD patients are most frequently found on the mitral valve, while the most significant clinical symptoms are caused by the affected aortic valve (26, 40). In a literature review conducted by Fenollar et al., valves from 26 out of 35 patients with Whipple's endocarditis showed at histology foamy macrophages associated with deposits of fibrin or inflammatory cells, while one patient had only foamy macrophages on the valves (40). Deposits of fibrin and platelets on the valves were present in 13 cases. The presence of polymorphonuclear neutrophils and lymphocytes was observed with 10 and 4 patients, respectively. In Whipple's endocarditis, compared to endocarditis due to other causes, it is more usual for more than one valve to be infected in the same patient.

Pericarditis occurs in more than half of the patients with WD (75). Myocarditis occurs far less often and is sometimes first evident with the onset of heart failure or sudden death (41).

Neurologic Involvement

A frequently overlooked area of involvement in WD is the CNS. Neurologic manifestations are diverse and can resemble any neurologic disease. Therefore, many cases of WD with CNS involvement are not diagnosed until postmortem (Table 2). Neurologic manifestations occur in three situations: neurologic involvement in classic WD, isolated neurologic symptoms due to *T. whipplei* infection without histologic evidence of intestinal involvement, and neurologic relapse of previously treated WD.

Neurologic symptoms have been reported in 6 to 63% of patients with intestinal WD. In some of these patients gastrointestinal involvement is minimally present (26, 45, 51). The typical symptomatology includes cognitive changes, present in 71% of these patients. The cognitive changes are associated with various psychiatric alterations in 47% of these patients (51, 68). Nearly every patient with CNS WD also has systemic signs. Other common clinical signs are ophtalmoplegia, nystagmus, and myoclonia, which are frequently noted in combination with disturbed sleep patterns, ataxia, seizures, or symptoms of cerebral compression (51, 98a). Various cranial nerve symptoms, such as hearing loss and blurred vision, have been reported. A specific oculomasticatory myorrhythmia and oculofacial skeletal myorrhythmia are considered to be characteristic for CNS WD and are always accompanied by supranuclear vertical gaze palsy (supranuclear ophtaloplegia). These symptoms occur in less than 20% of patients with CNS WD and have not yet been documented in other CNS diseases (68).

Neurological manifestations of cerebral WD very rarely include stroke-like symptoms. The pathogenesis of cerebral infarction is not well established, but cerebral vasculitis, arterial fibrosis, thrombosis, and thickening associated with the inflammation of adjacent brain parenchyma and leptomeninges, caused by the hematogenous spread of *T. whipplei* to the brain, may all be important triggers (36, 90). Recurrent stroke-like symptoms due to brain embolization caused by pedunculated vegetations on the mitral valve in Whipple's endocarditis has been reported in one case (87). Isolated neurologic symptoms have been described in 32 patients (1, 21, 26, 51, 62, 67, 68, 70, 84, 85, 88, 90, 91, 102, 105). Nineteen of these 32 patients had systemic symptoms such as fever, weight loss, articular pain, and peripheral lymphadenopathy, but no diarrhea. Of the 30 patients for whom follow-up data were available, 18 (60%) improved after treatment and 10 (33%) died (41). Therefore, neurologic manifestation is a major cause of deaths in WD. Earlier detection and treatment could probably improve the outcome, although the treatment of neurological alterations in WD patients is challenging. Treatment options are discussed below.

Patients with CNS involvement carry the highest risk for disease recurrence (44, 61), and those with a neurologic recurrence have poor prognosis (26, 99). Computer tomography or magnetic resonance imaging in CNS WD can show abnormalities like mild to moderate brain atrophy or focal lesions without a predilection for a specific site. However, these changes are not specific for WD but can be used for stereotactic biopsies that reveal a characteristic histology. Results of cerebrospinal fluid examination are normal or show a mild pleocytosis (26, 68). PAS-positive sickle-form particle-containing cells may be found with cerebrospinal fluid cytology, and PCR is often positive for *T. whipplei*, even in neurologically asymptomatic patients (105).

Table 2. Long-term consequences of infection with *Tropheryma whipplei*

Type of involvement	Manifestation
Neurologic	Progressive dementia and cognitive changes
	Supranuclear opthalmoplegia
	Altered level of consciousness
	Psychiatric symptoms
	Hypothalamic manifestations
	Cranial nerve abnormalities
Cardiovascular	Endocarditis, myocarditis, pericarditis
Musculoskeletal[a]	Oligo- and polyarthralgias
	Myalgias
Other[a]	Cachexia
	Lymphadenopathy
	Skin hyperpigmentation
	Possible association of malignant lymphomas

[a] Symptoms may be reversible.

Other Manifestations

Skin hyperpigmentation, particularly affecting light-exposed areas of the body (commonly misinterpreted as Addison's disease), has been observed with one-third of the patients with WD; the skin changes usually regress after treatment (26, 76). Hepatomegaly or splenomegaly can be present in some patients with this disorder. Less-frequent involvement has been reported for the kidney and the genitourinary and endocrine systems (26, 46). Chronic nonproductive cough or chest pain indicating lung involvement or pleuritis, polyserositis, ascites, hypotension, and edema are also among frequently found signs and symptoms, but only rarely do patients have persistent symptoms (26, 79).

Association of WD with Granulomatous Disease and Other Disorders

The inflammatory reaction in WD may be granulomatous. This was reported first in 1943 (4) and is described for approximately 9% of the patients (26) for various organs. Among the granulomas, sarcoid-like epitheloid noncaseating granulomas have been described frequently for patients with WD (9, 96, 97). These epitheloid cell granulomas are distinct from sickle-form particle-containing cells and WD macrophages (they are PAS negative) and are speculated to be a result of partially digested antigen, although no products of bacterial degradation have been observed. The sarcoid-like inflammation has also been described for various other organs, like bone marrow, kidneys, synovial tissue, liver, and lungs (19, 32, 97). In some patients, especially when WD affects the lung, sarcoidosis may be confused with WD (32). In a recent series of 40 patients in a randomized trial testing antibiotic treatment, two patients had sarcoid–like lesions (43a).

For several patients with WD, amyloidosis has been reported (26, 63), but it is unclear whether the amyloid deposits result from a chronic inflammatory response. It has to be pointed out that the amyloid deposits may be faintly PAS positive and thus may be misinterpreted with WD. An association of WD with malignancies has been described infrequently. There are reports of non-Hodgkin's lymphoma occurring after successful treatment of WD (53, 57), and clonal expansions simulating B-cell lymphoma have been found in patients' blood or bone marrow (42, 106). Besides personal observations in single patients, there are 3 patients out of 40 in the randomized trial (43a) who experienced a non-Hodgkin's or Hodgkin's lymphoma. Whether this is coincidence or whether B-cell transformation is a result of a chronic infectious stimulus (such as in the pathogenesis of MALT lymphoma) remains unclear.

Infections with nontuberculous mycobacteria (mostly *Mycobacterium avium-M. intracellulare*) in AIDS patients may histologically mimic WD (5, 28) and has been named "pseudo WD." However, this is quite rare and can be distinguished by a Ziehl-Neelsen stain. WD can be associated in rare instances with a number of opportunistic infections (26, 83). In addition, the intestinal symptoms may occur after the onset of immunosuppressive therapy (which is started in some patients due to unclear arthropathies) (71). The association of WD with giardiasis has been reported in more than 15 cases (39). In the recent series of a mostly German group of 40 patients, 10% had had giardiasis (Feurle, Marth et al., in preparation). It is speculated that an infection by one infectious mucosal agent may promote the infection with the other.

Laboratory Features

Laboratory abnormalities are nonspecific and can show evidence of malabsorption and protein-losing enteropathy, such as low beta carotene, vitamin deficiencies (B_{12}, D, K, and folic acid), low albumin and cholesterol concentration, raised stool fat excretion, and low D-xylose absorption. Many patients show (for unknown reasons) pronounced eosinophilia and serum immunoglobulin abnormalities (40, 76). Other nonspecific laboratory abnormalities are increased C-reactive protein, lymphocytopenia, thrombocytosis, and hypochromic anemia (46, 71). Several weeks after therapy initiation, these nonspecific laboratory findings usually normalize, while the immunologic parameters return to normal within months. In contrast, many features of the defective cellular immune response persist indefinitely (77).

DIAGNOSIS

The initial diagnostic procedure for a patient with clinical suspicion of WD is upper digestive endoscopy with small-bowel mucosal biopsy. The histological appearance of the biopsy samples reveals the diagnosis, since granular foamy macrophages stained purple with PAS are typical for WD. Biopsy samples should be taken from both the proximal and distal duodenum or jejunum. The proportion of macrophages among duodenal cells can range from under 5% (in the healthy host) to 50%. Infiltration of the bowel wall is associated with a widening and flattening of the villi and with dilated lacteals containing yellow lipid deposits because of the blockade of the villous lymphatics (26). However, PAS staining is not completely specific since patients with infection caused by *Mycobacterium avium-M. intracellulare, Rhodococcus equi, Bacillus cereus*, corynebacterium, histoplasma, or fungi also have PAS-positive macrophages. Biopsy samples from patients with melanosis coli, histiocytosis, and in rare instances, Crohn's disease can also be confused with WD (41, 79).

On endoscopy, the lesions of WD are commonly described as pale yellow shaggy mucosa alternating with an erythematous, erosive, or mildly friable mucosa in the postbulbar region of the duodenum or jejunum. Alternatively, whitish-yellow plaques can be seen in a patchy distribution (49, 81).

Bacteria can also be reliably visualized by electron microscopy, a technique which is used nowadays less frequently. WD is systemic disorder, and PAS-positive macrophages and electron-microscopically detectable bacilli have been shown in many cell types in almost all organs.

Culture is currently not yet a method of diagnosis and is carried out only in specialized laboratories. Major difficulties are the prolonged time necessary for primary culture, the high risk of contamination, and the fact that antibiotic pretreatment often precludes isolation of the bacterium (79). Immunohistochemical staining for antibodies against *T. whipplei* can detect the organism in various tissues, body fluids, and blood monocytes. This method provides direct visualization of the bacillus, has a greater sensitivity and specificity than PAS staining, and even can be used retrospectively on fixed samples (8, 29).

Autoimmunochemical staining in which anti-*T. whipplei* antibodies from the patients own serum were used enabled detection of *T. whipplei* in heart valve samples from patients with blood culture-negative endocarditis (64). PCR can be used to detect *T. whipplei* in samples from various tissue types and body fluids. For this method, it is critical to avoid contamination of the DNA sample and to include positive and negative controls to validate the test. On the basis of genome analysis, a new quantitative real-time PCR assay has been developed, offering substantially greater sensitivity and the same specificity, compared to earlier assays (38).

The proposed strategy for diagnosing WD is histologic examination of a small-bowel biopsy and PCR in parallel. The main limitation of this approach is that specificity of both techniques is less than optimal. In the absence of extraintestinal symptoms suggestive of WD, a normal intestinal histology practically rules out the diagnosis. Routine PCR testing of cerebrospinal fluid from patients with intestinal WD is obligatory, since around 50% have a positive PCR in the cerebrospinal fluid, even without neurologic or psychiatric symptoms (105). Depending on the clinical manifestations, it is necessary to perform PCR testing on extraintestinal samples (such as cardiac valve tissue, lymph nodes, and synovial tissue) from potentially affected sites.

TREATMENT AND CONTROL

WD was considered a fatal disorder before establishment of antibiotic therapy. Up to the early 1950s, there were approximately 30 case reports. The diagnosis of WD was established at autopsy or the patients died shortly after diagnosis (e.g., by laparatomy), although steroid treatment had some transient beneficial effects (59, 60). In 1961, in a series of nine patients for whom the diagnosis was established by lymph node biopsy, there were four lethal outcomes (18). In another review, all 4 untreated patients died with complications presumably related to WD, but only 1 out of 25 treated patients died due to CNS WD (3 others died later of other causes) (46). Antibiotic regimens were used on an empirical basis and led in many patients to rapid improvement and to long-lasting remission (89). Up to the 1980s, many patients were treated with penicillin, streptomycin, and tetracycline. Since tetracycline seems to be associated with a high frequency of relapse, trimpethoprim-sulfamethoxazole (160/800 mg orally twice daily) for 1 to 2 years is now recommended (44, 79).

Oral treatment should usually be preceded by a 2-week course of parenteral therapy with ceftriaxone (2 g daily), or alternatively with meropenem. This issue is to be clarified in a randomized controlled trial (SIMW) with 40 WD patients (43a). Another alternative, e.g., in cases of allergies, is a combination of streptomycin (1 g daily) together with penicillin G (1.2 million U daily).

The susceptibility of *T. whipplei* to various antimicrobial agents has been tested in vitro with the use of both cell and axenic cultures (13, 93). Doxycyline and sulfamethoxazole are active in vitro, but trimethoprim is not (12, 13, 15). In cell culture, cephalosporins, including ceftriaxone and fluoroquinolones, are not active, whereas in axenic medium, ceftriaxone and levofloxacin are active (12).

Vacuole acidification is critical to the survival of *T. whipplei* in phagosomes. Therefore, alkalizing agents like hydrochloroquine may increase the bactericidal effect of the antibiotics. The combination of doxycycline (200 mg daily) plus hydrochloroquine (200 mg three times daily) was the only successful treatment in vitro and was also successful in four treated patients: two with classic WD and two with blood culture-negative endocarditis (41). Based on the susceptibility tests and the previous results, the actual therapy recommendation for WD without neurologic involvement is trimpethoprim-sulfamethoxazole. Early contact with specialized centers for every newly diagnosed or refractory patient is important, and prospective trials are necessary to establish guidelines based on clinical evidence (for contacts, see www.whippledisease.info). In patients responding to treatment, diarrhea and fever resolve within 1 week. The other symptoms improve in many cases after a few weeks (44, 46, 61). Clinical improvement is accompanied by a normalization of laboratory findings and reconstitution of the villous architecture of the small intestine. Follow-up duodenal biopsies should be taken after 6 and 12 months. If no PAS-positive material is identified, antibiotic treatment can be stopped. In some patients, bacterial material persists and they have an antibiotic refractory disease. Others have relapses characterized by frequent occurrences of cerebral manifestations, and these patients have poor prognoses. In both groups, new treatment strategies are required.

CONCLUSIONS

Despite the recent advances, WD remains an enigmatic disease with many open questions. The reservoir of *T. whipplei* should be identified, the true prevalence of WD is yet to be determined, and the transmission mechanisms are to be elucidated. The role of asymptomatic carriers also remains unclear. Therapeutic recommendations are empirically based or based on in vitro susceptibility tests. Due to the rarity of the disorder, cooperative studies and clinical trials are necessary to clarify the unanswered questions and to establish evidence-based therapeutic recommendations.

REFERENCES

1. **Akar, Z., N. Tanriover, and S. Tuzgen.** 2002. Intracerebral Whipple disease: unusual location and bone destruction. *J. Neurosurg.* **97:**988–991.
2. **Altwegg, M., A. Fleisch-Marx, D. Goldenberger, S. Hailemariam, A. Schaffner, and R. Kissling.**1996. Spondylodiscitis caused by *Tropheryma whippelii. Schweiz. Med. Wochenschr.* **35:**1495–1499.
3. **Amsler, L., P. Bauernfeind, C. Nigg, R. C. Maibach, R. Steffen, and M. Altwegg.** 2003. Prevalence of *T. whipplei* DNA in patients with various gastrointestinal diseases and in healthy controls. *Infection* **31:**81–85.
4. **Apperly, F. L., and E. L. Copley.** 1943. Whipple's disease (lipophagia granulomatosis). *Gastroenterology* **1:**461–470.
5. **Autran, B., I. Gorin, M. Leibowitch, L. Laroche, J. P. Escande, J. Hewitt, and C. Marche.** 1983. AIDS in a Haitian woman with cardiac Kaposi's sarcoma and Whipple's disease. *Lancet* **i:**767–768.
6. **Ayoub, W. T., D. E. David, D. Torretti, and F. J. Viozzi.** 1982. Bone destruction and ankylosis in Whipple's disease. *J. Rheumatol.* **9:**930–931.
7. **Bai, J. C., A. H. Mota, E. Mauriño, S. Niveloni, F. Grossman, L. A. Boerr, and L. Fainboim.** 1991. Class I and class II HLA antigens in a homogeneous Argentinian population with Whipple's disease: lack of association with HLA-B 27. *Am. J. Gastroenterol.* **86:**992–994.
8. **Baisden, B. L., H. Lepidi, D. Raoult, P. Argani, J. H. Yardley, and J. S. Dumler.** 2002. Diagnosis of Whipple disease by immunohistochemical analysis: a sensitive and specific method for the detection of *T. whipplei* (the Whipple bacillus) in paraffin-embedded tissue. *Am. J. Clin. Pathol.* **118:** 742–748.
9. **Barbaryka, I., L. Thorn, and E. Langer.** 1979. Epithelioid cell granulomata in the mucosa of the small intestine in Whipple's disease. *Virchows Arch. A* **382:**227–235.
10. **Bassotti, G., M. A. Pelli, R. Ribacchi, M. Miglietti, M. L. Cavalletti, M. E. Rossodivita, P. Giovenali, and A. Morelli.** 1991. Giardia lamblia infestation reveals underlying Whipple's disease in a patient with longstanding constipation. *Am. J. Gastroenterol.* **86:**371–374.
11. **Benoit, M., F. Fenollar, D. Raoult, and J. L. Mege.** 2007. Increased levels of circulating IL-16 and apoptosis markers are related to the activity of Whipple's disease. *PLoS ONE* **6:** e494.
12. **Boulos, A., J. M. Rolain, M. N. Mallet, and D. Raoult.** 2005. Molecular evaluation of antibiotic susceptibility of *Tropheryma whipplei* in axenic medium. *J. Antimicrob. Chemother.* **55:**178–181.
13. **Boulos, A., J. M. Rolain, and D. Raoult.** 2004. Antibiotic susceptibility of *Tropheryma whipplei* in MRC5 cells. *Antimicrob. Agents Chemother.* **48:**747–52.
14. **Brouqui, P., H. Tissot-Dupont, and M. Drancourt.** 1993. Chronic Q fever: ninety-two cases from France, including 27 cases without endocarditis. *Arch. Intern. Med.* **153:**642–648.
15. **Cannon, W. R.** 2003. Whipple's disease, genomics, and drug therapy. *Lancet* **361:**1916.
16. **Célard, M., G. de Gevigney, and S. Mosnier.** 1999. Polymerase chain reaction analysis for diagnosis of *Tropheryma whippelii* infective endocarditis in two patients with no previous evidence of Whipple's disease. *Clin. Infect. Dis.* **29:**1348–1349.
17. **Chears, W. C., and C. T. Ashworth.** 1961. Electron microscopy study of the intestinal mucosa in Whipple's disease–demonstration of encapsulated bacilliform bodies in the lesion. *Gastroenterology* **41:**129–138.
18. **Chears, W. C., M. D. Hargrove, J. V. Verner, A. G. Smith, and J. M. Ruffin.** 1961. Whipple's disease; a review of twelve patients from one service. *Am. J. Med.* **30:**226–234.
19. **Cho, C., W. G. Linscheer, M. A. Hirschkorn, and K. Ashutosh.** 1984. Sarcoidlike granulomas as an early manifestation of Whipple's disease. *Gastroenterology* **87:**941–947.
20. **Cohen, A. S., E. M. Schimmel, P.R. Holt, and K. J. Isselbacher.** 1960. Ultrastructural abnormalities in Whipple's disease. *Proc. Soc. Exp. Biol. Med.* **105:**411–414.
21. **Coria, F., N. Cuadrado, and C. Velasco.** 2000. Whipple's disease with isolated central nervous system symptomatology diagnosed by molecular identification of *Tropheryma whippelii* in peripheral blood. *Neurologia* **15:**173–176.
22. **Desnues, B., M. Ihrig, D. Raoult, and J. L Mege.** 2006. Whipple's disease: a macrophage disease. *Clin. Vaccine Immunol.* **2:**170–178.
23. **Desnues, B., H. Lepidi, D. Raoult, and J. L. Mege.** 2005. Whipple disease: intestinal infiltrating cells exhibit a transcriptional pattern of M2/alternatively activated macrophages. *J. Infect. Dis.* **9:**1642–1646.
24. **Desnues, B., D. Raoult, and J. L. Mege.** 2005. IL-16 is critical for *T. whipplei* replication in Whipple's disease. *J. Immunol.* **175:**4575–4582.
25. **Dobbins, W. O., III.** 1981. Is there an immune deficit in Whipple's disease? *Dig. Dis. Sci.* **26:**247–252.
26. **Dobbins, W.O., III.** 1987. *Whipple's Disease.* Charles C. Thomas, Springfield, IL.
27. **Dobbins, W.O., III., and J. M. Ruffin.** 1967. A light- and electron-microscopic study of bacterial invasion in Whipple's disease. *Am. J. Pathol.* **51:**225–242.
28. **Dray, X., K. Vahedi, V. Delcey, A. Lavergne-Slove, L. Raskine, J. F. Bergmann, and P. Marteau.** 2007. *Mycobacterium avium* duodenal infection mimicking Whipple's disease in a patient with AIDS. *Endoscopy* **39**(Suppl. 1):E296–E297.
29. **Dumler, J. S., B. L. Baisden, J. H. Yardley, and D. Raoult.** 2003. Immunodetection of *T. whipplei* in intestinal tissues from Dr. Whipple's 1907 patient. *N. Engl. J. Med.* **348:** 1411–1412.
30. **Durand, D.V., C. Lecomte, P. Cathébras, H. Rousset, and P. Godeau.** 1997. Whipple disease: clinical review of 52 cases. *Medicine* (Baltimore) **76:**170–184.
31. **Dutly, F., and M. Altwegg.** 2001. Whipple's disease and "*Tropheryma whippelii.*" *Clin. Microbiol. Rev.* **14:**561–583.
32. **Dzirlo, L., M. Hubner, C. Mueller, B. Blaha, E. Formann, C. Dellinger, P. Petzelbauer, L. Muellauer, K. Huber, M. Kneussl, and M. Gschwantler.** 2007. A mimic of sarcoidosis. *Lancet* **369:**1832.

33. **Eck, M., H. Kreipe, D. Harmsen, and H. K. Müller-Hermelink.** 1997. Invasion and destruction of mucosal plasma cells by *Tropheryma whippelii*. *Hum. Pathol.* **28:**1424–1428.
34. **Ectors, N., K. Geboes, P. Rutgeerts, J. Delabie, V. Desmet, and J. Janssens.** 1992. RFD7-RFD9 coexpression by macrophages points to T cell–macrophage interaction deficiency in Whipple's disease. *Gastroenterology* **106:**A676.
35. **Enzinger, F. M., and E. B. Helwig.** 1963. Whipple's disease: a review of the literature and report of 15 patients. *Virchows Arch.* **336:** 238–268.
36. **Famularo, G., G. Minisola, and C. De Simone.** 2005. A patient with cerebral Whipple's disease and a stroke-like syndrome *Scand. J. Gastroenterol.* **40:**607–609.
37. **Fenollar, F., P. E. Fournier, D. Raoult, R. Gérolami, H. Lepidi, and C. Poyart.** 2002. Quantitative detection of *Tropheryma whipplei* DNA by real-time PCR. *J. Clin. Microbiol.* **3:** 1119–1120.
38. **Fenollar, F., P. E. Fournier, C. Robert, and D. Raoult.** 2004. Use of genome selected repeated sequences increases the sensitivity of PCR detection of *Tropheryma whipplei. J. Clin. Microbiol.* **42:**401–403.
39. **Fenollar, F., H. Lepidi, R. Gérolami, M. Drancourt, and D. Raoult.** 2003. Whipple disease associated with giardiasis. *J. Infect. Dis.* **188:**828–834.
40. **Fenollar, F., H. Lepidi, and D. Raoult.** 2001. Whipple's endocarditis: review of the literature and comparisons with Q fever, Bartonella infection, and blood culture-positive endocarditis. *Clin. Infect. Dis.* **33:**1309–1316.
41. **Fenollar, F., X. Puechal, and D. Raoult.** 2007. Whipple's disease. *N. Engl. J. Med.* **356:**55–66.
42. **Fest, T., B. Pron, M. P. Lefranc, C. Pierre, R. Angonin, B. de Wazières, Z. Soua, and J. L. Dupond.** 1996. Detection of a clonal BCL2 gene rearrangement in tissues from a patient with Whipple disease. *Ann. Intern. Med.* **8:**738–740.
43. **Feurle, G. E., B. Doerken, E. Schoepf, and V. Lenhard.** 1979. HLA-B27 and defects in the T-cell system in Whipples's disease. *Eur. J. Clin. Invest.* **9:**385–389.
43a. **Feurle, G. E., M. Maiwald, V. Moos, et al.** 2007. Randomized controlled trial of antimicrobial treatment in Whipple's disease (SIMW). Abstr. *Gastroenterology* **132**(Suppl. S1):639.
44. **Feurle, G. E., and T. Marth.** 1994. An evaluation of antimicrobial treatment for Whipple's disease: tetracycline versus trimethoprim-sulfomethoxazole. *Dig. Dis. Sci.* **39:**1642–1648.
45. **Feurle, G. E., B. Volk, and R. Waldherr.** 1979. Cerebral Whipple's disease with negative jejunal histology. *N. Engl. J. Med.* **300:**907–908.
46. **Fleming, J. L., R. H. Wiesner, and R. G. Shorter.** 1988. Whipple's disease: clinical, biochemical and histopathological features and assessment of treatment in 29 patients. *Mayo Clin. Proc.* **63:**539–551.
47. **Foreyard, A., C. Guglielminotti, and P. Berthelot.** 1996. Prosthetic joint infection caused by *Tropheryma whippelii* (Whipple's bacillus). *Clin. Infect. Dis.* **22:**575–576.
48. **Fredricks, D. N., and D. A. Relman. 2001.** Localization of *Tropheryma whippelii* rRNA in tissues from patients with Whipple's disease. *J. Infect. Dis.* **8:**1229–1237.
49. **Geboes, K., N. Ectors, H. Heidbuchel, P. Rutgeerts, V. Desmet, and G. Vantrappen.** 1992. Whipple's disease: the value of upper gastrointestinal endoscopy for the diagnosis and follow-up. *Acta Gastroenterol. Belg.* **2:**209–219.
50. **Geissdörfer, W., I. Wittmann, G. Seitz, R. Cesnjevar, M. Röllinghoff, C. Schoerner, and C. Bogdan.** 2001. A case of aortic valve disease associated with *Tropheryma whippelii* infection in the absence of other signs of Whipple's disease. *Infection* **29:**44–47.
51. **Gerard, A., F. Sarrot-Reynauld, and E. Liozon.** 2002. Neurologic presentation of Whipple disease: report of 12 cases and review of the literature. *Medicine* (Baltimore) **81:**443–457.
52. **Ghigo. E., C. Capo, M. Aurouze, J. P. Gorvel, D. Raoult, and J. L. Mege.** 2002. The survival of *Tropheryma whipplei*, the agent of Whipple's disease, requires phagosome acidification. *Infect. Immun.* **70:**1501–1506.
53. **Gillen, C. D., R. Coddington, P. G. Monteith, and R. H. Taylor.** 1993. Extraintestinal lymphoma in association with Whipple's disease. *Gut* **11:**1627–1629.
54. **Gisbertz, I. A., D. C. Bergmanns, J. A. van Marion-Kievit, and H. R. Haak.** 2001. Concurrent Whipple's disease and *Giardia lamblia* infection in a patient presenting with weight loss. *Eur. J. Intern. Med.* **12:**525–528.
55. **Gubler, J. G., M. Kuster, and F. Dutly.** 1999. Whipple endocarditis without overt gastrointestinal disease: report of four cases. *Ann. Intern. Med.* **31:**112–116.
56. **Groll, A., L. S. Valberg, J. B. Simon, D. Eidinger, D. Wilson, and D. R. Forsdyke.** 1972. Immunological defect in Whipple's disease. *Gastroenterology* **63:**943–950.
57. **Gruner, U., P. Goesch, A. Donner, and U. Peters.** 2001. Whipple disease and non-Hodgkin lymphoma. *Z. Gastroenterol.* **4:**305–309.
58. **Hargrove, J. R., J. V. Verner, A. G. Smith, R. R. Horswell, and J. M. Ruffin.** 1960. Whipple's disease. Report of two cases with intestinal biopsy before and after treatment. *Gastroenterology* **39:**619–622.
59. **Holt, P. R., K. J. Isselbacher, and C. M. Jones.** 1961. The reversibility of Whipple's disease. Report of a case, with comments on the influence of corticosteroid therapy. *N. Engl. J. Med.* **264:**1335–1339.
60. **Jones, C. M., J. A. Benson, Jr., and A. L. Roque.** 1953. Whipple's disease; report of a case with special reference to histochemical studies of biopsy material and therapeutic results of corticosteroid therapy. *N. Engl. J. Med.* **16:**665–670.
61. **Keinath, R. D., D. E. Merrell, and R. Vlietstra.** 1985. Antibiotic treatment and relapse in Whipple's disease: long term follow-up of 88 patients. *Gastroenterology.* **88:**1867–1873.
62. **Lee, A. G.** 2002. Whipple disease with supranuclear ophthalmoplegia diagnosed by polymerase chain reaction of cerebrospinal fluid. *J. Neuroophthalmol.* **22:**18–21.
63. **Leidig, P., M. Stolte, B. Krakamp, and S. Störkel.** 1994. Whipple's disease—a rare cause of secondary amyloidosis. *Z. Gastroenterol.* **2:**109–112.
64. **Lepidi, H., B. Coulibaly, J. P. Casalta, and D. Raoult.** 2006. Autoimmunohistochemistry: a new method for the histologic diagnosis of infective endocarditis. *J. Infect. Dis.* **193:** 1711–1717.
65. **Lepidi, H., F. Fenollar, R. Gerolami, J. L. Mege, M. F. Bonzi, M. Chappuis, J. Sahel, and D. Raoult.** 2003. Whipple's disease: immunospecific and quantitative immunohistochemical study of intestinal biopsy specimens. *Hum. Pathol.* **34:**589–596.
66. **LeVine, M. E., and W. O. Dobbins III.** 1973. Joint changes in Whipple's disease. *Semin. Arthritis Rheum.* **3:**79–93.
66a. **Li, W., F. Fenollar, J. M. Rolain, P. E. Fournier, G. E. Feurle, C. Müller, V. Moos, T. Marth, M. Altwegg, R. C. Calligaris-Maibach, T. Schneider, F. Biagi, B. La Scola, and D. Raoult.** 2008. Genotyping reveals a wide heterogeneity of *Tropheryma whipplei. Microbiology* **154:**521–527.
67. **Lohr, M., W. Stenzel, G. Plum, W. P. Gross, M. Deckert, and N. Klug.** 2004. Whipple's disease confined to the central nervous system presenting as a solitary frontal tumor: case report. *J. Neurosurg.* **101:**336–339.

68. **Louis, E. D., T. Lynch, P. Kaufmann, S. Fahn, and J. Odel.** 1996. Diagnostic guidelines in central nervous system Whipple's disease. *Ann. Neurol.* **40:**561–568.
69. Reference deleted.
70. **Lynch, T., J. Odel, and D. N. Fredericks.** 1997. Polymerase chain reaction-based detection of *Tropheryma whippelii* in central nervous system Whipple's disease. *Ann. Neurol.* **42:**120–124.
71. **Mahnel, R., A. Kalt, S. Ring, A. Stallmach, W. Strober, and T. Marth.** 2005. Immunosuppressive therapy in Whipple's disease patients is associated with the appearance of gastrointestinal manifestations. *Am. J. Gastroenterol.* **100:** 1167–1173.
72. **Maiwald, M., H. J. Ditton, A. von Herbay, F. A. Rainey, and E. Stackerbrandt.** 1996. Reassessment of the phylogenetic position of the bacterium associated with Whipple's disease and determination of the 16S–23S ribosomal intergenic spacer sequence. *Int. J. Syst. Bacteriol.* **46:**1078–1082.
73. **Maiwald, M., H. J. Ditton, A. von Herbay, F. A. Rainey, and E. Stackerbrandt.** 1999. Environmental occurrence of the Whipple's disease bacterium (*Tropheryma whippelii*). *Appl. Environ. Microbiol.* **64:**760–762.
74. **Maiwald, M., A. von Herbay, D. H. Persing, P. P. Mitchell, M. F. Abdelmalek, J. N. Thorvilson, D. N. Fredricks, and D. A. Relman.** 2001. *Tropheryma whippelii* DNA is rare in the intestinal mucosa of patients without other evidence of Whipple disease. *Ann. Intern. Med.* **2:**115–119.
75. **Maizel, H., J. M. Ruffin, and W. O. Dobbins III.** 1970. Whipple's disease: a review of 19 patients from one hospital and a review of the literature since 1950. *Medicine* (Baltimore) **72:**343–355.
76. **Marth, T.** 2005. Whipple's disease. p. 1306–1310. *In* G. Mandell, J. Dolin, and R. Bennett (ed.), *Principles and Practice of Infectious Disease*, 6th ed. Churchill Livingstone, Philadelphia, PA.
77. **Marth, T., N. Kleen, A. Stallmach, S. Ring, S. Aziz, C. Schmidt, W. Strober, M. Zeitz, and T. Schneider.** 2002. Dysregulated peripheral and mucosal Th1/Th2 response in Whipple's disease. *Gastroenterology* **123:**1468–1477.
78. **Marth, T., M. Neurath, B. A. Cuccherini, and W. Strober.** 1997. Defects of monocyte interleukin-12 production and humoral immunity in Whipple's disease. *Gastroenterology* **113:**442–448.
79. **Marth, T., and D. Raoult.** 2003. Whipple's disease. *Lancet* **361:**239–246.
80. **Marth, T., M. Roux, A. von Herbay, S. C. Meuer, and G. E. Feurle.** 1994. Persistent reduction of complement receptor 3 alpha-chain expressing mononuclear blood cells and transient inhibitory serum factors in Whipple's disease. *Clin. Immunol. Immunopathol.* **72:**217–226.
81. **Marth, T., and W. Strober.** 1996 .Whipple's disease. *Semin. Gastrointest. Dis.* **7:**41–48.
81a. **Martinetti, M., F. Biagi, C. Badulli, G. E. Feurle, C. Muller, V. Moos, T. Schneider, T. Marth, A. Marchese, L. Trotta, S. Sachetto, A. Pasi, A. De Silvestri, L. Salvaneschi, and G. R. Corazza.** 2009. The HLA alleles DRB1*13 and DQB1*06 are associated to Whipple's disease. *Gastroenterology*, 26 January 2009 [Epub ahead of print].
82. **Maxwell, J. D., A. Ferguson, A. M. McCay, R. C. Imrie, and W. C. Watson.** 1968. Lymphocytes in Whipple's disease. *Lancet* **i:**887–889.
83. **Meier-Willersen, H. J., M. Maiwald, and A. von Herbay.** 1993. Whipple's disease associated with opportunistic infections. *Dtsch. Med. Wochenschr.* **23:**854–860.
84. **Messori, A., P. Di Bella, and G. Polonara.** 2001. An unusual spinal presentation of Whipple disease. *Am. J. Neuroradiol.* **22:**1004–1008.
85. **Misbah, S. A., B. Ozols, A. Franks, and N. Mapstone.** 1997. Whipple's disease without malabsorption: new atypical features. *QJM* **90:**765–772.
86. **Moos, V., D. Kunkel, T. Marth, G. E. Feurle, B. LaScola, R. Ignatius, M. Zeitz, and T. Schneider.** 2006. Reduced peripheral and mucosal *T. whipplei*-specific Th1 response in patients with Whipple's disease. *J. Immunol.* **177:** 2015–2022.
87. **Naegeli, B., F. Bannwart, and O. Bertel.** 2000. An uncommon cause of recurrent strokes. *Tropheryma whippelii* endocarditis. *Stroke* **31:**2002–2003.
88. **Papadopoulou, M., M. Rentzos, C. Nicolaou, V. Ioannidou, A. Ioannidis, and S. Chatzipanagiotou.** 2003. Cerebral Whipple's disease diagnosed using PCR: the first case reported from Greece. *Mol. Diagn.* **7:**209–211.
89. **Paulley, D.** 1952. A case of Whipple's disease. *Gastroenterology* **22:**128–133.
90. **Peters, G., D. G. du Plessis, and P. R. Humphrey.** 2002. Cerebral Whipple's disease with a stroke-like presentation and cerebrovascular pathology. *J. Neurol. Neurosurg. Psychiatry* **73:**336–339.
91. **Posada, I. J., A. Ferreiro-Sieiro, E. Lopez-Valdes, A. Cabello, and F. Bermejo-Pareja.** 2004. Whipple's disease confined to the brain: a clinical case with pathological confirmation at necropsy. *Rev. Neurol.* **38:**196–198.
92. **Raoult, D., M. L. Birg, B. La Scola, P. E. Fournier, M. Enea, H. Lepidi, V. Roux, J. C. Piette, F. Vandenesch, D. Vital Durand, and T. J. Marrie.** 2000. Cultivation of the bacillus of Whipple's disease. *N. Engl. J. Med.* **342:**620–625.
93. **Raoult D., H. Ogata, S. Audic, C. Robert, K. Suhre, and M. Drancourt.** 2003. *Tropheryma whipplei* twist: a human pathogenic Actinobacteria with a reduced genome. *Genome Res.* **13:**1800–1809.
94. **Relman, D. A., T. M. Schmidt, R. P. Mac Dermot, and S. Falkow.** 1992. Identification of the uncultured bacillus of Whipple's disease. *N. Eng. J. Med.* **30:**293–301.
95. **Renesto. P., N. Crapoulet, H. Ogata, B. La Scola, G.Vestris, J. M. Claverie, and D. Raoult.** 2003. Genome-based design of a cell-free culture medium for *Tropheryma whipplei*. *Lancet* **362:**447–449.
96. **Rodarte, J. R., C. O. Garrison, K. E. Holley, and R. S. Fontana.** 1972. Whipple's disease simulating sarcoidosis. *Arch. Intern. Med.* **129:**479–482.
97. **Rouillon, A., C. J. Menkes, J. C. Gerster, I. Perez-Sawka, and M. Forest.** 1993. Sarcoid-like forms of Whipple's disease. Report of 2 cases. *J. Rheumatol.* **20:**1070–1072.
98. **Scheib, J. S., and R. J. Quinet.** 1990. Whipple's disease with axial and peripheral joint destruction. *South. Med. J.* **83:** 684–687.
98a. **Schneider, T., V. Moos, C. Loddenkemper, T. Marth, F. Fenollar, and D. Raoult.** 2008. Whipple's disease: new aspects of pathogenesis and treatment. *Lancet Infect. Dis.* **8:**179–190.
99. **Schnider, P. J., E. C. Reisinger, and W. Gerschlager.** 1996. Long-term follow-up in cerebral Whipple's disease. *Eur. J. Gastroenterol. Hepatol.* **8:**899–903.
100. **Schoedon, G., D. Goldenberger, R. Forrer, A. Gunz, F. Dutly, M. Höchli, M. Altwegg, and A. Schaffner.** 1997. Deactivation of macrophages with interleukin-4 is the key to the isolation of *Tropheryma whippelii*. *J. Infect. Dis.* **176:**672–677.

101. **Schöniger-Hekele, M., D. Petermann, B. Weber, and C. Müller.** 2007. *T. whipplei* in the environment: survey of sewage plant influxes and sewage plant workers. *Appl. Environ. Microbiol.* **73:**2033–2035.
102. **Schröter, A., J. Brinkhoff, and T. Günthner-Lengsfeld.** 2005. Whipple's disease presenting as an isolated lesion of the cervical spinal cord. *Eur. J. Neurol.* **12:**276–279.
103. **Trier, J. S., P. C. Phelps, S. Eidelmann, and C. E. Rubin.** 1965. Whipple's disease: light and electron microscope correlation of jejunal mucosal histology with antibiotic treatment and clinical status. *Gastroenterology* **48:**684–707.
104. **Upton, A. C.** 1952. Histochemical investigation of the mesenchymal lesions in Whipple's disease. *Am. J. Clin. Pathol.* **22:**755–764.
105. **Von Herbay. A., H. J. Ditton, F. Schuhmacher, and M. Maiwald.** 1997. Whipple's disease: staging and monitoring by cytology and polymerase chain reaction analysis of cerebrospinal fluid. *Gastroenterology* **113:**434–441.
106. **Wang, S., L. M. Ernst, B. R. Smith, G. Tallini, J. G. Howe, J. Crouch, and D. L. Cooper.** 2003. Systemic *Tropheryma whipplei* infection associated with monoclonal B-cell proliferation: a *Helicobacter pylori*-type pathogenesis? *Arch. Pathol. Lab. Med.* **12:**1619–1622.
107. **Watanakunakorn, C., and Burkert T.** 1993. Infective endocarditis at a large community teaching hospital, 1980–1990: a review of 210 episodes. *Medicine* (Baltimore) **72:** 90–102.
108. **Wilson, K. H., R. Blitchington, R. Frothingam, and J. A. Wilson.** 1991. Phylogeny of the Whipple's-disease-associated bacterium. *Lancet* **338:**474–475.
109. **Yardley, J. H., and T. R. Hendrix.** 1961. Combined electron and light microscopy in Whipple's disease—demonstration of "bacillary bodies" in the intestine. *Bull. Johns Hopkins Hosp.* **109:**80–98.

Sequelae and Long-Term Consequences of Infectious Diseases
Edited by Pina M. Fratamico, James L. Smith, and Kim A. Brogden

Chapter 12

Toxoplasma gondii

Jeffrey D. Kravetz

Toxoplasma gondii is an obligate intracellular protozoan that has the ability to infect all mammals, as well as birds and rodents, who serve as intermediate hosts. In immunocompetent hosts, 90% of primary infections caused by *T. gondii* are asymptomatic. The vast majority of symptomatic, primary infections cause a mild, mononucleosis-like illness with low-grade fever, malaise, headache, and cervical lymphadenopathy. Following this initial asymptomatic or symptomatic primary infection, the protozoan is usually contained by the immune system and remains dormant for the remainder of the host's life. However, if immunity wanes, the protozoan can resume its asexual life cycle and once again infect the host, though now without intact host defenses, causing cerebral toxoplasmosis, as well as myocarditis, pneumonitis, and chorioretinitis. Reactivation of *T. gondii* can thus lead to long-term consequences of a primary infection that occurred in the remote past.

In addition to reactivation of *T. gondii* causing long-term sequelae of a prior infection, primary infection of a pregnant individual can have dire consequences for a developing fetus. If the protozoan crosses the placenta, it can infect the fetus in utero, leading to a wide array of complications, ranging from chorioretinitis to mental retardation to miscarriage. The chorioretinitis can present at birth but can also present many years after an uneventful birth, as a direct result of infection or its resultant inflammatory response.

In order to completely understand the wide array of clinical manifestations as well as long-term consequences of *T. gondii* infection, a complete understanding of the protozoan's complex life cycle is imperative. Knowledge of this life cycle is also necessary to understand the epidemiology as well as appropriate preventive measures that lower the risk of primary infection in individuals at risk for long-term complications.

PATHOPHYSIOLOGY

T. gondii has a complex life cycle, with both asexual and sexual reproduction leading to the formation of three different forms of the protozoan. Sexual reproduction, which occurs in the small intestine of a cat, leads to the formation of oocysts. This portion of the life cycle occurs only in cats that have recently ingested infected meat (uncooked meat, including small rodents). Once a cat has acquired a primary infection, it develops immunity and thus rarely becomes reinfected. Thus, oocysts are identified in cat feces following their first exposure to meat containing infective tissue cysts. The majority of infective cats are thus outdoor cats who hunt for their food. Once a cat has ingested infected meat, several million oocysts are produced and excreted in the feces for 7 to 21 days (58). These oocysts become infective 1 to 5 days following defecation and can then be ingested by other hosts (including humans), leading to a continuation of the parasite's life cycle (53).

Bradyzoites are the slowly dividing or dormant form of *T. gondii* which has been contained by an immune response in various organs in an intermediate host. The bradyzoites are contained within tissue cysts and can remain dormant as long as the immune system remains intact.

Tachyzoites are the rapidly, asexually dividing form of *T. gondii* which disseminates within macrophages either prior to the development of an adequate immune response (primary infection) or following immunosuppression (reactivation). Primary infection results from the invasion of an intermediate host's intestinal wall via sporozoites (released from ingested oocysts) or bradyzoites (released from ingested tissue cysts). Once the sporozoites or bradyzoites cross the intestinal wall, they invade macrophages and begin the asexual portion of their life cycle. With an adequate immune response, the tachyzoites circulate for

Jeffrey D. Kravetz • Veterans Affairs Healthcare System, West Haven, CT 06516, and Yale University School of Medicine, New Haven, CT 06520.

7 to 10 days before being contained as bradyzoites within a tissue cyst. These tissue cysts can then remain dormant for the life of an intermediate host in various tissues, including the lymph nodes, muscle, brain, retina, myocardium, lungs, and liver (18).

There are three means of human infection with *T. gondii*. First, humans can ingest uncooked meat which contains tissues cysts. The prevalence of infective tissue cysts within different meats varies by location and method by which the meat was obtained. One study assessing the prevalence of viable *T. gondii* in meat using a bioassay revealed that only 7 out of 2,094 samples of pork obtained in retail stores in the United States contained viable *T. gondii* tissue cysts. The same study did not detect viable *T. gondii* tissue cysts in chicken or beef samples (26). However, meat obtained via noncommercial means may impart a higher risk of toxoplasmosis transmission. Ninety-three percent of pigs destined for human consumption on a farm in Massachusetts contained infective tissue cysts (24). Seventeen percent of chickens assayed for *T. gondii* in Ohio were found to have prior infection, and half of these caused infection when consumed by previously *T. gondii*-negative cats. Another small study showed 73% of chickens on a farm in Massachusetts to be infective (25). Thus, it appears that local meat sources may impart a higher risk of toxoplasmosis transmission.

In countries outside the United States, the prevalence of *T. gondii* tissue cysts in meat is also likely to be higher, given differences in processing techniques. A survey of fresh pork sausage obtained from a factory in Brazil revealed tissue cysts in 8.7% of samples (19). Free-range chickens studied in southern Brazil had a 65% seroprevalence for *T. gondii* antibodies, indicating prior *T. gondii* infection and probable carriage of tissue cysts (15). In order to lower the risk of transmission via consumption of tissue cysts, various methods are recommended. High-pressure processing of ground pork can kill tissue cysts prior to consumer distribution (50). In addition, cooking meat to an internal temperature of 67°C or freezing meat to below −12°C kills bradyzoites and thus eliminates this risk of transmission (22).

The second method of disease acquisition in humans is via the consumption of infective oocysts. These oocysts are produced by a *T. gondii*-seronegative (first exposure) cat that has recently ingested infective tissue cysts. As noted previously, the oocysts are not immediately infective and require 1 to 5 days to become infective (53). However, once oocysts are deposited by cats, they can remain infective for prolonged periods, depending on environmental conditions. In vitro studies show oocysts to remain infective for at least 200 days at temperatures ranging from 10°C to 25°C and for up to 54 months at 4°C (23). Thus, contact with soil contaminated with oocysts deposited by outdoor cats can be a source of disease transmission long after a cat has deposited its oocysts. Once ingested, the oocysts release sporozoites which invade the intestinal wall and circulate within macrophages, where asexual reproduction and tachyzoite formation occurs.

Congenital toxoplasmosis results from the transplacental transmission of infective tachyzoites from a mother with a primary toxoplasmosis infection. Assuming a normal immune system, congenital transmission occurs only in the 7 to 10 days after a pregnant woman acquires toxoplasmosis, when there are high levels of tachyzoites in the bloodstream. If a woman has already been infected with *T. gondii* prior to her pregnancy and has antibodies to *T. gondii*, she is unlikely to reacquire a primary infection during her pregnancy. The risk of congenital toxoplasmosis infection from a mother with primary toxoplasmosis increases during pregnancy, from 1% in the preconception period to 0% to 9% in the first trimester to 35% to 59% in the third trimester (Fig. 1) (56, 58, 71). Fortunately, the later in pregnancy that congenital toxoplasmosis infection occurs, the less severe the consequences. Infections during the first trimester can lead to miscarriage and severe malformations, including hydrocephalus and mental retardation. Preterm birth is more likely to occur with congenital infections occurring prior to 20 weeks of gestation, and the highest frequency of severe congenital malformations occurs with infection between the 10th and 24th gestational week (Fig. 2) (29, 71).

Hematogenous infection via blood transfusions is unlikely, given the short window of infectivity of tachyzoites during a primary infection. However,

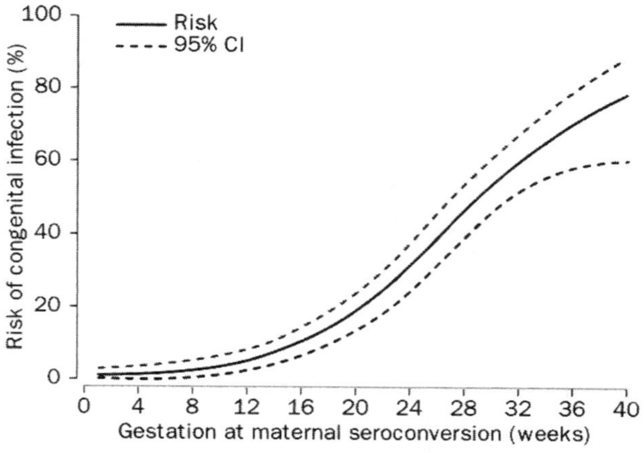

Figure 1. Risk of congenital infection according to duration of gestation at maternal seroconversion. (Reprinted from *The Lancet* [27] with permission from Elsevier.)

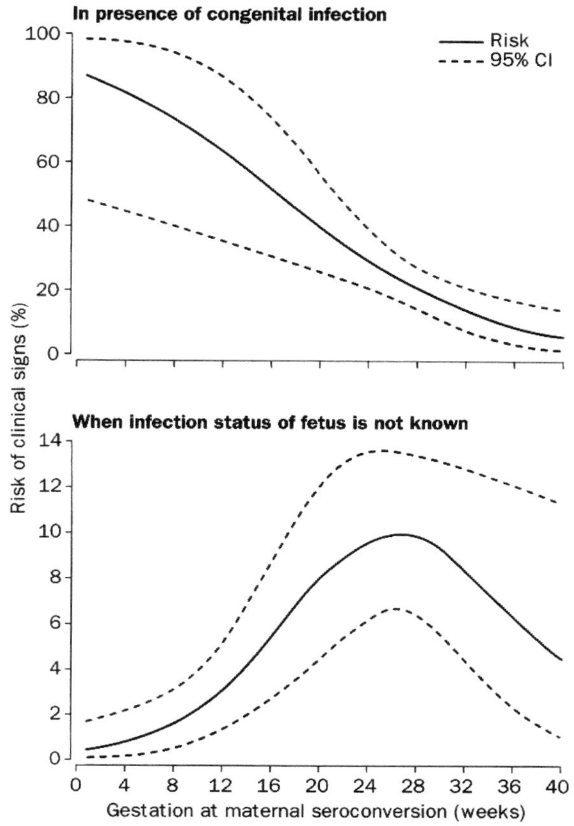

Figure 2. Risk of developing clinical signs (not necessarily symptomatic) before age 3 years according to gestational age. (Reprinted from *The Lancet* [27] with permission from Elsevier.)

screening of blood for tachyzoites is not performed, and cases of transmission have been reported with leukocyte transfusions (63, 72, 74). Leukoreduced blood is much less likely to transmit tachyzoites, since they circulate within macrophages. Though universal leukoreduction is not mandated in the United States, the American Red Cross has been attempting to ensure universal leukoreduction of platelet and red blood cell products in order to diminish the risk of disease transmission, as well as other transfusion reactions.

Finally, cases of toxoplasmosis infection following either solid-organ or hematopoietic stem cell transplantation and subsequent immunosuppression have been reported. Though most cases occurring in this setting are likely to be newly acquired primary infections in the setting of immunosuppression, there is also a risk of reactivation of a transplanted tissue cyst. Classically, the most commonly reported transplanted organ to be complicated by reactivation of a tissue cyst is the heart. However, virtually any solid organ can contain tissue cysts, due to the wide dissemination of tachyzoites during primary infection. Toxoplasmosis occurs in 0.3% to 7.6% of patients following hematopoietic stem cell transplantation, with a lower incidence occurring with trimethoprim-sulfamethoxazole prophylaxis (45).

EPIDEMIOLOGY AND RISK FACTORS

Toxoplasmosis has a worldwide distribution, with its prevalence directly related to risk factors associated with contact with *T. gondii* tissue cysts or oocysts. In a population of 35- to 45-year-old women in Jordan, where undercooked meat consumption and contact with contaminated soil is common, the seroprevalence (indicating prior infection) is up to 90% (42). On the other hand, the overall seroprevalence of pregnant women in Kent, United Kingdom, was 9.1%, and a similar population in Korea had a seroprevalence of only 0.79% (62, 78). In the United States, the overall age-adjusted seroprevalence from 17,658 serum samples obtained from participants in the Third National Health and Nutrition Examination Survey (NHANES III) was 22.5%. For women ages 15 to 44, the seroprevelance was 15% (Fig. 3) (40). In the United States, seroprevelance is unaffected by race, ethnicity, or socioeconomic class (54).

The relative contribution of risk factors for the acquisition of toxoplasmosis has been studied in both seroprevalence and incidence studies. *T. gondii* seroprevalence studies are inherently flawed since the time of acquisition is unclear and could have occurred decades prior to the study. Thus, the assessment of risk factors for *T. gondii* seropositivity in a general population is likely to have significant recall bias. A more accurate method of detecting risk factors for *T. gondii* infection is to survey risk factors associated with a primary infection. Since most primary infections are asymptomatic, laboratory evidence of a new

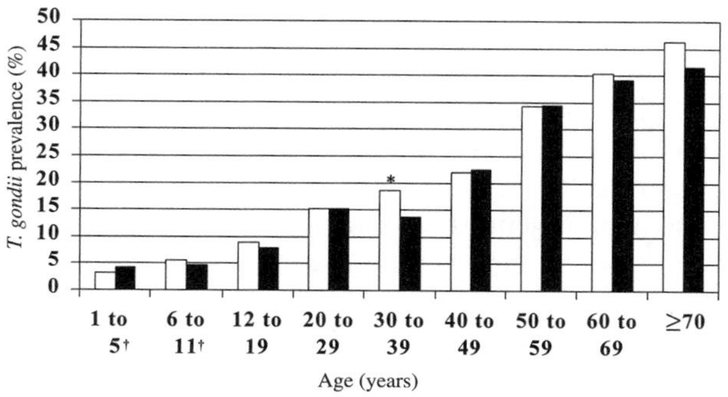

Figure 3. Seroprevalence of *Toxoplasma gondii*, by age and sex; Third National Health and Nutrition Examination Survey, 1988–1994. White bars represent males, black bars represent females. In the age group 30 to 39 years (*), seroprevalence was higher in males than in females ($P = 0.02$). Among children under 12 years (†), seroprevalence estimates are unstable because of low sample representation in these categories. (Reprinted from the *American Journal of Epidemiology* [40] with permission of Oxford University Press.)

seroconversion (development of anti-*T. gondii* immunoglobulin M [IgM]) is the gold standard for diagnosis of a primary infection. Most of the studies assessing seroconversion have been performed in seronegative, pregnant women, since primary infection in pregnancy can have severe consequences for a developing fetus.

The most significant risk factor to be identified in studies of *T. gondii* seroconversion is the consumption of raw meat. A prospective case-control study on primary toxoplasmosis infection in pregnancy in Norway revealed the following significant risk factors: eating raw or undercooked meat (including mutton and pork), eating unwashed vegetables or fruits, infrequent washing of kitchen knives after meat preparation, and cleaning the cat litter box (43). In another study in a high-risk population of women ages 15 to 45 in Yugoslavia, where the overall seroprevalence of *T. gondii* is 77%, the only risk factor identified was undercooked meat consumption (7). A case-control study in France involving 80 cases of primary toxoplasmosis infection in pregnancy revealed the following independent risk factors: poor hand hygiene, consumption of undercooked beef or lamb, and eating raw vegetables. Owning a pet cat was found to be of borderline significance (3). A large, multicenter, European case-control study with 252 cases of *T. gondii* seroconversion in pregnant women revealed contact with raw or undercooked beef, lamb, or other meat, as well as soil contact, to be independently associated with primary toxoplasmosis infection. Up to 63% of seroconversions were due to consumption of undercooked meat, while 17% were due to soil contact (13).

SYMPTOMS

Acute Infection in Immunocompetent Individuals

In immunocompetent individuals, 90% of primary toxoplasmosis infections are asymptomatic. In symptomatic patients with acute toxoplasmosis, the symptoms are mainly nonspecific and associated with hematogenous dissemination of the parasite. The most common symptomatic presentation is of a mononucleosis-like infection, with fever, headache, myalgia, bilateral lymphadenitis, and fatigue. In most patients, the constitutional symptoms are relatively mild. This syndrome does not require treatment and resolves spontaneously within 1 month in most patients. Rarely, acute cases can be complicated by pneumonitis (17), myocarditis with conduction system disease or congestive heart failure (12, 52), polymyositis (14, 57), hepatitis (76), or encephalitis (44).

Ocular Toxoplasmosis

Ocular toxoplasmosis can occur in both immunocompetent and immunocompromised hosts and can lead to wide array of symptoms, from asymptomatic retinal scars to blindness requiring enucleation. This infection has long been presumed to have been a result of a distant congenital infection, occurring with a peak incidence in the second through fourth decades of life (20). This theory was initially stated by Perkins, in the *British Journal of Ophthalmology*, in 1973, when he stated that "almost all cases of toxoplasmic chorioretinitis seen in the United Kingdom are the result of congenital infection" (66). However, more recent analysis has questioned this assumption, and it is now presumed that more cases of ocular toxoplasmosis are the result of postnatally acquired infections. This is based on a few observations. First, the clinical presentation of congenital and postnatally acquired ocular toxoplasmosis is different. Whereas bilateral eye disease is the norm in congenital disease, the most frequently seen manifestation of ocular toxoplasmosis is a focal area of retinitis occurring in one eye (20). In a retrospective review of 49 patients with ocular toxoplasmosis in Brazil (where the burden of ocular toxoplasmosis is higher than in the United States), 47 (95.9%) of the patients had unilateral involvement (28). Second, a case series published in 1996 by Montoya and Remington showed elevated levels of anti-toxoplasma IgM or IgE, in 22 out of 533 consecutive patients seen for toxoplasmic chorioretinitis, suggesting that acute, primary ocular toxoplasmosis was more common than previously assumed (59). Finally, analysis of seroprevalence data and documented rates of congenital toxoplasmosis infection led Gilbert and Stanford to argue that two-thirds of patients with ocular toxoplasmosis in the United Kingdom acquired their infections postnatally (32). In the United States, similar analysis has led Holland to conclude that the proportion of cases of postnatally acquired ocular toxoplasmosis is rising (36).

Despite the above observations, it is difficult to determine if a case of ocular toxoplasmosis occurred as a result of congenital infection or secondary to a postnatal infection. Since most cases of primary toxoplasmosis are asymptomatic in pregnant individuals, in the absence of congenital abnormalities or obvious birth defects, retinal lesions may not be identified until later in life, when the toxoplasmosis serology is difficult to interpret. However, both congenital and postnatally acquired ocular toxoplasmosis can lead to long-term consequences of a disease acquired in the remote past.

Clinically, ocular toxoplasmosis can cause a range of symptoms. Asymptomatic scars can be identified in a percentage of individuals. In 1972, a survey within a community in Maryland found retinochoroidal scars consistent with prior ocular toxoplasmosis in 0.6% of residents (77). In 1987, a survey in Alabama also identified 0.6% of individuals to have ocular toxoplasmosis (51). These individuals likely harbor tissue cysts in the retina and are at risk for recurrence of the disease, leading to eventual development of ocular symptoms.

Individuals who develop symptoms related to ocular toxoplasmosis may present with blurry vision, pain, photophobia, or scotoma. Most symptomatic infections cause a retinochoroiditis. In the United States, it is estimated that 35% of cases of retinochoroiditis in older children and adults are caused by *T. gondii* (49). *T. gondii* is also the most commonly identified cause of posterior uveitis and can be associated with elevated intraocular pressures in 38% of patients presenting with active retinochoroiditis (81) Optic nerve involvement has also been reported to occur in approximately five percent of individuals with active ocular toxoplasmosis (28). Severe cases of ocular toxoplasmosis can be complicated by retinal detachment, reported in 6% of patients in a case series of 150 patients with ocular toxoplasmosis by Bosch-Driessen et al. Five of the nine patients with retinal detachment developed legal blindness (8). The severity of ocular toxoplasmosis in an individual is affected by the patient's age and immune status and the virulence of the particular subtype of *T. gondii* causing the infection (37) Retinal lesions may heal spontaneously or with treatment, and leave an atrophic scar on the retina. In addition, multiple relapses have been reported and can occur for many years after the initial diagnosis of ocular toxoplasmosis. Over one quarter of patients with ocular toxoplasmosis present with recurrences within 2 years of the initial diagnosis (36).

Both the initial presentation of ocular toxoplasmosis and the subsequent relapses can occur years after the primary infection. This makes the timing of the initial infection difficult to determine and makes ocular toxoplasmosis a classic case of an infection with long-reaching, long-term consequences.

Congenital Toxoplasmosis

One of the most feared consequences of toxoplasmosis infection is the transmission of the parasite to a newborn, resulting in congenital toxoplasmosis. Fortunately, despite the prevalence of toxoplasmosis in the general population, congenital toxoplasmosis in the United States is still relatively rare. Based on newborn screening programs, it is estimated that there are between 400 and 4,000 cases of congenital toxoplasmosis in the United States per year (10). In the United States, only Massachusetts and New Hampshire have a neonatal screening program, where the incidence of congenital toxoplasmosis is approximately 1 in 10,000 to 1 in 12,000 (34). Further analysis of this screening program shows a strong association of the risk of congenital toxoplasmosis with the mother's country of birth, from 0 (mothers born in Vietnam) to 0.68 per 100,000 (mothers born in the United States) to 22.3 per 100,000 (mothers born in Laos) (38). However, since screening neonates for toxoplasmosis is not performed universally, the incidence in other parts of the United States is unknown.

In other countries with a higher seroprevalence of *T. gondii* than that in the United States, the incidence of congenital toxoplasmosis is greater. Worldwide, it is estimated that between 3 and 8 per 1,000 live births are infected in utero (71). In Europe, the incidence of congenital toxoplasmosis varies from country to country. In France, where the prevalence of toxoplasmosis in the adult population is relatively high, the incidence of congenital toxoplasmosis is 2 to 3 per 1,000 births, while in Switzerland, congenital toxoplasma infection is identified in 1 in 2,300 live births though only causes clinical symptoms in 1 in 16,250 births (75). Only 2.1 per 10,000 newborns in Denmark were diagnosed with congenital toxoplasmosis via a national neonatal screening program (73). In England and Wales, the incidence of congenital toxoplasmosis is extremely rare and estimated to be only 3.4 in 100,000 live births (31). In Brazil, the prevalence is estimated to be between 1 in 1,867 and 1 in 3,000 live births (64, 65). In Tanzania, a study of 849 pregnant women revealed evidence of congenital toxoplasma infection in 0.8% of newborns (21). Thus, though congenital toxoplasmosis in the United States is uncommon, its frequency in other countries makes it a worldwide newborn health problem.

The incidence of congenital toxoplasmosis in the United States remains low for a few reasons. First, only women who have a primary toxoplasmosis infection with circulating tachyzoites are able to transmit the parasite across the placenta. Thus, since the seroprevalence of toxoplasmosis among women of childbearing age (ages 15 to 44) is 15%, only 85% of pregnant individuals are at risk of acquiring a primary infection (40). Second, once infected, tachyzoites circulate for only 7 to 10 days, thus making for a narrow window for transmission to a developing fetus. In addition, transplacental transmission of toxoplasma tachyzoites in the first trimester is lower than later in pregnancy. Thus, during the most crucial stages of fetal development, the risk of infection is the lowest. Finally, as discussed previously, the prevalence of infective tissue cysts in commercial meat obtained in the United States is extremely low.

The diagnosis of congenital toxoplasmosis in utero is difficult in the absence of screening programs designed to detect *T. gondii* seroconversion. Since over 90% of immunocompetent individuals infected by *T. gondii* are asymptomatic, the only sign of primary infection is seroconversion by detection of IgG or IgM by the immunofluorescence antibody test, the immunosorbent agglutination assay, or other similar assays (47). IgG antibody levels increase 1 or 2 weeks after a primary infection and usually remain detectable for the life of the host. IgM antibody levels increase soon after infection and tend to remain elevated for 2 or 3 months (18). However, IgM antibodies detected via the immunosorbent agglutination method have been detected for up to 2 years after primary infection in up to 27% of women, making it difficult to determine the timing of infection (33). Thus, only new seroconversions (either IgG or IgM) detected during pregnancy place a developing fetus at risk for acquiring toxoplasmosis in utero. Currently, routine prenatal screening of mothers is performed in Austria, France, and Slovenia.

Congenital toxoplasmosis can also be diagnosed during the evaluation of an abnormal fetal ultrasound. Ultrasonographic findings of congenital toxoplasmosis in utero include hydrocephalus, intrauterine growth retardation, hepatomegaly, splenomegaly, cardiomegaly, and other placental abnormalities. Suspected cases of congenital toxoplasmosis can be evaluated for evidence of maternal seroconversion, though this is interpretable only if baseline serology is available. Amniocentesis and evaluation of the amniotic fluid via PCR is almost 100% sensitive and should be considered the gold standard for diagnosis of congenital toxoplasmosis in utero (67). In addition to prenatal diagnosis of congenital toxoplasmosis, neonatal screening is used to identify cases of congenital infection in Massachusetts and Rhode Island, Denmark, and portions of Brazil. Diagnosis is made by detection of IgM antibodies specific for *T. gondii* on blood samples obtained on Guthrie cards on day 5 postpartum (67).

There is a wide range of consequences of congenital toxoplasmosis for the developing fetus, from miscarriage, intrauterine growth retardation, or mental retardation to apparently asymptomatic cases presenting years after birth with ocular toxoplasmosis. Seventy to ninety percent of infants infected in utero are asymptomatic at birth (48). Of the symptomatic cases, most present with nonspecific symptoms, including rash, anemia, hepatosplenomegaly, hyperbilirubinemia, anemia, and thrombocytopenia. Neonates can also present with seizures related to intracranial calcifications and hydrocephalus. Chorioretinitis can be apparent at birth or can present many years later as a long-term consequence of the congenital infection. In a prospective study of 327 congenitally infected children followed for up to 14 years in France, 24% developed at least one retinochoroidal lesion. Of these individuals with ocular lesions, 29% of them developed either new lesions or reactivation of the initial retinochoroidal lesion up to 10 years after the initial presentation (80).

There are many long-term sequelae resulting from congenital toxoplasmosis in addition to ocular toxoplasmosis (discussed previously). Though it has been long presumed that congenital toxoplasmosis increases the risk of learning disabilities in children, this notion has been refuted by a recent prospective study of 178 children with congenital toxoplasmosis assessed at age 3. In comparison with uninfected children, 3- to 4-year-old children with congenital infection did not have evidence of developmental impairment or behavioral disturbances, though parents of these children were significantly more anxious (30). However, another case-control study involving over 12,000 live births did show an association between maternal exposure to toxoplasmosis and development of schizophrenia later in life. Compared with matched control subjects, the relative risk of developing schizophrenia (or other schizophrenia spectrum disorders, such as schizotypal personality disorder) was 2.61 (confidence interval [CI], 1.00 to 6.82) (9). Thus, many years after an asymptomatic maternal infection in utero, the offspring still appear to be at risk of long-term sequelae of toxoplasmosis.

It is difficult to assess the overall long-term impact of congenital toxoplasmosis on the population, since many infections are asymptomatic, while some complications manifest many years after the initial exposure. In a study performed in The Netherlands, Havelaar et al. attempted to provide an assessment of the disease burden by calculating disability-adjusted life years associated with congenital toxoplasmosis in the general population. This statistic takes into account the number of years of life lost and lived with a disability weighted by the severity of illness. According to their calculations, the estimated disease burden attributed to congenital toxoplasmosis was 620 disability-adjusted life years per year, which is similar to the effect of salmonellosis on the same population. Thirty-nine percent of the disability-adjusted life years was attributed to fetal loss, while 29% was attributed to chorioretinitis developing later in life (35). Thus, while it is difficult to assess the burden of congenital toxoplasmosis on the general population, long-term sequelae do play a significant role later in life.

Toxoplasma Encephalitis

During primary infection with *T. gondii*, tachyzoites disseminate for 7 to 10 days within macrophages prior to an immune response. Once an immune response develops, the tachyzoites are contained within tissue cysts (as bradyzoites), where they can remain dormant indefinitely, as long as the host's immune response remains intact. However, if cell-mediated immunity wanes, *T. gondii* can once again resume rapid growth and "reinfect" the same individual. The most common site of reactivation is the brain, where reactivation leads to toxoplasma encephalitis. Other sites of reactivation include the lungs, eyes, and myocardium.

Most cases of toxoplasma encephalitis occur in human immunodeficiency virus (HIV)-infected individuals with AIDS. Other risk factors associated with toxoplasma encephalitis include lymphoma (either Hodgkin's or non-Hodgkin's lymphoma), treatment with immunosuppressants for other malignancies or following organ transplantation, and use of high-dose steroids (49). In addition to these risk factors, a case series of 15 HIV-seronegative individuals with toxoplasma encephalitis showed the most common risk factor to be malnutrition (68). Nonetheless, most cases of toxoplasma encephalitis occur in HIV-infected individuals with AIDS.

In terms of the etiology of the infection, almost all cases are presumed to occur as a result of reactivation of a latent and remote infection. Thus, a typical case occurs in an individual who likely had an asymptomatic primary infection with *T. gondii* many years in the past. This is based on a few observations. First, almost all HIV-infected individuals who present with toxoplasma encephalitis already have IgG antibodies to *T. gondii* prior to the onset of symptoms. In one series of 75 patients with toxoplasma encephalitis, all patients had detectable levels of IgG against *T. gondii* prior to or immediately after diagnosis, suggesting a latent infection. In addition, the mean CD4 count was 78 cells/mm^3, showing that reactivation occurred in the setting of advanced immunodeficiency (70). In another larger series of 116 patients with toxoplasma encephalitis, 113 (97.4%) had detectable IgG titers to *T. gondii* prior to diagnosis. In addition, none of these individuals had detectable IgM antibodies at the time of diagnosis (4) Second, in multiple studies assessing risk factors for the development of toxoplasma encephalitis, multivariate analyses reveal only immune deficiency (specifically CD4 count of <200 cells/mm^3) and lack of appropriate antibiotic prophylaxis against *T. gondii* to be risk factors for toxoplasma encephalitis (1, 4, 61). Finally, in a study population of 1,699 patients with HIV infection who were followed for up to 8 years with *T. gondii* antibody determination every 6 months, only 14 individuals seroconverted during the follow-up and none of these individuals developed toxoplasma encephalitis (4). Another longitudinal study of 183 HIV-infected individuals revealed an annual incidence of new seroconversions of only 0.4% per year (69). Thus, toxoplasma encephalitis is a classic case whereby a remote infection presents years later as a long-term sequelae of the initial, asymptomatic infection.

Clinically, toxoplasma encephalitis has a varied presentation, depending on the location, number, size, surrounding edema, and subsequent mass effect associated with the underlying infection. Typically, toxoplasma encephalitis causes multiple ring-enhancing lesions to be visualized on magnetic resonance imaging (MRI) of the brain (Fig. 4). MRI has a better sensitivity for these lesions than computed tomography and is the imaging modality of choice for patients suspected of having toxoplasma encephalitis. Other presentations include solitary foci of infection with a single ring-enhancing lesion and diffuse toxoplasma meningoencephalitis. Most commonly, patients present with the subacute onset of nonspecific symptoms, including headache, fever, and altered mental status. As the lesions increase in size, multiple neurological symptoms develop, including focal motor weakness, sensory loss, cranial nerve paralysis, speech disturbances, visual field defects, cerebellar symptoms, and seizures. The onset of any focal neurological symptom, confusion, or new headache in an HIV-infected individual with known IgG antibody to *T. gondii* and a CD4 count of <200 cells/mm^3 (or even <400 cells/mm^3) warrants immediate imaging to evaluate for *T. gondii* infection. Even with the advent of highly active antiretroviral therapy, toxoplasma encephalitis remains the most prevalent neurological disorder occurring in patients with AIDS (2).

Diagnosis of toxoplasma encephalitis is based on a combination of clinical, radiological, and serological findings. Definitive diagnosis requires a compatible clinical syndrome, detectable IgG antibodies to *T. gondii*, typical computed tomography or MRI findings, and isolation of *T. gondii* from a brain biopsy specimen (5). Given the invasiveness of this technique, this is rarely performed, except in situations where differentiation from central nervous system lymphoma is difficult. Thus, most patients are treated for toxoplasma encephalitis based on a presumptive diagnosis. A presumptive diagnosis can be

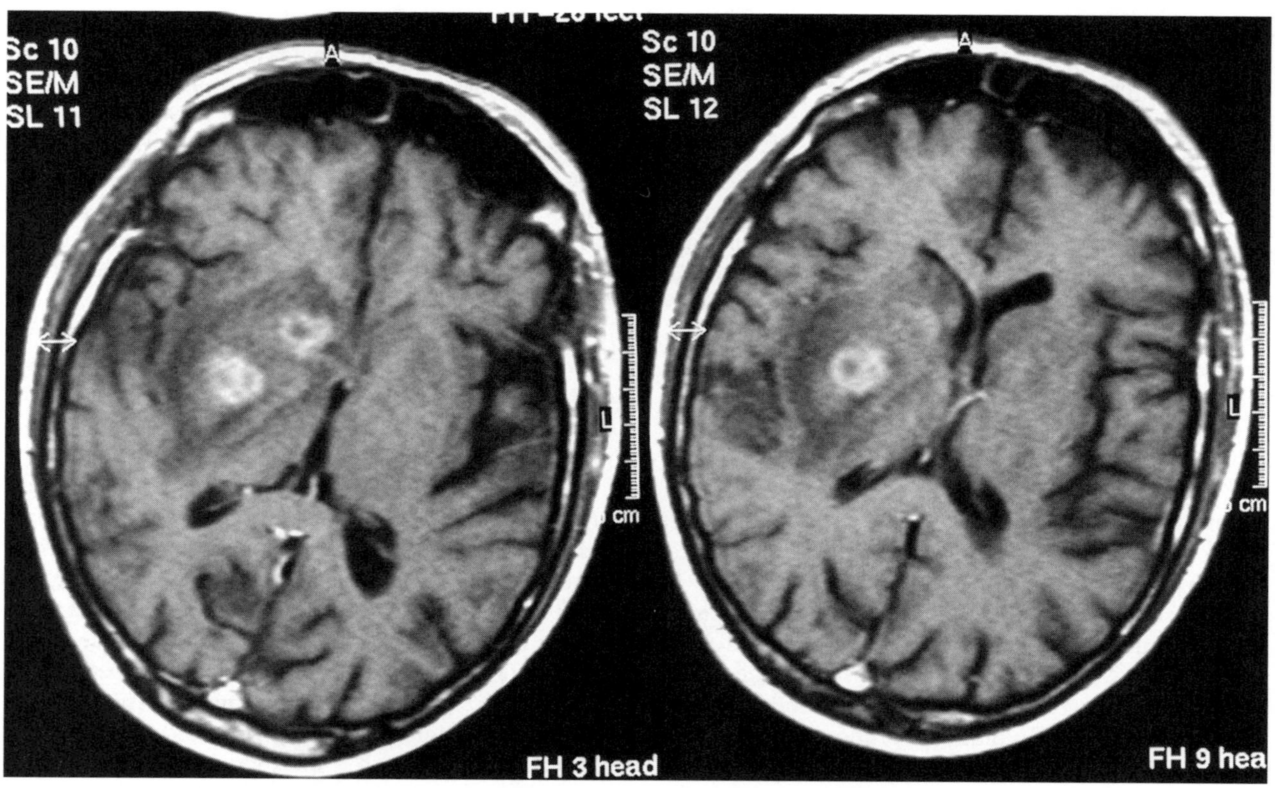

Figure 4. T1-weighted axial gadolinium-enhanced magnetic resonance image of toxoplasmosis encephalitis. (Image reprinted with permission from eMedicine.com, 2008; available at http://emedicine.medscape.com/article/344706-overview.)

made with a combination of clinical findings, detection of IgG antibodies to *T. gondii*, brain imaging, and a significant response to empiric anti-*T. gondii* chemotherapy. In this scenario, brain biopsy is thus reserved for those individuals who fail to show clinical improvement with empiric treatment.

According to the CDC guidelines, initial treatment of toxoplasma encephalitis should consist of a combination of pyrimethamine, sulfadiazine, and leucovorin (5). Alternative first-line regimens include pyrimethamine, clindamycin, and leucovorin or monotherapy with trimethoprim-sulfamethoxazole. A recent Cochrane Database review of the available randomized controlled trials on toxoplasma encephalitis therapy did not reveal any differences among the above three treatment regimens with regard to response rate and survival (16). Other regimens include atovaquone with pyrimethamine and leucovorin, atovaquone with sulfadiazine, and azithromycin with pyrimethamine and leucovorin. If no improvement occurs within the first 2 weeks, a brain biopsy should be strongly considered to make a definitive diagnosis. Typical treatment involves a 6-week course of antimicrobial regimen, followed by lifelong secondary prophylaxis, usually with continuation of the initial regimen at reduced doses. There is some evidence that either primary (instituted for a CD4 count of <200 cells/mm^3) or secondary prophylaxis can be discontinued with selected HIV-infected individuals with a significant response to highly active antiretroviral therapy with a sustained CD4 count of >200 cells/mm^3 (6, 55, 60). However, the decision to discontinue prophylaxis needs to be individualized, since the number of patients evaluated in these studies is still limited.

While reactivation of *T. gondii* clearly is the cause of toxoplasma encephalitis and thus a classic case of long-term sequelae of a remote infection, other central nervous system associations with *T. gondii* are less well defined. A study of 50 patients with cryptogenic epilepsy (normal brain MRI) revealed IgG antibodies to *T. gondii* in 52%, compared with 18% of healthy volunteers and 22% of epilepsy patients with a known cause (82). Though this finding is not proof of an association, it is possible that microscopic scars from a remote primary toxoplasmosis infection (not visible on MRI) could be a future epileptic focus.

Another association with seropositivity to *T. gondii* is schizophrenia (mentioned in the section above on congenital toxoplasmosis). A recent meta-analysis combining 23 studies on seropositivity to *T. gondii* revealed a combined odds ratio of 2.73 (CI, 2.1 to 3.6) for the prevalence of antibodies to *T. gondii* in patients diagnosed with schizophrenia (79). Most of the studies discussed above used patients without diagnosed mental illnesses as the control group. Another study of 50 patients with schizophrenia in Turkey, in comparison with patients with depressive disorders and healthy controls, showed seropositivity rates of 66% (for those with schizophrenia), 24% (for those with depressive disorders), and 22% (for healthy controls) (11). Thus, there is some possible association between prior *T. gondii* infection and the development of schizophrenia, though the direct connection is still unclear and not yet causal in nature.

PREVENTION OF TOXOPLASMOSIS

Since over 90% of primary infections with *T. gondii* are asymptomatic, and sequelae of the disease occur many years after the initial infection, primary prevention may offer the best chance to lower the risk of long-term sequelae. As outlined in the section on pathophysiology, toxoplasmosis is acquired by ingesting uncooked meat with tissue cysts, consuming infectious oocysts recently deposited by an infected cat, or from solid-organ or stem cell transplantation. The major risk factors identified for primary infection are undercooked meat consumption and eating unwashed fruit or vegetables (or other contact with soil). Whether changing a cat's litter box is a significant risk factor is unclear. Though cats with primary toxoplasma infection can deposit infectious oocysts with their feces, prompt cleaning of the litter box does not allow enough time (1 to 5 days) for the oocysts to become infectious. In addition, only outdoor cats that hunt (or indoor cats that ingest rodents living in a house) are a risk for acquiring toxoplasmosis. Thus, prevention of primary infection relies on appropriate counseling of individuals on risk factor reduction. The most important group of individuals to counsel on risk factor reduction are women of childbearing age who are attempting to become pregnant. In this population, primary infection can be devastating for a developing fetus and cause long-term sequelae for the unborn child. Methods to reduce reactivation of latent infection in immunocompromised individuals has been discussed previously.

Education about risk factor reduction should be provided prior to the diagnosis of pregnancy, since transmission of tachyzoites in the first trimester leads to the most severe complications for the fetus. All women of childbearing age should be counseled to avoid eating undercooked meat and should cook meat to an internal temperature of at least 67°C (153°F). In addition, freezing meat to below −12°C (10°F) also kills bradyzoites and thus eliminates this risk of transmission (22). It is also imperative to advise women to thoroughly wash hands and utensils used to prepare raw meat. When gardening, wearing gloves and thoroughly washing all fruit and vegetables obtained from a garden should eliminate the risk of contact with oocysts. Though the cat litter box is an unclear risk factor, when changing the litter, women should be counseled to either wear gloves or wash their hands following contact with cat litter. In addition, keeping a cat indoors, not feeding the cat undercooked meat, and changing the litter box on a daily basis should be advised. Table 1 provides a summary of appropriate risk factor counseling.

Unfortunately, knowledge of these risk factors among women of childbearing age is lacking. A survey of 403 pregnant women in the United States revealed that only 40% were aware that toxoplasmosis was an infection, and 21% believed that it was caused by a poison. Sixty percent of pregnant women surveyed believed that they could acquire toxoplasmosis from changing cat litter, while only 30% were aware that toxoplasmosis was found in raw or undercooked meat (41). Thus, education of women of childbearing age on risk factor reduction could be expected to have an impact on the risk of acquiring primary toxoplasma infection.

Both primary care physicians and obstetricians should counsel women on risk factor reduction. However, knowledge among these groups of physicians on appropriate risk factor reduction is also less than would be expected. In a survey of 364 obstetricians and gynecologists, only 83% responded that they advise pregnant women to avoid eating undercooked meat, while 100% advised against handling cat litter. Only 67.6% advised on proper gardening techniques. Surprisingly, 52.5% of respondents believed that keeping a cat outdoors would prevent toxoplasmosis (39). Another survey of 49 obstetricians and 53 internists or family practitioners revealed that both obstetricians (98%) and internists (88%) advised women to avoid changing the cat litter. However, while 98%

Table 1. Counseling for reduction of primary toxoplasmosis in women of childbearing age

Summary of appropriate risk factor counseling
1. Do not eat undercooked meat.
2. Wash hands and utensils after handling uncooked meat.
3. Wear gloves when gardening, or wash hands after gardening without gloves.
4. Wash all uncooked fruits and vegetables.
5. Wear gloves when changing the litter box of an outdoor cat.
6. Do not feed a cat uncooked meat.
7. Change the litter box daily.

of obstetricians advised women to avoid raw meat, only 65% of internists provided this advice. Both obstetricians (61%) and internists (41%) were less likely to advise women to avoid eating unwashed vegetables (46). Thus, both obstetricians and internists are less aware of appropriate risk factor modification than is needed and need to be better educated about these risks. Only with this knowledge can the risk of long-term consequences of toxoplasmosis infection for a developing fetus be reduced.

REFERENCES

1. **Abtrall, S., C. Rabaud, and D. Costagliola.** 2001. Incidence and risk factors for toxoplasmic encephalitis in human immunodeficiency virus-infected patients before and during the highly active antiretroviral therapy era. *Clin. Infect. Dis.* **33:**1747–1755.
2. **Antinori, A., D. Larussa, A. Cingolani, P. Lorenzini, S. Bossolasco, M. G. Finazzi, M. Bongiovanni, G. Guaraldi, S. Grisetti, B. Vigo, B. Gigli, A. Mariano, E. R. Dalle Nogare, M. De Marco, F. Moretti, P. Corsi, N. Abrescia, P. Rellecati, A. Castragna, C. Mussini, A. Ammassari, P. Cinque, A. D'Arminio Monforte, and Italian Registry Investigaive NeuroAIDS.** 2004. Prevalence, associated factors, and prognostic determinants of AIDS-related toxoplasmic encephalitis in the era of advanced highly active antiretroviral therapy. *Clin. Infect. Dis.* **39:**1681–1691.
3. **Baril, L., T. Ancelle, V. Goulet, P. Thulliez, V. Tirard-Fleury, and B. Carme.** 1999. Risk factors for *Toxoplasma* infection in pregnancy: a case-control study in France. *Scand. J. Infect. Dis.* **31:**305–309.
4. **Belanger, F., F. Derouin, L. Grangeot-Keros, and L. Meyer.** 1999. Incidence and risk factors of toxoplasmosis in a cohort of human immunodeficiency virus-infected patients: 1988–1995. *Clin. Infect. Dis.* **28:**575–581.
5. **Benson, C. A., J. E. Kaplan, H. Masur, A. Pau, and K. K. Holmes.** 2004. Treating opportunistic infections among HIV-infected adults and adolescents. Recommendations from CDC, the National Institutes of Health, and the HIV Medicine Association/Infectious Diseases Society of America. *MMWR Morb. Mortal. Wkly. Rep.* **53:**1–112.
6. **Bertschy, S., M. Opravil, M. Cavassini, E. Bernasconi, V. Schiffer, P. Schmid, M. Flepp, J.-P. Chave, A. Christen, and H. Furrer.** 2006. Discontinuation of maintenance therapy against toxoplasma encephalitis in AIDS patients with sustained response to anti-retroviral therapy. *Clin. Microbiol. Infect.* **12:**666–671.
7. **Bobic, B., I. Jevremovic, J. Marinkovic, D. Sibalic, and O. Djurkovic-Djakovic.** 1998. Risk factors for *Toxoplasma* infection in a reproductive age female population in the area of Belgrade, Yugoslavia. *Eur. J. Epidemiol.* **14:**605–610.
8. **Bosch-Driessen, L. H., S. Karimi, J. S. Stilma, and A. Rothova.** 2000. Retinal detachment in ocular toxoplasmosis. *Ophthalmology* **107:**36–40.
9. **Brown, A. S., C. A. Schaefer, C. P. Quesenberry, L. Liu, V. P. Babulas, and E. S. Susser.** 2005. Maternal exposure to toxoplasmosis and risk of schizophrenia in adult offspring. *Am. J. Psychiatry* **162:**767–773.
10. **Centers for Disease Control and Prevention.** 2000. CDC recommendations regarding selected conditions affecting women's health. *MMWR Morb. Mortal. Wkly. Rep.* **49:**59–68.
11. **Cetinkaya, Z., S. Yazar, O. Gecici, and M. N. Namli.** 2007. Anti-*Toxoplasma gondii* antibodies in patients with schizophrenia—preliminary findings in a Turkish sample. *Schizophren. Bull.* **33:**789–791.
12. **Chandenier, J., G. Jarry, D. Nassif, Y. Couadi, L. Paris, P. Thulliez, E. Bourges-Petit, and C. Raccurt.** 2000. Congestive heart failure and myocarditis after seroconversion for toxoplasmosis in two immunocompetent patients. *Eur. J. Clin. Microbiol. Infect. Dis.* **19:**375–379.
13. **Cook, A. J., R. E. Gilbert, W. Buffolano, J. Zufferey, E. Petersen, P. A. Jenum, W. Foulon, A. E. Semprini, and D. T. Dunn.** 2000. Sources of toxoplasma infection in pregnant women: European multicentre case-control study. *Br. Med. J.* **321:**142–147.
14. **Cuturic, M., G. R. Hayat, C. A. Vogler, and A. Velasques.** 1997. Toxoplasmic polymyositis revisited: case report and review of literature. *Neuromuscul. Disord.* **7:**390–396.
15. **da Silva, D. S., L. M. Bahia-Oliveira, S. K. Shen, O. C. Kwok, T. Lehman, and J. P. Dubey.** 2003. Prevalence of *Toxoplasma gondii* in chickens from an area in southern Brazil highly endemic to humans. *J. Parasitol.* **89:**394–396.
16. **Dedicoat, M., and N. Livesley.** 2006. Management of toxoplasmic encephalitis in HIV-infected adults (with an emphasis on resource-poor settings). *Cochrane Database Syst. Rev.* 3:CD005420.
17. **DeSalvador-Guillouet, F., D. Ajzenberg, S. Chaillou-Opitz, M. Saint-Paul, B. Dunais, P. Dellamonica, and P. Marty.** 2006. Severe pneumonia during primary infection with an atypical strain of *Toxoplasma gondii* in an immunocompetent young man. *J. Infect.* **53:**e47–e50.
18. **Despommier, D. D., R. W. Gwadz, and P. J. Hotez.** 1995. *Toxoplasma gondii*, p. 162–169. *In* D. D. Despommier, R. W. Gwadz, and P. J. Hotez (ed.), *Parasitic Diseases*, 3rd ed. Springer-Verlag, New York, NY.
19. **Dias, R. A. F., I. T. Navarro, B. B. Ruffolo, F. M. Bugni, M. V. Castro, and R. L. Freire.** 2005. *Toxoplasma gondii* in fresh pork sausage and seroprevalence in butchers from factories in Londrina, Parana State, Brazil. *Rev. Inst. Med. Trop. Sao Paulo.* **47:**185–189.
20. **Dodds, E. M.** 2006. Toxoplasmosis. *Curr. Opin. Ophthalmol.* **17:**557–561.
21. **Doehring, E., I. Reiter-Owona, O. Bauer, M. Kaisi, H. Hlobil, G. Quade, N. A. S. Hamudu, and H. M. Seitz.** 1995. *Toxoplasma gondii* antibodies in pregnant women and their newborns in Dar Es Salaam, Tanzania. *Am. J. Trop. Med. Hyg.* **52:**546–548.
22. **Dubey, J. P.** 1996. Strategies to reduce transmission of *Toxoplasma gondii* to animals and humans. *Vet. Parasitol.* **64:**65–70.
23. **Dubey, J. P.** 1998. *Toxoplasma gondii* oocyst survival under defined temperatures. *J. Parasitol.* **84:**862–865.
24. **Dubey, J. P., H. R. Gamble, D. Hill, C. Sreekumar, S. Romand, and P. Thuilliez.** 2002. High prevalence of viable *Toxoplasma gondii* infection in market weight pigs from a farm in Massachusetts. *J. Parasitol.* **88:**1234–1238.
25. **Dubey, J. P., D. H. Graham, E. Dahl, C. Sreekumar, T. Lehmann, M. F. Davis, and T. Y. Morishita.** 2003. *Toxoplasma gondii* isolates from free-ranging chickens from the United States. *J. Parasitol.* **89:**1060–1062.
26. **Dubey, J. P., D. E. Hill, J. L. Jones, A. W. Hightower, E. Kirkland, J. M. Roberts, P. L. Marcet, T. Lehmann, M. C. Vianna, K. Miska, C. Sreekumar, O. C. Kwok, S. K. Shen, and H. R. Gamble.** 2005. Prevalence of viable *Toxoplasma gondii* in beef, chicken, and pork from retail meat stores in the Unites States: risk assessment to consumers. *J. Parasitol.* **91:**1082–1093.

27. **Dunn, D., M. Wallon, F. Peyron, E. Petersen, C. Peckham and R. Gilbert.** 1999. Mother-to-child transmission of toxoplasmosis: risk estimates for clinical counseling. *Lancet* **353:**1829–1833.
28. **Eckert, G. U., J. Melamed, and B. Menegaz.** 2007. Optic nerve changes in ocular toxoplasmosis. *Eye* **21:**746–751.
29. **Freeman, K., L. Oakley, A. Pollak, W. Buffolano, E. Petersen, A. E. Semprini, A. Salt, and R. Gilbert.** 2005. Association between congenital toxoplasmosis and preterm birth, low birthweight and small for gestational age birth. *BJOG* **112:** 31–37.
30. **Freeman, K., A. Salt, A. Prusa, G. Malm, N. Ferret, W. Buffolano, D. Schmidt, H. K. Tan, and R. E. Gilbert.** 2005. Association between congenital toxoplasmosis and parent-reported developmental outcomes, concerns, and impairments, in 3 year old children. *BMC Pediatr.* **5:**23–33.
31. **Gilber, R., H. K. Tan, S. Cliffe, E. Guy, and M. Stanford.** 2006. Symptomatic toxoplasma infection due to congenital and postnatally acquired infection. *Arch. Dis. Child.* **91:** 495–498.
32. **Gilbert, R. E., and M. R. Stanford.** 2000. Is ocular toxoplasmosis caused by prenatal or postnatal infection? *Br. J. Ophthalmol.* **84:**224–226.
33. **Gras, L., R. E. Gilbert, M. Wallon, F. Peyron, and M. Cortina-Borja.** 2004. Duration of the IgM response in women acquiring *Toxoplasma gondii* during pregnancy: implications for clinical practice and cross-sectional incidence studies. *Epidemiol. Infect.* **132:**541–548.
34. **Guerina, N. G., H-W. Hsu, H. C. Meissner, J. H. Maguire, R. Lynfield, B. Stechenberg, I. Abroms, M. S. Pasternack, R. Hoff, R. B. Eaton, and G. F. Grady.** 1994. Neonatal serologic screening and early treatment for congenital *Toxoplasma gondii* infection. *N. Engl. J. Med.* **330:**1858–1863.
35. **Havelaar, A. H., J. M. Kemmeren, and L. M. Kortbeek.** 2007. Disease burden of congenital toxoplasmosis. *Clin. Infect. Dis.* **44:**1467–1474.
36. **Holland, G. N.** 2003. Ocular toxoplasmosis: a global reassessment. Part 1: epidemiology and course of disease. *Am. J. Ophthalmol.* **136:**973–988.
37. **Holland, G. N.** 2004. Ocular toxoplasmosis: a global reassessment. Part II: Disease manifestations and management. *Am. J. Ophthalmol.* **137:**1–17.
38. **Jara, M., H. W. Hsu, R. B. Eaton, and A. Demaria, Jr.** 2001. Epidemiology of congenital toxoplasmosis identified by population-based newborn screening in Massachusetts. *Pediatr. Infect. Dis. J.* **20:**1132–1135.
39. **Jones, J. L., V. J. Dietz, M. Power, A. Lopez, M. Wilson, T. R. Navin, R. Gibbs, and J. Schulkin.** 2001. Survey of obstetrician-gynecologists in the United States about toxoplasmosis. *Infect. Dis. Obstet. Gynecol.* **9:**23–31.
40. **Jones, J. L., D. Kruszon-Moran, M. Wilson, G. McQuillan, T. Navin, and J. B. McAuley.** 2001. *Toxoplasma gondii* infection in the United States: seroprevalence and risk factors. *Am. J. Epidemiol.* **154:**357–365.
41. **Jones, J. L., F. Ogunmodede, J. Scheftel, E. Kirkland, A. Lopez, J. Schulkin, and R. Lynfield.** 2003. Toxoplasmosis-related knowledge and practices among pregnant women in the United States. *Infect. Dis. Obstet. Gynecol.* **11:**139–145.
42. **Jumaian, N. F.** 2005. Seroprevalence and risk factors for *Toxoplasma* infection in pregnant women in Jordan. *East. Mediterr. Health J.* **11:**45–55.
43. **Kapperud, G., P. A. Jenum, B. Stray-Pedersen, K. K. Melby, A. Eskild, and J. Eng.** 1996. Risk factors for *Toxoplasma gondii* infection in pregnancy. Results of a prospective case-control study in Norway. *Am. J. Epidemiol.* **144:**405–412.
44. **Kaushik, R. M., S. K. Mahajan, A. Sharma, R. Kaushik, and R. Kukreti.** 2005. Toxoplasmic meningoencephalitis in an immunocompetent host. *Trans. R. Soc. Trop. Med. Hyg.* **99:**874–878.
45. **Kotton, C. N.** 2007. Zoonoses in solid-organ and hematopoietic stem cell transplant recipients. *Clin. Infect. Dis.* **44:**857–866.
46. **Kravetz, J. D., and D. G. Federman.** 2005. Prevention of toxoplasmosis in pregnancy: knowledge of risk factors. *Infect. Dis. Obstet. Gynecol.* **13:**161–165.
47. **Kravetz, J. D., and D. G. Federman.** 2005. Toxoplasmosis in pregnancy. *Am. J. Med.* **118:**212–216.
48. **Lebech, M., D. H. M. Joynson, H. M. Seitz, P. Thulliez, R. E. Gilbert, G. N. Dutton, B. Ovlisen, and E. Petersen.** 1996. Classification system and case definitions of *Toxoplasma gondii* infection in immunocompetent pregnant women and their congenitally infected offspring. *Eur. J. Clin. Microbiol. Infect. Dis.* **15:**799–805.
49. **Liesenfeld, O.** 2004. Toxoplasmosis. *In* L. Goldman and D. Ausiello (ed.), *Cecil Textbook of Medicine*, 22nd ed. Saunders, Philadelphia, PA.
50. **Lindsay, D. S., M. V. Collins, D. Holliman, G. J. Flick, and J. P. Dubey.** 2006. Effects of high-pressure processing on *Toxoplasma gondii* tissue cysts in ground pork. *J. Parasitol.* **92:**195–196.
51. **Maetz, H. M., R. N. Kleinstein, D. Federico, and J. Wayne.** 1987. Estimated prevalence of ocular toxoplasmosis and toxocariasis in Alabama. *J. Infect. Dis.* **156:**414.
52. **Mariani, M., M. Pagani, C. Inserra, and S. DeServi.** 2006. Complete atrioventricular block associated with toxoplasma myocarditis. *Europace* **8:**221–223.
53. **Markell, E. K., D. T. John, and W. A. Krotoski.** 1999. *Toxoplasma gondii*, p. 161–171. *In* K. Edwards, D. T. John, and W. A. Krotoski (ed.), *Markell and Voge's Medical Parasitology*, 8th ed. Saunders, Philadelphia, PA.
54. **McQuillan, G., D. Kruszon-Moran, B. J. Kottiri, L. R. Curtin, J. W. Lucas, and R. S. Kington.** 2004. Racial and ethnic differences in the seroprevalence of 6 infectious diseases in the United States: date from NHANES III, 1988-1994. *Am. J. Public Health* **94:**1952–1958.
55. **Miro, J. M., J. C. Lopez, D. Podzamczer, J. M. Peña, J. C. Alberdi, E. Martínez, P. Domingo, J. Cosin, X. Claramonte, J. R. Arribas, M. Santín, and E. Ribera.** 2006. Discontinuation of primary and secondary *Toxoplasma gondii* prophylaxis is safe in HIV-infected patients after immunological restoration with highly active antiretroviral therapy: results of an open, randomized, multicenter clinical trial. *Clin. Infect. Dis.* **43:**79–89.
56. **Mombro, M., C. Perathoner, A. Leone, V. Buttafuoco, C. Zotti, M. A. Lievre, C. Fabris.** 2003. Congenital toxoplasmosis: assessment of risk to newborns in confirmed and uncertain maternal infection. *Eur. J. Pediatr.* **162:**703–706.
57. **Montoya, J. G., R. Jordan, S. Lingamneni, G. J. Berry, and J. S. Remington.** 1997. Toxoplasmic myocarditis and polymyositis in patients with acute acquired toxoplasmosis diagnosed during life. *Clin. Infect. Dis.* **24:**676–683.
58. **Montoya, J. G., and O. Liesenfeld.** 2004. Toxoplasmosis. *Lancet* **363:**1965–1976.
59. **Montoya, J. G., and J. S. Remington.** 1996. Toxoplasmic chorioretinitis in the setting of acute acquired toxoplasmosis. *Clin. Infect. Dis.* **23:**277–282.
60. **Mussini, C., P. Pezzotti, A. Govoni, V. Borghi, A. Antinori, A. Monforte, A. De Luca, N. Mongiardo, M. C. Cerri, F. Chiodo, E. Concia, L. Bonazzi, M. Moroni, L. Ortona, R. Esposito, A. Cossarizza, and B. De Rienzo.** 2000. Discontinuation of primary prophylaxis for *Pneumocystis carinii*

pneumonia and toxoplasmic encephalitis in human immunodeficiency virus type 1-infected patients: the changes in opportunistic prophylaxis study. *J. Infect. Dis.* **181**:1635–1642.

61. **Nascimento, L. V., F. Stollar, L. B. Tavares, C. E. Cavasini, I. L. Maia, and J. A. Cordeiro.** 2001. Risk factors for toxoplasmic encephalitis in HIV-infected patients: a case-control study in Brazil. *Ann. Trop. Med. Parasitol.* **95**:587–593.
62. **Nash, J. Q., S. Chissel, J. Jones, F. Warburton, and N. Q. Verlander.** 2005. Risk factors for toxoplasmosis in pregnant women in Kent, United Kingdom. *Epidemiol. Infect.* **133**:475–483.
63. **Nelson, J. C., D. J. Kauffmann, D. Ciavarella, and W. J. Senisi.** 1989. Acquired toxoplasmic retinochoroiditis after platelet transfusions. *Ann. Ophthalmol.* **21**:253–254.
64. **Neto, E. C., E. Anele, R. Rubim, A. Brites, J. Schulte, D. Becker, and T. Tuuminen.** 2000. High prevalence of congenital toxoplasmosis in Brazil estimated in a 3-year prospective neonatal screening study. *Int. J. Epidemiol.* **29**:941–947.
65. **Neto, E. C., R. Rubin, J. Schulte, and R. Giugliani.** 2004. Newborn screening for congenital infectious diseases. *Emerg. Infect. Dis.* **10**:1069–1073.
66. **Perkins, E. S.** 1973. Ocular toxoplasmosis. *Br. J. Ophthalmol.* **57**:1–17.
67. **Petersen, E.** 2007. Toxoplasmosis. *Semin. Fetal Neonatal Med.* **12**:214–223.
68. **Pradhan, S., R. Yadav, and V. N. Mishra.** 2007. Toxoplasma meningoencephalitis in HIV-seronegative patients: clinical patterns, imaging features and treatment outcome. *Trans. R. Soc. Trop. Med. Hyg.* **101**:25–33.
69. **Reiter-Owona, I., R. Bialek, J. K. Rockstroh, and H. M. Seitz.** 1998. The probability of acquiring primary *Toxoplasma* infection in HIV-infected patients: results of an 8-year retrospective study. *Infection* **26**:20–25.
70. **Renold, C., A. Sugar, J.-P. Chave, L. Perrin, J. Delavelle, G. Pizzolato, P. Burkhard, V. Gabriel, and B. Hirschel.** 1992. *Toxoplasma* encephalitis in patients with the Acquired Immunodeficiency Syndrome. *Medicine* **71**:224–239.
71. **Rorman, E., C. S. Zamir, I. Rilkis, and H. Ben-David.** 2006. Congenital toxoplasmosis—prenatal aspects of *Toxoplasma gondii* infection. *Reprod. Toxicol.* **21**:458–472.
72. **Roth, J. A., S. E. Siegel, A. S. Levine, and C. W. Berard.** 1971. Fatal recurrent toxoplasmosis in a patient initially infected via a leukocyte transfusion. *Am. J. Clin. Pathol.* **56**:601–605.
73. **Schmidt, D. R., B. Hogh, O. Andersen, J. Fuchs, H. Fledelius, and E. Petersen.** 2006. The national neonatal screening programme for congenital toxoplasmosis in Denmark: results from the initial four years, 1999–2002. *Arch. Dis. Child.* **91**:661–665.
74. **Siegel, S. E., M. N. Lunde, A. H. Gelderman, R. H. Halterman, J. A. Brown, A. S. Levine, and R. G. Graw.** 1971. Transmission of toxoplasmosis by leukocyte transfusion. *Blood* **37**:388–394.
75. **Signorell, L. M., D. Seitz, S. Merkel, R. Berger, and C. Rudin.** 2006. Cord blood screening for congenital toxoplasmosis in northwestern Switzerland, 1982–1999. *Pediatr. Infect. Dis. J.* **25**:123–128.
76. **Sijpkens, Y. W., R. J. de Knegt, and S. D. van der Werf.** 1994. Unusual presentation of acquired toxoplasmosis in an immunocompetent adult. *Neth. J. Med.* **45**:174–176.
77. **Smith, R. E., and J. P. Ganley.** 1972. Ophthalmic survey of a community. 1: abnormalities of the ocular fundus. *Am. J. Ophthalmol.* **74**:1126–1130.
78. **Song, K. J., J. C Shin, H. J. Shin, and H. W. Nam.** 2005. Seroprevalence of toxoplasmosis in Korean pregnant women. *Korean J. Parasitol.* **2005**:69–71.
79. **Torrey, E. F., J. J. Bartko, Z.-R. Lun, and R. H. Yolken.** 2007. Antibodies to *Toxoplasma gondii* in patients with schizophrenia: a meta-analysis. *Schizophren. Bull.* **33**:729–736.
80. **Wallon, M., L. Kodjikian, C. Binquet, J. Garweg, J. Fleury, C. Quantin, and F. Peyron.** 2004. Long-term ocular prognosis in 327 children with congenital toxoplasmosis. *Pediatrics* **113**:1567–1572.
81. **Westfall, A. C., A. K. Lauer, E. B. Suhler, and J. T. Rosenbaum.** 2005. Toxoplasmosis retinochoroiditis and elevated intraocular pressure. A retrospective study. *J. Glaucoma* **14**:3–10.
82. **Yazar, S., F. Arman, S. Yalçin, F. Demirtaş, O. Yaman, and I. Şahin.** 2003. Investigation of probable relationship between *Toxoplasma gondii* and cryptogenic epilepsy. *Seizure* **12**:107–109.

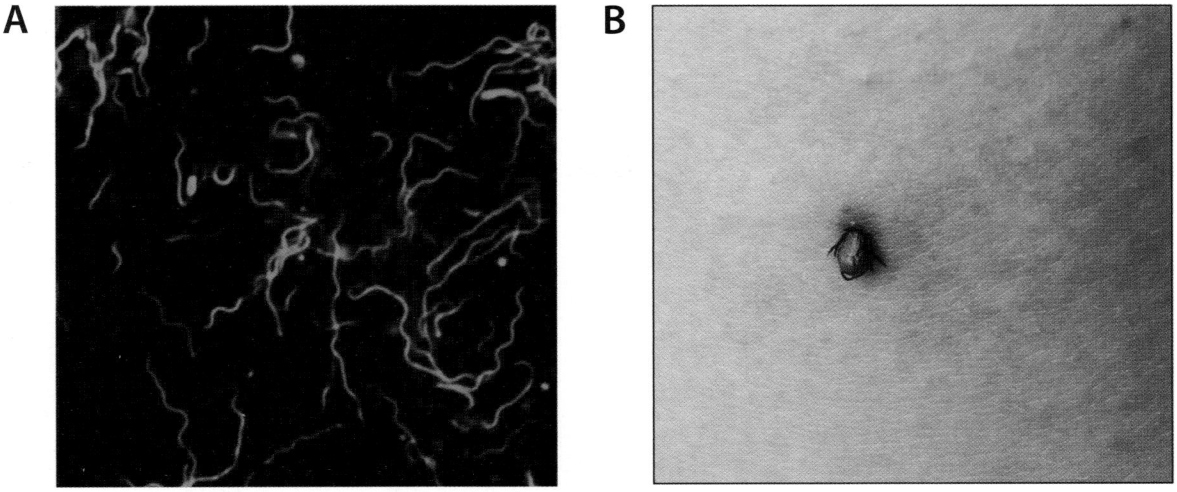

Color Plate 1. (A) Fluorescently labeled *B. burgdorferi* strain B31 visualized by fluorescent microscopy (magnification, ×250). (B) Picture of a semi-engorged attached female adult *Ixodes scapularis* tick (provided by K.A. de Groot).

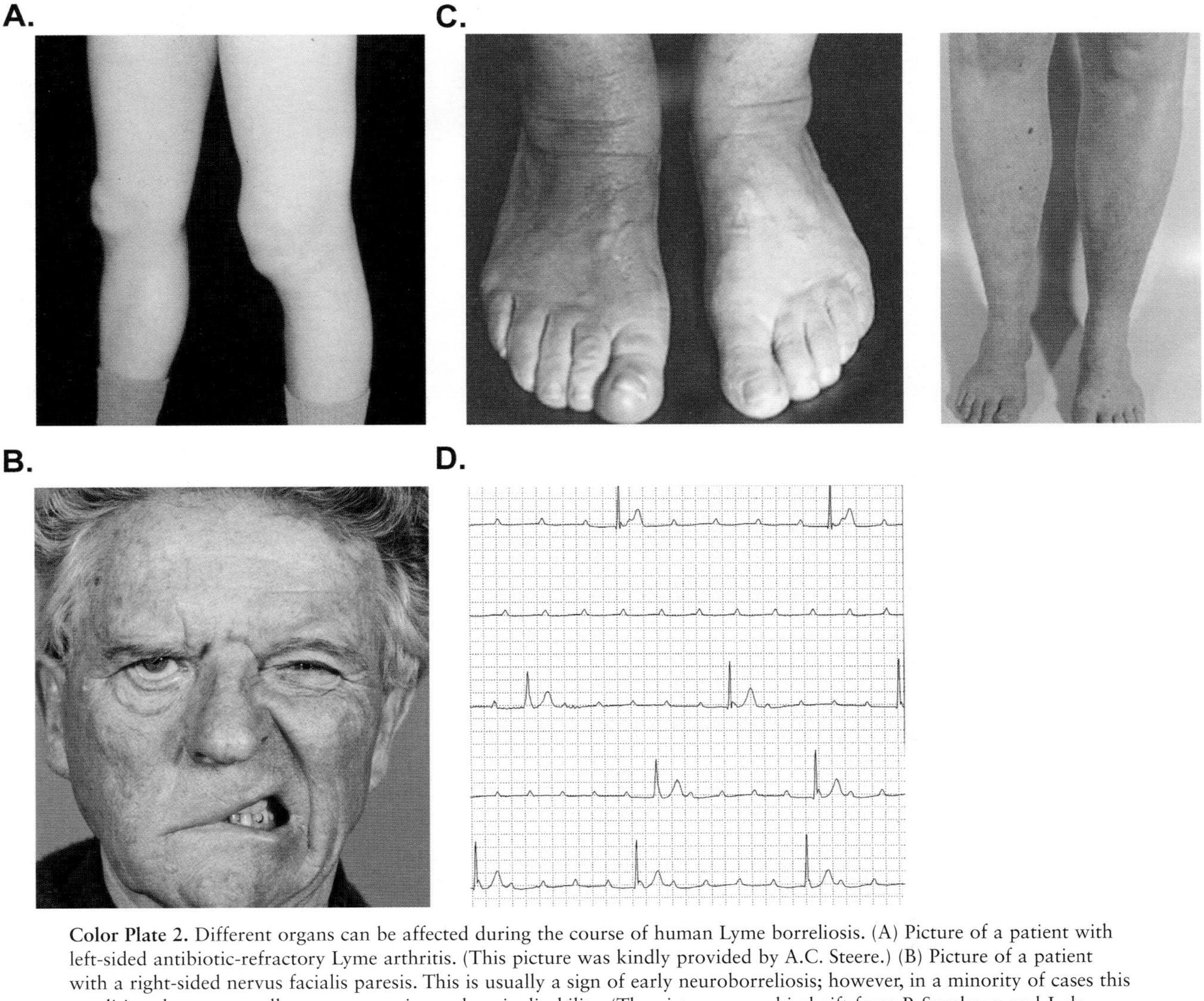

Color Plate 2. Different organs can be affected during the course of human Lyme borreliosis. (A) Picture of a patient with left-sided antibiotic-refractory Lyme arthritis. (This picture was kindly provided by A.C. Steere.) (B) Picture of a patient with a right-sided nervus facialis paresis. This is usually a sign of early neuroborreliosis; however, in a minority of cases this condition does not totally recover, causing a chronic disability. (The picture was a kind gift from P. Speelman and J. de Gans.) (C) Unilateral acrodermatitis chronica atrophicans in two European patients. (These pictures were kindly provided by D. J. Tazelaar.) (D) Holter registration of a total atrioventricular block in a patient with Lyme carditis (with an onset several years after the tick bite). (This picture was kindly provided by J. Verbunt.)

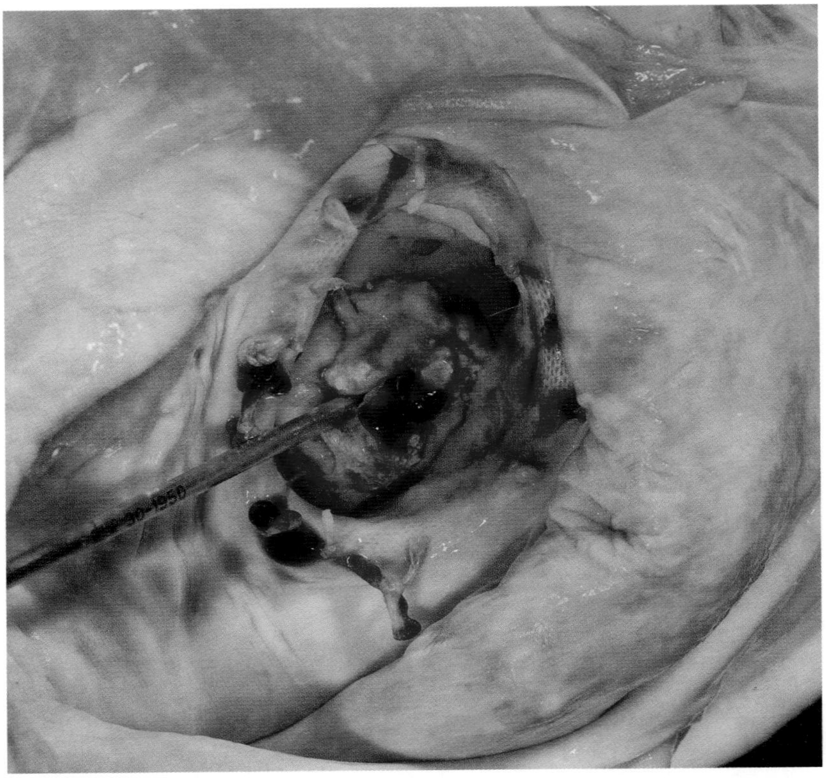

Color Plate 3. Rheumatic stenotic mitral valve status postring repair with moderate fibrosis and large vegetation (VGS) with anterior leaflet perforation. (Courtesy of Louis R. Dibernardo.)

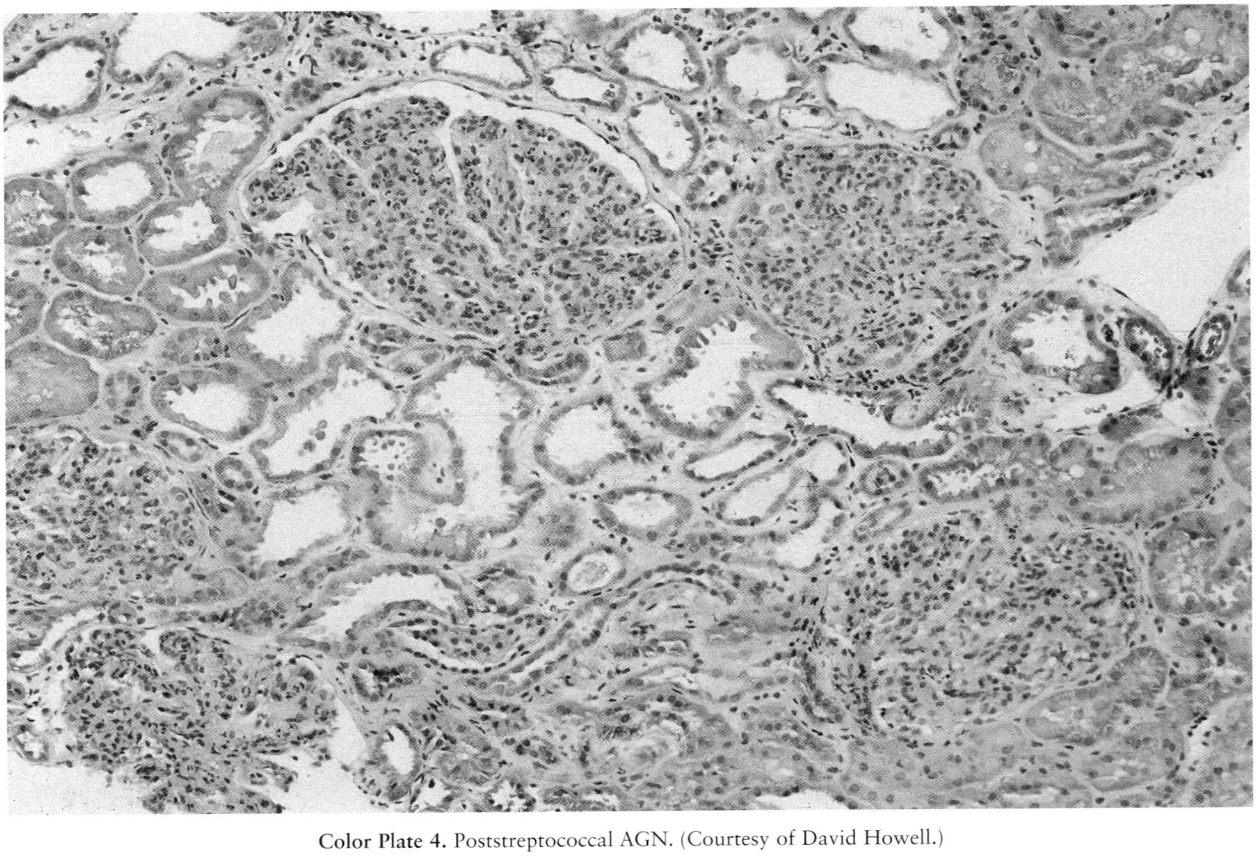

Color Plate 4. Poststreptococcal AGN. (Courtesy of David Howell.)

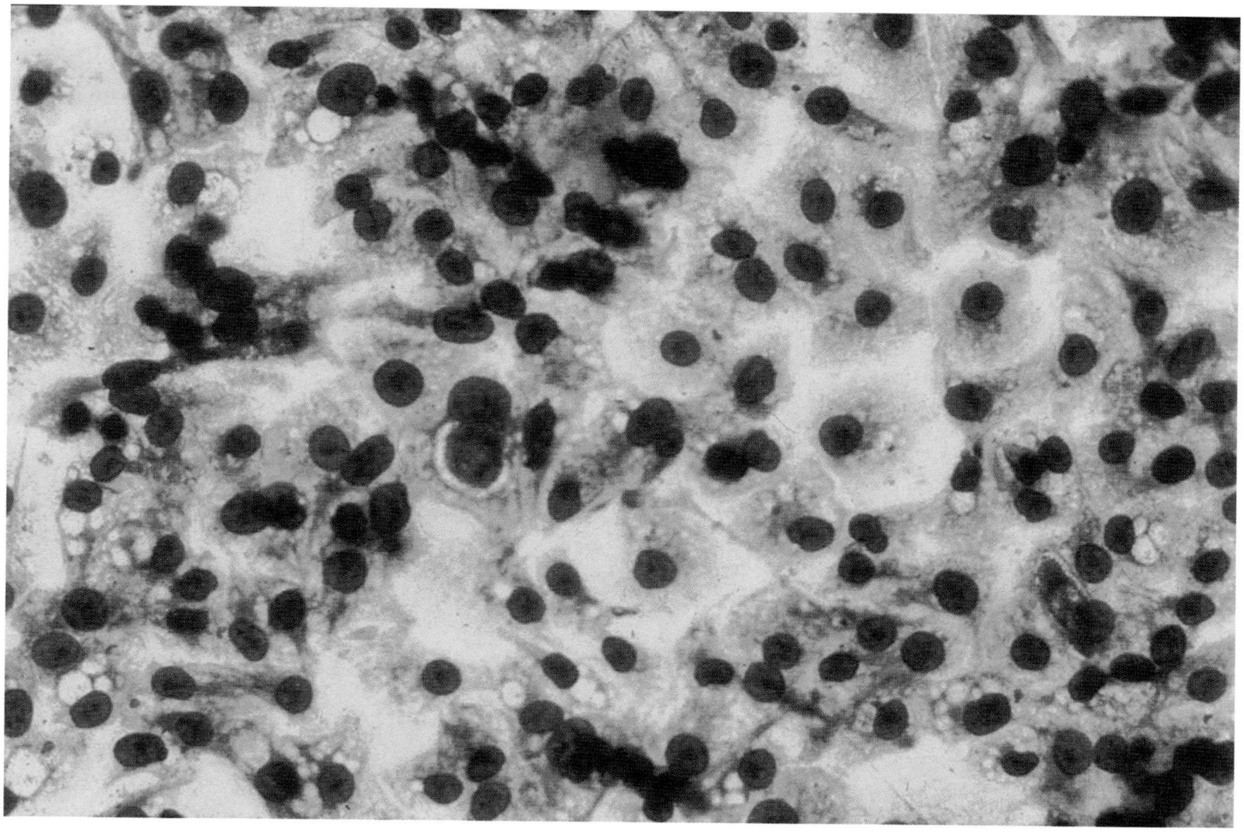

Color Plate 5. Section of an endometrial aspirate showing intensive infiltration with plasma cells scattered over the mucosa, a finding which can be seen with both gonococcal and chlamydial endometritis.

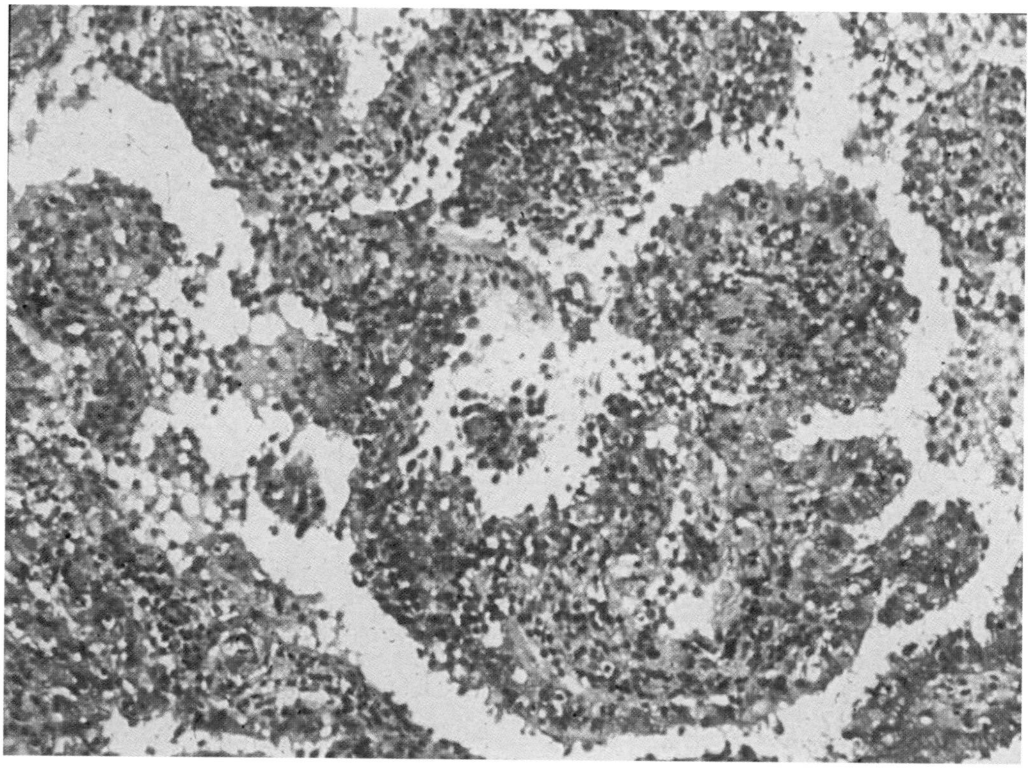

Color Plate 6. Total destruction of fallopian tube epithelium after an episode of salpingitis.

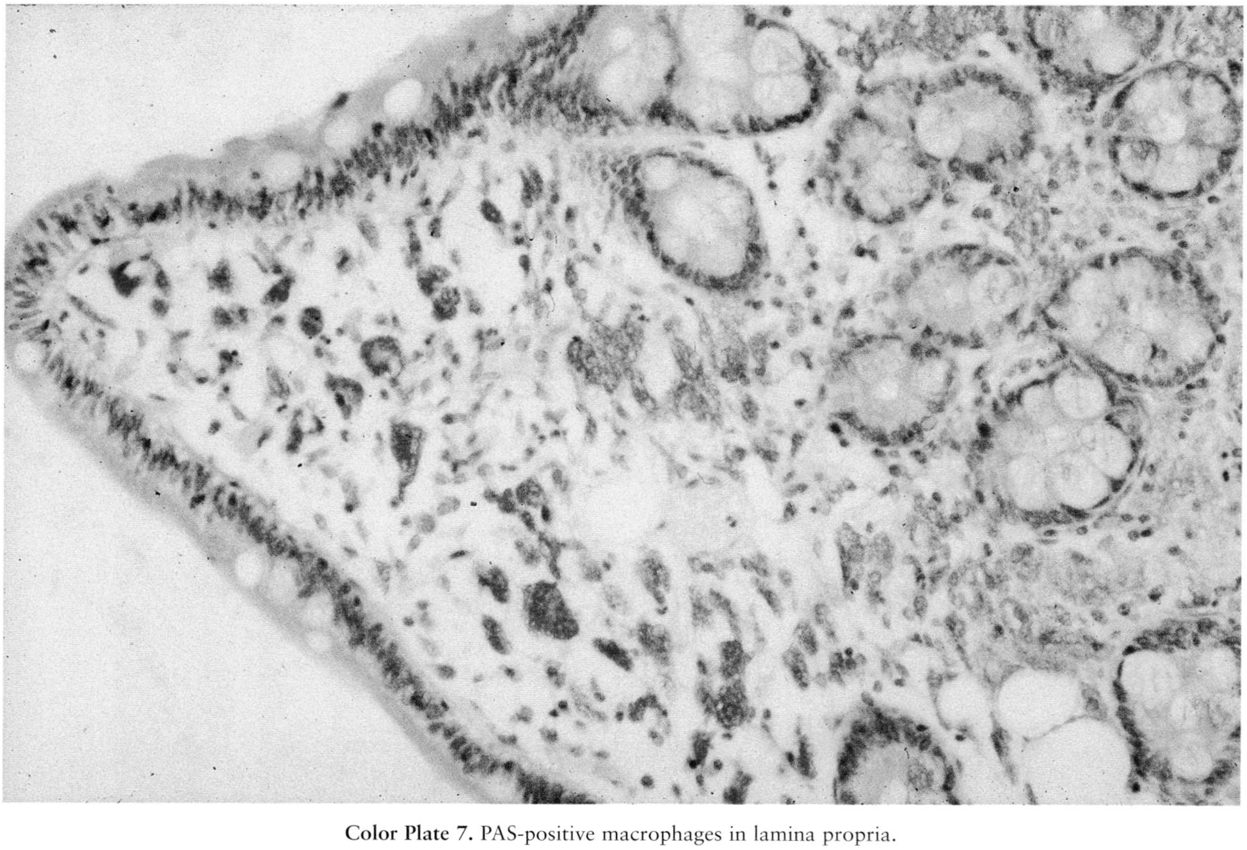

Color Plate 7. PAS-positive macrophages in lamina propria.

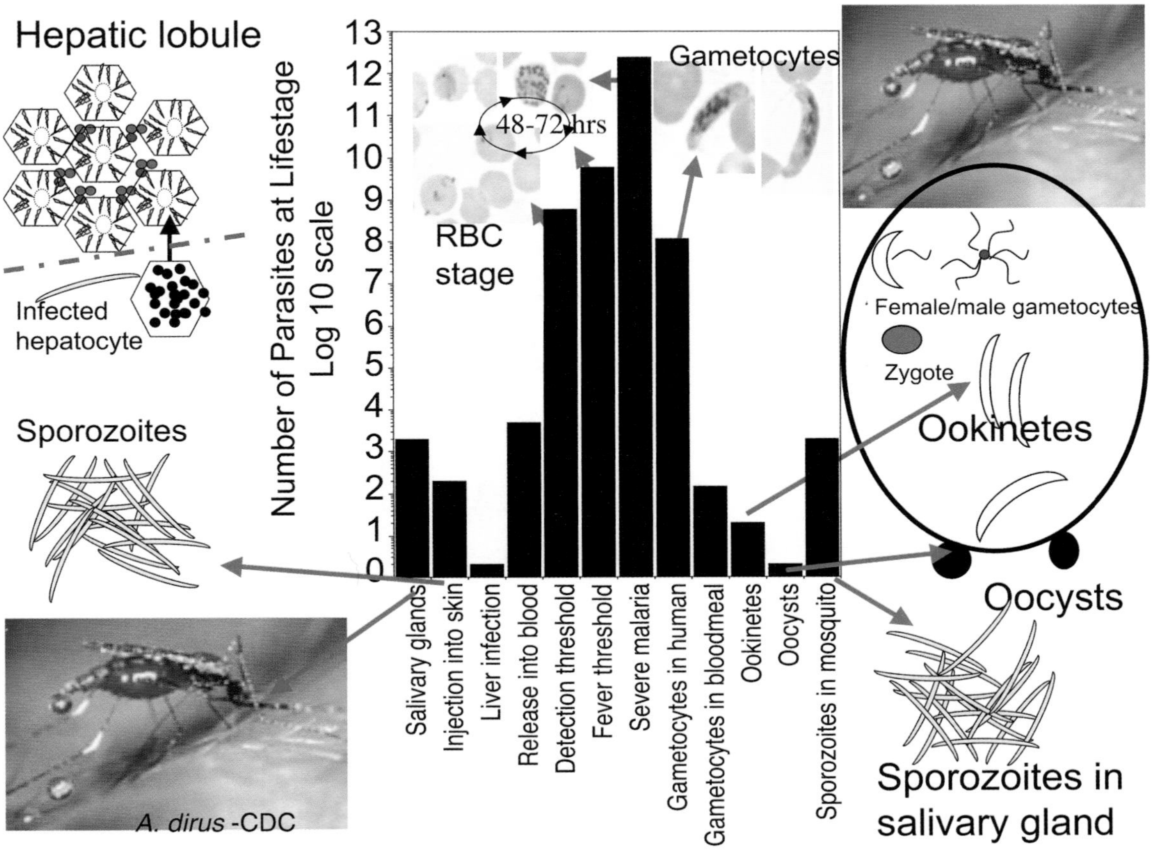

Color Plate 8. Malaria life cycle correlated to numbers of parasites at each stage. While the clinical manifestations of malaria correlate with the blood stages, the infection begins when a female mosquito injects hundreds of sporozoites into the dermis and only one or two invade hepatocytes. In a week, 5 to 10,000 progeny called merozoites burst from the single hepatocyte to start the cycle of erythrocyte invasion. In the case of *P. falciparum*, which multiplies at a rate of tenfold every 2 days, soon billions of parasites are circulating. Less than 0.1% differentiates into male and female gametocytes. The female mosquito again bites to imbibe 1 to 3 microliters of blood, containing 10 to 100 gametocytes. After fertilization, the zygote transforms into a ookinete, which penetrates through the stomach to the basement membrane. Only one or two oocysts develop per infectious bite. Each oocyst will produce thousands of sporozoites, which migrate to the salivary glands, ready for the cycle to begin again.

	P. falciparum	*P. vivax*	*P. ovale*	*malariae*
Hepatic Develop-ment Phase (days)	**5-6**	**8**	**9**	**15**
Erythrocytic Cycle (days)	**2**	**2**	**2**	**3**
Hypnozoites (relapses)	**No**	**Yes**	**Yes**	**No**
Merozoites per schizont	**30,000**	**10,000**	**15,000**	**2,000**
RBC preference	**All; prefers younger cells**	**Retics**	**Retics**	**Older RBCs**
Sporogony in Mosquito (days)	**9-10**	**8-10**	**12-14**	**14-16**
Ring Stage	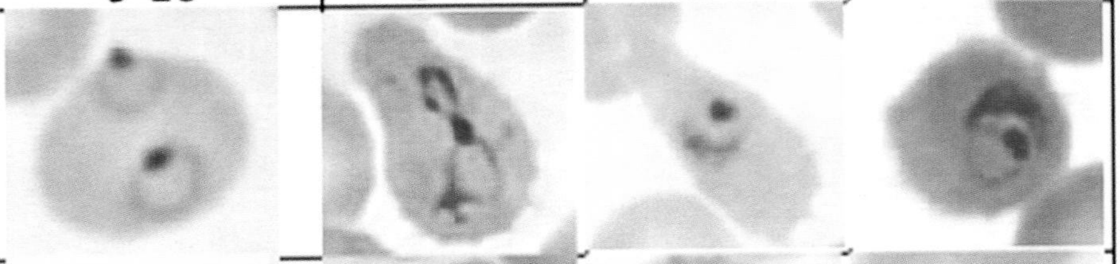			
Trophozoite Stage	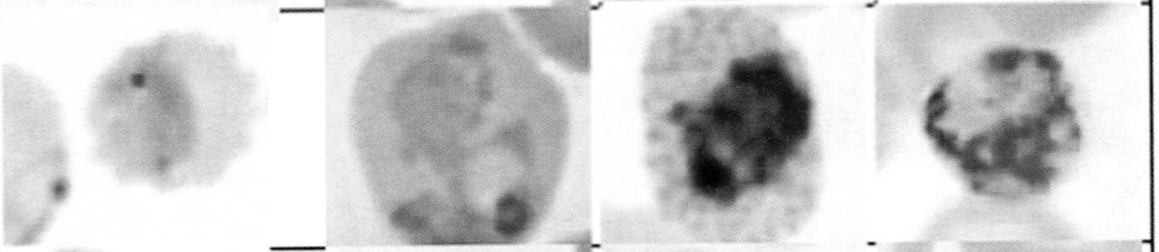			
Gametocyte Stage	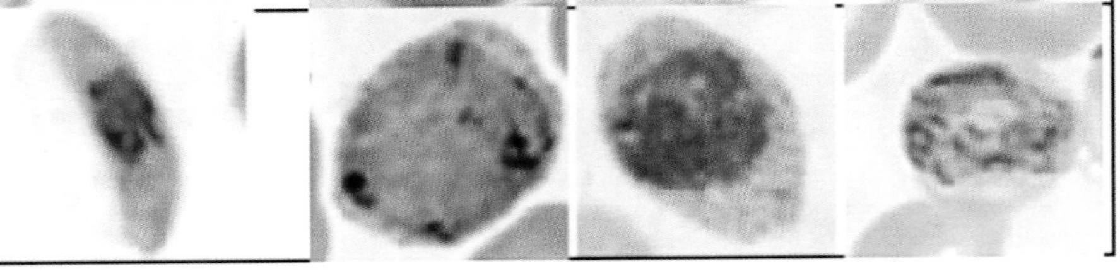			

Color Plate 9. Differentiation of human *Plasmodium* species. The four principal human malaria species can be separated on the basis of blood film examinations and the chronology of the different stages as well as the ability to be dormant in the liver to cause relapse months later, in the case of *P. vivax*.

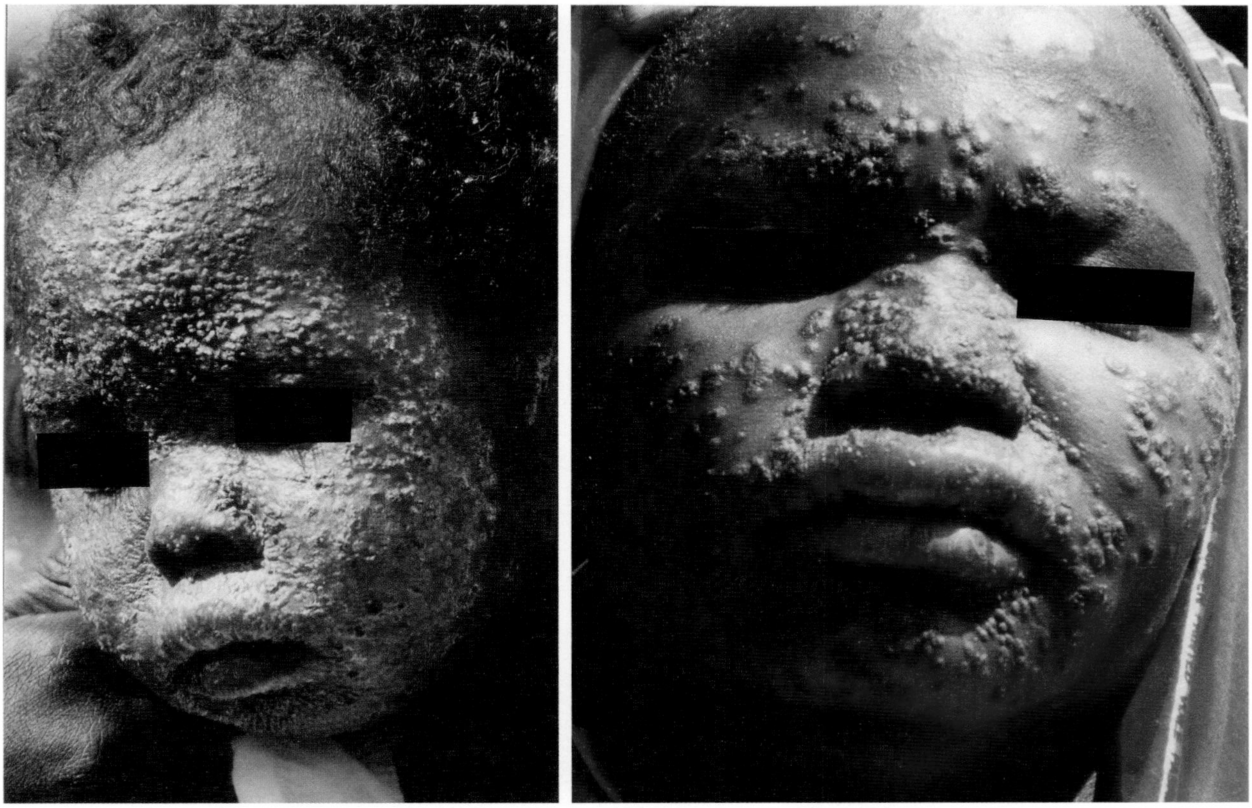

Color Plate 10. Two cases of post-kala-azar dermal leishmaniasis from Sudan, showing nodular eruption, with occasional confluence of the lesions. (Photographs courtesy of J. Dereure, with permission.)

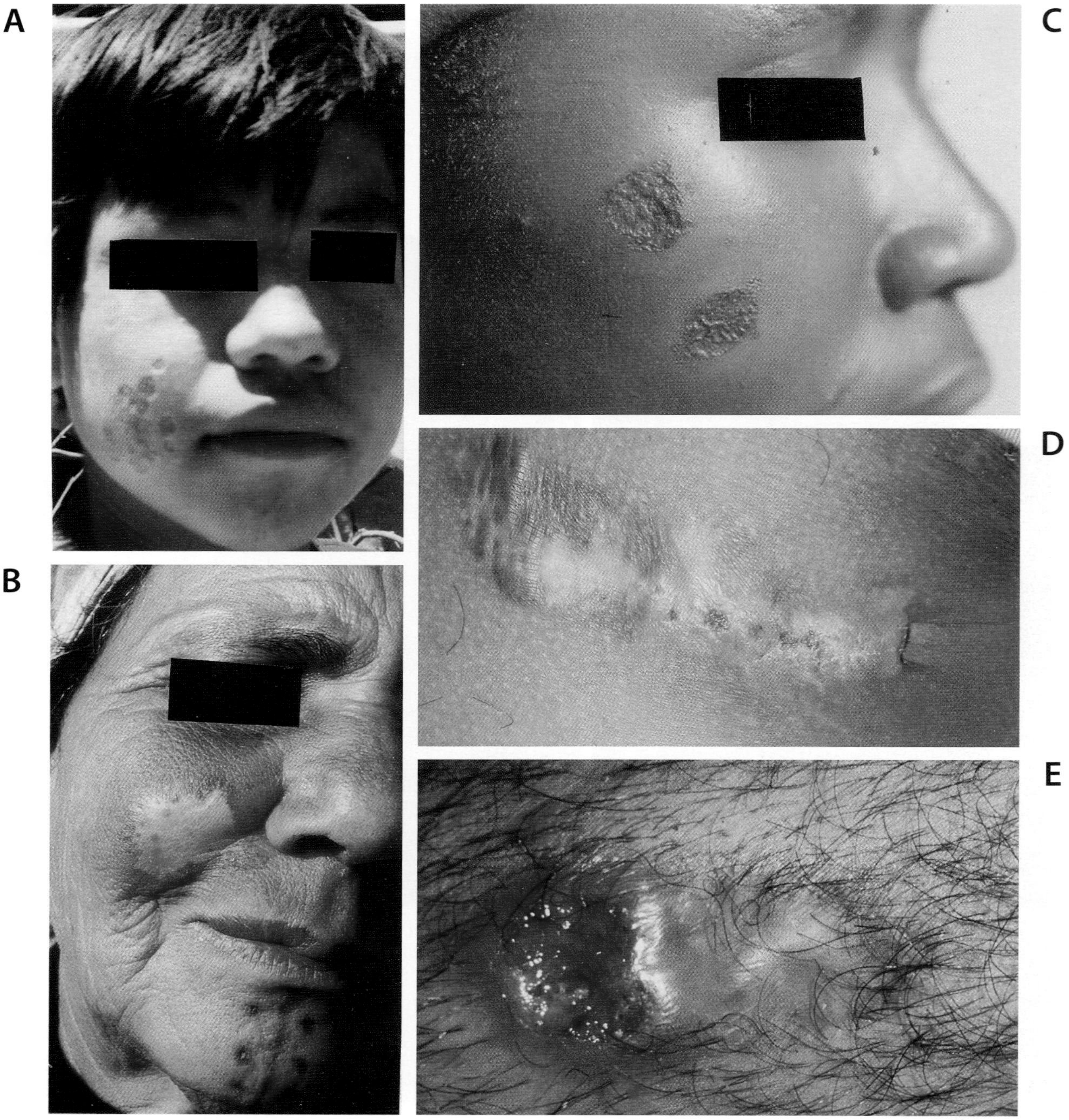

Color Plate 11. Scar patterns following the cures of various localized cutaneous leishmaniasis. (A) Multiple scars of an *L. peruviana* CL from Peru. (B) Large whitish scar following a *L. major* CL from Morocco (photograph courtesy of J. Dereure, with permission). (C) Hyperpigmented scar of an *L. major* CL from Senegal. (D and E) Reactivation of scars in *L. guyanensis* CL from French Guiana (photograph in panel D courtesy of P. Couppié, with permission, and photograph in panel E courtesy of E.R. Pradinaud, with permission).

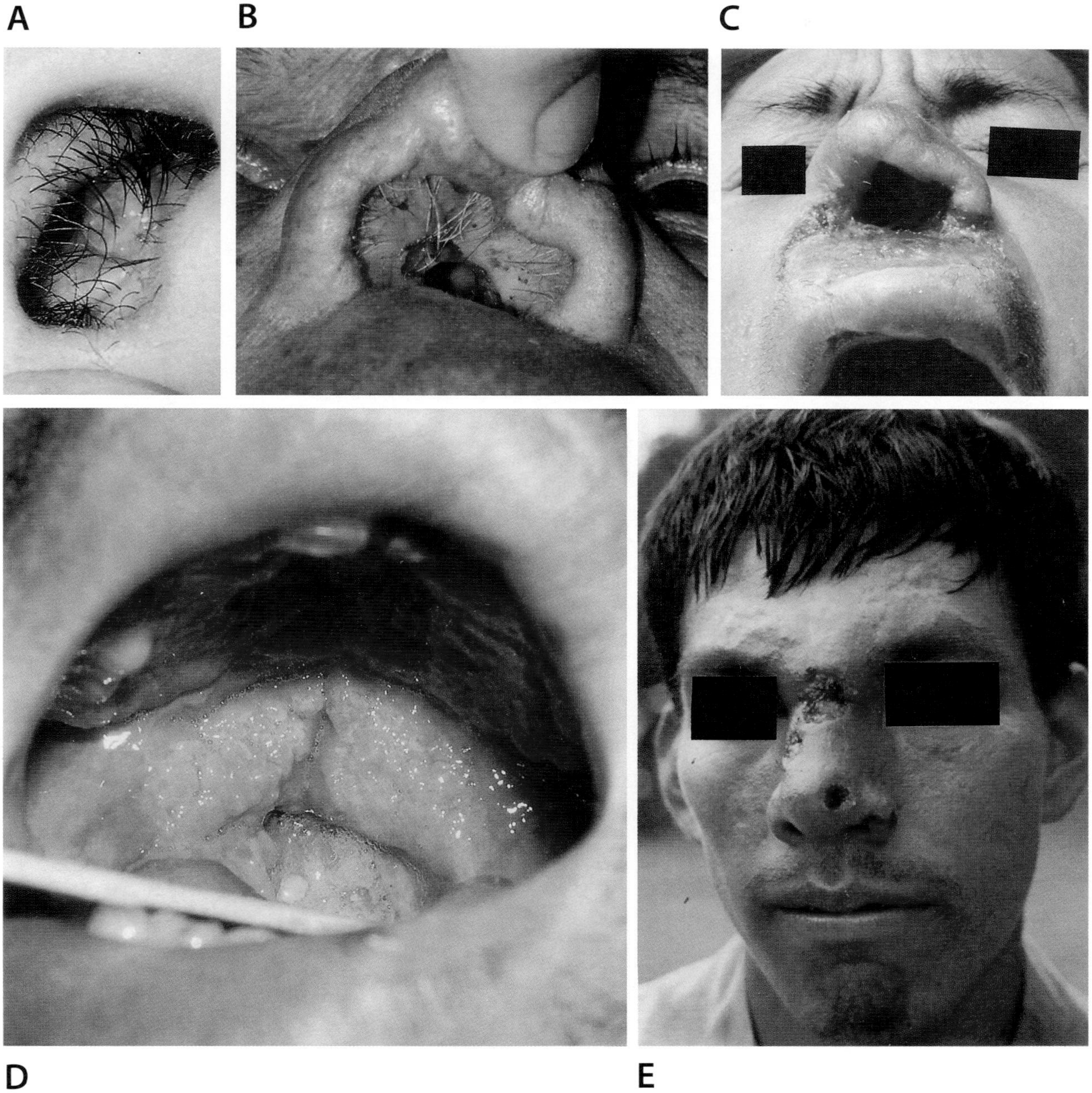

Color Plate 12. Mucosal lesions of MCL cases from Peru. The first granulomatous lesion of the anterior part of nasal septum (A) is rapidly destroying the nasal septum (B and C). (D) Pharyngeal granulomatous lesions. (E) External appearance of the nasal pyramid. (Photographs in panels A, B, C, and D courtesy of A. Llanos-Cuentas, with permission, and photograph in panel E courtesy of J.P. Guthmann, with permission.)

A

B

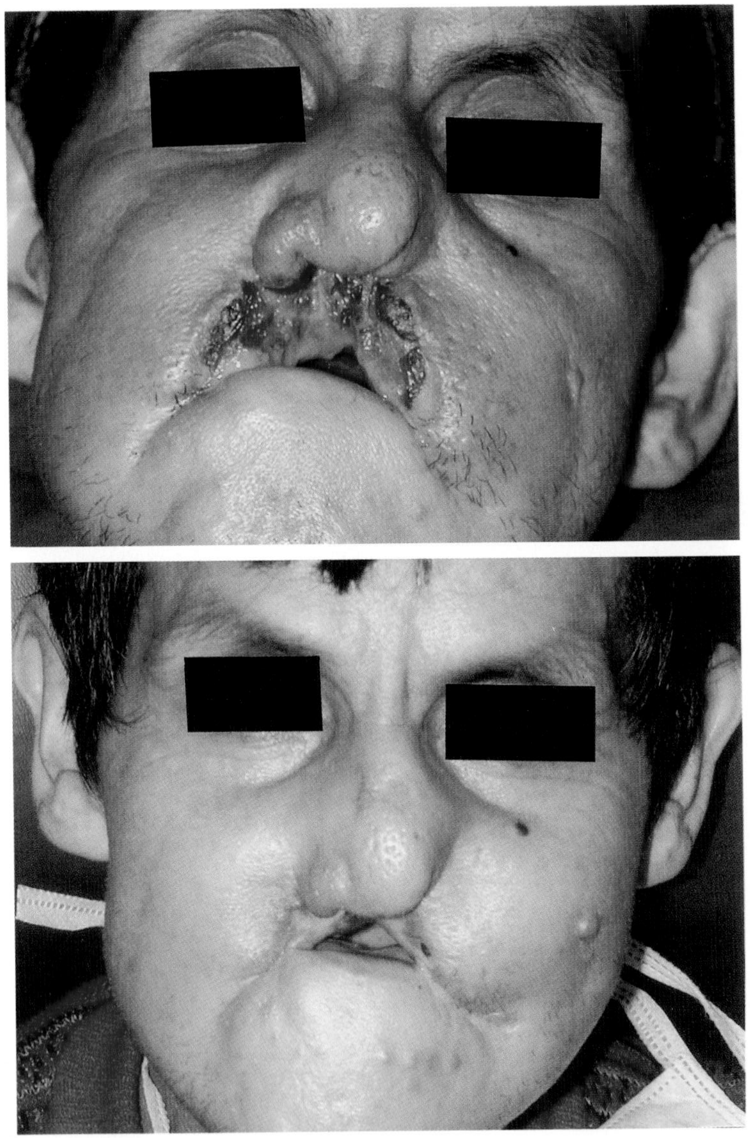

Color Plate 13. The mucosal lesions (A) and their subsequent sequelae, with retractive scars (B), are generally highly disfiguring, which has considerable socio-psychological impact for the patient. (Photographs courtesy of A. Llanos-Cuentas, with permission.)

A

B

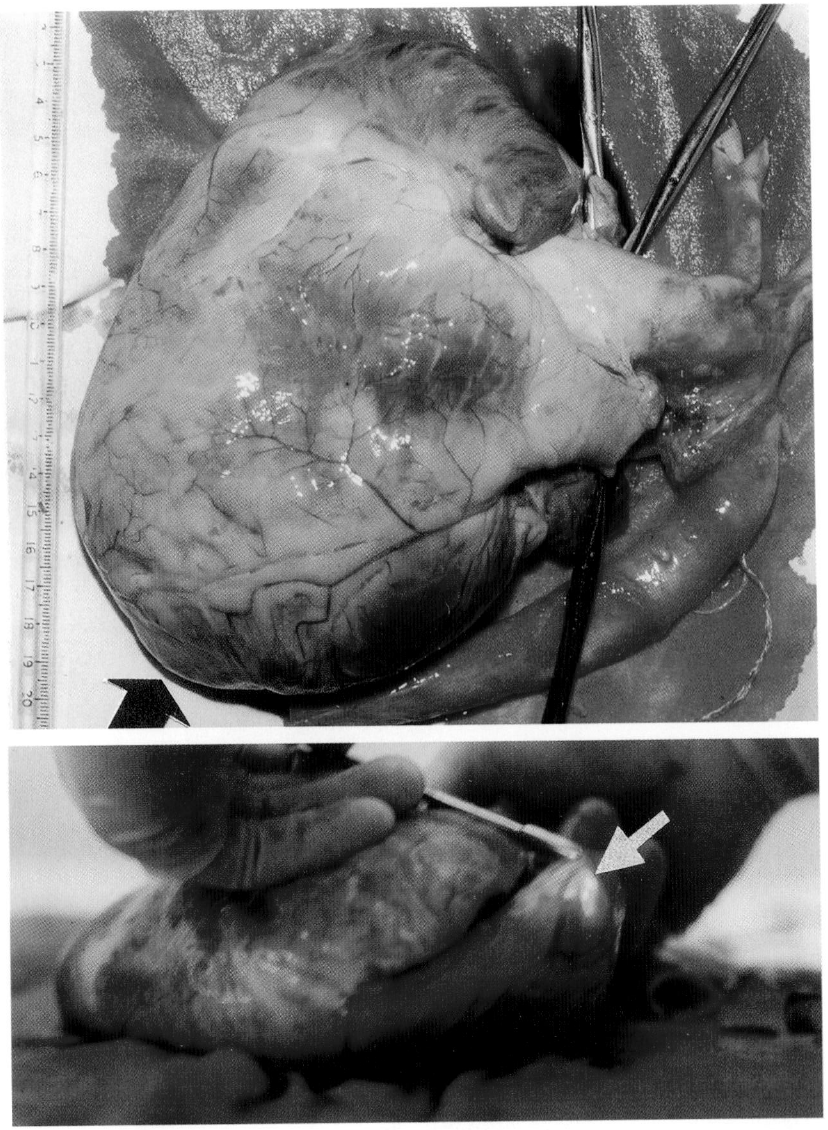

Color Plate 14. Necropsy aspect of a chronic Chagas cardiomyopathy. (A) External aspect with considerable dilatation of the heart. The small protrusion of the apex (arrow) corresponds to a ventricular apical aneurysm. (B) At the site of the aneurism, myocardium has disappeared, and only a thin membrane remains, consisting of pericardium and endocardium closely joined, as shown by transillumination.

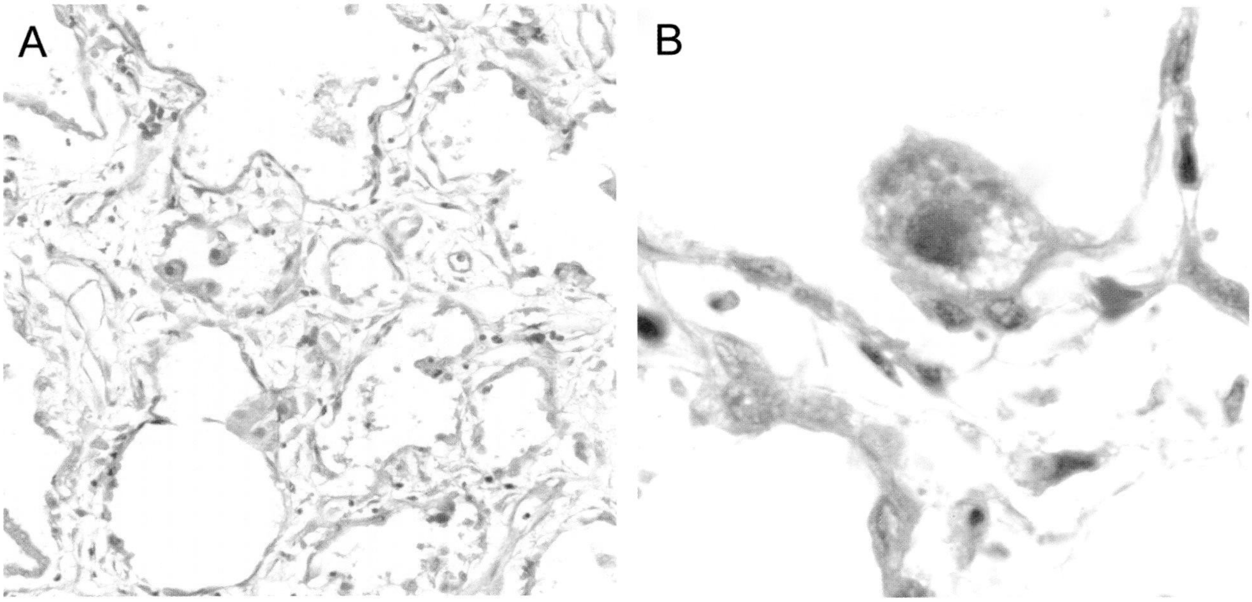

Color Plate 15. Photomicrographs of lung from an immunosuppressed patient who developed opportunistic infection by CMV. (A) Widening of the interstitium and occasional enlarged alveolar epithelial lining cells. Magnification, ×40. (B) The characteristic "owl's eye" intranuclear CMV inclusion in the cell at center (hematoxylin and eosin stains). Magnification, ×200.

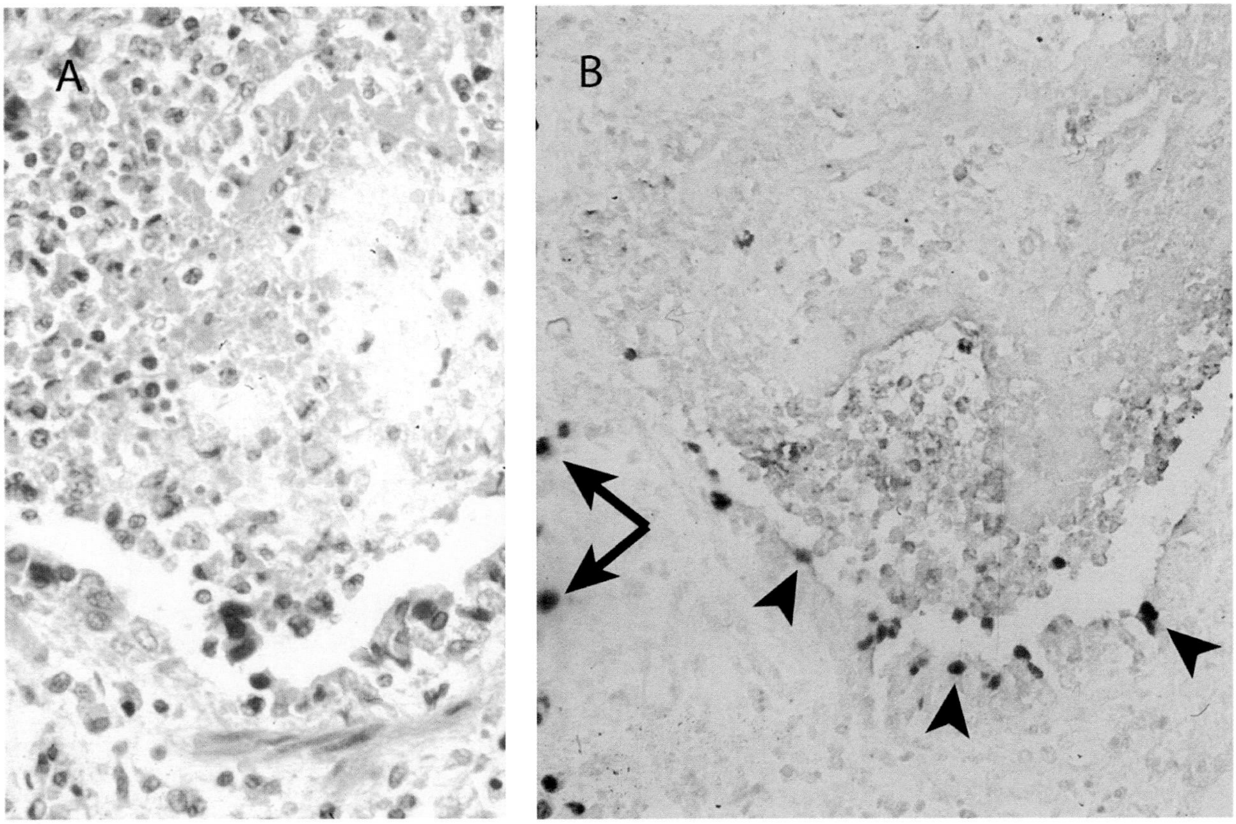

Color Plate 16. Histological preparations of adenovirus pneumonia in a pediatric patient. (A) Section stained with hematoxylin and eosin showing bronchial lumen partially filled with smudge cells. (B) In situ hybridization with an adenovirus probe of a serial section of the lung shown in panel A showing virus-positive epithelial cells lining the bronchioles (arrowheads) as well as in the parenchyma (arrows). Original magnification, ×250 (79).

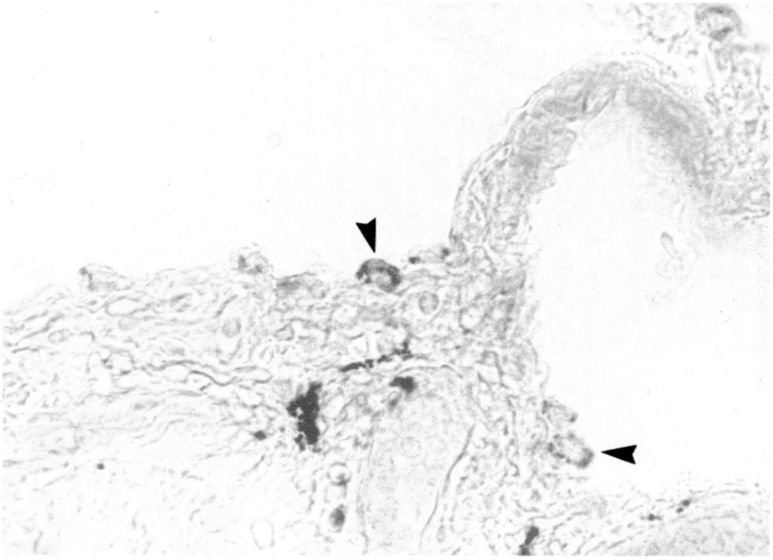

Color Plate 17. Immunohistochemical staining of a formalin-fixed paraffin-embedded section of human lung tissue with an antibody to adenovirus E1A. Arrows indicate alveolar epithelial cells that express adenovirus E1A protein. (Courtesy of Mark Elliott.)

Sequelae and Long-Term Consequences of Infectious Diseases
Edited by Pina M. Fratamico, James L. Smith, and Kim A. Brogden

Chapter 13

Taenia solium

AGNES FLEURY, ANA FLISSER, JOSÉ FLORES-RIVERA, AND TERESA CORONA

GENERAL FEATURES

Morphology and Life Cycle

Taenia solium is the parasite that causes human and swine cysticercosis. Human cysticercosis is a disease related to underdevelopment and poverty. It is found in countries and regions with inadequate sanitary infrastructure and insufficient health education. The life cycle of the parasite includes the adult stage, the egg, and the larval stage or cysticercus (Fig. 1). When a person ingests raw or semi-cooked pork meat with cysticerci, the scolex evaginates and attaches with its double row of 22 to 32 hooks and its four suckers to the mucosa in the upper third section of the small intestine, which is the duodenum-jejunum, and in 3 or 4 months transforms into a fully developed adult tapeworm. Intestinal taeniasis almost never induces symptoms. *T. solium* tapeworms measure 1 to 5 meters long; the scolex is followed by the neck, from which the strobila is formed, resembling a ribbon formed by 700 to 1,000 immature, mature, and gravid segments, properly named proglottids. The immature segments have not yet developed sexual organs, while the gravid segments resemble sacs full of eggs. Mature proglottids are found between immature and gravid ones; each mature segment contains 350 to 600 testes and three ovary lobes; therefore, tapeworms are hermaphroditic organisms. Gravid proglottids are released with feces, starting at 8 to 12 weeks after infection, each one containing between 50,000 and 60,000 eggs, located inside the multilobulated uterus. Since human beings can harbor two species of tapeworms, the number of lateral uterine branches allows identification of the species expelled by an infected person: *T. solium* has 7 to 14 branches, while *Taenia saginata* has 15 to 32. Although some books state that tapeworms can survive for about 25 years in the human intestine, recent experience indicates that *T. solium* remains only for short periods, releasing a few gravid proglottids in feces daily or 2 or 3 times per week. As proglottids are located farther away from the scolex, they become bigger; mature proglottids measure 2.1 to 2.5 mm long and 2.8 to 3.5 mm wide, while gravid segments measure 3.1 to 10 mm long and 3.8 to 8.7 mm wide. Eggs are spherical and have a radial appearance; they range in size from 26 to 34 μm, while cysticerci and adult worms are macroscopic and have a similar scolex, which measures 0.6 to 1.0 mm (9, 46, 53, 54, 63, 132).

Eggs are conformed by the oncosphere or hexacanth embryo and the embryophore that surrounds it (83). When swine ingest eggs, bile and enzymes disaggregate the embryophoric blocks and digest the oncospheral membrane. Yoshino published in 1933 histological images of the migration of *T. solium* oncospheres through the lamina propria and the circulation of swine; microscopic oncospheres and transitional forms were observed in the intestinal mucosa from 15 to 48 hours after infection. After penetration, larvae were transported through blood vessels, and postoncospheral development led to the formation of the metacestode or cysticercus. Macroscopic *T. solium* cysticerci were identified by Yoshino in liver, brain, and skeletal muscles of pigs 6 days after infection and measured around 0.3 mm, while 60 to 70 days afterwards, cysticerci had a fully developed scolex and measured between 6 to 9 mm (143–145). There is no explanation for the lack of descriptions of similar developmental stages in the many pathological reports of human brains.

Cysticerci establish primarily in skeletal and cardiac muscle, as well as in the brain of pigs, a process that takes approximately 12 weeks. They remain viable for at least 1 year, when pigs are usually sent to slaughter. Young cysticerci in pigs have minimal

Agnes Fleury, José Flores-Rivera, and Teresa Corona • Instituto Nacional de Neurología y Neurocirugía, Manuel Velasco Suarez SSA, México City, Mexico. **Ana Flisser** • Facultad de Medicina, Universidad Nacional Autónoma de México (UNAM), México City, Mexico.

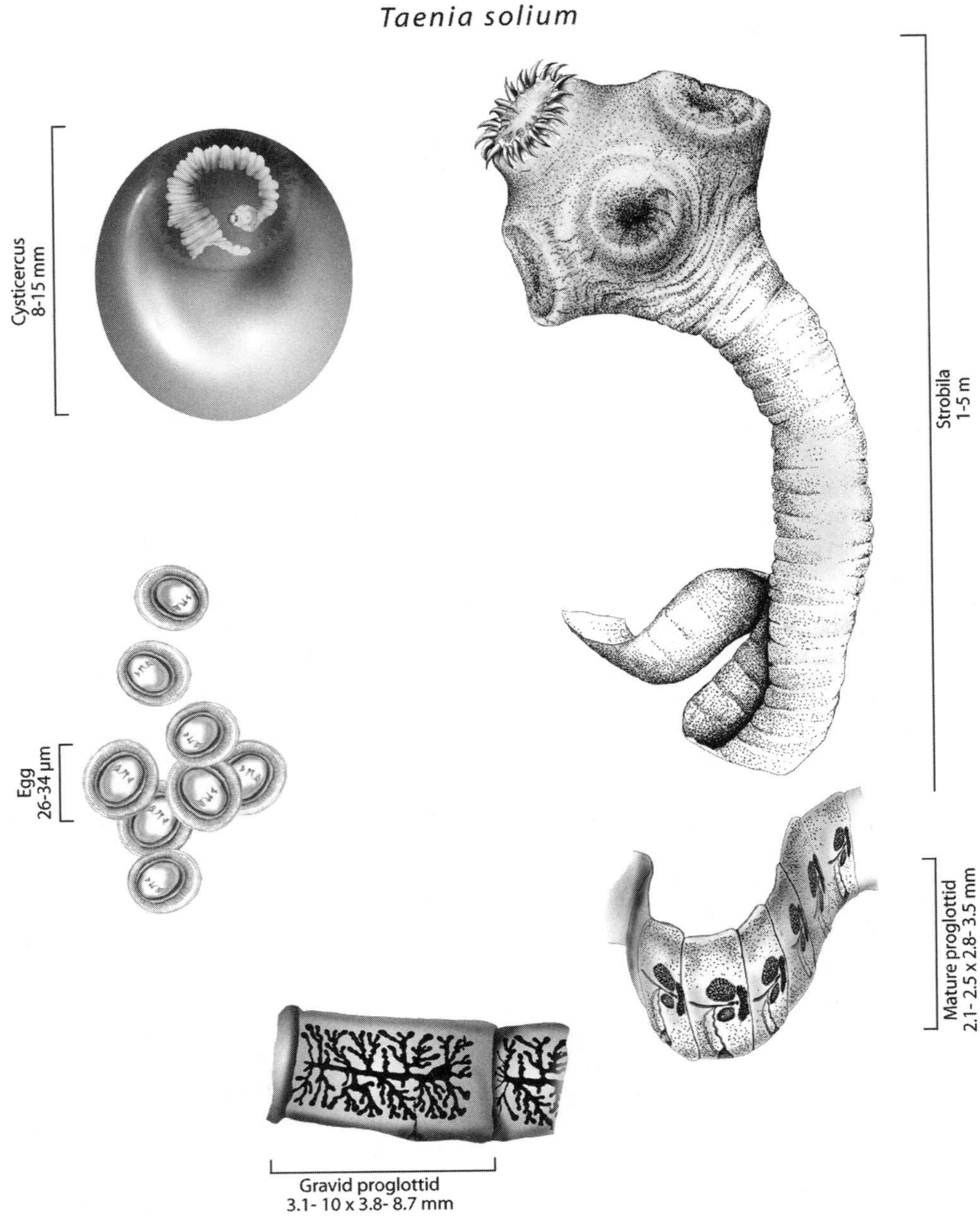

Figure 1. Drawing of the three life stages of *Taenia solium*: adult parasite showing the scolex, immature, mature, and gravid proglottids; microscopic eggs; and vesicular cysticercus.

inflammatory reaction surrounding them, while older parasites or those that have been treated with cestocidal drugs have an intense reaction that includes eosinophils, lymphocytes, and macrophages, the last engulf parasite remnants, eventually leaving a gliotic scar (4–6, 55, 58, 94, 140). Cysticerci are conformed by two chambers; the inner one contains the scolex and the spiral canal and is surrounded by the outer compartment that contains the vesicular fluid, usually less than 0.5 ml. When a living cysticercus is ingested by the definitive host, the first event that takes place is the widening of the pore of the bladder wall for the scolex and neck to emerge, leaving the bladder wall and vesicular fluid to disintegrate in the digestive tract (103).

The domestic pig is the intermediate host because it harbors the cysticercus; however, humans can acquire cysticercosis after accidentally ingesting *T. solium* eggs. Interestingly, the prevalence of taeniasis among patients with neurocysticercosis (NCC) is higher than previously reported. In addition, a clear association between the presence of taeniasis and the severity of NCC was seen, since most massive cerebral infections (with more than 100 cysticerci) were present in patients who harbored the adult tapeworm in the intestine. Therefore, the perception that tapeworms are silent guests, causing no harm to humans, is erroneous, and tapeworm carriers should be regarded as potential sources of contagion to themselves and to those living in their close environment (68). Consequently, an important risk factor is the presence of a tapeworm carrier in the household or neighborhood (55, 59). A study performed in a Mexican municipality with around 750,000 inhabitants showed that self-identification of tapeworm carriers is a feasible tool for control of *T. solium* (62). Also, previously identified tapeworm carriers can be treated with a high degree of efficacy (73).

The development of successful experimental models of taeniasis (89) allowed the analysis of histological and immunological aspects of the host-parasite relationship. Microscopic studies showed that the scolex anchors in the upper third part of the duodenum; it engulfs intestinal villi into its suckers and burrows its rostellum into Lieberkühn crypts of the subcutaneous mucosa (91). Histological analysis of the anchor site showed an intense inflammatory reaction surrounding the scolex; the most evident cells are goblet cells that increase from 20 to 80 per villous in hamsters and gerbils at 13 and 18 days postinfection, respectively, and mast cells that increase from 2 to 8 per villous in infected gerbils at 19 days, but not in hamsters. Specific antibodies and parasite antigens can be detected in serum and feces of infected hamsters (13–15).

T. solium cysticerci in humans develop mainly in the central nervous system, the eye, and striated and heart muscle and subcutaneous tissue. In the brain, parasites can be found in the parenchyma, the subarachnoid tissue, and the ventricles. Clinical manifestations depend on the location, number, and stages of the lesions as well as characteristics of the immune response of the host. In skeletal muscle, parasites can be palpated when superficial or seen in X-rays as white dots or nodules, but generally they do not interfere with muscle function, except after a massive infection, when they cause muscle pseudohypertrophy with intense inflammation and pain. In cardiac muscle, cysticerci may develop miocardiopathy. In the eye, parasites are found in the subretinian space, close to the macula, in the vitreous fluid or the anterior chamber; inflammation may cause blindness or decreased vision secondary to proliferative vitreo-retinopathy and retina detachment (23, 39, 53, 55, 87, 113, 125).

Presently, cysticercosis is still endemic in several countries of Latin America, Africa, and Asia; furthermore, due to migration there are many neurological cases in developed countries, such as the United States, and also recently, tapeworm carriers in the United States and Muslim countries have expanded interest in cysticercosis, which is proposed to be an emerging infectious disease (63, 118). Cysticercosis in dogs has recently come to awareness in countries such as Indonesia and China, where these animals are eaten, since they can be a source for humans to acquire taeniasis (72, 74).

Immune Responses Induced by *T. solium* during NCC

The immunology of human and porcine cysticercosis is particularly important because of its paradoxical relationship with disease pathogenesis. Living cysticerci may cause an asymptomatic infection through active evasion and suppression of immunity. Histological studies have shown that both in humans and pigs, live, viable cysticerci have little or no surrounding inflammation. In contrast, the immune-mediated inflammation around degenerating cysts may precipitate symptomatic disease. The humoral immune response is better understood than the cellular one. The fact that humans respond immunologically to antigens of *T. solium* cysticerci is well evident from the number of immunodiagnostic assays that have been developed using different types of antigens. The most frequent anti-cysticercus antibody is immunoglobulin G; it can be detected in serum, cerebrospinal fluid (CSF) and saliva and suggests that infection is of long duration. Antibodies have been found in most cases that have live or dying parasites, but only in few cases with calcified cysts. The humoral immune response in patients with NCC is quite heterogeneous, as evidenced by the number of antigens recognized. It has also been shown that the immune response may be transient in households of NCC patients and in apparently healthy individuals in the open population. Currently, the most frequently used techniques for immunodiagnosis of NCC are enzyme-linked immunosorbent assay and Western blotting. The use of such immunodiagnostic methods has shown that up to 15% of open population, rural and urban, has anti-cysticercus antibodies (31, 32, 40, 53, 55, 59, 61, 67, 92, 102, 121, 124).

Precise patterns and pathways of the cellular responses in human NCC are still under study. No clear hypothesis was available before demonstration of the Th1/Th2 duality of the T-helper cell response. Studies so far have addressed molecular components in the CSF, the serum, and the granuloma itself. Increased levels of interleukin (IL)-1 and IL-6 have been reported with CSF of patients with inflammatory NCC. High levels of IL-6 in the CSF of patients with subarachnoid NCC have also been reported, suggesting acute phase response. In addition, high levels of tumor necrosis factor alpha (TNF-α) have also been noted in the CSF of children with active NCC, which was undetectable in controls and children with inactive NCC. An immunological study of NCC patients treated with praziquantel (without major adverse effects) reported elevated soluble IL-2 in the CSF, suggesting a Th1-type immune response to therapy, in contrast with the Th2-type immune response found in animal models of viable cysticerci (2, 33, 90, 99, 119, 135).

Increased levels of eotaxin and IL-5, both eosinophil-selective mediators, have been found in the sera of patients with NC. These cytokines are involved in recruiting eosinophils locally as well as systemically. The presence of eosinophils as the first attack cells was reported with porcine cysticercosis after treatment and after vaccination. This suggests that eosinophils may play an important role in the degenerative phase in this parasitic infection. Very few immunohistochemical studies of the inflammatory response within cysticercus granulomas located in the human central nervous system are available, mainly due to limited available tissue specimens. The reports suggest an intermixture of Th1 and Th2 responses in brain granulomas (50, 58, 94, 109, 110, 116).

There is increasing evidence that many of the components and mechanisms of the immune response participate in the fight of the host against cysticerci and that the immune system is capable of both destroying the parasite and causing injury to the host. The outcome depends on which of the many possible combinations involving the immune and inflammatory responses is in operation against a given cysticercus in the brain of each patient at a given time and place. For therapeutic purposes, as a general rule, it is prudent not to interfere with the inflammatory response of an NCC patient. Anti-inflammatory drugs should be reserved for specific cases of persisting severity course with diffuse encephalitis and/or basal meningitis and intracranial hypertension (119).

One of the most interesting phenomena in immunoparasitology is the evasion of host immune response by the parasite (31, 52, 93, 119, 139). The mechanisms underlying this process are complex and involve survival of parasites lodged in immunologically privileged sites, masking of cysticercus antigens by host immunoglobulins, concomitant immunity, molecular mimicry, and suppression or deviation of host responses (8, 11, 58, 84, 95, 120, 122).

GENERAL FEATURES OF NCC

NCC is a disease with high morbidity and mortality (133) mainly because of the heterogeneity of the symptomatology caused by the parasites lodged in the brain, which makes diagnosis difficult. Most patients manifest their infection at 20 to 40 years of age, due to the prolonged period needed for the manifestation of the disease, from several months to up to 30 years, 4.8 years on average. The rate between adults and children is 8 to 1; patients 17 and younger represent 1 to 27% of the cases; thus, NCC is considered to have low-frequency pathology in children, (42, 112, 125, 137).

Most cysticerci lodge in the cerebral parenchyma and in the subarachnoidal space of the sulci (80%), followed by the meninges (18%) and other locations (around 2% of cases), such as the ventricles and spinal cord (Fig. 2). The variety in the locations of parasites is associated with the diversity of clinical symptomatology induced by cysticerci; practically any neurological sign can be present, similar to multiple sclerosis, in which the number and location of lesions will define clinical manifestations (39, 51, 126). Based on involution stage and location of the parasite, on the degree of inflammation and the clinical manifestations, several classifications of NCC have been proposed (48, 107, 126). Table 1 compiles the characteristics of NCC.

Two morphological types of metacestodes develop in humans: cellulose and racemose. A living cellulose cysticercus is a small, spherical or oval, white or yellow vesicle that measures between 0.5 and 1.5 cm and has a translucent bladder wall, through which the scolex can be seen as a small solid eccentric granule; usually there are no changes in size due to lack of growth. This type of cysticerci is generally separated from the host tissue by a thin collagenous capsule, within which it remains alive (47, 70, 104). The racemose cysticercus appears as a large, round or lobulated bladder circumscribed by a delicate wall, or it resembles a cluster of grapes, and it measures up to 10 or even 20 cm and may contain up to 60 ml of fluid. Cellulose cysticerci grow and transform into racemose ones in spacious areas. This feature is very common in basal cisterns, especially optic, carotid, Sylvian, and peduncular cisterns, forming degenerated vesicles grouped in clusters. The most important characteristic of this type of cysticerci is that the scolex cannot be seen; only detailed histological studies reveal its remains in some cases (19, 77, 104, 105). Symptoms occur usually after the cyst has initiated its degenerative process and are due mainly to the inflammatory response they induce. NCC seems to produce symptoms years after the initial invasion of

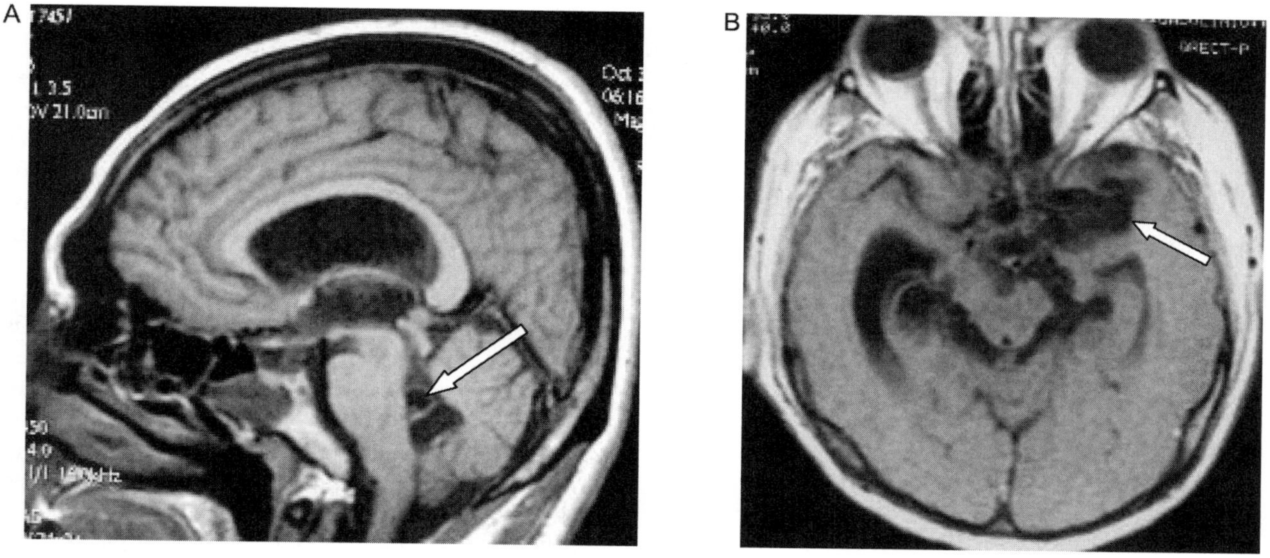

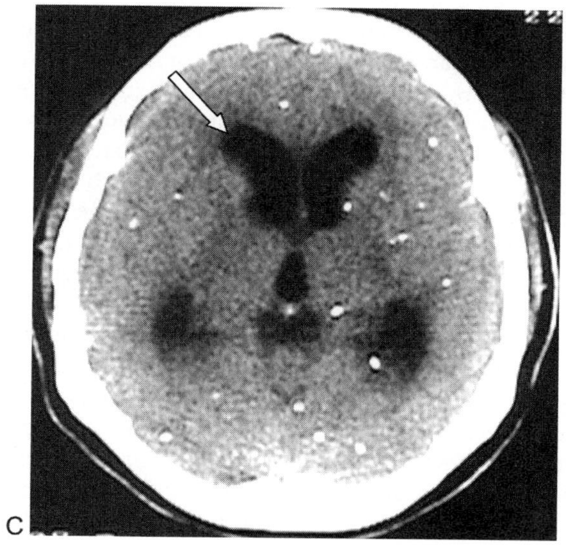

Figure 2. Images of NCC. (A) Sagittal T1-weighted magnetic resonance image showing a vesicular cysticercus in the IV ventricle (arrow). Ventricular cysticerci usually cause hydrocephalus and ependymitis. (B) Axial T1-weighted magnetic resonance image showing multiple racemose parasites located in basal cisterns. Subarachnoidal cysticerci usually cause arachnoiditis and hydrocephalus. (C) Computerized axial tomography showing multiple small and round calcified lesions in brain parenchyma associated with ventricular dilatation (arrow). This image is typical of chronic NCC.

the nervous system by the parasite, either by inflammation around the parasite, mass effect, or residual scarring. There is a clear association between inflammation around one or more cysts and development of symptoms, especially with regard to seizures (65). Ventricular parasites follow a progressive course and even after ventricular shunting, the membranes or inflammatory cells and proteins frequently block the shunt (88).

Living cysticerci induce minimal inflammation and can stay in this condition for several years because parasites evade the immune response. When the immune response becomes exacerbated, it generates a cascade of immunological mechanisms that causes parasite death but also severe damage to the neighboring structures in the host, especially to basal blood vessels. When cysticerci start to degenerate, they have an appearance of colloidal, whitish vesicles, with invaginated scolices, which cannot be identified due to a hydroptic degeneration caused by osmotic effects of the CSF that tends to enter the vesicle. The colloidal stage is followed by a granulomatous one, and finally parasites become calcified. In early stages the surrounding brain parenchyma shows minimal data of inflammation, with a connective tissue capsule surrounding and delimitating the parasite. When degeneration occurs, the intense inflammatory reaction that develops induces a dense collagen

Table 1. Characteristics of neurocysticercosis

Characteristic	Description
Location of cysticerci	Parenchyma
	Subarachnoidal space: cortical sulci, basal cisterns
	Ventricles: III, IV, lateral
	Spinal cord
Type of parasites	Cellulose cysticerci
	Racemose cysticerci
Number of parasites	Single cysticerci
	Multiple cysticerci
Involution of parasites	Living cysticerci (vesicular)
	Colloidal cysticerci
	Granuloma
	Calcifications
Inflammatory features	Arachnoiditis
	Ependymitis
	Edema
	Fibrosis
	Gliosis
	Arteritis
Main symptoms	Epilepsy
	Headache
	Intracranial hypertension
	Mass effect
	Psychiatric disorders
	Stroke

wall around cysticerci, with the presence of astrocitic gliosis, microglia and capillary vessel proliferation. Finally the calcified stage of the lesion is due to mineralization of the nodule, with intense gliosis and multinucleated giant cells, typical of a chronic inflammatory reaction to a foreign body surrounding it (47, 55, 104, 124). Parasites in different stages of involution are frequently found in the same brain, which suggests either recurrent infections, parasites with different survival abilities, or evasion versus exacerbation of the immune response in different parasites/sites of the brain.

Two types of techniques have been used for diagnostic support of NCC: imaging techniques (computed tomography [CT] and magnetic resonance [MR]) that allow the definition of the number, stage, location, and extension of the lesions and immunologic assays to identify anti-cysticercus antibodies and parasite antigens (53, 69, 113). Based on these techniques and on epidemiologic data, several criteria have been established for diagnosis: (i) absolute, when there is a histological demonstration of the parasite from biopsy of a brain or spinal cord lesion, cystic lesions showing the scolex on CT or MR, and direct visualization of subretinal parasites by funduscopic examination; (ii) major, when there are lesions highly suggestive of NCC on imaging studies, positive Western blotting of serum for the detection of anti-cysticercus antibodies, resolution of intracranial cystic lesions after therapy with praziquantel or albendazole, and spontaneous resolution of small single enhancing lesions; (iii) minor, when there are lesions compatible with NCC on imaging studies, clinical manifestations suggestive of NCC, positive enzyme-linked immunosorbent assay for detection of anti-cysticercus antibodies or cysticercus antigens, and cysticercosis outside the central nervous system; and (iv) epidemiologic, when there is evidence of a household contact with *T. solium*, individuals coming from or living in an area where cysticercosis is endemic, history of frequent travel to disease-endemic areas. Interpretation of these criteria allows two degrees of diagnostic certainty: (i) definitive diagnosis, in patients who have one absolute criterion or in those who have two major plus one minor and one epidemiologic criterion; and (ii) probable diagnosis, in patients who have one major plus two minor criteria, or one major plus one minor and one epidemiologic criterion, and in those who have three minor plus one epidemiologic criterion (40). In imaging studies, a parenchymal-living cysticercus generally is small, round, and hypodense (CT) or hypointense (MR). When the parasite is colloidal, an external ring of inflammation appears with contrast fluid. A hyperdense (CT) or hyperintense (MR) invaginated scolex can be seen in both cases. Big living or colloidal cysticerci, up to 5 cm long, can be found in the subarachnoidal space or in the ventricles. Calcified parasites are round (hyperdense) and are better detected by CT (7, 12, 42, 43, 53, 125, 138).

Treatment of NCC includes cestocidal drugs (praziquantel and albendazole) to kill living parasites and surgical procedures to remove intraventricular or subarachnoidal cysticerci or to place a ventricular shunt. Drugs to control symptoms are frequently used in order to reduce inflammation (corticoids), to control convulsive crisis (antiepileptics), or to reduce pain (analgesics). Pharmacokinetic and toxicologic studies performed in humans with either cestocidal drug have shown that these agents have a fast absorption and, in general, lack toxic effects. Efficacy of cestocidal treatment is measured by the reduction in the number and size of cysticerci seen in CT or MR, by clinical improvement, elimination of corticoids or anticonvulsants, and by the correction of ventricular dilatation. Risk of important secondary reactions to cestocidal drugs is probably related to the total number, size, and location of the parasites in the central nervous system, and degree of inflammatory reaction. The most frequent surgical intervention is placement of ventricular shunts to deviate CSF to the peritoneal cavity in order to control hydrocephalus. Solitary intraventricular cysticerci can be surgically removed, nowadays even by endoscopy, in order to promptly improve the patient's health (30, 38, 40–42, 53, 76, 125, 138).

LONG-TERM CONSEQUENCES OF NCC

Long-Term Consequences Due to the Presence of Cysticerci in Brain Parenchyma

Approximately 80 to 90% of patients with NCC have parasites lodged in brain parenchyma. Parasites located in the parenchyma frequently cause convulsive crisis or focal deficits to chronic manifestations with neurological deterioration. This location seems to be more frequent in children than in adults, and this fact explains, at least in part, why children frequently present with convulsive crises. Cysticercotic encephalitis, a rare and severe presentation characterized by the presence of multiple parenchymal cysts in colloidal stage, is seen mainly in children and young women. The inflammation generates intracranial hypertension without hydrocephalus and is manifested by headaches, vomiting, convulsive crisis, vision loss, papilledema, and conscience deterioration (24, 37, 51, 66).

Convulsive crises are present in 70% to 90% of the patients; they are mainly partial, secondarily generalized, and motor sensitive, due to a direct irritation of the parasite on the brain cortex or deeper routes. Less frequently generalized myoclonic crises and specific epileptic syndromes, such as complex partial crisis, are also detected. In countries where cysticercosis is endemic, late onset epilepsy is the main symptom of NCC, and this diagnosis must be considered for any adult patient with recent onset epilepsy. There are multiple ways how parenchymal cysticerci can cause seizures, most as direct or indirect effects of inflammation. Seizures occur early in the disease in the setting of intense inflammation associated with viable or degenerating cysts. Encephalomalacia and gliosis, end results of prior inflammation, have also been documented in cysticercosis and are other potential causes of seizure activity. A growing body of evidence suggests that chronic cysticercal granuloma is associated with seizure activity either before or after calcification (41, 97). Treatment is necessary, but how long the antiepileptic treatment should be applied is still in debate. Although most cases require treatment of at least 2 years, some of them will require longer treatment (134). Recurrent crises are frequent, and the presence of perilesional gliosis after parasite death is the factor that seems to be the most important in seizure recurrence (101). Direct mass effect is another clinical presentation of parenchymal NCC that behaves as any neoplasic process causing hemiparesia, dysphasia, blindness, and endocraneal hypertension (24, 37, 136). The most frequent long-term complications of this type of NCC are seen mainly in patients presenting epilepsy and include cognitive dysfunction, psychiatric and psychosocial disorders, and trauma.

Cognitive dysfunction may result from the combination of direct effects of seizures, traumatic brain injury secondary to seizures (including status epilepticus), influence of antiepileptic therapy on cognitive function, and psychosocial sequelae of diagnosis. The most frequent features are impaired attention, concentration, memory, and word finding. They can be sufficiently severe to interfere dramatically with the patient's everyday life, including employment, school, family relationships, and responsibilities, although the global intelligence quotient is generally not impaired. Regarding psychiatric and psychosocial disorders, different pathologies have been associated with epilepsy: psychosis that can be postictal, most commonly following prolonged tonic-clonic seizures and episodes of status, or interictal. The latter ones, which occur generally after a long duration of epilepsy, have been termed schizophrenic-like psychoses and have significantly worse outcome than functional schizophrenia. Depression is one of the most frequent mood disturbances in epilepsy; up to 80% of patients with epilepsy may report it. The cause is difficult to establish, since depression may develop as a reaction to having a chronic illness or may represent an endogeneous mood disturbance caused directly by epilepsy. Also, anxiety, phobias, panic disorders, fear, and attention deficit disorder are more frequent in epileptic patients than in normal subjects (20, 71, 78, 100, 114).

Patients with epilepsy have an increased risk of accidental injury and morbidity than the general population. This increased risk has various causes. (i) Seizures may lead to abrupt falls that occur without warning. (ii) Some type of seizures (absence or partial complex seizures) lead to loss of awareness, preventing the patient from performing and responding to dangerous situations. (iii) Antiepileptic medications may impair cognition, although this effect is probably minimal in most cases. (iv) Comorbid conditions, like attention deficits and cognitive or motor impairment, may also play an additional role in increasing injury risk. The main type of injuries is soft-tissue injuries. A prospective study showed that contusions, wounds, and abrasions accounted for 26%, 23%, and 11% of accidents, respectively, in persons with epilepsy. Less frequent but potentially much more serious injuries include drowning, severe burns, severe head injuries, and severe motor vehicle accidents (140).

Long-Term Consequences in Relation to the Presence of Cysticerci in Subarachnoidal Space and Ventricles

When parasites are located in the subarachnoidal space at the base of the brain or in the ventricles, the main pathologic mechanism involved in the long-term consequences and sequelae are inflammation of the arachnoids or of the ependymal lining that accompanies the parasite and its destruction. Degenerating cysticerci elicit an intense chronic immune inflammatory reaction in the subarachnoid space with participation of IL5, IL6, and IL10 and with the formation of dense exudates composed of collagen fibres, lymphocytes, plasma cells, multinucleated giant cells, eosinophils, and hyalinized parasitic membranes. This leads to abnormal thickening of the leptomeninges along the base of the brain from the optochiasmatic region to the foramen magnum. Ventricular parasites also elicit a local inflammatory reaction. Ependymal cells proliferate and protrude towards the ventricular cavities and may block the transit of CSF at the level of the cerebral aqueduct or Monro's foraminae. This process is called granular ependymitis. Arachnoiditis and ependymitis are chronic processes that can last years in spite of the use of anti-inflammatory treatments (26, 47, 55, 104, 112).

Three main complications can be seen. *Intracranial hypertension* in relation with hydrocephalus is the first cause of death in patients with NCC (35, 115). In the patients that survive, it is also the cause of complications, more frequently in relation with treatment, but also due to an increase of intracranial tension. The presentation can be acute, but it can also be more chronic with the development of a normal pressure hydrocephalus (98). The mechanisms of intracranial hypertension in these cases are the following: (i) a deficit in the absorption of CSF due to chronic arachnoiditis and fibrosis involving arachnoid villi, (ii) occlusion by thickened leptomeninges of Luschka's and Magendie's foraminae, (iii) the presence of granular ependymitis, and (iv) the presence of ventricular cysts (49).

Different structural and functional changes will happen when hydrocephalus occurs (137). At the beginning, much of the ependymal lining of the ventricles may be flattened but still intact. Afterwards, the subependymal tissue becomes edematous, CSF enters the periventricular tissue, and CSF absorption into the blood is increased. Periventricular edema remains confined mainly to white matter, and the central gray matter is usually spared. In case of severe hydrocephalus, the edematous fluid may spread throughout the white matter, separating cells and nerve fibers. Demyelinization and axonal degeneration will occur (44). The mechanisms by which hydrocephalus, first reversibly and then permanently, injures the brain are not understood completely, although increased intracranial pressure, decreased cerebral blood flow, tissue edema, tissue compression, and enlargement may all play a role (86). Neuron degeneration or death does not seem to be a major pathological feature (45), although some experimental studies demonstrate that cortical neurones are affected by structural as well as functional changes when hydrocephalus develops (10). A progressive damage in the cholinergic, dopaminergic, and noradrenergic systems may participate in development of symptomatology (130). Mainly, cognitive and psychiatric dysfunction, visual anomalies, and parkinsonism have been described (75). Cognitive and psychiatric dysfunction related to hydrocephalus in NCC patients, although mainly unstudied, are mentioned in some series of patients (64, 142) and are explained by the destruction of periventricular white matter tracts (36) and change in the cholinergic, dopaminergic, and noradrenergic contents (46, 130). One study performed in our institute showed that 21.5% of NCC patients were diagnosed with dementia that became reversible at 6 months after treatment (108).

Different mechanisms may be involved with visual loss, such as optic nerve damage, optic disc edema, secondary optic atrophy, and visual field constriction (25). The essential element in the pathogenesis of papilledema is an increase in pressure in the layers of the optic nerve, which communicate directly with the subarachnoid space. The pathogenesis of papilledema has also been ascribed to a blockage of axoplasmic flow in the optic nerve fibers and compression due to elevated CSF pressure. This resulted in swelling of axons behind the optic nerve head and leakage of their contents into the extracellular spaces of the disc, giving rise to optic disc edema. In other cases, pretectal affection by massive dilatation of the third ventricle with extension into the sella turcica occurs (79). Lesions in this area produce some of the most distinctive signs in neurology, named pretectal syndrome: abnormal pupils, vertical gaze limitation, and upper lid retraction, convergence-retraction of eye movements and paralysis of convergence, disjunctive eye positions, skew deviation, and nystagmus. Although most of these signs can disappear with treatment of hydrocephalus, a minority of patients remains with permanent residual signs. In a group of 206 patients presenting this syndrome, hydrocephalus due to NCC was the first cause (80).

Movement disorders in hydrocephalus patients are probably multifactorial. They generally include bradykinesia, rest and postural tremor, loss of postural reflexes, rigidity, and bradyphrenia. Dilatation of the lateral, third, and fourth ventricles exerts pressure effects on periventricular structures, including the upper midbrain and diencephalons, which may cause shear, torsion and ischemia of projections to the striatum or direct involvement of the striatum (34, 106).

Vascular complications, both ischemic or hemorrhagic, can occur when parasites are located close to vessels. As vascular events due to other causes, they represent an important source of motor and sensitive sequelae, with permanent disabilities. Vascular complications also occur in 3% of patients with parenchymatous cysticercosis. Different types of ischemic cerebrovascular diseases can be seen (21, 37). The most frequent are lacunar infarctions found in the lenticulostriate branches of the anterior or middle cerebral artery, which result from occlusive endarteritis secondary to the inflammatory reaction within the subarachnoid space, triggered by meningeal cysticerci. This leads to abnormal thickening of the leptomeninges at the base of the brain with subsequent entrapment and occlusion of blood vessels around the Willis Circle. Occlusive endarteritis affects mainly small penetrating arteries at the base of the brain, and thickening of the adventitia, fibrosis of the media, and endothelial hyperplasia leading to the occlusion of the lumen is found (1). Occlusion of the posterior limb of the internal capsule and of the corona radiate can cause pure motor hemiparesis and ataxic hemiparesis or sensorimotor stroke indistinguishable from those caused by atherosclerosis (17, 18). In these cases, CSF analysis shows generally an increased level of cells and proteins, although in some cases, CSF can remain normal. Cerebral angiography may be completely normal or may show segmental narrowing of major intracranial vessels. This syndrome generally occurs in patients with cysts confined to a focal area and is associated with mild arachnoiditis.

Also large infarcts involving deep and superficial sites of a major intracranial artery have occasionally been reported. In these cases, angiography demonstrates occlusion of anterior cerebral artery, middle cerebral artery, or sometimes of the supraclinoid segment of the internal carotid artery (85, 96, 111). In these cases, besides occlusive arteritis, atheroma-like deposits resulting from disruption of the endothelium may occur, which block the lumen of the major intracranial arteries (43, 111).

Another severe vascular complication is the so-called progressive midbrain syndrome in relation to multiple areas of ischemia in the midbrain and thalamus, which are the result of the occlusion of the paramedian thalamopeduncular branches of the mesencephalic artery (117). These branches are prone to develop inflammatory occlusion, as the interpeduncular and prepontine cisterns are where arachnoiditis is more intense. This syndrome occurs usually in patients with a history of shunted hydrocephalus due to arachnoiditis, and its mortality rate is 85%. In these cases, cysticerci are generally widely distributed in the subarachnoid space and are associated with an intense CSF inflammatory profile (21).

Hemorrhages are less frequent. They are usually due to the weakening of the arterial wall by the adherence of cysticerci to subarachnoid blood vessels with the formation of mycotic aneurism or to the rupture of an associated cerebral aneurysm. In these cases, the intense inflammatory infiltrate that surrounds the parasite immediately adjacent to the aneurysm suggests that inflammation might play an important role in its genesis (82, 127, 131). The frequency of vascular complications in these patients is not known with certainty. In different series of patients with symptomatic cysticercosis, the prevalence of stroke varies between 3 and 12% (3, 37). When angiography was performed on 28 patients with subarachnoid cysticercosis, 15 had angiographic evidence of cerebral arteritis (53%), Of these, 12 had a stroke syndrome ($P = 0.02$) and 8 (53%) had evidence of cerebral infarction on magnetic resonance imaging, compared to 1 patient without cerebral arteritis who had cerebral infarction ($P = 0.05$). The most commonly involved vessels were the middle cerebral artery and the posterior cerebral artery (16). The potential interest of using transcranial Doppler (TCD) in the evaluation of cysticercotic arteritis was demonstrated in nine patients with subarachnoidal cysticercosis and stroke. Arteritis of the main basal vessels was detected by TCD in 7 of 10 arterial lesions that were demonstrated by cerebral angiography. The Doppler pattern was occlusive in two cases and stenotic in five. With the three patients with lacunar infarcts, both cerebral angiography and TCD were normal. In six patients, arterial lesions were followed serially by TCD, and the stenotic pattern resolved within 4 to 6 months in three cases and remained in the stenotic range up to 12 months in one case, whereas an occlusive pattern persisted at 6 and 18 months in the other two cases (22).

Nerves and spinal cord entrapment can occur because different nerve structures are affected by arachnoiditis. The optic chiasm is frequently trapped within the dense exudates, leading to visual defects due to ischemic damage. Cranial nerves arising from the ventral side of the brainstem, mainly the occulomotor nerve, the trigeminal nerve, and the facial nerve, can also be affected with subsequent demyelination and dysfunction (29). At the spinal level, arachnoiditis can cause signs of spinal cord and/or cauda equina compression (27, 28). In these cases, surgical and medical treatments are generally insufficient and sequelae are very frequent.

Long-Term Consequences in Relation with Treatment

Placement of a ventricular shunt is one of the most frequent surgical acts in patients with NCC that live in countries where it is endemic (8, 123). It is frequently an emergency and can save lives. Approximately 13% of all patients with symptomatic NCC will develop hydrocephalus secondary to chronic arachnoiditis, intraventricular cysts or meningeal fibrosis. Although the placement of a shunt is mandatory in most cases, complications are frequent. Of these, dysfunctions and infections are the most frequent. Also, up to 80% of repetitive malfunctioning of shunts is due to persistent ependymitis, which is followed by invasive treatments that cause morbidity and frequent hospitalizations. A retrospective study that included 92 patients with cysticercotic arachnoiditis who underwent ventriculoperitoneal shunt placement, showed that half of the patients needed multiple surgical procedures for shunt obstruction. Also 11 patients (12%) developed bacterial meningitis, and 22% of the patients that survived had physical limitations with serious neurological complaints and were incapable of working (123). More recently, it has been shown that prognosis did not substantially improve, since out of 105 patients that underwent ventriculoperitoneal shunt placement, 53 (50.5%) required one or more shunt revisions (total of 164 procedures, 1.56 procedures/patients). These revisions were necessary due to shunt malfunctioning in 126 cases (77%) and secondary to infection in 23% of the cases (28). Another study reporting 21 NCC patients with hydrocephalus that required shunt placement also showed that 12 of them (57%) experienced shunt failures that required one or more revisions. A total of 23 shunt revisions were made; of those, 53% were due to obstruction in the distal segment, 26% to obstruction in the proximal segment, and 21% were due to obstruction at the valve; infection occurred only in 2 cases and 96% of the shunt failures occurred within 3 years after the original shunt placement (81). Shunt placement seems to be such a simple procedure that it is usually performed by residents of neurosurgery departments. Therefore, several recommendations have been defined (88): (i) trans-operative verification of the shunt's standards and functioning, (ii) adequate pressure when tying nuts to fasten connections, (iii) careful handling of the tubing material; (iv) proper angle given to the catheters; (v) verifying that the placement of the shunt is in the correct direction; (vi) precise implant in the ventricle and in the peritoneal cavity; and (vii) proper handling of the device in order to avoid bacterial colonization. Shunt dysfunction and infection generally require the placement of a new shunt. Malfunction of a shunt causes signs of intracranial hypertension. The occurrence of parkinsonian tremor was reported for a few patients as a sign of shunt dysfunction. This symptomatology usually disappeared within a few weeks of successful shunt revision. In patients that do not improve with shunt revision, levodopa therapy can be introduced (80).

Corticosteroid treatment is almost always necessary and often prolonged. Studies performed before the use of corticosteroids showed that without treatment, inflammation of subarachnoidal space lasted many years. Nine-year follow-up of NCC patients showed persistence of the original inflammation in 82% of the cases (123). To control inflammation, the use of corticosteroids for long periods and frequently in high doses diminishes inflammatory parameters, particularly when a ventricular shunt is needed (129). The chronic use of steroids provokes unwanted severe effects, particularly fluid and electrolyte abnormalities, hypertension, hyperglycemia, infections, osteoporosis, myopathy, behavioral alterations, cataracts, growth interruption, and redistribution of fat, added to the consequences of the suppression of the hypothalamic-hypophysis-suprarenal axis (128).

Antiepileptic treatment for antiepiletics may cause depression in cortical function, manifested as sedation and lethargy, personality changes, alteration of the intelligence quotient and of the peripheric nervous system, and, seldom, abnormal movements, and when epilepsy starts at a younger age, it is related to learning difficulty (24, 37, 65).

CONCLUSIONS

Cysticercosis is a chronic disease that involves mainly the central nervous system, where macroscopic parasites lodge in different numbers and sites, survive for different periods of time, and generate different types and degrees of inflammatory and immune responses. Although remarkable progress has been made during the last decades in relation to diagnosis, treatment, and prevention of NCC, mortality and morbidity are still high. This statement is all the more severe considering that the disease is preventable. Today, clinicians have effective drugs that in the majority of patients kill the parasite, but problems still exist in the control of the inflammatory reaction. As we have seen, long-term consequences are due mainly to inflammatory reactions that accompany parasite death; in cases of parenchymal cysticerci, inflammation participates in the genesis of gliosis and causes epilepsy, and in cases of subarachnoidal or ventricular parasites, inflammation is the major cause of CSF circulation dysfunction, vascular complications, and nerve entrapment. To control the inflammatory reaction, corticoids are employed, and although it is clear that their use has improved substantially the prognosis of NCC, it is also evident that this practice contains risks. As we have seen, their chronic use can be the cause of different complications, and it is possible that their immunosuppressive function can participate in some patients in the persistence of living cysticerci for long periods. Understanding better the immunological cascade that accompanies NCC will permit finding more specific anti-inflammatory molecules that would allow the reduction of long-term complications in these patients.

REFERENCES

1. **Aditya, G. S., A. Mahadevan, V. Santosh, Y. T. Chickabasaviah, C. B. Ashwathnarayanarao, and S. S. Krishna.** 2004. Cysticercal chronic basal arachnoiditis with infarcts, mimicking tuberculous pathology in endemic areas. *Neuropathology* **24:**320–325.
2. **Aguilar-Robolledo, F., R. Cedillo-Rivera, P. Llaguno-Violante, J. Torres-López, O. Muñoz-Hernandez, and J. A. Enciso-Moreno.** 2001. Interleukin levels in cerebrospinal fluid from children with neurocysticercosis. *Am. J. Trop. Med. Hyg.* **64:**35–40.
3. **Alarcón. F., F. Hidalgo, J. Moncayo, I. Viñán, and G. Dueñas.** 1992. Cerebral cysticercosis and stroke. *Stroke* **23:**224–228.
4. **Aluja, A. S., D. González, J. Rodríguez-Carbajal, and A. Flisser.** 1989. Histological description of tomographic images of *Taenia solium* cysticerci in pig brains. *Clin. Imaging* **13:**292–298.
5. **Aluja, A. S., J. J. Martinez, and A. N. M. Villalobos.** 1998. *Taenia solium* cysticercosis in young pigs: age of first infection, histological characteristics of the infection and antibody response. *Vet. Parasitol.* **76:**71–79.
6. **Aluja, A. S., and G. Vargas.** 1988. The histopathology of porcine cysticercosis. *Vet. Parasitol.* **28:**65–77.
7. **Amara, L., R. Maschietto-Maschietto, R. Cury, N. F. Ferreira, R. Mendoza, and S. S. Lima.** 2003. Unusual manifestations of neurocysticercosis in MR imaging: analysis of 172 cases. *Arq. Neuropsiquiatr.* **61:**533–541.
8. **Ambrosio, J., A. Landa, M. T. Merchant, and J. P. Laclette.** 1994. Protein uptake by cysticerci of *Taenia crassiceps*. *Arch. Med. Res.* **25:**325–330
9. **Andreassen, J.** 1998. *Intestinal tapeworms*, p. 521–537. *In* F. E. G. Cox, J. P. Kreier, and D. Wakelin (ed.), *Topley and Wilson's Microbiology and Microbial Infections*, 9th ed., vol. 5. Hodder Arnold, London, United Kingdom.
10. **Aoyama, Y., Y. Kinoshita, A. Yokota, and T. Hamada.** 2006. Neuronal damage in hydrocephalus and its restoration by shunt insertion in experimental hydrocephalus: a study involving the neurofilament-immunostaining method. *J. Neurosurg.* **104:**S332–S339.
11. **Arechavaleta, F., J. L. Molinari, and P. Tato.** 1998. A *Taenia solium* metacestode factor non-specifically inhibits cytokine production. *Parasitol. Res.* **84:**117–122.
12. **Arriada, M. N., L. M. Celis, C. J. Higuera, and T. Corona.** 2003. Imaging features of sellar cysticercosis. *Am. J. Neuroradiol.* **24:**1386–1389.
13. **Avila, G., L. Aguilar, S. Benitez, L. Yepez-Mulia, I. Lavenat, and A. Flisser.** 2002. Inflammatory response in the intestinal mucosa of gerbils and hamsters experimentally infected with the adult stage of *Taenia solium*. *Intl. J. Parasitol.* **32:**1301–1308.
14. **Avila, G., M. Benítez, L. Aguilar, and A. Flisser.** 2003. Kinetics of *Taenia solium* antibodies and antigens in experimental taeniosis. *Parasitol. Res.* **89:**284–289.
15. **Avila, G., N. Teran, L. Aguilar, P. Maravilla, P. Mata, and A. Flisser.** 2006. Laboratory animal models for human *Taenia solium*. *Parasitol. Intl.* **55**(Suppl.):S99–S103.
16. **Barinagarrementeria, F., and C. Cantú.** 1998. Frequency of cerebral arthritis in subarachnoid cysticercosis: an angiographic study. *Stroke* **29:**123–125.
17. **Barinagarrementeria, F., and O. H. Del Brutto.** 1988. Neurocysticercosis and pure motor hemiparesis. *Stroke* **19:**1156–1158.
18. **Barinagarrementeria, F., and O. H. Del Brutto.** 1989. Lacunar syndrome due to neurocysticercosis. *Arch. Neurol.* **46:** 415–417.
19. **Berman, J. D., P. C. Beaver, A. W. Cheever, and E. A. Quindlen.** 1981. Cysticercosis of 60 millilitre volume in human brain. *Am. J. Trop. Med. Hyg.* **30:**616–619.
20. **Brown, S.** 2006. Deterioration. *Epilepsia* **47**(Suppl. 2)**:**19–23.
21. **Cantú, C., and F. Barinagarrementeria.** 1996. Cerebrovascular complications of neurocysticercosis. Clinical and neuroimaging spectrum. *Arch. Neurol.* **53:**233–239.
22. **Cantú, C., J. Villarreal, J. L. Soto, and F. Barinagarrementeria.** 1998. Cerebral cysticercotic arthritis: detection and follow-up by transcranial Doppler. *Cerebrovasc. Dis.* **8:**2–7.
23. **Cardenas, F., H. Quiroz, A. Plancarte, A. Meza, A. Dalma, and A. Flisser.** 1992. *Taenia solium* ocular cysticercosis: findings in 30 cases. *Ann. Ophthalmol.* **24:**25–28.
24. **Carpio, A., and W. A. Hauser.** 2002. Prognosis for seizure recurrence in patients with newly diagnosed neurocysticercosis. *Neurology* **59:**1730–1734.
25. **Chang, G. Y., and J. R. Keane.** 2001. Visual loss in cysticercosis: analysis of 23 patients. *Neurology* **57:**545–548.
26. **Chavarria, A., A. Fleury, E. Garcia, C. Marquez, G. Fragoso, and E. Sciutto.** 2005. Relationship between the clinical heterogeneity of neurocysticercosis and the immune- inflammatory profiles. *Clin. Immunol.* **116:**271–278.
27. **Colli, B. O., J. A. Assirati, Jr., H. R. Machado, F. dos Santos, and O. M. Takayanagui.** 1994. Cysticercosis of the central nervous system. II. Spinal cysticercosis. *Arq. Neuropsiquiat.* **52:**187–199.
28. **Colli, B. O., C. G. Carlotti, Jr., J. A. Assirati, Jr., H. R. Machado, M. M. Valença, and M. C. Amato.** 2002. Surgical treatment of cerebral cysticercosis: long-term results and prognostic factors. *Neurosurg. Focus* **12:**e3.
29. **Colli, B. O., N. Martelli, J. A. Assirati, Jr., H. R. Machado, C. P. Salvarani, V. P. Sassoli, and S. V. Forjaz.** 1994. Cysticercosis of the central nervous system. I. Surgical treatment of cerebral cysticercosis: a 23 years experience in the Hospital das Clínicas of Ribeirão Preto Medical School. *Arq. Neuropsiquiat.* **52:**166–186.

30. **Colli, B. O., M. M. Valença, C. G. Carlotti, Jr., H. R. Machado, and J. A. Assirati, Jr.** 2002. Spinal cord cysticercosis: neurosurgical aspects. *Neurosurg. Focus* **12:**e9.
31. **Correa, D., and E. Medina-Escutia.** 1999. Host-parasite immune relationship in *Taenia solium* taeniasis and cysticercosis, p. 15–24. *In* H. H. Garcia and S. M. Martinez (ed.), *Taenia solium Taeniasis/Cisticercosis*, 2nd ed. Editorial Universo, Lima, Peru.
32. **Correa, D., A. Plancarte, M. A. Sandoval, E. Rodriguez-del Rosal, A. Meza, and A. Flisser.** 1989. Immunodiagnosis of human and porcine cysticercosis: detection of antibodies and parasite products. *Acta Leidensia* **57:**93–100.
33. **Cruz-Revilla, C., G. Rosas, G. Fragoso, G., F. Lopez-Casillas, A. Toledo, C. Larralde, and E. Sciutto.** 2000. *Taenia crassiceps* cysticercosis: protective effect and immune response elicited by DNA immunization. *J. Parasitol.* **86:** 67–74.
34. **Curran, T., and A. E. Lang.** 1994. Parkinsonian syndromes associated with hydrocephalus: case reports, a review of the literature, and pathophysiological hypotheses. *Mov. Disord.* **9:**508–520.
35. **DeGiorgio, C. M., I. Houston, S. Oviedo, and F. Sorvillo.** 2002. Deaths associated with cysticercosis. Report of three cases and review of the literature. *Neurosurg. Focus* **12:**e2.
36. **Del Bigio, M. R., M. J. Wilson, and T. Enno.** 2003. Chronic hydrocephalus in rats and humans: white matter loss and behavior changes. *Ann. Neurol.* **53:**337–346.
37. **Del Brutto, O. H.** 1992. Cysticercosis and cerebrovascular disease: a review. *J. Neurol. Neurosurg. Psychiat.* **55:**252–254.
38. **Del Brutto, O. H.** 1997. Clues to prevent cerebrovascular hazards of cysticidal drug therapy. *Stroke* **28:**1088.
39. **Del Brutto, O. H.** 2005. Neurocysticercosis. *Semin. Neurol.* **25:**243–251.
40. **Del Brutto, O. H., V. Rajshekhar, A. C. White, Jr., V. C. W. Tsang, T. E. Nash, O. M. Takayanagui, P. M. Schantz, C. A. W. Evans, A. Flisser, D. Correa, D. Botero, J. C. Allan, E. Sarti, A. E. Gonzalez, R. H. Gilman, and H. H. Garcia.** 2001. Proposed diagnostic criteria for neurocysticercosis. *Neurology* **57:**177–183.
41. **Del Brutto, O. H., R. Santibañez, C. A. Nobo, R. Aguirre, E. Díaz, and T. A. Alarcón.** 1992. Epilepsy due to neurocysticercosis: analysis of 203 patients. *Neurology* **42:**389–392.
42. **Del Brutto, O. H., and J. Sotelo.** 1989. Some unusual manifestations of neurocysticercosis. *Rev. Neurol. Neurosurg. Psychiat.* **29:**23–26.
43. **Del Brutto, O. H., J. Sotelo, and C. G. Roman.** 1998. Neuropathology, p. 37–46. *In* O. H. Del Brutto, J. Sotelo, and G. C. Roman (ed.), *Neurocysticercosis, a Clinical Handbook*. Swets and Zeitlinger, Lisse, The Netherlands.
44. **Ding, Y., J. P. McAllister II, B. Yao, N. Yan, and A. I. Canady.** 2001. Axonal damage associated with enlargement of ventricles during hydrocephalus: a silver impregnation study. *Neurol. Res.* **23:**581–587.
45. **Ding, Y., J. P. McAllister II, B. Yao, N. Yan, and A. I. Canady.** 2001. Neuron tolerance during hydrocephalus. *Neuroscience* **106:**659–667.
46. **Egawa, T., K. Mishima, N. Egashira, M. Fukuzawa, K. Abe, T. Yae, K. Iwasaki, and M. Fujiwara.** 2002. Impairment of spatial memory in kaolin-induced hydrocephalic rats is associated with changes in the hippocampal cholinergic and noradrenergic contents. *Behav. Brain Res.* **129:**31–39.
47. **Escobar, A.** 1983. The pathology of neurocysticercosis, p. 27–54. *In* E. Palacios, J. Rodriguez-Carbajal, and J. M. Taveras (ed.), *Cysticercosis of the Central Nervous System*. Charles C. Thomas, Springfield, IL.
48. **Estañol, B., T. Corona, and P. Abad.** 1986. A prognostic classification of cerebral cysticercosis: therapeutic implications. *J. Neurol. Neurosurg. Psychiat.* **49:**1131–1134.
49. **Estañol, B., E. Kleriga, M. Loyo, H. Mateos, L. Lombardo, F. Gordon, and A.F. Saguchi.** 1983. Mechanisms of hydrocephalus in cerebral cysticercosis: implications for therapy. *Neurosurgery* **13:**119–123.
50. **Evans, C. A. W., H. H. García, A. Hartnell, R. H. Gilman, P. J. Jose, M. Martinez, D. G. Remick, T. J. Williams, and J. S. Friedland.** 1998. Elevated concentration of eotaxin and interleukin-5 in human neurocysticercosis. *Infect. Immun.* **66:**4522–4525.
51. **Fleury, A., A. Dessein, M. Dumas, P. M. Preux, G. Tapia, C. Larralde, and E. Sciutto.** 2004. Symptomatic neurocysticercosis: host and exposure factors relating with disease heterogeneity. *J. Neurol.* **251:**830–837.
52. **Flisser, A.** 1989. *Taenia solium* cysticercosis: some mechanisms of parasite survival in immunocompetent hosts. *Acta Leidensia* **57:**259–263.
53. **Flisser, A.** 1994. Taeniasis and cysticercosis due to *Taenia solium*, p. 77–116. *In* T. Sun. (ed.), *Progress in Clinical Parasitology*, vol. 4. CRC, Boca Raton, FL.
54. **Flisser, A., D. Correa, G. Avila, and P. Maravilla.** 2005. Biology of *Taenia solium, Taenia saginata and Taenia saginata asiatica*, p. 1–9. *In* K. D. Murrell (ed.), *Manual on Taeniosis and Cysticercosis in Man and Animals: Detection, Treatment and Prevention*. WHO/FAO, OIE, Paris, France.
55. **Flisser, A., D. Correa, and C. A. W. Evans.** 2002. *Taenia solium* cysticercosis: new and revisited immunological aspects, p. 15–24. *In* G. Singh, and S. Prabhakar (ed.), *Taenia solium Cysticercosis: from Basic to Clinical Science*. CABI Publishing, Oxon, United Kingdom.
56. **Flisser, A., and P. S. Craig.** 2005. Larval cestodes, p. 677–712. *In* F. E. G. Cox, D. Wakelin, S. H. Gillespie, and D. D. Despommier (ed.), *Topley and Wilson's Microbiology and Microbial Infections*, 10th ed., vol 5. Hodder Arnold, London, United Kingdom.
57. **Flisser, A., D. Gonzalez, A. Plancarte, P. Ostrosky, R. Montero, A. Stephano, and D. Correa.** 1990. Praziquantel treatment of brain and muscle porcine *Taenia solium* cysticercosis. 2. Immunological and cytogenetic studies. *Parasitol. Res.* **76:**640–642.
58. **Flisser, A., D. Gonzalez, J. Rodriguez-Carbajal, M. Shkurovich, D. Correa, S. Cohen, M. Collado, I. Madrazo, E. Rodríguez-del Rosal, B. Fernández, F. Fernandez, and A. S. Aluja.** 1990. Praziquantel treatment of porcine brain and muscle *Taenia solium* cisticercosis. 1. Radiological, physiological and histopathological studies. *Parasitol. Res.* **76:**263–269.
59. **Flisser, A., and T. Gyorkos.** 2007. Contribution of immunodiagnostic tests to epidemiological/intervention studies of cysticercosis/taeniasis in Mexico. *Par. Immunol.* **29:**637–649.
60. **Flisser, A., R. Perez-Montfort, and C. Larralde.** 1979. The immunology of human and animal cysticercosis. A review. *Bull. W. H. O.* **57:**839–856.
61. **Flisser, A., A. Plancarte, and D. Correa.** 1991. *Taenia solium* cysticercosis: a review. *Res. Rev. Parasitol.* **51:**17–23.
62. **Flisser, A., A. Vázquez-Mendoza, J. Martínez-Ocaña, E. Gómez-Colín, R. Sánchez Leyva, and R. Medina-Santillán.** 2005. Evaluation of a self-detection tool for tapeworm carriers for use in public health. *Am. J. Trop. Med. Hyg.* **72:**510–512.
63. **Flisser, A., A. E. Viniegra, L. Aguilar-Vega, A. Garza-Rodriguez, P. Maravilla, G. Avila.** 2004. Portrait of human tapeworms. *J. Parasitol.* **80:**914–916.
64. **Forlenza, O. V., A. H. Filho, J. P. Nobrega, L. dos Ramos Machado, N. G. de Barros, C. H. de Camargo, and M. F. da**

Silva. 1997. Psychiatric manifestations of neurocysticercosis: a study of 38 patients from a neurology clinic in Brazil. *J. Neurol. Neurosurg. Psychiat.* **62**:612–616.

65. **Garcia, H. H., C. A. W. Evans, T. E. Nash, O. M. Takayanagui, A. C. White, Jr., D. Botero, V. Rajshekhar, V. C. W. Tsang, P. M. Schantz, J. C. Allan, A. Flisser, D. Correa, E. Sarti, J. S. Friedland, M. Martinez, A. E. Gonzalez, R. H. Gilman, and O. H. Del Brutto.** 2002 Current consensus guidelines for treatment of neurocysticercosis. *Clin. Microbiol. Rev.* **15**:747–756.
66. **Garcia, H. H., A. E. Gonzalez, C. A. W. Evans, and R. H. Gilman.** 2003. *Taenia solium* cysticercosis. *Lancet* **362**:547–556.
67. **Garcia, H. H., A. E. Gonzalez, R. H. Gilman, L. G. Palacios, I. Jimenez, S. Rodriguez, M. Verastegui, P. Wilkins, V. W. C. Tsang, and the Cysticercosis Working Group in Peru.** 2001. Short report: transient antibody response in *Taenia solium* infection in field conditions—a major contribution to high seroprevalence. *Am. J. Trop. Med. Hyg.* **65**:31–32.
68. **Gilman, R. H., O. H. Del Brutto, H. H. Garcia, M. Martinez, and the Cysticercosis Working Group in Peru.** 2000. Prevalence of taeniosis among patients with neurocysticercosis is related to severity of infection. *Neurology* **55**:1062.
69. **Ginier, B. L., and V. Poirier.** 1992. MR imaging of intraventricular cysticercosis. *Am. J. Neuroradiol.* **13**:1247.
70. **Gonzalez, D., J. Rodríguez-Carbajal, A. Aluja, and A. Flisser.** 1987. Cerebral cysticercosis in pigs studied by computed tomography and necropsy. *Vet. Parasitol.* **26**:55–69.
71. **Helmstaedter, C.** 2007. Cognitive outcome of status epilepticus in adults. *Epilepsia* **48**(Suppl. 8):85–90.
72. **Ito, A., M. I. Putra, R. Subahar, M. O. Sato, M. Okamoto, Y. Sako, M. Nakao, H. Yamasaki, K. Nakaya, P. S. Craig, and S. S. Margono.** 2002. Dogs as alternative intermediate hosts of *Taenia solium* in Papua (Irian Jaya), Indonesia confirmed by highly specific ELISA and immunoblot using native and recombinant antigens and mitochondrial DNA analysis. *J. Helminthol.* **76**:311–314.
73. **Jeri, C., R. H. Gilman, A. G. Lescano, H. Mayta, M. E. Ramirez, A. E. Gonzalez, R. Nazerali, and H. H. Garcia.** 2004. Species identification after treatment for human taeniasis. *Res. Lett. Lancet* **363**:949–950.
74. **Joshi, B. P., and C. G. Gupta.** 1970. A case of pressure syndrome due to *Cysticercus cellulosae* in the brain of the dog. *Ind. Vet. J.* **47**:366–367.
75. **Joubert, J.** 1990. Cysticercal meningitis, a pernicious form of neurocysticercosis, which responds poorly to praziquantel. *S. Afr. Med. J.* **77**:528–530.
76. **Jung, H., G. Cardenas, E. Sciutto, and A. Fleury.** 2008. Medical treatment for neurocysticercosis: drugs, indications and perspectives. *Curr. Top. Med. Chem.* **8**:424–433.
77. **Jung, R. C., M. A. Rodriguez, P. C. Beaver, J. E. Schenthal, and R. W. Levy.** 1981. Racemose cysticercus in human brain, a case report. *Am. J. Trop. Med. Hyg.* **30**:620–624.
78. **Kanner, A. M.** 2007. Epilepsy and mood disorders. *Epilepsia* **48**(Suppl. 9):20–22.
79. **Keane, J. R.** 1990. The pretectal syndrome: 206 patients. *Neurology* **40**:684–690.
80. **Keane, J. R.** 1995. Tremor as the result of shunt obstruction: four patients with cysticercosis and secondary parkinsonism: report of four cases. *Neurosurgery* **37**:520–522.
81. **Kelley, R., D. H. Duong, and G. E. Locke.** 2002. Characteristics of ventricular shunt malfunctions among patients with neurocysticercosis. *Neurosurgery* **50**:757–761.
82. **Kim, I. Y., T. S. Kim, J. H. Lee, M. C. Lee, J. K. Lee, and S. Jung.** 2005. Inflammatory aneurysm due to neurocysticercosis. *J. Clin. Neurosci.* **12**:585–588.
83. **Laclette, J. P., Y. Ornelas, M. T. Merchant, and K. Willms.** 1982. Ultrastructure of the surrounding envelopes of *Taenia solium* eggs, p. 375–387. *In* A. Flisser, K. Willms. J. P. Laclette, C. Larralde, C. Ridaura, and F. Beltrán (ed.), *Cysticercosis. Present State of Knowledge and Perspectives*. Academic Press, New York, NY.
84. **Laclette, J. P., C. Shoemaker, D. Richter, D., L. Arcos, N. Pante, C. Cohen, D. Bing, and A. Nicholson-Weller.** 1992. Paramyosin inhibits complement C1. *J. Immunol.* **148**:124–128.
85. **Levy, A. S., K. O. Lillehei, D. Rubinstein, and J. C. Stears.** 1995. Subarachnoid neurocysticercosis with occlusion of major intracranial vessels: case report. *Neurosurgery* **36**:183–188.
86. **Luciano, M. G., D. J. Skarupa, A. M. Booth, A. S. Wood, C. L. Brant, and M. J. Gdowski.** 2001. Cerebrovascular adaptation in chronic hydrocephalus. *J. Cereb. Blood Flow Metab.* **21**:285–294.
87. **Madiqubba, S., K. Vishwanath, G. Reddy, and G. K. Vemuqanti.** 2007. Changing trends in ocular cysticercosis over two decades: an analysis of 118 surgically excised cysts. *Ind. J. Med. Microbiol.* **25**:214–219.
88. **Madrazo, I., and A. Flisser.** 1992. Cysticercosis, p. 1419–1430. *In* M. L. J. Apuzzo (ed.), *Brain Surgery: Complication Avoidance and Management*. Churchill Livingstone, New York, NY.
89. **Maravilla, J. P., G. Avila, V. Cabrera, L. Aguilar, and A. Flisser.** 1998. Comparative development of *Taenia solium* in experimental models. *J. Parasitol.* **84**:882–886.
90. **Medina-Escutia, E., Z. Morales-Lopez, J. V. Proano, J. Vazquez, V. Bermudez, V. O. Navarrete, V. Madrid-Marina, J. P. Laclette, and D. Correa.** 2001. Cellular immune response and Th1/Th2 cytokines in human neurocysticercosis: lack of immune suppression. *Parasitology* **87**:587–590.
91. **Merchant, M. T., L. Aguilar, G. Avila, L. Robert, A, Flisser, and K. Willms.** 1998. *Taenia solium* description of the intestinal implantation sites in experimental hamster infections. *J. Parasitol.* **84**:681–685.
92. **Meza-Lucas, A., L. Carmona-Miranda, R. C. Garcia-Jeronimo, A. Torrero-Miranda, G. Gonzalez-Hidalgo, G. Lopez-Castellanos, and D. Correa.** 2003. Limited and short-lasting humoral response in *Taenia solium:* seropositive households compared with patients with neurocysticercosis. *Am. J. Trop. Med. Hyg.* **69**:223–227.
93. **Mitchell, G. F.** 1982. Genetic variation in resistance of mice to *Taenia taeniaeformis*: analysis of host-protective immunity and immune evasion, p. 575–584. *In* A. Flisser, K. Willms. J. P. Laclette, C. Larralde, C. Ridaura, and F. Beltran (ed.), *Cysticercosis. Present State of Knowledge and Perspectives*. Academic Press, New York, NY.
94. **Molinari, J. L., R. Meza, B. Suarez, S. Palacios, P. Tato, and A. Retana.** 1983. *Taenia solium*: immunity in hogs to the cysticercus. *Exp. Parasitol.* **55**:340–357.
95. **Molinari, J. L., P. Tato, O. A. Reynoso, and J. M. Cazares.** 1990. Depressive effect of a *Taenia solium* cysticercus factor on cultured human lymphocytes stimulated with phytohemaglutinin. *Ann. Trop. Med. Parasitol.* **84**:205–208.
96. **Monteiro, L., J. Almeida-Pinto, I. Leite, J. Xavier, and M. Correia.** 1994. Cerebral cysticercus arteritis: five angiographic cases. *Cerebrovasc. Dis.* **4**:125–133.
97. **Nash, T. E., O. Del Brutto, J. A. Butman, T. Corona, A. Delgado-Escueta, R. M. Duron, C. A. W. Evans, R. H. Gilman, A. E. Gonzalez, J. A. Loeb, M. T. Medina, S. Pietsch-Escueta, E. J. Pretell, O. M. Takayanagui, W. Theodore, V. C. W. Tsang, and H. H. Garcia.** 2004. Calcified neurocysticercosis and epileptogenesis. *Neurology* **62**:1934–1938.

98. **Oka, Y., K. Fukui, D. Shoda, T. Abe, Y. Kumon, S. Sakaki, and M. Torii.** 1996. Cerebral cysticercosis manifesting as hydrocephalus, case report. *Neurol. Med. Chir.* (Tokyo). **36:**654–658.
99. **Ostrosky-Zeichner, L., E. Garcia-Mendoza, C. Ríos, and J. Sotelo.** 1996. Humoral and cellular immune response within the subarachnoid space of patients with neurocysticercosis. *Arch. Med. Res.* **27:**513–517.
100. **Perrine, K., and S. Congett.** 1994. Neurobehavioral problems in epilepsy. *Neurol. Clin.* **12:**129–152.
101. **Pradhan, S., M. K. Kathuria, and R. K. Gupta.** 2000. Perilesional gliosis and seizure outcome: a study based on magnetization transfer magnetic resonance imaging in patients with neurocysticercosis. *Ann. Neurol.* **48:**181–187.
102. Proaño-Narvaez, J. V., A. Meza-Lucas, O. Mata-Ruiz, R. C. Garcia-Jeronimo, and D. Correa. **2002.** Laboratory diagnosis of human neurocysticercosis: double blind comparison of **enzyme-linked immunosorbent assay** and **electroimmunotransfer blot assay**. *J. Clin. Microbiol.* 40:2115–2118.
103. **Rabiela, M. T., Y. Ornelas, C. Garcia-Allan, E. Rodriguez del Rosal, and A. Flisser.** 2000. Evagination of *Taenia solium* cysticerci: a histologic and electron microscopy study. *Arch. Med. Res.* **31:**605–607.
104. **Rabiela, M. T., A. Rivas, S. Castillo, and F. Cancino.** 1982. Anatomopathologial aspects of human brain cysticercosis, p. 179–200. *In* A. Flisser, K. Willms. J. P. Laclette, C. Larralde, C. Ridaura, and F. Beltran (ed.), *Cysticercosis. Present State of Knowledge and Perspectives.* Academic Press, New York, NY.
105. **Rabiela, M. T., A. Rivas, and A. Flisser.** 1989. Morphological types of *Taenia solium* cysticerci. *Parasitol. Today* **5:**357.
106. **Racette, B. A., G. J. Esper, J. Antenor, K. J. Black, A. Burkey, S. M. Moerlein, T. O. Videen, V. Kotagal, J. G. Ojemann, and J. S. Perlmutter.** 2004. Pathophysiology of parkinsonism due to hydrocephalus. *J. Neurol. Neurosurg. Psychiatry* **75:**1617–1619.
107. **Rajshekhar, V.** 1991. Etiology and management of single small CT lesions in patients with seizures. Understanding a controversy. *Acta Neurol. Scand.* **84:**465–470.
108. **Ramirez-Bermudez, J., J. Higuera, A. L. Sosa, E. Lopez-Meza, M. Lopez-Gomez, and T. Corona.** 2005. Is dementia reversible in patients with neurocysticercosis? *J. Neurol. Neurosurg. Psychiatry* **76:**1164–1166.
109. **Restrepo, B. I., J. I. Alvarez, L. F. Castano, L. F. Arias, M. Restrepo, J. Trujillo, C. H. Colegial, and J. M. Teale.** 2001. Brain granulomas in neurocysticercosis are associated with a Th1 and Th2 profile. *Infect. Immunol.* **69:**4554–4560.
110. **Restrepo, B., P. Llaguno, P., M. A. Sandoval, M. A., J. A. Enciso, and J. M. Teale.** 1998. Analysis of immune lesions in neurocysticercosis patients: central nervous system response to helminth appears Th1-like instead of Th2. *J. Neuroimmunol.* **89:** 64–72.
111. **Rodriguez-Carbajal, J., O. H. Del Brutto, P. Penagos, J. Huebe, and A. Escobar.** 1989. Occlusion of the middle cerebral artery due to cysticercotic angiitis. *Stroke* **20:**1095–1098.
112. **Saenz, B., M. Ruiz-Garcia, E. Jimenez, J. Hernandez-Aguilar, R. Suastegui, C. Larralde, E. Sciutto, and A. Fleury.** 2006. Neurocysticercosis: clinical, radiologic, and inflammatory differences between children and adults. *Pediatr. Infect. Dis. J.* **25:**801–803.
113. **Salgado, P., R. Rojas, and J. Sotelo.** 1997. Cysticercosis: clinical classification based on imaging studies. *Arch. Intern. Med.* **157:**191.
114. **Salpekar, J. A., and D. W. Dunn.** 2007. Psychiatric and psychosocial consequences of pediatric epilepsy. *Semin. Pediatr. Neurol.***14:**181–188.
115. **Santo, A. H.** 2007. Cysticercosis-related mortality in the State of São Paulo, Brazil, 1985-2004: a study using multiple causes of death. *Cad. Saude Publ.* **23:**2917–2927.
116. **Sasaki, O., H. Suguya, K. Ishida, and K. Yoshimura.** 1993. Ablation of eosinophils with anti IL-5 antibody enhances the survival of intracranial worms of *Angiostrongylus cantonensis* in the mouse. *Parasite Immunol.* **15:**349–354.
117. **Sawhney, I. M., G. Singh, O. P. Lekhra, S. N. Mathuriya, P. S. Parihar, and S. Prabhakar.** 1998. Uncommon presentations of neurocysticercosis. *J. Neurol. Sci.* **154:**94–100.
118. **Schantz, P. M., P. P. Wilkins, and V. C. W. Tsang.** 1998. Immigrants, imaging and immunoblots: the emergence of neurocysticercosis as a significant public health problem, p. 213–242. *In* W. M. Scheld, W. A. Craig, and J. M. Hughes (ed.) *Emerging Infections* 2. ASM Press, Washington, DC.
119. **Sciutto, E., A. Chavarria, G. Fragoso, A. Fleury, and C. Larralde.** 2007. The immune response in *Taenia solium* cysticercosis: protection and injury. *Parasite Immunol.* **29:**621–636.
120. **Sciutto, E., G. Fragoso, M. Baca, V. De la Cruz, L. Lemus, E. Lamoyi.** 1995. Depressed T-cell proliferation associated with susceptibility to experimental infection with *Taenia crassiceps* infection. *Infect. Immun.* **63:**2277–2281.
121. **Sciutto, E., G. Fragoso, A. Fleury, J. P. Laclette, J. Sotelo, A. Aluja, L. Vargas, and C. Larralde.** 2000. *Taenia solium* disease in humans and pigs: an ancient parasitosis disease rooted in developing countries and emerging as a major health problem of global dimensions. *Microb. Infect.* **2:**1875–1890.
122. **Solano, S., I. M. Cortes, N. I. Copitin, P. Tato, and J. L. Molinari.** 2006. Lymphocyte apoptosis in the inflammatory reaction around *Taenia solium* metacestodes in porcine cysticercosis. *Vet. Parasitol.* **140:**171–176.
123. **Sotelo, J., and C. Marin.** 1987. Hydrocephalus secondary to cysticercotic arachnoiditis. *J. Neurosurg.* **66:**686–689.
124. **Sotelo, J., and O. H. Del Brutto.** 2000. Brain cysticercosis. *Arch. Med. Res.* **31:**3–14.
125. **Sotelo, J., and O. H. Del Brutto.** 2002. Review of neurocysticercosis. *Neurosurg. Focus* **12:**e1.
126. **Sotelo, J., V. Guerrero, and F. Rubio.** 1985. Neurocysticercosis: a new classification based on active and inactive forms. A study of 753 cases. *Arch. Intern. Med.* **145:** 442–445.
127. **Soto-Hernandez, J. L., S. Gomez-Llata, L. A. Rojas-Echeverri, F. Texeira, and V. Romero.** 1996. Subarachnoid hemorrhage secondary to a ruptured inflammatory aneurysm: a possible manifestation of neurocysticercosis: case report. *Neurosurgery* **38:**197–199.
128. **Stanbury, R. M., and E. M. Graham.** 1998. Systemic corticosteroid therapy—side effects and their management. *Br. J. Ophthalmol.* **82:**704–708.
129. **Suastegui-Roman, R. A., J. L. Soto-Hernandez, and J. Sotelo.** 1996. Effects of prednisone on ventriculoperitoneal shunt function in hydrocephalus secondary to cysticercosis: a preliminary study. *J. Neurosurg.* **84:**629–633.
130. **Tashiro, Y., and J. M. Drake.** 1998. Reversibility of functionally injured neurotransmitter systems with shunt placement in hydrocephalic rats: implications for intellectual impairment in hydrocephalus. *J. Neurosurg.* **88:**709–717.
131. **Tellez-Zenteno, J. F., O. Negrete-Pulido, C. Cantú, C. Márquez, F. Vega-Boada, and G. García-Ramos G.** 2003. Hemorrhagic stroke associated to neurocysticercosis. *Neurologia* **18:**272–275.

132. **Thornton, H.** 1979. Give yourself a tapeworm. *Vet. Rec.* **104:**287.
133. **Velasquez-Perez, L., and M. E. Jimenez-Marcial.** 2004. Hospital mortality at the Manuel Velasco Suarez National Institute of Neurology and Neurosurgery (1995-2001). *Gac. Med. Mex.* **140:**289–294.
134. **Verma, A., and S. Misra.** 2006. Outcome of short-term antiepileptic treatment in patients with solitary cerebral cysticercus granuloma. *Acta Neurol. Scand.* **113:**174–177.
135. **Wadia, N., S. Desai, and M. Bhatt.** 1988. Disseminated cysticercosis: new observations, including CT scan findings and experience with treatment by praziquantel. *Brain* **111:**597–614.
136. **Watson, N. F., M. J. Doherty, and J. R. Zunt.** 2005 Secondary narcolepsy following neurocysticercosis infection. *J. Clin. Sleep Med.* **15:**41–42.
137. **Weller, R. O., and J. Mitchell.** 1980. Cerebrospinal fluid edema and its sequelae in hydrocephalus. *Adv. Neurol.* **28:**111–123.
138. **White, A. C., Jr.** 2000. Neurocysticercosis: updates on epidemiology, pathogenesis, diagnosis and management. *Ann. Rev. Med.* **51:**187–206.
139. **White, A. C., Jr., P. Robinson, and R. Kuhn.** 1997. *Taenia solium* cysticercosis: host-parasite interaction and the immune response. *Chem. Immunol.* **66:**209–230.
140. **Willms, K., and M. T. Merchant.** 1980. The inflammatory reaction surrounding *Taenia solium* larvae in pig muscle: ultrastructural and light microscopic observations. *Parasite Immunol.* **2:**261–275.
141. **Wirrell, E. C.** 2006. Epilepsy-related injuries. *Epilepsia* **47**(Suppl. 1):79–86.
142. **Xie, S., G. Wei, and L. Zhao.** 1996. Intellectual status of patents cerebral cysticercosis. *Zhonghua Yi Xue Za Zhi.* **76:**440–442.
143. **Yoshino, K.** 1933. Studies on the post-embryonal development of *Taenia solium*. Part I. On the hatching of the egg of *Taenia solium*. *J. Med. Assoc. Formosa* **32:**139–141.
144. **Yoshino, K.** 1933. Studies on the post-embryonal development of *Taenia solium*. Part II. On the migration course of the oncosphere of *Taenia solium* within the intermediate host. *J. Med. Assoc. Formosa* **32:**155–158.
145. **Yoshino, K.** 1933. Studies on the post-embryonal development of *Taenia solium*. Part III. On the development of cysticercus cellulosae within the definite intermediate host. *J. Med. Assoc. Formosa* **32:**166–169.

Sequelae and Long-Term Consequences of Infectious Diseases
Edited by Pina M. Fratamico, James L. Smith, and Kim A. Brogden

Chapter 14

Long-Term Consequences of *Cryptosporidium* Infections in Immunocompetent and Immunodeficient Individuals

Simone M. Cacciò, Edoardo Pozio, Alfredo Guarino, and Fabio Albano

Protozoans of the genus *Cryptosporidium* are small coccidian parasites that infect the mucosal epithelium of a variety of vertebrate hosts, including humans. This parasite was first described in 1907 by Tyzzer in the gut of mice, but its pathogenic role was demonstrated only in 1955, when it was found to be associated with a diarrheal disease in turkeys (76). Although *Cryptosporidium* species were found in a broad range of farm animals, their impact was neglected until 1971, when they were found to be a common, serious primary cause of outbreaks of diarrhea in calves. The first cases of cryptosporidiosis in humans were documented in 1976, but it has been during the AIDS epidemics that the role of *Cryptosporidium* species as a serious pathogen has been established. The occurrence of massive waterborne outbreaks in developed countries and the recognition of the importance of pediatric infections in developing countries further indicate that cryptosporidiosis is a major public health problem at the global level (11, 28, 76, 81).

CHARACTERISTICS OF THE ORGANISM

The genus *Cryptosporidium* is classified in the phylum *Apicomplexa*, along with other parasites of great medical (e.g., the genera *Plasmodium* and *Toxoplasma*) and veterinary (the genus *Eimeria*) importance. The taxonomy of the genus *Cryptosporidium*, as is the case for many other protozoan parasites, is still unsatisfactory and is undergoing major revisions, specially in the light of new developmental, biochemical, and genetic data (76, 81). There are currently 16 recognized species within the genus (Table 1), as well as a number of *Cryptosporidium* genotypes, which appear to be host adapted and are thought to represent distinct species (81). From the public health perspective, the two major pathogens are *Cryptosporidium parvum* and *Cryptosporidium hominis*, which account for more than 90% of the infections. However, *Cryptosporidium meleagridis*, *C. felis*, *C. canis*, *C. muris*, and *C. suis* as well as the monkey and cervine genotypes of *Cryptosporidium* also cause infections in humans, particularly, but not exclusively, in immunocompromised individuals (10, 81).

The life cycle of most *Cryptosporidium* species is completed within the gastrointestinal tract (primarily the small intestine) of the host, with developmental stages being associated with the luminal surface of the mucosal epithelial cells (76). Infection results from the ingestion of parasite at the resistant and infective stages, i.e., the oocyst, which releases four sporozoites that invade the epithelial cells. In this process, the sporozoites induce the evagination of the host cell plasma membrane that surrounds the sporozoite and forms a parasitophorous vacuole. As a result, the parasite occupies an intracellular but extracytoplasmatic localization, which is unique to the genus *Cryptosporidium*. A feeder organelle allows the selective metabolic exchanges between the parasite and the cytoplasm of the host cell. The sporozoites then differentiate into trophozoites that undergo asexual replication to form type 1 meronts. The type 1 meronts rupture, releasing eight type 1 merozoites that invade new cells, resulting in a second cycle of asexual replication that culminates in the production of type 2 meronts, which contain four type 2 merozoites. These can again invade host cells and form the parasite at the sexual stages, the male microgamont or the female macrogamont. Fertilization precedes the development of sporulated oocysts that are either thick or thin walled. Thick-walled oocysts are excreted by the host into the environment, whereas thin-walled

Simone M. Cacciò and Edoardo Pozio • Department of Infectious, Parasitic and Immunomediated Diseases, Istituto Superiore di Sanità, Viale Regina Elena, 299, 00161 Rome, Italy. **Alfredo Guarino and Fabio Albano** • Department of Pediatrics, University Federico II of Naples, Via Sergio Pansini, 5, 80131 Naples, Italy.

Table 1. List of the currently recognized human pathogens in the genus *Cryptosporidium*

Species	Major hosts	Minor hosts	Site of infection
C. hominis	Humans	Dugongs, sheep	Small intestine
C. parvum	Humans, cattle, livestock	Deer, mice, pigs	Small intestine
C. suis	Pigs	Humans	Small and large intestine
C. felis	Cats	Humans, cattle	Small intestine
C. canis	Dogs	Humans	Small intestine
C. meleagridis	Humans, turkeys	Parrots	Small intestine
Cryptosporidium cervine genotype	Deer, cattle	Humans	Small intestine
C. muris	Rodents	Humans, rock hyrax, mountain goat	Stomach

oocysts can excyst endogenously, resulting in autoinfection, which helps to explain the mechanism of persistent infections.

There are several characteristics of *Cryptosporidium* parasites that markedly influence the epidemiology of the infection: (i) the infective dose is low (1 to 10 oocysts), (ii) oocysts are immediately infectious when excreted in feces, (iii) oocysts are remarkably stable and can survive for months in the environment, (iv) environmental dispersal can lead to the contamination of drinking water and food, and (v) some *Cryptosporidium* species have a zoonotic potential (11, 28, 76, 81).

The existence of multiple transmission routes (person-to-person, animal-to-person, waterborne, foodborne and, possibly, airborne transmission) and the difficulties in identifying the different species using conventional criteria, such as oocyst morphology, have made the epidemiology of human infection difficult to unravel (10, 81).

In humans, cryptosporidiosis has been reported from over 90 countries in six continents (29). From a review of over 130,000 immunocompetent people with diarrhea, it has been estimated that 6.1% (and up to 24% in human immunodeficiency virus (HIV)-positive people) and 2.1% (and up to 14% in HIV-positive people) in developing and developed countries, respectively, had *Cryptosporidium* infections on the basis of microscopic identification of the parasite (28). However, serosurveys indicated that up to 20% of individuals in the United States experience cryptosporidiosis by young adulthood, a figure that rises to 65% among children living in rural China and even to 90% among children living in urban shantytowns in Brazil (28). In Italy, 75% of a group of blood donors showed a specific cellular immunity against *Cryptosporidium* antigens, suggesting a large number of contacts between this parasite and humans, albeit only a very limited number of people developed the disease (35). Thus, cryptosporidiosis is common in developed regions and nearly universal in impoverished areas and is frequently underdiagnosed.

THE DISEASES

Cryptosporidiosis in the immunocompetent person is a self-limiting, acute gastroenteritis with a variety of presenting symptoms. In cases where the time of exposure has been known, the incubation period was about 5 to 7 days (range probably 2 to 14 days; wider limits have been suggested but are unlikely). There may be a prodrome of 1 to a few days, with malaise, abdominal pain, nausea, and loss of appetite. Gastrointestinal symptoms start suddenly, with the stools being described as watery, greenish with mucus in some cases, without blood or pus, and very offensive. Patients may evacuate their bowels more than 20 times a day but more usually 3 to 6 times. Other symptoms include colicky abdominal pain, especially after meals, anorexia, nausea and vomiting, abdominal distension, and marked weight loss. Flu-like systemic effects, including malaise, headache, myalgias, and fever, commonly occur. Gastrointestinal symptoms usually last about 7 to 14 days, but weakness, lethargy, mild abdominal pain, and intermittent loose bowels sometimes persist for up to a month longer (18, 29).

Symptoms of cryptosporidiosis are generally similar but often develop insidiously in immunocompromised patients. In those with late-stage AIDS with very low CD4 cell counts, or in some other profound deficiency states, diarrhea may be frequent, profuse, and watery, like cholera. Persistent nausea and vomiting is usually associated with severe diarrhea and suggests a poor prognosis (42). Associated symptoms include colicky abdominal pain often associated with meals, severe weight loss, weakness, malaise, anorexia, and low-grade fever. Cryptosporidial infection in immunocompromised patients may involve the pharynx, esophagus, stomach, duodenum, jejunum, ileum, appendix, colon, rectum, gallbladder, bile duct, pancreatic duct, and the bronchial tree. Cryptosporidial cholecystitis (presenting with severe right upper-quadrant abdominal pain), sclerosing cholangitis, pancreatitis, hepatitis, and respiratory-tract symptoms may occur, with or without diarrhea (42). The clinical picture may include other features of HIV infection, and there is often coinfection with other pathogens, such as cytomegalovirus, *Pneumocystis carinii*, and *Toxoplasma gondii*.

The fact that both immunocompetent and immunocompromised persons develop a diarrheal illness suggests that symptoms are not totally dependent on an intact immune response. On the other hand, not all *Cryptosporidium* infections in humans cause a diarrheal illness, and asymptomatic infections have been documented in some otherwise healthy individuals who have intact immune responses. These observations indicate that parasite replication is necessary, but not wholly sufficient, for the development of illness. It seems reasonable to state that the illness is the result of a combination of molecular events with contributions from parasite-derived products and the innate and/or acquired responses to them (18).

LONG-TERM CONSEQUENCES ASSOCIATED WITH THE ORGANISMS

The long-term morbidity impact of repeated or prolonged dehydrating and diarrheal illnesses in impoverished areas in the early critical formative years on child growth and development is only recently being addressed. In these areas, cryptosporidiosis is endemic and infection occurs early in life.

Based on pioneering studies of the impact of intestinal helminthic infections on physical fitness, physical activity, and cognitive function (3, 62, 75), long-term prospective surveillance studies have been performed to examine the potential effects of early childhood diarrhea and cryptosporidiosis on (i) nutritional status, (ii) physical fitness and activity, and (iii) cognitive function. Less compelling evidences suggest that *Cryptosporidium* may also play a role in inducing functional intestinal disorders, as well as micronutrient deficiencies, in a long-term prospective.

Long-Term Consequences for Nutritional Status

Studies in Peruvian children showed that cryptosporidial infections, with or without diarrhea, are associated with growth shortfalls, especially in very young or malnourished infants (19, 20) (Table 2). Younger age at *C. parvum* infection was related with a major effect on growth. Infants younger than 5 months infected with *C. parvum* gained weight significantly more slowly for the subsequent 2 months than did noninfected children of similar age. After infection, the children had an estimated weight deficit of approximately 500 g compared to age-matched noninfected children. Subsequently, these children gained weight more rapidly than did noninfected children of similar age, and catch-up weight was completed at 6 months after infection. A similar effect was observed on linear growth. The slower period of linear growth reached a plateau at 3 months after infection. These children had a height deficit of approximately 1 cm compared to noninfected children. No subsequent height catch-up occurred, and 1 year after infection, children still exhibited a height deficit compared with noninfected children of similar age. Children infected between ages 6 and 11 months and 12 and 17 months had a similar slowing of weight and height gain relative to noninfected children of similar age, but of smaller magnitude. These children were eventually able to cover the growth gap several months after infection. Stunting prior to *C. parvum* infection was associated with a more severe and protracted effect by *C. parvum* infection on growth (19).

A cohort study on 1,064 children from Guinea-Bissau suggested that cryptosporidiosis had persistent adverse effects on nutritional condition in children under age 2 years (57) (Table 2). Despite the fact that several studies (17, 44, 60) had shown increased carriage of *Cryptosporidium* species in malnourished children, without distinguishing between cause and effect, the authors of the Guinea-Bissau study support the hypothesis that it is the infection that induces malnutrition rather than the latter being a risk factor for cryptosporidiosis (57). Indeed, children who developed cryptosporidiosis were no different in weight or height before the infection than were children who did not. However, the cause-effect relationship between malnutrition and cryptosporidiosis is not clear. The association between malnutrition and cryptosporidiosis is supported by another study showing that more children with diarrhea and cryptosporidiosis than healthy controls are malnourished (47). As further evidence, low levels of serum mannose-binding lectin were found in Haitian children with cryptosporidiosis. Mannose-binding lectin is a key component of the innate immune system that circulates in the blood and binds to specific surface carbohydrates of a wide array of infectious agents. This study, like many others of children in developing countries, highlights the complexity of distinguishing the cause from the effect in the vicious cycle of immune derangement, malnutrition, intestinal malabsorption, and infection (46).

A recent paper analyzed the effect of the two major human pathogens, *C. hominis* and *C. parvum*, on oocyst shedding, symptoms, and long-term effects on growth (8). The authors found that infections due

Table 2. Summary of long-term functional and growth impairment in children with cryptosporidiosis

Study type	Setting	No. of children	Length of follow-up (yr)	Long-term consequence	Comment	Reference(s)
Longitudinal study	Peru	185	2	Impaired growth	Difficulty to separate the effect of age of infection on catch-up from that of stunting prior to infection	19, 20
Open study	Guinea Bissau	1,064	3	Impaired growth	Possible confounding and bias should be considered	57
Longitudinal study	Brazil	26	9	Impaired fitness	Sample size insufficient to control all possible confounders	38
Longitudinal study	Peru	143	9	Cognitive deficiency associated with *Giardia* infection but not with *C. parvum* infection	Good statistical analysis	6

to *C. hominis* were more common than those due to *C. parvum*. However, *C. hominis* infections, especially among asymptomatic children, as well as symptomatic *C. parvum* infections were associated with heavier infections, as evidenced by greater shortfalls in growth in the postinfection period.

In conclusion, *Cryptosporidium* species infection has a long-term impact on subsequent growth, especially when the infection is acquired during infancy, and is likely to be more severe in children who are already malnourished.

Long-Term Consequences for Physical Fitness and Activity

"Physical activity," and "physical fitness" are terms that describe different concepts. Physical activity is defined as any bodily movement produced by skeletal muscles that results in energy expenditure. The energy expenditure can be measured in kilocalories. Exercise is a subset of physical activity that is planned, structured, and repetitive and has as a final or an intermediate objective, i.e., the improvement or maintenance of physical fitness. Physical fitness is a set of attributes that are either health or skill related. The degree to which people have these attributes can be measured with specific tests.

The number of episodes of early childhood diarrhea and cryptosporidiosis was associated with diminished performance on physical and cognitive tests in a cohort of children 6 to 12 years old in Brazil (38). The physical fitness as judged by the Harward step test (HST) and cognitive function of 26 children who had complete surveillance for diarrhea in their first 2 years of life and who had continued surveillance until 6 to 9 years of age was investigated. Childhood diarrhea at 0 to 2 years of age correlated with reduced fitness by the HST at 6 to 9 years of age, even after controlling for anthropometric and muscle area effects, anemia, intestinal helminthes, *Giardia duodenalis* infections, respiratory illnesses, and socioeconomic variables. Early childhood cryptosporidial infections, either with or without diarrhea, were also associated with reduced fitness at 6 to 9 years of age, even when controlling for current nutritional status. Children with lower fitness scores were more likely to have experienced more days and more episodes of diarrhea and more cryptosporidial infection during early childhood. The magnitude and potential importance of the effect on fitness was illustrated by the 4% to 8% reductions in HST scores compared to the fitness score of a child with no diarrhea in the first 2 years of life. In contrast, there was no correlation of early childhood diarrhea with the activity scores or the activity scores with HST scores. In addition, early childhood diarrhea remained significantly correlated with fitness after controlling for activity scores.

Finally, pilot studies in these children suggest a prolonged impact of early childhood diarrhea on visual-motor coordination, auditory short-term memory and information processing, and cortical cognitive function.

Long-Term Consequences for Cognitive Function

Cognitive function in children is affected by environmental and health-related factors (7, 25). Risk factors that interfere with cognitive function are especially important during infancy because the first 2 years of life are essential for rapid growth and development. Chronic malnutrition during infancy may be associated with poor cognitive function (55, 65), although the cause-effect relationship and the mechanisms are not fully understood. Regardless of etiology, diarrhea is both a cause and an effect of malnutrition and can lead to linear growth retardation (38). The negative impact of early childhood diarrhea and malnutrition on school performance and cognitive function several years later have been well documented (6, 38, 61, 65). However, the pilot study by Guerrant et al. (38) noted that the correlation of early diarrhea with later cognitive impairment remained significant when controlling for early *Cryptosporidium* infection. In the latter study, neither environmental nor health-related factors were considered, thus raising the possibility that the observed association could be not true. Berkman et al. (6) showed that malnutrition in early childhood and potentially *G. duodenalis* infection were both associated with poor cognitive function at age 9 years. It is surprising that the investigators also found that infections with *G. duodenalis* had an adverse effect on cognitive scores, which was independent of the effects of diarrhea and growth retardation. *Cryptosporidium* species infection was not associated with impairment in cognitive function as assessed with the revised version of the full-scale intelligence quotient of the Wechsler intelligence scale for children. There is now consistent evidence that growth-retarded children have cognitive deficiencies. However, it would be a mistake to attribute cognitive deficiencies exclusively and entirely to poor nutrition or infection. A major problem with observational studies on developmentally regulated functions is the overlapping effects by environmental factors, growth retardation, and infections that also detrimentally affect IQ.

Long-Term Consequences for Functional Intestinal Disorders

Immune mechanisms may be involved in the long-term impact of human cryptosporidiosis on the development of functional intestinal disorders. Recent work in suckling rats explored the effects of early *C. parvum* gut infection on the subsequent development of jejunal hypersensitivity to distension in a rat model (52). The data suggest that neonatal cryptosporidiosis results in increased jejunal sensitivity to distension in adults. The infection model mimicked some key features of irritable bowel syndrome, in which visceral pain is a major symptom and increased sensitivity to gut distension is the putative mechanism.

Long-Term Consequences for Micronutrient Deficiency

The critical role of micronutrient malabsorption in the effects of cryptosporidiosis-related diarrhea on growth and physical and cognitive development and the importance of micronutrients in the effects of malnutrition on cryptosporidiosis remain largely to be fully defined. The complex interactions between micronutrient deficiency and infectious disease have potentially huge long-term developmental and societal impacts. These effects range from individual long-term functional impairment to effects on microbial virulence or antimicrobial resistance.

In conclusion, enteric cryptosporidiosis is generally a mild self-limited disease in healthy immunocompetent children. In immunodeficient children and in those malnourished, cryptosporidiosis may run a more severe and protracted course (37). However, in the latter condition, *Cryptosporidium* species infection may be associated with long-term clinically relevant problems, ultimately leading to growth deficiency and impaired physical and cognitive performances. The cause-effect relationship of such complex pathways and namely the specific role of *Cryptosporidium* species are yet to be defined.

CRYPTOSPORIDIOSIS IN CHILDREN WITH PIDs

Primary immunodeficiencies (PIDs) are rare inherited disorders of the innate, cellular, and/or humoral immune system. Among patients with PIDs, a particular susceptibility to *Cryptosporidium* species infection is observed in children with X-linked hyper-immunoglobulin M (IgM) syndrome (XHIM), resulting from CD40 ligand (CD40L) deficiency, hyper-IgM syndrome type 3 (HIGM3) caused by CD40 deficiency, primary CD4 lymphopenia, severe combined immunodeficiency syndrome, and gamma interferon deficiency (34, 40).

In these patients, who are unable to clear the infection, the bile tract is the most common site of extraintestinal infection, and this may result in chronic liver inflammation or even lead to liver cirrhosis. Colonization of the biliary system by *Cryptosporidium* species may also predispose to the development of sclerosing cholangitis (SC) and cholangiocarcinoma.

In particular, boys with XHIM-CD40L deficiency have a high incidence of life-threatening hepatic complications. Studies on experimentally infected mice have shown a more aggressive, often fatal liver injury in CD40L- and gamma interferon-knockout mice than in mice with severe combined immunodeficiency. This suggests that absent CD40-CD40L interaction and/or downregulation of gamma interferon-driven pathways may be directly involved in the development of *Cryptosporidium*-associated SC, bile duct dysplasia, and, possibly, neoplasms (53).

In a study of the association between XHIM and tumors of the pancreas, liver, and biliary tree, 14 of the 20 boys (70%) were found to be infected with *Cryptosporidium* species (39). In these patients, cholangiopathy and/or cirrhosis preceded the development of the tumors, suggesting that infection or inflammation of bile ducts caused by *Cryptosporidium* species may play an important role in the development of malignancy.

Another study, performed in Poland, found chronic cryptosporidiosis in three out of five patients with XHIM and in a single patient with primary CD4 lymphopenia and reported SC in these patients (80). Further support for the association between *Cryptosporidium* species infection and SC was found in a study in the United Kingdom that enrolled 35 children with clinical evidence of liver disease and found 12 of 27 children (44%) infected with the parasite, among which 9 had SC (70).

In a recent analysis of 126 patients with XHIM syndrome reported to the European Society for Immunodeficiency (ESID) registry, approximately 1/6 developed liver disease, and in more than 50% of cases this was associated with *Cryptosporidium* species infection (77). These figures may even be an underestimate, because more-sensitive molecular techniques reveal that a number of patients are colonized by *Cryptosporidium* species without evidence of its presence on conventional microbiology screening (53, 80).

In summary, unrecognized cases of cryptosporidiosis in children with PIDs may lead to serious consequences, with development of sclerosing cholangitis, liver cirrhosis, and cholangiocarcinoma. *Cryptosporidium* species, which are rarely found in humans, such as *C. meleagridis*, can play an important role in the pathogenesis of cholangitis and diarrhea in PID patients. Regular screening of these patients is therefore needed.

IMMUNOCOMPROMISED ADULTS

The determinants, clinical features, and response to treatment of cryptosporidiosis in immunocompromised adults are strongly related to the immune status of the host. In a study carried out in Italy, diarrhea lasting 15 days was observed only in HIV-positive individuals who had 300 CD4 cells/mm^3, but for six of them, the diarrhea lasted 30 days. Chronic diarrhea lasting 30 days was observed in persons who had 200 CD4 cells/mm^3 at the onset of infection. Most of them had severe symptoms (diarrhea, abdominal pain, gastritis, vomiting, pain at the right hypochondrium, and weight loss up to 18 kg). No case was observed among individuals with more than 300 CD4 cells/mm^3. The strong association between chronic disease and recurrent disease and the level of immunosuppression is further suggested by a model (using the individuals with 200 to 300 CD4 cells/mm^3 as the reference group) showing that the estimated odds ratio was 2.86 (95% confidence interval [CI], 0.24 to 33.90) for those with 100 to 199 CD4 cells/mm^3 and 15.0 (95% CI, 1.45 to 155.31) in those with less than 100 CD4 cells/mm^3. In addition, a percentage of HIV-positive individuals, all with less than 300 CD4 cells/mm^3 at the onset of symptoms, had diarrhea lasting for more than 15 but less than 30 days. The HIV-positive individuals with diarrhea for less than 30 days had mild symptoms (no pain at the right hypochondrium, no gastritis, no vomiting), and all of them showed clinical recovery. By contrast, among persons with more than 30 days of diarrhea, clinical and parasitological recovery occurred in 6 months to 1 year following paromomycin treatment (68).

The severity and duration of clinical symptoms is clearly associated with the CD4 cells/mm^3. The risk of clinical disease increases with a decrease in CD4 cells, so persons with 100 to 199 CD4 cells/mm^3 have a higher incidence of severe disease than those with 200 to 499 or more than 500 CD4 cells. With CD4 cell counts less than 200/mm^3, there is a dramatic increase in both the incidence and the severity of clinical manifestations.

The clinical picture of HIV-positive individuals with prolonged (more than 15 days) diarrhea was influenced by their CD4 cell count, even if individual variability among those in clinical recovery is great. A percentage of persons with low CD4 cell counts can develop severe gastric involvement (vomiting or gastritis, or both), and a percentage of them also develop pain at the right hypochondrium that, in some cases, requires the use of opiates. These individuals have a median CD4 cell count of 30 cells/mm^3 (68).

The contribution of the parasite genetic diversity to the clinical manifestations of cryptosporidiosis in HIV-infected people should not be underestimated. A recent cross-sectional study enrolled 2,490 HIV-infected people in Lima, Peru, and demonstrated *Cryptosporidium* species in 230 of them (14). Identification of the parasite at the species and subtype level allowed the authors to conclude that infections with *C. hominis*, *C. canis*, and *C. felis* were associated with diarrhea, while infection with *C. parvum* was associated with chronic diarrhea and vomiting (14).

Influence of the Highly Active Antiretroviral Therapy on Postinfection Sequelae

In a study carried out in London, cryptosporidiosis was detected in 12% of the HIV-positive individuals with a CD4 cell count of less than 200 cells/mm^3, in

2.6% of those with a CD4 cell count of 200 to 350 cells/mm^3, and in 1.4% of those with a CD4 cell count exceeding 350 cells/mm^3, although some of these individuals were undergoing highly active antiretroviral therapy (HAART) (27). In Italy, the relative hazard of death for cryptosporidiosis decreased by 74% among HIV-positive individuals in the period from 1997 to 1998, when HAART began to be widely used (26). In a London hospital, the prevalence of cryptosporidiosis in HIV-positive individuals decreased from 1.1% before the introduction of HAART to 0.3% after HAART, in which one proteinase inhibitor (PI) was included, with a 95% decrease in mortality (56). In a hospital in Alabama, the United States, the incidence of cryptosporidiosis in individuals with AIDS and a CD4 cell count of less than 200 cells/mm^3 decreased from 2% before HAART to 0.3% after HAART, in which four PIs were included (12). In the same hospital, cryptosporidiosis was detected in 2 of the 54 HIV-infected individuals who had undergone endoscopic diagnosis before the introduction of HAART and in only 1 of the 112 HIV-infected individuals taking HAART that included a PI (58). The importance of HAART in resolving cryptosporidiosis through an increase in the CD4 cell count has also been demonstrated by a plethora of case reports. In an HIV-positive person with severe cryptosporidiosis, the infection was rapidly eradicated after beginning HAART, with an increase in the CD4 cell count in peripheral blood and intestinal mucosa; moreover, the CD4 cell count in the intestinal mucosa showed a much more rapid increase and much higher CD4 cell count (73). Four individuals with cryptosporidiosis who had been unsuccessfully treated with paromomycin recovered 4 to 8 weeks after beginning HAART, with a mean 4.4-fold increase in the CD4 cell count. Only one person relapsed, 7 months after beginning HAART (16). Two studies have reported that the HAART-induced recovery from cryptosporidiosis was not associated with a consistent increase in the CD4 cell count. In one of these studies, an HIV-positive person with untreatable cryptosporidiosis and a CD4 cell count of 33 cells/mm^3 rapidly recovered from infection after beginning HAART, despite the fact that the CD4 cell count increased only to 84 cells/mm^3 (36). In another study, four HIV-positive individuals with cryptosporidiosis and a CD4 cell count of less than 100 cells/mm^3 showed clinical and parasitological resolution of cryptosporidiosis after beginning HAART, and no relapse was observed during the 6-month follow-up, despite the fact that their CD4 cell counts remained low, with a high viral load (50).

One study has shown that prognosis is independently related to two factors measured at the time of *Cryptosporidium* diagnosis: a CD4 count of less than 53 cells/mm^3 versus more than 53 cells/mm^3 (relative hazard 6.18; 95% CI, 2.99 to 12.76) and hematocrit of less than 37% versus more than 37% (relative hazard 2.27; 95% CI, 1.22 to 4.22) (23). The median survival in the subgroup with a CD4 cell count of more than 53 and hematocrit of more than 37% was 1,119 days compared to only 204 days in the subgroup with a CD4 cell count of less than 53 and hematocrit of less than 37%. This study also showed that an initial AIDS-defining diagnosis of cryptosporidiosis was a poor prognostic factor compared to other possible diagnoses (relative hazard of death, 2.01; 95% CI, 1.38 to 2.93). One aspect of chronic cryptosporidiosis in patients with AIDS is the large weight loss that many experience. One study from France reported that the severity of weight loss in such patients is independently associated with levels of nutrient intake ($P < 0.005$) and high stool frequency ($P > 0.01$) but not with nutrient malabsorption (5). As well as developing a more severe form of typical gastrointestinal disease, people with HIV infection can develop atypical disease presentations, affecting body systems not usually affected in immunocompetent individuals.

In chronic cryptosporidiosis, parasites can colonize other organs, such as the stomach, the biliary tract, the pancreas, and the respiratory tract. In an endoscopic study of 71 patients with AIDS and chronic diarrheal illness or other gastrointestinal disorders of unexplained origin, 24 individuals were positive for cryptosporidiosis. Of these 24 patients, 16 (67%) had parasites in the gastric epithelium (71). Few of the patients reported any symptoms that could be correlated with this gastritis, and the authors concluded that there was no clear correlation between gastric colonization and related clinical and pathological features. One particularly problematic complication of gastric involvement is antral narrowing and gastric outlet obstruction (31, 43, 59). Such gastric outlet obstruction can lead to nausea and vomiting and eventually may cause a severe reduction in nutrient intake. A further unusual complication of cryptosporidiosis in AIDS patients is pneumatosis cystoides intestinalis characterized by the presence of thin-walled, gas-containing cysts in the intestinal wall (24, 72, 74). Sometimes these cysts can rupture, resulting in a pneumoretroperitoneum and pneumomediastinum. There is a case report of cryptosporidiosis affecting the esophagus in a 2-year-old child and resulting in vomiting and dysphagia (45). Finally, there is also a case report of *Cryptosporidium* species infection causing appendicitis; the diagnosis was confirmed histologically after an appendectomy was performed (63).

In a British study, 65% of patients suffering from cholangitis had cryptosporidiosis (30). In a Spanish study, 18.6% of AIDS patients with chronic diarrhea due to *Cryptosporidium* species infection were reported to have this parasite in the common bile duct (48). In Milwaukee, WI (the United States), 29.3% patients with cryptosporidiosis documented biliary symptoms (78).

In the pre-HAART era, the presence of biliary symptoms in persons with AIDS and cryptosporidiosis was a strong indicator of the prognosis since most of patients with these symptoms die within 1 year, whereas only half of patients without these symptoms die. It is doubtful that this difference is due directly to the biliary involvement; it more likely reflects the point that more severely immunocompromised persons are more likely to experience biliary involvement.

It is difficult to assess the impact of cryptosporidiosis-related pancreatic disease. At autopsy, about one-third of patients with AIDS and cryptosporidiosis had parasites colonizing the pancreas (33). Histological changes were generally mild and were limited to hyperplastic squamous metaplasia. In an Italian study, three people with AIDS and cryptosporidiosis presented with acute or chronic pancreatitis, abdominal pain resistant to analgesics, increased serum amylase levels, and abnormalities at both sonography and computed tomography (13). Endoscopic retrograde cholangiopancreatography revealed papillary stenosis in all three patients.

In a study from Spain, 16.3% patients with chronic diarrhea due to *Cryptosporidium* species infection had oocysts detectable in the sputum; 71% had respiratory symptoms and an abnormal chest, but *Mycobacterium tuberculosis* or *Mycobacterium avium* was also detected, whereas the other patients had no respiratory symptoms and a normal chest (48). An additional 62 patients with respiratory cryptosporidiosis are reported in the literature, 40 of whom had another respiratory pathogen detected (22). Given the difficulty in diagnosing many respiratory pathogens and in the cases of multiple infections, what could be the etiological agent of the clinical disease? Consequently, it is not clear how relevant respiratory disease secondary to cryptosporidiosis is in the prognosis of and symptoms associated with AIDS. Neither of the works reported above can be taken to show that cryptosporidiosis causes respiratory disease.

Sequelae of Cryptosporidiosis in Immunocompetent People

In immunocompetent persons, the medium-term health effects of cryptosporidiosis is characterized by the recurrence of loss of appetite, vomiting, abdominal pain, and diarrhea, independently if the patients have been infected by *C. parvum* or by *C. hominis* (21, 41, 49). On the other hand, there are significant differences in the occurrence of nongastrointestinal symptoms as sequelae of cryptosporidiosis, i.e., joint pain, eye pain, headache, dizziness, and fatigue, following infections with *C. hominis* and *C. parvum*. Eye pain and recurrent headache are associated with *C. hominis* infection but not with *C. parvum* infection. Other symptoms, such as fatigue and joint pains, are present after infections with both species, but are significantly more common after *C. hominis* infection (41).

In the work of Hunter et al. (41), the relatively small number of case patients who reported joint pains (13 control subjects versus 36 case patients) means that firm conclusions about the nature and distribution of joint symptoms cannot be made. Symptom duration was significantly longer for case patients, and a greater proportion of case patients reported moderate and severe joint problems than did control subjects. However, this study shows some biases related to the people enrolled, their ages (most of them were young children), and the fact that only 33% of them had either already consulted a doctor about or were intending to arrange a consultation for their joint problems.

CRYPTOSPORIDIOSIS IN TRANSPLANT RECIPIENTS

Diarrhea can frequently be observed in solid-organ transplant (SOT) recipients as a result of infections, due to *Clostridium difficile* colitis, viral infections, and parasitic infections, including *Cryptosporidium* species, or to side effects of immunosuppressants. A handful of reports has described intestinal *Cryptosporidium* species infections in renal transplant patients. Some cases resulted in either mild disease or asymptomatic carriage; however, there have been reports of severe cryptosporidiosis in renal transplant patients, including biliary involvement treated with reduction of immunosuppression and a short course of antiparasitic agents (1, 40). About 10 cases of *Cryptosporidium* species infection in liver transplant recipients have been reported (15, 32, 51). In a study from Belgium of 461 children following liver transplantation, 3 (0.65%) developed diffuse cholangitis associated with intestinal *Cryptosporidium* species carriage (15). All three recipients required reoperation on the bile duct anastomosis, but biliary cirrhosis developed in one patient, requiring retransplantation. In a retrospective study from Pittsburgh, four (0.34%) pediatric cases of cryptosporidiosis were identified among 1,160 nonrenal, abdominal organ transplant recipients (32). Three of these four cases occurred in patients receiving liver transplants, and one occurred following a small bowel transplantation. All four patients spontaneously resolved their infections. Manz and Steuerwald (51) reported a case of cryptosporidiosis in an adult patient treated with interferon and ribavirin for recurrent hepatitis C after liver transplantation. The patient did not have HIV infection or immunoglobulin deficiency and recovered after the treatment was stopped and the dosage of immunosuppressant was lowered. A case of multiple infections with distinct *Cryptosporidium* species has been described for a transplanted ileum (67).

Albeit the experience with cryptosporidiosis in SOT is limited, the available data illustrate the need to have a high index of suspicion for cryptosporidiosis in any transplant patient who presents with severe diarrhea. Indeed, a recent survey on the etiology of diarrhea in 43 SOT recipients in Turkey (4) showed that in most cases (33 of 43, 76.7%) infectious agents were responsible for the diarrheal disease and demonstrated the presence of *Cryptosporidium* in 7 (21%) of them. Endoscopy and biopsies should be performed on all patients with clinically significant diarrhea and negative stool culture/stain. The disease course can be prolonged and may require a combination therapy for extended periods of time in conjunction with the reduction in immunosuppression. Supportive measures with a good nutrition are essential in the care of these patients.

TREATMENT AND CONTROL

A large number of antimicrobial drugs have been tested in animals and humans infected with *Cryptosporidium* species with no clear evidence of consistent effectiveness against this parasite (54). The first attempts to treat the infection focused, quite logically, on the use of anticoccidial and antiapicomplexan drugs, and over 200 compounds were tested, both in vitro and in vivo. Albeit several agents were found to have some activity, results of different studies have been inconsistent (54). Several factors may contribute to this lack of efficacy, including (i) the unique location of the parasite in the host cell (intracellular but extracytoplasmatic), which may affect drug concentration (transported from the host cell across to the parasite), (ii) the lack of specific targets or differences in targets either at the molecular or structural levels (e.g., the lack of the plastid in parasites of the genus *Cryptosporidium* could explain why macrolides show limited efficacy against them), (iii) differences in biochemical pathways, and (iv) existence of transport proteins or efflux pumps that transport drugs out of the parasite.

Treatment for Immunocompetent Patients

Since *Cryptosporidium* species infection in immunocompetent persons is a self-limiting disease, a symptomatic antidiarrheal treatment is usually sufficient. However, concomitant infections, stress, age, and other factors (e.g., malnutrition) can transitorily reduce the immunocompetence and increase the duration of the clinical symptoms. In addition, the infectious dose and the virulence of the parasite strain may also play a role in the severity and length of the infection. Thus, in case of persistent disease, the patients should be treated with an anti-*Cryptosporidium* therapy.

Today, the therapy of choice is nitazoxanide [2-acetyloxy-*N*-(5-nitro-2-thiazolyl) benzamide], a synthetic agent that has a demonstrated activity against a broad range of parasites as well as some bacteria. Nitazoxanide is rapidly hydrolyzed to its active desacetyl metabolite, named tizoxanide, which is further metabolized by glucuronidation to tizoxanide glucuronide. The exact mechanism of action on *Cryptosporidium* species remains unclear, but data from bacteria and anaerobic protozoa suggest that tizoxanide interferes with an enzyme (pyruvate; ferredoxin oxidoreductase) which is essential for anaerobic energy metabolism. Nitazoxanide has been approved in the United States in a suspension form for use in immunocompetent children aged 1 to 11 years with cryptosporidiosis (and giardiasis), whereas both suspensions and tablets are available in Latin America (79).

Treatment for Immunocompromised Patients

The treatment of cryptosporidiosis in immunocompromised patients can, in principle, be based on (i) the use of antimicrobial agents, (ii) passive immunotherapy, and (iii) immune reconstitution.

There have been a number of clinical trials over the last years, but in most cases results were mixed, contrasting, or difficult to reproduce, and very few were double-blind clinical trials, which enrolled a limited number of participants (9). Spiramycin, a macrolide antibiotic, produced encouraging results in pilot studies, but its efficacy in HIV-positive patients has not been demonstrated in controlled clinical trials. Azithromycin treatment was found to be effective in some studies (children and patients with chronic cryptosporidiosis), whereas other studies reported no significant response. Clarithromycin and rifabutin, alone or in combination, showed some efficacy as prophylactic agents, and a decrease in the risk of cryptosporidiosis was observed. Paromomycin, an aminoglycoside antibiotic that is poorly absorbed from the gastrointestinal tract, has been one of the most widely used agents to treat cryptosporidiosis in AIDS patients. Again, results of different trials were inconsistent (9). Here, the main problem is that many patients relapsed after an initial decrease in symptoms (lower frequency of stools and oocyst excretion).

A passive immunotherapy has also been investigated as a possible treatment in immunocompromised patients. It has been shown that for very young animals, which are exposed within hours of birth and typically become infected during the first week of life, a passive immunotherapy via maternal colostrum improves clinical symptoms and reduces oocyst shedding (69). Therefore, the use of bovine colostrum and colostral antibodies (from cows hyperimmunized with *C. parvum* oocysts) and chicken egg yolk antibodies (produced by vaccination of hens with *Cryptosporidium* species antigens and collection of eggs) have been evaluated for the treatment of the disease in humans. Results of these studies were quite variable and ranged from no improvement in clinical signs and parasite burden to resolution of diarrhea and cessation of oocyst shedding in others (69). The prophylactic effect of hyperimmune bovine colostrum was evaluated with 16 healthy adults challenged with *C. parvum*, but no significant difference in the duration and severity of the disease and time of onset of diarrhea was observed between volunteers who received hyperimmune bovine colostrum and those who received a nonfat milk placebo (64).

The advent of HAART has had a remarkable impact on many opportunistic viral, bacterial, and parasitic infections, resulting in a marked reduction in their occurrence and clinical course, at least in developed countries (66). HAART, which is based on a combination of nucleoside and nonnucleoside reverse transcriptase inhibitors and HIV PIs, results in immune restoration, which is characterized by an increase in memory and naïve $CD4^{+}C$ T cells and the recovery of $CD4^{+}C$ lymphocyte reactivity against opportunistic pathogens.

Three PIs, indinavir, saquinavir, and ritonavir, inhibit the development of *C. parvum* in both in vitro and in vivo models, and amprenavir, indinavir, nelfinavir, ritonavir, and saquinavir inhibit the in vitro development of *C. parvum*, suggesting that they exert a direct effect against *C. parvum* aspartyl proteases (66).

In summary, HAART is the treatment of choice for cryptosporidiosis in immunocompromised patients and can be used not only prophylactically but also as a treatment and secondary prophylaxis for established infections. It should, however, be remembered that cryptosporidiosis will remain a major problem for patients failing HAART, for most individuals living with AIDS in developing countries without access to HAART, and for severely malnourished children. Among these immunocompromised persons without the option of an effective treatment for the underlying disease, supportive management, including rehydration therapy, electrolyte replacement, and antimotility agents will remain the only alternatives for care until better drugs emerge.

CONTROL

Preventive measures are by far the most effective approach to control this parasite. Primary control is by limiting the opportunity for fecal-oral transmission, both direct and indirect. Symptom-free subjects not in contact with immunocompromised patients can normally be permitted to work if their hygiene is scrupulous. Spread via fomites is possible, but this route is limited by the susceptibility of oocysts to desiccation. Patients with AIDS are more susceptible to infection with uncommon species or genotypes, and advice may be needed to limit exposure.

Contamination of water supplies is inevitable, even in developed countries, and may be the source of some sporadic cases as well as outbreaks. When a public advisory notice is issued to boil water, raising the water just to boiling point is sufficient. In general, bottled water and water from point-of-use filters are unlikely to contain parasites but may carry an increased bacterial load, the health significance of which is uncertain for the immunocompromised. Patients with AIDS and others who are profoundly compromised should be advised never to drink water that has not been boiled or filtered through a suitable device. Users of filters should remember that these devices may concentrate potential pathogens and care is needed in replacing and disposing of filter elements.

Hospitals involved in the care of profoundly immunocompromised patients should be particularly vigilant in the management of patients with cryptosporidiosis. Long-term arrangements should be made for the provision of safe water for the immunocompromised to avoid difficulties when a notice to boil water is issued.

It is important, however, to remember that evidence for the effectiveness and cost-effectiveness of preventive interventions is lacking, as extensively discussed in a recent review (2). The paucity of evidence for an effective intervention also means that the published practice guidelines for the prevention and treatment of cryptosporidiosis rely mostly on studies that are of poor quality.

REFERENCES

1. **Abdo, A., J. Klassen, S. Urbanski, E. Raber, and M. G. Swain.** 2003. Reversible sclerosing cholangitis secondary to cryptosporidiosis in a renal transplant patient. *J. Hepatol.* **38:**688–691.
2. **Abubakar, I., S. H. Aliyu, C. Arumugam, P. R. Hunter, and N. K. Usman.** 2007. Prevention and treatment of cryptosporidiosis in immunocompromised patients. *Cochrane Database Syst. Rev.* **1:**CD004932.
3. **Adams, E. J., L. S. Stephenson, M. C. Latham, and S. N. Kinoti.** 1994. Physical activity and growth of Kenyan school children with hookworm, *Trichuris trichiura* and *Ascaris lumbricoides* infections are improved after treatment with albendazole. *J. Nutr.* **124:**1199–1206.
4. **Arslan, H., E. K. Inci, O. K. Azap, H. Karakayali, A. Torgay, and M. Haberal.** 2007. Etiologic agents of diarrhea in solid organ recipients. *Transpl. Infect. Dis.* **9:**270–275.
5. **Beaugerie, L., F. Carbonnel, F. Carrat, A. A. Rached, C. Maslo, J. P. Gendre, W. Rozenbaum, and J. Cosnes.** 1998. Factors of weight loss in patients with HIV and chronic diarrhea. *J. Acquir. Immune Defic. Syndr. Hum. Retrovirol.* **19:**34–39.
6. **Berkman, D. S., A. G. Lescano, R. H. Gilman, S. L. Lopez, and M. M. Black.** 2002. Effects of stunting, diarrhoeal disease, and parasitic infection during infancy on cognition in late childhood: a follow-up study. *Lancet* **359:**564–571.
7. **Brown, J. L., and E. Pollitt.** 1996. Malnutrition, poverty and intellectual development. *Sci. Am.* **274:**38–43.
8. **Bushen, O. Y., A. Kohli, R. C. Pinkerton, K. Dupnik, R. D. Newman, C. L. Sears, R. Fayer, A. A. Lima, and R. L. Guerrant.** 2007. Heavy cryptosporidial infections in children in northeast Brazil: comparison of *Cryptosporidium hominis* and *Cryptosporidium parvum*. *Trans. R. Soc. Trop. Med. Hyg.* **101:**378–384.
9. **Cacciò, S. M., and E. Pozio.** 2006. Advances in the epidemiology, diagnosis and treatment of cryptosporidiosis. *Expert Rev. Anti Infect. Ther.* **4:**429–443.
10. **Cacciò, S. M., R. C. Thompson, J. McLauchlin, and H. V. Smith.** 2005. Unravelling *Cryptosporidium* and *Giardia* epidemiology. *Trends Parasitol.* **21:**430–437.
11. **Cacciò, S. M.** 2005. Molecular epidemiology of human cryptosporidiosis. *Parassitologia* **47:**185–192.
12. **Call, S. A., G. Heudebert, M. Saag, and C. M. Wilcox.** 2000. The changing etiology of chronic diarrhea in HIV-infected patients with CD4 cell counts less than 200 cells/mm^3. *Am. J. Gastroenterol.* **95:**3142–3146.
13. **Calzetti, C., G. Magnani, D. Confalonieri, A. Capelli, S. Moneta, P. Scognamiglio, and F. Fiaccadori.** 1997. Pancreatite da *Cryptosporidium parvum* in pazienti con grave deficit immunitario correlato ad infezione da HIV. *Ann. Ital. Med. Int.* **12:**63–66.
14. **Cama, V. A., J. M. Ross, S. Crawford, V. Kawai, R. Chavez-Valdez, D. Vargas, A. Vivar, E. Ticona, M. Navincopa, J. Williamson, Y. Ortega, R. H. Gilman, C. Bern, and L. Xiao.** 2007. Differences in clinical manifestations among *Cryptosporidium* species and subtypes in HIV-infected persons. *J. Infect. Dis.* **195:**684–691.
15. **Campos, M., E. Jouzdani, C. Sempoux, J. P. Buts, R. Reding, J. B. Otte, and E. M. Sokal.** 2000. Sclerosing cholangitis associated to cryptosporidiosis in liver-transplanted children. *Eur. J. Pediatr.* **159:**113–115.
16. **Carr, A., D. Marriott, A. Field, E. Vasak, and D. A. Cooper.** 1998. Treatment of HIV-1-associated microsporidiosis and cryptosporidiosis with combination antiretroviral therapy. *Lancet* **351:**256–261.
17. **Cegielski, J. P., Y. R. Ortega, S. McKee, J. F. Madden, L. Gaido, D. A. Schwartz, K. Manji, A. F. Jorgensen, S. E. Miller, U. P. Pulipaka, A. E. Msengi, D. H. Mwakyusa, C. R. Sterling, and L. B. Reller.** 1999. *Cryptosporidium*, *Enterocytozoon*, and *Cyclospora* infections in pediatric and adult patients with diarrhea in Tanzania. *Clin. Infect. Dis.* **28:**314–321.
18. **Chappel, C. L., P. C. Okhuysen, and A. C. White, Jr.** 2003. *Cryptosporidium parvum*: infectivity, pathogenesis and the host-parasite relationship, p. 19–49. *In* R.C.A Thompson, A. Arnason, and U. M. Ryan (ed.), *Cryptosporidium: from Molecules to Disease*. Elsevier Press, Amsterdam, The Netherlands.
19. **Checkley, W., L. D. Epstein, R. H. Gilman, R. E. Black, L. Cabrera, and C. R. Sterling.** 1998. Effects of *Cryptosporidium parvum* infection in Peruvian children: growth faltering and subsequent catch-up growth. *Am. J. Epidemiol.* **148:**497–506.
20. **Checkley, W., R. H. Gilman, L. D. Epstein, M. Suarez, J. F. Diaz, L. Cabrera, R. E. Black, and C. R. Sterling.** 1997. Asymptomatic and symptomatic cryptosporidiosis: their acute effect on weight gain in Peruvian children. *Am. J. Epidemiol.* **145:**156–163.
21. **Cicirello, H. G., K. S. Kehl, D. G. Addiss, M. J. Chusid, R. I. Glass, J. P. Davis, and P. L. Havens.** 1997. Cryptosporidiosis in children during a massive waterborne outbreak in Milwaukee, Wisconsin: clinical, laboratory and epidemiologic findings. *Epidemiol. Infect.* **19:**53–60.
22. **Clavel, A., A. C. Arnal, E. C. Sanchez, J. Cuesta, S. Letona, J. A. Amiguet, F. J. Castillo, M. Varea, and R. Gomez-Lus.** 1996. Respiratory cryptosporidiosis: case series and review of the literature. *Infection* **24:**341–346.
23. **Colford, J. M., Jr., I. B. Tager, A. M. Hirozawa, G. F. Lemp, T. Aragon T, and C. Petersen.** 1996. Cryptosporidiosis among patients infected with human immunodeficiency virus. Factors related to symptomatic infection and survival. *Am. J. Epidemiol.* **144:**807–816.
24. **Collins, C. D., C. Blanshard, M. Cramp, B. Gazzard, and J. A. Gleeson.** 1992. Case report: pneumatosis intestinalis occurring in association with cryptosporidiosis and HIV infection. *Clin. Radiol.* **46:**410–411.
25. **Connolly, K. J., and J. D. Kvalsvig.** 1993. Infection, nutrition and cognitive performance in children. *Parasitology* **107:**187–200.
26. **Conti, S., M. Masocco, P. Pezzotti, V. Toccaceli, M. Vichi, S. Boros, R. Urciuoli, C. Valdarchi, and G. Rezza.** 2000. Differential impact of combined antiretroviral therapy on the survival of Italian patients with specific AIDS-defining illnesses. *J. Acquir. Immune Defic. Syndr.* **25:**451–458.
27. **Datta, D, B. Gazzard, and J. Stebbing.** 2003. The diagnostic yield of stool analysis in 525 HIV-1-infected individuals. *AIDS* **17:**1711–1713.
28. **Dillingham, R. A., A. A. Lima, and R. L. Guerrant.** 2002. Cryptosporidiosis: epidemiology and impact. *Microbes Infect.* **4:**1059–1066.
29. **Fayer, R.** 2003. *Cryptosporidium*: from molecules to disease, p. 11–18. *In* R. C. A. Thompson, A. Arnason, and U. M. Ryan (ed.), *Cryptosporidium: from Molecules to Disease*, Elsevier Press, Amsterdam, The Netherlands.
30. **Forbes, A., C. Blanshard, and B. Gazzard.** 1993. Natural history of AIDS related sclerosing cholangitis: a study of 20 cases. *Gut* **34:**116–121.
31. **Garone, M. A., B. J. Winston, and J. H. Lewis.** 1986. Cryptosporidiosis of the stomach. *Am. J. Gastroenterol.* **81:**465–470.
32. **Gerber, D. A., M. Green, R. Jaffe, D. Greenberg, G. Mazariegos, and J. Reyes.** 2000. Cryptosporidial infections after

solid organ transplantation in children. *Pediatr. Transplant.* **4**:50–55.

33. **Godwin, T. A.** 1991. Cryptosporidiosis in the acquired immunodeficiency syndrome: a study of 15 autopsy cases. *Hum. Pathol.* **22**:1215–1224.
34. **Gomez Morales, M. A., C. M. Ausiello, A. Guarino, F. Urbani, M. I. Spagnuolo, C. Pignata, and E. Pozio.** Severe, protracted intestinal cryptosporidiosis associated with interferon gamma deficiency: pediatric case report. *Clin. Infect. Dis.*, **22**:848–850.
35. **Gomez Morales, M. A., C. M. Ausiello, F. Urbani, and E. Pozio.** 1995. Crude extract and recombinant protein of *Cryptosporidium parvum* oocysts induce proliferation of human peripheral blood mononuclear cells in vitro. *J. Infect. Dis.* **172**:211–216.
36. **Grube, H., B. Ramratnam, C. Ley, and T, P. Flanigan.** 1997. Resolution of AIDS associated cryptosporidiosis after treatment with indinavir. *Am. J. Gastroenterol.* **92**:726.
37. **Guarino, A., A. Castaldo, S. Russo, M. I. Spagnolo, R. B. Canani, L. Tarallo, L. Di Benedetto, and A. Rubino.** 1997. Enteric cryptosporidiosis in pediatric HIV-infection. *J. Pediatr. Gastroenterol. Nutr.* **25**:182–187.
38. **Guerrant, D. I., S. R. Moore, A. A. Lima, P. D. Patrick, J. B. Schorling, and R. L. Guerrant.** 1999. Association of early childhood diarrhea and cryptosporidiosis with impaired physical fitness and cognitive function four-seven years later in a poor urban community in northeast Brazil. *Am. J. Trop. Med. Hyg.* **61**:707–713.
39. **Hayward, A. R., J. Levy, F. Facchetti, L. Notarangelo, H. D. Ochs, A. Etzioni, J. Y. Bonnefoy, M. Cosyns, and A. Weinberg.** 1997. Cholangiopathy and tumors of the pancreas, liver and biliary tree in boys with hyper IgM. *J. Immunol.* **158**:977–983.
40. **Hong, D. K., C. J. Wong, and K. Gutierrez.** 2007. Severe cryptosporidiosis in a seven-year-old renal transplant recipient. Case report and review of the literature. *Pediatr. Transplant.* **11**:94–100.
41. **Hunter, P. R., S. Hughes, S. Woodhouse, N. Raj, Q. Syed, R. M. Chalmers, N. Q. Verlander, and J. Goodacre.** 2004. Health sequelae of human cryptosporidiosis in immunocompetent patients. *Clin. Infect. Dis.* **39**:504–510.
42. **Hunter P. R., and G. Nichols.** 2002. Epidemiology and clinical features of *Cryptosporidium* infection in immunocompromised patients. *Clin. Microbiol. Rev.* **15**:145–154.
43. **Iribarren, J. A., A. Castiella, C. Lobo, P. Lopez, M. A. von Wichmann, J. Arrizabalaga, F. J. Rodriguez-Arrondo, and L. F. Alzate.** 1997. AIDS associated cryptosporidiosis with antral narrowing. A new case. *J. Clin. Gastroenterol.* **25**:693–694.
44. **Javier Enriquez, F., C. R. Avila, J. Ignacio Santos, J. Tanaka-Kido, O. Vallejo, and C. R. Sterling.** 1997. *Cryptosporidium* infections in Mexican children: clinical, nutritional, enteropathogenic, and diagnostic evaluations. *Am. J. Trop. Med. Hyg.* **56**:254–257.
45. **Kazlow, P. G., K. Shah, K. J. Benkov, R. Dische, and N. S. LeLeiko.** 1986. Esophageal cryptosporidiosis in a child with acquired immune deficiency syndrome. *Gastroenterology* **91**:1301–1303.
46. **Keusch, G. T.** 2003. The history of nutrition: malnutrition, infection and immunity. *J. Nutr.* **133**:336S–340S.
47. **Kirkpatrick, B. D., C. D. Huston, D. Wagner, F. Noel, P. Rouzier, J. W. Pape, G. Bois, C. J. Larsson, W. K. Alston, K. Tenney, C. Powden, J. P. O'Neill, and C. L. Sears.** 2006. Serum mannose-binding lectin deficiency is associated with cryptosporidiosis in young Haitian children. *Clin. Infect. Dis.* **43**:289–294.
48. **Lopez-Velez, R., R. Tarazona, A. Garcia Camacho, E. Gomez-Mampaso, A. Guerrero, V. Moreira, and R. Villanueva.** 1995. Intestinal and extraintestinal cryptosporidiosis in AIDS patients. *Eur. J. Clin. Microbiol. Infect. Dis.* **14**:677–681.
49. **MacKenzie, W. R., W. L. Schell, K. A. Blair, D. G. Addiss, D. E. Peterson, N. J. Hoxie, J. J. Kazmierczak, and J. P. Davis.** 1995 Massive outbreak of waterborne *Cryptosporidium* infection in Milwaukee, Wisconsin: recurrence of illness and risk of secondary transmission. *Clin. Infect. Dis.* **21**:57–62.
50. **Maggi, P., A. M. Larocca, N. Ladisa, S. Carbonara, O. Brandonisio, G. Angarano, and G. Pastore.** 2001. Opportunistic parasitic infections of the intestinal tract in the era of highly active antiretroviral therapy: is the $CD4^+$ count so important? *Clin. Infect. Dis.* **33**:1609–1611.
51. **Manz, M., and M. Steuerwald.** 2007. Cryptosporidiosis in a patient on PEG interferon and ribavirin for recurrent hepatitis C after living donor liver transplantation. *Transpl. Infect. Dis.* **9**:60–61.
52. **Marion, R., A. Baishanbo, G. Gargala, A. François, P. Ducrotté, C. Duclos, J. Fioramonti, J. J. Ballet, and L. Favennec.** 2006. Transient neonatal *Cryptosporidium parvum* infection triggers long-term jejunal hypersensitivity to distension in immunocompetent rats. *Infect. Immun.* **74**:4387–4389.
53. **McLauchlin J., C. F. Amar, S. Pedraza-Díaz, G. Mieli-Vergani, N. Hadzic, and E. G. Davies.** 2003. Polymerase chain reaction-based diagnosis of infection with *Cryptosporidium* in children with primary immunodeficiencies. *Pediatr. Infect. Dis. J.* **22**:329–335.
54. **Mead, J. R.** 2002. Cryptosporidiosis and the challenges of chemotherapy. *Drug Resist. Updat.* **5**:47–57.
55. **Mendez, M. A., and L. S. Adair.** 1999. Severity and timing of stunting in the first two years of life affect performance on cognitive tests in late childhood. *J. Nutr.* **129**:1555–1562.
56. **Miao, Y. M., F. M. Awad-El-Kariem, C. Franzen, D. S. Ellis, A. Müller, H. M. Counihan, P. J. Hayes, and B. G. Gazzard.** 2000. Eradication of cryptosporidia and microsporidia following successful antiretroviral therapy. *J. Acquir. Immune Defic. Syndr.* **25**:124–129.
57. **Molbak, K., M. Andersen, P. Aaby, N. Hojlyng, M. Jakobsen, M. Sodemann, and A. P. da Silva.** 1997. *Cryptosporidium* infection in infancy as a cause of malnutrition: a community study from Guinea-Bissau, West Africa. *Am. J. Clin. Nutr.* **65**:149–152.
58. **Mönkemüller, K. E., S. A. Call, A. J. Lazenby, and C. M. Wilcox.** 2000. Declining prevalence of opportunistic gastrointestinal disease in the era of combination antiretroviral therapy. *Am. J. Gastroenterol.* **95**:457–462.
59. **Moon, A., W. Spivak, and L. J. Brandt.** 1999. *Cryptosporidium*-induced gastric obstruction in a child with congenital HIV infection: case report and review of the literature. *J. Pediatr. Gastroenterol. Nutr.* **28**:108–111.
60. **Neira, P., M. T. Tardío, M. Carabelli, and L. Villalón.** 1989. Cryptosporidiosis in the V Region Chile: III. Study of malnourished patients, 1985-87. *Bol. Chil. Parasitol.* **44**:34–36.
61. **Niehaus, M. D., S. R. Moore, P. D. Patrick, L. L. Derr, B. Lorntz, A. A. Lima, and R. L. Guerrant.** 2002. Early childhood diarrhea is associated with diminished cognitive function 4 to 7 years later in children in a northeast Brazilian shantytown. *Am. J. Trop. Med. Hyg.* **66**:590–593.
62. **Nokes, C., S. M. Grantham-McGregor, A. W. Sawyer, E. S. Cooper, B. A. Robinson, and D. A. Bundy. 1994.** Parasitic helminth infection and cognitive function in school children. *Parasitology* **104**:539–547.
63. **Oberhuber, G., E. Lauer, M. Stolte, and F. Borchard.** 1991. Cryptosporidiosis of the appendix vermiformis: a case report. *Z. Gastroenterol.* **29**:606–608.

64. **Okhuysen, P. C., C. L. Chappell, J. Crabb, L. M. Valdez, E. T. Douglass, and H. L. DuPont.** 1998. Prophylactic effect of bovine anti-*Cryptosporidium* hyperimmune colostrum immunoglobulin in healthy volunteers challenged with *Cryptosporidium parvum*. *Clin. Infect. Dis.* **26:**1324–1329.

65. **Powell, C. A., S. P. Walker, J. H. Himes, P. D. Fletcher, and S. M. Grantham-McGregor.** 1995. Relationships between physical growth, mental development and nutritional supplementation in stunted children: the Jamaican study. *Acta Paediatr.* **84:**22–29.

66. **Pozio E., and M. A. Gomez Morales.** 2005. The impact of HIV-protease inhibitors on opportunistic parasites. *Trends Parasitol.* **21:**58–63.

67. **Pozio, E., F. Rivasi, and S. M. Cacciò.** 2004. Infection with *Cryptosporidium hominis* and reinfection with *Cryptosporidium parvum* in a transplanted ileum. *APMIS* **112:**309–313.

68. **Pozio, E., G. Rezza, A. Boschini, P. Pezzotti, A. Tamburrini, P. Rossi, M. Di Fine, C. Smacchia, A. Schiesari, E. Gattei, R. Zucconi, and P. Ballerini.** 1997. Clinical cryptosporidiosis and HIV-induced immunosuppression: findings from a longitudinal study of HIV-positive and negative former drug users. *J. Infect. Dis.* **176:**969–975.

69. **Riggs, M. W.** 2002. Recent advances in cryptosporidiosis: the immune response. *Microbes Infect.* **4:**1067–1080.

70. **Rodrigues, F., E. G. Davies, P. Harrison, J. McLauchlin, J. Karani, B. Portmann, A. Jones, P. Veys, G. Mieli-Vergani, and N. Hadzić.** 2004. Liver disease in children with primary immunodeficiencies. *J. Pediatr.* **145:**333–339.

71. **Rossi. P., F. Rivasi, M. Codeluppi, A. Catania, A. Tamburrini, E. Righi, and E. Pozio.** 1998. Gastric involvement in AIDS-associated cryptosporidiosis. *Gut* **43:**476–477.

72. **Samson, V. E., and W. R. Brown.** 1996. Pneumatosis cystoides intestinalis in AIDS-associated cryptosporidiosis. More than an incidental finding? *J. Clin. Gastroenterol.* **22:**311–312.

73. **Schmidt, W., U. Wahnschaffe, M. Schäfer, T. Zippel, M. Arvand, A. Meyerhans, E.O. Riecken, and R. Ullrich.** 2001. Rapid increase of mucosal CD4 T cells followed by clearance of intestinal cryptosporidiosis in an AIDS patient receiving highly active antiretroviral therapy. *Gastroenterology* **120:**984–987.

74. **Sidhu, S., S. Flamm, and S. Chopra.** 1994. Pneumatosis cystoides intestinalis: an incidental finding in a patient with AIDS and cryptosporidial diarrhea. *Am. J. Gastroenterol.* **89:**1578–1579.

75. **Stephenson, L. S., M. C. Latham, E. J. Adams, S. N. Kinoti, and A. Pertet.** 1993. Physical fitness, growth and appetite of Kenyan school children with hookworm, *Trichuris trichiura* and *Ascaris lumbricoides* infections are improved four months after a single dose of albendazole. *J. Nutr.* **123:**1036–1046.

76. **Thompson, R. C., M. E. Olson, G. Zhu, S. Enomoto, M. S. Abrahamsen, and N. S. Hijjawi.** 2005. *Cryptosporidium* and cryptosporidiosis. *Adv. Parasitol.* **59:**77–158.

77. **Toniati P., S. Giliani, A. Jones, G. de Saint Basile, P. Airo, G. Savoldi, M. Vihinen, and L. D. Notarangelo.** 2002. Report of the ESID collaborative study on clinical features and molecular analysis of X-linked hyper-IgM syndrome. *Eur. Soc. Immunodeficiencies Newsl.* **F9**(Suppl):40.

78. **Vakil, N. B., S. M. Schwartz, B. P. Buggy, C. F. Brummitt, M. Kherellah, D. M. Letzer, I. H. Gilson, and P. G. Jones.** 1996. Biliary cryptosporidiosis in HIV-infected people after the waterborne outbreak of cryptosporidiosis in Milwaukee. *N. Engl. J. Med.* **334:**19–23.

79. **White, C. A., Jr.** 2004. Nitazoxanide: a new broad spectrum antiparasitic agent. *Expert Rev. Anti Infect. Ther.* **2:**43–49.

80. **Wolska-Kusnierz, B., A. Bajer, S. M. Cacciò, E. Heropolitanska-Pliszka, E. Bernatowska, P. Socha, J. van Dongen, M. Bednarska, A. Paziewska, and E. Sinski.** 2007. *Cryptosporidium* infection in patients with primary immunodeficiencies. *J. Pediatr. Gastroenterol. Nutr.* **45:**458–464.

81. **Xiao, L., R. Fayer, U. Ryan, and S. J. Upton.** 2004. *Cryptosporidium* taxonomy: recent advances and implications for public health. *Crit. Rev. Microbiol.* **17:**72–97.

Sequelae and Long-Term Consequences of Infectious Diseases
Edited by Pina M. Fratamico, James L. Smith, and Kim A. Brogden

Chapter 15

Malaria

DAVID J. SULLIVAN, JR., AND NISHIENA GANDHI

CHARACTERISTICS OF *PLASMODIUM*

Malaria is classically known as a disease of fever, anemia, and splenomegaly, with clinical descriptions dating back 6,000 years (55). Protozoan *Plasmodium* species are apicomplexans named for the apical bodies or complexes specialized for invasion (5). Other pathogenic apicomplexans include *Toxoplasma gondii*, which as a single species is able to invade any cell type of almost any mammal; *Babesia*, which like *Plasmodium*, invades and thrives in erythrocytes; and *Cryptosporidium*, confined to the intestinal tract, which invades just beneath the surface of intestinal epithelium (67). *Plasmodium* species have distinct stages which invade hepatocytes, erythrocytes, mosquito intestinal cells, and salivary glands (77). The erythrocytic stage of *Plasmodium* is associated with the clinical signs and symptoms of malaria (124). The liver stage is completely asymptomatic, and there is debate whether mosquito stages alter fitness or survival in the mosquito (103).

There are over 100 species of *Plasmodium* which infect mammals, like mice (16), humans, and primates; birds, like ravens (73), canaries (119, 138), and penguins translocated to temperate zones (29); and reptiles, like snakes, lizards, and turtles (125, 126). Most species are unique to individual intermediate hosts, with the ubiquitous *Anopheles* female mosquito as the definitive host. As shown in Color Plate 8, in humans, infection begins with a mosquito bite delivering hundreds of sporozoites into the dermis. Then, tens of sporozoites enter the bloodstream via lymphatics and target the liver, where only a few cross the Kuppfer cells to reside in single heptocytes. In human malarias, approximately a week transpires in which the *Plasmodium* parasite produces thousands of progeny called merozoites (100). After release from the hepatocyte, the merozoites invade erythrocytes to begin a typically 48-h cycle defined by morphology into three stages: (i) the ring stage (like a signet ring); (ii) the trophozoite stage, which contains, as seen by light microscopy, the birefringent heme crystal, hemozoin; and (iii) the schizont stage, which has more than a single nucleus. (Schizogony, which refers to a type of nuclear division before cellular division, is also typical of *Toxoplasma* and *Babesia*.) The progeny merozoites reinvade additional erythrocytes, with a typical multiplication rate of approximately 10-fold per 48 h for *Plasmodium falciparum*. At this rate, the 10,000 merozoites released from the liver will multiply to 100 million in typically 8 days and to almost a trillion by 2 weeks. The *Plasmodium* parasites are entirely confined to the bloodstream, bone marrow, and spleen (77). They do not survive in tissues without a source of erythrocytes. Less than 1 out of 1,000 progeny will differentiate into male and female gametocytes, which are infective solely for the mosquito. In the case of ingestion of a blood meal without gametocytes, the parasite is unable to complete development in the mosquito (69). The protozoan *Plasmodium* parasites are haploid for their entire human life cycle, with sex, diploidy, and meiosis occurring in a brief interval in the definitive host of the female mosquito stomach (69). After the male gamete fertilizes the female gamete, the new zygote transforms into an ookinete which is capable of penetrating through a chitin-containing peritrophic matrix to cross the stomach epithelium and reside on or just within the basement membrane. The ookinete transforms into an oocyst which produces thousands of sporozoites that migrate and invade the salivary glands of the mosquito, ready to begin the cycle again (50, 133).

Principally four *Plasmodium* species infect and cause disease in humans, as shown in Color Plate 9.

David J. Sullivan, Jr. • Malaria Research Institute, Department of Molecular Microbiology and Immunology, Johns Hopkins University Bloomberg School of Public Health, Baltimore, MD 21205. **Nishiena Gandhi** • Department of Neurology/Neurosurgery, Johns Hopkins University School of Medicine, Baltimore, MD 21205.

Plasmodium malariae has a 72-h cycle in predominately older erythrocytes (25); *Plasmodium vivax* and *Plasmodium ovale* invade predominately reticulocytes with a 48-h cycle. They also have a hypnozoite stage in the liver, in which after sporozoite invasion, instead of replicating, the parasite lies dormant for weeks or months before commencement of nuclear multiplication. This late relapse into the bloodstream results in disease months or even years after the initial mosquito bite (53). *P. falciparum* can invade erythrocytes of all ages with a 48-h cycle and can reach high parasitemia. This is the species which causes most of the 1 to 2 million deaths each year (47, 49). *Plasmodium knowlesi*, a monkey species, has been identified on the basis of PCR to cause malaria cases in East Asia (27, 28, 63, 135, 137). This fifth human *Plasmodium* parasite is similar in morphology to *P. malariae*.

The genome of the most lethal human species, *P. falciparum*, along with that of murine malaria *Plasmodium yoelii*, was completed initially (16, 44). Genome sequences are largely available also for *P. vivax*. *P. falciparum* has 14 chromosomes with 23 Mb of DNA. The average gene size is approximately 2 kb, yielding approximately 5,300 open reading frames, which approximates the number of genes in yeast. More than half of the genome remains hypothetical. *P. falciparum* genes also typically have 0.5 to 1 kb of 5'or 3' untranslated regions flanking the genes. *P. falciparum* is very adenine- and thymine-rich, with almost 80% adenine-thymine content in exons and more than 90% within intergenic regions (44). However some other *Plasmodium* species, like *P. vivax*, have 60 to 70% adenine-thymine content. *Plasmodium* species have extrachromosomal DNA associated with the mitochondrion and apicoplast organelles.

Plasmodium has a single acristate mitochondrion necessary for heme synthesis and possible fatty acid metabolism (5, 127, 128). Energy production in erythrocytes is almost entirely from glycolysis. The intraerythrocytic *Plasmodium* ingests more than 75% of host cell hemoglobin as a source of amino acids and possibly effects a volume reduction (124). Interestingly, *Plasmodium* species have a plant-like, chloroplast-like organelle called the apicoplast, which is also single in number and localizes along with, but is separate from, the mitochondrion. In *Plasmodium* species, the apicoplast is surrounded by four membranes (139). The apicoplast functions in fatty acid synthesis, heme biosynthesis, and other essential, but undefined, functions (40). An additional organelle is the acidic lysosome-like digestive vacuole, where almost 75% of host erythrocyte hemoglobin is degraded into peptides by hemoglobinases, plasmepsins (aspartic proteases), and falcipains (cysteine proteases) (42, 45). The liberated heme is not degraded by heme oxygenase to yield carbon monoxide, iron, and biliverdin, but instead, the reactive heme species forms head-to-tail reciprocal dimers which crystallize into large 100- by 100- by 500-nm structures called hemozoin (85, 91). This unique intracellular crystallization prevents the reactive heme from inhibiting enzymes, damaging membranes, or producing oxygen radicals (106). Heme crystallization is the target of the widely used quinolines, like chloroquine or quinine (10, 95).

Another unique aspect of *P. falciparum* molecular biology is the ability to adhere to endothelial cells (77). The intraerythrocytic parasites send packets of proteins outside of its own plasma membrane, which translocate across the plasma membrane of the erythrocyte to form knobs on the otherwise smooth surface of the erythrocyte (114), as shown in Fig. 1. *P. falciparum* has more than 50 genes in the erythrocyte membrane protein family (123), which have multiple binding domains that attach to endothelial receptors like ICAM1 in the brain (115), chondroitin sulfate in the placenta (131), and CD36 in most other tissues (83). The parasite sticks like velcro in organs, thereby decreasing function. While the other human *Plasmodium* parasites do have *Plasmodium* proteins on the surface of the host erythrocyte, *P. falciparum* is unique in its ability to attach.

DISEASES CAUSED BY *PLASMODIUM*—ACUTE, CHRONIC, AND PERMANENT

Malaria is an acute self-limited disease which is entirely cured by drug treatment. It may persist by continued infective mosquito bites, resulting in chronic parasitemia. Chronic parasitemia causes chronic sequelae or permanently selects for genetic disorders which protect from severe malaria disease but cause other human disease, such as sickle cell anemia.

Acute Febrile Disease

All human *Plasmodium* species can cause cyclical fevers, anemia, and splenomegaly (24, 46). Typical fever curves of tertian malaria, *P. vivax* and *P. ovale*; quartan malaria, *P. malariae*; and aestivo autumnal or quotidian malaria, *P. falciparum*, are shown in Fig. 2. Malaria fevers are often a nonlocalizing, undifferentiated febrile illness similar to influenza or many other viral illnesses (62, 79, 122). Malaria parasitemia with fever often has a mild thrombocytopenia and the absence of eosinophilia in addition

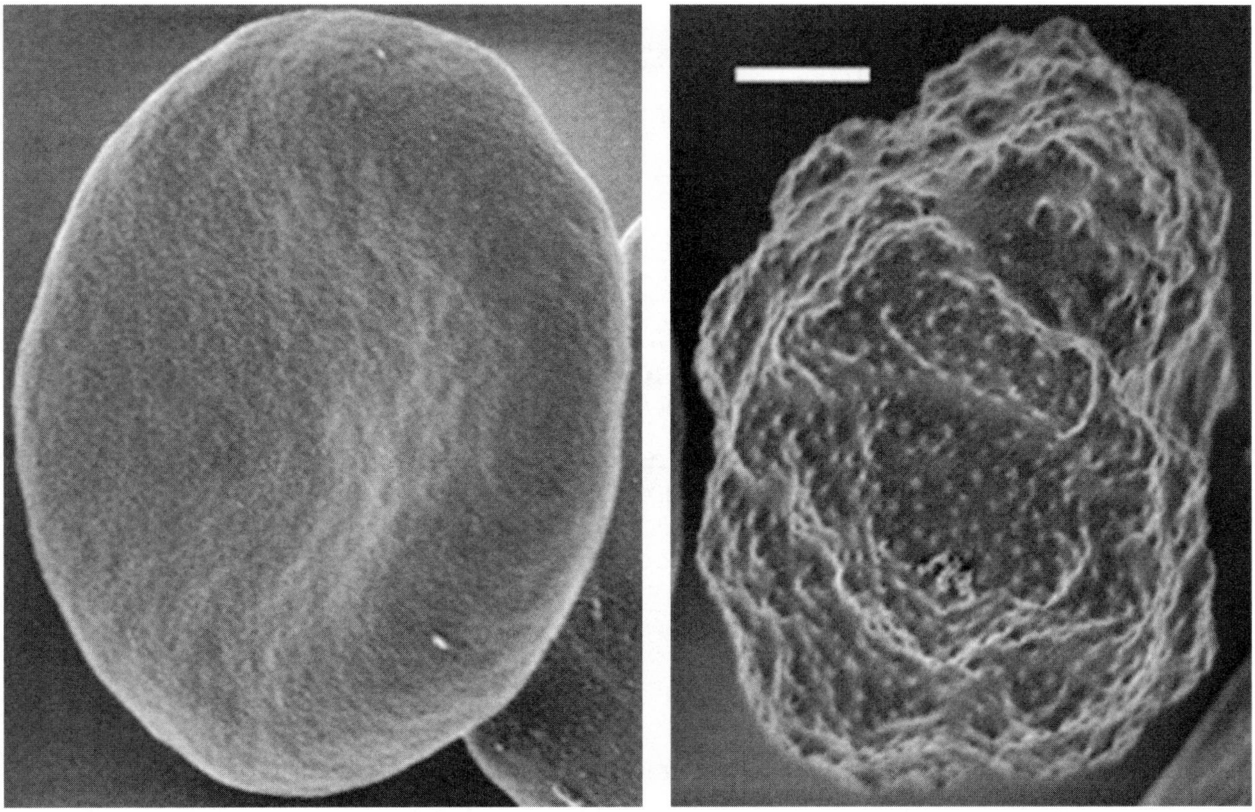

Figure 1. Surface changes of infected trophozoite-stage erythrocyte. The normal erythrocyte (left) has a smooth surface and minimizes its volume with the biconcave disc. In contrast, the infected trophozoite-stage erythrocyte has been transformed to contain knobs which act as ligands to host receptors on endothelial cells or leukocytes.

to mild anemia (46). The typical fever pattern consists of an initial cold stage in which a patient throws on blankets, then a hot stage where blankets are tossed off, and then peak temperature. After the peak temperature is reached, patients will sweat profoundly. Some have described the exhaustion of a malaria fever as similar to running a marathon. Most clinical malaria patients present with a mild splenomegaly, which can increase with chronic parasitemia. Anemia and mild thrombocytopenia are also characteristic. Acute *P. vivax* infection rarely causes death but presents with flu-like symptoms, muscle pains, and fever which are incapacitating for days. Often the patient will feel improved on the nonfebrile days. The rare deaths associated with *P. vivax* are secondary to splenic rupture (71, 146). *P. ovale* is geographically limited to small areas in Africa, with case presentations similar to those of *P. vivax* (8). *P. malariae* infection presents with classic symptoms but often can be asymptomatic or have relatively milder symptoms (25).

P. falciparum, in addition to the classic triad of fever, anemia, and spenomegaly, can cause reversible dysfunction of almost any organ, unless *P. falciparum* malaria progresses to death. Like *Neisseria meningitis* disease, *P. falciparum* malaria is a medical emergency with some patients dying within 24 h of presentation (11, 117). Death from *P. falciparum* malaria is usually associated with delay in patient presentation to healthcare, delay in diagnosis, and delay in initial drug treatment. Death from malaria is caused by severe anemia or cerebral malaria, with the precipitating pathophysiologic lethal event hard to define (57). Severe diseases with high parasitemias present with a reversible renal failure (78), liver dysfunction (68), or depressed myocardial function (46). A lactic acidosis is common (57, 96). *P. falciparum* malaria can also present as pneumonia (35) or gastrointestinal dysfunction with emesis predominating, (118) but also with diarrhea (102). Acute *P. falciparum* malaria is often associated with (12, 145) and/or is confused with acute bacterial sepsis (13).

Epidemiology of Malaria

Reasonable estimates of yearly malaria cases throughout the world number 300 to 500 million (116). Almost a third of the world's population lives in a region where malaria is endemic. Malaria is third behind tuberculosis and human immunodeficiency

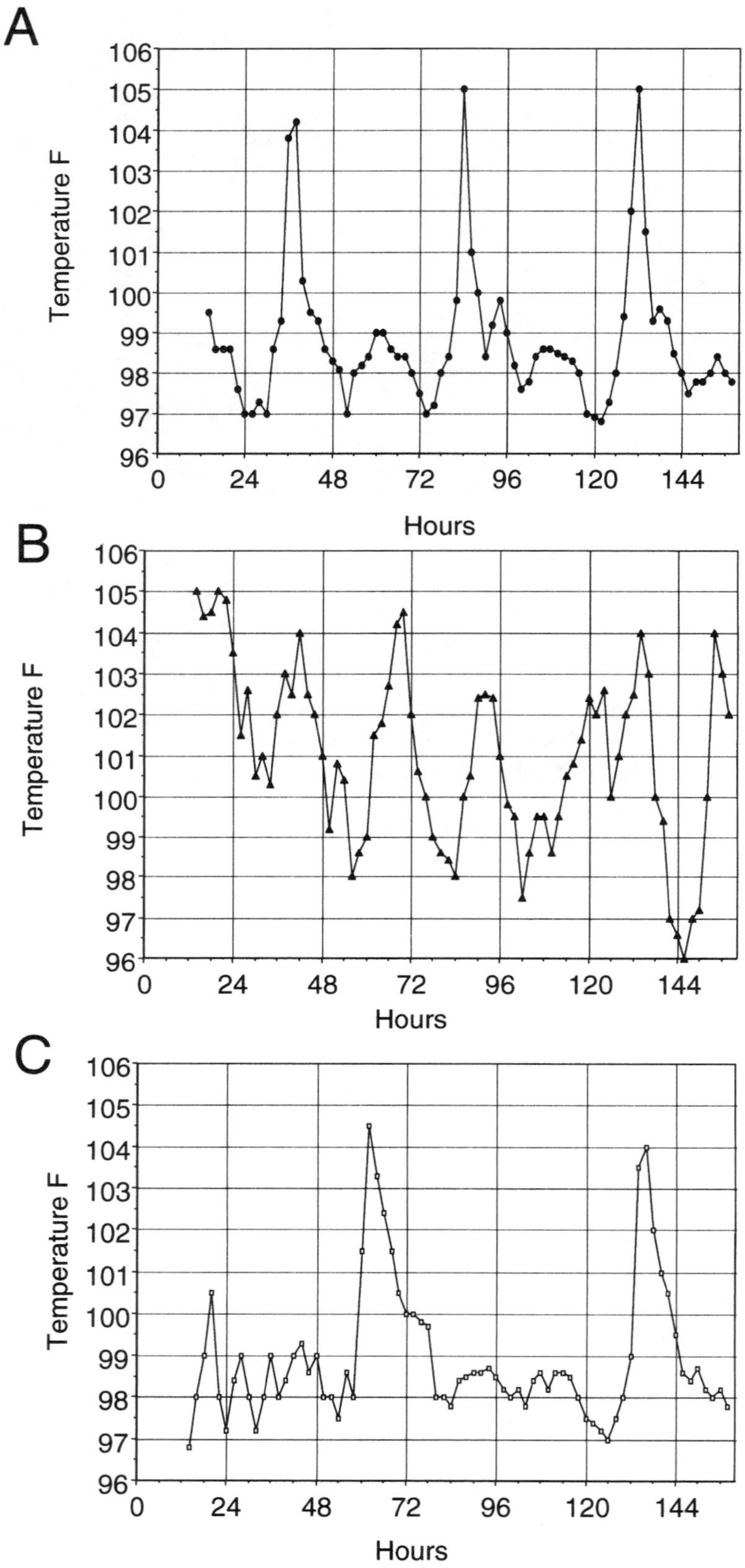

Figure 2. Malaria fever curves. Typical fever curves from patients with *P. vivax* or tertian malaria (A), *P. falciparum* or quotidian malaria (B), and *P. malariae or* quartan malaria (C), with temperatures every 48, 24 and 72 h.

virus as a single infectious disease killer, with 1 to 2 million deaths each year, predominantly in children under age 5 in sub-Saharan Africa (117). A hundred years ago, most of the United States was at risk for malaria, with individual cities such as Baltimore reporting more than a 1,000 cases a year. During the last decade, the United States has reported approximately 1,000 to 1,500 cases each year. The tiny island of Great Britain also reports as many cases of malaria as the United States (Fig. 3).

The Malaria Atlas Project aims "to develop the science of malaria cartography" (52). This needed project is starting on a global country level to map malaria prevalence year to year in an open-source accessible fashion. The data input are parasite prevalence rates based on laboratory diagnosis. The parasite prevalence can vary by age, which requires standardization, usually to prevalence in the 5- to 10-year-old age group (112).

Acute Malaria Anemia

The human *Plasmodium* parasites increase destruction and decrease production of erythrocytes (104). With *P. vivax* and *P. ovale*, which invade reticulocytes alone, peak parasitemia is restricted to 5 to 7%. However, *P. falciparum* can invade erythrocytes of all ages and can reach even past a 50% parasitemia (31, 33). A 10% parasitemia represents 400,000 parasites per ml or 400 million per ml or 400 billion per liter, which amounts to more than 2 trillion erythrocytes in an adult with 5 liters of blood volume. Every 2 days, a sustained 10% parasitemia would destroy a large number of erythrocytes. Also,

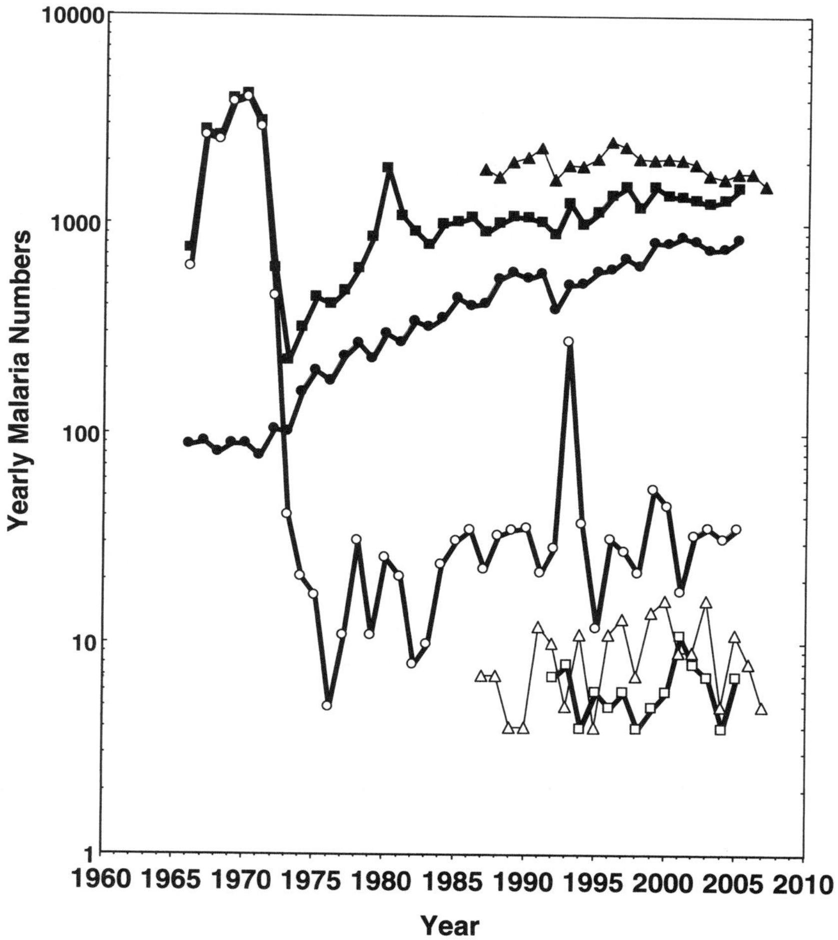

Figure 3. Imported malaria cases in the United States and the United Kingdom from 1966 to 2005. Total number of malaria cases from the United Kingdom (filled triangles) and the United States (filled squares) and total deaths in the United Kingdom (empty triangles) and the United States (empty squares). In the United States, total civilian cases (filled circles) outnumber military cases (empty circles) almost 10-fold.

the high parasite density results in the total biomass of parasite proteins approaching gram quantities per liter of blood (33), in contrast to nanogram quantities of endotoxin, which precipitate shock in bacterial sepsis (61, 72, 130). The enlarged spleen can also trap more erythrocytes. Compounding the anemia, uninfected erythrocytes have been shown to be more rapidly cleared by the spleen during acute malaria. Hydroxynonenal (110) and excess heme (90) have been separately implicated in increasing rigidity of uninfected erythrocytes. Despite mild elevations in erythropoietin, the marrow is unresponsive to erythrocyte production (20, 104). The phenomenon of rosetting infected erythrocytes to uninfected erythrocytes has been associated with severe malaria anemia (21). This rosetting is also mediated by the parasite knob proteins, PfEMP1, which also cause adherence to endothelial beds (83).

Acute Placental Malaria

A specific genotype of the knob proteins called var2CSA mediates binding to the chondroitin sulfate antigen present in high abundance in the placenta (36, 131). A primigravida pregnant women who has semi-immunity to parasites adherent to endothelium in other organs lacks this semiprotection to the parasites capable of binding to the placenta (77). A population of parasites then increases with high avidity to the placenta. This increases risk of severe malaria during pregnancy. Anemia, still births, and decreased birth weight result (64). Placental malaria can occur in up to 40% of pregnancies in endemic areas (121). An underestimated consequence of malaria is placental malaria causing low birth weight. This 1- or 2-kilogram deficit in infants increases morbidity and mortality from diarrhea or respiratory diseases (81).

Acute Cerebral Malaria

The pathogenesis of cerebral malaria is multi-factorial and begins with sequestration of parasitized erythrocytes to brain endothelial cells in postcapillary venules (98). The host immune system may still play a crucial role through cytokines and effector cells, like platelets (74, 120). The respective contribution of each process is still a matter for debate, but cerebral complications may result from concomitant microvessel obstruction, brain endothelial changes, and cytokine or metabolite perturbations. Severe malaria is associated with lactic acidosis 25 to 30% of the time. Lactate concentrations have been positively correlated with recovery time from coma (76). *N*-acetyl aspartate, detectable by magnetic resonance spectroscopy in murine experimental cerebral malaria, is a known marker of neuroglial injury (66, 92, 93, 144). Although a clear idea of the exact underlying mechanisms causing acute injury in cerebral malaria remains to be determined, it must be kept in mind that the majority of patients make a complete recovery, suggesting a largely reversible process in which only in some cases, a persistent neurologic injury produces long-term deficits.

Unfortunately, because most severe malaria cases are far from health centers with access to up-to-date imaging facilities, brain imaging and in particular, magnetic resonance imaging of cerebral malaria has been extremely limited. The few isolated cases of adults with cerebral malaria studied by imaging techniques have shown brain swelling, cortical and subcortical ischemic lesions, central pontine myelinolysis, small hemorrhagic lesions, and focal lesions in the cerebrum and brainstem (26, 43, 70). Although a few revealing studies have been conducted to shed light on the neuropathology of the disease, the subjects have been studied postmortem. It seems safe to assume, however, that some of these processes found to occur in fatal cerebral malaria cases are the same that lead to long-term neurologic sequelae in survivors.

A study by Medana et al. was performed of fatal cases of malaria in Vietnam, in which brain sections were analyzed for axonal injury by quantifying β-amyloid precursor protein (75). Axonal injury disrupts neural integrity and leads to faulty transportation, resulting in the accumulation of β-amyloid protein at axonal terminals. This study showed that both the frequency and extent of axonal injury correlated with patients who had cerebral malaria versus those with noncerebral malaria. Axonal injury was often accompanied by hemorrhages and demyelination. All these processes are potentially reversible and could thus explain a complete recovery as is seen in most cases. Although the axonal injury was diffuse in most cases, in others it showed predominance in the pons and internal capsule.

In addition to postmortem analysis and neuroimaging, cerebral spinal fluid (CSF) is a window for in vivo assessment of the central nervous system environment. In cerebral malaria, routine studies of CSF show no pleocytosis or increase in protein (60, 76). Cytokines are known to be important mediators in the pathogenesis of human malaria, but most studies correlating cytokines or other biomarkers have relied on serological sampling, which is removed from CSF. Other studies on CSF cytokines seem to show contrasting results for the serum levels. However, these previous studies strongly support the hypothesis that neuro-immune pathways are abnormally activated in cerebral malaria, and evaluation of CSF may be an avenue for assessment of neuro-inflammation, despite normal cell counts and protein.

In a study conducted by Dobbie et al. of the CSF of children with cerebral malaria in Kenya, quinolinic acid was found to be largely increased (32). This compound is an endogenous excitotoxin that is a selective agonist for *N*-methyl-D-aspartate glutamate receptors and can cause seizures, reversible neuronal swelling, and delayed neuronal disintegration in experimental animals. In another recent study by John et al., children with cerebral malaria had higher cerebrospinal fluid levels of interleukin (IL)-6, CXCL-8/IL-8, granulocyte-colony stimulating factor, tumor necrosis factor alpha, and IL-1 receptor antagonist. Elevated cerebrospinal fluid tumor necrosis factor alpha levels on admission were associated with an increased risk of neurologic deficits 3 months later and correlated negatively with age-adjusted scores for attention and working memory 6 months later (60).

As is evident from the above, a lot still remains to be learned about the mechanisms of central nervous injury in cerebral malaria. Studies need to be conducted on living patients using both structural and functional magnetic resonance imaging with correlation to cerebrospinal fluid cytokine and chemokine analysis and clinical exam. Additionally, prospective follow-up and repeated analysis using these parameters needs to be performed on those subjects who have known long-term neurologic sequelae.

LONG-TERM CONSEQUENCES ASSOCIATED WITH MALARIA

Because *P. vivax* and *P. ovale* can relapse from the liver, they may be able to cause multiple episodes of cyclic fevers, despite drug treatment targeted to the erythrocytic stages. In travelers returning from malarious regions, *P. vivax* can relapse even a year after exposure to infectious mosquito bites. The CDC has tracked the month of onset in returning travelers by species, showing that almost 80 to 90% of *P. falciparum* presents in the first 2 months, while *P. vivax* is evenly divided in timing of case presentation by monthly intervals up to a year (Fig. 4). Additionally, a case report exists in which a Greek immigrant to the United States, who had not lived for more than 30 years in an area where malaria was endemic, presented with dysplastic marrow. After chemotherapy, *P. malariae* was seen on smears and confirmed by PCR (132). This was believed to be secondary to chronic intermittent parasitemia. *P. malariae* has been additionally associated with a glomerular nephropathy from immune complex disease and focal glomerulosclerosis; however, this is rare (25).

Chronic *P. falciparum* disease results from multiple infective mosquito bites throughout the year ranging from 1 to 10 per year to hundreds per year. *P. falciparum* infections in the blood can persist on average 6 months (111). Severe malaria has an age-dependent incidence depending on intensity of mosquito transmission, also called entomologic inoculation rate (34). In high-transmission areas, children age 1 to 3 have most of the severe anemia, as shown in Fig. 5. Survival past age 5 results in reduced risk of deaths from semi-immunity, but peak parasitemia is actually from age 5 to 10. This translates to the fact that children performing well in school and out playing soccer will have a 60 to 70% rate of positive blood films. In moderate transmission settings, both severe anemia and cerebral malaria afflict young children, with protection from severe disease after age 5. In low transmission settings, both children and adults can present with severe malaria disease (111). Chronic malaria infection is associated with iron deficiency anemia and its associated consequences in development and cognition.

Chronic malaria antigen stimulation of the immune system by persistent parasitemia has been associated with oncogenic translocation by Epstein-Barr virus (EBV) to produce Burkitt's lymphoma. Denis Burkitt in the 1950s observed the frequent occurrence of large tumors of the jaw in areas of Uganda where malaria was holoendemic (14, 15). He shared some of the tumor with Epstein, who isolated the gamma-1 herpesvirus, now known as the Epstein-Barr virus, from all of the tumors. This was the first association of a virus with tumors (9, 65). Endemic Burkitt's lymphoma occurs in areas where malaria is holoendemic, with tumors of the jaw predominating rather than the abdomen, with a 100% association of Epstein-Barr virus. The pathology is the starry sky of monomorphic B cells in the background of macrophages. The tumor has a translocation of the c-myc oncogene to the transcriptional control of the immunoglobulin heavy or light chain. The epidemiology is 5 to 10 per 100,000 amongst children age 3 to 15 (65, 101). While malaria infection has been shown to affect T-cell subset levels, like T-cell receptor gamma omicron, the surface erythrocyte membrane protein CIDR alpha domain has been shown to induce EBV lytic cycles (22). Malaria separately has been shown to increase EBV viral loads (80). In a case control study in Africa, Burkitt's lymphoma was associated with more frequent malaria treatments in a year, and patients were less likely to have a bed net in the home (17, 101).

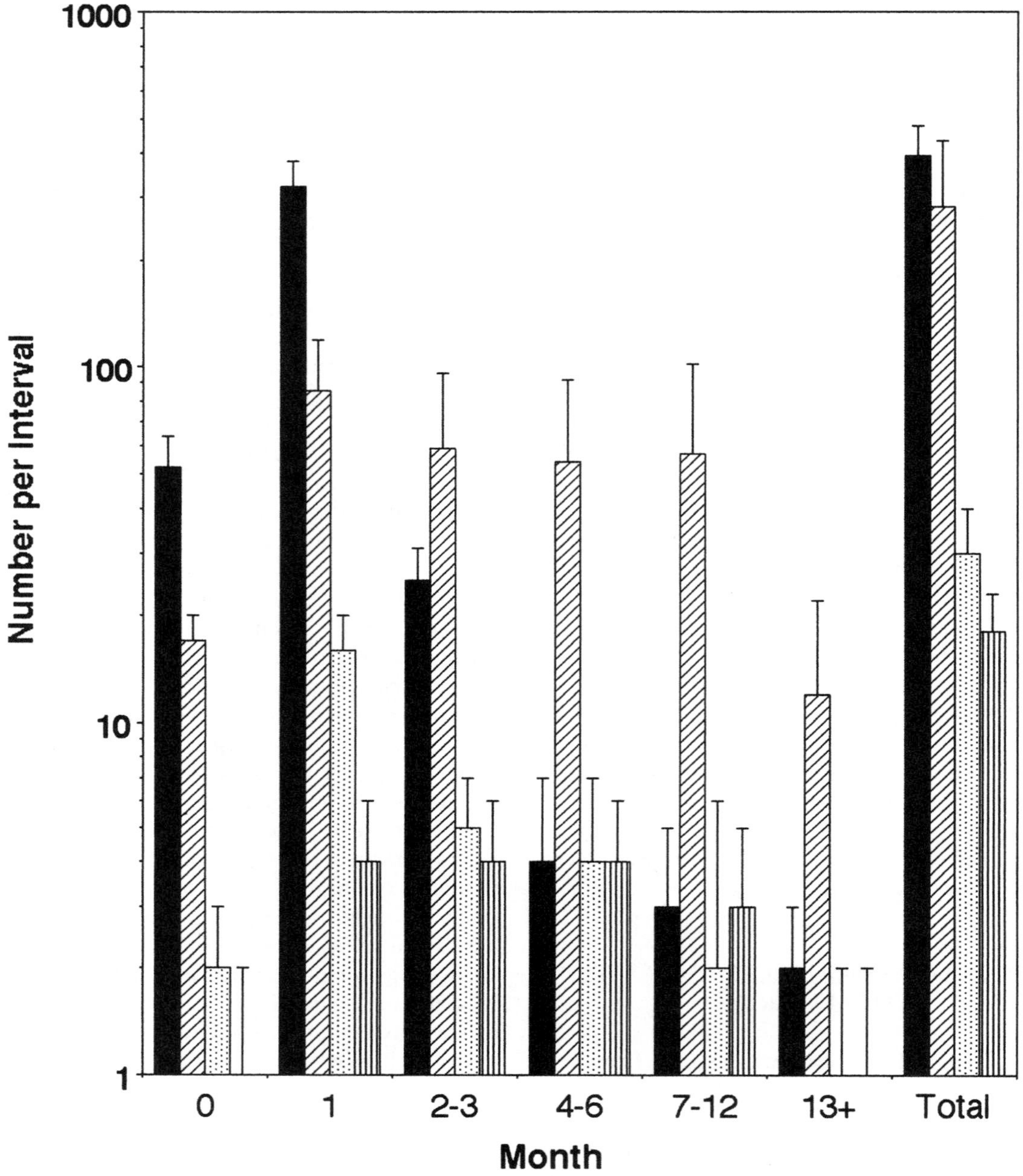

Figure 4. Onset of malaria case presentation, 1992 to 2005. The time to clinical presentation in months after travel by *Plasmodium* species, with *P. falciparum* (solid bar), *P. vivax* (hatched bar), *P. malariae* (stippled bar), and *P. ovale* (vertical bar). Values are averages of 12 years with standard deviations of the means.

Chronic Neurologic Sequelae

Acute seizures in the setting of cerebral malaria and/or as a consequence of high fevers from noncerebral malaria are a well-known and documented presentation of the disease (18, 129). However, although epilepsy has been a suspected long-term consequence of cerebral malaria, only more recently is this being confirmed via organized studies. Unfortunately, due to coinfection with neuro-cysticercosis in many affected populations, it has been difficult to tease out the direct implications of a history of *P. falciparum* infection to the epilepsy. However, data from a study conducted with a population in which cysticercosis was absent due to cultural reasons confirmed that epilepsy is more frequent among children who experience cerebral malaria (9.2%) or malaria with complicated seizures (11.5%) than among unexposed controls (2.2%) (84). The prevalence of epilepsy associated with this infection is similar to that reported

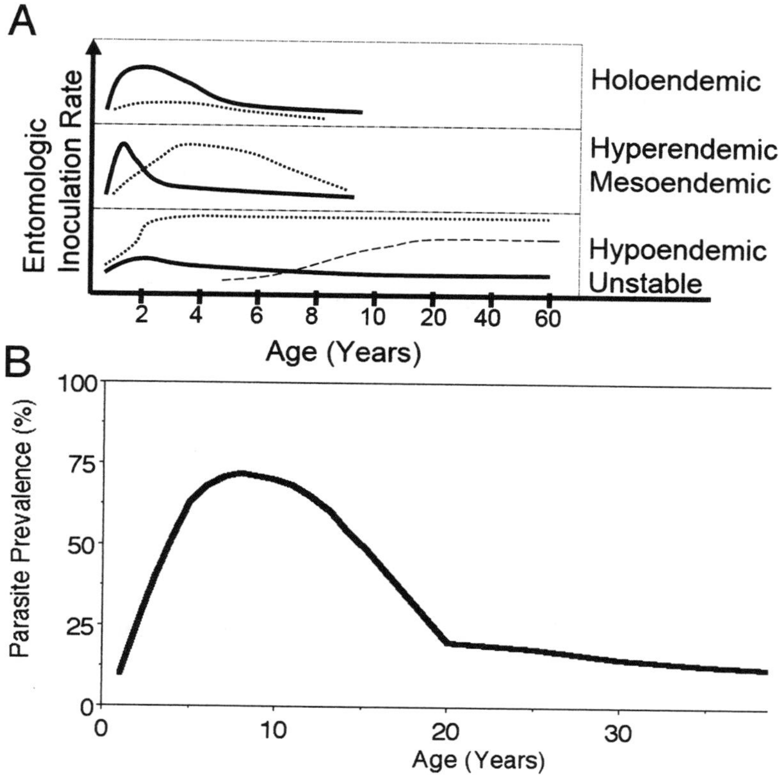

Figure 5. Age-dependent prevalence of severe malaria and deaths. (A) Increasing how often the mosquitoes deliver an infectious bite or the entomologic inoculation rate determines an age-dependent pattern for severe disease, anemia, cerebral malaria, or renal disease, varying from holoendemic (parasite prevalence greater than 60 to 70%), hyperendemic (parasite prevalence between 50 to 70%), mesoendemic (parasite prevalence between 20 and 50%), and hypoendemic (parasite prevalence less than 10%) forms of malaria. The entomologic inoculation rate can vary from 1 to over 1,000 each year. (B) Peak prevalence in a region where malaria is holoendemic follows by a few years the peak risk period for deaths, which is under age 5.

after other severe encephalopathies and to that twice reported after complicated febrile seizures.

The character of the epilepsy that occurs after cerebral malaria has been documented by several observers. After acute disease has passed, the first seizures occur just a few weeks thereafter and then continue at a relatively low frequency of about one per month. The most commonly reported seizure types were tonic-clonic (42%), focal becoming secondarily generalized (16%), and both (21%) (18). However, seizures associated with this infection tend to be easily controlled using phenobarbital, a widely and cheaply available antiepileptic medication in certain regions of the world where malaria is endemic.

The precise pathophysiology explaining this outcome remains poorly understood but is probably attributable to the cerebral damage that occurs during encephalopathy and due to the prolonged and repetitive seizures that occur in the acute phase of the disease that often convert to status epilepticus. Only about a quarter of these patients who develop epilepsy have electroencephalographic abnormalities at the time of acute illness. Whether mesial temporal sclerosis occurs in this setting, which then results in epilepsy (decades after the initial infection), is still unknown. Information is absent on this phenomenon due to limited periods of follow-up in many of the published studies.

Neurocognitive sequelae of cerebral malaria have increasingly been recognized, particularly with African children in the past 20 years (37, 58, 59, 82). These include both basic neurologic deficits and cognitive and behavioral problems (129). Neurologic deficits include cerebellar dysfunction, such as ataxia; motor dysfunction including hemiparesis, monoparesis, or complete paralysis; other motor deficits, such as spasticity and dysarthria; visual impairment from cortical blindness; and hearing problems. Cognitive and behavioral problems include clinically assessed learning and cognition disabilities, aggressive behavior, and scoring two or more standard deviations below the control groups in psychological testing. Currently it is thought that 24% of children have evidence of some neurocognitive impairment after cerebral malaria (82).

Due to the high incidence of this disease, this represents a substantial burden in malaria-endemic areas, suggesting that at least 250,000 children develop neurocognitive impairments from malaria in sub-Saharan Africa each year. Unfortunately, prior to this time, this huge public health burden had largely eluded documentation due to the paucity of relevant clinical data and problems with methodology used to describe deficits in cognitive domains in affected malaria-endemic cultures. However, within the last 10 years, impairment has been reported in a wide range of cognitive functions, including memory, attention, executive functions, and language. Risk factors for developing these persistent neurocognitive sequelae have been identified (58). Deep and persistent coma, hypoglycemia, and absence of hyperpyrexia as well as seizures were all associated with cognitive dysfunction. Risk factors for developing speech and language impairment include younger age (<3), hypoglycemia, severe malnutrition, and increased intracranial pressure during acute disease. Risk factors for developing motor impairments were the presence of prior seizures and focal neurologic signs during hospital admission.

Neurocognitive deficits after malaria in adults are not well documented. Both the prevalence and severity of these deficits are much less than in children (58). Cranial nerve lesions, neuropathies, and extra-pyramidal disorders have all been documented. There are some case reports of problems with memory and naming ability. A retrospective study suggests that cerebral malaria results in multiple neuropsychiatric symptoms, including problems with listening, personality change, and depression (129). Mixed anxiety-depression can occur after cerebral malaria infection (37).

Unfortunately, precise pathophysiology remains unknown besides neurologic damage secondary to the generalized encephalopathy and coma itself. However, due to differences in risk factors for impairment of specific neurologic areas, separate mechanisms may be responsible. One study showed that impairment of prostaglandin E2 metabolism, which in turn is reflected by absence of hyperpyrexia, may play a role in long-term sequelae (94). The concomitant prevalence of active epilepsy in this population may also offer partial explanation of the cognitive impairments which could be reflecting focal and/or recurrent seizures. This may be suggestive of hippocampal damage during acute disease, which can manifest as memory impairment and complex partial seizures at a later date.

Permanent Consequences of Malaria

Selection before reproductive potential is achieved leads to emergence of genotypes more capable of survival (51, 140). As malaria disease predominately occurs in young children in sub-Saharan Africa, falciparum malaria has exerted strong genetic selection to produce an altered erythrocyte resistant to severe disease or in the case of *P. vivax* to erythrocyte infection (88). Sabeti and colleagues have detected areas on human chromosomes which indicate recent selection by haplotype maps for malaria (105). Conversely, the chemotherapy of malaria with chloroquine has also induced a genetic sweep on the parasites' chromosome 7 (143). Other genetic sweeps are also evident on the *P. falciparum* genome by single-nucleotide polymorphism mapping (134).

Haldane is credited with the malaria hypothesis which explains a balanced polymorphism from endemic malaria (2). The sickle cell genotype was observed to occur at 20 to 40% incidence, geographically coincident with malaria in parts of Africa, with higher rates in malarious Greece. In 1949, Beet observed with some populations but not all, a difference in malaria prevalence in sicklers and nonsicklers (6). There were decreased numbers of palpable spleens in sicklers versus nonsicklers, with the observation that sicklers spent less time in the hospital. The data were criticized because of the heterogenous populations studied. In 1954, Allison provided the first empiric evidence for sickle cell trait producing a favorable outcome with malaria infection (3). In 290 children (age 5 months to 5 years), only 12/43 or 27.9% of sicklers had parasitemia, while 113/247 or 45% of nonsicklers had parasitemia. Comparing the geometric mean parasite density, 8/12 of the sicklers had the lowest grade with slight parasitemia, while three of the remaining four had *P. malariae* with moderate parasitemia. Of the 113 nonsicklers, only 34% were in the low grade with slight parasitemia. Allison (3) then recruited 15 sicklers and nonsicklers of the Luo tribe and used a combination of infected mosquito bites and injection of 15 ml of infected blood to test incidence of parasites. He did note that all had a level of semi-immunity with mild symptoms of infection, but 14/15 of the nonsicklers developed parasitemia, while only 2/15 of the sicklers developed parasitemia.

Revisiting this classic work, a group of 3,000 Kenyan children divided in two cohorts were followed to see if other diseases besides malaria were being selected by the heterozygote sickle trait (140). Results revealed that the heterozygote sickle trait had no effect on prevalence of asymptomatic parasitemia but had 50% protection against multiple clinical attacks of malaria, 75% protection against admission to the hospital, and 90% protection against severe malaria. Although there was no effect on geometric mean parasite density in the asymptomatic group, there was a 0.55 reduction in density with mild clinical malaria and a 0.77 reduction in density with severe malaria.

Other β-chain hemoglobinopathies associated with protection from malaria are hemoglobin C and E (1). Recently, Wellems, Fairhurst, and colleagues have demonstrated a reduced number and an abnormal organization of the knobs in hemoglobin AS genotypes as well as hemoglobin C individuals (4, 23, 39). This is predicted to reduce the number and location of adherent parasites sufficiently to reduce malarial disease. Disordered production of α- and β-chains known as α- and β-thalassemia also protect from severe malarial disease, with the mechanism still being debated (104, 136). In an interesting coincidence, the use of the malaria drug primaquine was associated with hemolytic anemias with an increased sequestration of erythrocytes in the spleen, resulting in hemoglobinuria and anemia (7). A human metabolite of primaquine is necessary to cause the abnormality, and it occurs only in individuals with less than 10% levels of glucose 6 phosphate dehydrogenase, important in oxidative damage protection via the Embden-Meyerhoff pathway. Interestingly fetal hemoglobin, which consists of α- and β-chains instead of α- and β-chains is also protective of high parasitemias and severe disease (108). Fetal hemoglobin persists for approximately 6 months from birth, when short asymptomatic *P. falciparum* infections are observed with infants. This also coincides with a waning of maternal antibodies, also postulated for protection.

MALARIA TREATMENT AND CONTROL

Malaria is an entirely preventable and curable disease. Control is divided into (i) mosquito measures, (ii) drugs, or (iii) the vaccine, present on the near horizon. Vector management starts with drying up watery mosquito larva habitats (109). An adult mosquito has an effective range limited to 2 km. Repellants based on DEET prevent mosquito landing for hours, while citronella and soy-based repellants are effective for tens of minutes (41, 97). The principles of insecticide nets are not only to interfere with biting but to decrease the life span of resting mosquitoes, which reduces transmission (30, 54). Most nets stun the mosquito rather than kill instantly. Multiple landings on nets with more insecticide accumulation will result in an earlier death. Indoor residual spraying has the same result of decreasing the lifetime of the female mosquito.

Chemotherapy aims to prevent infection, cure disease, and or decrease disease in populations with mass drug treatments (8, 107, 141). Only a few prophylactic medicines eradicate the liver stage of infection, while many rely upon inhibition of the erythrocyte stages after a 1- to 2-week incubation in the liver. Thus, quinolines like chloroquine, mefloquine, or tetracycline need to be taken for 4 weeks after leaving malaria-endemic areas to ensure adequate drug levels in case a mosquito bit on the last day of exposure and 10,000 parasites emerged from the liver 2 weeks later. The atovoquone/proguanil combination does eradicate actively replicating liver stages of *P. falciparum* and *P. vivax*, but not the hypnozoite of *P. vivax,* or *P. ovale*. Primaquine remains the sole drug clinically effective at eradicating all liver stages (53). Initial use of primaquine resulted in severe hemolytic anemia due to a glucose 6 phosphate dehydrogenase deficiency of less than 10% of normal levels.

The quinolines target hemozoin formation in the lipid environment of the acidic digestive vacuole and therefore are stage specific to the erythrocyte stages rather than to the gametocyte or liver stages (10). A contribution to the failure of the malaria eradication campaigns with dichlorodiphenyltrichloroethane and chloroquine in the 1950s and 1960s was that chloroquine rapidly killed the asexual erythrocyte stages but did not inhibit the gametocytes, thus having no impact on transmission because the patient was still infective to the mosquito. The present optimism with the artemisinin-based drugs are that they are able to kill gametocytes and therefore both cure disease and prevent transmission (55, 89). The peroxide bridge of the artemisinins are activated by either iron or heme to generate radicals (86, 99) which can target specific transporters like PfATPase 6, a calcium channel (38), or random proteins in close proximity to the activated molecules (87). The latter mechanism will minimize chances of drug resistance instead of the chance of a mutated drug target in the case of PfATPase 6. However, amplification of Pfmdr1 associated with the lipophilic mefloquine resistance may also lead to decreased accumulation of artemisinin, resulting in higher inhibition concentrations. In an interesting drug selection study, Paul Hunt and colleagues selected a mouse *Plasmodium chabaudi* for increased tolerance to artemisinin and found that a deubiquination enzyme was mutated (56). This suggests that the proteosome may be increasing clearance of damaged proteins in artemisinin-tolerant parasites. No alteration in the calcium transporting ATPase was seen. The antifolate drugs target the dihydrofolate reductase and dihydrooperate synthase genes, with high specificity to pyrimethamine that is altered by successive mutation in target genes, resulting in clinical resistance.

Trimethoprim, an antibacterial, retains therapeutic antiplasmodium activity, while pyrimethamine has no antibacterial activity. Preventive trimethoprim sulfisoxazole does decrease malaria parasitemia.

The malaria drugs differ in rapidity of clearance of parasites. A severely ill patient may have almost a trillion parasites or 10^{12}. Artemisinin, which clears 10^4 every 48-h cycle, is the most effective at parasite clearance, similar to quinine. Even with the rapid clearance, to reduce 10^{12} parasites to 10^0 necessitates 6 days of therapy. The less active quinolines and antifolates, while still rapidly parasiticidal, require almost 14 days or six cycles to clear parasites. Drugs such as azithromycin or tetracycline reduce parasitemia by a log each cycle so that it takes 24 days to clear the parasitemia. Many malaria drugs, while taken for a short 3-day period, have long half-lives, with effective drug concentrations for weeks.

Any control effort needs to be an integrated strategy which focuses on the vector and human host together (109). An obstacle to targeted control efforts is lack of an accurate understanding of the where and when of malaria epidemiology that could guide decision-making (48). Maps are the easiest and most information-rich way of representing this information. Malaria needs to be mapped on many different layers from country level to district level to village level to household level to inform control efforts. Spatial aspects of malaria risk and control have long been recognized (19). Malaria is focused around mosquito breeding sites with a limited transmission distance of a few kilometers. Mosquito breeding sites do not always follow higher human population densities. Compounding the local transmission is the diverse range of entomologic inoculation rates over 10 to 20 kilometers. In Sierra Leone, annual entomologic inoculation rates varied from 1 to 10 to 100 to 300 over a 3- to 4-sq-km area (19). Malaria can also be spatially clustered on household levels within villages, resulting in a small number of households with greater malaria burdens. The clustering can also occur around rivers or streams, which may not be apparent without a map. Many areas of malaria transmission appear to conform to the 20/80 rule where 20% of the host population contributes to approximately 80% of transmission potential (142). This implies that if control programs target the essential 20% core, they will be more effective. This heterogeneous pattern of malaria risk also makes untargeted control ineffective because it misses the high-risk individuals and locations, as well as overtreats areas that contribute little, if anything, to malaria maintenance (19). Because of the high basic infectious rates for malaria, which may be in the hundreds and sometimes thousands (113), missing these high-transmission individuals or locations can effectively negate costly malaria control efforts.

CONCLUSIONS

Acute malaria is entirely preventable and can be completely curable in settings with rapid accurate diagnosis and effective chemotherapy. In settings with endemic malaria characterized by constant infective mosquito bites, long-term carriage of persistent parasites somewhat tolerated by semi-immunity results. Chronic infection results in consequences of anemia or persistent neurologic deficits. The malaria parasites have permanently altered the human genome. These alterations will persist even after malaria is entirely eradicated.

REFERENCES

1. **Agarwal, A., A. Guindo, Y. Cissoko, J. G. Taylor, D. Coulibaly, A. Kone, K. Kayentao, A. Djimde, C. V. Plowe, O. Doumbo, T. E. Wellems, and D. Diallo.** 2000. Hemoglobin C associated with protection from severe malaria in the Dogon of Mali, a West African population with a low prevalence of hemoglobin S. *Blood* **96:**2358–2363.
2. **Akide-Ndunge, O. B., K. Ayi, and P. Arese.** 2003. The Haldane malaria hypothesis: facts, artifacts, and a prophecy. *Redox. Rep.* **8:**311–316.
3. **Allison, A. C.** 1954. Protection afforded by sickle-cell trait against subtertian malareal infection. *Br. Med. J.* **1:**290–294.
4. **Arie, T., R. M. Fairhurst, N. J. Brittain, T. E. Wellems, and J. A. Dvorak.** 2005. Hemoglobin C modulates the surface topography of *Plasmodium falciparum*-infected erythrocytes. *J. Struct. Biol.* **150:**163–169.
5. **Bannister, L. H., J. M. Hopkins, R. E. Fowler, S. Krishna, and G. H. Mitchell.** 2000. A brief illustrated guide to the ultrastructure of *Plasmodium falciparum* asexual blood stages. *Parasitol. Today* **16:**427–433.
6. **Beet, E. A.** 1949. The genetics of the sickle-cell trait in a Bantu tribe. *Ann. Eugen.* **14:**279–284.
7. **Beutler, E., and S. Duparc.** 2007. Glucose-6-phosphate dehydrogenase deficiency and antimalarial drug development. *Am. J. Trop. Med. Hyg.* **77:**779–789.
8. **Bottieau, E., J. Clerinx, E. Van Den Enden, M. Van Esbroeck, R. Colebunders, A. Van Gompel, and J. Van Den Ende.** 2006. Imported non-*Plasmodium falciparum* malaria: a five-year prospective study in a European referral center. *Am. J. Trop. Med. Hyg.* **75:**133–138.
9. **Brady, G., G. J. MacArthur, and P. J. Farrell.** 2007. Epstein-Barr virus and Burkitt lymphoma. *J. Clin. Pathol.* **60:**1397–1402.
10. **Bray, P. G., S. A. Ward, and P. M. O'Neill.** 2005. Quinolines and artemisinin: chemistry, biology and history. *Curr. Top. Microbiol. Immunol.* **295:**33–38.
11. **Breman, J. G., M. S. Alilio, and A. Mills.** 2004. Conquering the intolerable burden of malaria: what's new, what's needed: a summary. *Am. J. Trop. Med. Hyg.* **71:**1–15.
12. **Brent, A. J., J. O. Oundo, I. Mwangi, L. Ochola, B. Lowe, and J. A. Berkley.** 2006. *Salmonella* bacteremia in Kenyan children. *Pediatr. Infect. Dis. J.* **25:**230–236.

13. **Bronzan, R. N., T. E. Taylor, J. Mwenechanya, M. Tembo, K. Kayira, L. Bwanaisa, A. Njobvu, W. Kondowe, C. Chalira, A. L. Walsh, A. Phiri, L. K. Wilson, M. E. Molyneux, and S. M. Graham.** 2007. Bacteremia in Malawian children with severe malaria: prevalence, etiology, HIV coinfection, and outcome. *J. Infect. Dis.* **195:**895–904.
14. **Burkitt, D. P.** 1971. Epidemiology of Burkitt's lymphoma. *Proc. R. Soc. Med.* **64:**909–910.
15. **Burkitt, D. P.** 1969. Etiology of Burkitt's lymphoma--an alternative hypothesis to a vectored virus. *J. Natl. Cancer Inst.* **42:**19–28.
16. **Carlton, J. M., S. V. Angiuoli, B. B. Suh, T. W. Kooij, M. Pertea, J. C. Silva, M. D. Ermolaeva, J. E. Allen, J. D. Selengut, H. L. Koo, J. D. Peterson, M. Pop, D. S. Kosack, M. F. Shumway, S. L. Bidwell, S. J. Shallom, S. E. van Aken, S. B. Riedmuller, T. V. Feldblyum, J. K. Cho, J. Quackenbush, M. Sedegah, A. Shoaibi, L. M. Cummings, L. Florens, J. R. Yates, J. D. Raine, R. E. Sinden, M. A. Harris, D. A. Cunningham, P. R. Preiser, L. W. Bergman, A. B. Vaidya, L. H. van Lin, C. J. Janse, A. P. Waters, H. O. Smith, O. R. White, S. L. Salzberg, J. C. Venter, C. M. Fraser, S. L. Hoffman, M. J. Gardner, and D. J. Carucci.** 2002. Genome sequence and comparative analysis of the model rodent malaria parasite *Plasmodium yoelii yoelii. Nature* **419:**512–519.
17. **Carpenter, L. M., R. Newton, D. Casabonne, J. Ziegler, S. Mbulaiteye, E. Mbidde, H. Wabinga, H. Jaffe, and V. Beral.** 2008. Antibodies against malaria and Epstein-Barr virus in childhood Burkitt lymphoma: a case-control study in Uganda. *Int. J. Cancer* **122:**1319–1323.
18. **Carter, J. A., B. G. Neville, S. White, A. J. Ross, G. Otieno, N. Mturi, C. Musumba, and C. R. Newton.** 2004. Increased prevalence of epilepsy associated with severe falciparum malaria in children. *Epilepsia* **45:**978–981.
19. **Carter, R., K. N. Mendis, and D. Roberts.** 2000. Spatial targeting of interventions against malaria. *Bull. W. H. O.* **78:**1401–1411.
20. **Casals-Pascual, C., O. Kai, J. O. Cheung, S. Williams, B. Lowe, M. Nyanoti, T. N. Williams, K. Maitland, M. Molyneux, C. R. Newton, N. Peshu, S. M. Watt, and D. J. Roberts.** 2006. Suppression of erythropoiesis in malarial anemia is associated with hemozoin in vitro and in vivo. *Blood* **108:**2569–2577.
21. **Chen, Q., M. Schlichtherle, and M. Wahlgren.** 2000. Molecular aspects of severe malaria. *Clin. Microbiol. Rev.* **13:**439–450.
22. **Chene, A., D. Donati, A. O. Guerreiro-Cacais, V. Levitsky, Q. Chen, K. I. Falk, J. Orem, F. Kironde, M. Wahlgren, and M. T. Bejarano.** 2007. A molecular link between malaria and Epstein-Barr virus reactivation. *PLoS Pathog.* **3:**e80.
23. **Cholera, R., N. J. Brittain, M. R. Gillrie, T. M. Lopera-Mesa, S. A. Diakite, T. Arie, M. A. Krause, A. Guindo, A. Tubman, H. Fujioka, D. A. Diallo, O. K. Doumbo, M. Ho, T. E. Wellems, and R. M. Fairhurst.** 2008. Impaired cytoadherence of *Plasmodium falciparum*-infected erythrocytes containing sickle hemoglobin. *Proc. Natl. Acad. Sci. USA* **105:**991–996.
24. **Clark, I. A., and W. B. Cowden.** 2003. The pathophysiology of falciparum malaria. *Pharmacol. Ther.* **99:**221.
25. **Collins, W. E., and G. M. Jeffery.** 2007. *Plasmodium malariae*: parasite and disease. *Clin. Microbiol. Rev.* **20:**579–592.
26. **Cordoliani, Y. S., J. L. Sarrazin, D. Felten, E. Caumes, C. Leveque, and A. Fisch.** 1998. MR of cerebral malaria. *AJNR Am. J. Neuroradiol.* **19:**871–874.
27. **Cox-Singh, J., T. M. Davis, K. S. Lee, S. S. Shamsul, A. Matusop, S. Ratnam, H. A. Rahman, D. J. Conway, and B. Singh.** 2008. *Plasmodium knowlesi* malaria in humans is widely distributed and potentially life threatening. *Clin. Infect. Dis.* **46:**165–171.
28. **Cox-Singh, J., and B. Singh.** 2008. Knowlesi malaria: newly emergent and of public health importance? *Trends Parasitol.* **24:**406–410.
29. **Cranfield, M. R., T. K. Graczyk, F. B. Beall, D. M. Ialeggio, M. L. Shaw, and M. L. Skjoldager.** 1994. Subclinical avian malaria infections in African black-footed penguins (*Spheniscus demersus*) and induction of parasite recrudescence. *J. Wildl. Dis.* **30:**372–376.
30. **Curtis, C. F., C. A. Maxwell, S. M. Magesa, R. T. Rwegoshora, and T. J. Wilkes.** 2006. Insecticide-treated bed-nets for malaria mosquito control. *J. Am. Mosq. Control Assoc.* **22:**501–506.
31. **Desakorn, V., A. M. Dondorp, K. Silamut, W. Pongtavornpinyo, D. Sahassananda, K. Chotivanich, P. Pitisuttithum, A. M. Smithyman, N. P. Day, and N. J. White.** 2005. Stage-dependent production and release of histidine-rich protein 2 by *Plasmodium falciparum. Trans. R. Soc. Trop. Med. Hyg.* **99:**517–524.
32. **Dobbie, M., J. Crawley, C. Waruiru, K. Marsh, and R. Surtees.** 2000. Cerebrospinal fluid studies in children with cerebral malaria: an excitotoxic mechanism? *Am. J. Trop. Med. Hyg.* **62:**284–290.
33. **Dondorp, A. M., V. Desakorn, W. Pongtavornpinyo, D. Sahassananda, K. Silamut, K. Chotivanich, P. N. Newton, P. Pitisuttithum, A. M. Smithyman, N. J. White, and N. P. Day.** 2005. Estimation of the total parasite biomass in acute falciparum malaria from plasma PfHRP2. *PLoS Med.* **2:**e204.
34. **Dondorp, A. M., S. J. Lee, M. A. Faiz, S. Mishra, R. Price, E. Tjitra, M. Than, Y. Htut, S. Mohanty, E. B. Yunus, R. Rahman, F. Nosten, N. M. Anstey, N. P. Day, and N. J. White.** 2008. The relationship between age and the manifestations of and mortality associated with severe malaria. *Clin. Infect. Dis.* **47:**151–157.
35. **Duarte, M. I., C. E. Corbett, M. Boulos, and V. Amato Neto.** 1985. Ultrastructure of the lung in falciparum malaria. *Am. J. Trop. Med. Hyg.* **34:**31–35.
36. **Duffy, P. E., and M. Fried.** 2005. Malaria in the pregnant woman. *Curr. Top. Microbiol. Immunol.* **295:**169–200.
37. **Dugbartey, A. T., M. T. Dugbartey, and M. Y. Apedo.** 1998. Delayed neuropsychiatric effects of malaria in Ghana. *J. Nerv. Ment. Dis.* **186:**183–186.
38. **Eckstein-Ludwig, U., R. J. Webb, I. D. Van Goethem, J. M. East, A. G. Lee, M. Kimura, P. M. O'Neill, P. G. Bray, S. A. Ward, and S. Krishna.** 2003. Artemisinins target the SERCA of *Plasmodium falciparum. Nature* **424:**957–961.
39. **Fairhurst, R. M., D. I. Baruch, N. J. Brittain, G. R. Ostera, J. S. Wallach, H. L. Hoang, K. Hayton, A. Guindo, M. O. Makobongo, O. M. Schwartz, A. Tounkara, O. K. Doumbo, D. A. Diallo, H. Fujioka, M. Ho, and T. E. Wellems.** 2005. Abnormal display of PfEMP-1 on erythrocytes carrying haemoglobin C may protect against malaria. *Nature* **435:**1117–1121.
40. **Foth, B. J., and G. I. McFadden.** 2003. The apicoplast: a plastid in *Plasmodium falciparum* and other Apicomplexan parasites. *Int. Rev. Cytol.* **224:**57–110.
41. **Fradin, M. S., and J. F. Day.** 2002. Comparative efficacy of insect repellents against mosquito bites. *N. Engl. J. Med.* **347:**13–18.
42. **Francis, S. E., D. J. Sullivan, Jr., and D. E. Goldberg.** 1997. Hemoglobin metabolism in the malaria parasite *Plasmodium falciparum. Annu. Rev. Microbiol.* **51:**97–123.
43. **Gamanagatti, S., and H. Kandpal.** 2006. MR imaging of cerebral malaria in a child. *Eur. J. Radiol.* **60:**46–47.

44. **Gardner, M. J., N. Hall, E. Fung, O. White, M. Berriman, R. W. Hyman, J. M. Carlton, A. Pain, K. E. Nelson, S. Bowman, I. T. Paulsen, K. James, J. A. Eisen, K. Rutherford, S. L. Salzberg, A. Craig, S. Kyes, M. S. Chan, V. Nene, S. J. Shallom, B. Suh, J. Peterson, S. Angiuoli, M. Pertea, J. Allen, J. Selengut, D. Haft, M. W. Mather, A. B. Vaidya, D. M. Martin, A. H. Fairlamb, M. J. Fraunholz, D. S. Roos, S. A. Ralph, G. I. McFadden, L. M. Cummings, G. M. Subramanian, C. Mungall, J. C. Venter, D. J. Carucci, S. L. Hoffman, C. Newbold, R. W. Davis, C. M. Fraser, and B. Barrell.** 2002. Genome sequence of the human malaria parasite *Plasmodium falciparum*. *Nature* **419**:498–511.
45. **Gluzman, I. Y., S. E. Francis, A. Oksman, C. E. Smith, K. L. Duffin, and D. E. Goldberg.** 1994. Order and specificity of the *Plasmodium falciparum* hemoglobin degradation pathway. *J. Clin. Investig.* **93**:1602–1608.
46. **Grobusch, M. P., and P. G. Kremsner.** 2005. Uncomplicated malaria. *Curr. Top. Microbiol. Immunol.* **295**:83–104.
47. **Guerra, C. A., P. W. Gikandi, A. J. Tatem, A. M. Noor, D. L. Smith, S. I. Hay, and R. W. Snow.** 2008. The limits and intensity of *Plasmodium falciparum* transmission: implications for malaria control and elimination worldwide. *PLoS Med.* **5**:e38.
48. **Guerra, C. A., S. I. Hay, L. S. Lucioparedes, P. W. Gikandi, A. J. Tatem, A. M. Noor, and R. W. Snow.** 2007. Assembling a global database of malaria parasite prevalence for the Malaria Atlas Project. *Malar. J.* **6**:17.
49. **Guerra, C. A., R. W. Snow, and S. I. Hay.** 2006. Mapping the global extent of malaria in 2005. *Trends Parasitol.* **22**: 353–358.
50. **Haldar, K., S. C. Murphy, D. A. Milner, and T. E. Taylor.** 2007. Malaria: mechanisms of erythrocytic infection and pathological correlates of severe disease. *Annu. Rev. Pathol.* **2**:217–249.
51. **Harpending, H., and G. Cochran.** 2006. Genetic diversity and genetic burden in humans. *Infect. Genet. Evol.* **6**:154–162.
52. **Hay, S. I., and R. W. Snow.** 2006. The Malaria Atlas Project: developing global maps of malaria risk. *PLoS Med.* **3**:e473.
53. **Hill, D. R., J. K. Baird, M. E. Parise, L. S. Lewis, E. T. Ryan, and A. J. Magill.** 2006. Primaquine: report from CDC expert meeting on malaria chemoprophylaxis I. *Am. J. Trop. Med. Hyg.* **75**:402–415.
54. **Hill, J., J. Lines, and M. Rowland.** 2006. Insecticide-treated nets. *Adv. Parasitol.* **61**:77–128.
55. **Hsu, E.** 2006. Reflections on the 'discovery' of the antimalarial qinghao. *Br. J. Clin. Pharmacol.* **61**:666–670.
56. **Hunt, P., A. Afonso, A. Creasey, R. Culleton, A. B. Sidhu, J. Logan, S. G. Valderramos, I. McNae, S. Cheesman, V. do Rosario, R. Carter, D. A. Fidock, and P. Cravo.** 2007. Gene encoding a deubiquitinating enzyme is mutated in artesunate- and chloroquine-resistant rodent malaria parasites. *Mol. Microbiol.* **65**:27–40.
57. **Idro, R.** 2003. Severe anaemia in childhood cerebral malaria is associated with profound coma. *Afr. Health Sci.* **3**:15–18.
58. **Idro, R., J. A. Carter, G. Fegan, B. G. Neville, and C. R. Newton.** 2006. Risk factors for persisting neurological and cognitive impairments following cerebral malaria. *Arch. Dis. Child.* **91**:142–148.
59. **Idro, R., N. E. Jenkins, and C. R. Newton.** 2005. Pathogenesis, clinical features, and neurological outcome of cerebral malaria. *Lancet Neurol.* **4**:827–840.
60. **John, C. C., A. Panoskaltsis-Mortari, R. O. Opoka, G. S. Park, P. J. Orchard, A. M. Jurek, R. Idro, J. Byarugaba, and M. J. Boivin.** 2008. Cerebrospinal fluid cytokine levels and cognitive impairment in cerebral malaria. *Am. J. Trop. Med. Hyg.* **78**:198–205.
61. **Jonsson, B., A. Nyberg, and C. Henning.** 1993. Theoretical aspects of detection of bacteraemia as a function of the volume of blood cultured. *APMIS* **101**:595–601.
62. **Joshi, R., J. M. Colford, Jr., A. L. Reingold, and S. Kalantri.** 2008. Nonmalarial acute undifferentiated fever in a rural hospital in central India: diagnostic uncertainty and overtreatment with antimalarial agents. *Am. J. Trop. Med. Hyg.* 78:393–399.
63. **Kantele, A., H. Marti, I. Felger, D. Muller, and T. S. Jokiranta.** 2008. Monkey malaria in a European traveler returning from Malaysia. *Emerg. Infect. Dis.* **14**:1434–1436.
64. **Kaushik, A., V. K. Sharma, Sadhna, R. Kumar, and R. Mitra.** 1992. Malarial placental infection and low birth weight babies. *Mater. Med. Pol.* **24**:109–110.
65. **Kelly, G. L., and A. B. Rickinson.** 2007. Burkitt lymphoma: revisiting the pathogenesis of a virus-associated malignancy. *Hematology Am. Soc. Hematol. Educ. Program* **2007**:277–284.
66. **Kennan, R. P., F. S. Machado, S. C. Lee, M. S. Desruisseaux, M. Wittner, M. Tsuji, and H. B. Tanowitz.** 2005. Reduced cerebral blood flow and *N*-acetyl aspartate in a murine model of cerebral malaria. *Parasitol. Res.* **96**:302–307.
67. **Kim, K., and L. M. Weiss.** 2004. *Toxoplasma gondii*: the model apicomplexan. *Int. J. Parasitol.* **34**:423–432.
68. **Kochar, D. K., P. Singh, P. Agarwal, S. K. Kochar, R. Pokharna, and P. K. Sareen.** 2003. Malarial hepatitis. *J. Assoc. Physicians India* **51**:1069–1072.
69. **Lobo, C. A., and N. Kumar.** 1998. Sexual differentiation and development in the malaria parasite. *Parasitol. Today* **14**:146–150.
70. **Looareesuwan, S., P. Wilairatana, S. Krishna, B. Kendall, S. Vannaphan, C. Viravan, and N. J. White.** 1995. Magnetic resonance imaging of the brain in patients with cerebral malaria. *Clin. Infect. Dis.* **21**:300–309.
71. **Lubitz, J. M. 1949.** Pathology of the ruptured spleen in acute vivax malaria. *Blood* **4**:1168–1176.
72. **Marshall, J. C., P. M. Walker, D. M. Foster, D. Harris, M. Ribeiro, J. Paice, A. D. Romaschin, and A. N. Derzko.** 2002. Measurement of endotoxin activity in critically ill patients using whole blood neutrophil dependent chemiluminescence. *Crit. Care* **6**:342–348.
73. **Massey, J. G., T. K. Graczyk, and M. R. Cranfield.** 1996. Characteristics of naturally acquired *Plasmodium relictum capistranoae* infections in naive Hawaiian crows (*Corvus hawaiiensis*) in Hawaii. *J. Parasitol.* **82**:182–185.
74. **Medana, I. M., G. Chaudhri, T. Chan-Ling, and N. H. Hunt.** 2001. Central nervous system in cerebral malaria: 'innocent bystander' or active participant in the induction of immunopathology? *Immunol. Cell Biol.* **79**:101–120.
75. **Medana, I. M., N. P. Day, T. T. Hien, N. T. Mai, D. Bethell, N. H. Phu, J. Farrar, M. M. Esiri, N. J. White, and G. D. Turner.** 2002. Axonal injury in cerebral malaria. *Am. J. Pathol.* **160**:655–666.
76. **Medana, I. M., T. T. Hien, N. P. Day, N. H. Phu, N. T. Mai, L. V. Chu'ong, T. T. Chau, A. Taylor, H. Salahifar, R. Stocker, G. Smythe, G. D. Turner, J. Farrar, N. J. White, and N. H. Hunt.** 2002. The clinical significance of cerebrospinal fluid levels of kynurenine pathway metabolites and lactate in severe malaria. *J. Infect. Dis.* **185**:650–656.
77. **Miller, L. H., D. I. Baruch, K. Marsh, and O. K. Doumbo.** 2002. The pathogenic basis of malaria. *Nature* **415**:673–679.
78. **Mishra, S. K., K. Dietz, S. Mohanty, and S. S. Pati.** 2007. Influence of acute renal failure in patients with cerebral malaria - a hospital-based study from India. *Trop. Doct.* **37**: 10310–10314.
79. **Moody, A. 2002.** Rapid diagnostic tests for malaria parasites. *Clin. Microbiol. Rev.* **15**:66–78.

80. **Moormann, A. M., K. Chelimo, O. P. Sumba, M. L. Lutzke, R. Ploutz-Snyder, D. Newton, J. Kazura, and R. Rochford.** 2005. Exposure to holoendemic malaria results in elevated Epstein-Barr virus loads in children. *J. Infect. Dis.* **191:** 1233–1238.

81. **Moormann, A. M., A. D. Sullivan, R. A. Rochford, S. W. Chensue, P. J. Bock, T. Nyirenda, and S. R. Meshnick.** 1999. Malaria and pregnancy: placental cytokine expression and its relationship to intrauterine growth retardation. *J. Infect. Dis.* **180:**1987–1993.

82. **Mung'Ala-Odera, V., R. W. Snow, and C. R. Newton.** 2004. The burden of the neurocognitive impairment associated with *Plasmodium falciparum* malaria in sub-Saharan Africa. *Am. J. Trop. Med. Hyg.* **71:**64–70.

83. **Newbold, C. I., A. G. Craig, S. Kyes, A. R. Berendt, R. W. Snow, N. Peshu, and K. Marsh.** 1997. PfEMP1, polymorphism and pathogenesis. *Ann. Trop. Med. Parasitol.* **91:** 551–557.

84. **Ngoungou, E. B., J. Koko, M. Druet-Cabanac, Y. Assengone-Zeh-Nguema, M. N. Launay, E. Engohang, M. Moubeka-Mounguengui, P. Kouna-Ndouongo, P. M. Loembe, P. M. Preux, and M. Kombila.** 2006. Cerebral malaria and sequelar epilepsy: first matched case-control study in Gabon. *Epilepsia* **47:**2147–2153.

85. **Noland, G. S., N. Briones, and D. J. Sullivan, Jr.** 2003. The shape and size of hemozoin crystals distinguishes diverse *Plasmodium* species. *Mol. Biochem. Parasitol.* **130:**91–99.

86. **O'Neill, P. M., and G. H. Posner.** 2004. A medicinal chemistry perspective on artemisinin and related endoperoxides. *J. Med. Chem.* **47:**2945–2964.

87. **O'Neill, P. M., S. L. Rawe, K. Borstnik, A. Miller, S. A. Ward, P. G. Bray, J. Davies, C. H. Oh, and G. H. Posner.** 2005. Enantiomeric 1,2,4-trioxanes display equivalent in vitro antimalarial activity versus *Plasmodium falciparum* malaria parasites: implications for the molecular mechanism of action of the artemisinins. *Chembiochem* **6:**2048–2054.

88. **Oh, S. S., and A. H. Chishti.** 2005. Host receptors in malaria merozoite invasion. *Curr. Top. Microbiol. Immunol.* **295:** 203–232.

89. **Olliaro, P. L., and W. R. Taylor.** 2004. Developing artemisinin based drug combinations for the treatment of drug resistant falciparum malaria: a review. *J. Postgrad. Med.* **50:** 40–44.

90. **Omodeo-Sale, F., A. Motti, A. Dondorp, N. J. White, and D. Taramelli.** 2005. Destabilisation and subsequent lysis of human erythrocytes induced by *Plasmodium falciparum* haem products. *Eur. J. Haematol.* **74:**324–332.

91. **Pagola, S., P. W. Stephens, D. S. Bohle, A. D. Kosar, and S. K. Madsen.** 2000. The structure of malaria pigment beta-haematin. *Nature* **404:**307–310.

92. **Parekh, S. B., W. A. Bubb, N. H. Hunt, and C. Rae.** 2006. Brain metabolic markers reflect susceptibility status in cytokine gene knockout mice with murine cerebral malaria. *Int. J. Parasitol.* **36:**1409–1418.

93. **Penet, M. F., F. Kober, S. Confort-Gouny, Y. Le Fur, C. Dalmasso, N. Coltel, A. Liprandi, J. M. Gulian, G. E. Grau, P. J. Cozzone, and A. Viola.** 2007. Magnetic resonance spectroscopy reveals an impaired brain metabolic profile in mice resistant to cerebral malaria infected with *Plasmodium berghei* ANKA. *J. Biol. Chem.* **282:**14505–14514.

94. **Perkins, D. J., J. B. Hittner, E. D. Mwaikambo, D. L. Granger, J. B. Weinberg, and N. M. Anstey.** 2005. Impaired systemic production of prostaglandin E2 in children with cerebral malaria. *J. Infect. Dis.* **191:**1548–1557.

95. **Pisciotta, J. M., and D. Sullivan.** 2008. Hemozoin: oil versus water. *Parasitol. Int.* **57:**89–96.

96. **Planche, T., A. Dzeing, E. Ngou-Milama, M. Kombila, and P. W. Stacpoole.** 2005. Metabolic complications of severe malaria. *Curr. Top. Microbiol. Immunol.* **295:**105–136.

97. **Pollack, R. J., A. E. Kiszewski, and A. Spielman.** 2002. Repelling mosquitoes. *N. Engl. J. Med.* **347:**2–3.

98. **Pongponratn, E., G. D. Turner, N. P. Day, N. H. Phu, J. A. Simpson, K. Stepniewska, N. T. Mai, P. Viriyavejakul, S. Looareesuwan, T. T. Hien, D. J. Ferguson, and N. J. White.** 2003. An ultrastructural study of the brain in fatal *Plasmodium falciparum* malaria. *Am. J. Trop. Med. Hyg.* **69:**345–359.

99. **Posner, G. P., and S. R. Meshnick.** 2001. Radical mechanism of action of the artemisinin-type compounds. *Trends Parasitol.* **17:**266–268.

100. **Prudencio, M., A. Rodriguez, and M. M. Mota.** 2006. The silent path to thousands of merozoites: the *Plasmodium* liver stage. *Nat. Rev. Microbiol.* **4:**849–856.

101. **Rainey, J. J., W. O. Mwanda, P. Wairiumu, A. M. Moormann, M. L. Wilson, and R. Rochford.** 2007. Spatial distribution of Burkitt's lymphoma in Kenya and association with malaria risk. *Trop. Med. Int. Health.* **12:**936–943.

102. **Reisinger, E. C., C. Fritzsche, R. Krause, and G. J. Krejs.** 2005. Diarrhea caused by primarily non-gastrointestinal infections. *Nat. Clin. Pract. Gastroenterol. Hepatol.* **2:** 216–222.

103. **Riehle, M. A., P. Srinivasan, C. K. Moreira, and M. Jacobs-Lorena.** 2003. Towards genetic manipulation of wild mosquito populations to combat malaria: advances and challenges. *J. Exp. Biol.* **206:**3809–3816.

104. **Roberts, D. J., C. Casals-Pascual, and D. J. Weatherall.** 2005. The clinical and pathophysiological features of malarial anaemia. *Curr. Top. Microbiol. Immunol.* **295:**137–167.

105. **Sabeti, P. C., D. E. Reich, J. M. Higgins, H. Z. Levine, D. J. Richter, S. F. Schaffner, S. B. Gabriel, J. V. Platko, N. J. Patterson, G. J. McDonald, H. C. Ackerman, S. J. Campbell, D. Altshuler, R. Cooper, D. Kwiatkowski, R. Ward, and E. S. Lander.** 2002. Detecting recent positive selection in the human genome from haplotype structure. *Nature* **419:**832–837.

106. **Scholl, P. F., A. K. Tripathi, and D. J. Sullivan.** 2005. Bioavailable iron and heme metabolism in *Plasmodium falciparum*. *Curr. Top. Microbiol. Immunol.* **295:**293–324.

107. **Schwartz, E., M. Parise, P. Kozarsky, and M. Cetron.** 2003. Delayed onset of malaria--implications for chemoprophylaxis in travelers. *N. Engl. J. Med.* **349:**1510–1516.

108. **Shear, H. L., L. Grinberg, J. Gilman, M. E. Fabry, G. Stamatoyannopoulos, D. E. Goldberg, and R. L. Nagel.** 1998. Transgenic mice expressing human fetal globin are protected from malaria by a novel mechanism. *Blood* **92:**2520–2526.

109. **Shiff, C.** 2002. Integrated approach to malaria control. *Clin. Microbiol. Rev.* **15:**278–293.

110. **Skorokhod, A., E. Schwarzer, G. Gremo, and P. Arese.** 2007. HNE produced by the malaria parasite *Plasmodium falciparum* generates HNE-protein adducts and decreases erythrocyte deformability. *Redox Rep.* **12:**73–75.

111. **Smith, D. L., J. Dushoff, R. W. Snow, and S. I. Hay. 2005.** The entomological inoculation rate and *Plasmodium falciparum* infection in African children. *Nature* **438:**492–495.

112. **Smith, D. L., C. A. Guerra, R. W. Snow, and S. I. Hay.** 2007. Standardizing estimates of the *Plasmodium falciparum* parasite rate. *Malar. J.* **6:**131.

113. **Smith, D. L., F. E. McKenzie, R. W. Snow, and S. I. Hay.** 2007. Revisiting the basic reproductive number for malaria and its implications for malaria control. *PLoS Biol.* **5:**e42.

114. **Smith, J. D., and A. G. Craig.** 2005. The surface of the *Plasmodium falciparum*-infected erythrocyte. *Curr. Issues Mol. Biol.* **7:**81–93.
115. **Smith, J. D., A. G. Craig, N. Kriek, D. Hudson-Taylor, S. Kyes, T. Fagan, R. Pinches, D. I. Baruch, C. I. Newbold, and L. H. Miller.** 2000. Identification of a *Plasmodium falciparum* intercellular adhesion molecule-1 binding domain: a parasite adhesion trait implicated in cerebral malaria. *Proc. Natl. Acad. Sci. USA* **97:**1766–1771.
116. **Snow, R. W., M. Craig, U. Deichmann, and K. Marsh.** 1999. Estimating mortality, morbidity and disability due to malaria among Africa's non-pregnant population. *Bull. W. H. O.* **77:**624–640.
117. **Snow, R. W., E. L. Korenromp, and E. Gouws.** 2004. Pediatric mortality in Africa: *Plasmodium falciparum* malaria as a cause or risk? *Am. J. Trop. Med. Hyg.* **71:**16–24.
118. **Sowunmi, A., O. A. Ogundahunsi, C. O. Falade, G. O. Gbotosho, and A. M. Oduola.** 2000. Gastrointestinal manifestations of acute falciparum malaria in children. *Acta Trop.* **74:**73–76.
119. **Spencer, K. A., K. L. Buchanan, S. Leitner, A. R. Goldsmith, and C. K. Catchpole.** 2005. Parasites affect song complexity and neural development in a songbird. *Proc. Biol. Sci.* **272:**2037–2043.
120. **Srivastava, K., I. A. Cockburn, A. Swaim, L. E. Thompson, A. Tripathi, C. A. Fletcher, E. M. Shirk, H. Sun, M. A. Kowalska, K. Fox-Talbot, D. Sullivan, F. Zavala, and C. N. Morrell.** 2008. Platelet factor 4 mediates inflammation in experimental cerebral malaria. *Cell. Host Microbe* **4:**179–187.
121. **Steketee, R. W., B. L. Nahlen, M. E. Parise, and C. Menendez.** 2001. The burden of malaria in pregnancy in malaria-endemic areas. *Am. J. Trop. Med. Hyg.* **64:**28–35.
122. **Stephenson, I., J. Roper, M. Fraser, K. Nicholson, and M. Wiselka.** 2003. Dengue fever in febrile returning travellers to a UK regional infectious diseases unit. *Travel Med. Infect. Dis.* **1:**89–93.
123. **Su, X. Z., V. M. Heatwole, S. P. Wertheimer, F. Guinet, J. A. Herrfeldt, D. S. Peterson, J. A. Ravetch, and T. E. Wellems.** 1995. The large diverse gene family var encodes proteins involved in cytoadherence and antigenic variation of *Plasmodium falciparum*-infected erythrocytes. *Cell* **82:**89–100.
124. **Sullivan, D. J.** 2002. Theories on malarial pigment formation and quinoline action. *Int. J. Parasitol.* **32:**1645–1653.
125. **Telford, S. R., Jr.** 1977. The distribution, incidence and general ecology of saurian malaria in Middle America. *Int. J. Parasitol.* **7:**299–314.
126. **Telford, S. R., Jr.** 1986. Studies on African saurian malarias: *Plasmodium holaspi* n. sp. from the flying lacertid *Holaspis guentheri*. *J. Parasitol.* **72:**271–275.
127. **Vaidya, A. B.** 2004. Mitochondrial and plastid functions as antimalarial drug targets. *Curr. Drug Targets Infect. Disord.* **4:**11–23.
128. **Vaidya, A. B., and M. W. Mather.** 2005. A post-genomic view of the mitochondrion in malaria parasites. *Curr. Top. Microbiol. Immunol.* **295:**233–250.
129. **Varney, N. R., R. J. Roberts, J. A. Springer, S. K. Connell, and P. S. Wood.** 1997. Neuropsychiatric sequelae of cerebral malaria in Vietnam veterans. *J. Nerv. Ment. Dis.* **185:**695–703.
130. **Venet, C., F. Zeni, A. Viallon, A. Ross, P. Pain, P. Gery, D. Page, R. Vermesch, M. Bertrand, F. Rancon, and J. C. Bertrand.** 2000. Endotoxaemia in patients with severe sepsis or septic shock. *Intensive Care Med.* **26:**538–544.
131. **Viebig, N. K., E. Levin, S. Dechavanne, S. J. Rogerson, J. Gysin, J. D. Smith, A. Scherf, and B. Gamain.** 2007. Disruption of var2csa gene impairs placental malaria associated adhesion phenotype. *PLoS ONE* **2:**e910.
132. **Vinetz, J. M., J. Li, T. F. McCutchan, and D. C. Kaslow.** 1998. *Plasmodium malariae* infection in an asymptomatic 74-year-old Greek woman with splenomegaly. *N. Engl. J. Med.* **338:**367–371.
133. **Vlachou, D., T. Schlegelmilch, E. Runn, A. Mendes, and F. C. Kafatos.** 2006. The developmental migration of *Plasmodium* in mosquitoes. *Curr. Opin. Genet. Dev.* **16:**384–391.
134. **Volkman, S. K., P. C. Sabeti, D. DeCaprio, D. E. Neafsey, S. F. Schaffner, D. A. Milner, Jr., J. P. Daily, O. Sarr, D. Ndiaye, O. Ndir, S. Mboup, M. T. Duraisingh, A. Lukens, A. Derr, N. Stange-Thomann, S. Waggoner, R. Onofrio, L. Ziaugra, E. Mauceli, S. Gnerre, D. B. Jaffe, J. Zainoun, R. C. Wiegand, B. W. Birren, D. L. Hartl, J. E. Galagan, E. S. Lander, and D. F. Wirth.** 2007. A genome-wide map of diversity in *Plasmodium falciparum*. *Nat. Genet.* **39:**113–119.
135. **Vythilingam, I., Y. M. Noorazian, T. C. Huat, A. I. Jiram, Y. M. Yusri, A. H. Azahari, I. Norparina, A. Noorrain, and S. Lokmanhakim.** 2008. *Plasmodium knowlesi* in humans, macaques and mosquitoes in peninsular Malaysia. *Parasit. Vectors* **1:**26.
136. **Weatherall, D. J., L. H. Miller, D. I. Baruch, K. Marsh, O. K. Doumbo, C. Casals-Pascual, and D. J. Roberts.** 2002. Malaria and the red cell. *Hematology Am. Soc. Hematol. Educ. Program*:35–57.
137. **White, N. J.** 2008. *Plasmodium knowlesi*: the fifth human malaria parasite. *Clin. Infect. Dis.* **46:**172–173.
138. **Wiersch, S. C., W. A. Maier, and H. Kampen.** 2005. *Plasmodium (Haemamoeba) cathemerium* gene sequences for phylogenetic analysis of malaria parasites. *Parasitol. Res.* **96:**90–94.
139. **Wiesner, J., A. Reichenberg, S. Heinrich, M. Schlitzer, and H. Jomaa.** 2008. The plastid-like organelle of apicomplexan parasites as drug target. *Curr. Pharm. Des.* **14:**855–871.
140. **Williams, T. N., T. W. Mwangi, S. Wambua, N. D. Alexander, M. Kortok, R. W. Snow, and K. Marsh.** 2005. Sickle cell trait and the risk of *Plasmodium falciparum* malaria and other childhood diseases. *J. Infect. Dis.* **192:**178–186.
141. **Winstanley, P.** 2001. Modern chemotherapeutic options for malaria. *Lancet Infect. Dis.* **1:**242–250.
142. **Woolhouse, M. E., C. Dye, J. F. Etard, T. Smith, J. D. Charlwood, G. P. Garnett, P. Hagan, J. L. Hii, P. D. Ndhlovu, R. J. Quinnell, C. H. Watts, S. K. Chandiwana, and R. M. Anderson.** 1997. Heterogeneities in the transmission of infectious agents: implications for the design of control programs. *Proc. Natl. Acad. Sci. USA* **94:**338–342.
143. **Wootton, J. C., X. Feng, M. T. Ferdig, R. A. Cooper, J. Mu, D. I. Baruch, A. J. Magill, and X. Z. Su.** 2002. Genetic diversity and chloroquine selective sweeps in *Plasmodium falciparum*. *Nature* **418:**320–323.
144. **Yadav, P., R. Sharma, S. Kumar, and U. Kumar.** 2008. Magnetic resonance features of cerebral malaria. *Acta Radiol.* **49:**566–569.
145. **Zimmermann, O., R. de Ciman, and U. Gross.** 2005. Bacteremia among Kenyan children. *N. Engl. J. Med.* **352:**1379–1381.
146. **Zingman, B. S., and B. L. Viner.** 1993. Splenic complications in malaria: case report and review. *Clin. Infect. Dis.* **16:**223–232.

Sequelae and Long-Term Consequences of Infectious Diseases
Edited by Pina M. Fratamico, James L. Smith, and Kim A. Brogden

Chapter 16

Trypanosomatidae: *Leishmania* Species, *Trypanosoma cruzi* (Chagas Disease), and Associated Complications

JEAN-PIERRE DEDET

Trypanosomatidae is a family of flagellate protozoa belonging to the order Kinetoplastida (Protozoa and Mastigophora). As other members of the Kinetoplastida, trypanosomatids possess a highly characteristic large intracellular basophilic structure found close to the base of the flagellum, the kinetoplast, which contains a massive amount of mitochondrial DNA arranged as a complex network of maxi- and minicircles. Within the kinetoplastids, the trypanosomatids are distinguished by their single flagellum. Kinetoplast size, shape, and position in relation to other morphological features provide a basis for the recognition of different morphological stages in the life cycle of trypanosomatids (Fig. 1) and for recognition of the genera and subgenera (Table 1) (19).

All members of the family Trypanosomatidae are exclusively parasitic and have a large host spectrum, depending on the different genera. Trypanosomatids include parasites of plants (genus *Phytomonas*), insects (various genera, particularly *Crithidia, Blastocrithidia, Herpetomonas,* and *Leptomonas*), and vertebrates (*Sauroleishmania, Endotrypanum, Trypanosoma*, and *Leishmania*) (Table 1). These last two genera are of particular medical and veterinary interest, being parasites of mammals, including humans. The genus *Leishmania* includes a large number of species parasitizing a wide range of mammals, including humans, to which they are transmitted by the bite of a phlebotomine sandfly, an insect vector. They are responsible for a group of animal and/or human diseases called leishmaniasis. The genus *Trypanosoma* includes blood parasites of all the major classes of vertebrates. Those infecting aquatic vertebrates (fishes, amphibia, and chelonians) are transmitted by leeches, while those of terrestrial vertebrates (terrestrial amphibia, birds, and mammals) are transmitted by blood-sucking arthropods. The human diseases due to *Trypanosoma* species are the African human trypanosomiases, caused by *Trypanosoma brucei* subspecies, and American trypanosomiasis, or Chagas disease, due to *Trypanosoma cruzi.* Within the scope of this chapter we will consider the postinfectious sequelae and long-term consequences of leishmaniasis and Chagas disease.

LEISHMANIASES

Leishmaniases are parasitic diseases caused by protozoan flagellates of the genus *Leishmania*, parasites infecting numerous mammal species, including humans, and transmitted through the infective bite of an insect vector, the phlebotomine sandfly. The leishmaniases threaten 350 million people in 88 countries of four continents. The annual incidence of new cases is estimated between 1.5 and 2 million. In numerous underdeveloped countries, they remain a major public health problem (12).

Characteristics of *Leishmania*

Leishmania are dimorphic trypanosomatids, which present as two principal morphological stages (Fig. 1): the intracellular amastigote, which multiplies within the parasitophorous vacuoles of the mononuclear phagocytic cells of the mammalian host, and the flagellated promastigote within the intestinal tract of the insect vector and in culture medium.

Since the first *Leishmania* species was described (23), the number of species has increased steadily and currently stands around 30. As the different species are morphologically indistinguishable, other characters have been used for their taxonomy. Although DNA-based characters are increasingly being used, isoenzyme electrophoresis remains the gold-standard technique for taxonomic description and

Jean-Pierre Dedet • Université Montpellier 1, CHU de Montpellier, Laboratoire de Parasitologie-Mycologie, CNRS, UMR 2724 (CNRS, IRD, and Université Montpellier 1), Montpellier, France.

Shape	Kinetoplast position	Free flagellum	flagellum emergence	Undulating membrane	Name	Morphology
round	-	no	no	-	**amastigote**	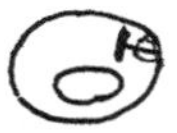
	anterior	yes	anterior	no	**choanomastigote**	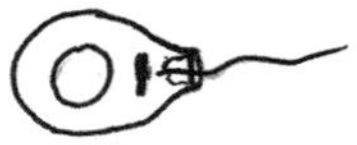
elongated		yes	anterior	no	**promastigote**	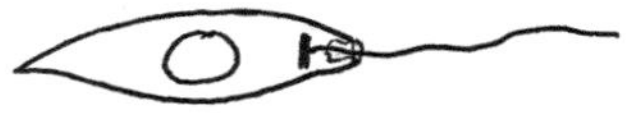
		yes	on side	yes	**epimastigote**	
	posterior	yes	on side	yes	**trypomastigote**	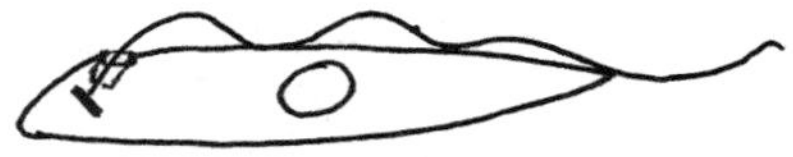
		yes	anterior	no	**opisthomastigote**	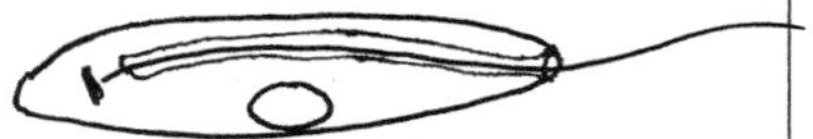

Figure 1. Schematic characteristics and representation of the principal morphological stages of the trypanosomatid flagellates.

identification and is the basis for the current classification. Various types of classification have been successively applied to the genus: monothetic Linnean classifications based on a few hierarchical characters (22), Adansonian phenetic classifications, and phylogenetic classification revealing a parental relationship between the different species of *Leishmania* (28) (Table 2).

In nature, *Leishmania* is alternately hosted by an insect acting as a vector (the phlebotomine sandfly) and by various mammals, including humans, acting as reservoir hosts. Sandflies are psychodid Diptera of the subfamily Phlebotominae. Their life cycle includes two different biological stages: the free-flying adult and the developmental stages (egg, four larval instars, and pupa). The adults are small flying insects about 2 to 4 mm in length, with a yellowish hairy body, active at dusk and during the night. Both sexes feed on plant juices, but females also need a blood meal, during which the *Leishmania* parasites are transmitted between the mammalian hosts. Among about 800 known species of sandflies, about 70, belonging to the genera *Phlebotomus* in the Old World and *Lutzomyia* in the New World, are proven or suspected vectors of *Leishmania*. Various species of seven different orders of mammals are the reservoir hosts responsible

Table 1. Main genera of the trypanosomatid family according to their respective morphological stages

Genus	Morphological stage					
	Amastigote	Choanomastigote	Epimastigote	Opisthomastigote	Promastigote	Trypomastigote
Blastocrithidia	+		+		+	
Crithidia	+	+				
Endotrypanum	+		+		+	+
Herpetomonas				+	+	
Leishmania	+				+	
Leptomonas	+				+	
Phytomonas					+	
Sauroleishmania	+				+	
Trypanosoma	+		+		+	+

Table 2. Simplified classification of the genus *Leishmania* derived from the phylogenetic analysis based on isoenzymes (28)

Classification
Subgenus *Leishmania*
L. donovani complex
L. donovani
L. infantum complex
L. infantum (syn. *L. chagasi*)
L. tropica complex
L. tropica
L. killicki complex
L. killicki
L. aethiopica complex
L. aethiopica
L. major complex
L. major
L. turanica complex
L. turanica
L. gerbilli complex
L. gerbilli
L. arabica complex
L. arabica
L. mexicana complex
L. mexicana (syn. *L. pifanoi*)
L. amazonensis complex
L. amazonensis (syn. *L. garnhami*)
L. aristidesi
L. enriettii complex
L. enriettii
L. hertigi complex
L. hertigi
L. deanei
Subgenus *Viannia*
L. braziliensis complex
L. braziliensis
L. peruviana
L. guyanensis complex
L. guyanensis
L. panamensis
L. shawi
L. naiffi complex
L. naiffi
L. lainsoni complex
L. lainsoni

for long-term maintenance of *Leishmania* in nature. Depending on the focus, the reservoir host can be either wild (carnivores, rodents, hyraxes, marsupials, and edentates) or domestic mammals (dog), or even, in particular situations, human beings (*Leishmania donovani* and *Leishmania tropica*).

The more than 88 countries in which leishmaniasis occurs range over the intertropical zones of America and Africa, extending into temperate regions of North and South America, southern Europe, and Asia. The limits of the disease are latitudes 45°N and 32°S. The geographical distribution is governed by those of the mammal or sandfly host species, their ecology, and their own distribution area. The leishmaniases include several "noso-epidemiological units," which can be defined as the conjunction of a particular *Leishmania* species, circulating in specific natural hosts, in a natural focus with specific ecological patterns, and having a particular spectrum of clinical expression.

Diseases Caused by *Leishmania*

The bite of an infected sandfly results in the intradermal inoculation of metacyclic promastigotes, whose establishment in the mammalian host is facilitated in a remarkable way by the sandfly saliva delivered at the same time (21). Within the dermis of mammalian skin, the metacyclic promastigotes are phagocytosed by macrophages within which they transform into amastigotes and have the capacity to resist intracellular digestion. When the intracellular development of the amastigotes remains localized at the inoculation site, this results in the development of a localized lesion of cutaneous leishmaniasis (CL). In other instances, the parasites spread to the organs of the mononuclear phagocytic system, giving rise to visceral leishmaniasis (VL). Amastigotes may also spread to other cutaneous sites, as in diffuse CL (DCL), or to mucosae, in the case of mucocutaneous leishmaniasis (MCL). The localization of the parasite to the various organs of the patient results in the clinical expression of the disease. It is directly related to the tropism of the parasite species (Table 3). In that sense, the genus *Leishmania* can be divided broadly into viscerotropic (*L. donovani* and *L. infantum*) and dermotropic species (roughly all other species). *L. braziliensis* and more rarely *L. panamensis* are known for their secondary mucosal spread. But the clinical expression of the leishmaniases depends not only on the genotypic potential of the different parasites but also on the immunological status of the patient. In particular, immunosuppression leads to particular clinical outcomes of the disease, both in VL and CL (see below).

VL

The incubation period is generally 2 to 6 months. The onset of the disease may be sudden or gradual, the most common symptom being irregular fever. In well-established VL, the patient presents a protuberant abdomen and muscle wasting of the limbs. Fever, the major symptom, is intermittent and irregular, with a double or triple rise per day, usually to 38 or 39°C. It lasts for some weeks, followed by an apyrexial period. Splenomegaly appears early and is almost invariably present. The spleen is firm, smooth,

Table 3. Usual tropisms and clinical expressions of the main anthropophilic species of *Leishmania*

Usual tropism	Species	Clinical expression[a]	
		Usual	Exceptional
Viserotropic species	*L. donovani*	VL, PKDL	LCL
	L. infantum	VL	LCL, DCL*
Dermotropic species	*L. aethiopica*	LCL, DCL	
	L. major	LCL	DCL*
	L. tropica	LCL	VL
	L. amazonensis	LCL, DCL	VL
	L. guyanensis	LCL	
	L. lainsoni	LCL	
	L. mexicana	LCL	DCL, VL*
	L. naiffi	LCL	
	L. peruviana	LCL	
	L. shawi	LCL	
	L. venezuelensis	LCL	
Dermo-mucotropic species	*L. braziliensis*	LCL, MCL	DCL*, VL*
	L. panamensis	LCL	MCL, DCL*

[a] VL, visceral leishmaniasis; LCL, localized cutaneous leishmaniasis; DCL, diffuse cutaneous leishmaniasis; MCL, mucocutaneous leishmaniasis. *, during immunosuppression.

mobile, and painless. Spleen size increases regularly, in relation to the duration of the disease. The liver is generally slightly enlarged and painless. The nodes are small, firm, painless, and mobile. Anemia is responsible for an extreme pallor of skin and mucosa. In India, patient skin has a greyish pigmentation, which gives rise to the local name of the disease (kala-azar). Asthenia and weight loss complete this classical presentation. Other symptoms can be found, such as digestive, pulmonary, and bleeding manifestations. VL is characterized by hemocytic changes and plasma protein alterations. Normochromic and normocytic anemia is the major and most frequent hematological sign. Leucopenia with neutropenia is frequently reported and can, when severe, be responsible for numerous associated infections. Platelet numbers are occasionally decreased. Severe thrombocytopenia, when associated with alterations of hepatic coagulation factors, is responsible for hemorrhages, which can be quite dramatic. The decrease of the three blood cell lines corresponds to the classical picture of pancytopenia, commonly associated with VL. The inflammation syndrome includes a raised erythrocyte sedimentation rate and increase of C-reactive protein. The plasma protein profiles are disturbed, with low albumin levels and hypergammaglobulinemia, corresponding to overproduction of polyclonal immunoglobulins (Ig), mainly IgG.

VL is a chronic disease, evolving slowly over many months or even a few years. The clinical and biological signs become progressively more severe, and body wasting reaches frank cachexia. Untreated, the disease is fatal in 90% of cases, mainly caused by intercurrent infection or hemorrhages. When administered in time, specific treatment generally leads to patient cure. However, relapses are more and more frequently reported and are attributed to the emergence of resistant parasite strains and/or to host characteristics, such as immunosuppression.

CL

CL presents as skin lesions, which are generally localized, without involvement of mucosae or generalized infection. They occur on exposed parts of the body surface accessible to sandflies, principally on the face, hands, forearms, and lower limbs. Rarely, dermotropic parasites may give rise to DCL, a special outcome related to a deficiency of the cell-mediated immune system of the patient, which will be considered in the next paragraph. All anthropophilic species of *Leishmania*, including the usually viscerotropic species *L. donovani* and *L. infantum,* can be responsible for localized CL (LCL), a mild self-healing infection. The incubation period varies between a week and several months, the mean duration being around 1 month. The cutaneous lesion starts as an erythematous papule which gradually enlarges, reaching its definitive size in a few weeks. The mature lesion has a regular outline and is generally round or oval in shape. Its dimensions are variable, usually a few centimeters in diameter. Depending on the number of infecting bites, the lesions can be single or multiple, 2 to 10 usually, but occasionally more. The lesions are painless, unless secondarily infected. The clinical types of cutaneous lesions are variable, depending on the species of parasite and the genetic and immunological background of the patient. The ulcerative lesion is the most common clinical feature of LCL. It resembles a volcano with sloping sides and a central ulcer, which has a variable depth and a more or less granulomatous bottom. A scab resulting from the coagulation of exudates can cover the ulceration. The outline of the lesion is more or less elevated, inflammatory, of reddish or purplish color on pale skin but hyperpigmented on darker skin. It can sometimes be slightly squamous and surrounded by smaller daughter papules. This type of lesion, classically known as "wet form," is characteristic of zoonotic CL, principally due to *L. major* (oriental sore and Biskra or Gafsa boils), *L. mexicana* (chiclero's ulcer), *L. guyanensis* (pian bois), *L. peruviana* (uta), and *L. braziliensis* (cutaneous lesion). More indolent "dry" lesions are characteristic of anthroponotic CL due to *L. tropica*.

More rarely, other clinical types of lesion are encountered, unrelated to *Leishmania* species: a dry type (papulo-nodular lesion, covered by superficial scales), a closed nodular type, an infiltrative plaque type, an eczematoid type, and a warty and pseudotumoural type. Whatever the clinical type of lesion, LCL evolution is chronic and leads most often to a spontaneous cure after a time, which varies, according to the species, from a few months (about 6 months for *L. major*, *L. mexicana*, or *L. peruviana* lesions) to a few years (more than 1 year for *L. aethiopica*, *L. infantum*, *L. tropica*, or *L. guyanensis* lesions). The cure, either spontaneous or following treatment, results in an permanent scar (see the following section below).

MCL

MCL, also named "espundia" since its early description (15), is a particular nosological entity mainly due to the species *L. braziliensis* and occasionally to *L. panamensis*. It is a wild zoonosis, of which the natural reservoir host(s) are not clearly established. It occurs from southern Mexico to the north of Argentina. This form of leishmaniasis evolves in two stages: a primary cutaneous lesion, eventually followed, after a variable time of latency, by secondary mucosal involvement. The initial cutaneous lesion does not fundamentally differ from the localized lesions caused by other dermotropic *Leishmania* species (see above), and it generally heals spontaneously. Following cure of the primary cutaneous lesion(s), the infection may remain asymptomatic for a variable period of time, which can be very long, sometimes indefinite. In some cases, secondary mucosal involvement occurs, which will be described in the following section (see below).

Long-Term Consequences Associated with *Leishmania*

We will consider in this section the long-term consequences and sequelae of leishmaniasis, with special emphasis on the long-term evolution of VL of immunosuppressed patients, post-kala-azar dermal leishmaniasis, the complications and scars resulting from LCL, some particularly long-lasting forms of CL (namely, leishmaniasis recidivans and DCL), and mucosal involvement of MCL and their disfiguring involvement and further sequelae.

Long-term evolution of immunosuppressed VL

The number of VL cases associated with immunosuppression has increased steadily over the past 20 or so years. All immunosuppressive states, whether resulting from human immunodeficiency virus (HIV) infection or from the use of immunosuppressive treatment of systemic diseases (hemopathies, systemic lupus erythematosus, Crohn's disease, etc.) or of organ transplantation (reviewed in reference 4), favor the development of VL. Cases of VL during HIV infection have been recorded in various foci in the world, particularly in southern Europe. By early 2001, out of more than 2,000 cases which had been reported to the WHO, 90% were from southern Europe: Spain, Italy, southern France, and Portugal (13). The spread of AIDS to rural areas where visceral leishmaniasis is endemic and of VL to suburban areas has resulted in a progressively increasing overlap between the two diseases, not only in Mediterranean Europe but also in the other foci of VL, such as North and East Africa, India, and Brazil. In southern Europe, coinfected patients are mainly adults and of male gender (85%), and 77.3% are 31- to 50-year-olds, while 70% of the cases belong to the risk group of intravenous drug users (13). The predominance of the coinfected cases in the intravenous drug user group has led to the postulate that direct interhuman transmission may occur via syringe sharing, an element with important epidemiological implications (1).

VL during HIV infection coincides with a serious state of immunosuppression, as 92% of patients have less than 200 CD4/ml. The clinical features are typical of VL in 87.6% of cases, but atypical symptoms are found in 12.4% of cases; these unusual symptoms are commonly of a cutaneous, pulmonary, or digestive nature, with the presence of parasites in lung, pleura, esophagus, stomach, duodenum, jejunum, colon, rectum, and healthy skin (13). The classical hematological abnormalities associated with VL in the immunocompetent host are frequently absent. These signs interfere with the alterations specific to AIDS and to other opportunistic infections, often associated with, or induced by, antiretroviral treatment. The prognosis of VL during HIV coinfection is different from that of VL for immunocompetent patients. During coinfection, relapse rates are high, reaching 60% during the first 12 months after treatment (10).

PKDL

Post-kala-azar dermal leishmanisis (PKDL) is an uncommon dermal manifestation occurring after apparent cure or during treatment of *L. donovani* VL. The pathogenesis of this VL complication remains unclear. PKDL was reported in 20% of cases in India (31) and 56% in Sudan (35). In India, PKDL appears after a latent period of approximately 1 year after kala-azar cure, while in Sudan it can start before symptoms of kala-azar have completely subsided. Beginning as depigmented macules, the PKDL skin lesions turn into papular and then nodular eruptions (Color Plate 10). Located initially on the face and the tips of upper limbs, they can extend to the whole body surface. The lesions normally do not ulcerate. They may contain numerous parasites, whatever their stage, and can play an important role in sandfly transmission and parasite dissemination. The lesions may self-cure within 6 months or last for many months or years.

Complications of CL and scars

Lesions of LCL can sometimes be complicated by a secondary bacterial infection, with possible lymphangitis progression. Superinfected lesions show higher inflammatory process with pain, which differs from a pure leishmanial lesion. Superinfection hinders the parasitological diagnosis of the lesion and needs specific antibiotic therapy. In countries where CL is endemic, topical applications of toxic products can lead to caustic or contact allergy reactions, with secondary eczematization. Whether cure is spontaneous or follows treatment, LCL results in a permanent scar. Depending on the clinical feature of the lesion, the scar is generally depressed, mainly following an ulcerative type lesion (Color Plate 11A). In certain patients, the scar can be cheloid and sometimes disfiguring. Its color, pinkish or whitish on pale skin (Color Plate 11B), can be hyperpigmented on dark skin (Color Plate 11C). The evolution of CL does not generally lead to mutilation, with the exception of chiclero's ulcer due to *L. mexicana*, which is occasionally responsible for partial destruction of the ear auricle. Clinical cure does not always lead to a complete disappearance of the parasites. In some cases, for example, in about 7% of *L. guyanensis* CL cases in French Guiana, the cure is followed by a resurgence of an active lesion directly on the scar (Color Plate 11D and E) (11). This reactivation can occur between a few months to a few years following the initial cure. This secondary lesion will also cure spontaneously.

Leishmaniasis recidivans

Leishmaniasis recidivans is a chronic form of leishmaniasis occurring mainly in some countries of the Middle East, such as Iran or Iraq, and essentially due to *L. tropica*. The lesion is located on the face and follows an acute lesion, after numerous months of evolution. The lesion shows a peripheral active zone around a central healing part. It extends continuously and can last for 20 to 40 years. The presentation mimics that of lupus vulgaris, which explains the name of lupoid leishmaniasis sometimes used. The lesion contains few parasites and is associated with an exaggerated cell-mediated immune response on the part of the host.

DCL

DCL, a particularly severe form of CL, was initially described from Venezuela (9). It is a peculiar and scarce clinical form, resulting from the parasitism of particular *Leishmania* species, *L. amazonensis* and occasionally *L. mexicana* (32) in the New World and *L. aethiopica* in the Old World (3), in patients with a specific defect in antileishmanial cell-mediated immunity (7). Since HIV infection has spread to leishmaniasis-endemic areas, DCL cases have occasionally been reported due to unusual species, such as *L. braziliensis* in the New World (29) and *L. infantum* (20) and *L. major* (16) in the Old World. A nonulcerated nodule rich in parasites represents the basic cutaneous lesion of this form of disease. The nodules are numerous, at first isolated and then joining to form large patches, disseminated over the whole of the body, to the face, as well as to the trunk and limbs. The general appearance of the patient mimics the presentation of lepromatous leprosy, with "leonine" face. The pathology of the lesion is characteristic, with a homogeneous epidermal and dermal infiltrate of vacuolated macrophages full of *Leishmania* amastigotes. The leishmanin skin test is negative. During the development of this condition, there is no ulceration or mucosal or visceral involvement, but there is a slow constant aggravation by successive relapses, interrupted with phases of remission. This form is resistant to therapy by classical antileishmanial drugs and especially to pentavalent antimonials and does not cure spontaneously.

MCL

The frequency of occurrence of secondary mucosal involvement appears variable, according to foci considered and authors. The period of time between cutaneous lesion and subsequent appearance of the mucosal involvement extends from several weeks to many years. Very long time intervals have occasionally been observed by several authors (33).

The mucosal involvement usually starts on the nasal mucosa. The patient suffers from nasal congestion, which causes nocturnal discomfort. Epistaxis can also be the initial symptom (33). The initial nasal lesion is generally limited to the anterior, cartilaginous part of the nasal septum. It appears as a small hyperemic inflammatory granuloma (Color Plate 12A), rapidly evolving to an ulcer (24). The septum is rapidly invaded and destroyed, which leads to the perforation of the nasal septum in its anterior part, a symptom generally considered pathognomonic of MCL (Color Plate 12B and C) (33). The involvement of nasal mucosa can be apparent from the exterior, even as early as the initial inflammatory stage, and manifests as congestion and edema of the nasal pyramid. At the stage of septum destruction, the nose is flattened and weighed down (Color Plate 12E) and is classically described as "tapir nose." The buccal mucosa is commonly affected at a later stage of the disease, with or without contiguous spread from the nasal lesions (Color Plate 13A). The mucosae of the palate (Color Plate 12D) and of the interior lips are the most frequently involved (Color Plate 13A), while the tongue generally remains uninjured. The palatal lesions are granulomatous and extensive and reach the velum. They produce the classical "Escomel cross." The lip lesions are inflamed and ulcerated, sometimes extending to the external part, with frequent tissue destruction. A palatal perforation can occur in the later stages and results in the interconnection of nasal fossae and the mouth cavity.

Laryngeal extension follows the rhino-buccal–pharyngeal localization of the parasites. The lesion is first infiltrative and manifests as dysphonia and metallic cough. When granulomatous, the laryngeal lesion can cause obstruction of the respiratory tract, with possible fatal consequences due to acute respiratory distress. Dysphagia and the resulting undernutrition have serious consequences for the physical condition of the patient. Tissue necrosis and disfigurement appear in the advanced stage of the condition and can be extremely severe. They result in disfiguring mutilations: the nose and lips can totally disappear, at which time the mouth and nasal cavity become connected by a single hole. Socio-psychological consequences are considerable for the patient, often leading to suicide. Death can occur following pulmonary superinfections consequent to false alimentary passages or acute respiratory obstruction. When treated and cured, patients exhibit disfiguring, sometimes retractile, scars (Color Plate 13B).

Treatment

Treatment of all the leishmaniases remains difficult, due to the multiplicity of the existing *Leishmania* species and their variable susceptibility to the available drugs, which are old, toxic, and expensive products. Resistance to the existing products is developing in some foci, such as India. There have been no significant changes in the treatment of leishmaniases for many years. Since the 1920s, treatment has been based on pentavalent antimonial compounds. Following the increasing incidence of VL cases in immunocompromised patients and the rise of acquired resistance to antimonials, amphotericin B, mainly in its liposomal form, has joined the antimonials as a first-line drug. Miltefosine, a new oral compound, has shown promising results and appears to be an efficient alternative for the treatment of Indian kala-azar. Other products, such as aminosidine or imidazoles, could find new applications, but there is no really new product in development at the present time.

Products

Pentavalent antimonials (Sb^V). Two closely related antimony derivatives are currently used: sodium stibogluconate (Pentostam; GlaxoSmithKline) and meglumine antimoniate (Glucantime; Aventis). They have distinct antimony rates of 100 and 85 mg Sb^V per ml, respectively. A generic antimonial (Albert David) is presently manufactured in India for local use.

In spite of a century of use, the mechanism of action of the antimonials remains unclear. It may involve inhibition of ATP synthesis. It is possible that antimonial salts have to be concentrated within the macrophage or parasite and transformed into active trivalent metabolites to be efficient. Antimonials are administered by the parenteral route and are rapidly excreted by the kidneys. Although numerous side effects have been attributed to antimonials, the scarcity of reported accidents and small number of available antileishmanial drugs justify their continued use. Some of the side effects of pentavalent antimonials are related to intolerance action and are of anaphylactic type, including shivers, fever, arthralgias, myalgias, skin rashes, abdominal symptoms, and headache. Other side effects seem to be linked to accumulation of product. They include reversible elevation of hepatocellular enzymes, subclinical pancreatitis, decrease in hemoglobin level and platelet count, and cardiac side effects. Exceptional sudden deaths have been reported for a few patients who received more than the recommended dose of Sb^V.

Pentavalent antimonial recommended dosage is 20 mg Sb^V /kg body weight/day, for 20 days for CL and 28 days for VL and MCL (17). They are currently injected by intravenous (IV) or intramuscular (IM) route. The IV route is preferred for the large volumes of drug required for most adults. In the case of a few localized cutaneous lesions, intralesional injections are used.

Amphotericin B. Amphotericin B is a polyene antibiotic, currently used in the treatment of systemic fungal infections. Amphotericin B action is targeted on ergosterol-like sterols, which are the major membrane sterols of *Leishmania* as well as fungi. It can also stimulate cytokine production of macrophages and enhance their phagocytic capacities. Efficient plasma concentrations are rapidly reached and persist beyond 24 hours. The product has slow renal elimination. Amphotericin B side effects are of two types. Intolerance signs occur during infusion and include chills, headache, cramps, hypotension, vertigo, paraesthesias, vomiting and, exceptionally, anaphylactic or cardiogenic shock. These manifestations are usually controlled by addition of corticoids within the liquid of suspension or by slowing down the infusion. Amphotericin B toxicity is mainly directed against renal function and hematological cell lines.

Amphotericin B is a powerful antileishmanial used in the treatment of severe leishmaniases (VL and MCL) or forms resistant to antimonials. Amphotericin B deoxycholate is formulated as a colloidal suspension (Fungizone; Bristol Myers Squibb), which is administered as a slow (6- to 8-hour) IV infusion (0.5 to 1 mg/kg dissolved in 500 ml dextrose 5%) on alternate days. The common regimens range from 14 to 20 infusions, for a total dose of 1.5 to 2 g. New lipid formulations of amphotericin B are the major advances of the last two decades.

Lipid-associated amphotericin B. When associated with lipids, amphotericin B is transported to the site of intracellular infection, which leads to more drug accumulation in infected cells, thereby increasing the therapeutic index. The three existing formulations are similar in some respects and globally less toxic than amphotericin B but have different tolerability and kinetics. Liposomal amphotericin B (AmBisome; Gilead Sciences) is a unilamellar formed from a variety of phospholipids in a membrane bilayer containing amphotericin B. This compound has a license for VL treatment in Europe and the United States. The two other formulations—amphotericin B phospholipid complex (Abelcet; Enzon Pharmaceuticals) and amphotericin B cholesterol dispersion (Amphocil; Zeneca Pharmaceuticals)—are not yet licensed for VL.

Liposomal amphotericin B has been used in several countries for VL treatment and has been shown to be less toxic than conventional amphotericin B and more efficient in both immunocompetent and immunocompromised patients (5). Short-course treatment is now currently used, including five daily injections of 3 or 4 mg/kg, plus a further injection of the same dose on the 10th day (total dose of 18 to 20 mg/kg). For immunocompromised patients, the number of injections is increased to 9 or 10.

Miltefosine. This alkyl phospholipid is an oral antineoplastic agent, which is a phosphocholine analogue affecting cell signaling pathways and membrane synthesis. It proved to be efficient in the treatment of experimental murine leishmaniasis. Several comparative and dose finding clinical trials have been carried out in India, with a total of about 700 patients, including antimonial-resistant VL cases (reviewed in reference 26). Initial cure rates were around 99%, and final cure rates were 92%. Miltefosine is widely acceptable, even if digestive side effects are frequent (about 50%), with mild vomiting or diarrhea in most patients. This product should not be used in pregnancy, due to teratogenic effects. Miltefosine is produced in India and Germany (Impavido; Zentaris), as 50-mg pills. It is recommended for treatment of VL in India.

Pentamidine. Pentamidine is an aromatic diamine first synthesized in the late 1930s. At present, the isethionate salt (Pentacarinat; Aventis) is the only form available for human use and is restricted to treatment of *L. guyanensis* CL. Pentamidine inhibits the synthesis of parasite DNA by blocking thymidine synthase and fixation of transfer RNA. In the absence of oral absorption, the drug is administered by the parenteral route, which provides a transient blood concentration, with rapid subsequent distribution and high tissue fixation. It is excreted slowly by the kidney.

Pentamidine can be responsible for immediate side effects, mainly in the case of rapid IV injection (hypotension, tachycardia, nausea, vomiting, facial erythema, pruritus, and syncope). Local reactions can also occur (urticaria, abcess formation, and phlebitis). Toxic side effects depend upon the dose and can affect pancreas, kidney, and blood cell lines. Alterations of glucose metabolism are directly linked to the product toxicity to pancreatic cells and can result in diabetes mellitus induction.

Pentamidine is given in doses of 4 mg/kg per injection. The IM or slow IV injections are made on alternate days, in patients confined to bed and having eaten nothing. Short courses (four doses) are currently used for treatment of certain forms of CL.

Aminosidine Aminosidine (paromomycin) is a wide-spectrum antibiotic of the aminoglycoside family. It showed powerful antileishmanial activity in vitro and in animal models. Like other aminoglycosides, paromomycin has renal and eighth cranial nerve toxicity. An injectable formulation of paromomycin was registered in India in 2006 and is being produced in that country (Gland Pharma). The recommended dose for administration by IM injection or IV infusion is 15 mg/kg per day, given for 10 days. Paromomycin has been efficiently used for VL treatment as monotherapy and in combination with pentavalent antimonials (reviewed in reference 26).

Several topical formulations have been tested for treatment of CL. An ointment formulation comprising 15% paromomycin sulfate and 12% methylbenzethonium chloride is licensed in Israel (Leshcutan; Teva Pharmaceutical Industries). It is effective for *L. major* CL, but with a local toxicity, which has led to investigations of other topical formulations.

Imidazoles. The antifungal azoles inhibit the sterol synthesis pathway of *Leishmania*. Some of them (ketoconazole, itraconazole, and fluconazole) have been tested in the treatment of CL, with contradictory results. Their low toxicity and the comfort of oral administration lead these products to be occasionally used for the treatment of CL, at doses of 200 to 400 mg/day for 1 to 3 months, for an adult.

Treatment regimens according to clinical features

The large variability of clinical forms of leishmaniasis, with their distinct evolution processes and different levels of severity, necessitate a decision on the drug regimen from case to case. This is all the more relevant, since the available classical antileishmanial drugs are not devoid of toxicity. VL may be treated as soon as diagnosis is completed. The efficiency of treatment is dependent on the stage of the disease, advanced stages being less responsive to antileishmanial drugs. Treatment requires confirmed first-line products, principally antimonials and amphotericin B. The conventional treatment is based on a 28-day course of pentavalent antimonial at a dose of 20 mg Sb^V/kg per day. Due to its excellent results, liposomal amphotericin B tends to be used as a first choice, with five daily injections (3 mg/kg per injection) and a final injection on the 10th day (total dose 18 mg/kg). Management of VL cases includes correcting nutritional deficiencies in severely wasted patients, blood transfusion in case of severe anemia, and treatment with appropriate antibiotics for any secondary bacterial infection.

Antimony resistance has reached impressive levels in some Indian foci, where antimony has become inadequate. Current treatment is carried out with miltefosine (100 mg/day for 28 days for adults weighing more than 25 kg, and 2.5 mg/kg/day for 28 days for children less than 25 kg).

For PKDL treatment in India, a combination of pentavalent antimonial (20 mg Sb^V/kg/day) and ketoconazole (200 mg twice daily) for 60 days was recommended (27). During pregnancy, liposomal amphotericin B appears to be the safest and most efficient product (25). For VL occurring in HIV-infected patients, liposomal amphotericin B is usually considered as the first-line drug, with a longer course, of five daily injections of 1.5 to 4 mg/kg, plus four further injections of the same dose on days 10, 17, 31, and 38 (total dose of 20 to 40 mg/kg). VL following organ transplantation poses apparent therapeutic problems resulting from the toxicity of the main antileishmanial drugs for transplanted organs. In reality, these cases need to be treated, as they are fatal in the absence of specific treatment. Despite the absence of controlled clinical studies, literature data show that the use of liposomal amphotericin B gives the best results with fewer side effects than antimonials (4). Once the antileishmanial treatment has been concluded, the problem with immunocompromised patients is that of secondary prophylaxis for prevention of relapses. Numerous schemes have been proposed, of which two are currently in use: a 3-mg/kg injection of liposomal amphotericin B every 3 to 6 weeks or a 2-mg/kg injection of pentamidine every 15 or 30 days.

Management of patients with LCL depends on the location and characteristics of the lesion(s), the *Leishmania* species involved, the risk of extension and the opinion of the patient. Briefly, three options are possible: therapeutic abstention or local or general treatment. Mild, rapidly self-healing forms of CL, such as those due to *L. major* or *L. peruviana*, can remain untreated, if the patient wishes. Various local treatments have been proposed, including diverse physical means (diathermy, cryotherapy, radiotherapy, and laser), surgical excision, or local applications of ointments. Trials of these methods have been limited, and without control groups, and the results were inconclusive. These procedures cannot be generalized.

Local infiltrations of pentavalent antomonials are recommended for the treatment of small numbers of lesions. Various protocols have been proposed consisting of a course of 5 to 10 infiltrations of 1 to 5 ml of antimonial, associated or not with cryotherapy. Infiltrations are done two or three times a week.

Systemic treatment is recommended for CL with large and/or multiple lesions; with lymphangitic dissemination, those of recidivans type; or with a risk of mucosal involvement. CL of immunocompromised patients should also be treated by systemic treatment. The currently used systemic treatment is a course of 20 days of pentavalent antimonial (20 mg Sb^V/kg per day). Oral imidazoles can occasionally be used as alternatives to antimonials in the case of *L. major* CL (fluconazole) or of *L. mexicana* CL (ketoconazole). A course of four or five IM injections of pentamidine (4 mg/kg per injection) on alternate days is the first-line treatment for CL due to *L. guyanensis* and *L. panamensis*.

Once established, DCL is resistant to treatment. All available antileishmanial products have been used for isolated case treatment: systematic pentavalent antimonials, pentamidine, immunotherapy, and combination of paromomycin and antimonial. At best, they temporarily improved the clinical evolution. There is an urgent need for the testing of various new molecules or formulations (liposomal amphotericin B and gamma interferon). But the scarcity of cases does not allow randomized clinical trials with control groups. A recent trial of 16 Venezuelan patients treated with miltefosine showed improvement during treatment but relapses after suspension of the treatment (34).

Systemic treatment of the *L. braziliensis* primary cutaneous lesion is recommended, with the hope of avoiding parasite extension to facial mucosae. The treatment currently used in areas where it is endemic is a 20-day course of pentavalent antimonial (20 mg Sb^V/kg per day). A recent study showed an efficacy of liposomal amphotericin B for treating cutaneous lesion of MCL (6), an observation which needs further confirmation. However, it has been shown that correct treatment does not consistently prevent the development of secondary mucosal lesions.

The treatment of mucosal lesions should be as early as possible, in order to avoid the extension of lesions and subsequent mutilation. The antimonials, at standard doses, are injected daily over 28 days. A comparative study showed the efficiency of meglumine antimoniate to be superior to that of sodium stibogluconate (2). The level of cure is variable according to country and the stage of the lesions. Amphotericin B deoxycholate is currently used for late-stage cases or those that respond poorly to antimonials. Cure was sometimes obtained from 1g, but larger doses (2 or 3 g) were often necessary.

Control and Prevention

Intervention strategies for prevention or control are hampered by the diversity of the structure of leishmaniasis foci, with many different reservoir hosts of zoonotic forms and a multiplicity of sandfly vectors, each with a different pattern of behavior. In 1990, a WHO Expert Committee described 11 distinct eco-epidemiological entities and defined control strategies for each one (33a).

The aim of prevention is to avoid host infection (human or canine) and subsequent disease. It includes means to prevent intrusion of people into natural zoonotic foci and protection against infective bites of sandflies. Prevention can be at an individual or collective level. It includes the use of repellents, pyrethroïd-impregnated bed nets, self- protection insecticides, indoor residual spraying, and forest clearance around human settlements. Control programs are intended to interrupt the life cycle of the parasite and to limit, or ideally, eradicate the disease. The structures and dynamics of natural foci of leishmaniasis are so diverse that a standard control program cannot be defined, and control measures must be adapted to local situations. The strategy depends on the ecology and behavior of the two main targets, the reservoir hosts and the vectors, which are not mutually exclusive.

Control measures will be very different depending on whether the disease is anthroponotic or zoonotic. In the New World, almost all the leishmaniases are sylvatic, and control is not usually feasible. Even removal of the forest itself may not be effective, as various *Leishmania* species have proved to be remarkably adaptable to environmental degradation.

Case detection and treatment are recommended when the reservoir host is human or dog, while massive destruction may be the chosen intervention if the reservoir host is a wild animal. The reduced efficacy of the current antileishmanial drugs and their toxicity limit their use for systematic treatment of cases. The high level of asymptomatic infection both in human and canine hosts affects the efficiency and the feasibility of systematic case detection and treatment programs.

As far as vectors are concerned, control of breeding sites is limited to the few instances where they are known (rodent burrows for *P. papatasi* and *P. duboscqi*). Anti-adult measures consist of insecticide spraying. Malaria control programs, based on indoor residual insecticide spraying, have had a side benefit for leishmaniasis incidence in several countries where a resurgence of leishmaniasis was observed after the ending of these campaigns: India, Italy, Greece and the Middle East, and Peru.

In practice, control programs include several integrated measures targeting not only the reservoir host and/or vector, but also associated environmental changes. Health education campaigns can improve considerably the efficiency of control programs. Leishmaniasis control programs have been developed in various countries to combat situations where it is endemic or epidemic (India, Nepal and Bangladesh, China, and Brazil for VL and Central Asian republics of the former USSR and Tunisia for CL).

CHAGAS DISEASE

Chagas disease is an infectious disease resulting from the parasitism of humans by *Trypanosoma cruzi*, a parasite of wild and domestic mammals, transmitted by blood-sucking triatomine bugs. Carlos Chagas, a Brazilian biologist, discovered the etiological agent in 1909, its vector, the domestic and wild reservoir hosts, susceptible laboratory animals, and the human disease (8).

This disease exists only in 21 countries of the American continents, extending from the south of the United States (states of Texas and California) to southern Argentina (state of Chubut, Patagonia). Within this territory, about 30 million people are at risk of being infected, the number of cases being estimated to be about 15 million (33b).

Characteristics of *T. cruzi*

Trypanosoma (*Schizotrypanum*) *cruzi* is a parasite of the intestinal tract of triatomine bugs and of the blood of several wild and domestic mammals, including humans. Triatomine bugs are large blood-sucking insects (Hemiptera and Reduviidae). Both sexes and all development stages (larvae, nymphs, and adult) are hematophagous. They are infected during a blood meal taken on an infected mammal. Within their midgut, the parasites actively multiply as epimastigotes (Fig. 1), which then migrate to the posterior part of the intestinal tract (Stercoraria section of the genus *Trypanosoma*, according to Hoare's classification [18]). Within the rectal ampullae of the bug, the parasites transform into infective penetrative slender forms (metacyclic trypomastigotes), which are eliminated in the feces of the infected bugs. As bugs often defecate on their host when taking a blood meal, the mammal becomes infected by passage of the metacyclic form through abraded skin, the wound caused by the insect's bite, or a mucous membrane.

In mammal blood, the trypomastigote has a characteristic "C" shape, with a large kinetoplast near a short, pointed posterior end, a free flagellum, and an undulating membrane (Fig. 1). The trypomastigotes penetrate phagocytic cell lines, and some nonphagocytic cells, in which they transform into the amastigote stage (Fig. 1), which multiplies intracellularly by binary division. Amastigotes emerging from ruptured cells transform into trypomastigotes, which penetrate new cells to renew the cycle of intracellular divisions. Tissue tropism of *T. cruzi* is directed preferentially to muscle cells, heart muscle, smooth muscles, and skeletal muscles. A proportion of trypomastigotes emerging from parasitized cells circulate in the blood, where they can be picked up by triatomine bugs taking a blood meal.

Genotypic characterization of *T. cruzi*, initially carried out by schizodeme analysis and more recently by various other molecular techniques, has shown a great diversity of parasite strains, which were consensually grouped into two distinct heterogeneous subpopulations, *T. cruzi* I and II (14).

T. cruzi is considered to be originally an enzootic parasite, circulating between wild mammals and sylvatic triatomine bugs. Human disease results from the intrusion of people within the wild cycle of the parasite. The colonization of human dwellings by some triatomine species and the adaptation of the parasite to domestic mammals (dogs, cats, guinea pigs, etc.) led to the establishment of domestic and peridomestic cycles. The poor rural habitat of the areas where the disease is endemic offers the ideal conditions for bugs to colonize houses. When established, the domestic cycles persist without further introduction of wild vectors or reservoir hosts. In this situation, the prevalence of human infection may be very high.

The intensive rural migrations into urban surroundings that occurred in Latin America in the 1970s and 1980s changed the epidemiological pattern of Chagas disease. In addition to the traditional vector-borne rural disease, it became an urban infection transmitted by blood transfusion. The prevalence of *T. cruzi*-infected blood banks in all countries where it is endemic is much higher than that of hepatitis or HIV infection, leading to massive human infection in the South American megapolises. Recently, cases of *T. cruzi* transmission by organ transplantation were also reported. The migration of persons infected by *T. cruzi* poses a public health problem, even for countries where the disease is not endemic, such as the United States and Canada.

Disease Caused by *T. cruzi*

Chagas disease includes three classical clinical stages of infection: an acute form, corresponding to a generalized infection; an intermediate asymptomatic stage;

and a late progressive stage, referred to as chronic Chagas disease. We will describe here the two first stages of the disease and keep the chronic phase for the next section.

Acute phase

The initial phase of Chagas disease corresponds to the period of circulation of trypomastigotes and multiplication of amastigotes in tissues. It may be undetected because of a lack of medical attention, absence of symptoms, or ignorance of the patient of a mild symptomatology.

In clinically apparent acute disease, there may be lesions at the portal of entry of the parasite after a short incubation period (4 or 5 days). The introduction of the parasite through the conjunctiva results in development of a painless, unilateral bipalpebral edema with conjunctivitis, the so-called Romaña's sign. In case of a cutaneous portal of entry, an edematous cutaneous lesion (chagoma) can develop. A lymphadenopathy can occur adjacent to the eye (oculoglandular complex) or to the cutaneous lesion (30).

Blood dissemination of the parasite can lead to general symptoms, the most common of which is fever, which is of variable intensity. Other general symptoms include generalized lymphadenopathies, myalgia, headache, hepato-splenomegaly, and facial or generalized edema.

Tachycardia shows the involvement of the heart early in the infection and regresses in the majority of patients. In a small proportion of cases (under 10% of the patients), congestive heart failure may occur and is fatal in less than 5% of these. Hypotension and arrhythmias are often apparent. Massive cardiomegaly on the chest radiograph indicates severe myocarditis. In nonfatal cases, the electrocardiographic and radiographic changes usually resolve within a year.

In congenital infections or in immunocompromised patients, meningoencephalitis is a complication carrying a poor prognosis. Irritability, lethargy, seizures, focal neurological deficits, and meningismus often lead within several days to a terminal coma. However, the majority of the patients show spontaneous clinical recovery, depending on the Th1 response of the T-helper immunity. Over 90 to 95% of untreated patients recover clinically within 2 to 4 months and enter in the intermediate phase.

Intermediate phase

This phase follows the asymptomatic or symptomatic acute phase. It corresponds to a stage when host immunity has curtailed intracellular replication of amastigotes and reduced the number of circulating trypomastigotes to subpatent levels.

The infection still exists, with blood trypomastigotes detectable by sensitive diagnostic methods, but is completely asymptomatic. Particularly, the electrocardiogram is normal, and contrasted radiographs of the digestive tract do not show any dilatation.

The majority of infected people in regions where the disease is endemic present with this form, which can last for many years, even for the whole life of the patient. But in about 30% of patients, a chronic phase occurs, with two kinds of clinical manifestation: cardiac involvement and digestive abnormalities. This chronic phase is considered below.

Long-Term Consequences Associated with *T. cruzi*

The major causes of morbidity and mortality at the chronic stage are cardiac involvement, referred as chronic Chagas heart disease, and the "mega"-syndromes of the gastrointestinal tract.

Chronic Chagas heart disease

Heart involvement during chronic Chagas is a consequence of the frequent involvement of the conducting tissue by parasite multiplication, with subsequent inflammatory, degenerative, and fibrotic changes, which are the base of conduction disorders. Lesions also affect the contractile myocardium.

In the first stage, asymptomatic patients show electrocardiographic alteration, such as right bundle branch block or anterior fascicular block. Physical examination is unremarkable, except for widened inspiratory splitting of the second heart sound due to right bundle branch block. Additional electrocardiographic abnormalities may appear, such as ventricular extrasystoles.

With time, the heart size increases (cardiomyopathy). Physical examination shows worsening exercise intolerance and palpitations. Chest radiographs show global cardiac enlargement. Sudden death may occur at this stage due to various causes that we analyze below.

Advanced Chagas heart disease is a form of congestive heart failure. The patient complains of dyspnea, weakness, palpitations, syncopal episodes, and chest pain. Physical examination shows a large and dilated heart, arterial hypotension, jugular venous distension, tender Hepatomegaly, and peripheral edema. On auscultation, the rhythm is irregular, with a third heart sound and murmurs of mitral and tricuspid insufficiency. The chest radiograph shows a massive enlargement of cardiac opacity. The main signs are those exhibited by electrocardiogram, consisting typically of ventricular conduction defects: ventricular arrhythmias, atrioventricular block, and sinus node dysfunction.

Chronic Chagas heart disease is generally a progressive disease, during which the patients experience several complications. About 65% of patients die within 2 years of the first episode of congestive heart failure. But sudden death can occur any time during the evolution, even in patients in whom disease has progressed silently. Sudden death in chronic Chagas can be due to several causes, including severe conduction abnormalities, such as sustained ventricular tachycardia or ventricular fibrillation, pulmonary or systemic thromboembolism, or rupture of a ventricular apical aneurysm (Color Plate 14).

Gastrointestinal forms of chronic Chagas disease

A small proportion of patients suffering from chronic Chagas disease have abnormalities of the digestive tract, due to denervation of autonomic ganglia in the walls of hollow organs, and subsequent motor dysfunction. The esophagus and colon are the most commonly affected.

Patients with mega-esophagus mainly present with dysphagia, regurgitation, and odynophagia, and occasionally with hiccough, belching, and excessive salivation. They frequently complain of food regurgitation, particularly during sleep. They progressively become malnourished and susceptible to pulmonary infections.

Colonic involvement is principally located in the rectosigmoid and descending colon (Fig. 2). Patients with megacolon suffer from severe constipation, gaseous distension, and abdominal pain. Constipation may worsen, bowel movements occurring only after weeks, or even a few months, resulting in complications including fecaloma, sigmoid volvulus, or even perforation. Involvement of other intestinal segments, such as the duodenum, ileum, and jejunum, are less frequent.

Treatment

Only two effective drugs are available for treatment of Chagas disease: a nitroimidazole derivative (benznidazole, Rochagan, or Radanil) and a nitrofurane compound (nifurtimox and Lampit). Both products are available only in countries where the disease is endemic, Brazil for Rochagan (Productos Roche Quimicos e Farmaceuticos, São Paulo) and Argentina for Lampit (Bayer).

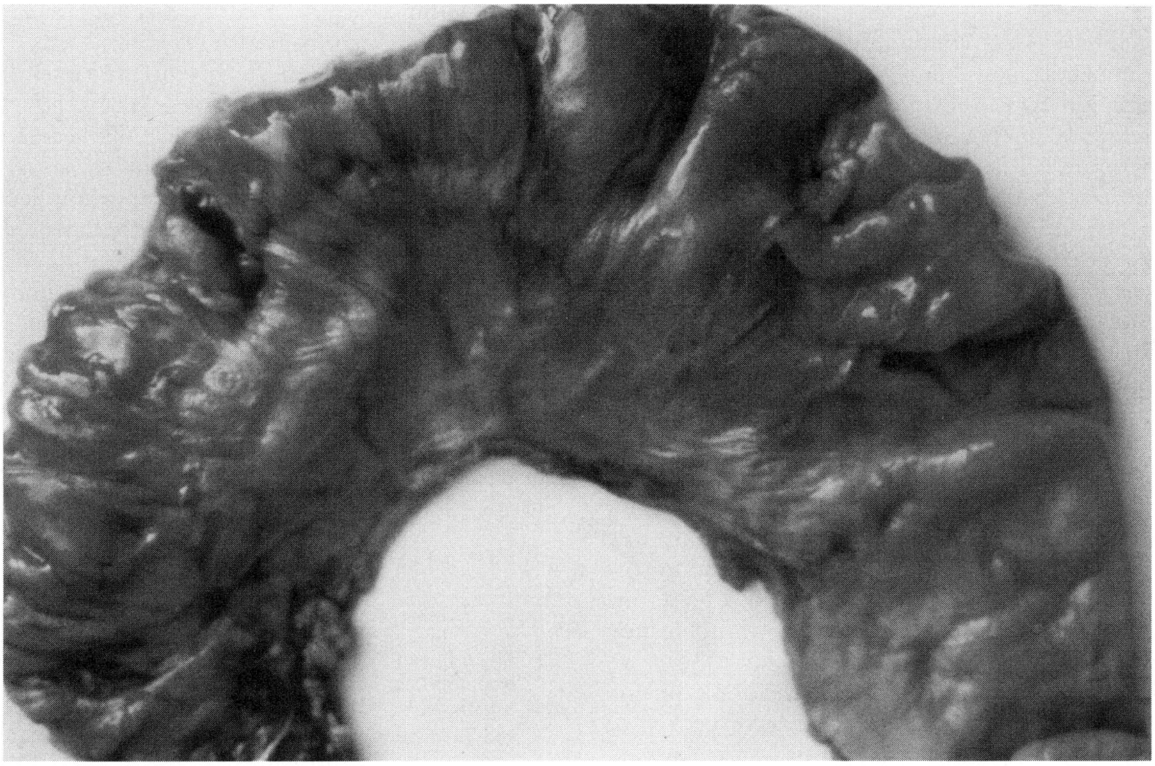

Figure 2. Postmortem megacolon, during digestive chronic Chagas disease.

Both drugs have trypanocidal effects on bloodstream trypomastigotes, by production of free radicals, and result in suppression of the parasitemia. They are administered orally and metabolized by the liver, and their metabolites are excreted renally. About two-thirds of patients experience side effects of digestive (anorexia, nausea, vomiting, and abdominal pain), neurological (peripheral polyneuritis), or cutaneous nature. About 15% of treated patients are unable to complete the treatment. The side effects resolve when treatment is interrupted.

The major indications of the two specific trypanocidal drugs are in the acute phase of Chagas disease when diagnosed, congenital infection and prevention of accidental laboratory infections. The current dosages for adults are 5 to 7 mg/kg/day in two oral doses for 60 days in the case of benznidazole, and 8 to 10 mg/kg/day in four oral doses for 90 days for nifurtimox. This treatment lowers the level of parasitemia and decreases the duration and severity of the infection. In some cases, early treatment may result in cure demonstrated by negative parasitemia and serological tests.

Because the available drugs are toxic, there is a general agreement to recommend not treating persons in the intermediate phase. Specific treatment has long been debated for declared chronic phase disease, but recent studies have emphasized the benefit of treating recent chronic phase in children aged less than 15 years. The possibility of cure during the chronic phase is not commonly admitted. Treatment is recommended for children under 10 years old (10 mg/kg/day in two oral doses of benznidazole, 15 to 20 mg/kg/day in four oral doses for nifurtimox), as they tolerate treatment better than older persons. Nonspecific treatment during the chronic phase includes the adequate treatment of the corresponding cardiac disorder. For digestive involvement, mild symptoms respond to dietary modifications and drug use. Advanced stages need surgical resection of the dilated segment and interposition of bowel segments for preserving digestive tract continuity.

Control

Neither vaccines to prevent *T. cruzi* infection nor drugs suitable for large-scale treatment are currently available. The control strategy for elimination of Chagas disease is based on the control of vectors, systematic screening in blood donors, and detection and treatment of congenital transmission (33b).

Control programs interrupting the domestic and peridomestic cycles of transmission have proven to be feasible by insecticide spraying of houses and annexes infested with triatomine bugs. But recolonization by the insects must be prevented by improvement of human dwelling and life conditions.

Control of Chagas disease is now given high priority by Latin American governments. A large national program was first established in Brazil in 1975, followed in 1991 by a regional program launched by the governments of the Southern Cone countries (Argentina, Bolivia, Brazil, Chile, Paraguay, and Uruguay). Similar programs were developed by the Andean countries (Colombia, Ecuador, Peru, and Venezuela) in 1997 and by Central American countries (Costa Rica, El Salvador, Guatemala, Mexico, Nicaragua, and Panama) in 1998. The attack phase of the vector control programs is based on massive insecticide spraying of houses, fumigant canisters, and insecticidal paints. This phase is followed by entomological surveillance, particularly with the "triatomine detection box."

Transmission through blood transfusion is preventable by screening of blood by serology and discarding positive units. In several American countries, serology of *T. cruzi* is mandatory for blood donors.

Congenital transmission unfortunately cannot be prevented during pregnancy because of toxicity and teratogenicity of available drugs. Serological surveillance of mothers and newborns is recommended. A positive serology in babies 6 months old, when maternal antibodies have disappeared, indicates the need for immediate treatment. All programs are placed within a primary health care context and have a strong component of health education.

In the last 20 years, Chagas disease has changed. Advances in diagnosis were made and a better understanding of the disease resulted. While treatment remains insufficient, national and international control programs have resulted in an important decrease in prevalence. The intervention programs carried out have contributed to interruption of disease transmission in some areas. Globally a reduction of 50% from infection rates in 1990 has been obtained. Brazil, Chile, and Uruguay have been declared free of Chagas disease transmission due to *Triatoma infestans*. But triatomine insects and Chagas disease will exist as long as poor housing conditions in the rural settings and urban poverty belts of the large cities exist.

REFERENCES

1. **Alvar, J., and M. Jimenez.** 1994. Could infected drug-users be potential *Leishmania infantum* reservoirs? *AIDS* **8**:854.
2. **Amato, V. S., F. F. Tuon, A. M. Siqueira, A. C. Nicodemo, and V. A. Neto.** 2007. Treatment of mucosal leishmaniasis in Latin America: systematic review. *Am. J. Trop. Med. Hyg.* 77:266–274.

3. **Balzer, R. J., P. Destombes, K. F. Schaller, and C. Sérié.** 1960. Leishmaniose cutanée pseudolépromateuse en Ethiopie. *Bull. Soc. Path. Exot.* **53**:293–298.
4. **Basset, D., F. Faraut, P. Marty, J. Dereure, E. Rosenthal, C. Mary, F. Pratlong, L. Lachaud, P. Bastien, and J. P. Dedet.** 2005. Visceral leishmaniasis in organ transplant recipients: 11 new cases and a review of the literature. *Microbes Infect.* **7**:1370–1375.
5. **Bern, C., J. Adler-Moore, J. Berenguer, M. Boelaert, M. De Boer, R. N. Davidson, C. Figueras, L. Gradoni, D. A. Kafetzis, K. Ritmeijer, E. Rosenthal, C. Royce, R. Russo, S. Sundar, and J. Alvar.** 2006. Liposomal amphotericin B for the treatment of visceral leishmaniasis. *Clin. Infect. Dis.* **43**:917–924.
6. **Brown, M., M. Noursadeghi, J. Boyle, and R. N. Davidson.** 2005. Successful liposomal amphotericin B treatment of *Leishmania braziliensis* cutaneous leishmaniasis. *Br. J. Dermatol.* **153**:203–205.
7. **Bryceson, A. D. M.** 1970. Diffuse cutaneous leishmaniasis in Ethiopia. III. Immunological studies. *Trans. R. Soc. Trop. Med. Hyg.* **64**:380–393.
8. **Chagas, C.** 1909. Nova tripanosomiaze humana. Estudos sobre a morfologia e o ciclo evolutivo do *Schizotrypanum cruzi* n. gen. n. species, ajente etiologico de nova entidade morbida do homen. *Mem. Inst. Oswaldo Cruz* **1**:159.
9. **Convit, J., and P. Lapenta.** 1948. Sobre un caso de leishmaniasis tegumentaria de forma disseminada. *Revta Policlin. Caracas* **17**:153–158.
10. **Cruz, I., J. Nieto, J. Moreno, C. Cañavate, P. Desjeux, and J. Alvar.** 2006. *Leishmania*/HIV co-infections in the second decade. *Indian J. Med. Res.* **123**:357–388.
11. **Dedet, J. P., R. Pradinaud, and F. Gay.** 1989. Epidemiological aspects of human cutaneous leishmaniasis in French Guiana. *Trans. R. Soc. Trop. Med. Hyg.* **83**:616–620.
12. **Desjeux, P.** 2004. Leishmaniasis: current situation and new perspectives. *Comp. Immun. Microbiol. Infect. Dis.* **27**:305–318.
13. **Desjeux, P., and J. Alvar.** 2003. *Leishmania*/HIV co-infections: epidemiology in Europe. *Ann. Trop. Med. Parasitol.* **97**:S3–S15.
14. **Devera, R., O. Fernandes, and J. R. Coura.** 2003. Should *Trypanosoma cruzi* be called "cruzi" complex? A review of the parasite diversity and the potential of selecting population after in vitro culturing and mice infection. *Mem. Inst. Oswaldo Cruz* **98**:1–12.
15. **Escomel, E.** 1911. La espundia. *Bull. Soc. Pathol. Exot.* **4**:489–492.
16. **Gillis, D., S. Klaus, L. F. Schnur, P. Piscopos, S. Maayan, E. Okon, and D. Engelhard.** 1995. Diffusely disseminated cutaneous *Leishmania major* infection in a child with acquired immunodeficiency syndrome. *Pediatr. Infect. Dis. J.* **14**:247–249.
17. **Herwaldt, B. L., and J. D. Berman.** 1992. Recommendation for treating leishmaniasis with sodium stibogluconate (Pentostam®) and review of pertinent clinical studies. *Am. J. Trop. Med. Hyg.* **46**:296–306.
18. **Hoare, C. A.** 1972. *The Trypanosomes of Mammals. A Zoological Monograph.* Blackwell Scientific, Edinburgh, United Kingdom.
19. **Hoare, C. A., and F. G. Wallace.** 1966. Developmental stages of trypanosomatid flagellates: a new terminology. *Nature* **212**:1385–1386.
20. **Jimenez, M. I., B. Guttierrez-Solar, A. Benito, A. Aguiar, E. Garcia, E. Cerceñado, and J. Alvar.** (1991). Cutaneous *Leishmania (L.) infantum* zymodemes isolated from bone marrow in AIDS patients. *Res. Rev. Parasitol.* **51**:91–94.
21. **Kamhawi, S.** 2000. The biological and immunomodulatory properties of sandfly saliva and its role in the establishment of *Leishmania* infections. *Microbes Infect.* **14**:1765–1773.
22. **Lainson, R., and J. J. Shaw.** 1987. Evolution, classification and geographical distribution, p. 1–120. *In* W. Peters and R. Killick-Kendrick (ed). *The Leishmaniases in Biology and Medicine*, vol.1. Academic Press, London, United Kingdom.
23. **Laveran, A., and F. Mesnil.** 1903. Sur un protozoaire nouveau (*Piroplasma donovani* Laveran et Mesnil) parasite d'une fièvre de l'Inde. *C. R. Acad. Sci.* **137**:957–961.
24. **Marsden, P. D., and R. R. Nonata.** 1975. Mucocutaneous leishmaniasis: a review of clinical aspects. *Rev. Soc. Bras. Med. Trop.* **9**:309–326.
25. **Mueller, M., M. Balasegaram, Y. Koummuki, K. Ritmeijer, M. R. Santana, and R. Davidson.** 2006. A comparison of liposomal amphotericin B with sodium stibogluconate for the treatment of visceral leishmaniasis in pregnancy in Sudan. *J. Antimicrob. Chemother.* **58**:811–815.
26. **Olliaro, P. L., P. J. Guerin, S. Gerst, A. A. Haaskjold, J. A. Rottingen, and S. Sundar.** 2005. Treatment options for visceral leishmaniasis: a systematic review of clinical sudies done in India, 1980-2004. *Lancet Infect. Dis.* **5**:763–774.
27. **Rathi, S. K., R. K. Pandhi, N. Khanna, and P. Chopra.** 2003. Therapeutic trial of sodium antimony gluconate alone and in combination with ketoconazole in post-kala-azar dermal leishmaniasis. *Indian J. Dermatol. Venereol. Leprol.* **69**:392–393.
28. **Rioux, J. A., G. Lanotte, E. Serres, F. Pratlong, P. Bastien, and J. Perieres.**1990. Taxonomy of *Leishmania*. Use of isoenzymes. Suggestions for a new classification. *Ann. Parasitol. Hum. Comp.* **65**:111–125.
29. **Rodrigues Coura, J., B. Galvao-Castro, and G. Grimaldi, Jr.** 1987. Disseminated American cutaneous leishmaniasis in a patient with AIDS. *Mem. Inst. Oswaldo Cruz* **82**:581–582.
30. **Romaña, C.** 1963. *Enfermedad de Chagas.* Lopez Libreros Editores, Buenos Aires, Argentina.
31. **Thakur, C. P., and K. Kumar.** 1992. Post kala-azar dermal leishmaniasis: a neglected aspect of kala-azar control programmes. *Ann. Trop. Med. Parasitol.* **86**:355–359.
32. **Velasco, O., S. J. Savarino, B. C. Walton, A. A. Gam, and F. A. Neva.**1989. Diffuse cutaneous leishmaniasis in Mexico. *Am. J. Trop. Med. Hyg.* **41**:280–288.
33. **Walton, B. C.** 1987. American cutaneous and mucocutaneous leishmaniasis, p. 637–664. *In* W. Peters and R. Killick-Kendrick (ed), *The Leishmaniases in Biology and Medicine*, vol. 2. Academic Press, London, United Kingdom.

33a. **WHO Expert Committee.** 1990. Control of leishmaniasis. WHO technical report no. 793. World Health Organization, Geneva, Switzerland.

33b. **WHO Scientific Working Group.** 2005. Report of the scientific working group on Chagas disease. TDR/SWG/09. World Health Organization, Geneva, Switzerland.

34. **Zerpa, O., M. Ulrich, B. Bianco, M. Polegre, A. Avila, N. Matos, I. Mendoza, F. Pratlong, C. Ravel, and J. Convit.** 2007. Diffuse cutaneous leishmaniasis responds to miltefosine but then relapses. *Br. J. Dermatol.* **156**:1328–1335.
35. **Zijlstra, E. E., A. M. El-Hassan, A. Ismael, and H. W. Ghalib.**1994. Endemic kala-azar in eastern Sudan: a longitudinal study on the incidence of clinical and subclinical infection and post-kala-azar dermal leishmaniasis. *Am. J. Trop. Med. Hyg.* **51**:826–836.

Sequelae and Long-Term Consequences of Infectious Diseases
Edited by Pina M. Fratamico, James L. Smith, and Kim A. Brogden

Chapter 17

Parasitic Helminths

AMAYA L. BUSTINDUY AND CHARLES H. KING

The helminthic parasites of humans are multicellular (metazoan) animal species that survive only by spending part of their lives infecting organ tissues or digestive spaces within the human body (Table 1). These helminth species, which are sometimes termed macroparasites (6), are considerably larger than the more familiar viruses, bacteria, and protozoa (microparasites) that also cause human infection. As a result, the helminths' interactions with host immunity and their consequent tissue pathology are substantially different in quality and quantity from those observed during typical viral, bacterial, or protozoan infections, as described in the other sections of this book. (NB: for a description of the helminthic disease cysticercosis (including neurocysticercosis) caused by the tapeworm *Taenia solium*, the reader is referred to Chapter 13.) In general, helminth parasites do not reproduce within the human body, so a patient's burden of helminthic infection only increases as he or she sustains repeated exposure to infectious forms of the parasite (e.g., embryonated eggs or mature larvae) (180). As a result, risk of helminth infection and disease is strongly tied to environmental factors, including socioeconomic status and local levels of sanitation (96).

By nature, helminth infections are long lasting, and the disease they cause is chronic in nature (180). If advanced disease occurs during the course of infection, it can result in permanent damage with significant patient disability (21, 38, 97). Although helminths cannot replicate within the human body, mostly all are long lived, with individual parasites surviving months to decades within the human host (6). Established helminth infection may take years to resolve, while at the same time, worm superinfection and reinfection are quite common events for people living within communities where helminth disease is endemic (3, 78, 166). It is important to note that helminth infection may persist long after a person leaves a disease transmission zone (169, 199). This leaves the affected patient with parasitic infection (and risk of its associated disease) for many years' duration (60). Ultimately, infection may last from one-third to one-half of a patient's lifetime, a process that results in continuing accumulation of parasite-mediated chronic tissue inflammation, with evolution of various organ-specific pathologies at all sites involved in the infection. Even after infection ends, the parasite-associated inflammation and tissue damage will persist for the remainder of a patient's lifetime (20, 60, 68, 85, 177). The long duration of parasite-associated inflammation may provoke local or systemic pathologies that might appear "atypical," given the expected localization of the parasite within the human body. However, these "aberrant" manifestations often contribute significantly to the health impact and local disease burden of these chronic parasitic infections (Table 2) (96).

The postinfectious clinical complications due to helminths are numerous, as different parasites generate different responses in the host and migrate to a variety of organs (Table 3). Historically, the disabling impact of chronic disease due to infection with these parasites has not been well addressed (96, 98). Fortunately, this is changing, as new research focuses on the overall health impact of these important etiologic agents and their substantial chronic disease burden (77). The "neglected" tropical diseases include three soil-transmitted helminths (*Ascaris*, hookworm, and *Trichuris*) as well as the helminthic parasites responsible for diseases like lymphatic filariasis, onchocerciasis, dracunculiasis, and schistosomiasis, among others. All of these parasitic diseases have long-term complications that result in disabilities, while also contributing to the perpetuation of poverty (79). In addition, in countries with high prevalence rates of helminth infection (Table 4), consideration is now being given to

Amaya L. Bustinduy • Department of Pediatrics, University Hospitals of Cleveland, Cleveland, OH 44106. **Charles H. King** • Center for Global Health and Diseases, Case Western Reserve University School of Medicine, Cleveland, OH 44106.

Table 1. Summary of clinically important helminths

Helminth	Transmission	Organs frequently affected	Age groups most affected (yr)	Severe chronic manifestations
Nematodes				
Onchocerca volvulus	Human to human through vector (*Simulium* black fly)	Eye Skin	5–60	Glaucoma, keratitis, retinitis Blindness Intractable pruritus Chronic skin changes (depigmentation [Leopard skin] or lichenification [Lizard skin]) Subcutaneous nodules
Wuchereria bancrofti *Brugia malayi* *Brugia timori*	Human to human through vector mosquito (*Culex, Anopheles, Aedes, Mansonia, Coquillettidia*)	Lymphatics Male genitalia Lungs Kidneys	>15	Lymphedema (Elephantiasis) Hydrocele, chronic GU obstruction Chronic interstitial lung disease, Tropical pulmonary eosinophilia Psychosocial stigma Nutritional deficiencies
Loa loa *Mansonella* species	Human to human through vector fly (*Chrysops*)	Subcutaneous migration to subconjunctiva, skin, lymphatics	>1	Lymphadenitis Endomyocardial fibrosis Psychiatric disturbances Renal failure Blindness Chronic dermatitis
Dracunculus medinensis (Dracunculiasis or guinea worm disease)	Ingestion of water containing intermediate host, copepods, known as "water-fleas" (*Cyclops*)	Skin	15–40	Incapacitation from pain and local tissue damage Arthritis Synovitis Ankylosis of limb Bacterial superinfections
Trichinella spiralis	Ingestion of contaminated meat (pork, boar, horse, wild mammals)	Muscle: voluntary, heart Nervous system	>3	Arrhythmias Electroencephalographic alterations Chronic muscle pain Early fatigability Chronic headaches
Angiostrongylus cantonensis	Ingestion of contaminated produce or freshwater snails(*Achatina fulica)*	GI tract CNS	>3	Eosinophilic meningitis Paresthesias Cranial nerve paralysis Peripheral nerve paralysis
Gnathostoma species	Ingestion of raw fish, slugs, or freshwater snails	GI tract CNS Skin Eye	>14	Eosinophilic meningitis Intracranial bleeding Intermittent chronic CNS symptoms Radicular pain Radiculomyelitis Paraplegia
Ascaris lumbricoides *Trichuris trichiura*	Human to human through oral-fecal ingestion of eggs	GI tract: intestine, biliary tract Lungs	.5–18	Intestinal obstruction Biliary tract obstruction Nutritional deficiencies Bronchial hyperreactivity
Necator americanus *Ancylostoma duodenale* (hookworms)	Human to human through fecal contamination of soil with eggs, emergence of infectious larvae; breast milk	Intestinal mucosa Lungs	All ages	Iron deficiency anemia Failure to thrive Intellectual and cognitive impairment Chlorosis Aberrant pregnancy outcomes: intrauterine growth retardation, fetal demise, miscarriage

Continued

Table 1. *Continued*

Helminth	Transmission	Organs frequently affected	Age groups most affected (yr)	Severe chronic manifestations
Strongyloides stercoralis	Human to human by soil contamination; filarial forms penetrate through skin; auto-infection	Intestinal mucosa Lung, disseminated	All ages	Chronic diarrhea alternating with constipation Hematochezia Chronic urticarial rashes Late dissemination with immunosuppression
Cestodes				
Echinococcus species	Contaminated food/water Animal reservoir (cattle, sheep, deer→ dog→ human)	Liver Lung Brain	>2	Hydatid cyst
Diphyllobothrium latum	Ingestion of undercooked fish Intermediate host: copepod, freshwater fish	Intestine Red blood cells Nervous system	>10	Vitamin B_{12} deficiency: Megaloblastic anemia Peripheral neuropathy Intestinal obstruction Subacute combined degeneration (SCD)
Waterborne trematodes				
Schistosoma mansoni	Through skin in waters contaminated by feces; Intermediate host: freshwater *Biomphalaria* snail	Intestine Liver CNS	>5	Liver fibrosis Portal hypertension Iron deficiency anemia Transverse myelitis
Schistosoma haematobium	Through skin in waters contaminated by urine; Intermediate host: freshwater *Bulinus* snail	Renal CNS Lungs	5–25	Renal failure Hydroureter/Hydronephrosis Anemia
			40+	Cor pulmonale Squamous cell bladder carcinoma
Schistosoma japonicum	Through skin in waters contaminated by feces; Intermediate host: freshwater *Oncomelania* snail	Intestine Liver CNS	>5	Grand mal epilepsy Portal hypertension Anemia
Food-borne trematodes				
Paragonimus westermani (lung fluke)	Undercooked crab/crayfish Intermediate host: freshwater snail	Lung Pleura CNS	All ages	Chronic cough Hemoptysis Pulmonary granulomas/calcifications Pleural thickening Pulmonary hemorrhages Seizures/visual disturbances Chronic headaches
Other *Paragonimus* species	Africa: undercooked crab; Japan: boar meat			
Fasciola hepatica (liver flukes)	Ingestion of aquatic plants (watercress, lettuce) Intermediate host: snail	Intestine Liver Biliary tract	All ages	Ascending cholangitis Gallbladder lithiasis Common bile duct lithiasis
Clonorchis sinensis *Opisthorchis* species	Ingestion of fish Intermediate host: snail	Intestine Liver Biliary tract	All ages	Ascending cholangitis Intrahepatic pigment stones
			50+	Cholangiocarcinoma

Table 2. Lesser-known chronic manifestations of parasitic infections

Chronic condition(s)	Helminth pathogen(s)
Growth stunting Undernutrition Cognitive impairment Anemia of chronic inflammation	*Schistosoma* spp./ *Trichuris*/ hookworms
Hyper-reactive dermatitis ('Sowda' in Yemen) Erisípelas de la costa or facial redness/swelling (Latin America) Mal morado: reddish discoloration of trunk/limbs (Latin America)	*Onchocerca volvulus*
Chyluria	*Wuchereria bancrofti* / *Brugia malayi*/ *Brugia timori*
Tropical pulmonary eosinophilia (TPE)	*Wuchereria bancrofti* / *Brugia malayi*/ *Brugia timori* *Ascaris lumbricoides*
Endomyocardial fibrosis (Loeffler's syndrome)	*Loa loa*
Pericarditis Hepatitis	*Mansonella* species of filaria
Limb contractures and joint ankylosis Ectopic parasite masses: pancreas, testis, lung, pericardium Spinal cord compression	*Dracuncula medinensis* (Guinea worm disease)
Myocarditis Encephalitis Pneumonitis	*Trichinella* species
Eosinophilic meningitis	*Angiostrongylus cantonensis* / *Gnathostoma* spp.
Ectopic masses: eye, lung, GI	*Gnathostoma* spp. *Toxocara* species (visceral larva migrans)
Hepatic abscesses Pancreatitis Asthma	*Ascaris lumbricoides*
Chlorosis: pasty appearance in severe infection Protein losing malnutrition: Kwashiorkor Pregnancy-related mortality Low birth weight	*Necator americanus, Ancylostoma duodenale* (hookworm)
Late dissemination during immunosuppression: 1. Cardiac arrhythmias: myocardial infiltration of larvae 2. Joints: arthritis 3. Cerebral/cerebellar abscesses 4. Bronchopneumonia with intra-alveolar hemorrhage	*Strongyloides stercoralis*
Cerebral cysts: increased intracranial pressure Kidney cysts: hematuria Bone cysts: pathological fractures Heart cysts: cardiac tamponade	*Echinococcus* spp.
Pernicious anemia Subacute combined degeneration (SCD) due to vitamin B_{12} deficiency	*Diphyllobothrium latum*
Transverse myelitis, seizures (neuroschistosomiasis)	*Schistosoma mansoni*
Pulmonary hypertension/cor pulmonale	*Schistosoma japonicum*
Squamous cell carcinoma of the bladder	*Schistosoma haematobium*
Meningitis Cerebral or spinal masses	*Paragonimus westermani* (lung fluke)
Ectopic infiltrations: spleen, liver, intestine, peritoneum Mesenteric lymphadenitis Cutaneous masses	Other *Paragonimus* spp.
Cryptic eosinophilia	*Fasciola hepatica*
Cholangiocarcinoma	*Clonorchis sinensis*/*Opisthorchis* species

the comorbid effects of parasitic helminths with infections such as human immunodeficiency virus (HIV), malaria, and tuberculosis in addressing the local and regional burden of disease (132).

In order to effectively pursue eradication of disease due to parasitic helminths, it is relevant to understand the pathogenesis and transmission of each one. In this chapter, parasite life cycles and vector ecology will be touched on only briefly, and we refer the reader seeking in-depth discussion of these topics to recent tropical medicine textbooks (65, 180).

Helminths are most easily classified according to their assigned phylogenetic class; there are nematodes (commonly known as roundworms), cestodes (also known as tapeworms), and trematodes (also referred to as flukes) (180). Chronic disease is classically associated with the final target destination of the parasite. Each one prefers to migrate to different end organs, including the bloodstream (*Schistosoma* species), the skin (*Onchocerca volvulus, Loa loa*), or the lymphatic system (*Wuchereria bancrofti, Brugia malayi*). Many helminths parasitize only the gastrointestinal (GI) tract (hookworm, tapeworms, foodborne flukes), causing localized chronic inflammation primarily at this site. Other parasites can migrate to multiple organs (164), resulting in multiple organ system pathologies.

NEMATODES (ROUNDWORMS)

A basic characteristic of this group of parasites is that their life cycles all involve molts through several larval stages, while maturing from eggs to adult worms. Typically they are infective at the third or fourth (L3 or L4) larval stages when they migrate into the body of the definitive human host, usually traveling through the bloodstream or lymphatic system in order to mature into adult parasites (128). Tissue damage and disease may be caused either by the migrating larval stages, the adult worms, or both.

Onchocerca volvulus

Epidemiology

O. volvulus is one of eight filarial nematodes that can infect humans and is best known as a causal agent for "river blindness" (53, 130). Onchocerciasis has enormous socioeconomic impact in affected communities, mostly due to the prevalence of parasite-related blindness (Fig. 1), which can be as high as 15% in some villages (53). There are an estimated 17.7 million people infected with *O. volvulus* worldwide. According to the WHO, an estimated 500,000 people experience secondary visual impairment and up to 270,000 become blind as a chronic complication of infection (207). Geographical distribution of onchocerciasis is limited to tropical Africa, Latin America, and the Arabian Peninsula. It is endemic in 37 countries, with an estimated 123 million people at risk living in these areas. The highest prevalence is found in sub-Saharan West African nations, such as Ghana, Nigeria, Liberia, Congo, and Mali (Table 4). Other known affected countries are Sudan, Yemen, and Oman in the Arabian Peninsula, Ecuador, Venezuela, Colombia, Brazil, southern Mexico, and Guatemala (188).

Life cycle and transmission

Humans are the only definitive host for *O. volvulus*. Human-to-human transmission occurs through an intermediate host or vector black fly of the genus *Simulium* (53). Transmission is focused near rivers and streams, because the female *Simulium* lays her eggs on rocks and foliage close to fast-flowing turbulent rivers and streams. Transmission occurs when the black fly bites an infected person and microfilariae that are present in the skin enter into the body of the fly with the blood meal. These microfilariae travel to the fly's thoracic muscles and mature to the next larval stages of the parasite over 7 to 9 days. Then the infective L3 larvae move to the head of the fly and are transmitted to the next human when the fly bites again to take its next blood meal (53).

Infecting third-stage microfilariae coming from an infectious bite require 1 to 3 years to develop into *Onchocerca* adults. These adults may then live up to 15 years inside the human host. One female worm can produce 0.5 to 1 million live microfilariae progeny in 1 year. The newborn, immature *O. volvulus* microfilaria migrates through connective tissues and skin to many different parts of the human body. Critical areas of involvement include the anterior and posterior segments of the eye, where microfilariae cause sclerosing keratitis, uveitis, chorioretinitis, and optic neuritis. The human inflammatory response to parasite antigens and to dying microfilaria causes, over the years, gradual sclerosal opacification of the anterior eye and (via autoimmune mechanisms) the posterior chamber of the eye, leading to irreversible blindness (69).

Clinical manifestations

The microfilariae of *O. volvulus* have a predilection for both the skin and the eyes. Their presence in these tissues results in a spectrum of disease. The profile of infection can range from asymptomatic infected persons in whom no clinical disease is evident (and

Table 3. Chronic helminth-related syndromes by organ system

Chronic syndrome	Helminths							
	Onchocerca volvulus	*W. bancrofti*, *B. malayi* (lymphatic filariasis)	*Loa loa*, *Mansonella* species	*Dracuncula medinensis* (guinea worm)	*Trichinella* species	*Angiostrongylus cantonensis*	*Gnathostoma* species	*Ascaris lumbricoides*, *T. trichiura*
Blindness	×		×					
Cancer								
Lymphedema/ lymphadenitis		×	×					
Chronic dermatitis	×		×	×				
Joint		×	×	×				
Muscle					×			
CNS					×	×	×	
Peripheral neuropathy						×	×	
Psychiatric disturbances			×					
Lung								×
Heart			×		×			
Intestinal obstruction								×
Chronic diarrhea								
Liver								
Biliary tract obstruction								×
Kidney		×	×					
Nutritional deficiencies	×	×						×
Anemia	×	×						×
Cognitive deficiencies								
Incapacitation	×	×	×	×	×	×	×	
Social isolation	×	×	×	×				
Pregnancy issues								

microfilariae are found in the dermis without any surrounding tissue reaction) to a severe inflammatory host response to microfilarial antigens which yields the classical pathology related to *O. volvulus* infection (53) (Table 1).

Dermatitis. Symptomatic skin inflammation is the most common clinical presentation of onchocerciasis (53). It is usually highly pruritic, resulting from tissue inflammation in reaction to motile larvae that migrate subcutaneously. This dermatitis is poorly responsive to conventional antipruritic therapy. It often affects the buttocks but can occur on other parts of the body. Abrasions due to patient scratching and skin excoriation are common findings. The spectrum of chronic onchodermatitis progresses from acute papular dermatitis, with a higher inflammatory response and recently linked to a T-helper cell 1 (Th1) immune response, to a chronic papular dermatitis and lichenified dermatitis (Sowda) that is associated with increased Th2-type responses (189). Classic depigmentation or "leopard skin" is associated with repeated episodes of skin inflammation that occur due to localized inflammation following death of microfilariae. Additional subcutaneous fibrosis and skin atrophy may give affected skin the clinical appearance of "lizard skin" (53) (Fig. 2).

Subcutaneous nodules. Also known as "onchocercomata," subcutaneous nodules containing adult *Onchocerca* worms occur most often over bony prominences of the hips, shoulders, or skull. These are mobile encapsulated nodules that contain coiled masses of two or more adult worms. Depending on

N. americanus, *A. duodenale* (hookworms)	*S. stercoralis*	*Echinococcus* species	*D. latum*	*Schistosoma mansoni*	*Schistosoma haematobium*	*Schistosoma japonicum*	*Paragonimus westermani*	*Fasciola hepatica*	*Opisthorchis* species, *C. sinensis*
					×				×
		×	×	×		×	×		
			×	×					
			×						
		×			×		×		
		×			×				
×		×	×						
	×								
×		×		×		×			
		×						×	×
				×	×				
×			×	×	×	×			
×	×		×	×	×	×			
×				×	×	×			
			×						
			×						
×				×	×	×			

geographic location (West Africa versus Central America), these will be found in different parts of the body, ranging from the torso and hips to the head and shoulders (53). The presence of nodules does not correlate with microfilarial load (138). If nodules become symptomatic, they may need to be surgically removed.

When onchocerciasis affects the eyes, typically both eyes are involved, and disease can include corneal, anterior chamber, posterior chamber, and retinal lesions. Animal models have recently shown that where neutrophil recruitment and activation into the cornea occur, they are part of a reaction to dead microfilariae shedding endosymbiotic *Wolbachia* bacteria (61). This reaction appears to be an important mechanism contributing to the pathogenesis of ocular onchocerciasis. In clinical examination, particularly with slit-lamp examination, if the patient is put in the prone position for a few minutes before examination, microfilariae and hypopyons may be seen in the anterior chamber of the eye(s). In the cornea, punctate keratitis with inflammatory cells accumulating around focal areas of inflammation will result in opacities. Symptoms of this form of the eye disease are, most often, a watering of the eyes and photosensitivity. Acute corneal inflammation can progress to sclerosing keratitis, with eventual total opacification of the cornea leading to irreversible blindness (53). Uveal and posterior chamber inflammation can also occur in chronic onchocerciasis. Of special note, treatment may aggravate inflammation during the period of microfilarial death and clearance that occurs 1 to 2 weeks posttherapy, with an important role likely played by *Wolbachia* antigens (61). The pathogenesis of all

Table 4. Geographic distribution

Helminth	Geographic distribution
Nematodes	
Onchocerca volvulus	Sub-Saharan Africa: Ghana, Nigeria, Liberia, Congo, Mali, Sudan Latin America: Brazil., Colombia, Ecuador, Venezuela, Arabian Peninsula: Yemen, Oman
Wuchereria bancrofti	Asia: India, Bangladesh Africa: Congo, Madagascar, Nigeria
Brugia malayi	Southeast Asia: Philippines, China, Indonesia, Malaysia
Brugia timori	East Timor
Loa loa	West Africa: Angola, southeastern Benin, Cameroon, Central African Republic, Chad, Democratic Republic of Congo, Gabon, Nigeria, Sudan, Equatorial Guinea
Dracunculus medinensis (guinea worm disease)	East and West Africa: Mauritania, Burkina Faso, Cote D'Ivoire, Ghana, Benin, Togo, Nigeria, Niger, southern Sudan, Ethiopia
Trichinella species	Cosmopolitan
Angiostrongylus cantonensis	Southeast Asia: Thailand, China, Australia, Japan Pacific Islands: Japan, Fiji, Island Reunion, Mauritius, Samoa, French Polynesia, Hawaii Caribbean: Jamaica United States: Louisiana
Gnathostoma species	Asia: Thailand, India, Japan, China, Malaysia, Philippines, Vietnam, Sri Lanka, Bangladesh Central and South America: Mexico and Ecuador Africa: Zambia
Ascaris lumbricoides	Cosmopolitan, but spares most of North America and northern Europe
Trichuris trichiura	United States: the Southeast
Necator americanus	South China, South India, sub-Saharan Africa, South America (Paraguay, northern Argentina, Brazil, Peru)
Ancylostoma duodenale	North China, North India, North Africa
Strongyloides stercoralis	Cosmopolitan in all tropical areas Europe: northern Italy, Spain, France, Switzerland, Poland United States: West Virginia (and any immunosuppressed population) Asia: Japan, Australia
Cestodes	
Echinococcus species	Cosmopolitan
Diphyllobothrium latum	United States: Alaska, Minnesota, Michigan, Florida, California Europe: Russia, Sweden, France, Finland, Ireland, Israel, Italy, Switzerland Africa: Madagascar Asia: China, Taiwan, Japan, Papua New Guinea, Philippines, Australia South America: Argentina, Chile
Trematodes, waterborne	
Schistosoma mansoni	Africa: most of the continent Middle East Caribbean South America
Schistosoma haematobium	Africa: most of the continent Middle East
Schistosoma japonicum	China, Southeast Asia, Philippines
Trematodes, foodborne	
Lung fluke, *Paragonimus westermani*	Asia: China, Korea, Japan, Vietnam
Other *Paragonimus* species	Africa: Cameroon South America: Ecuador, Peru
Liver flukes	61 countries, but most prevalent in the following:
Fasciola hepatica	South America: Bolivia, Peru Middle East: Iran, Egypt Europe: Portugal, France
Clonorchis sinensis/Opisthorchis species	China, Japan, Korea, Taiwan, Vietnam, Asian Russia

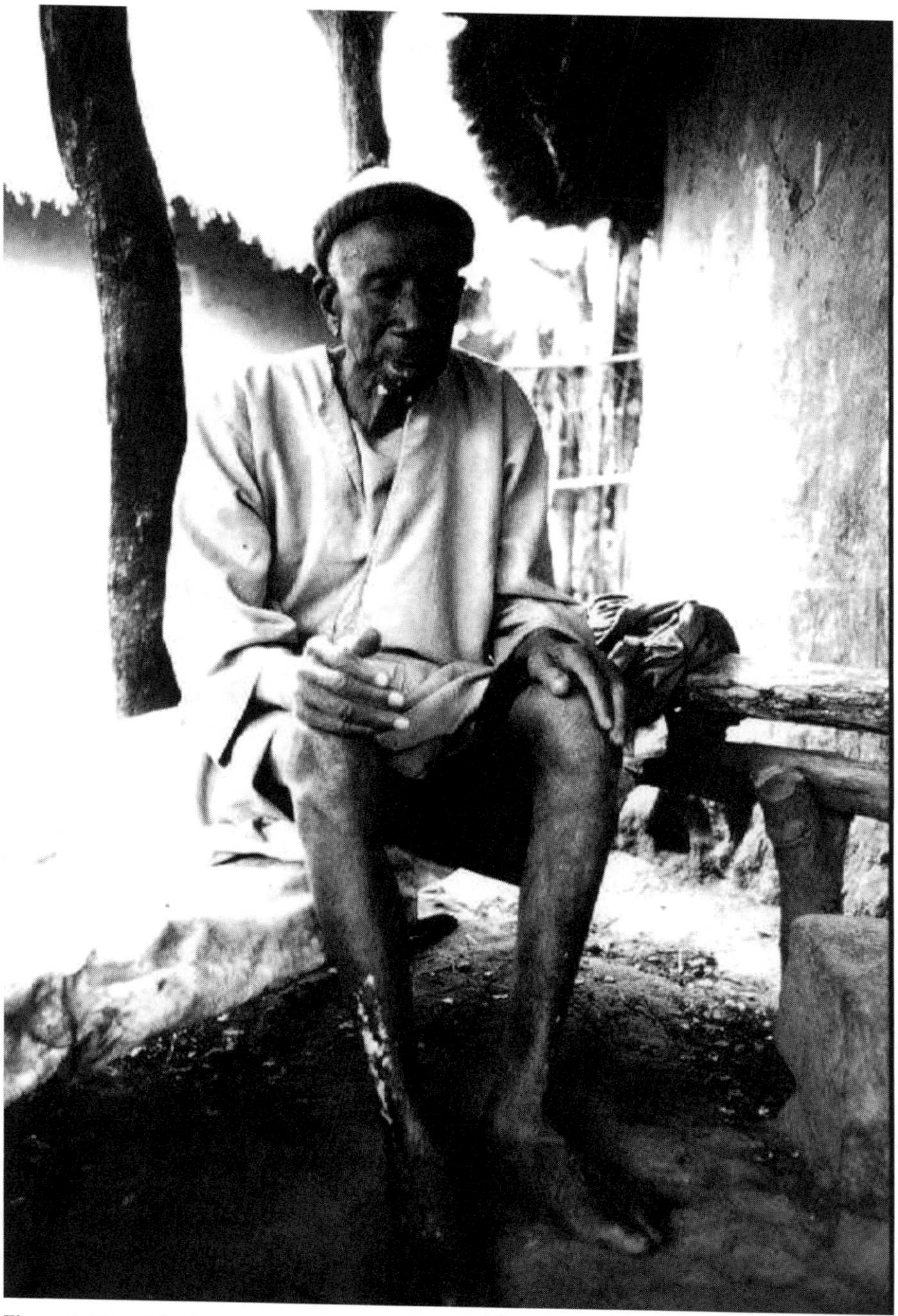

Figure 1. River blindness caused by *Onchocerca volvulus.* (Credit: World Health Organization.)

forms of *Onchocerca*-associated eye disease is believed to be immunologically mediated.

Immunology. Affected individuals with acute infection with *O. volvulus* have increased cellular immune responses compared to people with chronic infection, implying some immunomodulation or downregulation of immune response during prolonged infection (35).

Many filarial species, including *O. volvulus*, carry obligatory commensal bacteria of *Wolbachia* species as endosymbionts. Antigens of both *O. volvulus* and *Wolbachia* may therefore be presented to the human host during the course of infection. Skin disease (onchodermatitis) is mediated by reaction to specific *Onchocerca* antigens (189), whereas in corneal involvement, it appears that both *Wolbachia* and *Onchocerca* antigens are involved. Specifically, it

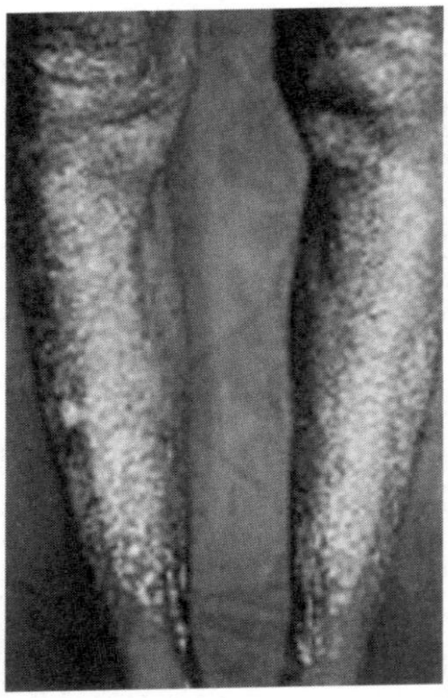

Figure 2. Leopard skin due to chronic onchocerciasis. (Credit: *Atlas of Tropical Medicine and Parasitology,* 6th ed., Elsevier.)

is believed that *Wolbachia* antigens released by microfilarial death are responsible for most of the local corneal inflammatory response that typically leads to blindness (162).

Coinfection with HIV. Patients with onchocerciasis appear to have a greater likelihood of converting to HIV positivity when exposed (62). Additionally, onchocercal dermatitis has been found to be significantly worse among HIV-infected patients (88).

Chronic complications. Chronic infection with *O. volvulus* is responsible for both severe disability and mortality (Tables 1 to 3). Little and coworkers (116) have recently established a clear association between *O. volvulus* microfilarial load and all-cause mortality.

Blindness. As a result of aggressive worldwide campaigns for onchocerciasis control, O. volvulus is no longer the most common infectious etiology of blindness in the world; it has been surpassed by trachoma. However, the long-term problem of infection-associated visual impairment and blindness still exists for many patients, such that onchocerciasis accounts for 0.8% of all blindness in the world (207). The repercussions of losing eyesight will vary depending on the socioeconomic context where it occurs. In less-developed communities that are highly dependent on physical labor in agriculture or fishing, blindness can be a devastating disability. Resources to adapt to blindness are typically limited within communities where it is endemic, which are often areas of significant rural poverty (152). Personal adaptation to blindness will often be substantially less than that available in wealthier societies.

Sleep deprivation. Chronic, intractable, pruritic dermatitis results in poor sleep patterns that can subsequently affect daily performance. Of particular long-term significance, disease can be associated with poor school performance and higher dropout rates from school, particularly among girls (207a).

Lymphadenopathy. Chronic inflammation in the pelvic region can result in damage and scarring of inguinal and femoral lymph nodes. These enlarged nodes may ultimately result in a "hanging groin" phenomenon, in which scarred, nontender, and fibrotic masses derived from affected lymph nodes go on to form pendulous folds in the affected areas (53).

Diagnosis

Traditionally, the gold-standard diagnosis of active onchocerciasis is made by bloodless superficial "skin snip" biopsy. Superficial skin tissue is obtained from the iliac crests, over the scapulae, and in some cases the scalp, and then cultured in physiologic saline and examined microscopically for the emergence of microfilariae (53). This skin-snip microscopy has lower sensitivity than several newer methods, including skin-snip PCR, enzyme-linked immunosorbent assays (ELISAs), and antigen detection, which are being evaluated in clinical trials. A recent review has compared the sensitivities and specificities of different methods (193). A rapid diagnostic card test has proven easy to use in the field, with 91% sensitivity and 100% specificity (202). It uses recombinant antigen from whole-blood from a finger prick to detect *O. volvulus*-specific immunoglobulin G4 (IgG4). Other diagnostic assays under development include a urine dipstick assay which is not yet commercially available. Antibody testing may be more useful for specific screening of populations for infection or exposure to *O. volvulus*, whereas PCR and antigen testing are potentially more useful for more sensitive diagnosis of infections in individuals and for monitoring the success of therapy (196).

Treatment

The standard treatment for onchocerciasis is ivermectin, which is a broad-spectrum antihelminthic agent that is active against a number of nematode species (8). Initially developed as a veterinary drug, ivermectin is now used as a potent antihelminthic agent for several different filarial diseases. Widespread use of ivermectin began in the 1980s in large trials in Africa. It is currently the treatment of choice for onchocerciasis, except in areas that also have *L. loa* (see below), and is given as a single dose of 150 µg/kg of body weight on a yearly basis. After treatment, microfilariae in the skin are killed within days, while ocular microfilariae may take up to 2 weeks to be killed (53). Recent studies have recommend optimal dosing every 3 months (instead of the standard yearly doses) on the basis of reduced risk of posttreatment inflammation (86). With fewer microfilariae dying after each of more-frequent treatments, there are likely to be fewer posttreatment side effects, such as edema, pruritus, and backache.

Ivermectin has no cidal activity against the adult worms of *O. volvulus*. However, repeated microfilaricidal treatments (as with ivermectin) can control or prevent chronic disease because morbidity is mainly associated with the presence of microfilariae in the skin and ocular tissues. There is an approved macrofilaricidal medication, suramin (8), but it requires parenteral injection, and its toxicity has made its use very limited (185). Because of the important role of immune response to the parasite's endosymbiont *Wolbachia* bacteria, new research is examining the possible value of doxycycline cotreatment to eradicate *Wolbachia*. The objective of this approach is to achieve long-term amicrofilaridermia. It appears that anti-*Wolbachia* treatment can result in the sterilization of female adult worms for up to 18 months posttreatment (71–73). This approach may prove highly valuable in terms of public health morbidity control and prevention in developing countries. There are limitations for its use, however, such as its photosensitizing and photo-onycholysis side effects (146).

Control measures

Effective suppression of *O. volvulus*-related disease has been obtained by suppression of *Simulium* black fly populations and by population-based drug programs (cf. the WHO-led Onchocerciasis Control Program (OCP) between 1974 and 2002) but at relatively high program cost. Originally the OCP was a vector control program that performed aerial larviciding over 50,000 km of rivers in West Africa. In later years, this was supplemented by annual ivermectin treatment campaigns. The present treatment-based African Program for Onchocerciasis Control has successfully replaced the OCP. It started in 1995, and it is due to end in 2009, when nation governments are expected to take over the initiative. Its intention, based on annual mass treatment with ivermectin in communities with high prevalence of *O. volvulus*, is to break the transmission cycle of the parasite (http://www.who.int/blindness/causes/priority/en/index3.html). In South America, the Onchocerciasis Control Program in the Americas is based on biannual ivermectin treatment. The countries involved are Brazil, Columbia, Venezuela, Mexico, Ecuador, and Guatemala.

Lymphatic Filariasis: *Wuchereria bancrofti*, *Brugia malayi*, *Brugia timori*

Collectively, these three filarial organisms are known to be the most common etiologic agents of lymphatic filariasis (LF). They are all thread-like nematodes transmitted from human to human by mosquito vectors (135). Chronic complications occur after prolonged parasite infection, usually initiated during early childhood, resulting in pronounced clinical manifestations from lymphatic dysfunction developing later in adulthood (135).

Epidemiology

According to the WHO, 120 million people around the world are infected with LF, while an estimated 1.3 billion people in 83 countries and territories (approximately 18% of the world's population) live in areas at risk of infection. The geographic distribution of LF is extensive (Table 4). About one-third of those at risk live in India, one-third in Africa, and the remainder live in Asia, the South Pacific, and in the Americas. Bangladesh, Democratic Republic of Congo, India, Indonesia, Madagascar, Nigeria, and the Philippines are among the most highly affected countries. In contrast to *Wuchereria bancrofti*, the *Brugia* parasites are confined to areas of east and south Asia, especially China, India, Indonesia, Malaysia, and the Philippines (204). The chronic complications attributed to infection with these parasites are dramatic, not only from a medical standpoint, but also because of their economic impact and psycho-sexual implications (210). Almost 25 million men suffer from LF-related genital disease (most commonly hydrocele), while an estimated 15 million people—the majority of them women—have lymphedema or elephantiasis of the leg (135).

Life cycle and transmission

About 90% of LF infections are due to *W. bancrofti* (Fig. 3), and most of the remaining 10% are due to *B. malayi*. *Brugia timori* is present only on the island of Timor in Indonesia (135). *W. bancrofti* has no known animal reservoir, while *B. malayi* is a zoonosis with feline and primate reservoirs (135).

The major vectors for *W. bancrofti* are (i) *Culex* mosquitoes in most urban and semi-urban areas,

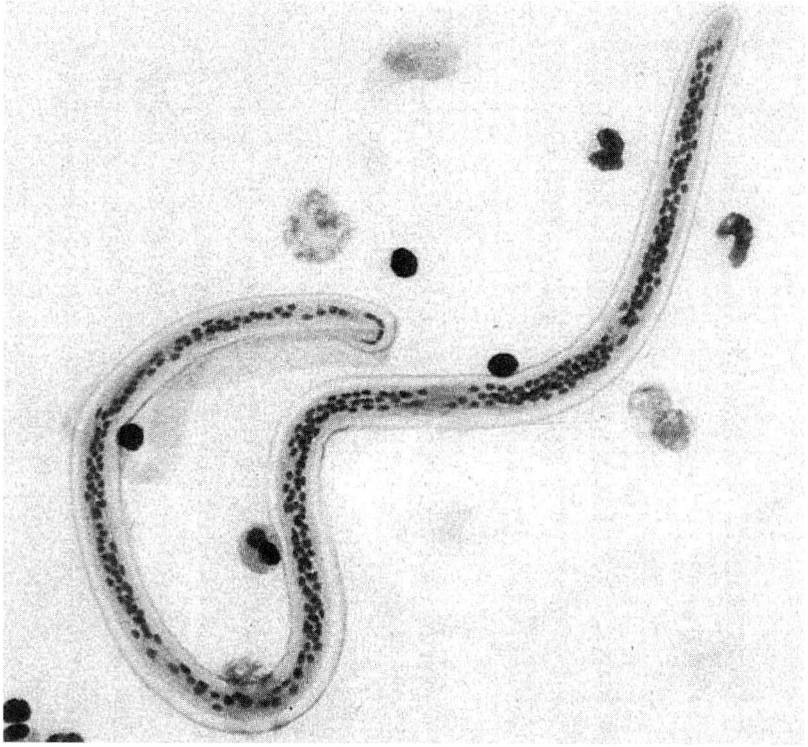

Figure 3. *Wuchereria bancrofti.* (Credit: *Atlas of Human Parasitology,* American Society of Clinical Pathologists.)

(ii) *Anopheles* in the more rural areas of Africa and elsewhere, and (iii) *Aedes* species in many of the Pacific islands where it is endemic. For *Brugia* parasites, *Mansonia* species mosquitoes serve as the major vector (174).

Filarial infection is initiated when humans are bitten by an infected hematophageous vector carrying L3 forms of parasite microfilariae. The mosquito punctures the skin and deposits the microfilariae into the skin. The larval form then migrates through the dermis into the lymphatic system, where they will mature into adult worms. Microfilarial transmission is not mechanical; larvae must mature within the mosquito in order to become infectious, and it can take up to 2 weeks before microfilariae can be transmitted human to human through a mosquito vector. Like *Onchocerca volvulus, W. bancrofti* carries the endosymbiotic rickettsia-like bacteria, *Wolbachia.* Its clinical relevance is that it seems to be important to parasite embryogenesis (70).

Clinical manifestations

There is a wide spectrum of disease from LF, ranging from very minimal clinical disease to severe lymphatic obstruction with elephantiasis of the limbs and edema of male genitalia (135) (Tables 1 to 3). Because the period of infection can last for decades, different clinical aspects of disease can arise during different periods of life.

Subclinical patent infection. It is important to consider the clinical relevance of the initial "asymptomatic" stages of LF, as they entail some degree of subclinical disease. Findings can range from microscopic hematuria and proteinuria to dilated lymphatics detected by ultrasound and lymphangectasia detected by lymphangioscintigraphy (54, 134, 140). Another transient, initial presentation is *filarial fever*; the acute, nonspecific fever presented by infected subjects may easily be confused with other diseases, such as malaria or dengue (depending on the area), as filarial lymphadenitis is often absent at this stage of LF (135).

Acute adenolymphangitis. The classic primary manifestation of LF occurs around adolescence, when it presents with sudden fever spikes and painful lymphadenopathy and lymphangitis, along with local edema. The lymphatic involvement is retrograde, and it can affect both upper and lower extremities. Genital involvement is seen almost exclusively during infection with *W. bancrofti* (143). Although the acute attack lasts only from 4 days to a week, it typically recurs one to three times a year, causing a great deal of suffering, along with a significant negative impact on the productivity of the affected individual.

Chronic lymphedema of the extremities. The most obvious chronic complication of LF infection is lymphedema of the extremities (106, 135) (Fig. 4). Typically, the lower extremities are more frequently affected. There are observed differences between the different LF parasites: *W. bancrofti* infection manifests with lymphedema of the entire leg, whereas brugian filariasis affects typically lymphatic vessels from the knee down. Asymmetry of limb involvement is the norm. The WHO has established a severity grading system for lymphedema that is dependent on its reversibility. Grade I corresponds to pitting edema that resolves with limb elevation. Grades II and III are better known as elephantiasis, which is an irreversible pitting edema of increasing severity. In the most severe cases there are also skin papillomatous changes and sclerosis (207b). Because other clinical entities may present with edema, conditions such as hepatic failure or cardiac failure need to be ruled out. Edema associated with LF may also present with an exudate of serous fluid from the overlying skin. With axillary involvement, the female breast is often affected by LF-related lymphedema (12, 110).

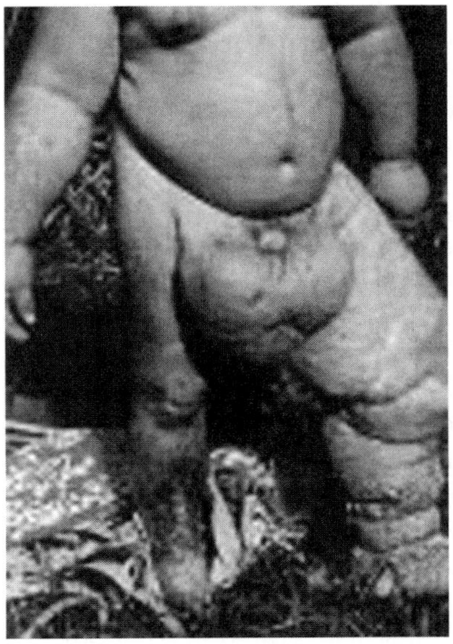

Figure 4. Elephantiasis from *Wuchereria bancrofti* infection. (Credit: *Atlas of Tropical Medicine and Parasitology*, 6th ed., Elsevier.)

Chronic obstruction in the genitourinary system. This complication is seen almost exclusively in *W. bancrofti* infection affecting the male. In some endemic areas, the prevalence of LF-associated hydrocele far surpasses that of peripheral lymphedema as a complication of infection. Hydroceles resulting from lymphatic obstruction are painless unless they are complicated by epididymitis or funiculitis. Other parts of the genitalia can also be affected, as when the penis becomes edematous and deformed with roughening of the overlying skin. In some severe cases, there may be lymph oozing from ruptured lymph ducts within the dermis (135).

Disability from the social impact of LF and chronic lymphedema

The social implications of the deformity caused by lymphedema are evident, in view of the fact that in many cases it leads to stigmatization that ostracizes the affected individual and delays medical care (77). The degree of stigmatization seems to be directly correlated with the severity of visible disease (210, 211). To date, the bulk of the LF literature is focused on the parasitological aspects of the disease, with the socioeconomic impact less well studied. According to the WHO, LF is the second most common cause of long-term disability after mental illness (203). Qualitative studies are now clarifying the correlation between poverty and poor outcomes of patients experiencing LF (149, 203, 211). As happens with many other disabling diseases, infected women, in particular, often carry an extra burden; their work productivity is decreased, while, through ostracism, their chances to marry and have children often become progressively limited as disease progresses (12, 106).

Chronic nutritional deficiencies

Weight loss often accompanies infection, probably occurring as a consequence of the increased energy cost associated with filarial fever, lymphangitis, and lymphadenitis. In onchocerciasis, we know that weight loss is associated with heavier worm loads, as assessed clinically by abundant nodules and large numbers of circulating microfilariae. For LF, it has been suggested that human protein-energy malnutrition may delay the development of stage-specific acquired immunity, with a corresponding prolongation of microfilarial patency (179). Filarial nematodes acquire certain nutrients directly from their hosts, particularly vitamin A, and symptoms of hypovitaminosis A can accompany infection, serve as an aggravating factor of disease, and worsen host response to intercurrent viral infections such as measles (179).

Less common chronic manifestations

Chyluria. Chyluria refers to urine with milkish appearance. It is the result of obstruction of the lymphatics-draining renal structures. There is great nutritional concern in the presence of chyluria due to the high content of fat and protein in the lymph that is lost in the urine (179). Fortunately, chyluria is not as prevalent as lymphedema or hydrocele (135).

Tropical pulmonary eosinophilia. Tropical pulmonary eosinophilia (TPE) is a clinical entity thought to be due to an exacerbated immunological response to the filarial parasites *W. bancrofti* and *B. malayi* (158, 195). It has been suggested that IL-4 induces this response and gamma interferon suppresses it (195). TPE affects males more than females. Usually TPE presents as an asthma-like illness, with paroxysmal nocturnal cough and wheezing and with systemic symptoms such as fever, weight loss, and fatigue. A characteristic finding of TPE is a peripheral blood eosinophilia of more than 3,000 eosinophils per microliter. The findings on chest radiograph may vary. On pulmonary function testing, a predominantly restrictive pattern is seen, but obstructive lung abnormalities may also occur (135). Studies indicate that the gamma-glutaryl transpeptidase found in the infective L3-stage larvae of *B. malayi* has been found to have similarities with the gamma-glutaryl transpeptidase present on the surface of human pulmonary epithelium (158). Thus, cross-reactivity of the host immune response may play an important role in the pathogenesis of TPE.

Chronic interstitial lung fibrosis. For many patients with TPE, despite the recommended standard 3-week course of antiparasite diethylcarbamazine therapy, low-grade alveolitis persists. This persistent inflammation is the most likely cause of the progressive interstitial fibrosis seen in many untreated or inadequately treated patients suffering from TPE (158, 195).

Immunity and host response

During chronic LF, there is a complex regulation of immune responses to *W. bancrofti* and *B. malayi*, with reduced responsiveness of T cells to antigens produced by microfilariae and decreased production of gamma interferon (122). There is a lack of clinical correlation between intensity of microfilaremia and risk of chronic lymphedema, suggesting that host immune responses may play a dominant role in determining infection-associated damage. Of note, prenatal sensitization to parasite antigens can occur in utero among babies born to mothers with microfilaremia. These children develop tolerance to filarial antigens, influencing their response to infection later in life (109, 176). Research has also focused on genetic polymorphisms predisposing to the development of chronic complications such as hydrocele. A cohort study in Ghana found increased risk of hydrocele with a genetic polymorphism of vascular endothelial growth factors. These growth factors are known to be major mediators of vascular permeability, which could logically play a role in hydrocele development (41).

Coinfection with HIV

Many aspects of the role of the coinfection with *W. bancrofti* or *B. malayi* in HIV disease remain unclear. A cross-sectional study in Tanzania has indicated a positive association between *W. bancrofti* infection and risk for HIV, but potential causes are still unknown (132).

A separate study has shown a positive association between maternal helminth infection and mother-to-child transmission of HIV (57). The proposed mechanism for this phenomenon is an activation of lymphocytes by parasite antigens in the placenta. Such results suggest the relevance of treating helminthic infections during pregnancy to reducing the impact on early childhood disease risk.

Diagnosis

In order to diagnose LF accurately at the species level, a parasite sample has to be obtained. This is often hard to do because adult worms lodge in lymphatics (with difficult access), and microfilariae may circulate only in a nocturnal pattern and may not be present in blood during the daytime. Often, the combination of epidemiologic history with classic physical findings is the best predictor of disease (135). Laboratory tests for the detection of microfilaremia from *W. bancrofti* and *B. malayi* include detection of microfilariae in blood smears with the use of a Giemsa stain, though this may still be negative in many active cases due to circadian variation in microfilaremia levels. In the absence of microfilaremia, detection of circulating filarial antigen may be used to establish the presence of active infection (127).

For detection of *W. bancrofti* antibodies, there is an available ELISA and a rapid card test with 96% sensitivity and 100% specificity (127, 201). No antibody test exists for *B. malayi*; however, a rapid test is available for field detection of this parasite (150). PCR testing is also available for both *W. bancrofti* and *B. Malayi* (124).

Imaging techniques such as ultrasonography of the scrotal area or the breast may offer substantial evidence in favor of an LF diagnosis. Ultrasound is able to detect adult *W. bancrofti* worms in scrotal lymphatic vessels of infected men, based on the characteristic pattern of adult worm movements, known as the "filarial dance sign" (123). This technique is able to delineate associated pathology, such as hydrocele and lymphedema, which can be diagnosed in early stages. Ultrasonography is also useful in the assessment of macrofilaricidal effects of antifilarial medication. Lymphoscintigraphy is also available as an imaging tool for diagnosis (54), but it is unlikely that it could be implemented on a large scale for the diagnosis of lymphatic filariasis.

Treatment

The recommended therapy is diethylcarbamazine, 6 mg/kg/day given 2 or 3 times daily for a total of 72 mg/kg over 10 to 14 days. For *W. bancrofti*, this leads to a 90% decrease in microfilariae in 1 month, with a sustained effect of up to 1 year. These responses are slower for infection with *B. malayi* (135). Yearly campaigns of treatment with diethylcarbamazine, or with combined ivermectin and albendazole, are proving to be both safe and effective in reducing LF-associated morbidity and new infection in affected areas (75). Surgical approaches to hydrocele are frequently curative, and many times provides symptomatic relief (84). Cellulitis caused by superinfection of the edematous tissues and skin breakage should be promptly addressed by proper hygiene and antibiotic therapy, as recurrent bacterial superinfection perpetuates and worsens lymphedema and elephantiasis formation (1). Ideally a wound culture should be sent to target superinfecting bacterial pathogens appropriately. In severe cases of lymphedema, fibrosis of the lymphatic vessels may impair irreversibly normal lymph drainage. There are surgical approaches like lymphatic-venous and nodal-venous anastomosis with different degrees of success (84). Access to such appropriate health care is often limited in resource-poor areas, and this poses a significant challenge to morbidity prevention campaigns.

Control of lymphatic filariasis

The Global Programme to Eliminate Lymphatic Filariasis was started in 1998 with two major goals: (ii) to interrupt transmission of the parasite and (ii) to provide care for those who suffer the devastating clinical manifestations of the disease (morbidity control). This latter goal addresses three filariasis-related conditions: acute inflammatory episodes, lymphedema, and hydrocele (1). By 2005, 42 of the 83 countries and territories classified as LF-endemic had benefited from mass drug administration (MDA) designed to eliminate transmission of LF as a public health problem. A total of 610 million people were targeted with MDA in 2005, of which 146 million were targeted with the WHO-recommended strategies of administering either diethylcarbamazine citrate (DEC) plus albendazole or DEC-fortified salt or, where onchocerciasis is coendemic with LF, ivermectin plus albendazole. The remaining at-risk population used DEC alone (75). In 2006, after up to 6 annual rounds of MDA and 10 rounds of DEC, the microfilaria prevalence was reduced to <1% in most risk areas, indicating substantial advances in disease prevention (204).

Loa loa

Human loiasis is an infection caused by the filarial nematode *L. loa*, an organism also known as the "eye worm" (103). Although it is not associated with high morbidity, in some areas where it is endemic, it is the third most common reason for a medical visit (133). Reasons for seeking care include the typical Calabar swelling of the skin and eye involvement with adult worms present in the conjunctiva. Complications of loiasis are rare but are nevertheless important due to their potential to cause substantial morbidity and mortality. Late, serious outcomes of loiasis include myocardiopathy, nephropathy, and encephalitis (103).

Epidemiology

Although *L. loa* is geographically restricted to West and Central Africa, it is highly endemic there, being responsible for 3 to 13 million chronic infections (103). Countries where it is endemic include Angola, southeastern Benin, Cameroon, Central African Republic, Chad, Democratic Republic of Congo, Gabon, Nigeria, Sudan, and Equatorial Guinea, with sporadic cases reported in Ghana, Uganda, Mali, and Ethiopia (Table 4). Risk of acquiring infection is related to the length of a patient's exposure, and infection typically requires at least 4 months of residence in a region where it is endemic (136). There are only a few case reports among short-stay visitors.

Life cycle and transmission

L. loa transmission occurs through vector flies of *Chrysops* species, which breed mainly in forested areas. Changes in the ecosystem due to human intervention are leading to changes in vector habitat, effecting either substantial increases or decreases in local transmission and prevalence. Transmission occurs when a fly bite introduces *Loa* microfilariae into the subcutaneous tissues. After 3 months, the larvae mature into adult worms that then migrate through the skin and other connective tissues, including the subconjunctiva, where the worms can often be seen with the unaided eye. Mature worms can survive in the host up to 17 years (187). Unlike other filariae, *L. loa* does not harbor the endosymbiotic bacteria *Wolbachia*, so there is no role of coadjuvant antibiotics in the treatment of loiasis (64).

Clinical manifestations

The classic clinical manifestations of loiasis are transit migratory angioedema (Calabar swelling) and migration of the adult worms across the conjunctiva, with an obvious "eye worm" visible without aid of magnification (Fig. 5) (103).

Calabar swelling. Classical Calabar swelling is caused by angioedema of uncertain etiology that is thought to represent a hypersensitivity response by the host to *Loa* microfilarial antigens. These swellings are evanescent and migratory and are most commonly seen on the face and extremities and after local trauma. Allergic symptoms of itching or pain can precede the nonpitting angioedema. Swelling duration is typically self limited and resolves in 2 to 4 days. It often recurs and thus can impair the patient's normal function (103).

Eye worm. As shown in Fig. 5, migration of the adult *L. loa* worm across the conjunctiva is obvious to the unaided vision of the examiner. Pruritus may occur with a transient edematous conjunctivitis that resolves spontaneously without sequelae (103).

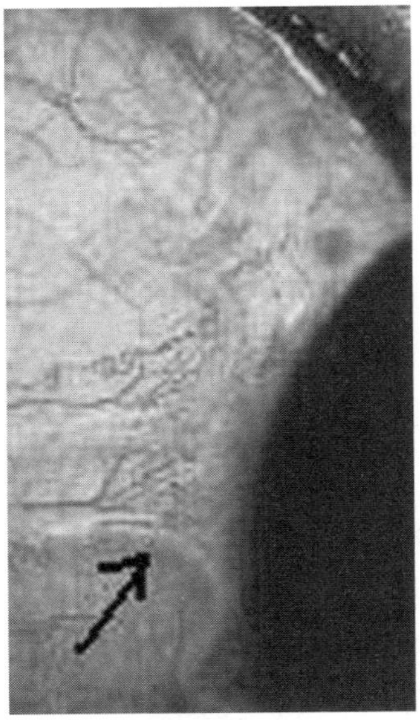

Figure 5. Eye worm of chronic *Loa loa* infection. (Credit: *Atlas of Tropical Medicine and Parasitology*, 6th ed., Elsevier.)

Chronic loiasis

After treatment with ivermectin, several complications may occur in cases of high intensity *L. loa* infection (58) (Tables 1 to 3). These include renal failure and an encephalopathy that may involve one of several degrees of mental impairment (18, 119). Such complications pose a significant problem in population-based mass campaigns of control of onchocerciasis in areas also where loiasis is endemic. The WHO has developed a new tool, RAPLOA (Rapid Assessment Procedure for Loiasis), that relates the prevalence of the key clinical manifestation of loiasis (history of eye worm) to the level of endemicity of the infection, which also reflects the local prevalence of high-intensity infection. As a screening mechanism, RAPLOA is a very useful tool for identifying areas with subjects at potential risk of *L. loa* encephalopathy related to ivermectin treatment (198).

Encephalitis is most commonly associated with people with high levels of microfilaremia (>5,000 microfilariae/ml of blood). In severe cases, microfilariae can often be observed in the cerebrospinal fluid (CSF). Patients can present with a variety of symptoms, ranging from mild headache, irritability, and insomnia to coma and death (194). Although it has historically been described after treatment, primarily with ivermectin, recent case reports of encephalitis unrelated to treatment point towards a poorly understood mechanism of central nervous system (CNS) disease in *L. loa*-infected patients (120, 183).

L. loa-related renal failure is the result of deposition of immune complexes in the glomerulus. Biopsy of affected kidneys shows sclerosed glomeruli (89, 142). It has been estimated that up to 30% of people infected with *L. loa* will have some form of renal involvement, as detected by microscopic hematuria or proteinuria (89, 142).

There is evidence of a linkage between loiasis and endomyocardial fibrosis. The strongest basis for this association is the clinical resolution of biopsy-proven endomyocardial fibrosis after anti-filarial treatment (7, 83). There are additional case reports *Loa*-associated complications of arthritis, posterior uveitis, and blindness (103).

Immunity and host response

There is a spectrum of disease in loiasis ranging from that seen in hosts who are asymptomatic with high-level microfilaremia (who are mostly long-term inhabitants of areas where loiasis is endemic) to symptomatic hosts with low levels of microfilaremia (who are frequently temporary visitors to loiasis-endemic sites). Clinical hyper-responsiveness is linked to hyperimmunoglobulinemia, eosinophilia, and increased levels of IgE. At the other end of the spectrum there are those hosts with suppressed response to filarial antigens (101). Filarial antigen-stimulated IgE production in the peripheral blood mononuclear cells is mediated by IL-4 and may be substantially downregulated by gamma interferon, with the two cytokines mediating a reciprocal regulation of IgE production (101).

Diagnosis

Loiasis should be included in the differential diagnosis of any person from an area where it is endemic who presents with urticaria, localized swelling, or sensation of a mass beneath the conjunctiva. It also needs to be considered in the presence of unexplained eosinophilia in a returned traveler or person from a *L. loa*-endemic area. A definite diagnosis can be made morphologically by extracting the worm from the eye or obtaining it from a blood sample. This should be done during the day due to the diurnal circulation of the microfilariae (103).

Serology can be obtained, but it is not specific and can cross-react with other filarial antigens of *W. bancrofti* and *B. malayi*. IgG4 antibodies to recombinant *L. loa* antigen Ll-SXP-1 are a highly specific marker of *L. loa* infection, with a sensitivity of 58% and specificity of 98% (105). The PCR assay, first used in 1991 (104), is more sensitive than the detection of IgG4 antibodies (191).

Treatment

The treatment of choice for loiasis is DEC at 80 to 100 mg/kg/day for 21 days (8). Treatment is curative in 45 to 50% of cases after the first dose, but even after full treatment, infection may recrudesce up to 8 years later. In such cases, several courses of treatment may be needed to eliminate infection (103).

In patients with heavy microfilarial loads, there is a risk of microfilarial lysis syndrome (59), entailing serious side effects, such as shock, renal failure, or fatal encephalitis. Plasmapheresis, or blood cell filtering to trap the microfilariae, has proven effective as a pretreatment intervention in heavily infected patients, in order to avoid side effects from lysis syndrome. Standard treatment with DEC then follows (17, 29, 161).

L. loa treatment with ivermectin reduces the microfilarial load, but it is ineffective against adult worms. In addition, there are high percentages of side effects, up to 70% among patients carrying high levels of microfilaremia. Many of the side effects are mild, including fever, headache, and pruritus, but some can include life-threatening events (47). The critical parasitemia level at which one could expect serious adverse effects seems to be 30,000 microfilariae/ml blood (47). Risk of ivermectin-related complications is an important consideration in areas where mass treatment is undertaken for onchocerciasis and in areas that are also *L. loa* endemic. Albendazole has been studied as an alternative to DEC and ivermectin. It has been shown to reduce microfilaremia, but its effect was not sustained over time (102, 182).

Control

There has been limited success in preventing *L. loa* with vector control due to the difficulty in gaining access to the *Chrysops* forest habitat. The only randomized, double-blind, placebo-controlled trial of DEC as a chemoprophylactic agent in temporary travelers to *L. loa*-endemic areas concluded that diethylcarbamazine given orally once weekly can be effective in preventing loiasis (137).

Mansonella Species Filariasis

The interest in *Mansonella* species is growing, as there is little understanding of host responses or host immunity among those infected with these less common filarial nematodes (103). It is known that *Mansonella*-related disease can range from asymptomatic up to advanced chronic complications, such as those seen with infections with *O. volvulus* and *L. loa*.

Mansonella streptocerca is a filarial nematode found in Central Africa. Streptocerciasis is a clinical entity that can be easily confused with onchocerciasis (103). It should be suspected in any person or traveler to a *Mansonella*-endemic area (103). Infected patients often present with inguinal lymphadenopathy, and/or chronic, intensely pruritic dermatitis. Whether elephantiasis can occur as a chronic complication of streptocerciasis is a subject of debate.

Mansonella perstans is another member of the same genus and is known to cause a disease similar to loiasis, with transient recurrent angioedema and urticaria of the extremities and face and other parts of the body (analogous to Calabar swellings seen in loiasis). Fever, arthralgias, and right upper quadrant pain can also be seen. Complications such as hepatitis and pericarditis may also occur (103). Geographic distribution of *M. perstans* includes Central Africa, several countries in Northern Africa, the Caribbean, and the northeastern basin of South America. The host response produced by *M. perstans* is granulomatous in nature (11, 103). Patients harboring *Mansonella* infections are mostly residents of areas where other filarial nematodes are endemic and where coinfections are the norm. As with other filariases, increased IgE and hypereosinophilia have been described (56). Treatment for all *Mansonella* species is with DEC (8, 103).

Dracunculus medinensis (Guinea Worm Disease)

Dracunculiasis, or guinea worm disease, is one of the earliest described parasitic infections and has been known since at least ancient Egyptian times (160). Dracunculiasis is a significantly disabling disease with great impact on childhood development and personal performance status. In endemic communities, disease symptom prevalence reemerges each year during the agricultural season, handicapping many farmers, mothers, and schoolchildren living in limited (subsistence) conditions.

Epidemiology

Since the full implementation of the Dracunculiasis Eradication Program by the WHO in 1986, at which time an estimated 3.5 million cases were reported from 20 countries and 120 million persons were at risk for the disease, the number of village units with endemic dracunculiasis has decreased from 23,165 in 1993 to 3,583 in 2006 (26). Currently, all of the remaining dracunculiasis-endemic areas, now down to nine countries, are in Africa. These are, in order of decreasing prevalence, Sudan, Ghana, Mali, Niger, Nigeria, Togo, Ethiopia, Burkina Faso, and Côte D'Ivoire (26).

Life cycle and transmission

The transmission takes place through ingestion of contaminated water that contains copepods (water fleas) carrying infectious *D. medinensis* larvae (L3) (160). When the copepods are lysed by the gastric juices of the host, the larvae that are released migrate to the small intestine, penetrate the bowel wall, and then these worms mature over the next 10 to 14 months in the thoracic and abdominal areas. Mature, 70- to 100-cm (gravid) female worms migrate peripherally towards the patient's limbs and erupt though areas of skin to release larvae that will enter freshwater and infect a new generation of copepods. Transmission usually occurs when a patient seeks to soak an affected limb in water to alleviate the pain and itching caused by the female worm. Stagnant sources of drinking water from ponds, dried-up river beds, and hand-dug or uncovered step wells most commonly harbor infected copepods (129).

Clinical manifestations

Infected people remain asymptomatic for up to 1 year, after which the mature gravid female worm migrates to the surface of the skin and produces a painful, then blistering papule (160) (Fig. 6). Blister rupture produces systemic symptoms of fever, pruritus, urticaria, nausea, diarrhea, and pain. The typical location of the worm appearance is the lower extremities, but worms can also emerge from other parts of the body, including the upper extremities, the head, buttocks, and genitalia. Traditional treatment for dracunculiasis involves a very painful process; as the worm emerges, the affected person pulls it out, winding a few centimeters of worm every day on a stick (160). During this multi-week process, there is a potential risk of breaking the worm and consequent exacerbation of local inflammation around the track of the worm. Cellulitis with secondary pyogenic infections is very common, aggravating the condition even more (160).

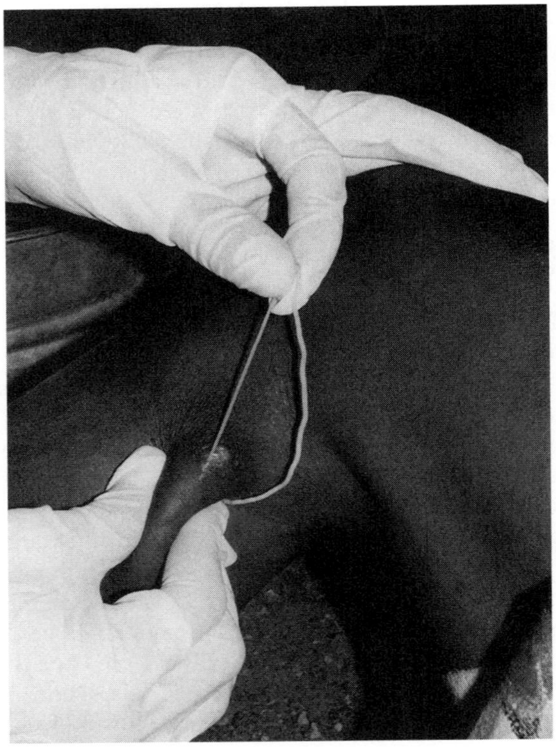

Figure 6. Dracunculiasis (guinea worm infection). (Credit: Centers for Disease Control and Prevention, http://phil.cdc.gov/phil/quicksearch.asp.)

Chronic incapacitation

During acute flares of dracunculiasis, the period of incapacitation generally ranges between 2 and 16 weeks, with an average of 8.5 weeks. Common chronic late complications include muscle contractures. During incapacitation, affected subjects may suffer joint and limb ankylosis. More severe disease is found when the migrating worms go to the retroperitoneum and on to critical tissues, such as the pericardium (91), orbital and palpebral areas (23), testicles (148), or spinal cord (46).

Diagnosis and treatment

The diagnosis of dracunculiasis is purely clinical and is generally made upon formation of the blister and emergence of the adult female worm (160). Secondary bacterial superinfections are not uncommon during treatment, with severe cellulitis and septic arthritis seen as common complications (157). Occlusive bandages can help keep the wound clean and dry and may prevent the patient from contaminating sources of drinking water. Applying topical antiseptics to help with the removal of the worm may help to prevent secondary bacterial infection. If secondary infection occurs, antibiotic therapy is imperative to prevent further spread that could lead to sepsis or irreversible muscle and tendon contractures from prolonged inflammation.

Control

Because curative options are limited, dracunculiasis control efforts are mainly geared towards prevention, focusing on community education. The most important behavior modification is the treatment of drinking water via cloth filtration in order to remove copepods. To this end, filters have also been developed from metal oil drums with filter cloth inserted in the top and spigots at the bottom. These have had better acceptance than traditional hand-sewn cloth filters (2). Abate larvicide can also be used in selected contaminated waters.

Soil-Transmitted Helminths: *Ascaris lumbricoides* (Roundworm), *Trichuris trichiura* (Whipworm), *Ancylostoma duodenale* and *Necator americanus* (Hookworms), and *Strongyloides stercoralis*

The three main soil-transmitted helminth infections, ascariasis, trichuriasis, and hookworm, are among the world's most prevalent infections and have a worldwide distribution (14). Strongyloidiasis is rarer but presents unique problems for management (169). Each parasite can produce acute and chronic clinical disease in humans. The so-called geohelminths share the common characteristic of being nematodes that are transmitted by fecal contamination of the soil, and they all colonize the intestinal tract of the affected human host (32, 76, 168, 169). A child living in poverty in a less-developed country is likely to be parasitized with at least one, and in many cases, all four soil-transmitted helminths, which can result in impairments in physical, intellectual, and cognitive development (14). This section focuses mainly on infections due to *Ascaris, Trichuris,* and hookworm, since these worms are currently responsible for the highest burden of disease.

Epidemiology

Hookworm infection is endemic in most developing areas of the subtropics and tropics, where sanitation is poor and environmental conditions, particularly moist and sandy soils, provide ideal parasite habitat. Less-developed coastal communities with intense agricultural activity are frequently the settings with the highest hookworm prevalence. In contrast, *Ascaris* and *Trichuris* infection are found both in urban slums and rural communities with poor sanitation (32, 168).

Ascariasis is the most prevalent parasitic infection in the world, with an estimated 25% of the world population infected with *Ascaris* (37). Local prevalence in developing communities frequently ranges from 12% up to 77% (25, 186). The intensity of worm burden explains many aspects of the severity of disease, and because worms do not reproduce in the human host, the efficiency of local transmission often determines the community prevalence of *Ascaris*-associated disease. Socioeconomic factors, mainly sanitation, play an important role in determining the degree of contamination of the human environment with fertile eggs. In a study conducted in 11 rural communities in Brazil, human crowding was found to be the best predictor of infection risk (25). Climate also has a large influence on the pattern of *A. lumbricoides* infection; in parts of Africa, low prevalence (5%) is found in areas with a short rainy season, in contrast to 70% prevalence in tropical monsoonal rainy areas (151). Pulmonary symptoms from worm migration often occur in affected areas of Saudi Arabia between March and May, after the rainy season (168).

An estimated 740 million people are infected with the hookworms *Ancylostoma duodenale, Necator americanus,* or both (76). *Necator americanus* is the predominant hookworm worldwide (39). Its high prevalence remains nearly constant in areas where it is endemic, even after mass treatment campaigns, due to a consistent pattern of reinfection (3). Overall, the highest prevalence and intensity of hookworm infections occur in sub-Saharan Africa, followed by China and Southeast Asia (76). The major health concern related to infection with hookworm is its ability to produce anemia. Unlike other soil-transmitted helminth infections (ascariasis and trichuriasis), in which high-intensity infections occur primarily among school-aged children, high-intensity hookworm infections frequently occur among adults (15). According to the WHO, hookworm infection is an important health threat to adolescent girls and women of reproductive age (4) because of the anemia-related impact on the outcomes in pregnancy, including low birth weight, impaired milk production, and increased risk of death for both the mother and the child (22). Up to 44 million pregnant women are estimated to be infected with hookworm.

Life cycle and transmission

A. lumbricoides, T. trichiura, and hookworm are all geohelminths, i.e., transmitted by ground contamination, but they have distinct differences in transmission. Both *A. lumbricoides* eggs and hookworm larvae must mature in a moist environment before they can infect the next human host (76, 168). *Ascaris* and *Trichuris* eggs contaminate food and fingers and infect humans when they are ingested and swallowed. Hookworm larvae crawl on the ground and low foliage and penetrate the skin directly. *Trichuris* larvae appear to migrate directly to their niche in the cecum (32). By contrast, hatched *Ascaris* and skin-penetrating hookworm larvae both migrate through the bloodstream to the lungs, where they mature and then ascend to the trachea and pharynx to be then swallowed in order to reach their final niche, the human small intestine (128). This common stage of migration through the lungs can cause a symptomatic allergic pulmonary syndrome, known as Loeffler's syndrome (168). The patient will typically present with a dry cough, dyspnea, and wheezing. Peripheral eosinophilia can be seen at that point, but it has its major peak when the larvae transits to the intestine via the pharynx. "Wakana disease" is a syndrome seen in adults, consisting of nausea, vomiting, cough, dyspnea, and eosinophilia associated with ingestion of a large number of *A. duodenale* L3 larvae (168).

Clinical manifestations

Ascariasis. There is a wide spectrum of disease that occurs with *A. lumbricoides* infection. This can range from asymptomatic infection to mild abdominal and pulmonary symptoms, or to an acute abdomen caused by overwhelming intestinal obstruction leading to death (168). The most common severe clinical syndromes are pneumonitis, intestinal obstruction, biliary obstruction, and pancreatic obstruction. These are due to the different stages of parasite migration to different organs (36, 40, 213). Children usually have the highest intensity of infection and tend to present with more severe clinical issues (213).

Lung manifestations in ascariasis are due to migration of newly infecting larvae hatched from eggs ingested in the previous 1 or 2 weeks. There is an immune-mediated hypersensitivity reaction to the presence of *Ascaris* antigens, which can be strongly allergenic. The clinical spectrum goes from mild cough with no radiological changes to Loeffler's syndrome, with pulmonary infiltrates, dyspnea, and eosinophilia. The burden of infection is one of the predictors of severity of presentation. During such an initial migratory stage of infection, no eggs may be detected in the stool (168). Intestinal manifestations correspond to the adult worm phase of infection. Intestinal obstruction can occur from aggregation of a large bolus of worms within the lumen of the intestine (Fig. 7). Because the diameter of a child's intestine is smaller, it is more prone to obstruction in this fashion (40). *Ascaris* migration into the biliary tree is also a common presenting symptom, leading to complications such as ascending cholangitis, acute pancreatitis, and obstructive jaundice (165).

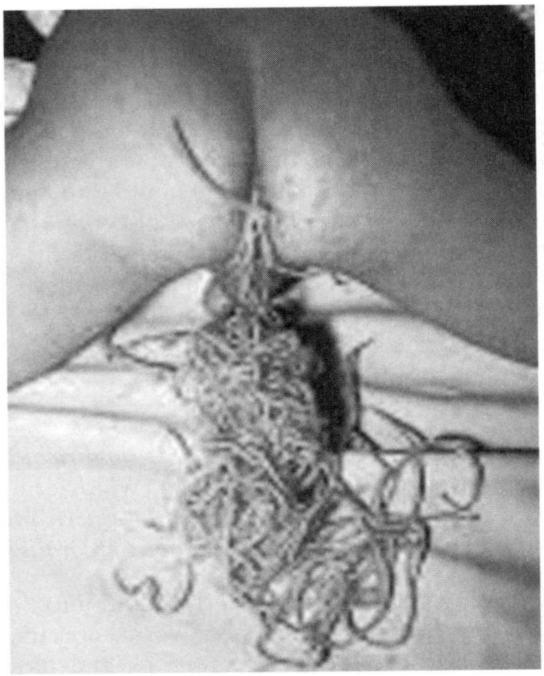

Figure 7. Heavy *Ascaris* infection with expelled worm ball. (Credit: *Atlas of Tropical Medicine and Parasitology*, 6th ed., Elsevier.)

Hookworm. Once established in the intestine, adult hookworms are approximately 1-cm-long parasites that cause host injury by attaching to the mucosa and submucosa of the small intestine and producing intestinal blood loss (76). The presence of between 40 and 160 adult hookworms in the human intestine results in blood loss sufficient to cause anemia and malnutrition. The term "hookworm disease" refers primarily to the iron-deficiency anemia with reduced host hemoglobin, serum ferritin, and protoporphyrin that results from moderate and heavy infections. Risk of this form of hookworm disease is in direct correlation with the number of resident parasites (as measured by quantitative egg counts in the stool).

Intestinal colonization by *A. duodenale* or *N. americanus* begins about 3 months after larval exposure. During the initial phase of intestinal involvement, clinical manifestations can include abdominal pain, nausea, and anorexia. The associated blood loss from hookworm infection can be as high as 0.3 ml per worm per day. The degree of iron deficiency anemia depends on the worm burden, the type of hookworm (*A. duodenale* causes more blood loss), iron reserves, and overall host nutrition (76).

Infantile ancylostomiasis is an extreme form of hookworm anemia with high mortality. It occurs in infants heavily infected with *A. duodenale,* typically presenting with diarrhea, melena, pallor, and failure to thrive (4). The majority of these severe cases present with eggs in their feces within 3 months of birth, supporting the theory that mother-to-child transmission may be responsible via transplacental and/or transmammary routes (213).

Whipworm (*Trichuris trichiura*). The main difference for early trichuriasis-related illness is the absence of pulmonary symptoms (32). Otherwise the clinical presentation can easily overlap with that of *Ascaris* infection. Rectal prolapse is a known complication of *Trichuris* infection (32). Growth stunting in childhood has been associated with severe *Trichuris* infection, manifesting as a "*Trichuris* dysentery syndrome" that includes pan-colitis, frequent bloody stools, malabsorption, and malnutrition.

Strongyloidiasis. *Strongyloides* stercoralis is an intestinal helminthic parasite of humans that is quite different from other GI worms (169). As part of its reproductive cycle, its eggs hatch to release living rhabditiform progeny within the lumen of the bowel. Ordinarily these larvae must pass out of the body and transform into filariform larvae in order to become infectious. However, in patients with delayed GI transit or with immunosuppression, this transformation and autoinfection may occur within the GI tract or perianal skin (131, 169). As a result, a patient's *S. stercoralis* infection may appear to persist for decades after he or she has left the area of endemic transmission. A complication of chronic strongyloidiasis is the "hyperinfection syndrome" known to occur in debilitated and critically ill patients (131). In this syndrome, infectious larvae migrate directly from the bowel lumen to the bloodstream and organs. As they migrate, they may carry bowel flora to the bloodstream, major organs, or meninges, introducing a severe, secondary bacterial infection that is frequently polymicrobial in nature and often fatal.

Geohelminth-associated severe anemia and nutritional deficiencies and impairment of growth and development. Infections with hookworm, *Trichuris,* and *A. lumbricoides* are all associated with anemia, with harmful consequences on the health of the parasitized hosts. Those who are most affected are chiefly children and pregnant women (4). The more insidious presentation of chronic anemia and malnutrition impacts growth and development of geohelminth-infected children (16, 38, 159, 163, 177). Findings suggest that hookworm infection can have a significant adverse effect on a child's working memory, which may have consequences for a child's reasoning ability and reading comprehension (163). Loss of schooling and learning opportunities often has an irreversible lifetime impact on productivity and personal performance. Chan estimated (by means of calculating disability-adjusted life years) that approximately 70% of the intestinal nematode health burden can be prevented by treating schoolchildren alone in high-prevalence communities (27).

Asthma. There is continuing controversy over whether geohelminths are protective or provocative in asthma. One large study concluded that there was an overall protection against asthma among patients infected with intestinal parasites (33). However, a meta-analysis of 30 studies concluded that *Ascaris lumbricoides* was associated with significantly increased odds of asthma, whereas hookworm infection was associated with a significantly strong reduction in asthma risk that was directly related to hookworm infection intensity (113). A recent case-control study in Bangladesh, which studied children with and without asthma symptoms, concluded that high titer anti-*Ascaris* IgE is associated with an increased risk of asthma symptoms among 5-year-olds who have a high helminthic infectious load (184).

Immunity and host response

The host's inflammatory process is similar in all geohelminth infections. When larvae migrate through human tissues, cells undergo mechanical trauma as well as lysis caused by larval enzymes (128). Granuloma formation can then be induced from mobilizing eosinophils, neutrophils, and macrophages. This is particularly true when *A. lumbricoides* larvae are present in pulmonary parenchyma, inducing a hypersensitivity reaction that induces bronchial spasm (168). Immune responses are typically polarized towards the production of T-helper cell type 2 (Th2) cytokines (34, 118, 128). In the case of infection with *A. lumbricoides*, IL-4 and IL-5 production are significantly augmented (34). Immune response has not been as well studied for hookworm infection, but there is increasing interest in the role of hookworm anti-clotting secretions. These appear to both prevent blood from clotting and downregulate host inflammatory response (42, 80).

Diagnosis

Microscopic examination and quantitative egg counts of fecal samples are most useful in determining the presence and intensity of geohelminth infection. The exception is *Strongyloides stercoralis,* which has living progeny and may require special culture techniques to detect (169). For all geohelminths, eggs may be absent in very early (migratory) stages of infection. A heavily infected patient may have eosinophilia, as well as normocytic or microcytic hypochromic anemia, as indicated from peripheral blood smears. Charcot-Leyden crystals in the sputum can aid in the diagnosis of pneumonitis associated with *A. lumbricoides* migration. Antibody testing for levels of parasite-specific and -nonspecific IgE is sometimes used to determine infection levels for research purposes.

Treatment

The treatments of choice for all geo-helminths are the benzimidazole drugs albendazole and mebendazole (8). Both act by disrupting the microtubules of the parasite. Cure rates may be as high as 100% for *Ascaris,* but the problem of rapid reinfection remains, since areas where it is endemic have little means to provide the hygiene measures needed to prevent transmission (170). Alternative drug treatment is available with levamisol or pyrantel (8). There is a global movement to provide treatment to pregnant women and adolescent girls, based on increasing evidence of the safety of these drugs during pregnancy (4, 67). Two randomized controlled clinical trials of mebendazole administered during pregnancy in Peru indicate that deworming with mebendazole can be safely included in antenatal care programs in hookworm-endemic areas (67, 111). Additionally, the WHO has concluded that albendazole and mebendazole may be used to treat children as young as 12 months if local circumstances show that relief from ascariasis and trichuriasis is justified (4, 125).

Surgical intervention is used for obstructive complications due to *Ascaris* infection. The mortality rate of late intervention for intestinal obstruction has been reported as high as 50% (200). For biliary obstruction, endoscopy has been reported to have excellent outcomes (214).

Control

Effective sanitation is the most important environmental intervention to interrupt transmission and prevent infection with geohelminths (170). Improvement in living standards, with the introduction of water pipelines, sewage systems, mechanized agriculture, and replacement of night soil (human feces) as fertilizer are the most effective methods. Due to the low cost of effective drugs, health education and sanitation have often been relegated to second place in helminth transmission control. However, education is the only effective tool for enabling both chemotherapy and sanitation measures (10).

Regular treatment of high-risk groups, particularly school-age children, has become the mainstay of helminth transmission control. As part of mass, age-targeted benzimidazole treatment for school-age children, teachers are asked to participate in drug administration, making it part of a community strategy (207c). There is a caveat in targeting school-age children in transmission control campaigns. Neglecting to include adults who are also infected with geohelminths, particularly hookworm, will fail to effectively stop transmission, and rates of infection in the community will continue to be high (3). Several hookworm vaccines are in different stages of development, which may make better prevention of infection a greater possibility (45).

Other tissue nematodes

Trichinellosis. Trichinellosis is caused by larval infection and tissue encystment by larvae of the animal nematode *Trichinella spiralis* (19). When humans ingest incompletely cooked meat containing encysted larvae, these forms hatch within the GI tract to become mature worms within 1 or 2 weeks. These in turn release living progeny (1,500 larvae/adult female worm), and these immature larvae penetrate the bowel wall and migrate to encyst within host tissues, with preference for the skeletal and cardiac muscles. Acute trichinosis is frequently characterized by GI discomfort, fever, headache, myalgias, subconjunctival hemorrhage and petechiae, and periorbital edema, along with marked eosinophilia (19). CNS involvement can be manifested as seizures, polyneuritis, meningitis, and psychotic symptoms (50). Cardiac involvement can lead to congestive heart failure and dysrhythmias. These last complications may prove fatal or result in long-term disabling sequelae (19).

Eosinophilic meningitis: *Angiostrongylus* and *Gnathostoma* species. Inadvertent human infection with parasites of domestic or wild animals can cause severe acute or subacute illness (66, 107, 126, 164). In this situation, humans cannot become patent hosts for these parasites because adult forms of these parasites never develop within the body. However, immature larvae of the invading parasite may migrate for weeks within patient organs before dying. Typically, the inflammatory response to this tissue invasion is much more severe than the inflammation seen in response to the common migratory human helminthic parasites, such as *Ascaris* or hookworm.

Human systemic or CNS disease is common following infection by the rat lungworm *Angiostrongylus cantonensis*, which is transmitted by food contamination via snails, slugs, or undercooked prawns or crab (117, 164). Angiostrongyliasis is found in Southeast Asia, Indonesia, Japan, the Philippines, Taiwan, southern areas of the Pacific, Egypt, Cuba, and Hawaii (107). Since 2000, a number of cases have been reported from Jamaica, and the disease may potentially be transmitted by snails in continental North America (171).

Nervous system disorders and eosinophilic meningitis are also common following infection caused by *Gnathostoma* species parasites of dogs and cats, which are transmitted by ingestion of undercooked freshwater fish or of frog, bird, or snake meat (28, 66) Gnathostomiasis has been reported in Japan, China, Malaysia, Indonesia, India, Bangladesh, Central America, and Israel.

With both types of infection, patient symptoms occur 1 to 3 weeks after exposure. These include creeping skin eruptions, abdominal and pleural symptoms, fever, and eosinophilia (31, 66). CNS invasion is marked by headache, meningismus, cranial nerve palsies, and paresthesias, which may be protracted and severe. Spinal cord involvement may present as radiculomyeloencephalitis. CSF examination is remarkable for intense eosinophilic pleocytosis (up to 90%), with mildly elevated CSF protein and normal or low-normal glucose concentrations. CSF cytology occasionally reveals parasite larvae (117), but the specific diagnosis is more frequently based on clinical presentation, exposure history, and serological evidence. Optimal therapy for this type of parasitic infection is not established. Benzimidazoles and corticosteroids have been used to alleviate symptoms of angiostrongyliasis (31); quinine and corticosteroids have been used to treat systemic gnathostomiasis. Both infections are self limited in nature, although neurological deficits may persist for months to years.

Visceral larva migrans. Visceral larva migrans is a common migratory parasitic infection caused by inadvertent ingestion of the eggs of animal roundworms, most frequently *Toxocara canis* and *Toxocara cati* (126). Infection is most frequent among children with pica who ingest contaminated soil. Developing larvae hatch within the gut and then may migrate into all tissues, including the CNS and eyes. Systemically, the subacute process of infection may be characterized by fever, hepatomegaly, eosinophilia, and symptoms of pulmonary infection. More chronic neurological symptoms may include absence attacks, generalized convulsions, focal sensorimotor deficits, and paraplegia, depending on the species of parasite (51). Focal retinal inflammation may be mistaken for retinoblastoma, leading to mistaken intervention for enucleation of the eye (126). Diagnosis is established by history of animal exposure and by serological studies, although by itself ocular disease may yield only low or nonspecific anti-*Toxocara* titers in the serum. A CSF eosinophilic pleocytosis may also be noted. Treatment with corticosteroids is frequently used to alleviate inflammatory symptoms. Specific antiparasitic therapy with albendazole, thiabendazole, or diethylcarbamazine has been associated with improvement of symptoms in some cases (126). The long-term outcome of most such infections is generally benign.

Cestodes (tapeworms)

The cestode tapeworms, which take their common name because of the flattened, tape-like appearance of their adult forms, are exclusively parasitic throughout their entire lives (180). Cestode parasites divide their life cycle between two or more different hosts; adult worms are found in the GI tract of vertebrate *definitive* hosts (92). Later, parasite eggs excreted in feces are transmitted into the local environment and ultimately hatch to form intermediate larval forms that infect either vertebrate or invertebrate *intermediate* hosts as tissue cysts. The tapeworm egg is the only stage that interacts with the external environment (209). There are health problems caused by cyst formation by the parasites *Echinococcus* and *Sparganum* (echinococcosis and sparganosis), as well as chronic health problems associated with infection by the "fish tapeworm," *Diphyllobothrium latum*. For a description of disease caused by *Taenia solium* infection and the outcomes of its associated condition, cysticercosis, the reader is referred to Chapter 13 of this book.

Echinococcus Species

Echinococcosis, caused by cestodes of the genus *Echinococcus,* is primarily a zoonotic tapeworm infection of dogs and other canids (167). Its medical importance lies in the potentially devastating consequences when humans become inadvertent intermediate hosts for the parasite. Infected patients often develop chronic cystic parasitic lesions within critical organs of the body. When this happens, complications can be severe and may prove lethal (167). Where echinococcosis is highly endemic, it can prove to be an enormous health and economic burden for the affected communities (20, 190).

The two species of greatest medical interest in human disease are *Echinococcus granulosus* and *Echinococcus multilocularis* (167). The former typically causes cystic echinococcosis (CE), and the latter causes alveolar echinococcosis (AE). Different genotypes have been identified recently for each species, with the sheep genotype, *E. granulosus* (G1), being the most widespread.

Life cycle and transmission

The definitive hosts of the *Echinococcus* species are carnivores. Domestic dogs are the primary reservoir for *E. granulosus,* whereas foxes and coyotes are the primary reservoir for *E. multilocularis* (167). In both settings, the canids carry the adult worms in their intestines and distribute parasite eggs into the environment in their feces. The canine carnivores acquire their tapeworm infection by ingesting immature tapeworm larval cysts in the organs of intermediate animal hosts that contain hydatid cysts (or protoscolices released from recently ruptured cysts). The usual intermediate hosts are sheep, cattle, pigs, deer, or caribou in the case of *E granulosus* and wild arvicolid rodents for *E. multilocularis*.

When humans ingest *Echinococcus* eggs, the eggs hatch in the small intestine, and larvae penetrate the bowel wall and then migrate through the bloodstream to encyst in various different viscera. Humans in contact with infected animals will ingest *Echinococcus* eggs either via directly contaminated water, soil, or contaminated vegetables or through foods indirectly contaminated by flies (167). Eggs of *E. granulosus* are capable of surviving in the soil throughout cold weather conditions, remaining viable for at least 1 year on pasture. However, they have high intolerance to desiccation by direct sunlight.

Epidemiology

Echinococcosis is distributed worldwide. The greatest prevalence of CE, in both animals and humans, is found in countries having temperate climates, such as those found in southern South America, the Mediterranean littoral, the southern and central republics of the former Soviet Union, Central Asia, China, Australia, and some areas of Africa (167). CE is an occupational hazard in populations who use dogs to raise sheep and cattle. In the United States, most CE infections are diagnosed in immigrants coming from areas where hydatid cyst disease is endemic. In the past, these patients were Italian and Greek primarily, but in more recent times more U.S. patients have originated from the Middle East and Asia. There is sporadic *E. granulosus* transmission with autochthonous CE in Alaska, Arizona, Utah, and New Mexico. Because prevalence was formerly high in parts of the United Kingdom, Australia, and New Zealand, sporadic late cases still present in these areas.

E. multilocularis is less common, being mostly a zoonosis of wild animals (167). Transmission is now most common in northern Eurasia and Turkey and in the highlands of Central Asia and western China (212). Past foci were described as Native American villages located in North American tundra (208). Transmission has also occurred in the northern plains section of the United States and Canada (167).

Clinical manifestations

Patients with echinococcosis have an extremely variable presentation in terms of both disease severity and the nature of their signs and symptoms. There is no pathognomonic clinical finding of the disease (92). Many infections remain asymptomatic for years and may even go undetected for the entire lifetime of the host, with only an incidental finding of hydatid cyst (CE) on autopsy or by an abdominal ultrasound obtained for other reasons.

CE (*E. granulosus*). Cysts most often localize in the liver or lung and can grow at different rates. The enlarging cystic mass displaces normal tissues and can start producing symptoms (based on location and size) after years to decades of growth. A single cyst is the norm in primary infections; however, multiple cysts or multiorgan involvement can be seen in up to 40% of patients. Liver is the most common location of the cysts (65%), followed by lung (25%). Unusual sites are bone, brain, spleen, and kidneys. In more sensitive critical organs, for example, hydatid cysts located in the brain or the eye, a cyst of only small size will produce symptoms. It is possible for secondary cysts to form from internal daughter cysts if the primary cyst is ruptured (spontaneously or induced by trauma) or if cyst contents spill during invasive procedures or surgery (92). Cyst rupture can cause a variety of host responses, including mild-to-severe anaphylactoid reactions, with risk of death. Ruptured cysts in the lungs might drain into the bronchi, or cysts may occlude airways, leading to secondary bacterial infections and severe pneumonia (167).

Liver disease. Hydatid cysts in the liver may grow for years before becoming symptomatic. This is partly because of the size and distensibility of the organ. Patients may present with an enlarged liver or a palpable mass, being symptomatic with anorexia, nausea, vomiting, difficulty with digestion, and/or epigastric pain. Urgent presentations might include cyst rupture, thoracobilia, or biliary fistula with signs of secondary bacterial infection or obstruction (115).

Lung disease. Intact cysts may be asymptomatic in the lungs, but leakage or rupture can lead to acute respiratory compromise with chest pain, coughing, and dyspnea. Occasionally, hydatid membranes may be coughed up, with a resolution of symptoms. About 40% of lung cysts present with concurrent liver cysts (5).

Unusual sites. The clinical manifestations of hydatid cysts in unusual anatomic locations are varied (Table 2). Cerebral cysts can present with increased intracranial pressure or focal epilepsy. Hematuria and loin pain can be the initial presentation of kidney cysts. Bone cysts can present with pathological fractures, which are frequently misdiagnosed as cancer or tuberculosis. The heart or pericardium can also develop CE, with potentially devastating consequences in the event of rupture, including cardiac tamponade with shock, complicated by systemic dissemination of daughter cyst protoscolices (167).

AE (*E. multilocularis*). For AE, the disease process is different from that of CE since organ damage is due to larval cystic infiltration rather than spherical enlargement (167). Typically the primary AE infection is in the liver, but direct extension to the contiguous organs, as well as hematogenous metastases to the lungs and brain, is also common. The AE larval mass (Fig. 8) very much resembles a malignancy in its appearance and metastatic behavior. Symptoms are often vague, with patients presenting with complaints of right upper quadrant discomfort or pain, weight loss, or malaise. At times, symptoms related to pulmonary or cerebral metastases can be the initial presentation (208). AE response to therapy is less good than that of CE; the mortality rate is high, ranging from 50 to 75% with and without surgery (82).

Socioeconomic impact of chronic disease

The morbidity associated with hydatid disease is considerable. Patients with hydatid cysts often require several surgical interventions, and if secondary spread occurs, disseminated hydatid disease often becomes inoperable. If livestock are heavily infected, this may also translate into economic devastation for the family (190). The economic burden is not only due to medical expenses but also to a loss of income. A study from Uruguay indicates that up to 60% of patients who have undergone surgery are unable to return to normal activity 4 months after intervention (167). Recent estimates of the combined losses resulting from human and livestock CE indicate an annual worldwide loss of US $193,529,740 due to this disease (20).

Diagnosis

The presence of a cystic mass in a person with a history of exposure to dogs in areas where *E. granulosus* is endemic should raise the suspicion of CE. Ultrasonography is now widely used for diagnosis due to its operability and low cost. The WHO/IWGE have proposed a standard classification (Fig. 9) to aid in the staging of CE (206). Computed tomography (CT) and magnetic resonance imaging (MRI) have also proven valuable for diagnosis and preoperative evaluation in staging the condition of the lesion (whether intact, unilocular, ruptured, complicated with daughter cysts, and/or calcified) as well as its anatomic extension.

For AE, the image often appears as indistinct solid tumors with central necrotic areas and calcifications. MRI and positron emission tomography scan are also being used for imaging diagnosis (153).

There is serologic testing available for both *E. granulosus* and *E. multilocularis*. ELISA and Western blot techniques are generally specific for these parasites (167); however, there are some confounding factors that may lead to false-positive results. These factors are coinfection with other helminthes, cancer, chronic immune disease, and the anatomic location of the cyst (lesions in the liver tend to be more immunogenic than cysts in other locations). For CE due to *E. granulosus*, there is a new latex agglutination test that can be performed for detection of circulating hydatid antigen in serum. This test has a sensitivity of 72% and a specificity of 98% (43). There is also a test for detecting hydatid antigen in

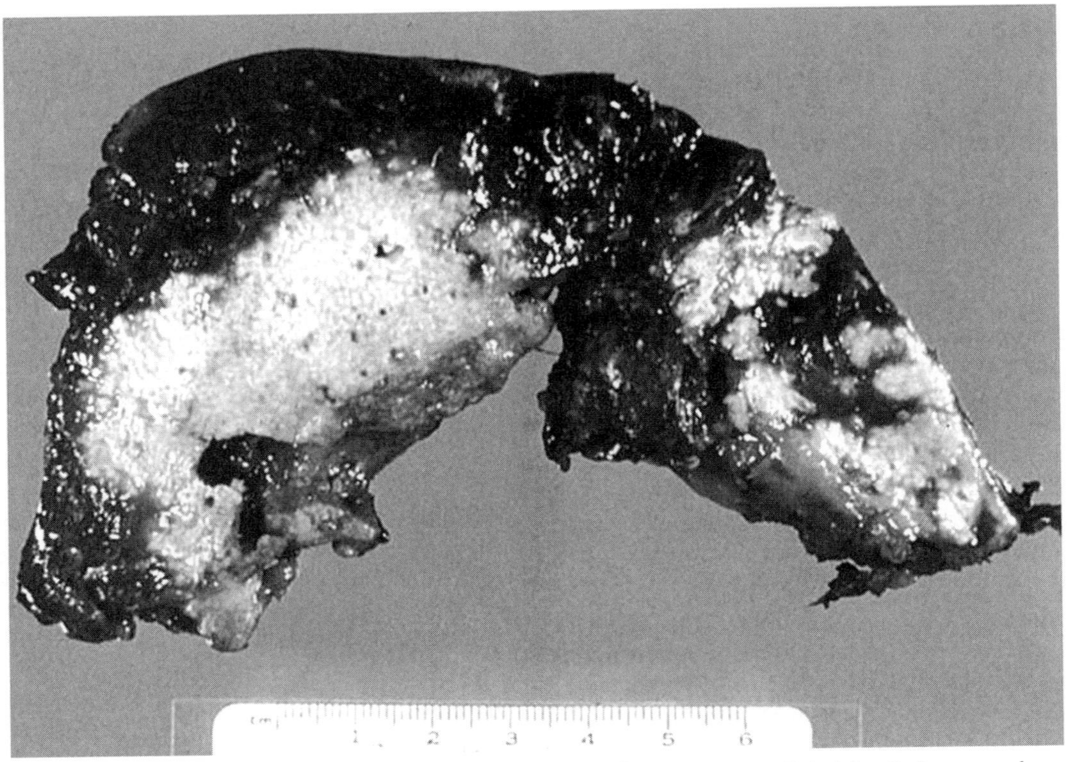

Figure 8. Alveolar echinococcosis of the liver. (Credit: *Tropical Infectious Diseases: Principles, Pathogens and Practice*, Elsevier.)

the urine, which may provide a simple, rapid, and noninvasive method of population-based surveys and diagnosis of hydatid disease (144). A PCR technique has also been developed that is useful for differentiating species and strains of *Echinococcus* (63).

Treatment

The ideal therapy for echinococcosis is removal of the infecting cyst. This is not always the optimal treatment, however, for a number of practical reasons.

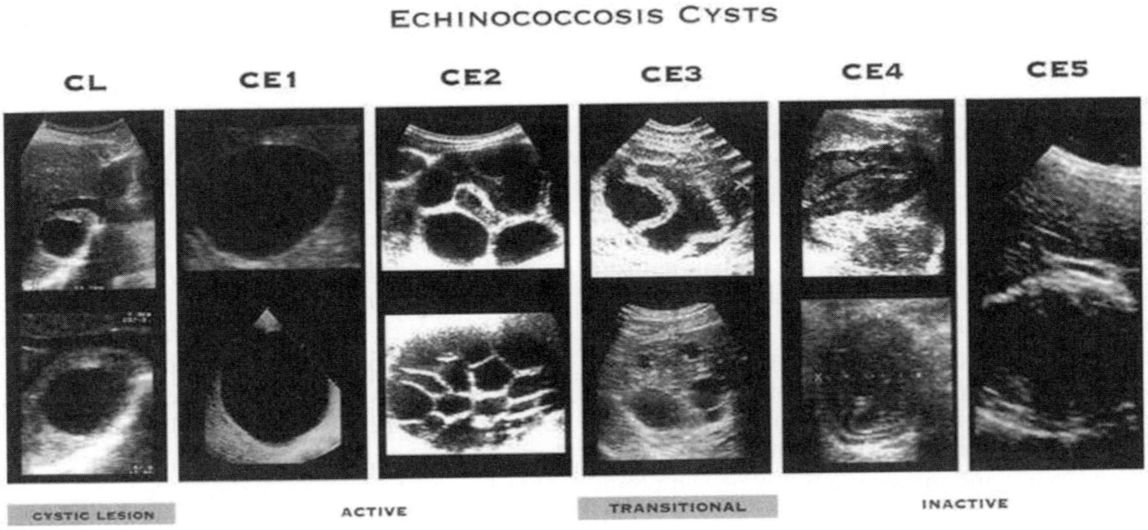

Figure 9. International classification of ultrasound images in cystic echinococcosis for application in clinical and field epidemiological settings. (Credit: World Health Organization.)

Many incidental cases of CE remain asymptomatic and can be observed and periodically monitored in a process of "watchful waiting." Invasive surgery runs the risk of cyst rupture, with the combined threat of acute anaphylaxis and cyst dissemination. Most often, a strategy of cysticidal therapy, combined with cyst aspiration or removal, provides a practical, effective resolution of infection and its associated symptoms.

Chemotherapy. Benzimidazole antihelminthics have been studied extensively for treatment of echinococcosis. For CE, albendazole has proven effective in treating liver cystic hydatidosis, in treatment courses ranging from 3 months to more than 1 year (52). Drug treatment alone has been much less effective in controlling AE.

Percutaneous aspiration and injection with reaspiration. As an alternative to surgical intervention, percutaneous aspiration and cysticidal injection appear to be an effective form of minimally invasive treatment (147), which has been used increasingly to supplement or even replace surgery (167).

Surgery. Surgery can cure the patient if the parasite is removed entirely. However, surgery involving cyst dissection is often painstakingly slow due to inflammatory adhesion of the cyst wall to adjacent tissues. Before cyst dissection, cyst contents must be sterilized with the use of a cysticidal agent, such as ethanol or hypertonic saline, that is *nontoxic* to humans (formaldehyde and antiseptics are no longer recommended due to their potential, systemic toxicity and local sclerosing effects [92]). For AE, the more aggressive form of echinococcosis, depending on parasite size and extension, different surgical modalities can include partial to total liver resection (with transplantation) or more limited intervention with a cystectomy or paracystectomy (24).

Control measures

CE can be eradicated with the use of aggressive control measures. The first country to eradicate *E. granulosus* was Iceland, over 130 years ago. It implemented measures of health education about exposure as well as strict prohibition of home slaughtering of sheep. In current public health practice, efforts are made to control the synanthropic cycle by providing anti-tapeworm praziquantel therapy to dogs (167). A vaccine against *E. granulosus* is being developed for sheep, and this will provide a further step in controlling transmission (114).

AE has been eradicated from most of Japan, to date the only country that has done so, by elimination of dogs and foxes harboring *E. multilocularis*. One northern island continues to have *E. multilocularis*, posing an obvious risk for reintroduction to the mainland (87).

Sparganosis

Sparganosis is an uncommon infection caused by tissue migration of larval tapeworms of the genus *Spirometra* (92, 209). Human sparganosis occurs by two mechanisms: following ingestion of procercoid-infected *Cyclops* species copepods in water or by direct tissue invasion from uncooked meat containing already developed, plerocercoid *Spirometra* cysts. Its geographical distribution is worldwide, with case series from China, Japan, Southeast Asia, and South and Central America and isolated reports from the United States and Europe (209).

Transmission

With *Cyclops* ingestion, the larval procercoid penetrates the intestinal wall and migrates to various sites, including subcutaneous tissues, the CNS, or muscle, where it develops into a second-stage larva or plerocercoid (209). Under natural conditions, plerocercoids will transfer from one aquatic or amphibious host to another. The alternative mechanism of acquiring sparganosis is if a human is exposed to the infected uncooked meat of an amphibian, reptile, bird, or mammal harboring plerocercoid larvae and the parasite cyst directly invades the adjacent human tissues. The latter occurs most frequently when raw meat is used as a poultice in traditional healing.

Disease

The infiltration of the plerocercoid into the subcutaneous tissues is associated with a nodular mass formation due to granulomatous inflammation involving lymphocytes, plasma cells, and eosinophils (192). Any part of the body may become involved, including neck, eye, breast, scrotum or pleura (81). Pain occurs due to edema of the tissues.

Chronic manifestations

Central nervous system. *Spirometra* larvae may migrate to unusual anatomic locations, such as the brain. There, it can provoke an intense inflammatory response, leading to chronic degenerative changes, such as cortical atrophy, white matter degeneration, ventricular dilatation, vasculitis, hemorrhage, or calcification (164). The clinical symptoms can vary from mild confusion to severe focal deficits or grand-mal seizures (74).

Sparganum proliferum. This progressive form of sparganosis is caused by larvae of an unknown species that proliferates within the tissues, creating multiple independent organisms and occasionally overwhelming tissue invasion (13).

Diagnosis

Diagnosis is usually done by biopsy identification of the parasite. MRI localization is most useful in this regard, when combined with stereotactic biopsies. Antibody testing is available but may yield false-positive results in the presence of *Clonorchis* and *Paragonimus* trematode infections.

Treatment and prevention

Surgical removal of the larvae is the treatment of choice. Instillation of ethanol as a larvicide can be curative. Oral therapy with the antihelminthic agent praziquantel has not proven effective. For public health prevention measures, water filtration will remove *Cyclops* from drinking water. Flash freezing of meat at −10°C is known to kill sparganum larvae and will remove the threat of plerocercoid infection.

Disease Caused by the "Fish Tapeworm," *Diphyllobothrium latum*

Infection with this tapeworm is associated with ingestion of dried, pickled, or undercooked freshwater fish (92, 209). The significant chronic complications of infection derive from the risk of associated vitamin B_{12} deficiency and the potentially severe clinical consequences that this entails.

Epidemiology

The tapeworm parasite *D. latum* is transmitted mostly in shallow freshwater littorals that have vegetation favoring the development of copepods and fish. High prevalence regions include areas of the northern temperate and subarctic zones, where freshwater fish is often consumed (44). Prevalence is decreasing worldwide, and it is not clear if the sources of infection are also in decline or if public health awareness has improved (44). Estimates of global burden are approximately 9 to 10 million human cases (209). In North America, diphyllobothriasis can be found among communities in Alaska, Canada, and the Great Lakes regions of Minnesota and Michigan, as well as some community foci in Florida and California.

Life cycle and transmission

D. latum requires three hosts. The *definitive* (tapeworm-bearing) hosts are humans and fish-eating carnivores, the first-level *intermediate* hosts are copepods, and the second-level intermediate hosts are freshwater fish. Transmission begins when the eggs passed in the feces of the human host reach freshwater and embryonate and are then ingested by small crustaceans (copepods). The ingested eggs hatch larvae that encyst inside this copepod host. If it, in turn, is ingested by a fish, the parasite cyst transfers to the muscle tissues of the fish. Then, when humans (or other animals) eat raw or undercooked fish meat containing the infectious plerocercoid larva, the cycle is completed when the immature cyst transforms into an adult tapeworm inside the vertebrate carnivore's intestine. Adults grow in length up to 10 meters, creating reproductive proglottid segments in their tail that result in egg release into the feces (209). Occasionally, infection is discovered when a long chain of proglottids is passed in the stool (Fig. 10).

Clinical manifestations

Uncomplicated presentation. Chronic infection with this parasite is often asymptomatic. When symptomatic, complaints focus on the GI tract, including vague abdominal pain with a report of "something moving inside," bloating, diarrhea, anorexia, and occasional reports of increased hunger, sore gums, or sore tongue (197).

Chronic complications. *D. latum* infection is associated with vitamin B_{12} deficiency through two mechanisms. The parasite uses substantial amounts of the vitamin directly. It also interferes with the action of host-derived intrinsic factor, which is required for vitamin B_{12} absorption by the human intestine. It has been estimated that up to 40% of persons infected with *D. latum* have vitamin B_{12} deficiency, and about 2% will go on to develop associated anemia. Diet is likely to be an important determinant of risk for B_{12} deficiency in the presence of *D. latum* infection (9). In addition to megaloblastic anemia, vitamin B_{12} deficiency is also associated with a multifocal metabolic neurological illness called subacute combined degeneration. This neurological disorder of the peripheral and CNS can occur entirely without manifestations of anemia and can occur with even mild vitamin B_{12} deficiency of any cause. It typically consists of degeneration of the lateral and dorsal columns of the spinal cord with concomitant peripheral nerve involvement. The clinical presentation is typically with paresthesia but may include loss of

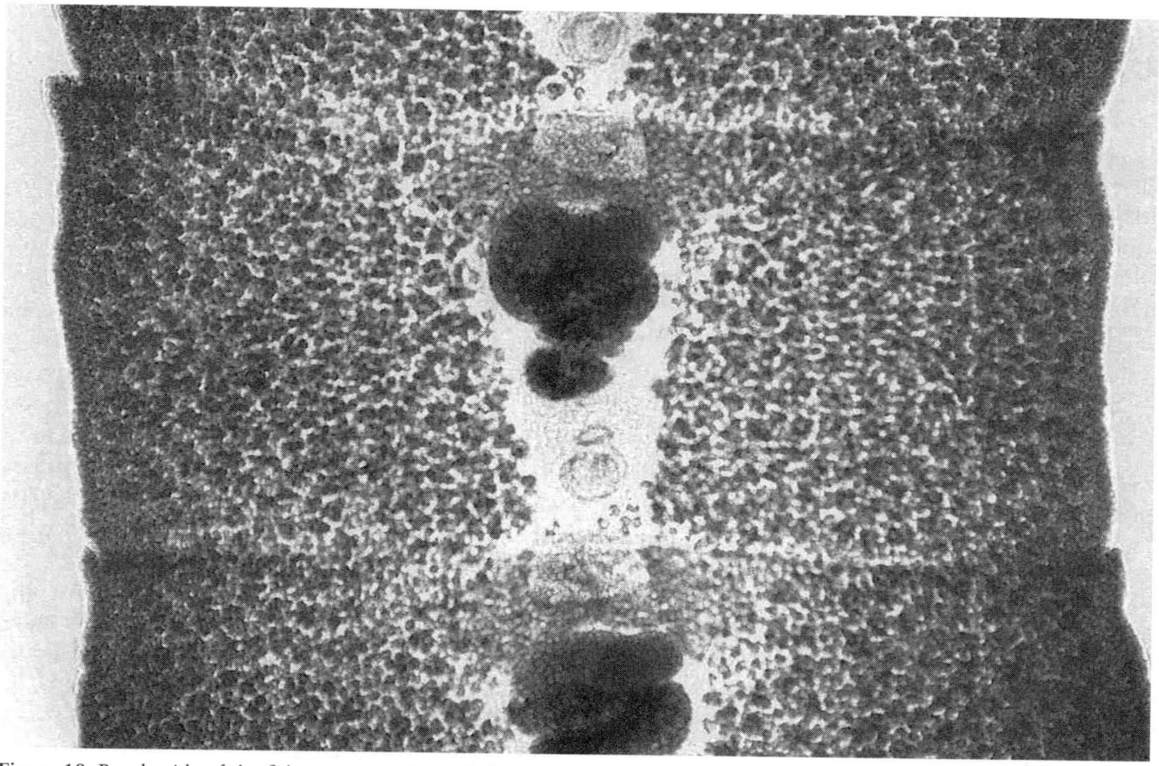

Figure 10. Proglottids of the fish tapeworm *Diphyllobothrium latum*. (Credit: *Atlas of Human Parasitology*, American Society of Clinical Pathologists.)

proprioception, ataxia, and muscle weakness, as well as changes in sensorium, including memory loss, dementia, personality change, and hallucinosis. Diagnosis is often made based on detection of multifocal lesions on MRI (175). Low or low-normal levels of serum B_{12}, combined with high serum levels of cysteine and methylmalonic acid and with *D. latum* eggs in stool, confirms the infectious etiology. Once the diagnosis is made, it is treated with parenteral vitamin B_{12} therapy, with generally good results (175).

Diagnosis

Diagnosis of *D. latum* is made by detection of eggs in the stool. When a proglottid has been expelled through the anus, it can also be morphologically identified based on vital staining of the uterine structure. There are no reliable serological tests to aid in the diagnosis of diphyllobothrosis. On peripheral blood examination, eosinophilia is present in only 5 to 10% of patients (209).

Treatment

Praziquantel is the drug of choice for elimination of adult tapeworm infection with *D. latum*. Doses of 5 to 10 mg/kg are used for both adults and children, given as a single dose (8).

Control measures

Avoidance of raw or undercooked fish consumption is the safest control measure. Freezing at −10°C for 24 h suffices to kill the plerocercoid larvae, which is the safest control measure for treating freshwater fish. Other control measures include education of cooks to prevent sampling of raw fish during preparation of foods (e.g., gefilte fish preparation) and community avoidance of sewage contamination into freshwater lakes in order to prevent viable *D. latum* eggs from infecting the water (209).

TREMATODES

Two different types of trematode parasites afflict humans. The *Schistosoma* parasites, known as "blood flukes," infect through the skin and colonize venules of the intestines or urinary tract (94). The "foodborne trematodes" are ingested as cysts within common foods (e.g., fish, crustaceans, vegetables) and go on to colonize the GI tract, biliary tree, liver, or lungs as adult worms (121). All trematodes go through an obligatory life-cycle stage within a specific freshwater snail intermediate host (181). Therefore, transmission of the parasites and risk of human infection is very closely linked to the distribution of habitat of these aquatic snails. Nevertheless, once established, infection commonly persists for years and may last for decades after a person has left the transmission zone (199). The fluke parasites can cause disease acutely, as larvae initially invade the human host, and all tend to cause some form of chronic pathology due to the inflammation provoked by the infecting adult forms or by their eggs, which are often trapped within host tissues. Even after infection is eliminated, disease pathology can persist due to the long-lasting damage caused by years of active infection (60, 85).

Schistosomiasis

Epidemiology

Approximately 207 million people are infected with schistosomiasis worldwide. Transmission occurs in at least 76 countries in Africa, the Middle East, South America, Asia, and the Philippines (94). Infection is typically most prevalent and most intense among school-age children (5 to15 years), and these individuals may manifest both acute and chronic forms of granulomatous pathology. Adults are more likely to manifest the "late" forms of pathology that develop though progressive fibrosis and scarring over many years of infection (172). Even with appropriate praziquantel therapy, reinfection can be common (166), and risk of advanced disease can increase with each additional year of infection (85).

Life cycle and transmission

Human schistosomiasis is most commonly caused by one of three major species, *Schistosoma haematobium*, *Schistosoma mansoni*, and *Schistosoma japonicum*. Infection is acquired when people wade or swim in freshwater containing the infectious cercariae of these specific parasites (181). This water-related transmission is mediated via the presence of particular intermediate snail hosts. These are *Bulinus* species snails for *S. haematobium*, *Biomphalaria* species snails for *S. mansoni*, and *Oncomelania* species snails for *S. japonicum*. Transmission is closely tied to poor sanitation, because parasite eggs released in human stool or urine must reach freshwater bodies to hatch and infect the intermediate snail host. Poverty is often a driving factor that causes people to come into frequent contact with high-risk transmission sites. However, developmental projects involving trench irrigation have often greatly contributed to transmission through creation of large areas of new snail habitat (48).

Clinical manifestations

Chronic disease due to schistosomiasis is caused by deposition of parasite eggs into local tissues, creating inflammation of critical organs, ultimately resulting in fibrotic scarring and organ dysfunction (94, 99). Usually, adult worms provoke limited immune response. However, each mating pair of adult schistosomes produces 300 to 3,000 eggs per day, and approximately half of these eggs become trapped in the body and never leave the human host. Schistosomes require host inflammatory response for their eggs to transit from the venous spaces, across the wall of the infected bladder or intestine, in order to reach the lumen and be released into the outside world. Even though there is some evidence that downregulation of host immune responses can occur that may limit host morbidity, the process of infection is essentially one of persistent, chronic inflammation and disease. Eggs typically are found in the bowel wall and liver for intestinal forms of schistosomiasis (*S. mansoni* and *S. japonicum*) and in the ureters and bladder in urinary schistosomiasis (*S. haematobium*). However, as disease progresses, eggs may be translocated to other areas of the body, including most abdominal organs, other pelvic organs, the lungs, and the brain and spinal cord, where they can cause significant local pathology (173). Chronic inflammation may have systemic metabolic effects that lead to poor growth and development in children and chronic anemias (55, 112, 145, 178).

Urinary schistosomiasis. Local inflammation of the ureters and bladder caused by eggs of *S. haematobium* can lead to polyp formation, local obstruction, hematuria, ulceration, tissue calcification, hydroureter, hydronephrosis, and obstructive uropathy accompanied by risk of ascending bacterial urinary tract infections, leading to renal failure (93). Long-term inflammation of the bladder is associated with risk of multifocal cancer formation. In *S. haematobium*-endemic areas of Africa, squamous cell carcinoma occurs at a rate of 1:100,000 population and typically occurs at a much younger age than is seen for bladder cancer in Europe and North America. The causative cancer link to *S. haematobium* infection is strong, and the parasite is listed as a definite carcinogen by the Internal Agency for Research on Cancer (IARC) (205).

Other, less well-known complications of urinary schistosomiasis result from "unusual" anatomic locations for egg deposition: hematospermia and infertility in men have been associated with prostate involvement and cervical and vaginal ulceration and infertility due to inflammatory fallopian obstruction have been well documented among affected women (97). When infection is heavy, *S. haematobium* may inflame the rectum, and eggs will be seen in the stool. Similarly, eggs may pass into the systemic venous circulation and become trapped in the lungs, where they can cause symptomatic respiratory disease (100). Some of the more insidious complications of chronic schistosomiasis, i.e., growth stunting, malnutrition, and anemia, have become better documented in recent years (55, 112, 145, 178). Because these outcomes are common among chronically infected populations, they represent a major health burden for the economies of developing countries where disease occurs (96).

Intestinal schistosomiasis. Disease caused by *S. mansoni* and *S. japonicum* is primarily focused on the walls of the intestines, while the most severe pathology occurs when eggs are flushed into the portal venules of the liver by normal portal flow (139, 141). The granulomatous inflammatory response to the trapped eggs leads to progressive presinusoidal fibrosis and portal hypertension. Hepatosplenomegaly due to inflammation, portal hypertension, or both is a common complication. Patients may suffer from abdominal pain, intermittent diarrhea, hematochezia, and, in heavy infection, iron loss. Portal hypertension may lead to varix formation, with recurrent esophageal variceal bleeding being the most lethal complication (156).

As with urinary schistosomiasis, the chronic inflammation caused by intestinal schistosomiasis contributes to anemia of chronic disease and growth and nutritional deficits (Fig. 11). Neuroschistosomiasis is another severe complication of infection, which involves inflammation or ischemia of the brain or spinal cord (49, 164). Aberrant migration of worms into the spinal circulation can cause catastrophic paraplegia. In a more subacute presentation, inflammation caused by deposition of eggs in the CNS can cause seizures, focal motor deficits, spinal cord compression, and cauda equina syndromes, or result in peripheral nerve damage within the spinal column. These syndromes can be irreversible or only partly reversible with therapy, resulting in lifetime disability.

Diagnosis

Routine diagnosis of schistosome infection is made by detection of parasite eggs in the urine (*S. haematobium*) or feces (*S. mansoni* and *S. japonicum*) (94). Following initial exposure, it can take 6 to 8 weeks for worms to mature sufficiently to release eggs, and standard parasitological testing may prove negative during this prepatent period. Light intensity infections (more common in adult age groups) may also not be detected well on standard parasitological testing of urine and stool. Where the travel and exposure history is positive and the index of suspicion of *Schistosoma* infection remains high, serology for anti-schistosome antibodies will establish prior exposure to the parasite. Eggs detected on tissue biopsy of inflamed rectum or bladder will also confirm the clinical diagnosis. Of note, eggs may persist in tissues for months to years after active infection has ended. The presence of viable (hatching) eggs suggests the presence of active infection. Nevertheless, symptomatic disease can persist or worsen after infection is resolved, and chronic complications must be diagnosed and treated symptomatically.

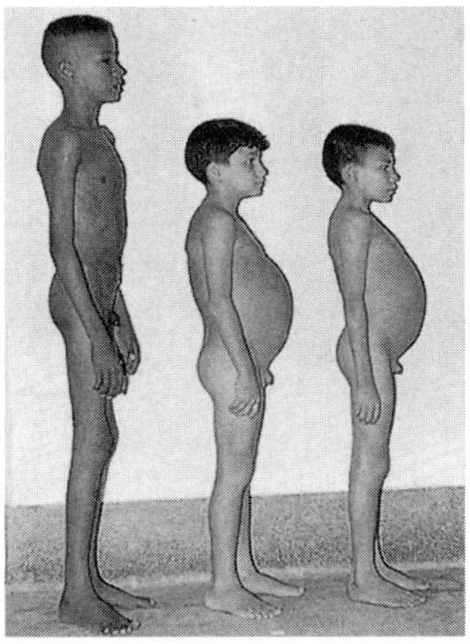

Figure 11. Growth retardation by chronic infection with *Schistosoma mansoni.* A combination of undernutrition and chronic infection with *S. mansoni*, especially around the time of puberty, can lead to significant retardation of growth. The boys seen here in the northeast of Brazil are (left to right) 14, 13, and 12 years old. The two on the right with hepatomegaly have schistosomiasis. Similar changes are seen in children infected with *S. japonicum.* (Credit: *Atlas of Tropical Medicine and Parasitology*, 6th ed., Elsevier.)

Ultrasound, CT, or MRI imaging of the urinary tract may show characteristic bladder thickening, polyp formation, and wall calcification in *S. haematobium* infection (95). Ureteral obstruction and hydronephrosis may take on several forms in urinary schistosomiasis (172). However, imaging may guide where surgical intervention would be most appropriate for late disease.

Imaging of intestinal schistosomiasis will often indicate a characteristic form of liver fibrosis around the portal radicals (Symmers fibrosis or "clay pipe stem" fibrosis). Signs of portal hypertension and ascites formation will help to gauge the extent of advanced portal circulatory disease (154).

In neuroschistosomiasis, CT or MRI imaging can indicate foci of CNS involvement, as well as levels of reactive inflammation surrounding the primary parasite-related lesion (worm or egg deposition) (49, 164).

Treatment and control

Specific anti-schistosomal therapy is obtained using the oral drug praziquantel (8). Treatment is 85 to 90% curative after a single dose. Treated patients should be rescreened 2 or 3 months after dosing and retreated if test results suggest continuing infection. The dose for *S. haematobium* and *S. mansoni* is 40 mg/kg body weight, given as a single dose. The dose for *S. japonicum* is higher, 60 mg/kg, and is typically given in 2 or 3 split doses at least 3 hours apart over a single day. Treatment is generally associated with improvement of signs and symptoms related to acute ongoing anti-parasite inflammation. Late fibrotic complications may not be reversible, however, due to the permanent scarring caused by long-term inflammation (30). Patients affected by such late disease may require surgical or other interventions to relieve their complications. Because anti-parasite inflammation may transiently increase after praziquantel treatment, patients with neuroschistosomiasis should receive anti-inflammatory (corticosteroid) treatment prior to praziquantel therapy.

Food-Borne Trematodes

This group of helminthic infections includes the "lung fluke," *Paragonimus westermani*, and the "oriental liver fluke," *Clonorchis sinensis*, as well as other liver (*Fasciola hepatica, Opisthorchis* species), intestinal (*Fasciola* species, *Fasciolopsis* species), and tissue (*Paragonimus* species) flukes that infect humans (90, 121).

Epidemiology

Food-borne trematodiases are now most common in Southeast Asia, although *Opisthorchis* infection is found throughout Eurasia (121). Tissue paragonimiasis, other than the lung fluke (*P. westermani*) is most common in West Africa (108). The liver fluke *Fasciola hepatica* is found worldwide as a veterinary pathogen and can infect humans in any country.

Life cycle and transmission

Transmission requires the presence of two or more intermediate hosts within the local environment. These are (i) an appropriate snail host that is susceptible to the particular fluke species and (ii) a suitable, secondary fish, crustacean, or plant host where the parasite cercariae can encyst (121). Human disease is acquired by eating raw, dried, pickled, or undercooked foods containing encysted larval forms of the parasite. Infection starts when host digestion activates and hatches the larvae, which emerge and start to mature into adult flukes. Some species (*P. westermani* and *F. hepatica*) migrate through the bowel wall to enter the cavities of the peritoneum or pleural spaces (108, 164). Others remain in the digestive tract to colonize the lumena of the biliary tree or intestines (121).

Clinical manifestations

Fluke infections that are limited to the intestine or biliary tree are often minimally symptomatic. Intestinal infection can result in localized inflammation in the bowel wall, leading to symptoms of cramping or diarrhea, and occasionally to local abscess formation. Liver flukes may present with right upper quadrant pain or paresthesias and be associated with symptoms of intermittent biliary obstruction that can be confused with cholelithiasis. Long-term infection with *Clonorchis sinensis* has been linked to the formation of multifocal biliary obstruction and enlargement of the biliary radicals. There is significant risk of cancer formation, with multifocal cholangiocarcinoma, a known complication of long-standing liver fluke-related disease (205).

The liver fluke *F. hepatica* often presents with more severe disease, because it migrates from the lumen of the intestine through the peritoneal cavity to reach the liver capsule directly. It penetrates the liver and establishes foci of inflammation that drain through the biliary tree. Adult worms may continue to move through the liver over time, causing more extensive tissue damage than other flukes. During the early migratory phases, *F. hepatica* may migrate into the pleural space, the pericardium, or CNS, causing localized inflammation and potentially life-threatening complications due to lung, heart, or CNS damage (121, 164).

The lung fluke *P. westermani* must similarly migrate from the intestine to its preferred niche in the bronchus of the lung. During early migration, it too can cause peritoneal, CNS, or cardiac disease due to "aberrant" migration (108). Once established in the lung, *Paragonimus* releases its eggs into the bronchial airspace, often provoking local inflammation, which may be associated with hematemesis. The presentation of lung fluke infection may be easily confused with active tuberculosis or primary bronchogenic carcinoma of the lung.

Diagnosis

Food-borne trematodes are usually diagnosed by detection of excreted eggs in the stool. In the case of the *Paragonimus* lung fluke, eggs may also be detected in the sputum. If endoscopy is performed, eggs may be seen in aspirates (bile or sputum), on cytology examination, or in endoscopic tissue biopsy specimens. When a histology of surgical biopsy specimens is performed, it is important to remember that flukes are relatively large in size (1 to 5 cm in length) and that multiple sections may be required to identify the infective species.

Treatment and control

Most food-borne trematode infections respond to praziquantel therapy (10 to 25 mg/kg body weight as a single dose). The one exception is *F. hepatica*, which is relatively resistant to praziquantel's effects. The preferred therapy for *F. hepatica* is triclabendazole (155).

As with schistosomiasis, elimination of the pathogen may resolve some, but not all, late complications of fluke infection. Treatment is expected to resolve symptoms caused by current inflammation but may not lead to regression of chronic fibrotic complications. Biliary reconstruction or partial lung resection may be required for liver or lung flukes, respectively, and continued follow-up for late cancer formation is appropriate after liver fluke infection.

REFERENCES

1. **Addiss, D. G., and M. A. Brady.** 2007. Morbidity management in the Global Programme to Eliminate Lymphatic Filariasis: a review of the scientific literature. *Filaria J.* **6**:2.
2. **Aikhomu, S. E., W. R. Brieger, and O. O. Kale.** 2000. Acceptance and use of communal filtration units in guinea worm eradication. *Trop. Med. Int. Health.* **5**:47–52.
3. **Albonico, M., P. G. Smith, E. Ercole, A. Hall, H. M. Chwaya, K. S. Alawi, and L. Savioli.** 1995. Rate of reinfection with intestinal nematodes after treatment of children with mebendazole or albendazole in a highly endemic area. *Trans. R. Soc. Trop. Med. Hyg.* **89**:538–541.
4. **Allen, H. E., D. W. Crompton, N. de Silva, P. T. LoVerde, and G. R. Olds.** 2002. New policies for using anthelmintics in high risk groups. *Trends Parasitol.* **18**:381–382.
5. **Amir-Jahed, A. K., R. Fardin, A. Farzad, and K. Bakshandeh.** 1975. Clinical echinococcosis. *Ann. Surg.* **182**:541–546.
6. **Anderson, R. M., and R. M. May.** 1991. *Infectious Diseases of Humans. Dynamics and Control.* Oxford University Press, New York, NY.
7. **Andy, J. J., F. F. Bishara, O. O. Soyinka, and W. O. Odesanmi.** 1981. Loasis as a possible trigger of African endomyocardial fibrosis: a case report from Nigeria. *Acta Trop.* **38**:179–186.
8. **Anonymous.** 2004, posting date. Drugs for parasitic infections. *Med. Lett. Drug Ther.* http://www.medletter.com/html_files/publicreading.htm#Parasitic.
9. **Anonymous.** 1976. Pathogenesis of the tapeworm anaemia. *Br. Med. J.* **2**:1028.
10. **Asaolu, S. O., and I. E. Ofoezie.** 2003. The role of health education and sanitation in the control of helminth infections. *Acta Trop.* **86**:283–294.
11. **Baird, J. K., R. C. Neafie, and D. H. Connor.** 1988. Nodules in the conjunctiva, bung-eye, and bulge-eye in Africa caused by *Mansonella perstans*. *Am. J. Trop. Med. Hyg.* **38**:553–557.
12. **Bandyopadhyay, L.** 1996. Lymphatic filariasis and the women of India. *Soc. Sci. Med.* **42**:1401–1410.
13. **Beaver, P. C., and F. A. Rolon.** 1981. Proliferating larval cestode in a man in Paraguay. A case report and review. *Am. J. Trop. Med. Hyg.* **30**:625–637.
14. **Bethony, J., S. Brooker, M. Albonico, S. M. Geiger, A. Loukas, D. Diemert, and P. J. Hotez.** 2006. Soil-transmitted helminth infections: ascariasis, trichuriasis, and hookworm. *Lancet* **367**:1521–1532.
15. **Bethony, J., J. Chen, S. Lin, S. Xiao, B. Zhan, S. Li, H. Xue, F. Xing, D. Humphries, W. Yan, G. Chen, V. Foster, J. M. Hawdon, and P. J. Hotez.** 2002. Emerging patterns of hookworm infection: influence of aging on the intensity of *Necator* infection in Hainan Province, People's Republic of China. *Clin. Infect. Dis.* **35**:1336–1344.
16. **Blumenthal, D. S., and M. G. Schultz.** 1976. Effects of *Ascaris* infection of nutritional status in children. *Am. J. Trop. Med. Hyg.* **25**:682–690.
17. **Bouree, P., N. Duedari, F. Bisaro, and F. Norol.** 1993. Value of filariopheresis in the treatment of *Loa loa* filariasis. *Pathol. Biol.* (Paris). **41**:410–414. (In French.)
18. **Boussinesq, M., J. Gardon, N. Gardon-Wendel, and J. P. Chippaux.** 2003. Clinical picture, epidemiology and outcome of *Loa*-associated serious adverse events related to mass ivermectin treatment of onchocerciasis in Cameroon. *Filaria J.* **2**(Suppl 1):S4.
19. **Bruschi, F., and K. D. Murrell.** 2006. Trichinellosis, p. 1217–1224. *In* R. L. Guerrant, D. H. Walker, and P. F. Weller (ed.), *Tropical Infectious Diseases, Principles, Pathogens and Practice*, 2nd ed. Churchill Livingstone, Philadelphia, PA.
20. **Budke, C. M.** 2006. Global socioeconomic impact of cystic echinococcosis. *Emerg. Infect. Dis.* **12**:296–303.
21. **Budke, C. M., Q. Jiamin, W. Qian, and P. R. Torgerson.** 2005. Economic effects of echinococcosis in a disease-endemic region of the Tibetan Plateau. *Am. J. Trop. Med. Hyg.* **73**:2–10.
22. **Bundy, D. A., M. S. Chan, and L. Savioli.** 1995. Hookworm infection in pregnancy. *Trans. R. Soc. Trop. Med. Hyg.* **89**:521–522.
23. **Burnier, M., Jr., A. A. Hidayat, and R. Neafie.** 1991. Dracunculiasis of the orbit and eyelid. Light and electron microscopic observations of two cases. *Ophthalmology* **98**: 919–924.
24. **Buttenschoen, K., and D. C. Buttenschoen.** 2003. *Echinococcus granulosus* infection: the challenge of surgical treatment. *Langenbecks Arch. Surg.* **388**:218–230.
25. **Carneiro, F. F., E. Cifuentes, M. M. Tellez-Rojo, and I. Romieu.** 2002. The risk of *Ascaris lumbricoides* infection in children as an environmental health indicator to guide preventive activities in Caparao and Alto Caparao, Brazil. *Bull. W. H. O.* **80**:40–46.
26. **CDC.** 2007. Progress toward global eradication of dracunculiasis, January 2005-May 2007. *MMWR Morb. Mort. Weekly Rept.* **56**:813–817.
27. **Chan, M. S.** 1997. The global burden of intestinal nematode infections: 50 years on. *Parasitol. Today* **13**:438–443.
28. **Chandenier, J., J. Husson, S. Canaple, C. Gondry-Jouet, P. Dekumyoy, M. Danis, G. Riveau, C. Hennequin, A. Rosa,

and C. P. Raccurt. 2001. Medullary gnathostomiasis in a white patient: use of immunodiagnosis and magnetic resonance imaging. *Clin. Infect. Dis.* **32:**E154–E157.

29. **Chandenier, J., C. Pillier-Loriette, A. Datry, M. Rosenheim, M. Danis, H. Felix, J. P. Nozais, and M. Gentilini.** 1987. Value of cytapheresis in the treatment of loaiasis with high blood microfilaria levels. Results in 7 cases. *Bull. Soc. Pathol. Exot. Filiales* **80:**624–633. (In French.)
30. **Chen, M. G., and K. E. Mott.** 1989. Progress in assessment of morbidity due to *Schistosoma haematobium* infection. *Trop. Dis. Bull.* **86:**R1–R36.
31. **Chotmongkol, V., K. Sawadpanitch, K. Sawanyawisuth, S. Louhawilai, and P. Limpawattana.** 2006. Treatment of eosinophilic meningitis with a combination of prednisolone and mebendazole. *Am. J. Trop. Med. Hyg.* **74:**1122–1124.
32. **Cooper, E.** 2006. Trichuriasis, p. 1252–1256. *In* R. L. Guerrant, D. H. Walker, and P. F. Weller (ed.), *Tropical Infectious Diseases, Principles, Pathogens and Practice*, 2nd ed. Churchill Livingstone, Philadelphia, PA.
33. **Cooper, P. J., M. E. Chico, L. C. Rodrigues, M. Ordonez, D. Strachan, G. E. Griffin, and T. B. Nutman.** 2003. Reduced risk of atopy among school-age children infected with geohelminth parasites in a rural area of the tropics. *J. Allergy Clin. Immunol.* **111:**995–1000.
34. **Cooper, P. J., M. E. Chico, C. Sandoval, I. Espinel, A. Guevara, M. W. Kennedy, J. F. Urban Jr, G. E. Griffin, and T. B. Nutman.** 2000. Human infection with *Ascaris lumbricoides* is associated with a polarized cytokine response. *J. Infect. Dis.* **182:**1207–1213.
35. **Cooper, P. J., T. Mancero, M. Espinel, C. Sandoval, R. Lovato, R. H. Guderian, and T. B. Nutman.** 2001. Early human infection with *Onchocerca volvulus* is associated with an enhanced parasite-specific cellular immune response. *J. Infect. Dis.* **183:**1662–1668.
36. **Crompton, D. W.** 2001. *Ascaris* and ascariasis. *Adv. Parasitol.* **48:**285–375.
37. **Crompton, D. W.** 1988. The prevalence of ascariasis. *Parasitol. Today* **4:**162–169.
38. **Crompton, D. W., and M. C. Nesheim.** 2002. Nutritional impact of intestinal helminthiasis during the human life cycle. *Annu. Rev. Nutr.* **22:**35–59.
39. **de Silva, N. R., S. Brooker, P. J. Hotez, A. Montresor, D. Engels, and L. Savioli.** 2003. Soil-transmitted helminth infections: updating the global picture. *Trends Parasitol.* **19:** 547–551.
40. **de Silva, N. R., H. L. Guyatt, and D. A. Bundy.** 1997. Morbidity and mortality due to *Ascaris*-induced intestinal obstruction. *Trans. R. Soc. Trop. Med. Hyg.* **91:**31–36.
41. **Debrah, A. Y., S. Mand, M. R. Toliat, Y. Marfo-Debrekyei, L. Batsa, P. Nurnberg, B. Lawson, O. Adjei, A. Hoerauf, and K. Pfarr.** 2007. Plasma vascular endothelial growth Factor-A (VEGF-A) and VEGF-A gene polymorphism are associated with hydrocele development in lymphatic filariasis. *Am. J. Trop. Med. Hyg.* **77:**601–608.
42. **Del Valle, A., B. F. Jones, L. M. Harrison, R. C. Chadderdon, and M. Cappello.** 2003. Isolation and molecular cloning of a secreted hookworm platelet inhibitor from adult *Ancylostoma caninum*. *Mol. Biochem. Parasitol.* **129:**167–177.
43. **Devi, C. S., and S. C. Parija.** 2003. A new serum hydatid antigen detection test for diagnosis of cystic echinococcosis. *Am. J. Trop. Med. Hyg.* **69:**525–528.
44. **Dick, T. A., P. A. Nelson, and A. Choudhury.** 2001. Diphyllobothriasis: update on human cases, foci, patterns and sources of human infections and future considerations. *Southeast Asian J. Trop. Med. Public Health.* **32**(Suppl 2)**:**59–76.
45. **Diemert, D. J., J. M. Bethony, and P. J. Hotez.** 2008. Hookworm vaccines. *Clin. Infect. Dis.* **46:**282–288.
46. **Donaldson, J. R., and T. A. Angelo.** 1961. Quadriplegia due to guineaworm abscess. *J. Bone Joint Surg. Am.* **43A:**1 97–198.
47. **Ducorps, M., N. Gardon-Wendel, S. Ranque, W. Ndong, M. Boussinesq, J. Gardon, D. Schneider, and J. P. Chippaux.** 1995. Secondary effects of the treatment of hypermicrofilaremic loiasis using ivermectin. *Bull. Soc. Pathol. Exot.* **88:**105–112. (In French.)
48. **Farley, J.** 1991. *Bilharzia. A History of Imperial Tropical Medicine*. Cambridge University Press, Cambridge United Kingdom.
49. **Ferrari, T. C.** 2004. Involvement of central nervous system in the schistosomiasis. *Mem. Inst. Oswaldo Cruz* **99:**59–62.
50. **Fourestie, V., H. Douceron, P. Brugieres, T. Ancelle, J. L. Lejonc, and R. K. Gherardi.** 1993. Neurotrichinosis. A cerebrovascular disease associated with myocardial injury and hypereosinophilia. *Brain* **116:**603–616.
51. **Fox, A. S., K. R. Kazacos, N. S. Gould, P. T. Heydemann, C. Thomas, and K. M. Boyer.** 1985. Fatal eosinophilic meningoencephalitis and visceral larva migrans caused by the raccoon ascarid *Baylisascaris procyonis*. *N. Engl. J. Med.* **312:**1619–1623.
52. **Franchi, C., B. Di Vico, and A. Teggi.** 1999. Long-term evaluation of patients with hydatidosis treated with benzimidazole carbamates. *Clin. Infect. Dis.* **29:**304–309.
53. **Freedman, D. O.** 2006. Onchocerciasis, p. 1176–1188. *In* R. L. Guerrant, D. H. Walker, and P. F. Weller (ed.), *Tropical Infectious Diseases, Principles, Pathogens and Practice*, 2nd ed. Churchill Livingstone, Philadelphia, PA.
54. **Freedman, D. O., P. J. de Almeida Filho, S. Besh, M. C. Maia e Silva, C. Braga, and A. Maciel.** 1994. Lymphoscintigraphic analysis of lymphatic abnormalities in symptomatic and asymptomatic human filariasis. *J. Infect. Dis.* **170:** 927–933.
55. **Friedman, J. F., H. K. Kanzaria, L. P. Acosta, G. C. Langdon, D. L. Manalo, H. Wu, R. M. Olveda, S. T. McGarvey, and J. D. Kurtis.** 2005. Relationship between *Schistosoma japonicum* and nutritional status among children and young adults in Leyte, the Philippines. *Am. J. Trop. Med. Hyg.* **72:** 527–533.
56. **Fux, C. A., B. Chappuis, B. Holzer, C. Aebi, G. Bordmann, H. Marti, and C. Hatz.** 2006. *Mansonella perstans* causing symptomatic hypereosinophilia in a missionary family. *Travel Med. Infect. Dis.* **4:**275–280.
57. **Gallagher, M., I. Malhotra, P. L. Mungai, A. N. Wamachi, J. M. Kioko, J. H. Ouma, E. Muchiri, and C. L. King.** 2005. The effects of maternal helminth and malaria infections on mother-to-child HIV transmission. *AIDS* **19:**1849–1855.
58. **Gardon, J., N. Gardon-Wendel, N. Demanga, J. Kamgno, J. P. Chippaux, and M. Boussinesq.** 1997. Serious reactions after mass treatment of onchocerciasis with ivermectin in an area endemic for *Loa loa* infection. *Lancet* **350:**18–22.
59. **Gentilini, M., and B. Carme.** 1981. Treatment of filariases in a hospital setting. Complications - results. *Ann. Soc. Belg. Med. Trop.* **61:**319–326. (In French.)
60. **Giboda, M., and N. R. Bergquist.** 1999. Post-transmission schistosomiasis. *Parasitol. Today* **15:**307–308.
61. **Gillette-Ferguson, I., A. G. Hise, H. F. McGarry, J. Turner, A. Esposito, Y. Sun, E. Diaconu, M. J. Taylor, and E. Pearlman.** 2004. *Wolbachia*-induced neutrophil activation in a mouse model of ocular onchocerciasis (river blindness). *Infect. Immun.* **72:**5687–5692.
62. **Gopinath, R., M. Ostrowski, S. J. Justement, A. S. Fauci, and T. B. Nutman.** 2000. Filarial infections increase susceptibility to human immunodeficiency virus infection in peripheral blood mononuclear cells in vitro. *J. Infect. Dis.* **182:** 1804–1808.

63. **Gottstein, B., and M. R. Mowatt.** 1991. Sequencing and characterization of an *Echinococcus multilocularis* DNA probe and its use in the polymerase chain reaction. *Mol. Biochem. Parasitol.* **44:**183–193.
64. **Grobusch, M. P., M. Kombila, I. Autenrieth, H. Mehlhorn, and P. G. Kremsner.** 2003. No evidence of *Wolbachia* endosymbiosis with *Loa loa* and *Mansonella perstans*. *Parasitol. Res.* **90:**405–408.
65. **Guerrant, R. L., D. H. Walker, and P. F. Weller (ed.).** 2006. *Tropical Infectious Diseases: Principles, Pathogens and Practice*, 2nd ed. Churchill Livingstone, Phildelphia, PA.
66. **Gutierrez, Y.** 2006. Other tissue nematode infections, p. 1231–1247. *In* R. L. Guerrant, D. H. Walker, and P. F. Weller (ed.), *Tropical Infectious Diseases, Principles, Pathogens and Practice*, 2nd ed. Churchill Livingstone, Philadelphia, PA.
67. **Gyorkos, T. W., R. Larocque, M. Casapia, and E. Gotuzzo.** 2006. Lack of risk of adverse birth outcomes after deworming in pregnant women. *Pediatr. Infect. Dis. J.* **25:** 791–794.
68. **Hall, A.** 2007. Micronutrient supplements for children after deworming. *Lancet Infect. Dis.* **7:**297–302.
69. **Hall, L. R., and E. Pearlman.** 1999. Pathogenesis of onchocercal keratitis (River blindness). *Clin. Microbiol. Rev.* **12:**445–453.
70. **Hise, A. G., I. Gillette-Ferguson, and E. Pearlman.** 2004. The role of endosymbiotic *Wolbachia* bacteria in filarial disease. *Cell. Microbiol.* **6:**97–104.
71. **Hoerauf, A., S. Mand, O. Adjei, B. Fleischer, and D. W. Buttner.** 2001. Depletion of *Wolbachia* endobacteria in *Onchocerca volvulus* by doxycycline and microfilaridermia after ivermectin treatment. *Lancet* **357:**1415–1416.
72. **Hoerauf, A., S. Mand, L. Volkmann, M. Buttner, Y. Marfo-Debrekyei, M. Taylor, O. Adjei, and D. W. Buttner.** 2003. Doxycycline in the treatment of human onchocerciasis: Kinetics of *Wolbachia* endobacteria reduction and of inhibition of embryogenesis in female *Onchocerca* worms. *Microbes Infect.* **5:**261–273.
73. **Hoerauf, A., S. Specht, M. Buttner, K. Pfarr, S. Mand, R. Fimmers, Y. Marfo-Debrekyei, P. Konadu, A. Y. Debrah, C. Bandi, N. Brattig, A. Albers, J. Larbi, L. Batsa, O. Adjei, and D. W. Buttner.** 2008. *Wolbachia* endobacteria depletion by doxycycline as antifilarial therapy has macrofilaricidal activity in onchocerciasis: a randomized placebo-controlled study. *Med. Microbiol. Immunol.* **197:** 295–311.
74. **Holodniy, M., J. Almenoff, J. Loutit, and G. K. Steinberg.** 1991. Cerebral sparganosis: case report and review. *Rev. Infect. Dis.* **13:**155–159.
75. **Horton, J., C. Witt, E. A. Ottesen, J. K. Lazdins, D. G. Addiss, K. Awadzi, M. J. Beach, V. Y. Belizario, S. K. Dunyo, M. Espinel, J. O. Gyapong, M. Hossain, M. M. Ismail, R. L. Jayakody, P. J. Lammie, W. Makunde, D. Richard-Lenoble, B. Selve, R. K. Shenoy, P. E. Simonsen, C. N. Wamae, and M. V. Weerasooriya.** 2000. An analysis of the safety of the single dose, two drug regimens used in programmes to eliminate lymphatic filariasis. *Parasitology* **121**(Suppl.): S147–S160.
76. **Hotez, P.** 2006. Hookworm infections, p. 1265–1273. *In* R. L. Guerrant, D. H. Walker, and P. F. Weller (ed.), *Tropical Infectious Diseases, Principles, Pathogens and Practice*, 2nd ed. Churchill Livingstone, Philadelphia, PA.
77. **Hotez, P., E. Ottesen, A. Fenwick, and D. Molyneux.** 2006. The neglected tropical diseases: the ancient afflictions of stigma and poverty and the prospects for their control and elimination. *Adv. Exp. Med. Biol.* **582:**23–33.
78. **Hotez, P. J., S. Brooker, J. M. Bethony, M. E. Bottazzi, A. Loukas, and S. Xiao.** 2004. Hookworm infection. *N. Engl. J. Med.* **351:**799–807.
79. **Hotez, P. J., D. H. Molyneux, A. Fenwick, J. Kumaresan, S. E. Sachs, J. D. Sachs, and L. Savioli.** 2007. Control of neglected tropical diseases. *N. Engl. J. Med.* **357:**1018–1027.
80. **Hotez, P. J., S. Narasimhan, J. Haggerty, L. Milstone, V. Bhopale, G. A. Schad, and F. F. Richards.** 1992. Hyaluronidase from infective *Ancylostoma* hookworm larvae and its possible function as a virulence factor in tissue invasion and in cutaneous larva migrans. *Infect. Immun.* **60:**1018–1023.
81. **Ishii, H., H. Mukae, Y. Inoue, J. I. Kadota, S. Kohno, F. Uchiyama, and Y. Nawa.** 2001. A rare case of eosinophilic pleuritis due to sparganosis. *Intern. Med.* **40:**783–785.
82. **Isik, N., G. Silav, A. Cerci, P. Karabagli, I. Elmaci, and M. Kalelioglu.** 2007. Cerebral alveolar echinococcosis. A case report with MRI and review of the literature. *J. Neurosurg. Sci.* **51:**145–151.
83. **Ive, F. A., A. J. Willis, A. C. Ikeme, and I. F. Brockington.** 1967. Endomyocardial fibrosis and filariasis. *Q. J. Med.* **36:**495–516.
84. **Jamal, S.** 1981. Lymphovenous anastomosis in filarial lymphedema. *Lymphology* **14:**64–68.
85. **Jia, T.-W., X.-N. Zhou, X.-H. Wang, J. Utzinger, P. Steinmann, and X.-H. Wu.** 2007. Assessment of the age-specific disability weight of chronic schistosomiasis japonica. *Bull. W. H. O.* **85:**458–465.
86. **Kamgno, J., J. Gardon, N. Gardon-Wendel, N. Demanga, B. O. Duke, and M. Boussinesq.** 2004. Adverse systemic reactions to treatment of onchocerciasis with ivermectin at normal and high doses given annually or three-monthly. *Trans. R. Soc. Trop. Med. Hyg.* **98:**496–504.
87. **Kamiya, Y., H. Sato, and Y. Ijama.** 2000. Epidemiology of echinococcosis in Aomori Prefecture, Japan. *Parasitol. Int.* **49**(Suppl.):83.
88. **Karp, C. L., and P. G. Auwaerter.** 2007. Coinfection with HIV and tropical infectious diseases. II. Helminthic, fungal, bacterial, and viral pathogens. *Clin. Infect. Dis.* **45:** 1214–1220.
89. **Katner, H., B. E. Beyt, Jr., and W. A. Krotoski.** 1984. Loiasis and renal failure. *South. Med. J.* **77:**907–908.
90. **Keiser, J., and J. Utzinger.** 2005. Emerging foodborne trematodiasis. *Emerg. Infect. Dis.* **11:**1507–1514.
91. **Kinare, S. G., G. B. Parulkar, and P. K. Sen.** 1962. Constrictive pericarditis resulting from dracunculosis. *Br. Med. J.* **1:**845.
92. **King, C. H.** 2005. Cestodes (tapeworms), p. 3285–3293. *In* G. L. Mandell, J. E. Bennett, and R. Dolin (ed.), *Principles and Practice of Infectious Diseases*, 6th ed. Churchill Livingstone, Philadelphia, PA.
93. **King, C. H.** 2001. Disease in schistosomiasis haematobia, p. 265–96. *In* A. A. F. Mahmoud (ed.), *Schistosomiasis*. Imperial College Press, London, United Kingdom.
94. **King, C. H.** 2006. Schistosomiasis, p. 1341–1348. *In* R. L. Guerrant, D. H. Walker, and P. F. Weller (ed.), *Tropical Infectious Diseases: Principles, Pathogens and Practice*, 2nd ed. Churchill Livingstone, Philadelphia, PA.
95. **King, C. H.** 2002. Ultrasound monitoring of structural urinary tract disease in *S. haematobium* infection. *Memorias do Instituto Oswaldo Cruz.* **97**(Suppl. 1)**:**149–152.
96. **King, C. H., and A.-M. Bertino.** 2008. Asymmetries of poverty: why global burden of disease valuations significantly underestimate the burden of neglected tropical diseases. *PLoS Negl. Trop. Dis.* **2:**e209.
97. **King, C. H., and M. Dangerfield-Cha.** 2008. The unacknowledged impact of chronic schistosomiasis *Chronic Illness* **4:**65–79.
98. **King, C. H., K. Dickman, and D. J. Tisch.** 2005. Reassessment of the cost of chronic helmintic infection: a meta-analysis of disability-related outcomes in endemic schistosomiasis. *Lancet* **365:**1561–1569.

99. **King, C. L.** 2001. Initiation and regulation of disease in schistosomiasis, p. 213–64. *In* A. A. F. Mahmoud (ed.), *Schistosomiasis*. Imperial College Press, London, United Kingdom.
100. **King, C. L.** 1997. Schistosomiasis, p. 135–55. *In* A. A. F. Mahmoud (ed.), *Parasitic Lung Diseases*, vol. 101. Marcel Dekker, New York, NY.
101. **King, C. L., C. C. Low, and T. B. Nutman.** 1993. IgE production in human helminth infection. Reciprocal interrelationship between IL-4 and IFN-gamma. *J. Immunol.* **150:**1873–1880.
102. **Klion, A. D., A. Massougbodji, J. Horton, S. Ekoue, T. Lanmasso, N. L. Ahouissou, and T. B. Nutman.** 1993. Albendazole in human loiasis: results of a double-blind, placebo-controlled trial. *J. Infect. Dis.* **168:**202–206.
103. **Klion, A. D., and T. B. Nutman.** 2006. Loiasis and *Mansonella* infections, p. 1163–1175. *In* R. L. Guerrant, D. H. Walker, and P. F. Weller (ed.), *Tropical Infectious Diseases, Principles, Pathogens and Practice*, 2nd ed. Churchill Livingstone, Philadelphia, PA.
104. **Klion, A. D., N. Raghavan, P. J. Brindley, and T. B. Nutman.** 1991. Cloning and characterization of a species-specific repetitive DNA sequence from *Loa loa*. *Mol. Biochem. Parasitol.* **45:**297–305.
105. **Klion, A. D., A. Vijaykumar, T. Oei, B. Martin, and T. B. Nutman.** 2003. Serum immunoglobulin G4 antibodies to the recombinant antigen, Ll-SXP-1, are highly specific for *Loa loa* infection. *J. Infect. Dis.* **187:**128–133.
106. **Krishna Kumari, A., K. T. Harichandrakumar, L. K. Das, and K. Krishnamoorthy.** 2005. Physical and psychosocial burden due to lymphatic filariasis as perceived by patients and medical experts. *Trop. Med. Int. Health.* **10:**567–573.
107. **Kuberski, T.** 2006. Angiostrongyliasis, p. 1225–1230. *In* R. L. Guerrant, D. H. Walker, and P. F. Weller (ed.), *Tropical Infectious Diseases, Principles, Pathogens and Practice*, 2nd ed. Churchill Livingstone, Philadelphia, PA.
108. **Kusner, D. J., and C. H. King.** 1993. Cerebral paragonimiasis. *Semin. Neurol.* **13:**201–208.
109. **Lammie, P. J., W. L. Hitch, E. M. Walker Allen, W. Hightower, and M. L. Eberhard.** 1991. Maternal filarial infection as risk factor for infection in children. *Lancet* **337:** 1005–1006.
110. **Lang, A. P., I. S. Luchsinger, and E. G. Rawling.** 1987. Filariasis of the breast. *Arch. Pathol. Lab. Med.* **111:**757–759.
111. **Larocque, R., M. Casapia, E. Gotuzzo, J. D. MacLean, J. C. Soto, E. Rahme, and T. W. Gyorkos.** 2006. A double-blind randomized controlled trial of antenatal mebendazole to reduce low birthweight in a hookworm-endemic area of Peru. *Trop. Med. Int. Health* **11:**1485–1495.
112. **Leenstra, T., H. M. Coutinho, L. P. Acosta, G. C. Langdon, L. Su, R. M. Olveda, S. T. McGarvey, J. D. Kurtis, and J. F. Friedman.** 2006. *Schistosoma japonicum* reinfection after praziquantel treatment causes anemia associated with inflammation. *Infect. Immun.* **74:**6398–6407.
113. **Leonardi-Bee, J., D. Pritchard, and J. Britton.** 2006. Asthma and current intestinal parasite infection: systematic review and meta-analysis. *Am. J. Respir. Crit. Care Med.* **174:** 514–523.
114. **Lightowlers, M. W., S. B. Lawrence, C. G. Gauci, J. Young, M. J. Ralston, D. Maas, and D. D. Health.** 1996. Vaccination against hydatidosis using a defined recombinant antigen. *Parasite Immunol.* **18:**457–462.
115. **Little, J. M.** 1976. Hydatid disease at Royal Prince Alfred Hospital, 1964 to 1974. *Med. J. Aust.* **1:**903–908.
116. **Little, M. P., L. P. Breitling, M. G. Basanez, E. S. Alley, and B. A. Boatin.** 2004. Association between microfilarial load and excess mortality in onchocerciasis: an epidemiological study. *Lancet* **363:**1514–1521.
117. **Lo Re, V., III, and S. J. Gluckman.** 2003. Eosinophilic meningitis. *Am. J. Med.* **114:**217–223.
118. **Loukas, A., and P. Prociv.** 2001. Immune responses in hookworm infections. *Clin. Microbiol. Rev.* **14:**689–703..
119. **Lukiana, T., M. Mandina, N. H. Situakibanza, M. M. Mbula, B. F. Lepira, W. T. Odio, J. Kamgno, and M. Boussinesq.** 2006. A possible case of spontaneous *Loa loa* encephalopathy associated with a glomerulopathy. *Filaria J.* **5:**6.
120. **Mackenzie, C., T. Geary, R. Prichard, and M. Boussinesq.** 2007. Where next with *Loa loa* encephalopathy? Data are badly needed. *Trends Parasitol.* **23:**237–238.
121. **MacLean, J. D., J. Cross, and S. Mahanty.** 2006. Liver, lung, and intestinal fluke infections, p. 1349–1369. *In* R. L. Guerrant, D. H. Walker, and P. F. Weller (ed.), *Tropical Infectious Diseases: Principles, Pathogens and Practice*, 2nd ed. Churchill Livingstone, Philadelphia, PA.
122. **Mahanty, S., H. E. Luke, V. Kumaraswami, P. R. Narayanan, V. Vijayshekaran, and T. B. Nutman.** 1996. Stage-specific induction of cytokines regulates the immune response in lymphatic filariasis. *Exp. Parasitol.* **84:**282–290.
123. **Mand, S., Y. Marfo-Debrekyei, M. Dittrich, K. Fischer, O. Adjei, and A. Hoerauf.** 2003. Animated documentation of the filaria dance sign (FDS) in bancroftian filariasis. *Filaria J.* **2:**3.
124. **McCarthy, J. S., M. Zhong, R. Gopinath, E. A. Ottesen, S. A. Williams, and T. B. Nutman.** 1996. Evaluation of a polymerase chain reaction-based assay for diagnosis of *Wuchereria bancrofti* infection. *J. Infect. Dis.* **173:**1510–1514.
125. **Montresor, A., S. Awasthi, and D. W. Crompton.** 2003. Use of benzimidazoles in children younger than 24 months for the treatment of soil-transmitted helminthiasis. *Acta Trop.* **86:**223–232.
126. **Moore, T. A., and J. S. McCarthy.** 2006. Toxocariasis and larva migrans syndromes, p. 1209–1216. *In* R. L. Guerrant, D. H. Walker, and P. F. Weller (ed.), *Tropical Infectious Diseases, Principles, Pathogens and Practice*, 2nd ed. Churchill Livingstone, Philadelphia, PA.
127. **More, S. J., and D. B. Copeman.** 1990. A highly specific and sensitive monoclonal antibody-based ELISA for the detection of circulating antigen in bancroftian filariasis. *Trop. Med. Parasitol.* **41:**403–406.
128. **Mulcahy, G., S. O'Neill, J. Fanning, E. McCarthy, and M. Sekiya.** 2005. Tissue migration by parasitic helminths - an immunoevasive strategy? *Trends Parasitol.* **21:**273–277.
129. **Muller, R.** 1971. *Dracunculus* and dracunculiasis. *Adv. Parasitol.* **9:**73–151.
130. **Nelson, G. S.** 1991. Human onchocerciasis: notes on the history, the parasite and the life cycle. *Ann. Trop. Med. Parasitol.* **85:**83–95.
131. **Newberry, A. M., D. N. Williams, W. M. Stauffer, D. R. Boulware, B. R. Hendel-Paterson, and P. F. Walker.** 2005. *Strongyloides* hyperinfection presenting as acute respiratory failure and gram-negative sepsis. *Chest* **128:**3681–3684.
132. **Nielsen, N. O., P. E. Simonsen, P. Magnussen, S. Magesa, and H. Friis.** 2006. Cross-sectional relationship between HIV, lymphatic filariasis and other parasitic infections in adults in coastal northeastern Tanzania. *Trans. R. Soc. Trop. Med. Hyg.* **100:**543–550.
133. **Noireau, F., B. Carme, J. D. Apembet, and J. P. Gouteux.** 1989. *Loa loa* and *Mansonella perstans* filariasis in the Chaillu mountains, Congo: parasitological prevalence. *Trans. R. Soc. Trop. Med. Hyg.* **83:**529–534.
134. **Noroes, J., D. Addiss, A. Santos, Z. Medeiros, A. Coutinho, and G. Dreyer.** 1996. Ultrasonographic evidence of abnor-

mal lymphatic vessels in young men with adult *Wuchereria bancrofti* infection in the scrotal area. *J. Urol.* **156:** 409–412.
135. **Nutman, T. B., and J. W. Kazura.** 2006. Filariasis, p. 1152–1162. *In* R. L. Guerrant, D. H. Walker, and P. F. Weller (ed.), *Tropical Infectious Diseases, Principles, Pathogens and Practice*, 2nd ed. Churchill Livingstone, Philadelphia, PA.
136. **Nutman, T. B., K. D. Miller, M. Mulligan, and E. A. Ottesen.** 1986. *Loa loa* infection in temporary residents of endemic regions: recognition of a hyperresponsive syndrome with characteristic clinical manifestations. *J. Infect. Dis.* **154:**10–18.
137. **Nutman, T. B., K. D. Miller, M. Mulligan, G. N. Reinhardt, B. J. Currie, C. Steel, and E. A. Ottesen.** 1988. Diethylcarbamazine prophylaxis for human loiasis. Results of a double-blind study. *N. Engl. J. Med.* **319:**752–756.
138. **Okulicz, J. F., A. S. Stibich, D. M. Elston, and R. A. Schwartz.** 2004. Cutaneous onchocercoma. *Int. J. Dermatol.* **43:**170–172.
139. **Olveda, R. M.** 2001. Disease in schistosomiasis japonica, p. 361–390. *In* A. A. F. Mahmoud (ed.), *Schistosomiasis.* Imperial College Press, London, United Kingdom.
140. **Ottesen, E. A.** 1992. The Wellcome Trust Lecture. Infection and disease in lymphatic filariasis: an immunological perspective. *Parasitology* **104**(Suppl.)**:**S71–79.
141. **Ouma, J. H., T. El-Khoby, A. Fenwick, and R. E. Blanton.** 2001. Disease in Schistosomiasis Mansoni in Africa, p. 333–360. *In* A. A. F. Mahmoud (ed.), *Schistosomiasis.* Imperial College Press, London, United Kingdom.
142. **Pakasa, N. M., N. M. Nseka, and L. M. Nyimi.** 1997. Secondary collapsing glomerulopathy associated with *Loa loa* filariasis. *Am. J. Kidney Dis.* **30:**836–839.
143. **Pani, S. P., J. Yuvaraj, P. Vanamail, V. Dhanda, E. Michael, B. T. Grenfell, and D. A. Bundy.** 1995. Episodic adenolymphangitis and lymphoedema in patients with bancroftian filariasis. *Trans. R. Soc. Trop. Med. Hyg.* **89:**727–4.
144. **Parija, S. C., P. T. Ravinder, and K. S. Rao.** 1997. Detection of hydatid antigen in urine by countercurrent immunoelectrophoresis. *J. Clin. Microbiol.* **35:**1571–1574.
145. **Parraga, I. M., A. M. Assis, M. S. Prado, M. L. Barreto, M. G. Reis, C. H. King, and R. E. Blanton.** 1996. Gender differences in growth of school-aged children with schistosomiasis and geohelminth infection. *Am. J. Trop. Med. Hyg.* **55:**150–156.
146. **Passier, A., A. Smits-van Herwaarden, and E. van Puijenbroek.** 2004. Photo-onycholysis associated with the use of doxycycline. *Br. Med. J.* **329:**265.
147. **Pelaez, V., C. Kugler, M. del Carpio, D. Correa, E. Lopez, E. Larrieu, M. Guangiroli, and J. Molina.** 1999. Treatment of hepatic hydatid cysts by percutaneous aspiration and hypertonic saline injection: results of a cooperative work. *Bol. Chil. Parasitol.* **54:**63–69. (In Spanish.)
148. **Pendse, A. K., B. M. Soni, R. Omprakash, and S. P. Gupta.** 1982. Testicular dracunculosis--a distinct clinical entity. *Br. J. Urol.* **54:**56–58.
149. **Perera, M., M. Whitehead, D. Molyneux, M. Weerasooriya, and G. Gunatilleke.** 2007. Neglected patients with a neglected disease? A qualitative study of lymphatic filariasis. *PLoS Negl. Trop. Dis.* **1:**e128.
150. **Rahmah, N., S. Taniawati, R. K. Shenoy, B. H. Lim, V. Kumaraswami, A. K. Anuar, S. L. Hakim, M. I. Hayati, B. T. Chan, M. Suharni, and C. P. Ramachandran.** 2001. Specificity and sensitivity of a rapid dipstick test (Brugia Rapid) in the detection of *Brugia malayi* infection. *Trans. R. Soc. Trop. Med. Hyg.* **95:**601–604.
151. **Ratard, R. C., L. E. Kouemeni, M. M. Ekani Bessala, C. N. Ndamkou, M. T. Sama, and B. L. Cline.** 1991. Ascariasis and trichuriasis in Cameroon. *Trans. R. Soc. Trop. Med.* **85:**84–88.
152. **Reidpath, D. D., P. A. Allotey, A. Kouame, and R. A. Cummins.** 2003. Measuring health in a vacuum: examining the disability weight of the DALY. *Health Policy Plan.* **18:**351–356.
153. **Reuter, S., K. Nussle, O. Kolokythas, U. Haug, A. Rieber, P. Kern, and W. Kratzer.** 2001. Alveolar liver echinococcosis: a comparative study of three imaging techniques. *Infection* **29:**119–125.
154. **Richter, J., C. Hatz, G. Campagne, N. R. Bergquist, and J. M. Jenkins.** 2000. Ultrasound in schistosomiasis: a practical guide to the standardized use of ultrasonography for the assessment of schistosomiasis-related morbidity TDR/STR/SCH/00.1. World Health Organization, Geneva, Switzerland.
155. **Richter, J., M. Knipper, K. Gobels, and D. Haussinger.** 2002. Fascioliasis. *Curr. Treat. Options Infect. Dis.* **4:**313–317.
156. **Richter, J., E. de Monteiro, R. M. Braz, M. Abdalla, I. M. Abdel-Rahim, U. Fano, U. Huntgeburth, and H. Feldmeier.** 1992. Sonographic organometry in Brazilian and Sudanese patients with hepatosplenic schistosomiasis mansoni and its relation to the risk of bleeding from oesophageal varices. *Acta Trop.* **51:**281–290.
157. **Rohde, J. E., B. L. Sharma, H. Patton, C. Deegan, and J. M. Sherry.** 1993. Surgical extraction of guinea worm: disability reduction and contribution to disease control. *Am. J. Trop. Med. Hyg.* **48:**71–76.
158. **Rom, W. N., V. K. Vijayan, M. J. Cornelius, V. Kumaraswami, R. Prabhakar, E. A. Ottesen, and R. G. Crystal.** 1990. Persistent lower respiratory tract inflammation associated with interstitial lung disease in patients with tropical pulmonary eosinophilia following conventional treatment with diethylcarbamazine. *Am. Rev. Respir. Dis.* **142:** 1088–1092.
159. **Rousham, E. K., and C. G. Mascie-Taylor.** 1994. An 18-month study of the effect of periodic anthelminthic treatment on the growth and nutritional status of pre-school children in Bangladesh. *Ann. Hum. Biol.* **21:**315–324.
160. **Ruiz-Tiben, E., and D. R. Hopkins.** 2006. Dracunculiasis, p. 1204–1208. *In* R. L. Guerrant, D. H. Walker, and P. F. Weller (ed.), *Tropical Infectious Diseases, Principles, Pathogens and Practice*, 2nd ed. Churchill Livingstone, Philadelphia, PA.
161. **Saeed, A. A., P. J. Green, M. Naoroz, H. A. Lee, and G. V. Raman.** 1984. *Loa loa*: the use of a blood cell separator to reduce microfilaraemia before specific chemotherapy. *J. Infect.* **9:**161–166.
162. **Saint Andre, A., N. M. Blackwell, L. R. Hall, A. Hoerauf, N. W. Brattig, L. Volkmann, M. J. Taylor, L. Ford, A. G. Hise, J. H. Lass, E. Diaconu, and E. Pearlman.** 2002. The role of endosymbiotic *Wolbachia* bacteria in the pathogenesis of river blindness. *Science* **295:**1892–1895.
163. **Sakti, H., C. Nokes, W. S. Hertanto, S. Hendratno, A. Hall, D. A. Bundy, and Satoto.** 1999. Evidence for an association between hookworm infection and cognitive function in Indonesian school children. *Trop. Med. Int. Health* **4:** 322–334.
164. **Salata, R. A., and C. H. King.** 2008. Parasitic infections of the central nervous system, p. 921–946. *In* M. J. Aminoff (ed.), *Neurology and General Medicine.* Churchill Livingstone, Philadelphia, PA.
165. **Sandouk, F., S. Haffar, M. M. Zada, D. Y. Graham, and B. S. Anand.** 1997. Pancreatic-biliary ascariasis: experience of 300 cases. *Am. J. Gastroenterol.* **92:**2264–2267.

166. **Satayathum, S. A., E. M. Muchiri, J. H. Ouma, C. C. Whalen, and C. H. King.** 2006. Factors affecting infection or reinfection with *Schistosoma haematobium* in coastal Kenya: survival analysis during a nine-year, school-based treatment program. *Am. J. Trop. Med. Hyg.* **75:**83–92.
167. **Schantz, P. M., P. Kern, and E. Brunetti.** 2006. Echinococcosis, p. 1304–1326. *In* R. L. Guerrant, D. H. Walker, and P. F. Weller (ed.), *Tropical Infectious Diseases, Principles, Pathogens and Practice*, 2nd ed. Churchill Livingstone, Philadelphia, PA.
168. **Seltzer, E., M. Barry, and D. W. Crompton.** 2006. Ascariasis, p. 1257–1264. *In* R. L. Guerrant, D. H. Walker, and P. F. Weller (ed.), *Tropical Infectious Diseases, Principles, Pathogens and Practice*, 2nd ed. Churchill Livingstone, Philadelphia, PA.
169. **Siddiqui, A. A., R. M. Genta, and S. L. Berk.** 2006. Strongyloidiasis, p. 1274–1285. *In* R. L. Guerrant, D. H. Walker, and P. F. Weller (ed.), *Tropical Infectious Diseases, Principles, Pathogens and Practice,* 2nd ed. Churchill Livingstone, Philadelphia, PA.
170. **Singer, B. H., and C. D. Ryff.** 2007. Neglected tropical diseases, neglected data sources, and neglected issues. *PLoS Negl. Trop. Dis.* **1:**e104.
171. **Slom, T. J., M. M. Cortese, S. I. Gerber, R. C. Jones, T. H. Holtz, A. S. Lopez, C. H. Zambrano, R. L. Sufit, Y. Sakolvaree, W. Chaicumpa, B. L. Herwaldt, and S. Johnson.** 2002. An outbreak of eosinophilic meningitis caused by *Angiostrongylus cantonensis* in travelers returning from the Caribbean. *N. Engl. J. Med.* **346:**668–675.
172. **Smith, J. H., and J. D. Christie.** 1986. The pathobiology of *Schistosoma haematobium* infection in humans. *Hum. Pathol.* **17:**333–345.
173. **Smith, J. H., I. A. Kamel, A. Elqi, and R. von Lichtenberg. 1974.** A quantitative post-mortem analysis of urinary schistosomiasis in Egypt. I. Pathology and pathogenesis. *Am. J. Trop. Med. Hyg.* **23:**1054–1071.
174. **Southgate, B. A.** 1992. Intensity and efficiency of transmission and the development of microfilaraemia and disease: their relationship in lymphatic filariasis. *J. Trop. Med. Hyg.* **95:**1–12.
175. **Srikanth, S. G., P. N. Jayakumar, M. K. Vasudev, A. B. Taly, and H. S. Chandrashekar.** 2002. MRI in subacute combined degeneration of spinal cord: a case report and review of literature. *Neurol. India* **50:**310–312.
176. **Steel, C., A. Guinea, J. S. McCarthy, and E. A. Ottesen.** 1994. Long-term effect of prenatal exposure to maternal microfilaraemia on immune responsiveness to filarial parasite antigens. *Lancet* **343:**890–893.
177. **Stephenson, L. S.** 1994. Helminth parasites, a major factor in malnutrition. *World Health Forum* **15:**169–172.
178. **Stephenson, L. S., M. C. Latham, K. M. Kurz, S. N. Kinoti, M. L. Oduori, and D. W. Crompton.** 1985. Relationships of *Schistosoma haematobium*, hookworm and malarial infections and metrifonate treatment to growth of Kenyan school children. *Am. J. Trop. Med. Hyg.* **34:**1109–1118.
179. **Storey, D. M.** 1993. Filariasis: nutritional interactions in human and animal hosts. *Parasitology* **107**(Suppl.): S147–S158.
180. **Strickland, G. T.** 2000. Helminth infections- general principles, p. 713–716. *In* G. T. Strickland (ed.), *Hunter's Tropical Medicine and Emerging Infectious Diseases*, 8th ed. W. B. Saunders, Philadelphia, PA.
181. **Sturrock, R. F.** 2001. The schistosomes and their intermediate hosts, p. 7–83. *In* A. A. F. Mahmoud (ed.), *Schistosomiasis*. Imperial College Press, London, United Kingdom.
182. **Tabi, T. E., R. Befidi-Mengue, T. B. Nutman, J. Horton, A. Folefack, E. Pensia, R. Fualem, J. Fogako, P. Gwanmesia, I. Quakyi, and R. Leke.** 2004. Human loiasis in a Cameroonian village: a double-blind, placebo-controlled, crossover clinical trial of a three-day albendazole regimen. *Am. J. Trop. Med. Hyg.* **71:**211–215.
183. **Taiwo, S. S., and M. O. Tamiowo.** 2007. *Loa loa* meningoencephalitis in Southwestern Nigeria. *West Afr. J. Med.* **26:**156–159.
184. **Takeuchi, H., K. Zaman, J. Takahashi, M. Yunus, H. R. Chowdhury, S. E. Arifeen, A. Baqui, S. Wakai, and T. Iwata.** 2008. High titre of anti-*Ascaris* immunoglobulin E associated with bronchial asthma symptoms in 5-year-old rural Bangladeshi children. *Clin. Exp. Allergy* **38:** 276–282.
185. **Taylor, M. J., W. H. Makunde, H. F. McGarry, J. D. Turner, S. Mand, and A. Hoerauf.** 2005. Macrofilaricidal activity after doxycycline treatment of *Wuchereria bancrofti*: a double-blind, randomised placebo-controlled trial. *Lancet* **365:**2116–2121.
186. **Thein, H., S. Than, A. Htay Htay, L. Myint, and M. Thein Maung.** 1984. Epidemiology and transmission dynamics of *Ascaris lumbricoides* in Okpo village, rural Burma. *Trans. R. Soc. Trop. Med. Hyg.* **78:**497–504.
187. **Thomson, M. C., V. Obsomer, M. Dunne, S. J. Connor, and D. H. Molyneux.** 2000. Satellite mapping of *Loa loa* prevalence in relation to ivermectin use in west and central Africa. *Lancet* **356:**1077–1078.
188. **Thylefors, B.** 2004. Eliminating onchocerciasis as a public health problem. *Trop. Med. Int. Health* **9:**A1–A3.
189. **Timmann, C., R. S. Abraha, C. Hamelmann, D. W. Buttner, B. Lepping, Y. Marfo, N. Brattig, and R. D. Horstmann.** 2003. Cutaneous pathology in onchocerciasis associated with pronounced systemic T-helper 2-type responses to *Onchocerca volvulus*. *Br. J. Dermatol.* **149:**782–787.
190. **Torgerson, P. R.** 2003. Economic effects of echinococcosis. *Acta Trop.* **85:**113–8.
191. **Toure, F. S., E. Mavoungou, P. Deloron, and T. G. Egwang.** 1999. Comparative analysis of 2 diagnostic methods of human loiasis: IgG4 serology and nested PCR. *Bull. Soc. Pathol. Exot.* **92:**167–170. (In French.)
192. **Tsou, M. H., and T. W. Huang.** 1993. Pathology of subcutaneous sparganosis: report of two cases. *J. Formos. Med. Assoc.* **92:**649–653.
193. **Udall, D. N.** 2007. Recent updates on onchocerciasis: diagnosis and treatment. *Clin. Infect. Dis.* **44:**53–60.
194. **Van Bogaert, L., A. Dubois, P. G. Janssens, J. Radermecker, G. Tverdy, and M. Wanson.** 1955. Encephalitis in *Loa-loa* filariasis. *J. Neurol. Neurosurg. Psychiatry* **18:**103–119.
195. **Vijayan, V. K.** 2007. Tropical pulmonary eosinophilia: pathogenesis, diagnosis and management. *Curr. Opin. Pulm. Med.* **13:**428–433.
196. **Vincent, J. A., S. Lustigman, S. Zhang, and G. J. Weil.** 2000. A comparison of newer tests for the diagnosis of onchocerciasis. *Ann. Trop. Med. Parasitol.* **94:**253–258.
197. **Von Bonsdorff, B.** 1977. *Diphyllobothriasis in Man.* Academic Press, London, United Kingdom.
198. **Wanji, S., N. Tendongfor, M. Esum, S. S. Yundze, M. J. Taylor, and P. Enyong.** 2005. Combined utilisation of rapid assessment procedures for Loiasis (RAPLOA) and onchocerciasis (REA) in rain forest villages of Cameroon. *Filaria J.* **4:**2.
199. **Warren, K. S., A. A. F. Mahmoud, P. Cummings, D. J. Murphy, and H. B. Houser.** 1974. *Schistosomiasis mansoni* in Yemeni in California: duration of infection, presence of disease, therapeutic management. *Am. J. Trop. Med. Hyg.* **23:**902–909.

200. **Wasadikar, P. P., and A. B. Kulkarni.** 1997. Intestinal obstruction due to ascariasis. *Br. J. Surg.* **84:**410–412.

201. **Weil, G. J., P. J. Lammie, and N. Weiss.** 1997. The ICT filariasis test: a rapid-format antigen test for diagnosis of bancroftian filariasis. *Parasitol. Today* **13:**401–404.

202. **Weil, G. J., C. Steel, F. Liftis, B. W. Li, G. Mearns, E. Lobos, and T. B. Nutman.** 2000. A rapid-format antibody card test for diagnosis of onchocerciasis. *J. Infect. Dis.* **182:** 1796–1799.

203. **WHO.** 1999. Building partnerships for lymphatic filariasis: strategic plan. WHO/FIL/99.198. World Health Organization, Geneva, Switzerland.

204. **WHO.** 2007. Global programme to eliminate lymphatic filariasis: Annual report on lymphatic filariasis 2006. *Weekly Epidemiol. Rec.* **82:**361–380.

205. **WHO.** 1994. *IARC Monographs on the Evaluation of Carcinogenic Risks to Humans. Schistosomes, Liver Flukes and Helicobacter pylori*, vol. 61. World Health Organization, Geneva, Switzerland.

206. **WHO.** 2003. Informal working group. International classification of ultrasound images in cystic echinococcosis for application in clinical and field epidemiological settings. *Acta Trop.* **85:**253–261.

207. **WHO.** 2001. Onchocerciasis (river blindness). Report from the Tenth InterAmerican Conference on Onchocerciasis, Guayaquil, Ecuador. *Weekly Epidemiol. Rec.* **76:**205–212.

207a. **WHO.** 1998. *TDR News* **55:**5.

207b. **WHO.** 1984. Lymphatic filariasis. WHO technical report series no. 702. World Health Organization, Geneva, Switzerland.

207c. **WHO.** 2002. Prevention and control of schistosomiasis and soil-transmitted helminthiasis: report of a WHO expert committee. Technical report series no. 912. World Health Organization, Geneva, Switzerland.

208. **Wilson, J. F., and R. L. Rausch.** 1980. Alveolar hydatid disease. A review of clinical features of 33 indigenous cases of *Echinococcus multilocularis* infection in Alaskan Eskimos. *Am. J. Trop. Med. Hyg.* **29:**1340–1355.

209. **Wittner, M., and H. Tanowitz.** 2006. *Taenia* and other tapeworms, p. 1327–1340. *In* R. L. Guerrant, D. H. Walker, and P. F. Weller (ed.), *Tropical Infectious Diseases, Principles, Pathogens and Practice*, 2nd ed. Churchill Livingstone, Philadelphia, PA.

210. **Wynd, S., D. N. Durrheim, J. Carron, B. Selve, J. P. Chaine, P. A. Leggat, and W. Melrose.** 2007. Socio-cultural insights and lymphatic filariasis control--lessons from the Pacific. *Filaria J.* **6:**3.

211. **Wynd, S., W. D. Melrose, D. N. Durrheim, J. Carron, and M. Gyapong.** 2007. Understanding the community impact of lymphatic filariasis: a review of the sociocultural literature. *Bull. W. H. O.* **85:**493–498.

212. **Yang, Y. R., T. Sun, Z. Li, J. Zhang, J. Teng, X. Liu, R. Liu, R. Zhao, M. K. Jones, Y. Wang, H. Wen, X. Feng, Q. Zhao, Y. Zhao, D. Shi, B. Bartholomot, D. A. Vuitton, D. Pleydell, P. Giraudoux, A. Ito, M. F. Danson, B. Boufana, P. S. Craig, G. M. Williams, and D. P. McManus.** 2006. Community surveys and risk factor analysis of human alveolar and cystic echinococcosis in Ningxia Hui Autonomous Region, China. *Bull. W. H. O.* **84:**714–721.

213. **Yu, S. H., Z. X. Jiang, and L. Q. Xu.** 1995. Infantile hookworm disease in China. A review. *Acta Trop.* **59:** 265–270.

214. **Zargar, S. A., B. A. Khan, G. Javid, G. N. Yattoo, A. H. Shah, G. M. Gulzar, J. Singh, M. A. Khan, and N. A. Shah.** 2004. Endoscopic management of early postoperative biliary ascariasis in patients with biliary tract surgery. *World J. Surg.* **28:**712–715.

Sequelae and Long-Term Consequences of Infectious Diseases
Edited by Pina M. Fratamico, James L. Smith, and Kim A. Brogden

Chapter 18

Acute Viral Infections with Rare Late Complications

E. David McIntosh

Attributing an illness to a long-past infection retrospectively requires a degree of evidence, at least a lingering serological marker, a molecular fingerprint, or an acknowledgment that the illness has been observed in other similar patients. Prospective cohort studies have the potential to provide stronger evidence, although the follow-up period may need to be very long and the attribution tenuous. There is always the possibility that a confounder has intervened and the original insult is wrongly blamed for the outcome.

Pediatricians generally hand over their chronic patients at an appropriate point between adolescence and adulthood. The progression of disease is continuous, while there is not necessarily continuity of care. Infants and children who sustain acute infections, and recover completely, are unlikely to be handed on to adult physicians. Those who bear stigmata are at least likely to draw attention to themselves as adults. If the stigmata are external, visible, and identifiable, then it is possible to say, "He had chickenpox as a child; she had polio."

EARLY MANIFESTATIONS OF VIRAL INFECTIONS

Acute viral infections may result in early complications. These include rubella in arthritis; measles and influenza in bacterial pneumonia; mononucleosis in autoimmune hemolytic anemia; influenza and varicella in Reye syndrome; influenza and Epstein-Barr virus in Guillain-Barré syndrome (28); and measles, mumps, rubella, varicella, influenza, and Epstein-Barr virus in acute disseminated encephalomyelitis.

Congenital and neonatal viral infections usually display their acute manifestations in highly recognizable ways. The association between congenital cataracts and congenital rubella virus infection was first described by the Australian ophthalmologist Norman Gregg (10). The full congenital rubella syndrome includes heart, eye, hearing, and central nervous system defects, along with intrauterine growth retardation. Congenital cytomegalovirus (CMV) and varicella infection may also present with distinctive clinical features in the neonate, circumferential scarring being associated with the latter. Perinatal herpes simplex virus infection may present with devastating encephalitis, while untreated congenital human immunodeficiency virus (HIV) infection presents with early severe infections in infancy.

ACUTE VIRAL INFECTIONS WITH RARE LATE COMPLICATIONS

The long-term or late rare complications of acute viral infections will be the main focus in this chapter. Both congenital and acquired viral infections will be covered.

CMV

An incentive for following up patients long-term is the opportunity to document the natural history of an infection. Another incentive is to detect late-onset effects as early as possible and to do something to either treat or prevent them. Deafness is common after congenital CMV infection and may become manifest many months after birth. The Congenital CMV Longitudinal Study Group documented the duration of CMV excretion in the urine as a surrogate marker of persistent viral replication in children who had been congenitally infected (23). In particular, the group wished to study the relationship between persistent viral replication and child growth, cognitive function and the progression of sensorineural hearing loss. The results are shown in Table 1. There was no significant difference in the duration of CMV urinary excretion between children born with asymptomatic and symptomatic congenital CMV infection, nor was

E. David McIntosh • Imperial College, Faculty of Medicine, London SW7 2AZ, United Kingdom.

Table 1. Duration of CMV urinary excretion according to the presence of outcome in children with congenital CMV infection (23)

Growth measurements on or after 6 yr of age	Duration of excretion[a] with presence of outcome		*P* value
	Yes	No	
Ht Z score <−1	4.06 (10)[b]	4.02 (60)	0.64
Wt Z score <−1	3.99 (6)	4.08 (64)	0.64
Wt for ht Z score <−1	4.85 (8)	3.90 (62)	0.32
Head circumference Z score <−1	3.15 (11)	4.10 (59)	0.26
Intelligence/development quotient <85 on or after 6 yr of age	4.10 (7)	4.06 (63)	0.73
Sensorineural hearing loss at 6 yr of age	3.30 (21)	4.59 (49)	0.19
Progressive sensorineural hearing loss	3.30 (15)	4.59 (55)	0.12

[a]Median duration of urinary excretion (years).
[b]Numbers in parentheses indicate number of subjects in each group.

there an association between long-term growth or cognitive outcome and duration of excretion. However, there was a significant association between sensorineural hearing loss and a shorter duration of CMV excretion. The reason for this is not known. Ganciclovir did not have a significant effect on viral excretion.

A long-term longitudinal study was performed of congenitally infected infants in Sweden, born between 1977 and 1985, followed up for 7 years (1). The 76 infants identified (39 female/37 male) were discovered through screening 16,474 newborns (around 1:1,000). Table 2 shows that the average CMV excretion rate decreased from 100% at birth to 57% at 4 years of age (the controls had been selected randomly among normal births). This means that the likelihood of associating a neurological abnormality with a congenital CMV infection diminishes with time and that a constellation of symptoms in later life may only suggest a viral origin. The neurological status was abnormal in 11/60 (18%) patients at 7 years versus 1/39 (3%) of controls, as well as in 2 patients followed up for a shorter period of time. The congenitally infected patients had various combinations of microcephaly, cerebral palsy, intellectual handicap, deafness, developmental delay, and epilepsy. This means that the majority of congenitally infected infants were in fact asymptomatic on long-term follow-up. Chronic disease was observed in two patients: type 1 diabetes with onset at 6 years of age and celiac disease diagnosed at 2 years of age.

Cranial ultrasound scanning has been used in an attempt to predict neurological outcome in children. Cranial ultrasound scanning was used to follow up infants infected with congenital CMV for a minimum of 12 months (mean age ± standard deviation at last follow-up visit 42.3 ± 11.3 months) (2). Of 57 patients diagnosed at birth, 56 were available for follow-up in this way. Of the 11 surviving neonates who had had abnormal ultrasound results, only 1, who had moderate ventriculomegaly and a hyperechoic lesion, had a normal outcome at follow-up. Strabismus had developed in one infant, and another developed strabismus plus sensorineural hearing loss. Various combinations of ventriculomegaly, diffuse calcification, cerebellar hypoplasia, and periventricular cysts which had been found at birth were present in the other eight and were associated with poor psychomotor development, sensorineural hearing loss, and/or motor delay. The individual risks for sequelae are shown in Table 3.

Congenital Rubella Syndrome

An opportunity was provided by the description of the congenital rubella syndrome by Gregg and his documentation of the cohort of his "original" patients (10). This group of 50 patients was followed

Table 2. Thirty-five congenitally CMV-infected infants and 50 control infants, followed up by virus isolation testing in urine (1)

Infant group (*n*)	No. positive/no. tested (%) in virus isolation test at age:							
	<1 Wk	3 Mo	6 Mo	9 Mo	12 Mo	18 Mo	30 Mo	4 Yr
Patients (35)	35/35 (100)	28/29 (97)	24/26 (92)	21/22 (95)	22/27 (81)	14/21 (67)	12/17 (71)	4/7 (57)
Controls (50)	0/50 (0)	10/42 (24)	15/43 (35)	11/35 (31)	12/36 (33)	12/36 (33)	6/22 (27)	4/11 (36)

Table 3. Value of cranial ultrasound scanning in predicting outcome in 57 patients with congenital CMV infection (2)

Parameter	No. of newborns with poor outcome/total no. (%)		Odds ratio (95% CI)[b]	P value	Positive predictive value (%)	Negative predictive value (%)
	Normal ultrasound results	Pathological ultrasound results[a]				
Developmental quotient ≤85	0/45	8/11 (72.7)	NE	<0.001	72.7	100
Motor delay	0/45	6/11 (54.5)	NE	<0.001	54.5	100
Sensorineural hearing loss	3/45 (6.7)	6/11 (54.5)	16.8 (3.2 to 89.0)	<0.001	54.5	93.3
Sequela	3/45 (6.7)	11/12 (91.7)	154 (17.3 to 1219.6)	<0.001	91.7	93.3

[a]One newborn had pathological ultrasound results during the neonatal period but had a normal outcome. Follow-up data were available for 11 of the 12 patients who lived.
[b]CI, confidence interval; NE, could not be estimated.

up when they were 25 years of age (20). These patients had been born between 1939 and 1944. Menser noted: "25 were below the tenth percentile for weight and/or height. Six seemed prematurely aged, particularly the undiagnosed diabetic. Many of the patients had a distinctive facial appearance, reminiscent of that described previously. Five had generalised muscular hypotonia." Apart from a high frequency of ocular, hearing, and speech defects, cardiovascular defects were detected in 11 patients, only 2 of whom had had the defects detected in the first year of life. As mentioned, diabetes mellitus was diagnosed at the 25-year follow-up and, by 1971 when they were around 27 to 32 years of age, 5 of the 50 had diabetes mellitus and 4 had latent diabetes. The mechanism underlying the development of diabetes may be the induction by the rubella virus of an autoimmune reaction against the pancreatic beta cells (27).

The 50 "original" patients were again followed up at 50 years of age (18). Of those 40 available for a full clinical assessment (3 declined this assessment), 6 were under the third percentile for height. Hearing was impaired in all 40, severely so in 36. Twenty-three subjects had eye defects related to congenital rubella, 7 cases being due to microphthalmia and cataracts which had been treated surgically in infancy, while 5 had glaucoma. Eight had congenital cardiovascular defects. Of the five who had been diagnosed with diabetes mellitus in 1971, four remained so, while one appeared to have had a remission. An additional patient had become diabetic by the time of the 50-year follow-up. Seven of the 50 had died (Table 4). In addition to the three deaths from malignancy, an additional patient had recently been treated for malignant melanoma, and while the overall incidence rate for malignant disease was not increased compared to that of the general population, the death rate from malignancy was. When followed up at the 60-year milestone, an additional 10 had died, but by then the four deaths from malignancy did not demonstrate a statistically significant increase over that of the general population (14). However, the prevalence of diabetes (22%), thyroid disease (19%), early menopause (73%), and osteoporosis (12.5%) was increased compared with that of the general population.

What was also discovered at that 60-year follow-up was that the frequencies of HLA-A1 (44%) and HLA-B8 (34%) were increased, and the haplotype HLA-A1, B8, DR3, said to be highly associated with many autoimmune conditions, was present in 25%. Whether or not these are associated with an increased likelihood of congenital rubella could only be elucidated by a study of newborns. The importance of rubella vaccination is highlighted by the recent rise in congenital rubella after a rubella epidemic in Brazil (15).

Congenital and Early HIV Infection

With improved treatment, infants born with or contracting HIV infection are maturing into adults. There is a developing interest in their long-term outcome, which, of course, can be confounded by the treatment itself, not to mention other environmental factors. The Pediatric AIDS Clinical Trials Group

Table 4. Causes of death in 50 subjects with congenital rubella followed up for 50 years (18)

Cause of death	Sex	Age (yr)
Testicular cancer	Male	34
Stomach cancer	Female	43
Breast cancer	Female	50
Eisenmenger syndrome	Female	30
Eisenmenger syndrome	Female	32
Hypertension, ruptured cerebral aneurysm	Female	38
AIDS	Male	49

(PACTG) is a prospective cohort study following long-term outcomes in HIV-infected infants and children (9). A total of 2,298 HIV-infected and 1,021 HIV-exposed, uninfected infants, children, and adolescents were enrolled in PACTG 219C between September 2000 and December 2002. The median age of those infected was 10 years, while for those uninfected, it was 1 year. Among 1,808 HIV-infected participants who were <15 years of age at the last visit date, 25 children had been hospitalized for psychiatric manifestations, 8 before enrollment in PACTG 219C. Regardless of age, 32 children were hospitalized for psychiatric manifestations. No psychiatric admissions were observed in the noninfected cohort.

The study concluded that children with HIV/AIDS are at increased risk for psychiatric hospitalizations during childhood and early adolescence compared with the general pediatric population. It was also postulated that the more severely affected children may not have been eligible for enrollment in the study. The results provide compelling reasons for doctors treating such patients to be sensitive and responsive towards mental changes in their patients. It is possible that congenitally infected women surviving into adulthood will give birth to babies with a "congenital HIV syndrome," although HIV therapy will again be a confounder.

Hepatitis B and Hepatitis C

The extraordinary ability of hepatitis B virus (HBV) vaccination to reduce hepatocellular carcinoma has been demonstrated clearly in Taiwan (6). With vaccination, the average annual incidence of hepatocellular carcinoma in children in Taiwan 6 to 14 years of age decreased from 0.70 per 100,000 children between 1981 and 1986 to 0.57 per 100,000 between 1986 and 1990, and to 0.36 between 1990 and1994 ($P < 0.01$). This was associated with a significant decrease in mortality from hepatocellular carcinoma as well. Maternally acquired HBV and HBV acquired horizontally early in life are much more likely to lead to long-term liver disease than infection acquired in adulthood. In Australia, a high rate of hepatitis B surface antigen carriage in unvaccinated immigrant families suggests that there will be an increase in hepatocellular carcinoma at some point in the future (19). The molecular mechanisms responsible for hepatocellular carcinogenesis are gradually being elucidated (3). For hepatitic C virus (HCV) in Australia, modeling predicts that the prevalence of HCV-related cirrhosis and the incidence of HCV-related liver failure and hepatocellular carcinoma will more than triple by the year 2020 (16). The pathogenesis of chronic HCV infection is most likely based on the ability of the virus to escape from humoral and cellular immunity (12). Histological studies of children with chronic HCV indicate that children often have mild histological forms, possibly with some degree of immunological tolerance, suggesting that the natural history of HCV in children is commonly a very prolonged one with clinically silent persistence of virus and with progression to clinically apparent chronic liver disease delayed until adulthood (12).

Other Viruses

Nipah virus (NiV) is an emerging zoonosis causing outbreaks of encephalitis (26). Twenty-two serologically confirmed survivors of NiV outbreaks which occurred in Bangladesh in 2003, 2004, and 2005 were followed up between mid-2005 and mid-2006. While 12 patients were healthy neurologically, 7 (32%) had moderate-to-severe objective neurological dysfunction that had persisted since, or developed subsequent to, the onset of acute NiV encephalitis. The abnormalities included cognitive dysfunction or developmental delay ($n = 4$), ataxia/gait disturbance ($n = 2$) and persistent focal weakness ($n = 2$). Delayed onset neurological abnormalities, such as cranial nerve dysfunction and acute cervical dystonia, occurred months to years later in four patients. It is this delay in onset which causes the most concern, in that patients who have seemingly recovered are at risk of developing neurological problems later in life.

West Nile virus (WNV) is also an emerging cause of epidemics, and the mortality and morbidity are well known, including the persistence of neurological sequelae after acute meningo-encephalitis. However, the appearance of West Nile flaccid paralysis or "poliomyelitis" is becoming increasingly recognized as a serious, longer-term outcome of acute infection (25). There is also emerging evidence that WNV infection may be associated with the subsequent development of parkinsonism, as are possibly other viruses, such as Bunyavirus, coxsackie virus, Japanese encephalitis virus, and influenza (5, 13, 21, 24). It is also possible that with WNV, a "post-polio" syndrome will develop in the same way that it develops following classical poliovirus poliomyelitis (29). In adults, followed up at a mean of 13 months after acute infection in a study performed in North Dakota, multiple somatic complaints, tremor, and abnormalities in motor skills and executive functions were common long-term problems among these patients, regardless of how mild or how severe their original infection had been (4).

A seemingly innocent childhood infection, "hand, foot and mouth disease" caused by enteroviruses may also be associated with long-term neurological sequelae (7). These infections are sometimes associated with encephalitis and the development of a poliomyelitis-like syndrome and thus could be expected on rare occasions to cause persistent or new problems. A group in Taiwan followed up 142 children following enterovirus 71 infection; 71 of them had had initial neurological involvement. They were followed up at a median age of 2.9 years, and the results are shown in Table 5. Not only was enterovirus 71 infection associated with long-term neurological sequelae, but it was also associated in some cases with neurodevelopmental delay and reduced cognitive function. It would be advisable to submit children previously affected by enterovirus encephalitis to neurodevelopmental screening in order to anticipate and treat dysfunction.

Another enterovirus, the coxsackie virus, may have a similar role as rubella virus and CMV in causing placental infection, fetal mortality, and long-term morbidity (8). Seven infants were shown to have been born with neonatal coxsackie virus infection by means of identification of the virus in the placenta (8). One of those infants died, and the remaining six, with an age range of 4 to 15 years, were examined. Each of the six living children experienced marked, global cognitive defects evident soon after birth, which required intensive physical therapy, occupational therapy, and on occasions, anti-seizure therapy and institutionalization. Only one had evidence of cerebral palsy. The clinical findings are shown in Table 6, which highlights the fact that nearly all the neurological sequelae were cognitive. When the placentas had been examined at the time of birth, there were no distinguishing external features. The most common histological finding was Hofbauer cell hyperplasia with focal calcification and chronic villitis evident in some. Isolation of a virus from the placenta and confirmation of a viral etiology are highly specialized endeavors which would be undertaken only if there is a compelling clinical reason and certainly if there is hope that treatment of the neonate/infant may result in amelioration of the condition.

Staying with long-term neurological sequelae, latent and/or chronic influenza virus has long been thought to be associated with parkinsonism, but there is little if any solid evidence for that. It should be noted, for example that the 1917 pandemic of von Economo's disease, which led to parkinsonism (encephalitis lethargica), preceded the 1918–1919 influenza pandemic, and many studies since have failed to provide conclusive evidence (5). That is not to say the influenza virus infection cannot lead to long-term neurological sequelae—it can. For example, influenza virus B encephalitis was reviewed by a group in Nebraska after the hospitalization of several children with this condition (22). For 10 of 14 patients (both children and adults) for whom clinical outcome could

Table 5. Clinical and neurological outcomes of 142 patients after enterovirus 71 infection with central nervous system involvement (7)[a]

Variable	Group 1 (n = 61)	Group 2 (n = 53)	Group 3 (n = 28)	P value[b]
Demographic characteristics				
Male sex (no.)	45	28	15	0.04
Age at onset (yr)				<0.001
Median	2.0	2.3	0.7	
Range	0.1 to 7.7	0.2 to 13.5	0.2 to 4.3	
Age at assessment (yr)				<0.001
Median	4.7	6.7	3.1	
Range	1.3 to 12.4	2.2 to 20.8	1.5 to 5.9	
Outcome				
Recovery (no. [%])	61 (100)	42 (79)	7 (25)	<0.001
Focal limb weakness and atrophy (no. [%])	0	10 (19)[c]	18 (64)	
Dysphagia with tube feeding (no. [%])	0	0	17 (61)	
Central hypoventilation with ventilator support (no. [%])	0	0	16 (57)	
Facial nerve palsy (no. [%])	0	1 (2)[d]	7 (25)	
Seizure (no. [%])	0	0	4 (14)	
Hypoxia-related psychomotor retardation (no. [%])	0	0	5 (18)	

[a]Group 1 comprises patients with mild central nervous system (CNS) involvement (aseptic meningitis); group 2 comprises patients with severe CNS involvement (encephalitis [32 patients], a poliomyelitis-like syndrome [16 patients], or encephalomyelitis [5 patients]; group 3 comprises patients with cardiopulmonary failure after CNS involvement.
[b]P values for the overall comparisons were calculated with the Krustal-Wallis test for continuous variables or Fisher's exact test for categorical variables.
[c]Sequelae of focal limb weakness and atrophy were found in 1 of 5 patients with encephalomyelitis (20%) and in 9 of 16 patients with poliomyelitis-lime syndrome (56%).
[d]Facial nerve palsy was seen with 1 of 32 patients with encephalitis (3%).

Table 6. Clinical findings in six of seven children aged between 4 and 15 years, after intrauterine infection with coxsackie virus (8)[a]

Case	EGA (yr)	BW (g)	Apgar at 1 min/5 min	Pregnancy complication	Status
1	37	3,220	5/9	Gestational diabetes	Neutropenic and thrombocytopenic at birth; respiratory distress; neurological delays
2	39	3,610	5/7	Multiple upper respiratory infections	Respiratory failure; viral exanthema at birth; neonatal seizure; neurological delays
3	43	4,280	4/7	Viral prodrome, second trimester	Respiratory failure, persistent pulmonary hypertension; neonatal seizures; severe mental retardation; blindness
4	27	1,335	2/4	New onset diabetic ketoacidosis; preterm labour	Grade III intraventricular hemorrhage; neurological delays
5	37	1,988	2/8	Intrauterine growth retardation	Thrombocytopenia; macular rash at birth; mental retardation
6	25	850	5/7	Viral prodrome, second trimester	Respiratory distress; intraventricular hemorrhage and retardation
7	28	1,120	5/7	Preterm rupture of membranes; fetal pericardial effusion; coxsackie titre positive in pregnancy	Expired day 1 due to respiratory insufficiency

[a]EGA, estimated gestational age; BW, birth weight.

be obtained, neurological abnormalities resolved completely. However, for three patients, long-term sequelae ensued: paresis of extra-ocular muscles, ataxia, new-onset cognitive difficulties, and difficulties with rhythmic speech, with one patient dying (of concurrent respiratory syncytial virus [RSV] infection). Furthermore, prenatal exposure to influenza may be a neurodevelopmental risk factor for schizophrenia in adult life (17).

As for RSV infection, it is often associated with the development of recurrent wheezing and asthma, but it is also associated with future obstructive airways disease (11). The current evidence is not in favor of a causal link, although the majority of studies indicate that the infant who develops RSV and subsequent wheezing has abnormalities which predate the RSV infection, and the link may be merely by association (31). What is needed to prove causation would be a controlled clinical trial which randomizes to some form of intervention or a successful RSV vaccination program, which could show a subsequent reduction in obstructive airways disease.

One infection for which there is a successful vaccination program is varicella-zoster virus. The success of this program in the United States in reducing the incidence of childhood chickenpox has been remarkable (30), but its effectiveness in reducing future herpes zoster (shingles) remains to be assessed. Another successful vaccination program, that against measles, is associated with a dramatic reduction in subacute sclerosing panencephalitis, the rare late-onset consequence of measles.

CONCLUSIONS

Congenital, neonatal, and childhood viral infections usually display their acute manifestations in highly recognizable ways. Their immediate complications are easily linked to the viral antecedent. By contrast, maternally acquired HBV infection or HBV infection acquired horizontally during early childhood may go undetected for years. Maternally and horizontally acquired HBV infection predisposes to carriage, liver cirrhosis, and hepatocellular carcinoma in older children and in adults. Neonatal HBV vaccination prevents hepatocellular carcinoma.

The long-term consequences of congenital and acquired infections include endocrine, immunological, and cardiovascular disease, deafness, visual problems, intellectual handicap, developmental delay, cerebral palsy, and other neurological problems, such as parkinsonism and poliomyelitis-like syndromes. With the survival of HIV-infected infants into adulthood, the long-term consequences are now being described. The long-term benefits arising from the diagnosis, treatment, and prevention of pediatric viral infections are considerable and should not be underestimated in the designing of screening and immunization programs.

REFERENCES

1. **Ahlfors, K., S.-A. Ivarsson, and S. Harris.**1999. Report on a long-term study of maternal and congenital cytomegalovirus infection in Sweden. Review of prospective studies available in the literature. *Scand. J. Infect. Dis.* **31**:443–457.

2. **Ancora, G., M. Lanari,,T. Lazzarotto, V. Venturi, E.Tridapalli, F. Sandri,, M. Menarini, E. Ferretti, and G. Faldella.** 2007. Cranial ultrasound scanning and prediction of outcome in newborns with congenital cytomegalovirus infection. *J. Pediatr.* **150:**157–161.
3. **Butel, J. S.** 2000. Viral carcinogenesis: revelation of molecular mechanisms and etiology of human disease. *Carcinogenesis* **21:**405–426.
4. **Carson, P. J., P. Konewko, K. S. Wold, P. Mariani, S. Goli, P. Bergloff, and R. D. Crosby.** 2006. Long-term clinical and neuropsychological outcomes of West Nile infection. *Clin. Infect. Dis.* **43:**723–730.
5. **Casals, J., T. S. Elizan, and M. D. Yahr.** 1998. Postencephalitis parkinsonism – a review. *J. Neural Transm.* **105:**645–676.
7. **Chang L.-Y., L.-M., Huang, S. S.-F. Gau, Y.-Y. Wu, S.-H. Hsia, T.-Y. Fan, K.-L. Lin, Y.-C. Huang, C.-Y. Lu, and T.-Y. Lin.** 2007. Neurodevelopment and cognition in children after enterovirus 71 infection. *N. Engl. J. Med.* **356:**1226–1234.
8. **Euscher, E., J. Davis, I. Holzman, and G. J. Nuovo.** 2001. Coxsackie virus infection of the placenta associated with neurodevelopmental delays in the newborn. *Obstet. Gynecol.* **98:**1019–1026.
9. **Gaughan, D. M., M. D. Huges, J. M. Oleske, K. Malee, C. A. Gore, S. Nachman, and the Pediatric AIDS Clinical Trials Group 219C Team.** 2004. Psychiatric hospitalizations among children and youths with human immunodeficiency virus infection. *Pediatrics* **113:**e544–e551.
10. **Gregg, N. M. C. A.** 1941. Congenital cataract following German measles in the mother. *Trans. Ophthalmol. Soc. Aust.* **3:**35–46.
11. **Hogg, J. C.** 1999. Childhood viral infection and the pathogenesis of asthma and chronic obstructive lung disease. *Am. J. Respir. Crit. Care Med.* **160:**S26–S28.
12. **Kesson, A. M.** 2002. Diagnosis and management of paediatric hepatitis C virus infection. *J. Paediatr. Child Health* **38:**213–218.
13. **Kuno, G.** 2001. Persistence of arboviruses and antiviral antibodies in vertebrate hosts: its occurrence and impacts. *Rev. Med. Virol.* **11:**165–190.
14. **Forest, J. M., F. M. Tujrnbull, G. F. Sholler, R. E. Hawker, F. J. Martin, T. T. Doran, and M. A. Burgess.** 2002. Gregg's congenital rubella patients 60 years later. *Med. J. Aust.* **177:**664–667.
15. **Lanzieri, T. M., C. Segatto, M. M. Siqueira, E. C. De Oliveira Santos, L. Jin, and R. Prevots.** 2001. Burden of congenital rubella syndrome after a community-wide rubella outbreak, Rio Branco, Acre, Brazil, 2000 to 2001. *Pediatr. Infect. Dis. J.* **22:**323–329.
16. **Law, M. G., G. J. Dore, N. Bath, S. Thompson, N. Crofts, K. Dolan, W. Giles, P. Gow, J. Kaldor, S. Lovesday, E. Powell, J. Spencer, and A. Wodak.** 2001. Modelling hepatitis C virus incidence, prevalence and long-term sequelae in Australia, 2001. *Int. J. Epidemiol.* **32:**717–724.
17. **Limosin, F., F. Rouillon, C. Payan, J.-M.Cohen, and N. Strub.** Prenatal exposure to influenza as a risk factor for adult schizophrenia. *Acta Psychiatr. Scand.* **107:**331–335.
18. **McIntosh, E. D. G., and M. A. Menser.** 1992. A fifty-year follow-up of congenital rubella. *Lancet* **340:**414–415.
19. **McIntosh, E. D. G., R. C. Givney, J. Zhang, M. A. Burgess, and Y. E. Cossart.** 1998. Molecular epidemiology and variation of hepatitis B virus in recent immigrant families to Australia. *J. Med. Virol.* **56:**10–17.
20. **Menser, M. A., L. Dodd, and J. D. Harley.** 1967. Twenty-five-year follow-up of congenital rubella. *Lancet* **ii:**1347–1350.
21. **Mitsuyama, Y., H. Fukunaga, and S. Takayama.** 1983. Parkinson's disease of post-encephalitic type following general paresis – an autopsied case. *Folia Psychiat. Neurol. Jpn.* **37:**85–93.
22. **Newland, J. G., J. R. Romero, M. Varman, C. Drake, A. Holst, T. Safranek, and K. Subbarao.** 2003. Encephalitis associated with influenza B virus infection in 2 children and a review of the literature. *Clin. Infect. Dis.* **36:**e87–e95.
23. **Noyola, D. E., G. J. Demmler, W. D. Williamson, C. Griesser, S. Sellers, A. Llorente, T. Littman, S. Williams, L. Jarrett, and M. D. Yow.** 2000. Cytomegalovirus urinary excretion and long term outcome in children with congenital cytomegalovirus infection. *Pediatr. Infect. Dis. J.* **19:**505–510.
24. **Rail, D., C. Scholtz, and M. Swash.** 1981. Post-encephalitic parkinsonism: current experience. *J. Neurol. Neurosurg. Psychiatry* **44:**670–676.
25. **Sejvar, J. J.** 2007. The long-term outcomes of human West Nile virus infection. *Clin. Infect. Dis.* **44:**1617–1624.
26. **Sejvar, J. J., J. Hossain, S. K. Saha, E. S. Gurley, S. Banu, J. D. Hamadani, M. A. Faiz, F. M. Siddiui, Q. D. Mohammad, A. H. Mollah, R. Uddin, R. Alam, R. Rahman, C. T. Tan, W. Bellini, P. Rota, R. F. Breiman and S. P. Luby.** 2007. Long-term neurological and functional outcome in Nipah virus infection. *Ann. Neurol.* **62:**235–242.
27. **Szopa, T. M., P. A. Titchener, N. D. Portwood, and K. W. Taylor.** 1993. Diabetes mellitus due to viruses – some recent developments. *Diabetologia* **36:**687–695.
28. **Tam, C. C., S. J. O'Brien, I. Petersen, A. Islam, A. Hayward, and L. C. Rodrigues.** 2007. Guillain-Barré Syndrome and preceding infection with campylobacter, influenza and Epstein-Barr virus in the General Practice Research Database. *PLoS ONE* **2:**e344.
29. **Trojan, D. A., and N. R. Cashman.** 2005. Post-poliomyelitis syndrome. *Muscle Nerve* **31:**6–19.
30. **Vázquez, M., and E. D. Shapiro.** 2005. Varicella vaccine and infection with varicella-zoster virus. *N. Engl. J.Med.* **352:**439–440.
31. **Wennergren, G., and S. Kristjánsson.** 2001. Relationship between respiratory syncytial virus bronchiolitis and future obstructive airway diseases. *Eur. Respir. J.* **18:**1044–1058.

Sequelae and Long-Term Consequences of Infectious Diseases
Edited by Pina M. Fratamico, James L. Smith, and Kim A. Brogden

Chapter 19

Latent Viral Infections

SHIZU HAYASHI, RICHARD G. HEGELE, AND JAMES C. HOGG

Latent viral infections can be defined by the following series of events. As with most viral infections, the virus first successfully infects the host cells at the primary site of infection and produces mild to moderate injury as viral progeny are released. For viruses that develop latent infections, these progeny infect secondary cells which may become the site of latency where replication is restricted until virus-specific external stimuli reactivate the latent genome to replicate and cause further injury. Multiple rounds of this sequence result in recurrent disease which may differ from that caused by the initial primary infection. Latency, therefore, differs from chronic infection, where, in the latter, infectious progeny are always present. Besides complete viral genomes being involved in latency, it is also possible that key sequences of the viral genome are retained within the host cell and cause problems when the appropriate inciting agent is presented to this cell. This possibility, in the case of adenovirus infection, will be discussed separately at the end of this chapter.

Virus pathogens that establish latent infections (Table 1) have double-stranded DNA genomes that are replicated in the host nucleus and include herpesvirus, polyomavirus, papillomavirus, and adenovirus. Members of the *Poxviridae*, such as vaccinia or variola, that causes smallpox also have double-stranded DNA genomes but have evolved to replicate in the cytoplasm of host cells and, as such, might not occupy the cellular compartment required for latency. Human immunodeficiency virus (HIV) is a retrovirus with an RNA genome that is reverse transcribed into DNA before it is integrated into the host genome as proviral DNA. While viral progeny is subsequently produced from RNA transcribed from the integrated viral DNA, the integrated proviral DNA continues to be maintained in a latent form that eludes immune detection. The initiating primary infection with its associated high levels of viremia stimulates a robust immune response, but one which fails to eliminate the latent proviral forms. As this leads to a prolonged period of clinical latency, HIV is more appropriately included in Chapter 21 with the slow viral infections.

For any virus to persist in the host cell, it is imperative that it possess a mechanism to evade immune detection, initially to allow adequate spread of virus, particularly in appropriate host cells, then to conceal viral products required to maintain latency, and finally to permit virus production during reactivation. All viruses that form latent infections have evolved one or many methods to avoid elimination by the host immune system. Some strategies used by latent viruses to evade immune detection and the viruses that employ them are listed in Table 2. Also in the section on human cytomegalovirus (CMV) below, some of the many mechanisms employed by this virus to circumvent host cell immunity are discussed in greater detail.

HERPESVIRIDAE

General Characteristics

As reviewed in reference 171, human herpesviruses include herpes simplex virus type 1 (HSV-1) and -2, CMV, varicella-zoster virus (VZV), Epstein-Barr virus (EBV), and human herpesvirus 6A (HHV-6A), -6B, -7, and -8. Herpesviruses have a linear double-stranded DNA genome, and for the human viruses the DNA are 129 and 236 kilobase pairs for VZV and CMV, respectively. Replication of the viral DNA and the assembly of the icosadeltahedral capsid around this DNA occur in the nucleus of the host cell. The capsid is surrounded by a tegument and then an envelope from the host cell membrane that carries viral glycoprotein spikes on its surface as the virus emerges from the host cell. Destruction of the host cell follows virus production. Virion size ranges from 120 to 200 nm. The viral genome specifies genes required for producing viral progeny, including those of enzymes of nucleic acid metabolism, DNA synthesis, and protein processing. All are able to form

Shizu Hayashi, Richard G. Hegele, and James C. Hogg • James Hogg iCAPTURE Centre for Cardiovascular and Pulmonary Research, University of British Columbia, Vancouver, BC V6Z 1Y6, Canada.

Table 1. General classification and features of the latent human viruses

Family or subfamily	Envelope	Double-stranded DNA	Virus	Genome size (kilobase pairs)[a]
Herpesviridae α	Yes	Linear	Herpes simplex virus 1 (HHV-1)	152
			Herpes simplex virus 2 (HHV-2)	155
			Varicella-zoster virus (HHV-3)	129
Herpesviridae β			Cytomegalovirus (HHV-5)	236
			HHV-6A	160
			HHV-6 B	159
			HHV-7	154
Herpesviridae γ			Epstein-Barr virus (HHV-4)	172
			HHV-8	139
Polyomaviridae	No	Circular	JC virus	5.1
			BK virus	5.1
			Simian virus 40 (nonhuman)	5.2
Papillomaviridae	No	Circular	Human papillomavirus (HPV)	7–8
Adenoviridae	No	Linear	Human adenovirus	36

[a]Based on http://www.ncbi.nlm.nih.gov/sites/entrez.

latent infections in which the viral genome takes the form of a closed circular molecule. Also, the cell type in which each virus becomes latent is specific but varies between viruses and is thus the basis for the differences in clinical diseases that each causes.

The organization of the genes of many of the herpesviruses resembles those of the majority of mammalian genes. They have a promoter upstream of the TATA box; transcription initiation downstream of the TATA box; and a short untranslated leader sequence, followed by an open reading frame initiated with a classic AUG methionine codon; and end with a short 3′ untranslated sequence and the polyadenylation signal. Besides genes required for viral replication, herpesviruses possess genes to allow them to establish latent infections and, equally important, to allow reactivation from the latent state. A single gene product may have multiple but possibly unrelated functions, and some are involved in establishing latency. Besides the bona fide viral genes, many herpesvirus genomes encode at least one gene from the host, and these retain the original cellular function or are altered to fit viral needs.

In the following sections on herpesviruses, which uses HSV as a representative of the family, the molecular aspects of herpes simplex genome organization and its regulation of gene expression will be described in greater detail than the other herpesviruses.

HSV-1 AND HSV-2

General Features

The HSV are members of the α subfamily of herpesviruses. The general features of the two serotypes,

Table 2. Strategies used by latent virus to avoid immune detection[a]

Mechanism	Selected examples
Restricted gene expression	HSV, VZV in latently infected neurons; EBV in B cells
Infection of immune privilege sites or sites inaccessible to immune system	HSV, VZV persistence in neurons; CMV in kidney
Antigenic variation: mutation of antigenic sites required for immune recognition	EBV T-cell escape variants
Interference with antigen processing or presentation	HSV ICP47, HCMV US6, Ad E3-19K proteins interfere with TAP; HCMV pp65 inhibits processing of IE proteins; EBV EBNA-1 inhibits proteasome-mediated processing
Altered MHC expression or trafficking	HCMV US3, Ad E3-19K retention of MHC-I in ER; HCMV US2 reverse translocation of MHC-I from ER to cytoplasm
Suppression of cell surface molecules required for T-cell recognition of MHC class I	Ad E3-19K protein
Inhibition of cytokine expression or function	HCMV, Ad E1A block JAK/STAT signal transduction; EBV EBER, Ad VA RNAs inhibit interferon function; EBV BCRF1 (IL-10 homologue) inhibits IL-2, IFN synthesis, and TAP1 expression.

[a]Modified from reference 214.

HSV-1 and HSV-2, as reviewed in reference 170, are very similar, so they will be discussed together, with any specific and relevant differences in these features that impact on the diseases they cause being noted. The 120-nm-diameter virion consists of a core of double-stranded DNA of about 150 kilobases wrapped as a toroid, an icosahedral capsid around the core, a tegument surrounding the core, and an outer envelope consisting of a lipid bilayer with spikes of viral glycoproteins embedded in it. Since the viral capsid does not contain highly basic proteins to neutralize the negative charges of the viral DNA, polyamine spermidine and spermine bound to the DNA allow its proper folding into the capsule. The virion lipids are similar to those of the cytoplasmic membrane of the host cell.

The viral genome is organized into two regions of unique sequences, designated U_L (long) and U_S (short), bracketed by inverted repeats (223) that are made up of unique sequences and of direct repeats, including multiple copies of these, in which copy numbers can vary. The L and S regions can be inverted relative to each other to give four genomic isomers designated the prototype (no inversion), I_L (inversion of L), I_S (inversion of S), and I_{SL} (inversion of both) (72). Of the about 90 identified transcriptional units, at least 84 encode proteins. Viral transcripts encode single proteins, except in three cases. The exceptions include a single transcript from which open reading frame (ORF) P and ORF O proteins are synthesized from the same methionine but diverge between the 1st and 35th codons; the U_L26 gene that encodes a polypeptide that cleaves itself to yield an amino terminal protease product and the carboxy-terminal ICP35a,b product, which is a component of the capsid scaffolding; and an mRNA that contains the ORFs of U_L1, U_L2, and U_L3 (but the proteins U_L1 and U_L2 are from mRNAs distinct from U_L3) (192). Many clusters of transcriptional units are 3′ coterminal, some ORFs are antisense to each other, and a few instances in which transcripts arise from alternative splicing of an RNA have been identified. Of the two alternatively spliced transcripts, two involve introns within a coding domain. The transcripts that are not expressed as proteins include the latency-associated transcripts. Viral genes are classed as α (immediate early), β (early), and γ (late), depending on their general temporal sequence of expression. The α components are found near the termini of the L and S regions, and the β and γ genes are scattered in both, with the exception of two functional clusters. A β gene cluster that flanks the L origin of DNA synthesis includes genes for DNA polymerase and single-stranded DNA binding protein and a γ gene cluster mapping next to each other in the S sequence specify membrane glycoproteins (gD, gE, gG, gI, and gJ).

Primary Infection and Viral Replication

Primary infection as reviewed in reference 233 occurs through contact, usually in the oropharyngeal region in the case of HSV-1 and through genital contact in the case of HSV-2, of a susceptible seronegative individual with one excreting HSV, in which the virus replicates in the corresponding mucosal cells. It subsequently infects the sensory nerve endings for retrograde transport to a dorsal route ganglion, specifically to the trigeminal for HSV-1 and a sacral ganglion for HSV-2, to establish a latent infection.

Viral entry into the host cell, best described with nonpolarized cells, begins with attachment of a viral envelope glycoprotein, most often gC, to glycosaminoglycans, usually heparin sulfate, on the cell surface (reviewed in reference 170). This is followed by gD binding to a coreceptor, which can be one of several cellular molecules, including nectins, which are immunoglobulin superfamily members expressed by many cell types. Another identified coreceptor is a member of the tumor necrosis factor family, HveA, but it is expressed only by lymphoid cells, while the third is 3-O-sulfated heparin sulfate. Whether the last can mediate entry into humans remains to be determined. Finally, the virus gains entry into the cell by fusion of the viral envelope with the host cell plasma membrane in which participation of gD and the gH-gL heterodimer is implicated. In less studied polarized cell systems, as is the case with human tissues, the same proteins are involved, but differences in participating members are found, depending on whether entry is apical or basolateral. The released capsid along with some of the associated tegument proteins is transported through the microtubular network to the nuclear pores, whereupon interaction with the nuclear pore complex, the capsid together with the tegument components releases the DNA into the nucleus. This DNA rapidly circularizes without the need for additional protein synthesis.

Viral gene transcription by host RNA polymerase II is coordinately regulated in a sequential order by participating viral factors, starting with the α immediate early (1E) genes, where a viral tegument protein VP16 complexed with host cell factors stimulates their transcription. Many of these, in turn, are required for transcription of the β genes, such as those involved in viral DNA replication, for example, the viral DNA polymerase; and in nucleotide metabolism, for example, thymidine kinase; as well as in γ gene expression, which is also stimulated by viral DNA replication. In particular, ICP4 functions in a nonclassical manner as a transcriptional activator but can also function as a repressor, and its multiple posttranscriptionally modified forms might dictate how this protein behaves. The thymidine kinase activity is thought to provide nucleoside triphosphate precursors for DNA synthesis in resting cells, such as neurons, where the homologous cellular enzyme is not expressed. In parallel with this hierarchy of transcriptional control of the viral genome by the viral products, promoters of α genes, in general, contain many binding sites for cellular transcription factors; β promoters possess fewer, and the γ promoters even fewer. Upon infection, HSV inhibits transcription, splicing, and transport of host RNA as well as host protein synthesis. At the same time, many of the other modifications of the viral proteins, other than the aforementioned cleavage and glycosylation, for example phosphorylation, sulfation, myristolylation, ribosylation, and nucleotidylation, rely on host enzymes, but some are virally encoded.

Viral DNA synthesis initiated on circular molecules relies on viral proteins, including DNA polymerase, its processivity factor, an origin-binding protein, the single-stranded DNA binding protein, and a helicase-primase complex of three proteins, as well as unidentified host factors. There are three origins of HSV DNA replication, where the two *oriS* sequences are located in the two inverted repeats, respectively, that bracket the S unique sequence and the third origin, the *oriL* sequence, is located in the L sequence. The bulk of the DNA is synthesized by a rolling-circle mechanism resulting in head-to-tail concatamers. These are then cleaved into full-length monomer genomes and encapsidated by the γ capsid proteins that were transported to the nucleus for capsid assembly. Homologous recombination is very efficient in HSV-infected cells, and recombination between terminal repeats and internal inverted repeats produces the four alignments of the genomic L and S segments.

Preassembled capsids bud through the inner nuclear membrane where the tegument layer is added, and although the details are not clear at this point, this nuclear membrane is eventually replaced by the plasma membrane with the viral glycoproteins. In addition to spreading from one cell to the next through the extracellular space, HSV can spread directly from cell to cell, likely through cell junctions. The gE and gI glycoproteins are required for this mode of spread (42).

For the infected cell, a productive infection results in an enlarged nucleolus that can subsequently fragment. At the same time that the chromatin becomes compacted and marginates, intranuclear inclusion bodies form that are thought to be the viral replication compartments, the nucleus becomes multilobed, the microtubular network undergoes changes, and the cells round up and adhere to each other. In specific cell types, the Golgi fragments (26). Of the host functions, DNA synthesis is shut off, protein synthesis reduced, and glycosylation ceased. Not only is host cell transcription and transcript processing turned off, but existing mRNA is degraded, and cellular proteins can be selectively degraded, or by imposing posttranslational modifications, stabilized or redirected to perform other tasks. Also, HSV infection blocks cell cycle progression even before the stage of host DNA synthesis. The final outcome of productive herpesvirus infection is host cell death. Although primary viral replication can sometimes cause clinical disease and can infrequently lead to more severe central nervous system (CNS) infection, the interaction between virus and host predominantly has subclinical consequences and leads to latent infection.

Latent Infection and Reactivation

Latent infection of HSV (reviewed in references 170 and 233) entails the following sequence of events. The virus enters nerve endings of sensory nerves innervating the infected mucosal epithelium that is producing virus. From the nerve endings, the virus is transported retrograde along the axon in the form of the unenveloped nucleocapsid to the nucleus of these nerve cells where the virus replicates for several days before becoming latent. In latently infected neurons, viral genomes acquire the characteristics of circular DNA (53, 135, 167, 168), and once latent, no replicating virus can be detected in sensory ganglia innervating the site of inoculation (170). This implicates a host immune response that is effective in eliminating virus at the primary site of infection. Latency in the majority of infected neurons could be attributed to the lack of nuclear host factors required for the expression of α genes in the "quiescent" sensory neurons, together with the expression of the transcriptional unit encoding the latency-associated transcripts, which most likely downregulate the α, subsequent β, and γ lytic gene expression. Only a fraction of neurons harboring latent HSV periodically reactivate upon injury or stimulation of cells innervated by latently infected neurons. This is different from the reactivation of VZV where all latently infected cells reactivate at once. Reactivation results in infectious virus that is carried anterogradely to peripheral tissues by axonal transport, usually to cells at or near the site of initial infection (169). It has been shown that the severity of lesions caused by the first infection is reflected in the frequency of reactivations resulting in recrudescences of lesion (170). Although replication of HSV results in destruction of the infected cell, reactivation of latent virus in the sensory neuron does not destroy the host cell. Depending on several factors, including the host immune status, the reactivation may be asymptomatic or lead to a recurrent lesion, which may vary considerably in severity from punctate lesions that are invisible to the naked eye to severe, debilitating lesions in immunosuppressed individuals. Reactivation relies on a cellular cofactor that resides in the cytoplasm and is translocated into the nucleus only under conditions of reactivation to enhance α gene expression (107). Besides recurrence of disease from a reactivated latent infection, reinfection from an external source, also called initial infection, although of low frequency, has been identified by molecular techniques that allow the differentiation of strains of virus.

Host Immunological Response

Virus-specific host humoral responses develop 2 to 6 weeks after the onset of disease and persist for the lifetime of the host (reviewed in reference 233). However, this humoral immunity, together with the associated cell-mediated response by cytotoxic T lymphocytes does not prevent reactivation and disease recurrences or exogenous reinfection. In newborns, the host response to infection is compromised by a host defense mechanism that is not fully mature and consequently, the severity of infection in this population is greater. Transplacentally acquired antibodies from the mother do not totally protect the newborn, and this is consistent with the inadequacies of immune protection from previous infections in preventing recurrence of disease in adults.

Epidemiology of Disease

Neurovirulence and latency are two properties of HSV that influence the human disease which this virus causes (reviewed in reference 233). Infection results most commonly in asymptomatic or mild illness, but in a few cases severe and life-threatening disease ensue. While HSV-1 and -2 are transmitted by different routes and affect different areas of the body, a great deal of overlap is found in the diseases they cause. Infections occur worldwide; humans are the only reservoir of this virus, and transmission is through close physical contact. Since over half the world's population experiences recurrent infections, they are consequently potential transmitters of virus, and no seasonal variations in infection rates are found.

Primary HSV-1 infections occur at a young age (less than 5 years), at which mouth and lips are the most common sites of infection and gingivostomatitis is the usual clinical manifestation. Virus is shed from the mouth and in stool in about 20% of children, ranging in age from 7 months to 2 years, for an average of 7 to 10 days, and neutralizing antibodies appear between 4 and 7 days after the onset of disease and peak at about 3 weeks (24). Virus shedding decreases with age. The most common form of recurrent infections, those caused by reactivation of latent virus, is herpes labialis, with predicted average frequency of recurrence of about 33% per year, and recurrent excretion in the absence of symptoms occurs.

Since HSV-2 infections are usually acquired through sexual contact, primary infections rarely occur before onset of sexual activity. While genital HSV infections can also be attributed to HSV-1, it is less severe and less prone to reoccur. In otherwise healthy women, genital HSV infection occurs in 0.09 to 0.24%; women have higher rates of infection than men, and promiscuity adds further increases. In monogamous relationships, the risk of transmission of HSV-2 from seropositive male to seronegative woman is 20% annually, but 50% from respective female to male, and the risk decreases if the seronegative individual is positive for HSV-1 (21). In the United States, seroprevalence increased 30% in the period from 1976 to 1994, to 22%. As with HSV-1 infection, viral shedding occurs, decreases with age, and can be asymptomatic. Some studies have shown that HSV-2 infections increase infection by HIV-1 and human T-cell lymphotrophic virus type 1.

As with HSV-1 orolabial infections, recurrent HSV-2 infections are frequently asymptomatic. In cases where reactivation of a latent infection occurs in pregnant women, there is the possibility of virus transmission to their infants. Although recurrent infections occurred in 84% of these pregnant women (220), the incidence of cervical viral shedding is low (0.56% and 0.66% in symptomatic and asymptomatic infections, respectively), with rates of transmission of 3% or lower, and transmission from a recurrent infection does not result in neonatal HSV disease. On the other hand, although uncommon, primary and initial (reinfection from external source) infection can become widely disseminated to visceral sites during pregnancy and lead to life-threatening maternal diseases, such as necrotizing hepatitis and encephalitis, with mortality approaching 50% (156). Fetal death, not always associated with maternal death, occurs with equal frequency. With the advent of a safe antiviral acyclovir therapy, treatment is possible if HSV disease is progressive in these women. In primary infections before 20 weeks gestation, spontaneous abortion is reported to be as high as 25% compared to the 20% routine rate of fetal loss. At later times in gestation, primary infections are not associated with spontaneous abortions. The consequences to a fetus born to a mother with primary infection could be either neonatal HSV disease (see below) or severe intrauterine growth retardation (22).

Symptoms and Pathology of Disease

Symptoms and pathology of HSV disease are reviewed in reference 233.

Oropharyngeal disease

Symptoms of a primary infection in children vary greatly from completely asymptomatic, which is most common, to combinations of symptoms, including fever; sore throat; vesicular lesions with a fluid-containing cavity within or beneath the epidermis that is less than 5 mm in diameter and ulcerative lesions; gingivostomatitis with the inside of the mouth and gums affected; edema; localized lymphadenopathy; anorexia, most likely due to the edema of the mucosal membranes and associated pain, and as a result, an inability to eat; and malaise. Primary infections later in life present with pharyngitis associated with a mononucleosis syndrome. (The symptoms and pathology of disease are reviewed in reference 233.)

The vesicular lesions that are found around the mouth and on the junction of the lips and skin (orolabial) ulcerate on an erythematous base and eventually crust over and heal and are indicative of recurrent infections, also popularly called cold sores. On the other hand, the gingival lesions that do not form a scab result from primary infections. Recurrent orolabial lesions are preceded by pain, burning, tingling, and itching for less than 6 hours, followed by the appearance of vesicles for up to 48 hours before they progress to an ulcerative, then crusting, stage, with complete healing in 8 to 10 days.

Genital disease

Genital disease is different from the oropharyngeal form, in that the primary infection causes the most severe disease, while the recurrent form is the mildest. Primary infection is associated with greater numbers of replicating virus and a longer period of viral excretion (3 weeks). Vesicles, pustules, and ulcers appear at the site of infection and last on average for 3 weeks. In women, lesions appearing on the vulva with involvement of the cervix are excruciatingly painful and are associated with possible extragenital lesions of the perineum, buttocks, and vagina. A urinary retention syndrome in 10 to 15% of female patients and aseptic meningitis in 25% occur. In men, lesions appear on the glans penis or the penile shaft with extragenital lesions of the thigh, buttocks, and perineum. Systemic complications are uncommon in men. In both, paresthesias and dysethesias of the lower extremities, fever, localized inguinal adenopathy and dysuria, and malaise can occur. Complications include sacral radioculomyelitis, neuralgias, and meningoencephalitis. In male homosexuals, perianal and anal infections with associated procitis are common.

Exogenous reinfection or initial infections, those occurring despite preexisting antibodies, are less severe, with the number of lesions, severity of pain, and likelihood of complications decreased and quicker healing (within 2 weeks) than that of primary infections. Interestingly, preexisting antibodies to HSV-1 reduce severity of HSV-2 disease, although they do not prevent reinfection.

Recurrent disease is preceded by a prodome and local irritation, limited to a smaller number of vesicles, in men, on the shaft of the penis, and in women, as a vulvar irritation, and these last for 7 to 10 days (3). Virus shedding is limited to 2 to 5 days, with lower concentrations of virus compared to a primary infection. Neurological and systemic complications are uncommon, but paresthesias and dysathesis can occur. Recurrence of genital herpes is frequent and correlates with the severity of the primary infection, although rates of recurrence vary between individuals. Recurrences, whether asymptomatic or symptomatic, are frequent—with one-third of patients experiencing recurrences over nine times per year, another third 4 to 7 times, and the last third, 2 to 3 times—and raise the issue of transmission of infection to the sexual partner.

Neonatal HSV infections

Neonatal HSV infection occurs in 1 of 3,000 to 5,000 deliveries a year (143, 144). Factors affecting transmission of infection to fetus include (i) the type of maternal infection (for which the duration and quantity of viral excretion, as well as the total time to heal, are highest for primary infections and lowest for recurrent infections, and the risk of transmission is 30% and 3%, respectively); (ii) the presence of maternal antibody to HSV, which decreases transmission; (iii) an increasing duration of ruptured membranes, which increases risk of transmission; and (iv) certain forms of medical intervention, for example, the use of fetal monitor scalp electrodes. Transmission can happen in utero from transplacental or ascending infection; intrapartum, which accounts for 75 to 80% of all transmissions to neonates; and postnatally.

Neonatal HSV infections most often are symptomatic and frequently lethal. Intrauterine infections are most severe. Intrapartum or postnatal HSV infection can result in three degrees of increasing disease severity: (i) disease of the skin, eye, and mouth; (ii) encephalitis with or without skin involvement; and (iii) disseminated infection involving multiple organs. The first of these is associated with lower mortality but not without significant morbidity. In infections localized to the skin, vesicle clusters appear in the part of the body in direct contact with virus during birth, and subsequently the rash can spread to other areas of the body. These children and those with eye or mouth infection, present at 10 or 11 days after birth, and those with skin lesions have recurrent infections over the next 6 months. Infections of the eye result in keratoconjuctivitis, or later, chorioretinitis. If the eye is the only site of infection, microphthalmia or retinal dysplasia results. About 30% of children with disease of the skin, eye, and/or mouth develop long-term neurological problems, including spastic quadriplegia, microencephaly, and blindness, and these present between 6 months and 1 year of life. A subclinical infection of the CNS is implied by HSV DNA detectable in the cerebrospinal fluid.

Encephalitis results as a consequence of CNS infection alone or in combination with disseminated disease. About one-third of babies with neonatal HSV have the encephalitis component alone, and infection results most likely from retrograde axonal transport of virus, as opposed to infection by a bloodborne route. Clinical manifestations of encephalitis include seizures, lethargy, irritability, tremors, poor feeding, temperature instability, bulging fontanelle, and pyramidal tract signs. When untreated, death results in 50% of infants with localized CNS disease. The long-term prognosis of CNS infection or disseminated disease is poor, with severe neurological impairment, including psychomotor retardation associated with microencephaly, hydranencephaly, porencephalic cysts, spasticity, blindness, chorioretinitis, or learning disabilities.

Disseminated disease results in the worst prognosis for both morbidity and mortality and accounts for one-half to two-thirds of neonatal HSV infections, although introduction of antiviral therapy has reduced this to 23%. The main organs infected are the liver and adrenals, but most other organs, including the brain as a result of encephalitis, can be affected. Without therapy and as a result of HSV pneumonitis or disseminated intravascular coagulopathy, death occurs in greater than 80%.

Other HSV diseases beyond the newborn age

HSV-1 infection of the eye results in herpetic keratoconjuctivitis associated with photophobia, tearing, eyelid edema, and cheomis, with branching dendritic lesions that are pathognomonic for this disease. Advanced disease is associated with geographic corneal ulcers. Recurrent infections are common, and progressive disease can result in loss of vision.

Skin infections of the digits, known as herpetic whitlow and most common in health care professionals (173) at 2.4 cases in 100,000 individuals per year, could be caused by HSV-1 or -2 (60). In patients with atopic dermatitis, HSV can cause eczema herpeticum, with lesions either localized or disseminated.

Immunocompromised individuals, either as a result of immunotherapy, for example, for organ transplant, an underlying disease such as AIDS, or malnutrition, are at an increased risk for HSV infection. Transplant recipients are at risk for increased severity of infection and may develop progressive disease involving the respiratory tract, esophagus, and even the gastrointestinal tract (103, 141). Reactivation of latent infections can occur at multiple sites (234), and transfer of infection from a transplanted organ has been reported (141).

Infection of the CNS resulting in herpes simplex encephalitis is one of the most common causes of sporadic fatal encephalitis in the western world ((186)). Focal encephalitis is associated with fever, altered consciousness, bizarre behavior, disordered state of mind, and localized neurological findings. In untreated patients, mortality is over 70%, and only 2.5% of all patients regain normal neurological function. With respect to the viral origin, in patients with virologically confirmed encephalitis, 65% of the viral isolates from the brain and orolabial regions were identical, and these were from patients with a primary infection (232). The remaining patients could have recurrent infections.

Besides encephalitis, HSV infections in other areas of the nervous system cause meningitis, myelitis, and radiculitis (reviewed in reference 36). Whether HSV infection of the brain causes chronic degenerative diseases and psychiatric disorders requires further study. A similar situation exists for idiopathic peripheral facial nerve palsy or Bell's palsy, in which the possibility of HSV as an etiological agent was reported in 1972 (132). Since then varicella-zoster infections have been ascribed to the most severe form of palsy, know as the Ramsay-Hunt syndrome, as well as to a subgroup of zoster sine herpete patients in whom no cutaneous abnormality is present but serological evidence of asymptomatic VZV reactivation is present (reviewed in reference 197). About half of the more recent studies of Bell's palsy patients support HSV as a possible causative agent. For example, reactivation of HSV-1 was determined by virological examination in 15% of the patients (94); HSV-1/HSV-2 DNA was determined by PCR in tear and saliva samples from 31% of the patients, with an increase in viral DNA after the onset of disease in 29% (1); in samples collected 5 days after the onset of palsy, PCR of saliva together with serology showed HSV-1 reactivation in 32% patients, excluding those diagnosed with Ramsay-Hunt syndrome or zoster sine herpete (57); and a significantly higher prevalence of shed HSV-1 was found in saliva of palsy patients than in that of healthy volunteers, and a significantly higher prevalence of shed HSV-1 was found in saliva of palsy patients collected within 2 weeks after the onset of disease than in that of healthy volunteers, as well as compared to patients with Ramsay Hunt syndrome when palsy patients' saliva samples were tested within 7 days after the onset of palsy (56). Recent investigations of Bell's palsy patients that do not support this viral etiology include the inability to identify HSV-1/HSV-2 nucleic acid by PCR in cerebral spinal fluid from these patients (91, 200), in the postauricular muscle (200), or in facial muscle biopsy specimens and tear samples, while controls without facial palsy, although negative in the aforementioned tissues and the ganglion scarpae, were HSV-1/HSV-2 positive (82%) with respect to the geniculate ganglion (115). Results from the above studies, both supporting and not supporting HSV, should be evaluated in the light of studies on cranial nerve ganglia (trigeminal, geniculate, vestibular, spiral, and vagal ganglia) from a random population sample in which 42% were positive for HSV by PCR (221).

VZV

General Features

Like HSV, VZV (reviewed in reference 30) is a member of the α subfamily of herpesviruses and shares the property of replicating and spreading efficiently, of destroying the host cell upon replication, and of establishing a life-long latent infection of sensory nerve ganglia from which it can reactivate one or more times. However, unlike HSV, VZV has a much narrower host range that is limited to cells of human and simian origin. This virus infects the skin, mucous membranes, viscera, and nervous system. Virus particles are similar to that of other herpesviruses and consist of the core, with a linear double-stranded DNA of approximately 129 kilobase pairs; the nucleocapsid; the tegument; and the envelope. Each of the four components shares features with those found in HSV. Furthermore, like HSV, the genome is organized into unique long and short sequences, each bracketed by terminal repeats and internal repeats, and while inversions of the unique sequences also occur, inversions of the shorter of them predominate, to yield two isomeric forms. At least 70 unique genes are encoded in the genome; many are 3′ coterminal, 11 have overlapping reading frames, and the large tracts that are collinear with HSV support the many homologous genes between the two viruses. The proteins from many of these common genes, however, have strikingly different properties. VZV also shares at least 40 conserved genes with the other human herpesviruses.

Infection of cells parallels HSV infection and begins with the attachment of viral envelope glycoproteins to the receptors on the plasma membrane, followed by fusion with the plasma membrane, release of the capsid and its transport to the nuclear membrane where the DNA is released into the nucleus, and replication of the viral DNA as a result of the transcriptional repertoire that regulates sequential expression of immediate early, early, and late genes. It culminates in capsid assembly and subsequent release of the enveloped virus. Also, the consequence of productive infection is lysis of the infected cell. However, unlike HSV, VZV does not shut off host protein synthesis.

Primary Infection

As reviewed in reference 8, varicella, also called chicken pox, results from a multistep primary infection initiated by exposure of the mucous membranes of the respiratory tract to respiratory droplets or from contact with vesicular fluid from an infected individual. The virus is thought to spread to regional lymph nodes and subsequently to liver and other cells of the reticuloendothelial system, where a primary viremia results after viral replication. A secondary viremia occurs as a result of replication in peripheral blood mononuclear cells, possibly T lymphocytes, and allows the infection to spread hematogenously to cutaneous epithelial cells. Therefore, unlike HSV, VZV has the potential to disseminate throughout the body during a primary infection. This highly contagious infection, which mainly occurs in childhood, results in febrile illness and produces a generalized pruritic vesicular rash. VZV-specific host immune response prevents further viral replication. However, if viral replication from a primary infection is not controlled adequately, a progressive disseminated infection involving the lungs, liver, CNS, and other organs can lead to pneumonia (lungs), hepatic failure (liver), and encephalitis or cerebellar ataxia (CNS).

Latent Infection and Reactivation

VZV is thought to spread from mucocutaneous lesions by anterograde neural transport to the sensory nerve ganglia innervating the affected site, including the trigeminal, geniculate, and many dorsal root ganglia as well as the olfactory bulbs to establish latency. The virus resides predominantly in neuronal cells in the ganglia, but the possible involvement of both neuronal and nonneuronal cells (121, 225) suggests a difference between VZV latency and that of HSV. Also, VZV latency which involves multiple genes is different from latency-associated transcript-based HSV latency and raises questions concerning avoidance of immune surveillance by VZV. Reactivation is usually observed with elderly or immunocompromised patients. Herpes zoster is a vesicular rash restricted to a dermatomal distribution which reflects transport along multiple axons of a single sensory nerve. In immunocompetent individuals, second episodes of herpes zoster, unlike HSV reactivation, are rare, most likely due to a robust and immediate immune response. Acute VZV reactivation produces severe, acute pain and may progress to the chronic syndrome called *postherpetic neuralgia* (229). Inflammation of the dorsal root ganglia, motor and sensory roots, neuritis, and segmental myelitis occurs. Further spread of virus in the CNS can lead to encephalitis. Other complications of herpes zoster result from reactivation in specific nerves. Reactivation in the trigeminal ganglion can cause conjunctivitis, dendritic keratitis, anterior uveitis, iridocyclitis with secondary glaucoma, retinitis and panophthalmitis, and a loss of vision but not blindness, as a result of retrobulbar neuritis and optic atrophy. Reactivation in the geniculate ganglion of the seventh and eight cranial nerve causes the Ramsay-Hunt syndrome of facial palsy and in the second branch of the fifth cranial nerve produces oral lesions. Lumbosacral herpes zoster can cause neurogenic bladder dysfunction or ileus with intestinal obstruction, and chronic paralysis of an extremity can result from herpes zoster. In immunocompromised individuals, VZV reactivation results in a more extensive dermatomal rash, and cutaneous replication is often accompanied by cell-associated viremia. Subsequent spread hematogenously (215) can lead to the same pathologic consequences as those in patients with progressive varicella.

Treatment

Live attenuated varicella vaccine, the first human herpesvirus vaccine licensed for clinical use and offering protection against disease in 85 to 95% of exposures, is recommended for routine vaccination in childhood and for susceptible older children and adults. For treatment of complications of varicella and herpes zoster, nucleoside analogues, for example acyclovir, are effective in reducing clinical severity in many cases.

CMV

General Features

Human CMV (reviewed in reference 138) is a member of the β subfamily of herpesviruses. Characteristics it shares with other herpes viruses are those of virion structure, including the core with a linear double-stranded DNA of 236 kilobase pairs, an icosahedral nucleocapsid, the tegument, and the envelope; the ability to establish life-long latent infections; and amino acid homology in 46 viral ORFs controlling DNA replication, genome packaging, and virion morphogenesis. Shared features, more specifically with the β viruses, include salivary gland tropism, strict species specificity, slow growth in cultured cells, and amino acid homology in a core set of 70 to 80 common ORFs, despite divergent nucleotide sequences. Its genome can be divided into terminal repeats and internal repeats that bracket the long and short unique regions which can undergo inversion, as in HSV. Besides the single copy of genomic DNA, the virion contains two classes of RNA, one which forms a hybrid with the origin of replication and the other which is found within the tegument and is expressed after entry into host cells. Two other forms of viral particles, besides the infective virion, are produced: a noninfectious enveloped capsid lacking an electron-dense DNA core and dense bodies that comprise several tegument proteins within an envelope without nucleocapsid or DNA. At least 213 or so known genes have had functional assignments, and the 46 that are dispensable for viral replication may contribute to optimizing growth, dissemination, tissue tropism, immune evasion, and pathogenesis in the host.

The human CMV replication cycle, especially the early events, are only partially understood but, as with other herpesviruses discussed above, relies on attachment of viral envelope glycoproteins to the receptors on the plasma membrane of the host cell, which includes interaction with heparin sulfate, then fusion of the membranes and penetration of the cell surface, transport of the released nucleocapsid to the nuclear membrane where the DNA is released into the nucleus, and replication of the viral DNA as a result of the coordinated expression of immediate early, early, and late viral genes. The viral genome is replicated via a rolling circle type of replication process from the single origin of replication that carries the stably hybridized RNA. The DNA is then cleaved and packaged into capsids. The nucleocapsids that accumulate in the nucleus form the inclusions observable by light microscopy as the typical "owl's eye" (Color Plate 15). Envelopment occurs at the nuclear membrane or by a de-envelopment and re-envelopment process involving budding into cytoplasmic vesicles. Virions are released by exocytosis of these vesicles.

Primary Infection

Primary infections of CMV, mainly in childhood, result from direct contact of the mucosal epithelium of the genitourinary tract, upper alimentary tract, or respiratory tract with secretions from an infected individual. Replication in the mucosal epithelium leads to a systemic infection in which virus is absent in the blood but replicates in leukocytes (164, 240). The virus is further distributed to hematopoietic cells, endothelium, and epithelium, including ductal epithelium, so that virus, shed in all bodily secretions, including breast milk, can be transmitted. The primary infection with its accompanying viremia continues for at least 6 months in adults (164, 240) to several years in young children (154), despite a robust host immune response. Recent popular use of day care centers, taken together with this extended secretion of virus from infected individuals, renders these facilities a major source of infection (4). After this long period of persistence, the primary infection is cleared but the virus remains latent in hematopoietic cells of the myeloid lineage. The primary infection, which is usually restricted to a mild disease by host innate and adaptive immunity, primes a lifelong latency from which reactivation can occur, again with little disease consequence.

Human CMV has evolved numerous intricate and effective strategies to evade and modulate the host immune response, particularly cell-mediated immunity provided by natural killer cells and cytotoxic T lymphocytes, but these will not be presented in detail in this chapter. The importance of these viral functions, nonetheless, should be emphasized since they allow the virus to prolong the primary infection by impeding viral clearance, to establish latency, to reactivate successfully from latency, and, also, to alter the course of disease. At the same time, many of the genes that provide these functions are dispensable for viral replication. Several genes downregulate major histocompatibility complex (MHC) class I expression (238), each affecting different steps in the pathway that leads to mature cell surface MHC expression, while others downregulate interferon-induced MHC class II expression (137) and do so, again, by targeting different steps in the process of class II expression. Among the mechanisms employed by the virus is expression of a number of cellular homologues, for example, a functional viral interleukin 10 (IL-10) (106), an anti-inflammatory molecule; an MHC class I heavy-chain homologue (23) that prevents effective natural killer cell responses; and virus-encoded chemokines directed at leukocytes (158) and chemokine receptors (27), to name a few.

While CMV primary infections are, as a rule, clinically considered asymptomatic, they account for about 8% of all cases of mononucleosis. Like the EBV-induced disease, malaise, headache, and fatigue are common, with clinical findings of fever that lasts on average for 2 weeks, cervical adenopathy, pharyngitis, splenomegaly, elevated liver enzymes, and lymphocytosis with atypical lymphocytes (153). Complications such as Guillain-Barré syndrome, peripheral neuropathy, meningoencephalitis, Rasmussen encephalitis, myocarditis, hemolytic anemia, thrombocytopenia, retinitis, gastrointestinal ulceration, hepatitis, and pneumonitis have been reported.

Latent Infection and Reactivation

CMV remains latent in the nucleus of a small percentage of lineage-committed myeloid cells in the form of closed circular viral DNA, from which latency-associated transcripts are known to be expressed. However, it is not known whether these transcripts or their expected protein products, for which antibodies can be detected in sera of healthy CMV seropositive individuals (111), are required for the establishment or maintenance of latency. Viral latent gene expression changes as the host cells differentiate as a consequence of proinflammatory stimuli, and this maturation process supports reactivation of latent virus. Reactivation, which causes more serious disease than a primary infection in immunocompromised individuals, results in an interplay of the following: differentiation of latently infected cells by cytokine stimulation to a more permissive phenotype, reduced immune surveillance to allow viral replication and subsequent systemic spread, and compromising disease states that can develop in these patients. The possibility that a persistent infection of replication-competent virus, albeit at a low level and possibly in a different cell type, could exist alongside a latent infection needs to be investigated further.

CMV Infection in the Immunocompromised Host

CMV is distributed widely, but recent improvements in hygiene have limited the virus to only 40 to 60% of the population in developed countries. This raises the risk of congenital transmission and its consequences. Of similar clinical relevance, the ever increasing numbers of immunosuppressed individuals in recent years, mainly after transplantation but also as a result of AIDS, have increased the number of those predisposed to primary infections or reactivation of CMV with much more serious consequences. In the case of organ transplantations, the source of the virus could be the donor organ, possibly after reactivation of a latent infection. Infection with CMV is common in any population because it can occur from a primary infection, by reactivation of latent virus, or by reinfection in those with a previous infection. Infection in immunocompromised individuals is equally, if not more, frequent, especially in transplant or transfusion recipients exposed to donor tissue with either a primary or latent infection. However, depending on the degree of immunosuppression, the infection can be clinically undetected, and when disease occurs, it can be self limited to minor illness or progress to involve multiple organs and be life threatening.

CMV infection of the fetus (153) is most likely from hematogenous spread from infected placental cells either from a recurrent or primary infection of the mother; the rate of fetal infection from mothers who were infected with CMV more than a year prior to conception is 2.2%. The ability of the virus to disseminate to multiple developing organs and to infect many cell types is especially critical in the CNS, where infection of most cell types could damage the developing brain by lysis of infected cells, including stem cells; by interference of neuronal migration; or by vascular compromise. The majority (50 to 90%) of symptomatic newborns are affected by a combination of mental retardation, cerebral palsy, sensorineural hearing loss and impaired vision, while only 7 to 25% of asymptomatic infants are affected. Congenital CMV infection has been estimated to be the leading cause of sensorineural deafness and the leading infectious cause of brain damage in children. Infection-inflicted damage of the liver, kidney, and glandular epithelial cells and, although cytomegalic cells are not found in spleen and bone marrow, hemolytic anemia and thrombocytopenia are observed in cases of congenital CMV infection. Although abnormalities of jaundice, hepatitis, hepatosplenomegaly, petechiae, and thrombocytopenia, due to the reticuloendothelial system, clear within a few weeks, disease can be severe and results in neonatal death in about 10% of symptomatic infections. In contrast to the morbidity and mortality of congenital CMV infections, the infection from intrapartum transmission that occurs at birth (165) and postnatal infection that can be attributed to exposure to maternal secretions, most likely in mother's milk (44), are rarely associated with clinical disease.

In solid organ transplantations (153), primary infection from the transplanted organ is generally more severe than that of reactivation or reinfection. The most common symptoms are fever, leucopenia, malaise, arthalgias, and macular rash. Patients in whom these symptoms do not resolve can develop pneumonitis, gastrointestinal ulceration, severe hepatic dysfunction, or opportunistic fungal infection, and, most consistently, impaired graft function.

As with solid-organ transplantation, the main source of CMV in bone marrow transplant patients is reactivation of endogenous virus or transplanted cells or blood products from the donor, so that the seropositivity for CMV of the recipient and donor are significant risk factors (153). Pneumonitis is the most common CMV disease of clinical relevance, while gastrointestinal disease alone or together with pneumonia also occur as well as hepatitis, encephalitis, and retinitis, but less frequently. Deaths from CMV infection have continued to decrease in recent times to very low levels, most likely due to recent efforts to prevent transfusion-acquired CMV infection in seronegative patients, reduce graft-versus-host disease, improve rapid and effective CMV diagnosis and prediction of patients at risk, and apply timely and effective antiviral agents.

The possibility that CMV infection and/or reactivation play a role in atherosclerosis has been suggested. CMV seropositivity in coronary angioplasty patients was associated with posttransplant coronary artery restenosis (241), and CMV infection in immunosuppressed cardiac transplant patients, with higher rates of graft rejection, more severe graft atherosclerosis, higher mortality (67), and greater risk of coronary artery disease in the cardiac graft (133). However, the role of CMV in this disease needs to be reevaluated in light of the high number of patients with coronary artery disease but without CMV infection and the fact that the age of most patients requiring cardiac transplants is long past the early age of viral acquisition (153).

CMV is an important opportunistic infectious agent in both adults and children with HIV infection, particularly those with AIDS, and the risk of developing CMV disease is linked to immune status, as reflected in low $CD4^+$ T-lymphocyte counts (153). Diseases caused by CMV in these patients are, in order of decreasing frequency, retinitis, esophagitis, and colitis, with the combination of retinitis and esophagitis also occurring. Less common are encephalitis, peripheral neuropathy, polyradiculoneuritis, pneumonitis, gastritis, and hepatitis. The question of whether CMV advances the progression of AIDS remains unsettled, but it is clearer that reduction of HIV-1 viral load by antiretroviral agents is associated with a reduction in CMV viremia and disease (40, 150).

HHV-6 (VARIANTS A AND B) AND -7

General Features

HHV-6A, -6B, and -7 are members of the *Roseolovirus* genus of the β subfamily of herpesviruses (157). The properties they share with other members of the herpesviruses include virion structure; a linear double-stranded genome, in this case of 154 to 160 kilobase pairs; genes conserved among the other herpesviruses; high prevalence in their natural host; the general features of the lytic replication cycle; and the ability to establish latent infections. Properties that they share with the more extensively studied member of the β subfamily, CMV, are genomes that are genetically collinear, with several of the genes found only in this subfamily, and a generally prolonged replication cycle. They are, however, distinct from their relatives, with a genome organization comprising one central unique segment bracketed by a pair of direct repeat sequences, instead of the usual long and short unique regions, and the direct repeats of HHV-6 contain sequences similar to those found at the telomeres of mammalian chromosomes. These telomere-like sequences could mediate site-specific integration of HHV-6 genomes into host chromosomes at their telomeres (38). Other differences are a cluster of genes unique to roseoloviruses; their growth mainly in T lymphocytes, although the viruses are detected in other cell types (see below); high prevalence; and association with a febrile rash illness. The HHV-6A and -B variants are closely related but show differences with respect to cell tropism, interactions with cells and with the signaling pathways of the immune system, DNA sequence, and epidemiology (157). HHV-6B and HHV-7 cause exanthema subitum, also known as roseola (207, 237).

Replication of Virus

One of the cellular receptors for HHV-6 is CD46 (182), which is also the receptor for measles virus, although it alone does not confer infectivity in all human cell types. One of the receptors for HHV-7 is CD4 (123). Gene expression patterns follow those of other herpesviruses and include sequential expression of immediate early genes that do not require de novo protein synthesis, then the early genes required for DNA replication, and finally the late genes that encode among others, viral structural proteins. DNA replication is initiated at one origin that is more similar to other β viruses. After the rolling-circle type of viral replication, unit length genomes are packaged into nucleocapsid in the nucleus. By a process of envelopment, de-envelopment, and re-envelopment, the virion proceeds from the nucleus, through the endoplasmic reticulum to the Golgi, where viral glycoproteins are acquired and are, thereafter, released by exocytosis or cell lysis (211). Both HHV-6 and -7 induce a cytopathic effect on infected cells.

Primary Infection and Disease

Infections by these ubiquitous viruses occur mainly in childhood, primarily in the first 6 months after birth (149, 208), through close contact with infected individuals, mainly by transmission through saliva; as well as during pregnancy, when newborns are infected by intrauterine or transvaginal transmission; and during pediatric transplantation (236). In the very few cases of exanthema subitum in which HHV-7 was isolated, virus was found in peripheral blood mononuclear cells (207). Exanthema subituma is caused by HHV-6B and HHV-7 and has features of sudden fever that lasts a few days and a rash appearing on the trunk and face that spreads to the lower extremities; HHV-6A infections are rare. Asymptomatic primary infections do occur. Associated symptoms and complications (reviewed in reference 236) include febrile convulsions associated with HHV-6 or HHV-7 persistence in the CNS and a risk of developing meningitis and encephalitis and, for HHV-6, mild liver dysfunction, although fatal or chronic hepatitis has also been reported. Primary infections in adults can cause a mononucleosis-like illness and hemophagocytic syndrome.

Latent Infection, Reactivation, and Disease

Various cells types have been implicated as harboring latent virus. For HHV-6, these are peripheral blood mononuclear cells, particularly in monocytes (102), and early bone marrow progenitors (122). The salivary glands, CNS, kidneys, lungs, and cervix of pregnant women are also HHV-6 positive. HHV-7 latently infects cells similar to HHV-6 and includes $CD4^+$ lymphocytes. Clinical diseases, as a consequence of latent virus reactivation, occur primarily in immunosuppressed individuals. Asymptomatic HHV-6 reactivation is common after allogeneic bone marrow transplantation (34), but febrile illness, rash, bone, marrow suppression, encephalitis (43), pneumonitis, and increased severity of acute graft-versus-host disease (33) are reported. Also, primary infections that are self limiting occur (34). With respect to solid-organ transplantation, HHV-6 is associated with transplant rejection after kidney transplantation (148, 222); with skin rash, severe cytopenia, interstitial pneumonitis, febrile illness with life-threatening thrombocytopenia and progressive encephalopathy after liver transplantation (193, 194); and, along with HHV-7, with concurrent CMV disease complications after kidney and liver transplantation (reviewed in reference 236). Evidence has been presented that HHV-6 is possibly associated with interstitial pneumonia (99), encephalitis (180), and retinitis (160) in AIDS patients and that this virus plays an enhancing role in HIV disease (48, 104). Whether HHV-6 is the causative agent in pityriasis rosea, a common papulosquamous skin disorder (29, 105, 228); any malignancies (reviewed in reference 236); chronic fatigue syndrome (100, 224); or multiple sclerosis (2, 213) remains unresolved. With respect to drug-induced hypersensitivity syndrome, a recent study demonstrates that reactivation of other members of the herpesviruses beside HHV-6 may contribute to this disease (188).

EBV

General Features

EBV, also known as HHV-4, is a member of the γ subfamily of potentially oncogenic herpesviruses (98) and was the first candidate human tumor virus described (50). Like other herpesviruses, it has a virion structure that includes a core with a linear double-stranded DNA of 172 kilobase pairs, an icosahedral nucleocapsid, the tegument, and an outer envelope with external glycoprotein spikes; and the ability to establish life-long latent infections as well as expression of several glycoproteins that are homologous to those of well-conserved glycoproteins of other herpesviruses. Its genome organization is reminiscent of that of other herpesviruses and consists of one short and one long mostly unique sequence bounded by terminal and internal repeats. Unlike HSV with three origins of replication, in lytic infections EBV uses two origins of viral DNA replication located at either end of the long unique sequence.

Primary Infection

Most children in the developing world are infected with EBV within the first 3 years of life, and seropositivity reaches 100% by the time they are 10 years old compared to 50% in developed countries (166). These early, usually asymptomatic primary infections are most likely transmitted from parents by the oral route (66), while later acquisition is from intimate oral contact during adolescence, which can result in infectious mononucleosis. Many of the following details of EBV infection are based on studies of infectious mononucleosis and as such may not reflect viral infection in asymptomatic individuals. Also, the events of a primary infection are not completely resolved, with, on one hand, the oropharyngeal epithelium as the primary target (195) and subsequent transfer to B lymphocytes where latency is established, and with on the other, B cells as the targets (51) in an environment that supports their lytic infection from which virus establishes latency. The primary lytic infection is resolved by a robust and primarily $CD8^+$ T-lymphocyte response, but residual viral shedding can continue.

Latent Infection

EBV colonizes the B-lymphoid system, and its expression of six Epstein-Barr nuclear antigens (EBNAs), two latent integral membrane proteins (LMPs), two small nonpolyadenylated RNAs (or EBERs), and highly spliced BamHI A rightward transcripts maintains the latent state of nonpermissive lytic viral replication—that is, the presence of the latent episomal circular form of the viral genome—and, particularly in lymphoid tissue, transforms the previously resting B lymphocytes to cells capable of continuous proliferation (166). Reactivation from latency can occur at mucosal epithelium infiltrated by these B cells, now expressing only EBERs, LMP2A, and the BamHI A transcripts in a reversion to the resting memory B-cell phenotype when they circulate in the peripheral blood and lymphoid tissues of asymptomatic carriers. Most adults have been infected with EBV, intermittently shed virus in their saliva, and carry the virus in the latent state in their peripheral blood B lymphocytes (146).

Viral Evasion Strategies

The strategies that EBV has evolved to evade host immune responses are as varied as those of CMV, except that they are targeted to B-lymphocyte host cells. They include, among others, mechanisms to downregulate expression of viral antigens on circulating infected B cells, expression of soluble receptor for a host ligand required for alpha interferon release (202), and expression of a viral homologue of IL-10 (116). One of the functions of viral LMP-1 is to upregulate expression of HLA class I and the transporters that supply these HLA molecules with viral peptides (176) and thus enhance immune detection, appearing contradictory to viral survival.

On the other hand, it can be viewed as advantageous since immune recognition of virally infected cells is necessary to prevent the fatal consequences to the host of the latency-induced lymphoproliferative disease.

Diseases Caused by EBV

Nonmalignant diseases

Primary EBV infections in adolescence or early adult life manifest as infectious mononucleosis in up to 50% of these individuals (166). Symptoms including mild transient fever for several weeks with pharyngitis, lymphadenopathy, and general malaise are not considered emanating from viral replication but from proinflammatory cytokines produced by a large number of reactive T cells. The disease almost always resolves to an asymptomatic carrier state, but complications from the combined effects of infiltrating B cells and reactive T cells can occur and include interstitial nephritis, hepatitis, and pneumonia. Symptoms of recurrent fever, lymphadenopathy, and hepatosplenomegaly over several years can occur in younger children as a result of a primary infection, most likely one that is not resolved.

Other nonmalignant diseases associated with EBV include the X-linked lymphoproliferative syndrome (XLP), a rare familial condition, in which the mutated XLP gene whose product normally functions in the cell-mediated response to EBV no longer confers this immunity. Thus, affected boys are extremely sensitive to EBV, with a hyperacute infectious mononucleosis-like syndrome that culminates in liver failure and death as a result of widespread lymphocytic infiltration and hepatic necrosis. EBV-associated hemophagocytic syndrome is also a rare condition that leads to a common outcome with XLP, but the primary infection, in this case, leads to a virus-driven T-cell proliferation. Oral leukoplakia is a wart-like lesion on the lateral borders of the tongue that develops when lytic cycle antigens from replicating EBV either prolong the life of the infected cells through anti-apoptotic mechanisms (74) or disrupt epithelial cell differentiation (39). These lesions, which occur in immunocompromised HIV carriers, transplant patients, and occasionally in healthy individuals, respond well to treatment with acyclovir but can recur on withdrawal of treatment.

Whether EBV is associated with the lung disease idiopathic pulmonary fibrosis is still controversial. Expression of viral capsid antigen and glycoprotein gp340/220 in type II alveolar epithelial cells in 70% of patients but only in 2% of controls (45) was confirmed in another study along with a demonstration of viral DNA (199). In contrast, results of immunostaining for three different viral antigens, in situ hybridization for EBV RNA and PCR for EBV DNA, did not support the previous results (226). Of patients with lymphocytic interstitial pneumonia, a diffuse lymphoid proliferation affecting the interstitial space on the lung, 64% were positive for EBV by in situ hybridization of lung samples compared to 20% of patients with idiopathic pulmonary fibrosis. The interstitial infiltrate in the former were primarily made up of B lymphocytes (11). Since it has been shown that infected B cells traffic to the lung (6), whether these cells could be the source of viral transmission to the lung needs further investigation.

Malignancies associated with EBV

EBV is now firmly linked to seven types of human malignancies (Table 3) in which the viral genome is detected in a significant proportion of tumors of the relevant histological subtype and the genome is present in every tumor cell in virus-positive cases (166). Burkitt's lymphoma (125) has a B-lymphoid origin, most likely germinal center B cells. The endemic form with a very high incidence of 5 to 10 cases/10^5 per year is geographically distributed in areas with intense *Plasmodium falciparum* malaria, namely equatorial Africa and New Guinea. This form of Burkitt's lymphoma is a childhood malignancy with an unusual pattern of presentation at extranodal sites. All tumors carry monoclonal EBV episomes, are monoclonal with respect to rearrangement of the immunoglobulin (Ig) locus, and carry one of three translocations between the c-myc locus on chromosome 8 and either the Ig locus on chromosome 14 or the light-chain locus on chromosome 2 or 22. The sporadic form of Burkitt's lymphoma is a rare childhood lymphoma that occurs worldwide. Compared to the endemic form, its incidence is 50- to 100-fold lower, its association with the EBV genome is less consistent, and the tumors occur in older children and appear more frequently as an abdominal mass, and occasionally as a leukemia. A third form appears in HIV-infected individuals, has a presentation more akin to the sporadic type, and although it has a much higher incidence in this population than those of either childhood forms, its association with EBV is lower.

Hodgkin's disease is a lymphoma with a reactive infiltrate of nonmalignant cells making up 98% of the mass, and the remaining cells are malignant mononuclear Hodgkin and multinuclear Reed-Sternberg cells that have a postgerminal center B-cell origin (108). Based on the ratio of malignant to reactive cells and the composition of the infiltrate, four histologic subtypes, nodular sclerosing (ns), mixed cellularity (mc),

Table 3. Summary of EBV-associated malignancies[a]

Tumor	Subtype	Latent period	EBV genome +ve (%)	Cell origin
Burkitt's lymphoma	Endemic	3–8 yr post-EBV	100	Lymphoid B cell
	Sporadic	3–8 yr post-EBV	15–85	
	AIDS associated	3–8 yr post-HIV	30–40	
Hodgkin's disease	Mixed cell, lymphocyte depleted	>10 yr post-EBV	60–80	Postgerminal center B cell
	Nodular sclerosing	>10 yr post-EBV	20–40	
Posttransplant lymphoma	Immunodeficiency	<3 mo post-EBV	100	B cell
	Posttransplant	<1 yr posttransplant	>90	
	AIDS associated	>8 yr post-HIV	>80	
T-cell lymphoma	Virus-associated hemophagocytic syndrome	1 or 2 yr post-EBV	100	CD4+ or CD8+ T cells
	Nasal NK/T-cell lymphoma	>30 yr post-EBV	100	NK or T cells
Nasopharyngeal carcinoma	Nonkeratinizing	>30 yr post-EBV	100	Epithelial
	Keratinizing	>30 yr post-EBV	30–100	
Gastric carcinoma	UCNT[b]	>30 yr post-EBV	100	Epithelial
	Adenocarcinoma	>30 yr post-EBV	5–15	
Leiomyosarcoma	Immunodeficiency	Not available	≥50	Smooth muscle
	Posttransplant	<5.5 yr posttransplant	≥50	
	AIDS-associated	<5 yr post-AIDS diagnosis	100	

[a]Modified from reference 166.
[b]UCNT, undifferentiated carcinomas of the nasopharyngeal type.

lymphocyte depleted (ld), and lymphocyte predominant (lp), are used to classify this disease, and the first three are referred to as classic Hodgkin's. Classic Hodgkin's disease has a worldwide distribution, but in the western world disease incidence is low in childhood, with a peak of the ns form of disease in young adults. This difference suggests a delayed exposure in the West to an infectious agent in young adults (124), as seen with EBV in infectious mononucleosis. Indeed, monoclonal EBV genomes in tumor biopsy samples (231) and localization of EBV DNA to the malignant cells (230), as well as the viral genome in every malignant cell in virus-positive cases and the same viral episome at every site in a patient with multiple lesions (230) have been reported. Although the frequency of tumor cells with the EBV genome is high in Hodgkin's disease, the role of this virus in the pathogenesis of this disease is not completely understood. Also, the existence of EBV-negative Hodgkin's implies that other etiologies can produce lymphomas with similar phenotypes.

Other B-cell lymphomas that are EBV positive include those arising at sites of long-term inflammation (35, 183). Another association involves rare cases of chronic lymphocytic leukemia in which cells are transformed to a Hodgkin's–Reed-Sternberg-like phenotype and have the potential to progress to classic EBV-positive Hodgkin's disease (140).

Several T-cell lymphomas associated with EBV have been identified. Virus-associated hemophagocytic T-cell lymphoma originates from mature CD4+ and CD8+ lymphocytes, most frequently in Southeast Asian children after an acute primary EBV infection or with chronic active EBV infection (90, 204). The extranodal nasal NK/T-cell lymphoma, again most common in Southeast Asia, presents in the nasal cavity, causes erosion of bone tissue and is EBV positive (71, 151). Some of these tumors are of T-cell origin, while others have characteristics of NK cells. Other EBV-positive T- or NK cell tumors have been reported and reviewed in reference 203.

Nasopharyngeal carcinoma is a tumor of the nasopharyngeal epithelium and is classified as either keratinizing with clear evidence of squamous differentiation or nonkeratinizing with poorly differentiated or undifferentiated epithelial cells (reviewed in reference 86). While nasopharyngeal carcinoma is a rare tumor in Europe and North America with an incidence of 0.5 cases/10^5 per year, it can be 50 times more common in Southeast Asia, among the Inuit, and in some North and East African populations. In the higher-incidence populations, the tumors are of the nonkeratinizing type and preferentially affect middle-aged men. All tumors of the nonkeratinizing form have been found to be EBV positive, as are most of the rarer keratinizing forms of tumors in Southeast Asia and about 30% of these in European populations. An example of EBV-positive cells in nasopharyngeal carcinoma is shown in Fig. 1. Although antibody titers to lytic cycle antigens increase in proportion to tumor

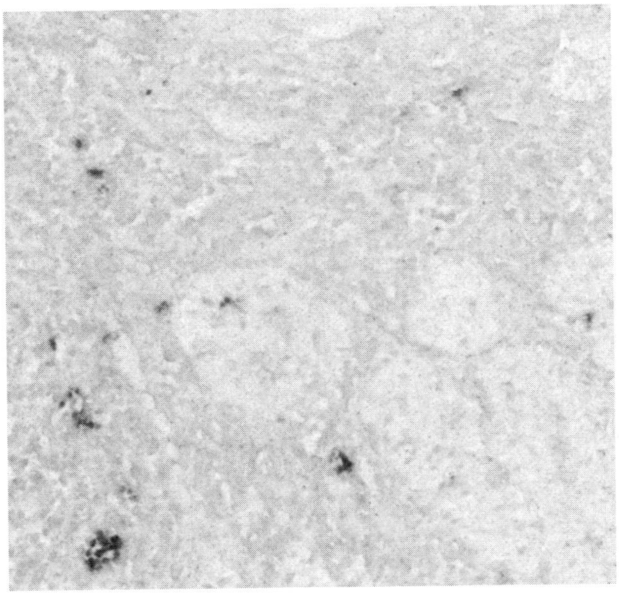

Figure 1. In situ hybridization with an EBV probe in tumor tissue from a patient with nasopharyngeal carcinoma. Scattered EBV-positive single cells and groups of cells are evidence of a lytic infection. Magnification, ×40. (Courtesy of Joan A. Barbera.)

burden, only the episomal circular, and thus latent, form of viral DNA is found in the tumors. Questions concerning genetic susceptibility and environmental exposure and the combination of these risk factors for nasopharyngeal carcinoma (86), as well of the role of EBV at the molecular and cellular levels in tumor progression, are currently being assessed.

Other tumors that are EBV positive are the rare lymphoepthelialomas and gastric carcinoma, both of epithelial origin. Tumors of other lineages associated with EBV are follicular dendritic cell tumors (190), and, although hepatitis B and C viruses may play a more dominant role, EBV DNA and expression of EBNA1 are reported for a number of hepatocellular carcinomas (205).

Malignancies associated with EBV in immunocompromised patients are the fatal B-cell lymphoproliferations. In the category of congenitally immunodeficient patients, some of those with XLP, described above (206), and others with Wiskott-Aldrich syndrome (46) are at risk for EBV-driven B-lymphoproliferative disease. Sustained immunosuppression in transplant recipients increases their risk of EBV-associated posttransplant lymphoproliferative disease in which higher levels of immunosuppression, seronegativity, and age are risk factors (reviewed in reference 145). Viral genome load and replication as other factors that influence disease need further evaluation. Compared to transplant patients, the risk of developing B-cell lymphomas in HIV patients is increased and the tumor types are more diverse (14). About half of these AIDS lymphomas are associated with EBV compared to 90% in transplant recipients. There are two types of EBV genomes in most populations, with type 1 being by far the most common. The two are distinguished only by differences of 16 to 47% in the amino acid sequence of the EBV nuclear antigens. Of these two types about one-third of the EBV-positive lymphomas of AIDS carry type 2 (17). This is different from transplant patients, of which most carry type 1 (52). Other EBV-associated malignancies in AIDS patients are classic Hodgkin's disease (177) in which the tumors are EBV positive in 90% of cases and leiomyosarcoma, especially in HIV-positive children (131) but also in young transplant recipients (113).

POLYOMAVIRUSES

General Features

Polyomaviruses (reviewed in references 31 and 126) are nonenveloped but encapsidated viruses with covalent closed circular superhelical double-stranded DNA genomes of only 5 kilobase pairs that are organized into chromatin. Two human polyomaviruses, BK virus and JC virus, have been identified. As they show closest homology to SV40, a simian polyomavirus that, along with the mouse polyomavirus, has been studied most extensively, much of the information concerning these human viruses are based on information from SV40. Recently, two other human polyomaviruses, KIPpy V and WUPyV, have been identified in patients' respiratory tract samples but little as yet is known about their pathologic potential.

Virus infection of the cell proceeds with attachment and penetration of virion; its migration to the nucleus, which in the case of SV40 is facilitated by nuclear localization signals on the capsid proteins; and viral genome uncoating, possibly in the nucleus, followed by transcription. The viral genome is organized into an early region, that is, the portion from which regulatory proteins, also called tumor antigens, are expressed from entry to late times, and a late region from which three capsid proteins are expressed after viral DNA replication. The genome contains a single unique origin of replication, with promoters and enhancers of transcription located close to the origin. Transcription by RNA polymerase II is bidirectional from this site, with transcription on one strand of a common precursor RNA from which early mRNAs for large and small T antigens in SV40 and related human viruses are generated by alternative splicing, and similar transcription on the other strand for late mRNAs.

Viral DNA replication (31) occurs in the nucleus where expression of only one viral gene product, large T antigen, is required, with the remaining proteins being provided by the host replication machinery. Therefore, polyomaviruses rely on the host cell being in S phase, and large T antigen promotes entry into S phase. Viral DNA synthesis proceeds from the origin of replication bidirectionally in a manner similar to host DNA replication, except that the viral origin is used for DNA synthesis multiple times, while the cellular origin is used only once per S phase. Once viral DNA replication begins, T antigen-stimulated late gene expression follows with subsequent encapsulation of viral chromatin. Virions are released either from disintegrating cells or from membranes of intact cells.

Polyomavirus infection can be productive when viral replication and assembly of progeny virus is followed by release of virions and cell death in cells that allow permissive growth or are nonproductive when infection does not result in viral DNA replication, since large T antigen is unable to interact with host factors to promote S phase but instead promotes cell transformation. The resulting nonpermissive infection occurs in hosts not related to the species of origin. In most of these cells the viral genome is subsequently lost, and the cells revert to normal growth; in a few, the viral DNA becomes integrated into host cell genomes and, with continued expression of large T antigen, cells become transformed. Even in the case of a permissive infection, these human viruses can induce mutations, such as chromosomal damage and translocations, leading to chromosomal abnormalities and even cell death. SV40 can replicate in primate cells but can transform or even immortalize them if mutations occur in the relevant cellular genes.

Human BK and JC Viruses

JC virus isolated by inoculating fetal brain cells with extracts of brains of patients with progressive multifocal leukoencephalopathy (PML) is mainly neurotrophic; BK virus was isolated from urine of an immunosuppressed renal transplant patient (both viruses reviewed in reference 126). The human viruses show closest homology to SV40. Most individuals become infected in childhood, likely through respiratory inhalation, and stromal cells in tonsillar tissue become infected, and antibodies are acquired. B lymphocytes in the peripheral blood appear to be the principal carrier of virus, and virus is found in multiple organs besides brain and kidney, suggesting hematogenous spread. Cell specificity of the two human viruses depends on differences in the noncoding sequence located between the early and late coding sequences, which is the regulatory region of the viral genome and is hypervariable. Latency probably occurs in most infected individuals.

Diseases Caused by Polyomaviruses

Both viruses are associated with diseases affecting immune-compromised hosts, suggesting that the human polyomaviruses remain latent in tissues and can be reactivated during times of immune suppression. They are also considered potential tumor viruses since they induce malignant tumor histotypes when administered to rodents (10) or brain tumors in New World monkeys (117). More recently, sequences of a previously unknown polyomavirus that is most closely related to African green monkey virus were found integrated into the tumor genome of human Merkel cell carcinoma (51a). This virus may potentially be the first example of a human cancer caused by a human polyomavirus; however, further studies are required before an etiological link with Merkel cell carcinoma is accepted.

Diseases caused by JC virus

PML is a demyelinating disease caused by JC virus lytic infection of oligodendrocytes, which are the myelin-producing cells in the white matter. Symptoms include muscle weakness, cognitive abnormalities, and sensory and visual defects. It is probable that JC virus remains latent, either integrated into host DNA or as an episome, at several sites and becomes reactivated by an as-yet unknown mechanism during immunosuppression to infect the brain. This disease was rare before but now, particularly with immunosuppression associated with HIV, has become more common. Why the increased incidence of PML in AIDS patients is not clear, but the fact that JC virus can be found in lymphocytes opens the possibility for a direct interaction between this polyomavirus and HIV in a common host cell (28, 49, 59)

Although JC virus has not been found in brain tumors in PML patients (58), it has been identified in an unusual oligoastrocytoma (162) and an xantoastrocytoma (15) in non-PML and immunocompetent patients. It has also been found outside the nervous system in leukemias and lymphomas (196) as well as in colon tumors and colorectal cancers in which the copy number of virus is higher than in the noninvolved colon tissue from the same patient (110).

Diseases caused by BK virus

BK virus has been identified in kidney diseases and cystitits in renal allograft recipients for which transfer from donor kidney has been documented, in bone marrow transplant recipients (7), and in a more limited number of cases of retinitis, pneumonia, and encephalitis (73, 181, 219). BK virus has been identified in human tumors, but as it has also been found in nontumor tissue, its relevance to human cancers is not completely clear. This is supported by a more recent study in which low copy numbers of BK virus DNA were found in 6 of 76 bladder carcinomas, but these were negative for BK virus T-antigen staining, and one of two available paired normal tissues was also positive (172)

Diseases caused by SV40

Since the mid 1950s when many lots of poliovirus vaccines were contaminated with SV40 (189), the concern regarding its oncogenic potential in humans has been raised. A statement from the U.S. Food and Drug Administration in 2003 rejected a causal relationship between SV40-containing polio vaccines and cancer (http://www.fda.gov/ola/2003/simianvirus1113.html), but SV40 antigens have been detected in rare cancers in the general population (reviewed in reference 25). In some studies, no association between SV40 exposure and increased risk for the rare tumors was found (128, 201), while in others, SV40 DNA and T antigen continue to be identified in malignant mesotheliomas (37, 41, 127, 209) as well as other tumors (127).

PAPILLOMAVIRUS

General Features

Papillomaviruses (reviewed in reference 83) are small DNA tumor viruses that can induce warts and, in humans, cause cervical cancers and other epithelial tumors. They were originally grouped as one family with the polyomaviruses since they shared common properties of small size (160- to 200-nm diameter), a nonenveloped virion, an icosahedral capsid, a double-stranded 7- to 8-kilobase pair circular DNA genome that is packaged as chromatin, and viral replication and virion assembly in the nucleus, which in the case of papillomavirus was in squamous epithelial cells, as well as activation of the cellular genes necessary for the replication of their own DNA. Based on molecular biological findings, differences between the two groups of viruses have placed them in two distinct viral families. These differences include a larger genome for papillomaviruses (8 versus 5 kilobases) as well as more ORFs which encode different numbers of structural and nonstructural proteins, transcription of papillomavirus genes from the same DNA strand as opposed to both strands for polyomavirus, and conserved family-specific epitopes in the major capsid protein.

The papillomavirus viral genome is organized so that all ORFs are found on one strand of the viral DNA with the early genes which encode the regulatory proteins, including those required for viral DNA replication that are located together but transcribed from multiple promoters with alternate and multiple splicing patterns of their mRNA products. The protein products of these genes can have multiple functions. The early genes are separated from the late genes which encode the two viral capsid proteins that are expressed only in productively infected cells. There is also a region devoid of genes which has regulatory functions, since it contains constitutive enhancer elements that respond to both cellular and viral transcription factors, thus conferring tissue or cell-type specificity, as well as facilitating initial gene expression after virus infection or maintenance of viral latency. This region also contains the origin of viral DNA replication.

Attachment, entry, and uncoating of the virus are thought to be similar to that of the polyomaviruses with α_6 integrins being strong candidates for viral receptors on squamous epithelial cells as well as many other cell types. The steps in the viral replicative cycle are linked to the differentiation stages of the squamous epithelium cells that the virus infects. Initially, the virus infects the basal cells which are capable of dividing, and the early genes are expressed at this stage. Late gene expression occurs only as these cells become terminally differentiated and viral DNA is synthesized and virions are assembled. Assembly and release of virions has not been well characterized, but release is thought to occur in the cornified layers of the keratinized epithelium without any cytolytic effect.

Papillomavirus DNA replication occurs at three stages of differentiation of the host cell. The first takes place in the basal epithelial cells where the viral genome is amplified 50 to 100 times. The second occurs in synchrony with the DNA replication of the host basal cell, and the products are distributed to the daughter cells equally to maintain a stable copy number. The association of the viral DNA to host mitotic chromosomes (88) suggests a mechanism to couple virus DNA replication and partitioning to that of the host. The third is a vegetative replication which occurs in the terminally differentiated cells of the papilloma where the viral DNA is packaged as virions.

Whether papillomaviruses establish true latent infections typical of the herpesviruses or whether they persist with very low levels of viral replication is not clear.

Pathology and Diseases Caused by Papillomaviruses

There are more than 100 human papillomavirus (HPV) genotypes (types). They are broadly classified into three groups, depending on preferential site of infection: the cutaneous types that cause nongenital skin warts in otherwise healthy individuals; the EV type which causes nongenital skin lesions in those with a rare condition, epidermodysplasia verruciformis (EV) characterized by susceptibility to widespread chronic infection of HPV or in immunosuppressed individuals; and the genital-mucosal type which infects the genital skin and mucosa or nongenital mucosa (reviewed in reference 118). The cutaneous types cause papillomas (reviewed in reference 118), usually called warts, on the skin which are benign epithelial lesions that develop on stratified epithelium. The virus must first gain access through traumatized upper layers of the epithelium to gain access to basal proliferative cells where they replicate at a low level. Virions formed in the upper differentiated epithelium are shed as the cells are desquamated. Cells of the thickened epidermis, a characteristic of papillomas, have abnormal nuclei that are eccentric, pyknotic, and surrounded by a halo. These lesions arise after a variable period of latency, remain for months to years, and then regress spontaneously. Although they are a result of viral infection, how the virus induces these changes is poorly understood. Skin warts are caused by HPV type 1 (HPV-1) to -4 and -7, -10, -28, and -41.

The EV types cause warts in children which, in susceptible individuals, become widespread, do not tend to regress, and, in one-third of EV patients, progress to squamous cell cancers, usually on sun-exposed areas. HPV-3 and -10, in EV patients as in the general population, cause flat warts, and HPV-5 and -8, which are EV specific, are most oncogenic. An autosomal recessive pattern of inheritance is found in half of affected individuals.

More than 25 genital-mucosal HPV types infect the anogenital tract, and most of the infections are sexually transmitted. These types are subdivided into high risk (HPV-16, -18, and -45), intermediate risk (HPV-31, -33, -35, -51, and -52), or low risk (HPV-6, -11, -42, -43, and -44), depending on the risk for malignant progression to cervical cancer of the lesion they induce. The low-risk group causes papillomas, referred to as condylomas or genital warts and, like the cutaneous types, the lesions they cause are self limited, regress spontaneously or with treatment but may persist for years. However, even the low-risk types may infrequently be associated with cancer after their genomes have undergone sequence rearrangements in the noncoding regulatory region (65). Recurrent respiratory papillomatosis of childhood is a rare condition in which the papillomas can block the airways. The low-risk genital types HPV-6 and -11 are most commonly involved, and intrapartum transmission of HPV from mother to child is suggested as a source of infection (93), with a long and variable period of latency, up to 5 years, before symptoms occur. Patients with HPV-11 and those younger than 3 years of age at diagnosis are prone to develop more aggressive disease (235), and in some laryngeal and bronchogenic carcinomas that develop in patients with a history of early onset recurrent respiratory papillomatosis, integration of the HPV-11 genome was found (161). Other lesions caused by these viruses include those of the oral cavity, laryngeal papillomas that develop after childhood, and nasal and conjunctival papillomas.

Cervical cancer is the third most common cancer among women worldwide (152), although a more recent estimate of it in European women is lower (19). Squamous cell cancers are the most common histological type, while others are adenocarcinomas and those of neuroendocrine origin. The squamous cell cancers develop through a progression of dysplastic changes, although most dysplasias resolve spontaneously. Also, identification of most premalignant lesions by Pap smear screening followed by appropriate treatment can interrupt the progression to an invasive cancer. HPV-16, -18, -31, and -45 are implicated in cervical carcinomas, of which more than 90% contain HPV DNA (16). These viruses are also implicated in anal cancers. The oncogenic potential of HPV-16 and -18 is supported by the oncogenes that they express. E6 of the high-risk HPV associates with p53 tumor suppressor protein and induces ubiquitin-dependent degradation of p53; E6 of the low-risk types does not bind p53. E7 of the high-risk type binds and inactivates the underphosphorylated form of the retinoblastoma tumor suppressor; binding by the low-risk counterpart is 10 times lower. E7 of the high-risk type interacts with other host proteins that regulate cell transformation and proliferation (reviewed in reference 83). Compared to benign papillomas in which the viral DNA remains as an episome, in cervical cancers integration of the partially deleted genome with the retention of the E6 and E7 viral oncogenes is common (187).

Other malignancies associated with HPV (reviewed in reference 118) include vulvular and vaginal cancer; penile cancer; oral cancer, especially that of the tonsils; esophageal cancer; and nonmelanoma skin cancers. The last of these are divided into basal or squamous cell carcinomas, with HVP-5 and -8 identified in the latter. These cancers develop many years after the initial infection and progress from either a benign papilloma or mild dysplasia, although even the high-risk HPV types mostly have benign outcomes and the progression to an invasive cancer can be interrupted. Host immune status is an important parameter in cancer progression, since impaired immune status is associated with greater risk of a persistent infection and consequently of progression to higher grades of dysplasia (184). Related to immune status, some HLA class II polymorphisms are associated with increased cervical cancer risk, while others are protective (reviewed in references 20 and 198). Exposure to cocarcinogens, for example, sun exposure of skin in malignant tumors that arise in EV as noted above, also increases malignant progression. That HIV infection is a risk factor for malignancies associated with HPV infection, particularly those of the anogenital tract (54), is compatible with the immunosuppression associated with HIV infection as well as the sexual route of transmission of both viruses.

ADENOVIRUS

General Features

Adenoviruses are nonenveloped DNA viruses with a double-stranded DNA genome of 36 kilobase pairs (63, 81). The human adenoviruses comprise 51 serotypes that are classified into six groups, A to F, according to sequence homology and oncogenicity when injected into rats. The icosahedral capsid of the 70- to 10-nm-diameter virion is composed of the hexon and penton proteins (63, 81, 82). The fiber protein which protrudes from the twelve vertices formed by the penton bases has a knob domain which serves as a ligand for receptors on the host cell. The knob domain of groups A, C, D, E, and F adenoviruses attaches to the coxsackie B virus and adenovirus receptor (CAR) on the host cell surface, while that of group B viruses, except for serotypes 3 and 7, attaches to CD46 (129). This binding facilitates further interactions between the penton base and members of the integrin family, mainly $\alpha_V\beta_{1,3,5}$, which are required for internalization of the virus. The details of adenovirus internalization, including fiber shedding, endocytosis, release from endosomes with loss of the penton bases are reviewed in references 63 and 191. The viral capsid is then directed by microtubules to the nuclear pore where nuclear import of the hexons results in the release of the viral DNA into the nucleus for its transcription, replication, and packaging. Once in the nucleus, E1A, the product of one of the five early transcription units, is the first viral protein to be expressed, since its gene has a constitutive promoter. E1A activates the expression of other viral genes required for viral replication and does so, not by binding directly to the promoters of these genes, but by interacting with cellular transcription factors and other regulatory proteins necessary for the transcription of the genes (191). This capacity of E1A to bind host transcriptional regulators and thus regulate not only viral genes but also genes of the host cell (191) will be relevant to its role in the pathogenesis of chronic obstructive pulmonary disease (COPD) (see below). The genes of the early unit, the two delayed early units, and one late unit are all transcribed by the host RNA polymerase II, and each gene gives rise to multiple mRNAs as a consequence of alternative splicing and the use of different polyadenylation sites. The early genes modify the host cell environment for optimal viral replication, antagonize host antiviral defenses, and provide viral gene products needed for viral DNA replication.

Viral DNA replication (191) relies on the virally encoded polymerase that binds to the origins of replication located in the inverted terminal repeats of the viral chromosome. There are two types of replication events. In the first, one of the double strands serves as a template to replicate a complementary daughter strand, and this can happen from either end of the linear DNA. In the second, the now displaced parental strand circularizes by means of its complementary termini to generate the same terminus as in the duplex genome and thus can support synthesis of a daughter strand. The late genes which encode, among others, the viral structural proteins are expressed from one major late promoter when viral DNA replication begins. Once late mRNAs are synthesized, host mRNA, although synthesized, is blocked from nuclear export and viral mRNA is preferentially translated. This blockage of host protein synthesis leads to the degeneration of the host cell. Subsequent virion assembly occurs in the nucleus, and its release from the cell is facilitated by a disruption of specific components of the cytoskeleton to make the cell more susceptible to lysis. This process is further supported by expression of a virally encoded death protein that accumulates to kill the cell.

Primary Infections

Adenovirus enters the host by the mouth, nasopharynx, or the ocular conjunctiva from airborne or contaminated water sources. The different groups of human adenovirus have preferred sites of infection and, in immunocompetent individuals, mainly cause mild disease at these sites (63, 81, 82) (Table 4), where the epithelial cells are the main target of infection, although limited replication and persistence occurs in lymphocytes in the lymphoid tissue at these sites (reviewed in reference 119). The most common human adenoviruses are those that belong to group C (185), which predominantly infects the upper re-

Table 4. Classification of human adenoviruses and the diseases they cause[a]

Group	Serotypes	Major site(s) of infection	Associated disease
A	12, 18, 31	Intestine	Gastroenteritis
B	3, 7, 11, 14, 16, 21, 34, 35, 50	Lung, urinary tract	Acute respiratory disease, pharyngitis, pneumonia, pharyngoconjunctival fever, acute hemorrhagic cystitis
C	1, 2, 5, 6	Upper respiratory tract	Pharyngitis, pneumonia
D	8–10, 13, 15, 17, 19, 20, 22–30, 32, 33, 36–39, 42–49, 51	Eye	Epidemic keratoconjunctivitis
E	4	Respiratory tract	Acute respiratory disease, conjunctivitis
F	40, 41	Intestine	Gastroenteritis

[a]Based on references 81 and 82.

spiratory tract. This group, along with groups B and E, which infect the lower respiratory tract, causes clinical symptoms ranging from mild pharyngitis to acute respiratory disease. In the case of an adenovirus pneumonia, some of the infected respiratory cells have enlarged nuclei that are often referred to as smudge cells (Color Plate 16).

Persistent and Latent Infections

Persistent adenovirus infections with shedding of replication-competent virus, particularly in the stool, account for its spread by the fecal-oral route. Latent infections, particularly in lymphocytes, where viral DNA in the absence of infectious virus was detected, have been reported (reviewed in reference 81). In contrast to the herpesviruses, little is known about the mechanism of adenovirus latency. Whether the genes of the E3 region that are also expressed early in the viral life cycle and assist in subverting the host immune response against the virus (82, 191) affect this persistence has not been tested in vivo in humans, nor have other possible mechanisms been investigated.

Adenovirus and Disease

Adenovirus infections occur frequently in approximately 50% of infants and nearly 100% of adults (9, 18, 85). In the face of these infections, disease in immunocompetent individuals is uncommon and rarely fatal due to potent innate and adaptive immune responses. In the susceptible minority, however, particularly those in the pediatric age group, those who are military recruits, and those who are immunosuppressed for transplantation and cancer or by HIV infection, disease is more common (see below). Adenovirus has also been identified in epidemic keratoconjunctivitis; acute hemorrhagic cystitis; gastrointestinal diseases, such as diarrhea, intussusception, and celiac disease; and myocarditis.

In childhood

In children younger than 5 years of age, who are more vulnerable since this is likely a primary infection, adenovirus causes up to 5% of acute respiratory disease. The symptoms include nasal congestion, coryza, and cough. Exudative tonsillitis, accompanied by generalized malaise, fever, chill, myalgia, and headache is clinically indistinguishable from group A streptococcus infections. Conjunctivitis, either alone or in combination with the above, can occur. The ubiquitous serotypes 1, 2, 5, and 6 from group C are commonly found, as well as serotype 3 from group B (18, 185). Adenovirus accounts for 10% of pneumonias in this population (81), and the serotypes isolated from the lungs include 1, 2, 3, 5, 7 (175), and 21 (12, 112). In situ hybridization showed that alveolar and bronchiolar epithelial cells are infected by adenovirus in pneumonias (79) (Color Plate 16). Other, less common, respiratory consequences of adenovirus infection reported for this age group include bronchiolitis (5, 12, 159), postinfectious bronchiolitis obliterans (32), and, when combined with or preceded by measles infection, bronchiectasis (92, 227).

In military recruits

Adenovirus infections were reported for military recruits soon after the discovery of this virus (77, 85). Fatigue, stress, and crowded living conditions contribute to the spread of an epidemic form of infection, and the serotypes most prominent are 4 and 7 and less frequently 3 and 21 (68, 84, 139, 174). Susceptibility to these serotypes reflects immunity to group C adenovirus acquired in early childhood. Effective vaccines against adenovirus 4 and 7 were developed (210) but discontinued after 1996, so that infections continue to be a problem in this population to the present day (178, 179).

In immunocompromised patients

Adenovirus infections and the associated morbidity and mortality in immunocompromised patients are a growing concern, particularly with increases in solid-organ and bone marrow transplantations, as well as in those with AIDS and malignancies (reviewed in references 89, 101, and 114). In transplant patients, vulnerability to adenovirus infection is greatest in the pediatric population, and incidents of infection and severity of disease are higher in allogeneic versus autologous transplants. The source of virus can be a primary infection, reactivation of a persistent or latent infection (see above) in the recipient, or possibly, in the case of transplant patients, transmission from the donor. Pneumonitis, which develops from infection mainly by group C adenoviruses (Table 4), has the worst prognosis for survival, along with hepatitis and meningoencephalitis. In lung transplant recipients, adenovirus was associated with respiratory failure leading to death or graft loss and with the diagnosis of necrotizing bronchocentric pneumonia or obliterative bronchiolitis. While most patients eventually clear the virus, treatment for those with adenoviremia, a predictor of a fatal outcome, is limited to antiviral drugs, of which cidofovir, an inhibitor of the viral DNA polymerase, and its lipid ester show some promise. Various modes of immunotherapy, including adenovirus-specific cytotoxic lymphocytes, are currently being investigated.

Malignancies

Group A adenoviruses were found to be highly oncogenic in animal models (reviewed in 120; 212). Adenoviral nucleic acid or protein, however, has not been demonstrated in most human tumors studied (69, 70). The identification of adenoviral nucleic acid in cancers of potential neuroendocrine origin (87, 109) that have been reported requires confirmation.

Adenovirus E1A and COPD

COPD (155) is defined by the irreversible airflow limitation measured by the volume of air that can be forcibly expired from the lungs in 1 second and its ratio to the forced vital capacity. The key determinants limiting airflow are an increase in resistance in the small conducting airways less than 2 mm in diameter (80, 216, 239) and emphysematous destruction of the lung elastic recoil force available to drive expiratory flow (134). COPD is currently the fourth leading cause of death in the world (WHO global burden of disease study [http://www.who.int/mip/2003/other_documents/en/globalburdenofdisease.pdf]), and further increases in its prevalence and mortality are predicted (142). The major risk factor is the inhalation of toxic particles and gases, primarily from the tobacco smoking habit (155). Respiratory infections in early childhood are also associated with reduced lung function and increased respiratory problems later in life (62), which could lead to COPD.

Childhood respiratory infections as a potential risk factor for COPD led to investigations of adenovirus because it is a common respiratory virus of early childhood and because, unlike other common childhood respiratory viruses, namely rhinovirus, respiratory syncytial virus, the parainfluenza viruses, influenza, and coronavirus, which are all RNA viruses, adenovirus with its double-stranded DNA genome has the potential to persist in the nuclei of infected cells, as supported by the persistent or latent infections reported above. Also, a possibility of the stable integration of the viral DNA, particularly the E1 region, into the chromosomes of the host cell is supported by evidence in adenovirus-transformed cells (reviewed in reference 64) and preliminary results from human lungs (71a). Similarly, the possibility of the integration of double-stranded DNA papillomavirus genomes into chromosomes of human host cells has been reported above. Furthermore, group C adenovirus was chosen as a target of study because these serotypes (types 1, 2, 5, and 6) are ubiquitous, mainly in children (81, 185). Besides predominance of this group in upper respiratory tract infections in general (Table 4), its association with pneumonias in infants (see above) is evidence that it also infects the lower respiratory tract.

Studies showed that lungs of COPD patients who were asymptomatic for viral infections harbored more group C adenovirus E1A DNA than those of controls with similar smoking history (130), that in these lungs the E1A protein was expressed mainly in alveolar (Color Plate 17), but also in bronchiolar epithelial cells (47), and that E1A protein expression, as well as the expression of the inflammatory marker intercellular adhesion molecule (ICAM)-1 and the number of inflammatory cells, increased with disease severity in these patients (163). A role for adenovirus infections in COPD was further supported by studies of guinea pigs in which, after the initial acute infection with adenovirus 5 had subsided and viral replication ceased, E1A DNA and protein continued to be detected in alveolar and airway epithelial cells, and bronchiolitis persisted (217). Short-term (218) and chronic exposure (136) to cigarette smoke at this time increased the number of inflammatory cells and caused emphysema-like changes, respectively, compared to uninfected animals.

The ability of E1A to regulate gene transcription of the host cell has been documented above. To determine whether this capacity to modulate host gene expression is the basis of the relationship between E1A and increased lung inflammation in COPD, A549 cells (95), as a model of alveolar epithelial cells, and primary bronchiolar epithelial cells expressing adenovirus 5 E1A (75) were developed. In response to LPS stimulation of these cells, the presence of E1A increased ICAM-1 (75, 95) and IL-8 expression (75, 96), and these increases were accompanied by increased binding activity of the transcription factor nuclear factor (NF)-κB (75, 97), which has binding sites in the promoters of the two genes. Support that E1A is affecting the promoters of these genes came from studies showing that E1A increased ICAM-1 promoter driven reporter gene expression in these cells (75, 76). These results suggest that E1A regulates the expression of specific mediators in response to LPS by a common mechanism. Importantly, these are mediators that promote increases in the number of neutrophils in lungs of COPD patients (reviewed in reference 75), with IL-8 serving as a potent neutrophil chemoattractant and ICAM-1, a ligand for the adhesion receptor on neutrophils. Site-directed mutagenesis studies showed that of the two NF-κB binding sites in the ICAM-1 promoter, the one most proximal to the transcription start site was essential for increased expression by E1A (147a). More recently, chromatin immunoprecipitation assays were designed to investigate whether E1A participates with the proteins of the transcription complex that assembles at this site to promote transcription of the ICAM-1 gene. In both A549 and bronchiolar epithelial cells stimulated with LPS, the presence of E1A increased the binding of NF-κB, the coactivator p300, and RNA polymerase II to this promoter, and E1A was also present at this site (K. Morimoto et al., unpublished data). Besides the E1A-induced increases in response to LPS, expression of both ICAM-1 and IL-8 genes was increased by E1A in response to stimulation with environmental particulate matter <10 μm, and again increased gene expression was associated with activation of NF-κB (55, 61). Taken together, these results suggest that in lung epithelial cells, adenovirus E1A regulates the expression of mediators relevant to the pathogenesis of COPD by interacting with transcriptional regulators at the promoters of these genes and that the regulation of this response to inflammatory stimuli, whether from bacteria or environmental pollutants, may play a role in the emphysematous destruction of the lung in COPD.

Besides modulating inflammatory mediator expression in lung epithelial cells, adenovirus E1A upregulates the expression transforming growth factor-β1 and connective tissue growth factor (147), two growth factors that are important in extracellular matrix deposition. These results suggest that E1A can also promote the process of peripheral airway remodeling that occurs in COPD (78). Studies of guinea pig cells demonstrated that E1A transforms peripheral lung epithelial cells to cells with a more mesenchymal phenotype (13), possibly to myofibroblasts that are active in tissue repair, and further support a role for E1A in airway remodeling. In summary, our results support a role for adenovirus infection in the pathogenesis of COPD in which expression of the viral E1A enhances the inflammatory response of lung epithelial cells to noxious stimuli, be they cigarette smoke products, bacterial products, or environmental pollutants.

REFERENCES

1. **Abiko, Y., M. Ikeda, and R. Hondo.** 2002. Secretion and dynamics of herpes simplex virus in tears and saliva of patients with Bell's palsy. *Otol. Neurotol.* **23:**779–783.
2. **Ablashi, D. V., H. B. Eastman, C. B. Owen, M. M. Roman, J. Friedman, J. B. Zabriskie, D. L. Peterson, G. R. Pearson, and J. E. Whitman.** 2000. Frequent HHV-6 reactivation in multiple sclerosis (MS) and chronic fatigue syndrome (CFS) patients. *J. Clin. Virol.* **16:**179–191.
3. **Adams, H. G., E. A. Benson, E. R. Alexander, L. A. Vontver, M. A. Remington, and K. K. Holmes.** 1976. Genital herpetic infection in men and women: clinical course and effect of topical application of adenine arabinoside. *J. Infect. Dis.* **133**(Suppl):A151–A159.
4. **Adler, S. P.** 1988. Cytomegalovirus transmission among children in day care, their mothers and caretakers. *Pediatr. Infect. Dis.* J 7:279–285.

4a. **Allander, T., K. Andreasson, S. Gupta, A. Bjerkner, G. Bogdanovic, M. A. A. Persson, T. Dallianis, T. Ramqvist, and B. Andersson.** 2007. Identification of a third human polyomavirus. *J. Virol.* **81:**4130–4136.

5. **Al-Shehri, M. A., A. Sadeq, and K. Quli.** 2005. Bronchiolitis in Abha, Southwest Saudi Arabia: viral etiology and predictors for hospital admission. *West Afr. J. Med.* **24:**299–304.
6. **Andiman, W. A., R. Eastman, K. Martin, B. Z. Katz, A. Rubinstein, J. Pitt, S. Pahwa, and G. Miller.** 1985. Opportunistic lymphoproliferations associated with Epstein-Barr viral DNA in infants and children with AIDS. *Lancet* **ii:**1390–1393.
7. **Apperley, J. F., S. J. Rice, J. A. Bishop, Y. C. Chia, T. Krausz, S. D. Gardner, and J. M. Goldman.** 1987. Late-onset hemorrhagic cystitis associated with urinary excretion of polyomaviruses after bone marrow transplantation. *Transplantation* **43:**108–112.
8. **Arvin, A. M.** 2001. Varicella-zoster virus, p. 2731–2767. *In* D. M. Knipe, P. M. Howley, D. E. Griffin, R. A. Lamb, M. A. Martin, B. Roizman, and S. E. Straus (ed.), *Fields Virology*, 4th ed., vol. 2. Lippincott Williams & Wilkins, Philadephia, PA.
9. **Badger, G. F., C. Curtiss, J. H. Dingle, H. S. Ginsberg, E. Gold, and W. S. Jordan, Jr.** 1956. A study of illness in a group of Cleveland families. X. The occurrence of adenovirus infections. *Am. J. Hyg.* **64:**336–348.

10. **Barbanti-Brodano, G., F. Martini, M. De Mattei, L. Lazzarin, A. Corallini, and M. Tognon.** 1998. BK and JC human polyomaviruses and simian virus 40: natural history of infection in humans, experimental oncogenicity, and association with human tumors. *Adv. Virus. Res.* **50:**69–99.
11. **Barbera, J. A., S. Hayashi, R. G. Hegele, and J. C. Hogg.** 1992. Detection of Epstein-Barr virus in lymphocytic interstitial pneumonia by in situ hybridization. *Am. Rev. Respir. Dis.* **145:**940–946.
12. **Becroft, D.** 1967. Histopathology of adenovirus infection of the respiratory tract in young children. *J. Clin. Pathol.* **20:**561–569.
13. **Behzad, A. R., K. Morimoto, J. Gosselink, J. Green, J. C. Hogg, and S. Hayashi.** 2006. Induction of mesenchymal cell phenotypes in lung epithelial cells by adenovirus E1A. *Eur. Respir. J.* **28:**1106–1116.
14. **Beral, V., T. Peterman, R. Berkelman, and H. Jaffe.** 1991. AIDS-associated non-Hodgkin lymphoma. *Lancet* **337:**805–809.
15. **Boldorini, R., R. Caldarelli-Stefano, G. Monga, M. Zocchi, M. Mediati, A. Tosoni, and P. Ferrante.** 1998. PCR detection of JC virus DNA in the brain tissue of a 9-year-old child with pleomorphic xanthoastrocytoma. *J. Neurovirol.* **4:**242–245.
16. **Bosch, F. X., M. M. Manos, N. Munoz, M. Sherman, A. M. Jansen, J. Peto, M. H. Schiffman, V. Moreno, R. Kurman, and K. V. Shah.** 1995. Prevalence of human papillomavirus in cervical cancer: a worldwide perspective. International biological study on cervical cancer (IBSCC) Study Group. *J. Natl. Cancer Inst.* **87:**796–802.
17. **Boyle, M. J., W. A. Sewell, T. B. Sculley, A. Apolloni, J. J. Turner, C. E. Swanson, R. Penny, and D. A. Cooper.** 1991. Subtypes of Epstein-Barr virus in human immunodeficiency virus-associated non-Hodgkin lymphoma. *Blood* **78:**3004–3011.
18. **Brandt, C. D., H. W. Kim, A. J. Vargosko, B. C. Jeffries, J. O. Arrobio, B. Rindge, R. H. Parrott, and R. M. Chanock.** 1969. Infections in 18,000 infants and children in a controlled study of respiratory tract disease. I. Adenovirus pathogenicity in relation to serologic type and illness syndrome. *Am. J. Epidemiol.* **90:**484–500.
19. **Bray, F., R. Sankila, J. Ferlay, and D. M. Parkin.** 2002. Estimates of cancer incidence and mortality in Europe in 1995. *Eur. J. Cancer* **38:**99–166.
20. **Breitburd, F., N. Ramoz, J. Salmon, and G. Orth.** 1996. HLA control in the progression of human papillomavirus infections. *Semin. Cancer Biol.* **7:**359–371.
21. **Brown, Z. A., S. Selke, J. Zeh, J. Kopelman, A. Maslow, R. L. Ashley, D. H. Watts, S. Berry, M. Herd, and L. Corey.** 1997. The acquisition of herpes simplex virus during pregnancy. *N. Engl. J. Med.* **337:**509–515.
22. **Brown, Z. A., L. A. Vontver, J. Benedetti, C. W. Critchlow, C. J. Sells, S. Berry, and L. Corey.** 1987. Effects on infants of a first episode of genital herpes during pregnancy. *N. Engl. J. Med.* **317:**1246–1251.
23. **Browne, H., G. Smith, S. Beck, and T. Minson.** 1990. A complex between the MHC class I homologue encoded by human cytomegalovirus and beta 2 microglobulin. *Nature* **347:**770–772.
24. **Buddingh, G. J., D. I. Schrum, J. C. Lanier, and D. J. Guidry.** 1953. Studies of the natural history of herpes simplex infections. *Pediatrics* **11:**595–610.
25. **Butel, J. S., and J. A. Lednicky.** 1999. Cell and molecular biology of simian virus 40: implications for human infections and disease. *J. Natl. Cancer Inst.* **91:**119–134.
26. **Campadelli, G., R. Brandimarti, C. Di Lazzaro, P. L. Ward, B. Roizman, and M. R. Torrisi.** 1993. Fragmentation and dispersal of Golgi proteins and redistribution of glycoproteins and glycolipids processed through Golgi following infection with herpes simplex virus 1. *Proc. Natl. Acad. Sci. USA* **90:**2798–2802.
27. **Chee, M. S., S. C. Satchwell, E. Preddie, K. M. Weston, and B. G. Barrell.** 1990. Human cytomegalovirus encodes three G protein-coupled receptor homologues. *Nature* **344:**774–777.
28. **Chowdhury, M., J. P. Taylor, C. F. Chang, J. Rappaport, and K. Khalili.** 1992. Evidence that a sequence similar to TAR is important for induction of the JC virus late promoter by human immunodeficiency virus type 1 Tat. *J. Virol.* **66:**7355–7361.
29. **Chuh, A. A., S. S. Chiu, and J. S. Peiris.** 2001. Human herpesvirus 6 and 7 DNA in peripheral blood leucocytes and plasma in patients with pityriasis rosea by polymerase chain reaction: a prospective case control study. *Acta Derm. Venereol.* **81:**289–290.
30. **Cohen, J. I., and S. E. Straus.** 2001. Varicella-zoster virus and its replication, p. 2707–2730. *In* D. M. Knipe, P.M. Howley, D. E. Griffin, R. A. Lamb, M. A. Martin, B. Roizman, and S. E. Straus (ed.), *Fields Virology*, 4th ed., vol. 2. Lippincott Williams & Wilkins, Philadelphia, PA.
31. **Cole, C. N., and S. D. Conzen.** 2001. Polyomaviridae: the viruses and their replication, p. 2141–2174. *In* D. M. Knipe, P.M. Howley, D. E. Griffin, R. A. Lamb, M. A. Martin, B. Roizman, and S. E. Straus (ed.), *Fields Virology*, 4th ed., vol. 2. Lippincott Williams & Wilkins, Philadelphia, PA.
32. **Colom, A. J., A. M. Teper, W. M. Vollmer, and G. B. Diette.** 2006. Risk factors for the development of bronchiolitis obliterans in children with bronchiolitis. *Thorax* **61:**503–506.
33. **Cone, R. W., R. C. Hackman, M. L. Huang, R. A. Bowden, J. D. Meyers, M. Metcalf, J. Zeh, R. Ashley, and L. Corey.** 1993. Human herpesvirus 6 in lung tissue from patients with pneumonitis after bone marrow transplantation. *N. Engl. J. Med.* **329:**156–161.
34. **Cone, R. W., M. L. Huang, L. Corey, J. Zeh, R. Ashley, and R. Bowden.** 1999. Human herpesvirus 6 infections after bone marrow transplantation: clinical and virologic manifestations. *J. Infect. Dis.* **179:**311–318.
35. **Copie-Bergman, C., G. Niedobitek, D. C. Mangham, J. Selves, K. Baloch, T. C. Diss, D. N. Knowles, G. Delsol, and P. G. Isaacson.** 1997. Epstein-Barr virus in B-cell lymphomas associated with chronic suppurative inflammation. *J. Pathol.* **183:**287–292.
36. **Craig, C. P., and A. J. Nahmias.** 1973. Different patterns of neurologic involvement with herpes simplex virus types 1 and 2: isolation of herpes simplex virus type 2 from the buffy coat of two adults with meningitis. *J. Infect. Dis.* **127:**365–372.
37. **Cristaudo, A., R. Foddis, A. Vivaldi, R. Buselli, V. Gattini, G. Guglielmi, F. Cosentino, F. Ottenga, E. Ciancia, R. Libener, R. Filiberti, M. Neri, P. Betta, M. Tognon, L. Mutti, and R. Puntoni.** 2005. SV40 enhances the risk of malignant mesothelioma among people exposed to asbestos: a molecular epidemiologic case-control study. *Cancer Res.* **65:**3049–3052.
38. **Daibata, M., T. Taguchi, T. Sawada, H. Taguchi, and I. Miyoshi.** 1998. Chromosomal transmission of human herpesvirus 6 DNA in acute lymphoblastic leukaemia. *Lancet* **352:**543–544.
39. **Dawson, C. W., A. G. Eliopoulos, J. Dawson, and L. S. Young.** 1995. BHRF1, a viral homologue of the Bcl-2 oncogene, disturbs epithelial cell differentiation. *Oncogene* **10:**69–77.

40. **Deayton, J., A. Mocroft, P. Wilson, V. C. Emery, M. A. Johnson, and P. D. Griffiths.** 1999. Loss of cytomegalovirus (CMV) viraemia following highly active antiretroviral therapy in the absence of specific anti-CMV therapy. *AIDS* **13**:1203–1206.
41. **De Luca, A., A. Baldi, V. Esposito, C. M. Howard, L. Bagella, P. Rizzo, M. Caputi, H. I. Pass, G. G. Giordano, F. Baldi, M. Carbone, and A. Giordano.** 1997. The retinoblastoma gene family pRb/p105, p107, pRb2/p130 and simian virus-40 large T-antigen in human mesotheliomas. *Nat. Med.* **3**:913–916.
42. **Dingwell, K. S., C. R. Brunetti, R. L. Hendricks, Q. Tang, M. Tang, A. J. Rainbow, and D. C. Johnson.** 1994. Herpes simplex virus glycoproteins E and I facilitate cell-to-cell spread in vivo and across junctions of cultured cells. *J. Virol.* **68**:834–845.
43. **Drobyski, W. R., K. K. Knox, D. Majewski, and D. R. Carrigan.** 1994. Brief report: fatal encephalitis due to variant B human herpesvirus-6 infection in a bone marrow-transplant recipient. *N. Engl. J. Med.* **330**:1356–1360.
44. **Dworsky, M., M. Yow, S. Stagno, R. F. Pass, and C. Alford.** 1983. Cytomegalovirus infection of breast milk and transmission in infancy. *Pediatrics* **72**:295–299.
45. **Egan, J. J., J. P. Stewart, P. S. Hasleton, J. R. Arrand, K. B. Carroll, and A. A. Woodcock.** 1995. Epstein-Barr virus replication within pulmonary epithelial cells in cryptogenic fibrosing alveolitis. *Thorax* **50**:1234–1239.
46. **Elenitoba-Johnson, K. S., and E. S. Jaffe.** 1997. Lymphoproliferative disorders associated with congenital immunodeficiencies. *Semin. Diagn. Pathol.* **14**:35–47.
47. **Elliott, W. M., S. Hayashi, and J. C. Hogg.** 1995. Immunodetection of adenoviral E1A proteins in human lung tissue. *Am. J. Respir. Cell. Mol. Biol.* **12**:642–648.
48. **Emery, V. C., M. C. Atkins, E. F. Bowen, D. A. Clark, M. A. Johnson, I. M. Kidd, J. E. McLaughlin, A. N. Phillips, P. M. Strappe, and P. D. Griffiths.** 1999. Interactions between betaherpesviruses and human immunodeficiency virus in vivo: evidence for increased human immunodeficiency viral load in the presence of human herpesvirus 6. *J. Med. Virol.* **57**:278–282.
49. **Enam, S., T. M. Sweet, S. Amini, K. Khalili, and L. Del Valle.** 2004. Evidence for involvement of transforming growth factor beta1 signaling pathway in activation of JC virus in human immunodeficiency virus 1-associated progressive multifocal leukoencephalopathy. *Arch. Pathol. Lab. Med.* **128**:282–291.
50. **Epstein, M. A., G. Henle, B. G. Achong, and Y. M. Barr.** 1965. Morphological and biological studies on a virus in cultured lymphoblasts from Burkitt's lymphoma. *J. Exp. Med.* **121**:761–770.
51. **Faulkner, G. C., S. R. Burrows, R. Khanna, D. J. Moss, A. G. Bird, and D. H. Crawford.** 1999. X-Linked agammaglobulinemia patients are not infected with Epstein-Barr virus: implications for the biology of the virus. *J. Virol.* **73**:1555–1564.
51a. **Feng, H., M. Shuda, Y. Chang, and P. S. Moore.** 2008. Clonal integration of a polyomavirus in human Merkel cell carcinoma. *Science* **319**:1096–1100.
52. **Frank, D., E. Cesarman, Y. F. Liu, R. E. Michler, and D. M. Knowles.** 1995. Posttransplantation lymphoproliferative disorders frequently contain type A and not type B Epstein-Barr virus. *Blood* **85**:1396–1403.
53. **Fraser, N. W., A. M. Deatly, D. M. Mellerick, M. I. Muggeridge, and J. G. Spivack.** 1986. Molecular biology of latent HSV-1, p. 39–54. *In* C. Lopez, B. Roizman (ed.), *Human Herpesvirus Infections: Pathogenesis, Diagnosis, and Treatment.* Raven, New York, NY.
54. **Frisch, M., R. J. Biggar, and J. J. Goedert.** 2000. Human papillomavirus-associated cancers in patients with human immunodeficiency virus infection and acquired immunodeficiency syndrome. *J. Natl. Cancer Inst.* **92**:1500–1510.
55. **Fujii, T., J. C. Hogg, N. Keicho, R. Vincent, S. F. Van Eeden, and S. Hayashi.** 2003. Adenoviral E1A modulates inflammatory mediator expression by lung epithelial cells exposed to PM10. *Am. J. Physiol. Lung Cell. Mol. Physiol.* **284**:L290–297.
56. **Furuta, Y., S. Fukuda, E. Chida, T. Takasu, F. Ohtani, Y. Inuyama, and K. Nagashima.** 1998. Reactivation of herpes simplex virus type 1 in patients with Bell's palsy. *J. Med. Virol.* **54**:162–166.
57. **Furuta, Y., F. Ohtani, H. Kawabata, S. Fukuda, and T. Bergstrom.** 2000. High prevalence of varicella-zoster virus reactivation in herpes simplex virus-seronegative patients with acute peripheral facial palsy. *Clin. Infect. Dis.* **30**:529–533.
58. **Gallia, G. L., J. Gordon, and K. Khalili.** 1998. Tumor pathogenesis of human neurotropic JC virus in the CNS. *J. Neurovirol.* **4**:175–181.
58a. **Gaynor, A. M., M. D. Nissen, D. M. Whiley, I. M. MacKay, S. B. Lambert, G. Wu, D. C. Brennan, G. A. Storch, T. P. Sloots, and D. Wang.** 2007. Identification of a novel polyomavirus from patients with acute respiratory tract infections. *PLoS Pathogens* **3**:595–604.
59. **Gendelman, H. E., W. Phelps, L. Feigenbaum, J. M. Ostrove, A. Adachi, P. M. Howley, G. Khoury, H. S. Ginsberg, and M. A. Martin.** 1986. Trans-activation of the human immunodeficiency virus long terminal repeat sequence by DNA viruses. *Proc. Natl. Acad. Sci. USA* **83**:9759–9763.
60. **Gill, M. J., J. Arlette, and K. Buchan.** 1988. Herpes simplex virus infection of the hand. A profile of 79 cases. *Am. J. Med.* **84**:89–93.
61. **Gilmour, P. S., I. Rahman, S. Hayashi, J. C. Hogg, K. Donaldson, and W. MacNee.** 2001. Adenoviral E1A primes alveolar epithelial cells to PM(10)-induced transcription of interleukin-8. *Am. J. Physiol. Lung Cell. Mol. Physiol.* **281**:L598–L606.
62. **Gold, D. R., I. B. Tager, S. T. Weiss, T. D. Tosteson, and F. E. Speizer.** 1989. Acute lower respiratory illness in childhood as a predictor of lung function and chronic respiratory symptoms. *Am. Rev. Respir. Dis.* **140**:877–884.
63. **Goncalves, M. A., and A. A. de Vries.** 2006. Adenovirus: from foe to friend. *Rev. Med. Virol.* **16**:167–186.
64. **Graham, F. L.** 1984. Transformation by and oncogenicity of human adenoviruses, p. 339–398. *In* H. S. Ginsberg (ed.), *The Adenoviruses.* Plenum Press, New York, NY.
65. **Grassmann, K., S. P. Wilczynski, N. Cook, B. Rapp, and T. Iftner.** 1996. HPV6 variants from malignant tumors with sequence alterations in the regulatory region do not reveal differences in the activities of the oncogene promoters but do contain amino acid exchanges in the E6 and E7 proteins. *Virology* **223**:185–197.
66. **Gratama, J. W., M. A. Oosterveer, G. Klein, and I. Ernberg.** 1990. EBNA size polymorphism can be used to trace Epstein-Barr virus spread within families. *J. Virol.* **64**:4703–4708.
67. **Grattan, M. T., C. E. Moreno-Cabral, V. A. Starnes, P. E. Oyer, E. B. Stinson, and N. E. Shumway.** 1989. Cytomegalovirus infection is associated with cardiac allograft rejection and atherosclerosis. *JAMA* **261**:3561–3566.
68. **Gray, G. C., J. D. Callahan, A. W. Hawksworth, C. A. Fisher, and J. C. Gaydos.** 1999. Respiratory diseases among U.S.

military personnel: countering emerging threats. *Emerg. Infect. Dis.* **5**:379–385.

69. **Green, M., W. S. M. Wold, and K. H. Brachmann.** 1980. Human adenovirus transforming genes: group relationships, integration, expression in transformed cells and analysis of human cancers and tonsils, p. 373–397. *In* M. Essex, , G. Todaro, and H. zur Hausen (ed.), *Cold Spring Harbor Conference on Cell Proliferation Viruses in Naturally Occurring Tumors.* Cold Spring Harbor Laboratory, Cold Spring Harbor, NY.
70. **Green, M., W. S. Wold, J. K. Mackey, and P. Rigden.** 1979. Analysis of human tonsil and cancer DNAs and RNAs for DNA sequences of group C (serotypes 1, 2, 5, and 6) human adenoviruses. *Proc. Natl. Acad. Sci. USA* **76**:6606–6610.
71. **Harabuchi, Y., N. Yamanaka, A. Kataura, S. Imai, T. Kinoshita, F. Mizuno, and T. Osato.** 1990. Epstein-Barr virus in nasal T-cell lymphomas in patients with lethal midline granuloma. *Lancet* **335**:128–130.

71a. **Hayashi, S., T. Harris, I. C. Gillam, and E. G. Sedgwick.** 2000. Adenovirus E1A DNA integration into chromosomes of lung epithelial cells of COPD patients. *Eur. Resp. J.* **16**:17S. (Abstract.)

72. **Hayward, G. S., R. J. Jacob, S. C. Wadsworth, and B. Roizman.** 1975. Anatomy of herpes simplex virus DNA: evidence for four populations of molecules that differ in the relative orientations of their long and short components. *Proc. Natl. Acad. Sci. USA* **72**:4243–4247.
73. **Hedquist, B. G., G. Bratt, A. L. Hammarin, M. Grandien, I. Nennesmo, B. Sundelin, and S. Seregard.** 1999. Identification of BK virus in a patient with acquired immune deficiency syndrome and bilateral atypical retinitis. *Ophthalmology* **106**:129–132.
74. **Henderson, S., D. Huen, M. Rowe, C. Dawson, G. Johnson, and A. Rickinson.** 1993. Epstein-Barr virus-coded BHRF1 protein, a viral homologue of Bcl-2, protects human B cells from programmed cell death. *Proc. Natl. Acad. Sci. USA* **90**:8479–8483.
75. **Higashimoto, Y., W. M. Elliott, A. R. Behzad, E. G. Sedgwick, T. Takei, J. C. Hogg, and S. Hayashi.** 2002. Inflammatory mediator mRNA expression by adenovirus E1A-transfected bronchial epithelial cells. *Am. J. Respir. Crit. Care Med.* **166**:200–207.
76. **Higashimoto, Y., N. Keicho, W. M. Elliott, J. C. Hogg, and S. Hayashi.** 1999. Effect of adenovirus E1A on ICAM-1 promoter activity in human alveolar and bronchial epithelial cells. *Gene Expr.* **8**:287–297.
77. **Hilleman, M. R., and J. H. Werner.** 1954. Recovery of new agent from patients with acute respiratory illness. *Proc. Soc. Exp. Biol. Med.* **85**:183–188.
78. **Hogg, J. C., F. Chu, S. Utokaparch, R. Woods, W. M. Elliott, L. Buzatu, R. M. Cherniack, R. M. Rogers, F. C. Sciurba, H. O. Coxson, and P. D. Pare.** 2004. The nature of small-airway obstruction in chronic obstructive pulmonary disease. *N. Engl. J. Med.* **350**:2645–2653.
79. **Hogg, J. C., W. L. Irving, H. Porter, M. Evans, M. S. Dunnill, and K. Fleming.** 1989. In situ hybridization studies of adenoviral infections of the lung and their relationship to follicular bronchiectasis. *Am. Rev. Respir. Dis.* **139**:1531–1535.
80. **Hogg, J. C., P. T. Macklem, and W. M. Thurlbeck.** 1968. Site and nature of airway obstruction in chronic obstructive lung disease. *N. Engl. J. Med.* **278**:1355–1360.
81. **Horowitz, M. S.** 2001. Adenoviruses, p. 2301–2326. *In* D. M. Knipe, P. M. Howley, D. E. Griffin, R. A. Lamb, M. A. Martin, B. Roizman, and S. E. Straus (ed.), *Fields Virology*, 4th ed., vol. 2. Lippincott Williams & Wilkins, Philadelphia, PA.
82. **Horwitz, M. S.** 2004. Function of adenovirus E3 proteins and their interactions with immunoregulatory cell proteins. *J. Gene. Med.* **6**(Suppl. 1):S172–S183.
83. **Howley, P. M., and D. R. Lowy.** 2001. Papillomaviruses and their replication, p. 2197–2229. *In* D. M. Knipe, P. M. Howley, D. E. Griffin, R. A. Lamb, M. A. Martin, B. Roizman, and S. E. Straus (ed.), *Fields Virology*, 4th ed., vol. 2. Lippincott Williams & Wilkins, Philadelphia, PA.
84. **Huebner, R. J., W. P. Rowe, and R. M. Chanock.** 1958. Newly recognized respiratory tract viruses. *Annu. Rev. Microbiol.* **12**:49–76.
85. **Huebner, R. J., W. P. Rowe, T. G. Ward, R. H. Parrott, and J. A. Bell.** 1954. Adenoidal-pharyngeal-conjunctival agents: a newly recognized group of common viruses of the respiratory system. *N. Engl. J. Med.* **251**:1077–1086.
86. **IARC (International Agency for Research on Cancer).** 1998. Epstein-Barr virus and Kaposi sarcoma, herpesvirus/human
herpesvirus 8. *IARC Monographs on the Evaluation of Carcinogenic Risks to Humans.* Vol. 70. World Health Organization, Geneva, Switzerland. http://monographs.lars.fr/ENG/Monographs/vol70/volume70.pdf. Accessed 3 June 2008.
87. **Ibelgaufts, H., K. W. Jones, N. Maitland, and J. F. Shaw.** 1982. Adenovirus-related RNA sequences in human neurogenic tumours. *Acta Neuropathol.* **56**:113–117.
88. **Ilves, I., S. Kivi, and M. Ustav.** 1999. Long-term episomal maintenance of bovine papillomavirus type 1 plasmids is determined by attachment to host chromosomes, which is mediated by the viral E2 protein and its binding sites. *J. Virol.* **73**:4404–4412.
89. **Ison, M. G.** 2006. Adenovirus infections in transplant recipients. *Clin. Infect. Dis.* **43**:331–339.
90. **Jones, J. F., S. Shurin, C. Abramowsky, R. R. Tubbs, C. G. Sciotto, R. Wahl, J. Sands, D. Gottman, B. Z. Katz, and J. Sklar.** 1988. T-cell lymphomas containing Epstein-Barr viral DNA in patients with chronic Epstein-Barr virus infections. *N. Engl. J. Med.* **318**:733–741.
91. **Kanerva, M., L. Mannonen, H. Piiparinen, M. Peltomaa, A. Vaheri, and A. Pitkaranta.** 2007. Search for herpesviruses in cerebrospinal fluid of facial palsy patients by PCR. *Acta Otolaryngol.* **127**:775–779.
92. **Kaschula, R. O., J. Druker, and A. Kipps.** 1983. Late morphologic consequences of measles: a lethal and debilitating lung disease among the poor. *Rev. Infect. Dis.* **5**:395–404.
93. **Kashima, H. K., P. Mounts, and K. Shah.** 1996. Recurrent respiratory papillomatosis. *Obstet. Gynecol. Clin. North Am.* **23**:699–706.
94. **Kawaguchi, K., H. Inamura, Y. Abe, H. Koshu, E. Takashita, Y. Muraki, Y. Matsuzaki, H. Nishimura, H. Ishikawa, A. Fukao, S. Hongo, and M. Aoyagi.** 2007. Reactivation of herpes simplex virus type 1 and varicella-zoster virus and therapeutic effects of combination therapy with prednisolone and valacyclovir in patients with Bell's palsy. *Laryngoscope* **117**:147–156.
95. **Keicho, N., W. M. Elliott, J. C. Hogg, and S. Hayashi.** 1997. Adenovirus E1A gene dysregulates ICAM-1 expression in transformed pulmonary epithelial cells. *Am. J. Respir. Cell Mol. Biol.* **16**:23–30.
96. **Keicho, N., W. M. Elliott, J. C. Hogg, and S. Hayashi.** 1997. Adenovirus E1A upregulates interleukin-8 expression induced by endotoxin in pulmonary epithelial cells. *Am. J. Physiol.* **272**:L1046–L1052.
97. **Keicho, N., Y. Higashimoto, G. P. Bondy, W. M. Elliott, J. C. Hogg, and S. Hayashi.** 1999. Endotoxin-specific NF-

kappaB activation in pulmonary epithelial cells harboring adenovirus E1A. *Am. J. Physiol.* **277:**L523–L532.

98. **Kieff, E., and A. B. Rickinson.** 2001. Epstein-Barr virus and its replication, p. 2511–2573. *In* D. M. Knipe, P. M. Howley, D. E. Griffin, R. A. Lamb, M. A. Martin, B. Roizman, and S. E. Straus (ed.), *Fields Virology*, 4th ed., vol. 2. Lippincott Williams & Wilkins, Philadelphia, PA.
99. **Knox, K. K., and D. R. Carrigan.** 1994. Disseminated active HHV-6 infections in patients with AIDS. *Lancet* **343:**577–578.
100. **Koelle, D. M., S. Barcy, M. L. Huang, R. L. Ashley, L. Corey, J. Zeh, S. Ashton, and D. Buchwald.** 2002. Markers of viral infection in monozygotic twins discordant for chronic fatigue syndrome. *Clin. Infect. Dis.* **35:**518–525.
101. **Kojaoghlanian, T., P. Flomenberg, and M. S. Horwitz.** 2003. The impact of adenovirus infection on the immunocompromised host. *Rev. Med. Virol.* **13:**155–171.
102. **Kondo, K., T. Kondo, T. Okuno, M. Takahashi, and K. Yamanishi.** 1991. Latent human herpesvirus 6 infection of human monocytes/macrophages. *J. Gen. Virol.* **72:**1401–1408.
103. **Korsager, B., E. S. Spencer, C. H. Mordhorst, and H. K. Andersen.** 1975. Herpesvirus hominis infections in renal transplant recipients. *Scand. J. Infect. Dis.* **7:**11–19.
104. **Kositanont, U., C. Wasi, N. Wanprapar, P. Bowonkiratikachorn, K. Chokephaibulkit, S. Chearskul, K. Chimabutra, R. Sutthent, S. Foongladda, R. Inagi, T. Kurata, and K. Yamanishi.** 1999. Primary infection of human herpesvirus 6 in children with vertical infection of human immunodeficiency virus type 1. *J. Infect. Dis.* **180:**50–55.
105. **Kosuge, H., K. Tanaka-Taya, H. Miyoshi, K. Amo, R. Harada, T. Ebihara, Y. Kawahara, K. Yamanishi, and T. Nishikawa.** 2000. Epidemiological study of human herpesvirus-6 and human herpesvirus-7 in pityriasis rosea. *Br. J. Dermatol.* **143:**795–798.
106. **Kotenko, S. V., S. Saccani, L. S. Izotova, O. V. Mirochnitchenko, and S. Pestka.** 2000. Human cytomegalovirus harbors its own unique IL-10 homolog (cmvIL-10). *Proc. Natl. Acad. Sci.* USA **97:**1695–1700.
107. **Kristie, T. M., J. L. Vogel, and A. E. Sears.** 1999. Nuclear localization of the C1 factor (host cell factor) in sensory neurons correlates with reactivation of herpes simplex virus from latency. *Proc. Natl. Acad. Sci. USA* **96:**1229–1233.
108. **Kuppers, R., and K. Rajewsky.** 1998. The origin of Hodgkin and Reed/Sternberg cells in Hodgkin's disease. *Annu. Rev. Immunol.* **16:**471–493.
109. **Kuwano, K., M. Kawasaki, R. Kunitake, N. Hagimoto, Y. Nomoto, T. Matsuba, Y. Nakanishi, and N. Hara.** 1997. Detection of group C adenovirus DNA in small-cell lung cancer with the nested polymerase chain reaction. *J. Cancer Res. Clin. Oncol.* **123:**377–382.
110. **Laghi, L., A. E. Randolph, D. P. Chauhan, G. Marra, E. O. Major, J. V. Neel, and C. R. Boland.** 1999. JC virus DNA is present in the mucosa of the human colon and in colorectal cancers. *Proc. Natl. Acad. Sci. USA* **96:**7484–7489.
111. **Landini, M. P., T. Lazzarotto, J. Xu, A. P. Geballe, and E. S. Mocarski.** 2000. Humoral immune response to proteins of human cytomegalovirus latency-associated transcripts. *Biol. Blood Marrow Transplant.* **6:**100–108.
112. **Lang, W. R., C. W. Howden, J. Laws, and J. F. Burton.** 1969. Bronchopneumonia with serious sequelae in children with evidence of adenovirus type 21 infection. *Br. Med. J.* **1:**73–79.
113. **Lee, E. S., J. Locker, M. Nalesnik, J. Reyes, R. Jaffe, M. Alashari, B. Nour, A. Tzakis, and P. S. Dickman.** 1995. The association of Epstein-Barr virus with smooth-muscle tumors occurring after organ transplantation. *N. Engl. J. Med.* **332:**19–25.
114. **Leen, A. M., C. M. Bollard, G. D. Myers, and C. M. Rooney.** 2006. Adenoviral infections in hematopoietic stem cell transplantation. *Biol. Blood Marrow Transplant.* **12:**243–251.
115. **Linder, T., W. Bossart, and D. Bodmer.** 2005. Bell's palsy and herpes simplex virus: fact or mystery? *Otol. Neurotol.* **26:**109–113.
116. **Liu, Y., R. de Waal Malefyt, F. Briere, C. Parham, J. M. Bridon, J. Banchereau, K. W. Moore, and J. Xu.** 1997. The EBV IL-10 homologue is a selective agonist with impaired binding to the IL-10 receptor. *J. Immunol.* **158:**604–613.
117. **London, W. T., S. A. Houff, D. L. Madden, D. A. Fuccillo, M. Gravell, W. C. Wallen, A. E. Palmer, J. L. Sever, B. L. Padgett, D. L. Walker, G. M. ZuRhein, and T. Ohashi.** 1978. Brain tumors in owl monkeys inoculated with a human polyomavirus (JC virus). *Science* **201:**1246–1249.
118. **Lowy, D. R., and P. M. Howley.** 2001. Papillomaviruses, p. 2231–2264. *In* D. M. Knipe, P. M. Howley, D. E. Griffin, R. A. Lamb, M. A. Martin, B. Roizman, and S. E. Straus (ed.), *Fields Virology*, 4th ed., vol. 2. Lippincott Williams & Wilkins, Philadelphia, PA.
119. **Lukashok, S., and M. S. Horwitz.** 1997. Adenovirus persistence, p. 147–164. *In* R. Ahmed, and I. Chen (ed.), *Persistent Viral Infections*. John Wiley & Sons, Chichester, United Kingdom.
120. **Lukashok, S. A., and M. S. Horwitz.** 1998. New perspectives in adenoviruses. *Curr. Clin. Top. Infect. Dis.* **18:**286–305.
121. **Lungu, O., P. W. Annunziato, A. Gershon, S. M. Staugaitis, D. Josefson, P. LaRussa, and S. J. Silverstein.** 1995. Reactivated and latent varicella-zoster virus in human dorsal root ganglia. *Proc. Natl. Acad. Sci. USA* **92:**10980–10984.
122. **Luppi, M., P. Barozzi, C. Morris, A. Maiorana, R. Garber, G. Bonacorsi, A. Donelli, R. Marasca, A. Tabilio, and G. Torelli.** 1999. Human herpesvirus 6 latently infects early bone marrow progenitors in vivo. *J. Virol.* **73:**754–759.
123. **Lusso, P., P. Secchiero, R. W. Crowley, A. Garzino-Demo, Z. N. Berneman, and R. C. Gallo.** 1994. CD4 is a critical component of the receptor for human herpesvirus 7: interference with human immunodeficiency virus. *Proc. Natl. Acad. Sci. USA* **91:**3872–3876.
124. **MacMahon, B.** 1966. Epidemiology of Hodgkin's disease. *Cancer Res.* **26:**1189–1201.
125. **Magrath, I.** 1990. The pathogenesis of Burkitt's lymphoma. *Adv. Cancer Res.* **55:**133–270.
126. **Major, E. O.** 2001. Human polyomavirus, p. 2175–2196. *In* D. M. Knipe, P. M. Howley, D. E. Griffin, R. A. Lamb, M. A. Martin, B. Roizman, and S. E. Straus (ed.), *Fields Virology*, 4th ed., vol. 2. Lippincott Williams & Wilkins, Philadelphia, PA.
127. **Malkin, D., S. Chilton-MacNeill, L. A. Meister, E. Sexsmith, L. Diller, and R. L. Garcea.** 2001. Tissue-specific expression of SV40 in tumors associated with the Li-Fraumeni syndrome. *Oncogene* **20:**4441–4449.
128. **Manfredi, J. J., J. Dong, W. J. Liu, L. Resnick-Silverman, R. Qiao, P. Chahinian, M. Saric, A. R. Gibbs, J. I. Phillips, J. Murray, C. W. Axten, R. P. Nolan, and S. A. Aaronson.** 2005. Evidence against a role for SV40 in human mesothelioma. *Cancer Res.* **65:**2602–2609.
129. **Marttila, M., D. Persson, D. Gustafsson, M. K. Liszewski, J. P. Atkinson, G. Wadell, and N. Arnberg.** 2005. CD46 is a cellular receptor for all species B adenoviruses except types 3 and 7. *J. Virol.* **79:**14429–144436.

130. **Matsuse, T., S. Hayashi, K. Kuwano, H. Keunecke, W. A. Jefferies, and J. C. Hogg.** 1992. Latent adenoviral infection in the pathogenesis of chronic airways obstruction. *Am. Rev. Respir. Dis.* **146:**177–184.

131. **McClain, K. L., C. T. Leach, H. B. Jenson, V. V. Joshi, B. H. Pollock, R. T. Parmley, F. J. DiCarlo, E. G. Chadwick, and S. B. Murphy.** 1995. Association of Epstein-Barr virus with leiomyosarcomas in children with AIDS. *N. Engl. J. Med.* **332:**12–18.

132. **McCormick, D. P.** 1972. Herpes-simplex virus as a cause of Bell's palsy. *Lancet* **i:**937–939.

133. **McDonald, K., T. S. Rector, E. A. Braulin, S. H. Kubo, and M. T. Olivari.** 1989. Association of coronary artery disease in cardiac transplant recipients with cytomegalovirus infection. *Am. J. Cardiol.* **64:**359–362.

134. **Mead, J., J. M. Turner, P. T. Macklem, and J. B. Little.** 1967. Significance of the relationship between lung recoil and maximum expiratory flow. *J. Appl. Physiol.* **22:**95–108.

135. **Mellerick, D. M., and N. W. Fraser.** 1987. Physical state of the latent herpes simplex virus genome in a mouse model system: evidence suggesting an episomal state. *Virology* **158:**265–275.

136. **Meshi, B., T. Z. Vitalis, D. Ionescu, W. M. Elliott, C. Liu, X. D. Wang, S. Hayashi, and J. C. Hogg.** 2002. Emphysematous lung destruction by cigarette smoke. The effects of latent adenoviral infection on the lung inflammatory response. *Am. J. Respir. Cell Mol. Biol.* **26:**52–57.

137. **Miller, D. M., and D. D. Sedmak.** 1999. Viral effects on antigen processing. *Curr. Opin. Immunol.* **11:**94–99.

138. **Mocarski, E. S., Jr., and C. T. Courcelle.** 2001. Cytomegaloviruses and their replication, p. 2629–2673. *In* D. M. Knipe, P. M. Howley, D. E. Griffin, R. A. Lamb, M. A. Martin, B. Roizman, and S. E. Straus (ed.), *Fields Virology*, 4th ed., vol. 2. Lippincott Williams & Wilkins, Philadelphia, PA.

139. **Mogabgab, W. J.** 1968. Acute respiratory illnesses in university (1962-1966), military and industrial (1962-1963) populations. *Am. Rev. Respir. Dis.* **98:**359–379.

140. **Momose, H., E. S. Jaffe, S. S. Shin, Y. Y. Chen, and L. M. Weiss.** 1992. Chronic lymphocytic leukemia/small lymphocytic lymphoma with Reed-Sternberg-like cells and possible transformation to Hodgkin's disease. Mediation by Epstein-Barr virus. *Am. J. Surg. Pathol.* **16:**859–867.

141. **Montgomerie, J. Z., D. M. Becroft, M. C. Croxson, P. B. Doak, and J. D. North.** 1969. Herpes-simplex-virus infection after renal transplantation. *Lancet* **ii:**867–71.

142. **Murray, C. J., and A. D. Lopez.** 1996. Evidence-based health policy—lessons from the Global Burden of Disease Study. *Science* **274:**740–743.

143. **Nahmias, A. J., H. L. Keyserling, and G. M. Kerrick.** 1983. Herpes simplex, p. 636–678. *In* J. S. Remington and J. O. Klein (ed.), *Infectious Diseases of the Fetus and Newborn Infant.* WB Saunders, Philadelphia, PA.

144. **Nahmias, A. J., F. K. Lee, and S. Bechman-Nahmias.** 1990. Sero-epidemiological and sociological patterns of herpes simplex virus infection in the world. *Scand. J. Infect. Dis.* **69:**19–36.

145. **Nalesnik, M. A.** 1998. Clinical and pathological features of post-transplant lymphoproliferative disorders (PTLD). *Springer Semin. Immunopathol.* **20:**325–342.

146. **Nilsson, K., G. Klein, W. Henle, and G. Henle.** 1971. The establishment of lymphoblastoid lines from adult and fetal human lymphoid tissue and its dependence on EBV. *Int. J. Cancer* **8:**443–450.

147. **Ogawa, E., W. M. Elliott, F. Hughes, T. J. Eichholtz, J. C. Hogg, and S. Hayashi.** 2004. Latent adenoviral infection induces production of growth factors relevant to airway remodeling in COPD. *Am. J. Physiol. Lung Cell. Mol. Physiol.* **286:**L189–197.

147a. **Ogawa, E., A. Kartono, J. C. Hogg, S. Hayashi.** 2003. The mechanism of ICAM-1 gene regulation by adenovirus E1A in transfected human bronchial epithelial cells. *Am. J. Respir. Crit. Care Med.* **167:**A401. (Abstract.)

148. **Okuno, T., K. Higashi, K. Shiraki, K. Yamanishi, M. Takahashi, Y. Kokado, M. Ishibashi, S. Takahara, T. Sonoda, K. Tanaka,** K. Baba, H. Yabuuchi, and T., Kurata. 1990. Human herpesvirus 6 infection in renal transplantation. *Transplantation* **49:**519–522.

149. **Okuno, T., K. Takahashi, K. Balachandra, K. Shiraki, K. Yamanishi, M. Takahashi, and K. Baba.** 1989. Seroepidemiology of human herpesvirus 6 infection in normal children and adults. *J. Clin. Microbiol.* **27:**651–653.

150. **O'Sullivan, C. E., W. L. Drew, D. J. McMullen, R. Miner, J. Y. Lee, R. A. Kaslow, J. G. Lazar, and M. S. Saag.** 1999. Decrease of cytomegalovirus replication in human immunodeficiency virus infected-patients after treatment with highly active antiretroviral therapy. *J. Infect. Dis.* **180:**847–849.

151. **Pallesen, G., S. J. Hamilton-Dutoit, and X. Zhou.** 1993. The association of Epstein-Barr virus (EBV) with T cell lymphoproliferations and Hodgkin's disease: two new developments in the EBV field. *Adv. Cancer Res.* **62:**179–239.

152. **Parkin, D. M., P. Pisani, and J. Ferlay.** 1999. Estimates of the worldwide incidence of 25 major cancers in 1990. *Int. J. Cancer* **80:**827–841.

153. **Pass, R. F.** 2001. Cytomegalovirus, p. 2675–2705. *In* D. M. Knipe, P. M. Howley, D. E. Griffin, R. A. Lamb, M. A. Martin, B. Roizman, and S. E. Straus (ed.), *Fields Virology*, 4th ed., vol. 2. Lippincott Williams & Wilkins, Philadelphia, PA.

154. **Pass, R. F., C. Hutto, R. Ricks, and G. A. Cloud.** 1986. Increased rate of cytomegalovirus infection among parents of children attending day-care centers. *N. Engl. J. Med.* **314:**1414–1418.

155. **Pauwels, R. A., A. S. Buist, P. Ma, C. R. Jenkins, and S. S. Hurd.** 2001. Global strategy for the diagnosis, management, and prevention of chronic obstructive pulmonary disease: National Heart, Lung, and Blood Institute and World Health Organization Global Initiative for Chronic Obstructive Lung Disease (GOLD): executive summary. *Respir. Care* **46:**798–825.

156. **Peacock, J. E., Jr., and F. A. Sarubbi.** 1983. Disseminated herpes simplex virus infection during pregnancy. *Obstet. Gynecol.* **61:**13S–18S.

157. **Pellett, P. E., and G. Dominguez.** 2001. Human herpesviruses 6A, 6B, and 7 and their replication, p. 2769–2784. *In* D. M. Knipe, P. M. Howley, D. E. Griffin, R. A. Lamb, M. A. Martin, B. Roizman, and S. E. Straus (ed.), *Fields Virology*, 4th ed., vol. 2. Lippincott Williams & Wilkins, Philadelphia, PA.

158. **Penfold, M. E., D. J. Dairaghi, G. M. Duke, N. Saederup, E. S. Mocarski, G. W. Kemble, and T. J. Schall.** 1999. Cytomegalovirus encodes a potent alpha chemokine. *Proc. Natl. Acad. Sci. USA* **96:**9839–9844.

159. **Pichler, M. N., J. Reichenbach, H. Schmidt, G. Herrmann, and S. Zielen.** 2000. Severe adenovirus bronchiolitis in children. *Acta Paediatr.* **89:**1387–1389.

160. **Qavi, H. B., M. T. Green, G. K. SeGall, and R. L. Font.** 1989. Demonstration of HIV-1 and HHV-6 in AIDS-associated retinitis. *Curr. Eye Res.* **8:**379–387.

161. **Reidy, P. M., H. H. Dedo, R. Rabah, J. B. Field, R. H. Mathog, L. Gregoire, and W. D. Lancaster.** 2004. Integration of human papillomavirus type 11 in recurrent respira-

tory papilloma-associated cancer. *Laryngoscope* **114:**1906–1909.

162. **Rencic, A., J. Gordon, J. Otte, M. Curtis, A. Kovatich, P. Zoltick, K. Khalili, and D. Andrews.** 1996. Detection of JC virus DNA sequence and expression of the viral oncoprotein, tumor antigen, in brain of immunocompetent patient with oligoastrocytoma. *Proc. Natl. Acad. Sci. USA* **93:**7352–7357.
163. **Retamales, I., W. M. Elliott, B. Meshi, H. O. Coxson, P. D. Pare, F. C. Sciurba, R. M. Rogers, S. Hayashi, and J. C. Hogg.** 2001. Amplification of inflammation in emphysema and its association with latent adenoviral infection. *Am. J. Respir. Crit. Care Med.* **164:**469–473.
164. **Revello, M. G., M. Zavattoni, A. Sarasini, E. Percivalle, L. Simoncini, and G. Gerna.** 1998. Human cytomegalovirus in blood of immunocompetent persons during primary infection: prognostic implications for pregnancy. *J. Infect. Dis.* **177:**1170–1175.
165. **Reynolds, D. W., S. Stagno, T. S. Hosty, M. Tiller, and C. A. Alford, Jr.** 1973. Maternal cytomegalovirus excretion and perinatal infection. *N. Engl. J. Med.* **289:**1–5.
166. **Rickinson, A. B., and E. Kieff.** 2001. Epstein-Barr virus, p. 2575–2627. *In* D. M. Knipe, P. M. Howley, D. E. Griffin, R. A. Lamb, M. A. Martin, B. Roizman, and S. E. Straus (ed.), *Fields Virology*, 4th ed., vol. 2. Lippincott Williams & Wilkins, Philadelphia, PA.
167. **Rock, D. L., and N. W. Fraser.** 1983. Detection of HSV-1 genome in central nervous system of latently infected mice. *Nature* **302:**523–525.
168. **Rock, D. L., and N. W. Fraser.** 1985. Latent herpes simplex virus type 1 DNA contains two copies of the virion DNA joint region. *J. Virol.* **55:**849–852.
169. **Roizman, B.** 1966. An inquiry into the mechanisms of recurrent herpes infection of man, p. 283–304. *In* M. Pollard (ed.), *Perspectives in Virology*, vol. 4. Harper-Row, New York, NY.
170. **Roizman, B., and D. M. Knipe.** 2001. Herpes simplex viruses and their replication, p. 2399–2509. *In* D. M. Knipe, P. M. Howley, D. E. Griffin, R. A. Lamb, M. A. Martin, B. Roizman, and S. E. Straus (ed.), *Fields Virology*, 4th ed., vol. 2. Lippincott Williams & Wilkins, Philadelphia, PA.
171. **Roizman, B., and P. E. Pellett.** 2001. The family *Herpesviridae*: brief introduction, p. 2381–2397. *In* D. M. Knipe, P. M. Howley, D. E. Griffin, R. A. Lamb, M. A. Martin, B. Roizman, and S. E. Straus (ed.), *Fields Virology*, 4th ed., vol. 2. Lippincott Williams & Wilkins, Philadelphia, PA.
172. **Rollison, D. E., W. J. Sexton, A. R. Rodriguez, L. C. Kang, R. Daniel, and K. V. Shah.** 2007. Lack of BK virus DNA sequences in most transitional-cell carcinomas of the bladder. *Int. J. Cancer* **120:**1248–1251.
173. **Rosato, F. E., E. F. Rosato, and S. A. Plotkin.** 1970. Herpetic paronychia—an occupational hazard of medical personnel. *N. Engl. J. Med.* **283:**804–805.
174. **Rosenbaum, M. J., E. A. Edwards, P. F. Frank, W. E. Pierce, Y. E. Crawford, and L. F. Miller.** 1965. Epidemiology and prevention of acute respiratory disease in naval recruits. I. Ten years' experience with microbial agents isolated from naval recruits with acute respiratory disease. *Am. J. Public Health Nations Health* **55:**38–46.
175. **Rosman, F. C., A. S. Mistchenko, H. S. Ladenheim, J. P. do Nascimento, H. N. Outani, K. Madi, and H. L. Lenzi.** 1996. Acute and chronic human adenovirus pneumonia: cellular and extracellular matrix components. *Pediatr. Pathol. Lab. Med.* **16:**521–541.
176. **Rowe, M., R. Khanna, C. A. Jacob, V. Argaet, A. Kelly, S. Powis, M. Belich, D. Croom-Carter, S. Lee, S. R. Burrows, J. Trowsdale, D. J. Moss, and A. B. Rickinson.** 1995. Restoration of endogenous antigen processing in Burkitt's lymphoma cells by Epstein-Barr virus latent membrane protein-1: coordinate up-regulation of peptide transporters and HLA-class I antigen expression. *Eur. J. Immunol.* **25:**1374–1384.
177. **Rubio, R.** 1994. Hodgkin's disease associated with human immunodeficiency virus infection. A clinical study of 46 cases. Cooperative Study Group of Malignancies Associated with HIV Infection of Madrid. *Cancer* **73:**2400–2407.
178. **Russell, K. L., M. P. Broderick, S. E. Franklin, L. B. Blyn, N. E. Freed, E. Moradi, D. J. Ecker, P. E. Kammerer, M. A. Osuna, A. E. Kajon, C. B. Morn, and M. A. Ryan.** 2006. Transmission dynamics and prospective environmental sampling of adenovirus in a military recruit setting. *J. Infect. Dis.* **194:**877–885.
179. **Russell, K. L., A. W. Hawksworth, M. A. Ryan, J. Strickler, M. Irvine, C. J. Hansen, G. C. Gray, and J. C. Gaydos.** 2006. Vaccine-preventable adenoviral respiratory illness in US military recruits, 1999-2004. *Vaccine* **24:**2835–2842.
180. **Saito, Y., L. R. Sharer, S. Dewhurst, B. M. Blumberg, C. B. Hall, and L. G. Epstein.** 1995. Cellular localization of human herpesvirus-6 in the brains of children with AIDS encephalopathy. *J. Neurovirol.* **1:**30–99.
181. **Sandler, E. S., V. M. Aquino, E. Goss-Shohet, S. Hinrichs, and K. Krisher.** 1997. BK papova virus pneumonia following hematopoietic stem cell transplantation. *Bone Marrow Transplant.* **20:**163–165.
182. **Santoro, F., P. E. Kennedy, G. Locatelli, M. S. Malnati, E. A. Berger, and P. Lusso.** 1999. CD46 is a cellular receptor for human herpesvirus 6. *Cell* **99:**817–827.
183. **Sasajima, Y., H. Yamabe, Y. Kobashi, K. Hirai, and S. Mori.** 1993. High expression of the Epstein-Barr virus latent protein EB nuclear antigen-2 on pyothorax-associated lymphomas. *Am. J. Pathol.* **143:**1280–1285.
184. **Schiffman, M. H.** 1994. Epidemiology of cervical human papillomaviruses. *In* H. Hausen (ed.), *Human Pathogenic Papillomaviruses*. Springer-Verlag, Heidelberg, Germany.
185. **Schmitz, H., R. Wigand, and W. Heinrich.** 1983. Worldwide epidemiology of human adenovirus infections. *Am. J. Epidemiol.* **117:**455–466.
186. **Schmutzhard, E.** 2001. Viral infections of the CNS with special emphasis on herpes simplex infections. *J. Neurol.* **248:**469–477.
187. **Schwarz, E., U. K. Freese, L. Gissmann, W. Mayer, B. Roggenbuck, A. Stremlau, and H. zur Hausen.** 1985. Structure and transcription of human papillomavirus sequences in cervical carcinoma cells. *Nature* **314:**111–114.
188. **Seishima, M., S. Yamanaka, T. Fujisawa, M. Tohyama, and K. Hashimoto.** 2006. Reactivation of human herpesvirus (HHV) family members other than HHV-6 in drug-induced hypersensitivity syndrome. *Br. J. Dermatol.* **155:**344–349.
189. **Shah, K., and N. Nathanson.** 1976. Human exposure to SV40: review and comment. *Am. J. Epidemiol.* **103:**1–12.
190. **Shek, T. W., F. C. Ho, I. O. Ng, A. C. Chan, L. Ma, and G. Srivastava.** 1996. Follicular dendritic cell tumor of the liver. Evidence for an Epstein-Barr virus-related clonal proliferation of follicular dendritic cells. *Am. J. Surg. Pathol.* **20:**313–324.
191. **Shenk, T. E.** 2001. Adenoviridae: the viruses and their replication, p. 2265–2300. *In* D. M. Knipe, P. M. Howley, D. E. Griffin, R. A. Lamb, M. A. Martin, B. Roizman, and S. E. Straus (ed.), Fields Virology, 4th ed., vol. 2. Lippincott Williams & Wilkins, Philadelphia, PA.

192. **Singh, J., and E. K. Wagner.** 1993. Transcriptional analysis of the herpes simplex virus type 1 region containing the TRL/UL junction. *Virology* **196:**220–231.

193. **Singh, N., D. R. Carrigan, T. Gayowski, and I. R. Marino.** 1997. Human herpesvirus-6 infection in liver transplant recipients: documentation of pathogenicity. *Transplantation* **64:**674–678.

194. **Singh, N., D. R. Carrigan, T. Gayowski, J. Singh, and I. R. Marino.** 1995. Variant B human herpesvirus-6 associated febrile dermatosis with thrombocytopenia and encephalopathy in a liver transplant recipient. *Transplantation* **60:**1355–1357.

195. **Sixbey, J. W., J. G. Nedrud, N. Raab-Traub, R. A. Hanes, and J. S. Pagano.** 1984. Epstein-Barr virus replication in oropharyngeal epithelial cells. *N. Engl. J. Med.* **310:**1225–1230.

196. **Smith, M.** 1997. Considerations on a possible viral etiology for B-precursor acute lymphoblastic leukemia of childhood. *J. Immunother.* **20:**89–100.

197. **Steiner, I., and Y. Mattan.** 1999. Bell's palsy and herpes viruses: to (acyclo)vir or not to (acyclo)vir? *J. Neurol. Sci.* **170:**19–23.

198. **Stern, P. L.** 1996. Immunity to human papillomavirus-associated cervical neoplasia. *Adv. Cancer Res.* **69:**175–211.

199. **Stewart, J. P., J. J. Egan, A. J. Ross, B. G. Kelly, S. S. Lok, P. S. Hasleton, and A. A. Woodcock.** 1999. The detection of Epstein-Barr virus DNA in lung tissue from patients with idiopathic pulmonary fibrosis. *Am. J. Respir. Crit. Care Med.* **159:**1336–1341.

200. **Stjernquist-Desatnik, A., E. Skoog, and E. Aurelius.** 2006. Detection of herpes simplex and varicella-zoster viruses in patients with Bell's palsy by the polymerase chain reaction technique. *Ann. Otol. Rhinol. Laryngol.* **115:**306–311.

201. **Strickler, H. D., J. J. Goedert, M. Fleming, W. D. Travis, A. E. Williams, C. S. Rabkin, R. W. Daniel, and K. V. Shah.** 1996. Simian virus 40 and pleural mesothelioma in humans. *Cancer Epidemiol. Biomarkers Prev.* **5:**473–475.

202. **Strockbine, L. D., J. I. Cohen, T. Farrah, S. D. Lyman, F. Wagener, R. F. DuBose, R. J. Armitage, and M. K. Spriggs.** 1998. The Epstein-Barr virus BARF1 gene encodes a novel, soluble colony-stimulating factor-1 receptor. *J. Virol.* **72:**4015–4021.

203. **Su, I. J., and J. Y. Chen.** 1997. The role of Epstein-Barr virus in lymphoid malignancies. *Crit. Rev. Oncol. Hematol.* **26:**25–41.

204. **Su, I. J., Y. H. Hsu, M. T. Lin, A. L. Cheng, C. H. Wang, and L. M. Weiss.** 1993. Epstein-Barr virus-containing T-cell lymphoma presents with hemophagocytic syndrome mimicking malignant histiocytosis. *Cancer* **72:**2019–2027.

205. **Sugawara, Y., Y. Mizugaki, T. Uchida, T. Torii, S. Imai, M. Makuuchi, and K. Takada.** 1999. Detection of Epstein-Barr virus (EBV) in hepatocellular carcinoma tissue: a novel EBV latency characterized by the absence of EBV-encoded small RNA expression. *Virology* **256:**196–202.

206. **Sullivan, J. L., and B. A. Woda.** 1989. X-linked lymphoproliferative syndrome. *Immunodefic. Rev.* **1:**325–347.

207. **Tanaka, K., T. Kondo, S. Torigoe, S. Okada, T. Mukai, and K. Yamanishi.** 1994. Human herpesvirus 7: another causal agent for roseola (exanthem subitum). *J. Pediatr.* **125:**1–5.

208. **Tanaka-Taya, K., T. Kondo, T. Mukai, H. Miyoshi, Y. Yamamoto, S. Okada, and K. Yamanishi.** 1996. Seroepidemiological study of human herpesvirus-6 and -7 in children of different ages and detection of these two viruses in throat swabs by polymerase chain reaction. *J. Med. Virol.* **48:**88–94.

209. **Testa, J. R., M. Carbone, A. Hirvonen, K. Khalili, B. Krynska, K. Linnainmaa, F. D. Pooley, P. Rizzo, V. Rusch, and G. H. Xiao.** 1998. A multi-institutional study confirms the presence and expression of simian virus 40 in human malignant mesotheliomas. *Cancer Res.* **58:**4505–4509.

210. **Top, F. H., Jr., E. L. Buescher, W. H. Bancroft, and P. K. Russell.** 1971. Immunization with live types 7 and 4 adenovirus vaccines. II. Antibody response and protective effect against acute respiratory disease due to adenovirus type 7. *J. Infect. Dis.* **124:**155–160.

211. **Torrisi, M. R., M. Gentile, G. Cardinali, M. Cirone, C. Zompetta, L. V. Lotti, L. Frati, and A. Faggioni.** 1999. Intracellular transport and maturation pathway of human herpesvirus 6. *Virology* **257:**460–471.

212. **Trentin, J. J., Y. Yabe, and G. Taylor.** 1962. The quest for human cancer viruses. *Science* **137:**835–841.

213. **Tuke, P. W., S. Hawke, P. D. Griffiths, and D. A. Clark.** 2004. Distribution and quantification of human herpesvirus 6 in multiple sclerosis and control brains. *Mult. Scler.* **10:**355–359.

214. **Tyler, K. L., and N. Nathanson.** 2001. Pathogenesis of viral infections, p. 199–243. *In* D. M. Knipe, P. M. Howley, D. E. Griffin, R. A. Lamb, M. A. Martin, B. Roizman, and S. E. Straus (ed.), *Fields Virology*, vol. 1. Lippincott Williams & Wilkins, Philadelphia, PA.

215. **Vafai, A., M. Wellish, and D. H. Gilden.** 1988. Expression of varicella-zoster virus in blood mononuclear cells of patients with postherpetic neuralgia. *Proc. Natl. Acad. Sci. USA* **85:**2767–2770.

216. **Van Brabandt, H., M. Cauberghs, E. Verbeken, P. Moerman, J. M. Lauweryns, and K. P. Van de Woestijne.** 1983. Partitioning of pulmonary impedance in excised human and canine lungs. *J. Appl. Physiol.* **55:**1733–1742.

217. **Vitalis, T. Z., N. Keicho, S. Itabashi, S. Hayashi, and J. C. Hogg.** 1996. A model of latent adenovirus 5 infection in the guinea pig (*Cavia porcellus*). *Am. J. Respir. Cell Mol. Biol.* **14:**225–31.

218. **Vitalis, T. Z., I. Kern, A. Croome, H. Behzad, S. Hayashi, and J. C. Hogg.** 1998. The effect of latent adenovirus 5 infection on cigarette smoke-induced lung inflammation. *Eur. Respir. J.* **11:**664–669.

219. **Voltz, R., G. Jager, K. Seelos, L. Fuhry, and R. Hohlfeld.** 1996. BK virus encephalitis in an immunocompetent patient. *Arch. Neurol.* **53:**101–103.

220. **Vontver, L. A., D. E. Hickok, Z. Brown, L. Reid, and L. Corey.** 1982. Recurrent genital herpes simplex virus infection in pregnancy: infant outcome and frequency of asymptomatic recurrences. *Am. J. Obstet. Gynecol.* **143:**75–84.

221. **Vrabec, J. T., and D. A. Payne.** 2001. Prevalence of herpesviruses in cranial nerve ganglia. *Acta Otolaryngol.* **121:**831–835.

222. **Wade, A. W., A. T. McDonald, P. D. Acott, S. Lee, and J. F. Crocker.** 1998. Human herpes virus-6 or Epstein-Barr virus infection and acute allograft rejection in pediatric kidney transplant recipients: greater risk for immunologically naive recipients. *Transplant. Proc.* **30:**2091–2093.

223. **Wadsworth, S., R. J. Jacob, and B. Roizman.** 1975. Anatomy of herpes simplex virus DNA. II. Size, composition, and arrangement of inverted terminal repetitions. *J. Virol.* **15:**1487–1497.

224. **Wallace, H. L., II, B. Natelson, W. Gause, and J. Hay.** 1999. Human herpesviruses in chronic fatigue syndrome. *Clin. Diagn. Lab. Immunol.* **6:**216–223.

225. **Wang, K., T. Y. Lau, M. Morales, E. K. Mont, and S. E. Straus.** 2005. Laser-capture microdissection: refining estimates of the quantity and distribution of latent herpes

simplex virus 1 and varicella-zoster virus DNA in human trigeminal Ganglia at the single-cell level. *J. Virol.* **79:**14079–14087.

226. **Wangoo, A., R. J. Shaw, T. C. Diss, P. J. Farrell, R. M. du Bois, and A. G. Nicholson.** 1997. Cryptogenic fibrosing alveolitis: lack of association with Epstein-Barr virus infection. *Thorax* **52:**888–891.
227. **Warner, J. O., and W. C. Marshall.** 1976. Crippling lung disease after measles and adenovirus infection. *Br. J. Dis. Chest* **70:**89–94.
228. **Watanabe, T., T. Kawamura, S. E. Jacob, E. A. Aquilino, J. M. Orenstein, J. B. Black, and A. Blauvelt.** 2002. Pityriasis rosea is associated with systemic active infection with both human herpesvirus-7 and human herpesvirus-6. *J. Invest. Dermatol.* **119:**793–7.
229. **Watson, P. N., and R. J. Evans.** 1986. Postherpetic neuralgia. A review. *Arch. Neurol.* **43:**836–840.
230. **Weiss, L. M., L. A. Movahed, R. A. Warnke, and J. Sklar.** 1989. Detection of Epstein-Barr viral genomes in Reed-Sternberg cells of Hodgkin's disease. *N. Engl. J. Med.* **320:**502–506.
231. **Weiss, L. M., J. G. Strickler, R. A. Warnke, D. T. Purtilo, and J. Sklar.** 1987. Epstein-Barr viral DNA in tissues of Hodgkin's disease. *Am. J. Pathol.* **129:**86–91.
232. **Whitley, R., A. D. Lakeman, A. Nahmias, and B. Roizman.** 1982. DNA restriction-enzyme analysis of herpes simplex virus isolates obtained from patients with encephalitis. *N. Engl. J. Med.* **307:**1060–2.
233. **Whitley, R. J.** 2001. Herpes simplex viruses, p. 2461–2509. *In* D. M. Knipe, P. M. Howley, D. E. Griffin, R. A. Lamb, M. A. Martin, B. Roizman, and S. E. Straus (ed.), *Fields Virology*, 4th ed., vol. 2. Lippincott Williams & Wilkins, Philadelphia, PA.
234. **Whitley, R. J., M. Levin, N. Barton, B. J. Hershey, G. Davis, R. E. Keeney, J. Whelchel, A. G. Diethelm, P. Kartus, and S. J. Soong.** 1984. Infections caused by herpes simplex virus in the immunocompromised host: natural history and topical acyclovir therapy. *J. Infect. Dis.* **150:**323–329.
235. **Wiatrak, B. J., D. W. Wiatrak, T. R. Broker, and L. Lewis.** 2004. Recurrent respiratory papillomatosis: a longitudinal study comparing severity associated with human papilloma viral types 6 and 11 and other risk factors in a large pediatric population. *Laryngoscope* **114:**1–23.
236. **Yamanishi, K.** 2001. Human herpesviruses 6 and human herpesviruses 7, p. 2785–2801. *In* D. M. Knipe, P. M. Howley, D. E. Griffin, R. A. Lamb, M. A. Martin, B. Roizman, and S. E. Straus (ed.), *Fields Virology*, 4th ed., vol. 2. Lippincott Williams & Wilkins, Philadelphia, PA.
237. **Yamanishi, K., T. Okuno, K. Shiraki, M. Takahashi, T. Kondo, Y. Asano, and T. Kurata.** 1988. Identification of human herpesvirus-6 as a causal agent for exanthem subitum. *Lancet* **i:**1065–1067.
238. **Yamashita, Y., K. Shimokata, S. Mizuno, H. Yamaguchi, and Y. Nishiyama.** 1993. Down-regulation of the surface expression of class I MHC antigens by human cytomegalovirus. *Virology* **193:**727–736.
239. **Yanai, M., K. Sekizawa, T. Ohrui, H. Sasaki, and T. Takishima.** 1992. Site of airway obstruction in pulmonary disease: direct measurement of intrabronchial pressure. *J. Appl. Physiol.* **72:**1016–1023.
240. **Zanghellini, F., S. B. Boppana, V. C. Emery, P. D. Griffiths, and R. F. Pass.** 1999. Asymptomatic primary cytomegalovirus infection: virologic and immunologic features. *J. Infect. Dis.* **180:**702–707.
241. **Zhou, Y. F., M. B. Leon, M. A. Waclawiw, J. J. Popma, Z. X. Yu, T. Finkel, and S. E. Epstein.** 1996. Association between prior cytomegalovirus infection and the risk of restenosis after coronary atherectomy. *N. Engl. J. Med.* **335:**624–630.

Sequelae and Long-Term Consequences of Infectious Diseases
Edited by Pina M. Fratamico, James L. Smith, and Kim A. Brogden

Chapter 20

Sequelae of Chronic Viral Hepatitis

PAOLO SACCHI, RAFFAELE BRUNO, GIUSEPPE BARBARO, AND GIORGIO BARBARINI

Chronic liver diseases are a major cause of morbidity and mortality worldwide. Viral chronic hepatitis accounts for a great proportion of liver cirrhosis, end-stage liver disease (ESLD), and related deaths, and it is linked to the development of hepatocellular carcinoma and to the increased need for liver transplantation. Recently, the availability of new antiviral drugs has profoundly changed the characteristics of these diseases, giving the physician the possibility to slow or stop their natural histories.

Viral hepatitis can be defined as a disease in which the necroinflammatory process of the liver accounts for the majority of the clinical and laboratory features. Etiologic agents include at least five taxonomically different viral agents: hepatitis A virus (HAV), hepatitis B virus (HBV), hepatitis C virus (HCV), hepatitis delta virus (HDV), and hepatitis E virus (HEV). Hepatitis caused by other viruses, such as Epstein-Barr or cytomegalovirus, is part of clinical manifestations of extrahepatic diseases and will not be discussed here. In this chapter, we will review the natural history of chronic viral hepatitis, including a focus on pathogenesis, and outline the characteristics of the complications and the management.

CHARACTERISTICS OF HEPATITIS VIRUSES

HAV

HAV is a nonenveloped 27-nm and heat-, acid-, and ether-resistant RNA virus in the *Hepatovirus* genus of the picornavirus family. HAV has an incubation period of approximately 4 weeks. Its replication is limited to the liver, but the virus is present in the liver, bile, stool, and blood during the late incubation period and acute preicteric phase of illness. Despite the persistence of virus in the liver, viral shedding in feces, viremia, and infectivity diminish rapidly once jaundice becomes apparent. Antibodies to HAV (anti-HAV) can be detected during acute illness when serum aminotransferase activity is elevated. HAV-immunoglobulin M (IgM) antibody persists for up to 6 to 12 months and is followed by the appearance of IgG antibodies during the convalescence phase. The diagnosis of HAV is made during acute illness by demonstrating anti-HAV IgM antibodies. Anti-HAV IgG antibodies remain detectable indefinitely, and patients with serum anti-HAV antibodies are immune to reinfection. HAV is generally a self-limiting disease resolving without sequelae. In some (very rare) cases it may cause a clinical picture of fulminant hepatitis requiring the need for orthotopic liver transplantation (13).

HBV

HBV is a member of the *Hepadnaviridae* family and is a small, double-stranded, enveloped DNA virus with a genome maintained in a circular pattern. The HBV genome encodes its own proteins from four overlapping genes: S, C, P, and X. HBV is recognized as one of a family of animal viruses called hepadnaviruses (hepatotropic DNA viruses) and is classified as hepadnavirus type 1.

HBV exists as three morphologic forms. Each of them replicates in the liver, contains its own endogenous DNA polymerase, has partially double-stranded and partially single-stranded genomes, and has a replicative strategy different from that of other DNA viruses but similar to that of retroviruses. Hepadnaviruses rely on reverse transcription (effected by the DNA polymerase) of minus-strand DNA from a "pregenomic" RNA intermediate. Plus-strand DNA is transcribed from the minus-strand DNA template by the DNA-dependent DNA polymerase and converted in the hepatocyte nucleus to a covalently

Paolo Sacchi, Raffaele Bruno, and Giorgio Barbarini • Division of Infectious and Tropical Disease, Foundation IRCCS San Matteo Hospital, University of Pavia, Via Taramelli 5, 27100 Pavia, Italy. **Giuseppe Barbaro** • Department of Medical Pathophysiology, University La Sapienza, Rome, Italy.

closed circular DNA, which serves as a template for messenger RNA and pregenomic RNA. Viral proteins are translated from the messenger RNA, and the proteins and genome are packaged into virions and secreted from the hepatocyte. The envelope protein expressed on the outer surface of the virion is defined as *hepatitis B surface antigen* (HBsAg). Hepatitis B isolates fall into one of at least eight subtypes and seven genotypes (A to G).

The intact virion contains a nucleocapsid core particle. Nucleocapsid proteins are coded for by the C gene. The antigen expressed on the surface of the nucleocapsid core is referred to as *hepatitis B core antigen* (HBcAg), and its corresponding antibody is anti-HBc. A third HBV antigen is *hepatitis B e antigen* (HBeAg), which is a nucleocapsid protein that is immunologically distinct from intact HBcAg produced by the same C gene. The C gene has two initiation codons, a precore and a core region. Also packaged within the nucleocapsid core is a DNA polymerase, which directs replication and repair of HBV DNA. HBcAg particles remain in the hepatocyte and are exported after encapsidation by an envelope particle containing HBsAg. The secreted nucleocapsid protein, HBeAg, provides a convenient, readily detectable, qualitative marker of HBV replication and relative infectivity (13).

HCV

HCV, which before its identification was labeled "non-A, non-B hepatitis virus," is a linear, single-stranded, positive-sense, RNA virus, with a genome similar to that of flaviviruses. HCV belongs to the genus *Hepacivirus* in the family *Flaviviridae*. At least six distinct genotypes, as well as subtypes within genotypes, of HCV have been identified by nucleotide sequencing. Genotypes differ one from another in sequence homology by about 30%. Because divergence of HCV isolates within a genotype or subtype and within the same host may vary insufficiently to define a distinct genotype, these intragenotypic differences are referred to as *quasispecies* and differ in sequence homology by only a few percent. HCV infection does not induce lasting immunity against reinfection with different virus genotypes or even the same virus genotype. Some HCV genotypes are distributed worldwide, while others are more geographically confined. In addition, differences exist among genotypes in responsiveness to antiviral treatment (13).

HDV

The delta hepatitis agent, or HDV, is a defective RNA virus that coinfects with and requires the helper function of HBV (or other hepadnaviruses) for its replication and expression. Its nucleocapsid expresses delta antigen and contains the virus genome. The delta core is "encapsidated" by an outer envelope of HBsAg, indistinguishable from that of HBV. The genome is a small, circular, single-stranded RNA (minus strand) that is nonhomologous with HBV DNA. HDV RNA requires host RNA polymerase II for its replication. Delta antigens have been shown to bind directly to RNA polymerase II, resulting in stimulation of transcription. Although complete hepatitis D virions and liver injury require the cooperative helper function of HBV, intracellular replication of HDV RNA can occur without HBV. HDV can either infect a person simultaneously with HBV (*coinfection*) or superinfect a person already infected with HBV (*superinfection*). When HDV infection is transmitted from a donor with one HBsAg subtype to an HBsAg-positive recipient with a different subtype, the HDV agent assumes the HBsAg subtype of the recipient, rather than the donor. Because HDV relies absolutely on HBV, the duration of HDV infection is determined by the duration of (and cannot outlast) HBV infection. In self-limited infection, anti-HDV antibodies are present at low titer and transiently. In chronic HDV infection, anti-HDV antibodies circulate in high titer, and both IgM and IgG anti-HDV can be detected. HDV antigen in the liver and HDV RNA in serum and liver can be detected during the HDV replicative phase (13).

HEV

HEV is transmitted by the enteric route, with a geographic distribution involving primarily India, Asia, Africa, and Central America. This agent, with epidemiologic features resembling those of HAV, has a single-stranded, positive-sense RNA genome. All HEV isolates appear to belong to a single serotype. The virus has been detected in stool, bile, and liver and is excreted in the stool during the late incubation period. Both IgM anti-HEV and IgG anti-HEV can be detected, but both fall rapidly after acute infection, reaching low levels within 9 to 12 months (13).

HBV

Epidemiology and Route of Transmission

Rates of acute HBV infection have declined from 9.2/100,000 persons in 1981 to 1.8/100,000 in 2005 in the United States. There were 5,494 acute cases of hepatitis B reported for 2005, with 51,000 estimated when asymptomatic cases and underreporting are factored in. Approximately 1.2 million individuals in the United States are infected with HBV, with the 25-to-45 age group having the greatest prevalence (3.6/100,000).

Approximately 400 million individuals are infected with HBV worldwide, and 50 million individuals are diagnosed each year. Areas of high endemicity have a lifetime risk of HBV infection of greater than 60%, with the major determinant of infection being exposure to an infected sibling or perinatal transmission. Perinatal transmission rates are 70% to 90% for mothers who are positive for both HBsAg and HBeAg and drops to 10% for those positive only for HBsAg. Areas of greatest endemicity are found in most of Asia (except Japan and India), most of the Middle East, the Amazon Basin in South America, most of the Pacific Islands, Africa, Native Alaskans, Australian Aborigines, and Maoris. The lifetime risk for HBV infection is 20% to 60% in areas of moderate endemicity and less than 20% in areas of low endemicity.

HBV is spread by percutaneous or mucosal contact with infectious body fluids, by sexual contact, and perinatally. Viral concentrations are highest in blood and serous fluids and are lowest in semen, saliva, and cervical fluids. HBV may be transmitted by needles, which includes intravenous drug use, tattooing, piercing, acupuncture, and needle sticks. Re-use of medical instruments and disposable needles, along with contamination from multidose vials, are risk factors in underdeveloped countries. Although Caucasians in the United States and British populations are usually infected in adolescence or adulthood (by means of sexual contact or sharing of intravenous needles), nearly every Asian person with this infection (whether born in or outside Asia) acquires it at birth from an infected mother or within 2 years of age by means of close contact with infected relatives (22).

Natural History of HBV Infection

Clinical manifestations

The incubation period for HBV lasts from 6 weeks to 6 months (average, 90 days), and development of symptoms is inversely proportional to age. Newborns are usually asymptomatic; 5% to 15% of children aged 1 to 5 years may have symptoms, and 33% to 50% of older children and adults become symptomatic (Fig. 1) (13). The preicteric phase ranges from 3 to 10 days. Clinical and extrahepatic

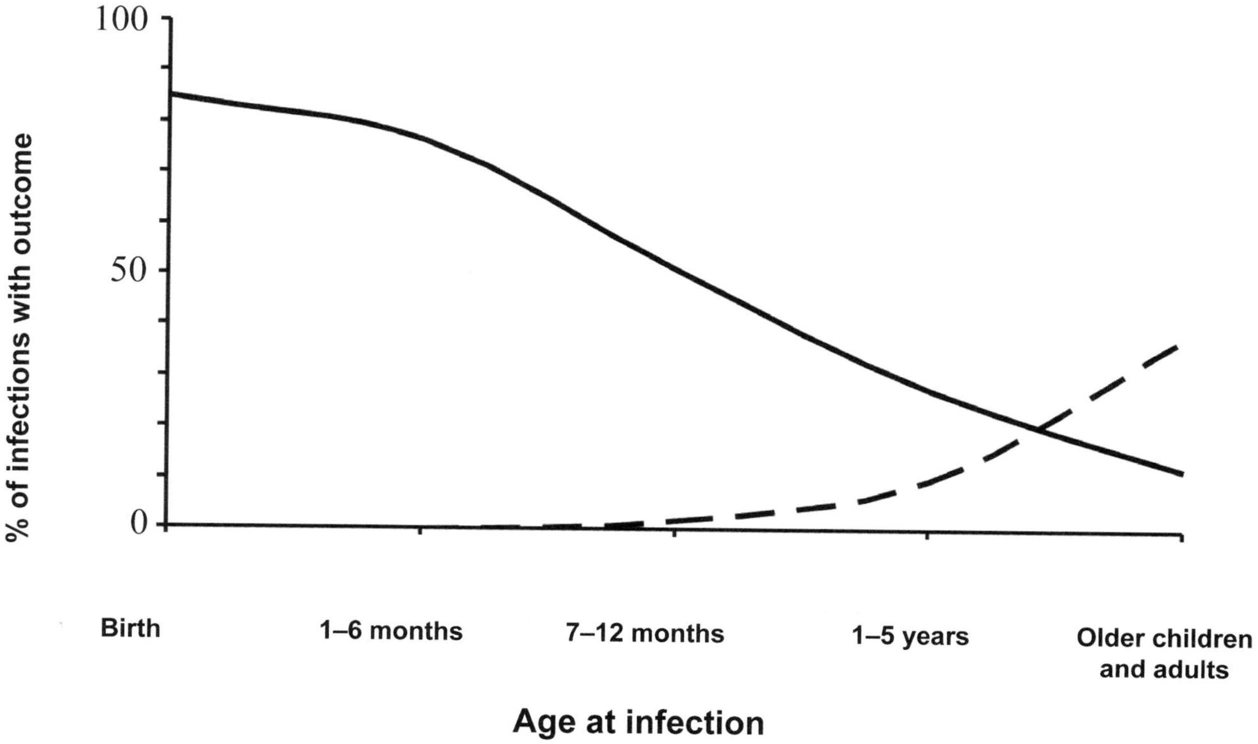

Figure 1. Outcome of HBV infection based on age at time of infection. Solid line, risk of chronicity; dashed line, percentage presenting with symptoms.

manifestations are similar to HAV infection. The icteric phase lasts 1 to 3 weeks, with hepatic tenderness and enlargement and light stools. Liver transaminases can be elevated into the thousands. Bilirubin and prothrombin times can also be elevated. Fatigue may persist for weeks or months. One percent to 2% of individuals develop fulminant hepatitis; 20 to 30% of these individuals die (26).

Serologic markers of HBV infection

After a person becomes infected with HBV, the first virologic marker detectable in serum is HBsAg. The appearance of HBsAg precedes the onset of clinical symptoms and remains detectable during the entire icteric or symptomatic phase of acute hepatitis B and beyond. Normally, HBsAg becomes undetectable 1 to 2 months after the onset of jaundice and rarely persists beyond 6 months. After HBsAg disappears, antibody to HBsAg (anti-HBs) becomes detectable in serum and remains detectable indefinitely thereafter. While HBcAg is not detectable routinely in the serum of infected patients, anti-HBc is readily demonstrable in serum, beginning within the first 1 or 2 weeks after the appearance of HBsAg and preceding detectable levels of anti-HBs by weeks to months. Anti-HBc may represent serologic evidence of current or recent HBV infection; however, in some persons, anti-HBc may persist in the circulation longer than anti-HBs and detection of anti-HBc represents hepatitis B infection in the remote past. Rarely, however, detection of anti-HBc represents low-level hepatitis B viremia, with HBsAg below the detection threshold. Recent and remote HBV infections can be distinguished by determination of the immunoglobulin class of anti-HBc. Anti-HBc IgM antibodies predominate during the first 6 months after acute infection, whereas anti-HBc IgG antibodies predominate beyond 6 months. Therefore, patients with current or recent acute hepatitis B have IgM anti-HBc antibodies in their serum. In patients who have recovered from hepatitis B in the remote past, as well as those with chronic HBV (CHB) infection, anti-HBc antibodies are predominantly IgG. Generally, in persons who have recovered from hepatitis B, anti-HBs and anti-HBc persist indefinitely. The temporal association between the appearance of anti-HBs antibodies and resolution of HBV infection, as well as the observation that persons with anti-HBs antibodies in serum are protected against reinfection with HBV suggests that *anti-HBs antibodies are the protective antibody*. Therefore, strategies for prevention of HBV infection are based on providing susceptible persons with circulating anti-HBs.

The other readily detectable serologic marker of HBV infection, HBeAg, appears concurrently with or shortly after HBsAg. Its appearance coincides temporally with high levels of virus replication and reflects the presence of circulating intact virions and detectable HBV DNA. In self-limited HBV infections, HBeAg becomes undetectable shortly after peak elevations in aminotransferase activity, before the disappearance of HBsAg, and anti-HBe then becomes detectable.

In CHB infection, HBsAg remains detectable beyond 6 months, anti-HBc is primarily IgG, and anti-HBs antibodies are either undetectable or detectable at low levels. During early CHB infection, HBV DNA can be detected both in serum and in hepatocyte nuclei. This *replicative stage* of HBV infection is the time of maximal infectivity and liver injury; HBeAg is a qualitative marker, and HBV DNA is a quantitative marker of this replicative phase. Over time, the replicative phase of CHB infection gives way to a relatively *nonreplicative phase*. This occurs at a rate of approximately 10% per year and is accompanied by seroconversion from HBeAg positive to anti-HBe positive. Most of these patients would be characterized as *inactive HBV carriers*. In reality, the designations *replicative* and *nonreplicative* are only relative. Even in the so-called nonreplicative phase, HBV replication can be detected with highly sensitive amplification probes, for example, by PCR. Occasionally, nonreplicative HBV infection converts back to replicative infection. Such spontaneous reactivations are accompanied by reexpression of HBeAg, HBV DNA, and sometimes anti-HBc IgM, as well as by exacerbations of liver injury (11).

Risk factors for chronicization

The risk of the HBV infection becoming chronic after acute infection depends greatly on the age when contracting the virus. For infants infected either at birth or within the first year of life, the risk is over 90%. The reason for this high rate of chronicization is unknown but may be related to the immunological immaturity of the infants. For children acquiring the infection between the age of 1 and 5 years, the risk is around 30%, whereas for subjects over the age of 6 years and for immunocompetent adults, the risk is estimated at <2% (Fig. 1).

The time of the infection has a great impact not only on the risk of chronicity but on the disease profile of chronic carriers. Patients infected during adolescence or adulthood, such as the majority of Caucasian carriers, do not have an immune tolerance phase but go toward the immune clearance phase of the disease immediately after the infection. Their disease is therefore of a short duration. Disease activity becomes quiescent after HBeAg seroconversion to anti-HBe. These patients have been labeled "healthy" carriers of HBV. In contrast, the patients acquiring the infection at birth or within the first 2 years of life have a prolonged immune tolerance phase followed by a prolonged immune clearance phase before HBeAg seroconversion. Each of these phases may last for several decades. The disease does continue, at least in a proportion of patients, after HBeAg seroconversion.

With "healthy" hepatitis B carriers, HBeAg seroconversion is usually preceded by a marked decrease in HBV DNA levels, from the range of 10^7 to 10^{10} copies to $<10^5$ genome copies/ml, followed by a decrease in alanine aminotransferase (ALT) levels into the normal range but persistence of HBsAg. In a follow-up study from northern Italy of 296 blood donors for a mean period of 30 years, there was no clinically significant liver disease or mortality compared to 157 uninfected controls (30). The authors attributed this favorable prognosis to the lack of comorbidity, inactive HBV infection (normal ALT and low HBV DNA levels), and abstaining from alcohol intake. One major factor for this excellent outcome is the probable age when acquiring the infection. Indeed, northern Italians are much more likely to have the infection later in life. This is supported by the fact that 32.2% of the 296 carriers lost HBsAg during follow-up, an event that is far less frequent for patients having the infection early in life.

A second study was carried out for long-term follow-up of HBeAg-positive patients who received alpha interferon (IFN-α) and untreated controls in Germany (34). Patients who had clearance of HBeAg, irrespective of whether this was after interferon therapy or occurred spontaneously, had much better survival than those who continued to be positive for HBeAg (though the patients receiving interferon continued to have a higher rate of HBeAg clearance). The situation is completely different for patients who acquire the infection at birth or early childhood. In a prospective follow-up of 22,707 Taiwan male civil servants, the relative risk of hepatocellular carcinoma (HCC) in persons who were positive for HBsAg compared with noncarriers was 217 (3). Further analyses showed that, compared to that of noncarriers, the relative risk of HCC development for HBsAg carriers without cirrhosis was 201 and for those with cirrhosis as high as 961. It has been estimated that 50% of male patients and 14% of female patients with CHB will die of liver diseases (i.e., complications of cirrhosis and HCC) (2).

Emergence of precore and core promoter mutations

The HBV core (preC/C) gene is divided into precore and core regions with two in-phase initiation codons separated by about 90 nucleotides. The preC/C gene encodes the HBeAg (precore mRNA) and the core protein and polymerase (pregenomic RNA). Mutations arise in the HBV genome at a rate 10-fold higher than that of other DNA viruses due to the lack of a proofreading function in the HBV reverse transcriptase (47). It has commonly been assumed that precore and core promoter mutations emerge as a result of selection under immune pressure at the time of HBeAg seroconversion. In 376 Chinese CHB patients, precore and core promoter mutations were detected in 44.2% and 69.1% of HBeAg-positive patients, respectively. Fifty percent of patients under 30 years of age had precore mutations. Precore mutations probably develop because of immune pressure early during the phase of immune clearance of HBV, well before actual HBeAg seroconversion. Another study comparing 79 Chinese CHB patients with cirrhosis-related complications and 158 matched patients without complications showed that precore mutations had no relationship with HBV DNA levels or complications (51). Core promoter mutations had no relationship with HBV DNA levels but were associated with more complications, including HCC.

Significance of HBeAG and anti-HBe positivity

For patients acquiring HBV infection during adolescence/adulthood, HBeAg seroconversion to anti-HBe status signifies stable nonprogressive disease in the majority of patients. For patients acquiring the HBV infection in early life, the disease continues to progress in some patients after HBeAg seroconversion. In an earlier study from Taiwan of 683 patients followed up for an average of 35.3 months, the annual rate for the development of new cirrhosis (diagnosed by follow-up liver biopsies or laparoscopy) for HBeAg-positive and anti-HBe-positive patients were 2.4% and 1.3% , respectively (*P* was not significant) (48, 49). Thus, new cirrhosis continues to develop after HBeAg seroconversion. In a recent study of the natural history of CHB in 3,233 Asian patients, the median age of HBeAg seroconversion was 35 years, whereas the median age for the development of cirrhosis complications was 57.2 years (23). It is not surprising that 73.5% of the patients are anti-HBe positive when cirrhosis complications develop. Thus, in subjects acquiring HBV infection in the first years of life, the disease tends to progress and the majority of cirrhosis complications and HCC occurs after HBeAg seroconversion.

Factors Associated with Disease Progression after HBeAg Seroconversion

A proportion of patients demonstrate a persistence of detectable HBV DNA and elevation of ALT after HBeAg seroconversion. These individuals carry a naturally occurring mutant form of HBV not producing HBeAg because of the presence of a mutation in the precore or core promoter region. The most frequent precore mutation is a G-A change at nucleotide 1896 (G1896A); the most common core promoter mutation involves two nucleotide substitutions at nucleotides 1762 and 1764.

Precore and core promoter mutations

Patients from the Mediterranean countries acquiring HBV infection in early childhood have HBeAg-negative disease predominantly (>90%) associated with precore mutations and genotype D. For HBeAg-negative Asian patients, 45 to 57% have precore mutations and 41 to 70% have core promoter mutations.

HBV DNA levels

The Risk Evaluation of Viral Load Elevation and Associated Liver Disease/Cancer-Hepatitis B Virus (REVEAL-HBV) cohort study of 3,653 hepatitis B carriers from Taiwan found that there was a dose-proportional relationship between HBV DNA levels and the risk for the development of cirrhosis and HCC (10). This is especially prominent for patients who were HBeAg negative with normal ALT levels and no cirrhosis on enrollment. The study showed that an elevated HBV DNA level of ~10^4 copies/ml (~2,000 IU/ml) was a strong risk predictor of HCC and cirrhosis. For the subjects of the REVEAL-HBV study followed up for HCC development with available repeat serum samples at follow-up, the hazard ratio for the development of HCC compared with subjects with HBV DNA levels <10^4 copies/ml (<2,000 IU/ml) on enrollment was highest at 10.1 for subjects whose HBV DNA remained above 10^5 copies/ml (<20,000 IU/mL). However, for subjects whose HBV DNA was 10^5 copies/mL (<20,000 IU/ml) on enrollment but had decreased to <10^4 copies/ml (<2,000 IU/ml) during follow-up, the hazard ratio was 3.8, still a substantial risk factor. In patients who acquired the HBV infection in early childhood, disease progression was dependent on HBV DNA levels (i.e., level of viral replication) but could still occur when the HBV DNA level had decreased to <10^4 copies/ml (10).

ALT levels

The role of ALT levels in predicting the clinical course of HBV infection has also been investigated. In a prospective cohort study of 94,533 men and 47,522 women with no known liver or other diseases (selected from a Korean medical insurance corporation), it was found that mortality from liver disease was increased for men and women with ALT levels between 0.5 and 1 × upper limit of normal (ULN) compared to people with ALT levels <0.5 × ULN, and the same was true for serum aspartate aminotransferase. For Asian patients with CHB, the abovementioned study of 3,233 patients stratified the risk of developing complications of cirrhosis and HCC according to the ALT levels both on presentation and during follow-up into five groups: <0.5 × ULN, 0.5 to 1 × ULN, >1 to 2 × ULN, >2 to 6 × ULN and >6 × ULN. Patients with ALT levels <0.5 × ULN had the lowest risk of developing complications. Patients with ALT levels of 0.5 to 1 × ULN already had a significantly increased risk of complications compared with patients with ALT levels <0.5 × ULN. The highest risk occurred in patients with ALT levels between 1 and 2 × ULN (21).

Coinfection: HCV, HDV, and HIV

Coexistent HCV and HBV infections have been estimated to be present in 10% to 15% of patients with CHB and are more common among injecting drug users. Acute coinfection with HBV and HCV may show a shorter duration of HBs antigenemia and a lower peak for transaminases. Acute coinfection of HCV and HBV or acute HCV with preexisting CHB has also been reported to increase the risk of severe hepatitis and fulminant hepatic failure. Patients with dual HBV and HCV infection show an increased risk of cirrhosis and HCC development.

HDV is a satellite virus, which is dependent on HBV for the production of envelope proteins. HBV/HDV coinfection most commonly occurs in the Mediterranean area and parts of South America. HDV infection usually presents in two forms. The first is due to the coinfection of HBV and HDV. This usually results in a more severe acute hepatitis with a higher mortality rate but has a low tendency to chronicization. The second is a superinfection of HDV in a HBV carrier and can manifest as a severe "acute" hepatitis in previously asymptomatic HBV carriers or as an exacerbation of underlying CHB. Unlike coinfection, HDV superinfection in HBV carriers almost always results in chronic infection with both viruses. A higher proportion of persons with CHB/HDV coinfection develop cirrhosis, hepatic decompensation, and HCC.

Studies have found that between 6% and 13% of persons infected with human immunodeficiency virus (HIV) are also coinfected with HBV. Coinfection with HIV is more common in persons from regions where both viruses are endemic, such as sub-Saharan Africa. Coinfected HBV and HIV patients tend to have higher levels of HBV DNA, lower rates of spontaneous HBeAg seroconversion, more-severe liver disease, and increased rates of liver-related mortality. In addition, severe flares of hepatitis can occur in HIV coinfected patients with low CD4 counts who experience immune reconstitution after initiation of highly active antiretroviral therapy.

Patients with HIV infection may have high levels of HBV DNA and hepatic necroinflammation with anti-HBc but not HBsAg, so called "occult HBV." Therefore, it is prudent to test all HIV-infected persons for both HBsAg and anti-HBc, and positive subjects for at least one of these markers should be tested for HBV DNA. Persons who are negative for all HBV seromarkers should receive the hepatitis B vaccine. If feasible, the hepatitis B vaccine should be given when CD4 cell counts are >200/μl, as response to the vaccine is poor below this level. Persons with CD4 counts below 200 should receive highly active antiretroviral therapy first and the HBV vaccine when CD4 counts rise above 200/μl (27).

Control of HBV Infection

Antiviral therapy

The aims of treatment for CHB are to achieve sustained suppression of HBV replication and remission of liver disease. The ultimate goal is to prevent cirrhosis, hepatic failure, and HCC. Parameters used to assess treatment response include normalization of serum ALT, decrease in the serum HBV DNA level, loss of HBeAg with or without detection of anti-HBe, and improvement in liver histology. While IFNs are administered for predefined durations, nucleoside analogues (NA) are usually administered until specific end points are achieved. The different approach is related to the additional immune modulatory effects of IFN. For HBeAg-positive patients, viral suppression with currently approved treatments can be sustained in 50 to 90% of patients if treatment is stopped after HBeAg seroconversion is achieved. For HBeAg-negative patients, relapse is frequent even when HBV DNA has been suppressed to levels undetectable by PCR assays for more than a year; therefore, the end point for stopping treatment is unclear. Tables 1 and 2 summarize the results obtained with commercially available NA. In HBeAg-negative patients, a better response rate is obtained with entecavir, but the therapy would probably be administered indefinitely. In HBeAg-positive patients, a better response could be obtained with polyethylene glycol-IFN-α-2a for 48 weeks.

Antiviral resistance

A major concern with long-term NA treatment is the selection of antiviral-resistant mutations. The rate at which resistant mutants are selected is related to the pretreatment serum HBV DNA level, rapidity of viral suppression, duration of treatment, and prior exposure to NA therapies. The incidence of genotypic resistance also varies with the sensitivity of the methods used for detection of resistant mutations and the patient population being tested. Lamivudine is associated with the highest and entecavir with the lowest rate of drug resistance in NA-naive patients. The first manifestation of antiviral resistance is virologic breakthrough, which is defined as a $>1\text{-log}_{10}$ (10-fold) increase in serum HBV DNA from the nadir during treatment in a patient who had an initial virologic response. Up to 30% of virologic breakthrough observed in clinical trials is related to medication noncompliance; thus, compliance should be ascertained before testing for genotypic resistance. Serum HBV DNA levels tend to be low initially because most antiviral-resistant mutants have decreased replication fitness compared with wild-type HBV.

Judicious use of NA in patients with CHB is the most effective prophylaxis against the development of antiviral-resistant HBV. Thus, patients with minimal disease and those who are unlikely to achieve a sustained response should not be treated with NA, particularly if they are young (<30 years). When possible, the most potent NA with the lowest rate of genotypic resistance should be administered and compliance reinforced. Once antiviral-resistant HBV mutants have been selected, they are archived (retained in the virus population) even if treatment is stopped, and lamivudine-resistant HBV mutants have been detected up to 4 years after withdrawal of lamivudine (27).

Prevention

Prevention of hepatitis B is possible with currently available vaccines. Universal vaccination of school-age children has been encouraged and is already a requirement for entry into school in many countries. This kind of vaccination program has been demonstrated to reduce the incidence of HCC at the population level in Taiwan. Hepatitis B vaccination is also recommended for patients with chronic liver disease because of the increased risk for complications from hepatitis B infection, including the development of HCC.

New vaccines against hepatitis B

Despite the success of universal hepatitis B vaccination in many countries, HBV remains a major public

Table 1. Responses to approved antiviral therapies among treatment-naive patients with HBeAg-positive CHB

Response	% with indicated response to[b]:							
	Lamivudine, 100 mg q.d.,, 48–52 wk	Placebo	Adefovir, 10 mg q.d., 48 wk	Placebo	Entecavir, 0.5 mg q.d., 48 wk	Telbivudine, 600 mg q.d., 52 wk	PEG, 180 mcg q.w., 48 wk	PEG + lamivudine, 180 mcg q.w. + 100 mg q.d., 48 wk
Loss of serum HBV DNA[a]	40–44	16	21	0	67	60	25	69
Loss of HBeAg	17–32	6–11	24	11	22	26	30/34[c]	27/28[c]
HBeAg seroconversion	16–21	4–6	12	6	21	22	27/32[c]	24/27[c]
Loss of HBsAg	<1	0	0	0	2	0	3	3
Normalization of ALT	41–75	7–24	48	16	68	77	39	46
Histologic improvement	49–56	23–25	53	25	72	65	38[e]	41[e]
Durability of response	50–80[d]		~90[d]		69[d]	~80	NA	

[a]Hybridization or branched-chain DNA assays (lower limit of detection 20,000 to 200,000 IU/ml or 5 or 6 log copies/ml) in standard IFN-α studies, some lamivudine studies, and PCR assays (lower limit of detection approximately 50 IU/ml or 250 copies/ml) in other studies.
[b]NA, not available; q.d., once a day; q.w., once a week.
[c]Responses at week 48/week 72 (24 weeks after stopping treatment).
[d]No or short duration of consolidation treatment (lamivudine and entecavir), or most patients had consolidation treatment (adefovir and telbivudine).
[e]Posttreatment biopsy samples obtained at week 72.

health problem, leading to about 1 million deaths per year. Prevention of hepatitis B remains the cornerstone in reduction of the incidence of disease and its complications. As hyporesponsiveness of HBV-specific T cells to antigen stimulation is considered an important determinant of virus persistence during CHB infection, therapeutic strategies have been aimed at correcting or overcoming this deficiency. Basically, four types of therapeutic vaccines are being developed to fight CHB infection. They include vaccines based on injection of recombinant HBV proteins or HBV envelope subviral particles, naked DNA combined with viral vectors, and vaccines based on T-cell peptide epitopes derived from different HBV proteins. Below, we will outline the principal findings on the development of these types of vaccines (20).

Protein-based vaccines

Many studies using the currently available recombinant anti-hepatitis B vaccines suggest that standard protein vaccination has a specific but transient effect on viral replication in HBsAg chronic carriers. One alternative to protein vaccination combines recombinant HBsAg with anti-HBs antibodies, which results in the formation of antigen-antibody immune

Table 2. Responses to approved antiviral therapies among treatment-naive patients with HBeAg-negative CHB

Response	% with indicated response to[b]:							
	Lamivudine, 100 mg q.d., 48–52 wk	Placebo	Adefovir, 10 mg q.d., 48 wk	Placebo	Entecavir, 0.5 mg q.d., 48 wk	Telbivudine, 600 mg q.d., 52 wk	PEG, 180 mcg q.w., 48 wk	PEG, 180 mcg q.w. + lamivudine, 100 mg q.d., 48 wk
Loss of serum HBV DNA[a]	60–73	NA	51	0	90	88	63	87
Normalization of ALT	60–79	NA	72	29	78	74	38	49
Histologic improvement	60–66	NA	64	33	70	67	48[c]	38[c]
Durability of response	<10		~5		NA	NA	~20	~20

[a]Hybridization or branched-chain DNA assays (lower limit of detection 20,000 to 200,000 IU/ml or 5 or 6 log copies/ml) in standard IFN-α studies, some lamivudine studies, and PCR assays (lower limit of detection approximately 50 IU/ml or 250 copies/ml) in other studies.
[b]NA, not available.
[c]Posttreatment biopsy samples obtained at week 72.

complexes. These complexes enhance the immunogenic effects of HBsAg by increasing the likelihood of this antigen being captured and taken up by antigen-presenting cells, thereby increasing proliferation of HBs-specific T cells. This approach has been used in a double-blind placebo-controlled clinical trial (41). For the 10 chronic HBV carriers in the group receiving immune complexes, half showed a 2 or 3 log decrease of HBV DNA load, seroconversion to anti-HBeAg, and elevated transaminase activities.

DNA vaccines

DNA vaccines have been shown to activate HBV-specific Th1 T-cell responses in healthy or infected individuals. Ten HBV chronic carriers with active HBV replication, nonresponders to antiviral treatments, were injected intramuscularly with a DNA vaccine encoding small and middle HBV envelope proteins (28). This vaccine was shown to activate not only T-cell HBV-specific responses but also natural killer (NK) cells. Specific modifications in the NK cell repertoire have been observed after HBV DNA vaccination, with a specific subset of NK cells secreting increased levels of IFN-γ without cytotoxic activity. Another clinical trial based on DNA vaccination was performed with 12 previously nontreated CHB carriers who were injected 12 times with an HBV DNA vaccine in combination with lamivudine (49). The authors showed that memory T-cell responses were induced and persisted for at least 40 weeks after therapy. These responses correlated with virological responses that were observed for half of the patients.

Prime-boost therapeutic vaccines

In a phase IIa study, Schneider et al. (41) investigated the efficacy of a therapeutic vaccine comprising a "prime" with DNA and two modified vaccinia Ankara "boosts." Patients were randomized into three groups receiving the vaccine alone, the vaccine plus lamivudine as antiviral treatment, or lamivudine alone. Twenty of the 53 patients studied developed IFN-γ-secreting T-cell responses, but these were of low frequencies. HBeAg-to-anti-HBe seroconversion was observed more frequently with patients receiving the vaccine alone than with patients treated with lamivudine.

T-cell epitope-based vaccines

In a dose escalation trial carried out in 26 normal subjects, a T-cell epitope-based vaccine was shown to be safe and capable of inducing a primary HBV core-specific cytotoxic T lymphocyte response. Administration of this single-epitope vaccine initiates cytotoxic T lymphocyte activity in CHB carriers but with a magnitude being well below that seen with patients following resolution of acute hepatitis B. A more recent phase I trial, performed with healthy volunteers, showed that intramuscular injection of a vaccine consisting of DNA, administered every 4 weeks over a period of 12 weeks (a total of four doses), was safe and well tolerated in all healthy volunteers.

HEPATITIS C

Epidemiology and Route of Transmission

Globally, 3% of the population, or 170 million people, are infected with blood-borne HCV infection, including nearly 5 million in the United States, 85% of whom have chronic disease. HCV infection spread widely before measures were implemented to screen for the virus. In Fig. 2 and 3, the global burden of disease and HCV genotype distribution are shown. Estimates in the United States of HCV prevalence were based on data obtained from the Third National Health and Nutrition Examination Survey (NHANES III), which sampled 21,000 noninstitutionalized civilian people between 1988 and 1994 (1); 1.8% of this population had antibodies to HCV, and 74% had detectable HCV RNA. The projection of this to the entire U.S. population suggested that nearly 4 million individuals in the United States were infected. These data also identified demographic, ethnic, and geographic variations. Non-Hispanic blacks and men were most likely to have been exposed, and 65% of all HCV antibody-positive persons were between the ages of 30 and 49 years. Other data derived from a survey of 1,032 outpatient veterans found that 18% had evidence of HCV exposure, whereas in a screening of homeless veterans, 40% were found to have evidence of HCV exposure. Screening in prison systems showed even higher rates of HCV exposure, with a prevalence of 39% among 6,536 male inmates and 54% among 977 female inmates in a California correction system (39).

After the identification of the virus in 1989 and the recognition of potential risk factors for exposure, implementation of universal precautions, screening of blood products, and educational and needle-exchange programs led to a dramatic decrease in the incidence of hepatitis C. The Centers for Disease Control and Prevention estimates that the annual incidence of acute HCV infection has decreased from 240,000 new cases per year in the United States in the 1980s to

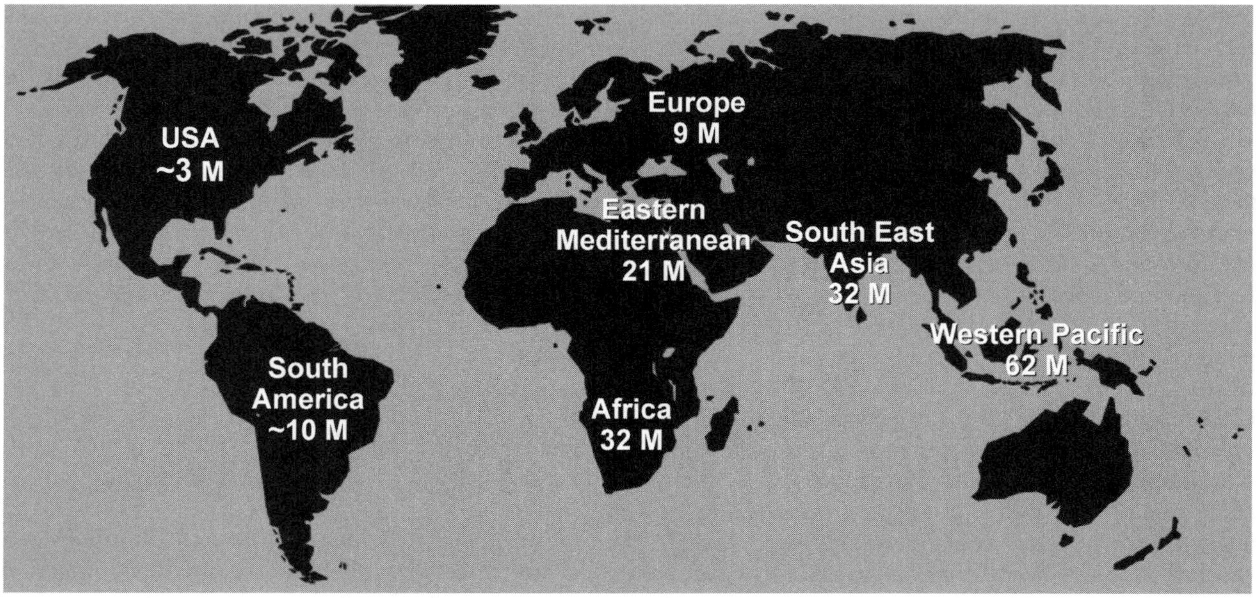

Figure 2. Epidemiology of HCV infection: 170 million (M) people are chronically infected with HCV (1, 9).

26,000 in 2004 (http://www.cdc.gov/ncidod/diseases/hepatitis/c/fact.htm). This decrease in disease acquisition will unfortunately not translate to a decrease in disease burden for decades. In most individuals, the disease is clinically silent, remaining unrecognized for 20 years or more before the liver disease becomes symptomatic. Although the prevalence of HCV infection has decreased since the 1990s, the prevalence of liver disease is not expected to peak until after the year 2030 and to plateau until around 2040 (1, 8).

Natural History

As indicated previously, hepatitis C is a major public health problem. It is currently both the leading cause of liver disease-related death and the most common indication for liver transplantation in the United States. Hepatitis C is also one of the leading causes of HCC. A population-based study of cancer epidemiology (the Surveillance, Epidemiology and End Results program]) revealed that over the last 10 years

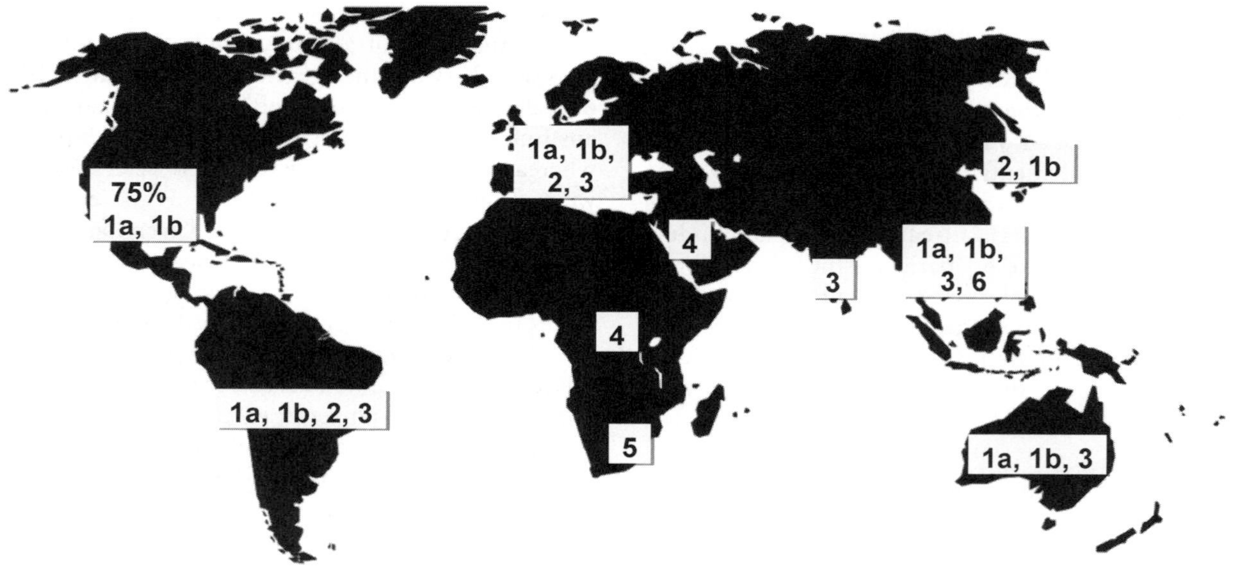

Figure 3. Genotype prevalence of HCV varies according to geographic region (1, 9).

in the United States, the incidence of liver cancer has increased more than that of any other malignancy, with HCV directly responsible for the majority of cases (8).

There are significantly different rates for developing cirrhosis among patients. A retrospective survey of chronic hepatitis C acquired through blood transfusion found that the mean time to the onset of cirrhosis was 18 years after exposure. It has been postulated that approximately 20% of HCV-infected patients develop cirrhosis after 20 years. Variables independently related to risk for disease progression are male sex, older age at acquisition (>40 years), daily alcohol consumption (≥50 g per day), and HIV or HBV coinfection. Also the degree of hepatic inflammation determines the development of cirrhosis. One study found that up to one-third of HCV-infected patients had severe hepatic inflammation on biopsy and thus risk rapid progression to cirrhosis in 20 to 30 years, whereas those with mild disease on liver biopsy had a lower rate of progression of cirrhosis in the same time period (43). Another study by Yano and colleagues found that aggressive histology was associated with a 50% chance of progression to cirrhosis in less than 10 years (50).

Poynard and colleagues applied mathematical modeling to a large cross-sectional study of HCV-infected patients with known histology. They found that after acquiring disease, cirrhosis did progress linearly but at different rates over different time periods. There was minimal progression during the first 10 years after infection, although disease progression accelerated during each subsequent decade, with the most rapid phase occurring in the last 5 of 40 years. Disease was significantly more virulent in those patients who acquired hepatitis C after the age of 50. After histological diagnosis, the asymptomatic phase of cirrhosis is generally well tolerated, with excellent survival until symptoms of decompensation occur. Approximately 4% of compensated cirrhotic patients decompensate per year, and this drastically affects survival. Once complications arise, there is more than a 50% chance of succumbing to disease manifestations within 5 years (8, 35).

Control of Hepatitis C

Current treatment paradigm

The goal of treatment is to prevent disease complications. This is best accomplished through disease eradication, defined as sustained virologic response (SVR) (continued undetectable HCV RNA by a sensitive PCR-based assay 24 weeks after discontinuation of treatment). Therapeutic options for hepatitis C have changed significantly since the introduction of interferon monotherapy. The current standard of care is combination pegylated interferon (PEG) and weight-based ribavirin (RBV). This regimen doubled the SVR compared with interferon monotherapy but still leaves much to be desired (17, 18, 21, 31).

Monitoring of on-treatment response

For the majority of patients, PEG-RBV therapy is associated with many side effects (flu-like symptoms, hemolytic anemia, irritability, and depression), some of which may result in dose adjustments or discontinuation. It would be ideal to administer the appropriate amount of medication for the shortest effective duration to minimize toxicity. Integral to this strategy is the ability to recognize patients who are most likely to respond, as well as those who are least likely to respond, so that adherence can be encouraged or treatment can be stopped (17, 18, 22).

Need to treat patients with liver cirrhosis

Much evidence suggests that an increased risk of HCC is observed even in subjects who have cleared HCV. Viral clearance needs to be achieved prior to the development of cirrhosis to have a marked impact on the development of HCC. A recent collaborative study with >10 years of follow-up with 883 individuals with cirrhosis caused by hepatitis C showed a significant difference in the rate of HCC following viral clearance, as well as a significant reduction in hepatic decompensation compared with that seen with nonresponders (7).

Antiviral therapy for those individuals with decompensated cirrhosis caused by hepatitis C is fraught with complications and frequently requires the use of adjunctive therapy to support the various blood components, and in some series a high risk of septicemia has been reported. Tolerance of antiviral therapy is considerably even less after liver transplantation, with adherence rates to full-dose therapy as low as 30% being reported, leading to a reduced efficacy of treatment. Thus, whenever possible, viral clearance needs to be achieved pretransplant. This indicates that all those with cirrhosis who may be suitable transplant candidates in the future should be treated whenever possible (6).

Liver transplantation

Liver transplantation is the best option for an individual with hepatic decompensation due to end-stage liver disease or early HCC. Currently, there are 17,227 people actively waiting for approximately 7,000 liver donations per year, according to the UNOS Organ Procurement and Transplantation Network (www.optn.org/data, accessed 16 January 2007). Hepatitis C is the most common indication for liver transplantation. In addition, hepatitis C universally recurs posttransplant for HCV infection, with reinfection at the time of hepatic reperfusion. By the fourth day posttransplant, the viral load has reached pretransplant levels, peaking 1 to 3 months after surgery at levels that are frequently 10 to 100 times greater than the original baseline.

Although not predictable, posttransplant hepatitis C is generally more cytotoxic, with the median interval from hepatic replacement to development of cirrhosis only 10 years. Thirty percent of patients will develop cirrhosis 5 years after transplantation, and the time until manifesting symptoms of decompensation and death is significantly shorter than in immunocompetent hosts. Up to one-fourth of transplanted patients with hepatitis C will die or require retransplantation within 5 years. Ideally, HCV should be eradicated prior to transplantation. However, very few patients are able to tolerate the therapy without dose reductions or interruptions, and therefore, few clear the virus or achieve SVR. HCV genotype 2/3 and the ability to tolerate full-dose therapy were associated with a more favorable response. These patients also remained virus-free after transplant. HCV treatment after liver replacement is just as challenging as pretransplant treatment. Several strategies exist for management of HCV posttransplantation. Some advocate for preemptive HCV therapy as soon as the patient is clinically able to tolerate treatment. Ideally, this would eliminate disease while the viral load is still low and prior to histologic damage. Unfortunately, therapy immediately post-liver transplant is poorly tolerated, with only 10% to 25% achieving SVR. Few would debate that those patients with recurrent disease and evidence of at least stage 2 cirrhosis should be considered for combination PEG-RBV therapy. This approach posttransplant is particularly challenging because it requires serial protocol liver biopsies to identify patients with progressive cirrhosis, and results remain suboptimal, with SVR rates ranging between 9% and 45% in case series (31, 37a).

Prevention of Hepatitis C

HCV vaccines

Prevention of hepatitis C is more difficult, given the lack of an effective vaccine. Although recent publications describe the development of in vitro replication systems leading to the production of infectious viral particles (46), there is currently no cell culture model suitable for synthesizing vaccines based on killed or attenuated virus. Three types of vaccine approaches have been pursued: those based on induction of specific B-cell immunity, those based on induction of specific cellular immunity, and those based on attempting to modulate, in a nonspecific manner, existing immunity in already infected hosts (19).

Leading B- and T-cell vaccine studies

The earliest vaccine developed was based on recombinant HCV glycoproteins E1 and E2 adjuvanted with MF59 (HCV E1E2MF59C.1). Preclinical studies performed in chimpanzees have shown that the development of a carrier state after experimental challenge was a rare event in vaccinated compared with nonvaccinated individuals (14% versus 70%; D. Rosa, unpublished data). Results of a phase I study performed with healthy volunteers who received the vaccine showed that the vaccine was well tolerated in the 16 subjects tested. Maximal vaccine effects were observed after three injections (16). CD8 1-neutralizing antibodies were detected in 70 to 83% of patients, while pseudo-type neutralizing antibodies directed at genotype 1a- and 1b-derived particles could be detected in 40 to 80% of patients.

The second B cell-based vaccine consists of a recombinant E1 glycoprotein of an HCV genotype 1b isolate expressed in mammalian cells and adjuvanted with alum. Original clinical trials (phase 1 and 2) were performed using an *Escherichia coli*-derived protein, while the more recent extended phase II trial is being conducted with a yeast-derived antigen. The second trial included 24 chronically infected HCV patients, previous nonresponders to standard therapy (33). The results are promising, showing an association between vaccination and regression of liver inflammation. Other vaccines are currently being tested, and the results of the trials will become available soon.

New Drugs for Hepatitis C

Given the multitude of patients who need effective HCV therapy, research and development have yielded several attractive approaches that are likely to transform current practice. These new therapeutic strategies have been based on the development of oral antivirals, the so-called specifically targeted antiviral therapies for HCV agents. These drugs target specific viral enzymes important in the replication of HCV. Two classes of compounds are actually under development in this setting: protease inhibitors and polymerase inhibitors.

Protease inhibitors

Although several protease inhibitors are in various stages of development, two compounds, telaprevir (VX-950) and boceprevir (SCH 503034), have generated considerable excitement, as very favorable results from phase 1 and phase 2 trials have been reported. Telaprevir (VX-950) was initially administered to genotype 1 treatment-naive HCV-infected subjects as a 14-day monotherapy in a phase 1 dose-escalation study. Treatment with telaprevir resulted in dramatic decreases in HCV viral load. The optimal dose, 750 mg every 8 hours, led to a 4- to 4.5-$\log_{10}$ decline in viral load in nearly all patients after 14 days of dosing, with some becoming HCV RNA-undetectable. However, some patients had a rapid decline in viral load followed by viral rebound, offering the first insight into the growing concern of viral resistance.

The efficacy of telaprevir as either monotherapy or in combination with PEG was subsequently assessed in treatment-naive genotype 1 patients without cirrhosis. Again, rapid viral reduction was achieved with telaprevir treatment. This reduction was greatest in the PEG combination (i.e., PEG + telaprevir) treatment arm, with a median viral load reduction of 5.5 $\log_{10}$s from baseline. Some patients on telaprevir monotherapy experienced plateaus or rebounds associated with resistance mutations, and some patients on combination therapy had resistant virus, although HCV RNA continued to decline throughout therapy. Even though they are resistant to telaprevir, viral variants remained fully susceptible to subsequent PEG-RBV treatment. The addition of RBV to the combination of PEG and telaprevir offered additional viral suppression. After 28 days of dosing with this triple-therapy regimen, 100% of 12 genotype 1 HCV-infected patients had HCV RNA levels <10 IU/ml (32) in a phase 2 trial of telaprevir given in combination with PEG and RBV (PROVE 1). Interim analysis found that 88% of patients receiving the triple combination regimen achieved rapid virological response (i.e., HCV RNA undetectable at week 4) compared with 16% receiving the current standard of care (i.e., PEG + RBV + placebo). However, side effects (primarily pruritus, rash, and gastrointestinal-related symptoms) were common and frequently led to treatment discontinuation. Virologic breakthrough was also higher in the telaprevir treatment arms (7% versus 2%), 75% of which occurred in patients who never achieved undetectable HCV RNA. All patients with breakthrough had drug-resistant virus. Among those patients who achieved rapid virological response and discontinued treatment at week 12, two-thirds remained HCV RNA-undetectable at week 20 posttreatment.

SCH 503034 (boceprevir) is another NS3 serum protease inhibitor. In contrast to the initial investigations with telaprevir, boceprevir was introduced into a prior PEG nonresponder population to assess the safety, antiviral activity, and emergence of strains resistant to this agent when given in combination with PEG. HCV genotype 1 nonresponder patients received treatment in three stages: boceprevir monotherapy for 7 days, weight-based PEG-2b for 14 days, or both drugs for 14 days (40). Crossover among groups occurred between each phase. Boceprevir monotherapy resulted in a less than 3-$\log_{10}$-decline in viral load in the majority of patients; however, combination treatment (boceprevir + PEG) was significantly more effective, with several patients becoming HCV RNA-negative after 14 days. One patient did develop resistance mutations. Side effects were minimal with boceprevir monotherapy, and in combination, they were typical of interferon therapy.

Polymerase inhibitors

The RNA-dependent RNA polymerase (NS5B) and the 3′ end of the infective virus' positive RNA bind to the replication complex, resulting in the synthesis of a complementary negative-strand RNA that serves as a template for the subsequent production of genomic RNA. This process represents an appealing target for antiviral therapy. Recently, investigation of two HCV polymerase inhibitors (NM283 and HCV-796) has been halted due to tolerability concerns. Several other compounds in this class are in various stages of development, with patients actively enrolled in phase 2 investigations involving R1 626. Given the issues of drug resistance seen with the protease inhibitors, most experts believe that the most effective therapeutic strategies will involve multidrug regimens utilizing PEG-RBV in combination with both protease and polymerase inhibitors.

R1 626 is the prodrug of a nucleoside analogue (R1 479) that targets the HCV RNA polymerase. In a phase 1, multicenter, observer-blinded, randomized, placebo-controlled, multiple ascending-dose study, R1 626 was administered at doses ranging from 500 mg to 1,500 mg twice daily for 14 days in treatment-naive HCV genotype 1 patients (37). This initial dose-escalation study demonstrated a clinically significant mean 1.2-$\log_{10}$ decline in HCV RNA with the dosing regimen of 1,500 mg twice daily. Additional studies found dose-dependent inhibition, with undetectable HCV RNA, after 15 days in five of nine patients receiving 4,500 mg R1 626 twice daily. Viral rebound was noted with lower doses of R1 626 given as monotherapy but was not associated with phenotypic or genotypic evidence of resistance. Similar to what has been observed with other specifically targeted antiviral therapies for HCV agents, interim analysis of a 48-week study assessing the efficacy of combination therapy with R1 626 + PEG ± RBV in treatment-naive patients with chronic hepatitis C genotype 1 showed that this triple-therapy regimen further suppressed the virus. HCV RNA was undetectable at week 4 in 80% of patients treated with triple therapy (using R1 626 at a dose of 1,500 mg twice daily) versus in only 5% of patients who received the standard of care (PEG + RBV) and in 33% of patients who received the same dose of R1 626 (1,500 mg twice daily) + PEG but without RBV.

HCC

HCC is the fifth most common cancer in the world, with over 600,000 new diagnoses per year. In the United States, it was projected that there would be 19,160 new cases and 16,780 deaths related to HCC in 2007. The incidence of HCC in the United States is increasing, and infection with the hepatitis C virus is thought to be the major cause. Indeed, HCC is the fastest growing cause of cancer-related death in the United States. HCC generally occurs in association with cirrhosis, particularly due to hepatitis C, hepatitis B, alcohol, hereditary hemochromatosis, and primary biliary cirrhosis (6). This malignancy is recognized as an early complication and the most frequent cause of death in persons with viral-associated cirrhosis (3, 20).

Results of previous prospective controlled studies showed that the annual incidence of HCC in hepatitis B carriers was 0.5% (2). The annual incidence increased with age, so that at age 70 the incidence was 1%. The incidence in patients with known cirrhosis was 2.5% per year. The relative risk of HCC was about 100; hepatitis B carriers were 100 times more likely to develop HCC than uninfected individuals.

The risk of HCC in patients with chronic hepatitis C is highest and has been best studied in patients who have established cirrhosis, for whom the incidence of HCC is between 2 and 8% per year. It should be noted that these data come from clinic-based studies. There is a single prospective population-based study of the risk of HCC in patients with hepatitis C (44). In this study of 12,008 men, being anti-HCV positive conferred a 20-fold increased risk of HCC compared to being anti-HCV negative. The presence or absence of cirrhosis was not evaluated. Hepatitis C-infected individuals who do not have cirrhosis have a much lower risk of developing HCC (44).

Despite recent advances in the management of HCC, median survival is less than 1 year. However, it is highly variable and depends on both the biologic aggressiveness of the tumor (currently defined by the size and number of tumors and presence of vascular invasion) and the underlying hepatic function. Liver transplantation remains the most effective treatment because it removes the tumor and eliminates the risk for new tumors, and it prevents liver failure. Survival after liver transplantation is similar to that for other indications, if Milan criteria (no evidence of extrahepatic tumor and unifocal tumor mass less than 5 cm in diameter or multifocal tumors up to three in number, each less than 3 cm in diameter) are followed (6). For individuals with small tumors and intact hepatic function without portal hypertension, resection provides nearly equivalent outcomes as orthotopic liver transplantation. Thus, where possible, resection is favored over transplantation for these patients. Patients with more advanced disease can have prolonged survival with chemoembolization.

Epidemiology

The incidence of HCC in the United States is increasing, with the Surveillance, Epidemiology, and End Results database showing an incidence of 3.0 cases per 100,000 in 1998. An analysis of the Northern Kaiser Permanente Medical Care Program, which has more than 3 million members, revealed a continuing increase in HCC incidence (14, 31a). The cases per 100,000 increased from 3.1 in 1997 to 4.6 in 2005. The cases of HCC attributed to nonalcoholic fatty liver disease (NAFLD) increased 10-fold, from 0.03 to 0.46 per 100,000 between 1997 and 2005. Thus, the incidence of HCC continues to rise, with an increasing but still relatively small proportion due to NAFLD. This increase in HCC incidence will likely continue because as the peak in HCV-related HCC wanes, there will probably be an increase in HCC related to NAFLD.

Prevention

Based on the epidemiology data listed above, preventive strategies remain the best way to reduce the incidence of HCC and its complications. HBV vaccination is still the best strategy to reduce the incidence of HCC. Treatment of hepatitis B-associated cirrhosis with the oral antiviral agent lamivudine has been shown to reduce the risk of developing HCC. However, lamivudine is no longer recommended as a first-line therapy for HBV infection because of the high rate of resistance with prolonged treatment. Using a matched case-controlled methodology, a Korean group showed a marked reduction in the incidence of HCC in patients treated with lamivudine (24); however, after the emergence of lamivudine resistance, stopping treatment with lamivudine and switching to adefovir monotherapy after viral breakthrough was recommended (25). The identification of a risk gradient for HCC based on HBV DNA levels has already had a marked impact on the latest AASLD recommendations for hepatitis B treatment. The abovementioned REVEAL-HBV study showed that HBV DNA levels >10,000copies/ml, age, male sex, HBeAg positivity, the presence of cirrhosis, and alcohol consumption were strong and independent predictors for HCC (5). A further analysis of the group with HBsAg positivity, no cirrhosis, and HBV DNA levels <10,000 copies/ml (inactive carriers) showed a 2.7-fold increased risk for HCC, even after correcting for other known risk factors. These patients are not usually treated unless a biopsy shows significant inflammation, but they should be considered for HCC screening. Another analysis showed that spontaneous reductions over time in HBV DNA levels from 300 to 100,000 copies/ml to <300 copies/ml, after controlling for other risks, eliminated the additional risk of developing HCC, based on the baseline HBV DNA level. This suggests that reducing HBV DNA levels can decrease future cancer risk (10).

Prevention of hepatitis C-associated HCC is more difficult given the lack of an effective vaccine. Successful achievement of a sustained SVR to treatment with the current standard of care, PEG in combination with RBV, in patients with chronic hepatitis C infection may prevent the development of HCC. Unfortunately, if cirrhosis has already been established, the risk of HCC, although likely decreased, does not appear to be eliminated. This impression was confirmed in a French study of 244 patients in which the cumulative incidence of HCC was lower in the group that achieved an SVR than in the non-SVR group (8). Nevertheless, there were still four cases of HCC that developed in SVR patients. The better results in the SVR group may also be confounded by the improved SVR rate in milder liver disease. Five additional case reports of HCC occurring 3 to 6 years after achieving SVR were presented, and this included two patients with only minor levels of cirrhosis. Thus, it appears to be prudent to continue surveillance for HCC after SVR. Unfortunately, nearly half of patients with HCV infection will be nonresponders to standard care antiviral therapy. The Hepatitis C Antiviral Long-Term Treatment Against Cirrhosis study was established to answer the question of whether suppressive doses of PEG given to patients with advanced cirrhosis and cirrhosis could prevent the development of decompensated cirrhosis and HCC (12). This well-designed, randomized, controlled trial enrolled 1,050 patients with chronic hepatitis C and advanced cirrhosis who were nonresponders to prior therapy with PEG and RBV; approximately half were treated for 3.5 years with PEG alfa-2a. There were no differences in the rates of decompensated liver disease or HCC between the treatment and control groups. Thus, maintenance therapy with PEG is not effective and should not be used for nonresponders to previous interferon-based therapy. The annual incidence of HCC was close to 1% (control, 3.2%; and treated, 2.8%) over the 3.5-year study, which is lower than the generally reported rate of 3.2% to 4.7 % for HCV-infected patients (15). The rate may be underestimated for cirrhotic patients in general because two-thirds of patients in the Hepatitis C Antiviral Long-Term Treatment Against Cirrhosis study had only bridging cirrhosis, and the patients included in the study had to have compensated liver disease. However, the annual incidence of HCC was only slightly lower in the bridging cirrhosis group, which raises the issue of whether these patients should also be in a surveillance program (3, 6, 34).

Management of HCC

Liver transplantation

Since the institution of the model for end-stage liver disease (MELD) score, HCC has become the primary indication in up to 22% of all liver transplantations in the United States. For those patients who meet Milan criteria, results are excellent, with a 75%, 5-year survival and <10% tumor recurrence rates (4, 42). MELD exception points (i.e., priority MELD score) are automatic if the patients meet Milan criteria. Despite this success, patients on the waiting list for transplantation may still drop out because of tumor progression or because of death before being transplanted. The Michigan group analyzed the UNOS (United Network for Organ Sharing) database from 1998 to 2006 for causes of dropout among HCC candidates for liver transplant (38). In multivariate analysis, the most important risk factors for dropout included Child's class C (hazard ratio of 4.4) and meeting Milan criteria (hazard ratio of 0.37). This suggests that we may be underestimating the priority of patients with HCC and significant hepatic dysfunction (3, 35).

The University of California at San Francisco (UCSF) group has published a prospective study of patients transplanted under UCSF criteria (unifocal tumor masses less than 6.5 cm in diameter or multifocal tumors less than four in number, each less than

4.5 cm in diameter, with total tumor diameter less than 8 cm) with long-term survival and recurrence rates equal to those in published studies adhering to Milan criteria. The authors presented their results from a prospective study of 61 patients who were "downstaged" with chemoembolization, radiofrequency ablation, or resection. "Downstaging" was successful in 70% of patients, and 57% of patients have been transplanted so far. Four-year intention to treat survival was 69%, and posttransplant survival was 92%, with no recurrences (3).

Systemic chemotherapy

Advanced HCC patients are defined as having large tumors and either portal vein invasion, metastasis, or performance status of 1 to 2. They can have Child's class A or B cirrhosis. Systemic chemotherapy for advanced HCC has limited response rates and no clear impact on survival. Thus, current treatment guidelines suggest participation in clinical trials for these patients. Sorafenib should be considered first-line therapy for advanced HCC. This suggestion is based on results showing an improvement in overall survival (10.7 versus 7.9 months) in a large placebo-controlled trial (26). All patients in the trial were Child's class A, and the drug was reasonably well tolerated. Sorafenib is a multikinase inhibitor with activity against the Raf/vascular endothelial growth factor receptor and platelet-derived growth factor receptor and is one of several new agents that target pathways thought to be important in the pathogenesis of HCC.

REFERENCES

1. **Alter, M. J., D. Kruszon-Moran, O. V. Nainan, G. M. McQuillan, F. Gao, L. A. Moyer, R. A. Kaslow, and H. S. Margolis.** 1999. The prevalence of hepatitis C virus infection in the United States, 1988 through 1994. *N. Engl. J. Med.* **341**:556–562.
2. **Beasley, R. P.** 1982. Hepatitis B virus as the etiologic agent in hepatocellular carcinoma. *Hepatology* **2**(Suppl):21S–26S.
3. **Beasley, R. P., L. Y. Hwang, C. C. Lin, and C. S. Chien.** 1981. Hepatocellular carcinoma and hepatitis B virus. A prospective study of 22,707 men in Taiwan. *Lancet* **2**:1129–1133.
4. **Befeler, A. S., and A. M. Di Bisceglie.** 2002. Hepatocellular carcinoma: diagnosis and treatment. *Gastroenterology* **55**:1609–1619.
5. **Benvegnù, L., M. Gios, S. Boccato, and A. Alberti.** 2004. Natural history of compensated viral cirrhosis: a prospective study on the incidence and hierarchy of major complication. *Gut* **53**:744–749.
6. **Bruix, J., and M. Sherman.** 2005. Management of hepatocellular carcinoma. *Hepatology* **42**:1208–1236.
7. **Bruno, S., T. Stroffolini, M. Colombo, S. Bollani, L. Benvegnù, G. Mazzella, A. Ascione, T. Santantonio, F. Piccinino, P. Andreone, A. Mangia, G. B. Gaeta, M. Persico, S. Fagiuoli, P. L. Almasio, and Italian Association of the Study of the Liver Disease (AISF).** 2007. Sustained virological response to interferon-alpha is associated with improved outcome in HCV-related cirrhosis: a retrospective study. *Hepatology* **45**:579–587.
8. **Cardoso, A. C., R. Moucari, N. Boyer, T. Asselah, A. Laatar, M.-P. Ripault, M. Martinot-Peignoux, S. Maylin, P. Bedossa, and P. Marcellin.** 2007. Positive impact of antiviral therapy on the long term outcome of chronic hepatitis C patients with cirrhosis. *Hepatology* **46**(Suppl. 1):346A. (Abstract.)
9. Reference deleted.
10. **Chen, C.-F., H.-I. Yang, U. Iloeje, C.-F. Chen, H.-I. Yang, U. Iloeje, J. Su, C.-L. Jen, S.-L. You, and C.-J. Chen.** 2007. Changes in serum HBV DNA level using a trajectory model predict the risk of HCC in chronic hepatitis B patients: the REVEAL-HBV study. *Hepatology* **46**(Suppl. 1):639A. (Abstract.)
11. **Chen, C.-J., H.-I. Yang, J. Su, C. L. Jen , S. L. You, S. N. Lu, G. T. Huang, U. H. Iloeje, and the REVEAL-HBV Study Group.** 2006. Risk of hepatocellular carcinoma across a biological gradient of serum hepatitis B virus DNA level. *JAMA* **295**:65–73.
12. **Di Bisceglie, A. M., M. L. Shiffman, G. T. Everson, K. L. Lindsay, J. E. Everhart, E. C. Wright, W. M. Lee, A. S. Lok, H. Bonkovsky, T. R. Morgan, J. L. Dienstag, M. Ghany, C. Morishima, and K. K. Snow.** 2007. Prolonged antiviral therapy with peginterferon to prevent complications of advanced liver disease associated with hepatitis C: results of the hepatitis C antiviral long-term treatment against cirrhosis (HALT-C) trial. *Hepatology* **46**(Suppl. 1):80A. (Abstract.)
13. **Dienstag, J. L., and K. J. Isselbacher.** 2005. Acute viral hepatitis, p. 1882–1937. *In* D. L. Casper, A. S. Fauci, L. Longo, E. Braunwald, S. L. Hauser, and J. L. Jameson (ed.), *Harrison's Principles of Internal Medicine.* McGraw-Hill, New York, NY.
14. **El-Serag, H. B., and A. C. Mason.** 1999. Rising incidence of hepatocellular carcinoma in the United States. *N. Engl. J. Med.* **340**:745–750.
15. **Fattovich, G., T. Stroffolini, I. Zagni, and F. Donato.** 2004. Hepatocellular carcinoma in cirrhosis: incidence and risk factors. *Gastroenterology* **127**(Suppl. 1):S35–S50.
16. **Frey, S. E., G. J. Gorse, A. M. DiBisceglie, D. Rosa, Z. Stamataki, J. McKeating, R. Ray, S. Coates, V. Schultze, S. Abrignan, M. Houghton, H. Hill, and R. B. Belshe.** 2006. A phase 1 trial of a novel E1E2/MF59C.1 hepatitis C vaccine candidate in healthy HCV-negative adults (DMID 01-002). *J. Clin. Virol.* **36**(Suppl. 2):S5. (Abstract.)
17. **Fried, M. W., M. L. Shiffman, K. R. Reddy, C. Smith, G. Marinos, F. L. Gonçales, Jr., D. Häussinger, M. Diago, G. Carosi, D. Dhumeaux, A. Craxi, A. Lin, J. Hoffman, and J. Yu.** 2002. Peginterferon alfa-2a plus ribavirin for chronic hepatitis C virus infection. *N. Engl. J. Med.* **347**:975–982.
18. **Hadziyannis, S. J., H. Sette, Jr., T. R. Morgan, V. Balan, M. Diago, P. Marcellin, G. Ramadori, H. Bodenheimer, Jr., D. Bernstein, M. Rizzetto, S. Zeuzem, P. J. Pockros, A. Lin, A. M. Ackrill, and the PEGASYS International Study Group.** 2004. Peginterferon-alpha2a and ribavirin combination therapy in chronic hepatitis C: a randomized study of treatment duration and ribavirin dose. *Ann. Intern. Med.* **140**:346–355.
19. **Heathcote, J. E.** 2007. Antiviral therapy: chronic hepatitis C. *J. Viral Hepat.* **14**(Suppl. 1):82–88.
20. **Inchauspé, G., and M. L. Michel.** 2007. Vaccines and immunotherapies against hepatitis B and hepatitis C viruses. *J. Viral Hepat.* **14**(Suppl. 1):97–103
21. **Jensen, D. M., T. R. Morgan, P. Marcellin, P. J. Pockros, K. R. Reddy, S. J. Hadziyannis, P. Ferenci, A. M. Ackrill, and B.**

Willems. 2006. Early identification of HCV genotype 1 patients responding to 24 weeks peginterferon alpha-2a (40 kd)/ribavirin therapy. *Hepatology* **43:**954–960.

22. **Lai, C.-L., and M.-F. Yuen.** 2007. The natural history of chronic hepatitis B. *J. Viral Hepat.* **14**(Suppl. 1):6–10.
23. **Liaw, Y. F., D. I. Tai, C. M. Chu, and T. J. Chen.** 1988. The development of cirrhosis in patients with chronic type B hepatitis: a prospective study. *Hepatology* **8:**493–496.
24. **Liaw, Y. F., J. J. Sung, W. C. Chow, G. Farrell, C. Z. Lee, H. Yuen, T. Tanwandee, O. M. Tao, K. Shue, O. N. Keene, J. S. Dixon, D. F. Gray, J. Sabbat, and the Cirrhosis Asian Lamivudine Multicentre Study Group.** 2004. Lamivudine for patients with chronic hepatitis B and advanced liver disease. *N. Engl. J. Med.* **351:**1521–1531.
25. **Liaw, Y. F., C. M. Lee, R. N. Chien, and C. T. Yeh.** 2006. Switching to adefovir monotherapy after emergence of lamivudine-resistant mutations in patients with liver cirrhosis. *J. Viral Hepat.* **13:**250–255.
26. **Llovet, J., S. Ricci, V. Mazzaferro, P. Hilgard, E. Gane, J. F. Blanc, A. C. de Oliveira, A. Santoro, J. L. Raoul, A. Forner, M. Schwartz, C. Porta, S. Zeuzem, L. Bolondi, T. F. Greten, P. R. Galle, J. F. Seitz, I. Borbath, D. Häussinger, T. Giannaris, M. Shan, M. Moscovici, D. Voliotis, J. Bruix, and the SHARP Investigators Study Group.** 2008. Sorafenib in advanced hepatocellular carcinoma. *N. Engl. J. Med.* **359:** 378–90.
27. **Lok, A. S., and B. J. McMahon.** 2007. Chronic hepatitis B. *Hepatology* **45:**507–539.
28. **Mancini-Bourgine, M., H. Fontaine, D. Scott-Algara, S. Pol, C. Brechot, and M. L. Michel.** 2004. Induction or expansion of T-cell responses by a hepatitis B DNA vaccine administered to chronic HBV carriers. *Hepatology* **40:**874–882.
29. Reference deleted.
30. **Manno, M., C. Camma, F. Schepis, F. Bassi, R. Gelmini, F. Giannini, F. Miselli, A. Grottola, I. Ferretti, C. Vecchi, M. De Palma, and E. Villa.** 2004. Natural history of chronic HBV carriers in northern Italy: morbidity and mortality after 30 years. *Gastroenterology* **127:**756–763.
31. **Manns, M. P., J. G. McHutchison, S. C. Gordon, V. K. Rustgi, M. Shiffman, R. Reindollar, Z. D. Goodman, K. Koury, M. Ling, and J. K. Albrecht.** 2001. Peginterferon alfa-2b plus ribavirin compared with interferon alfa-2b plus ribavirin for initial treatment of chronic hepatitis C: a randomised trial. *Lancet* **358:**958–965.

31a. **Manos, M., and R. C. Murphy.** 2007. Viral hepatitis registry, Kaiser Permanente Northern California, Oakland, California. Trends in the incidence and etiology of hepatocellular carcinoma in a managed care population: The roles of viral hepatitis and fatty liver disease. *Hepatology* **46**(Suppl. 1): 400A. (Abstract.).

32. **McHutchison, J. G., G. T. Everson, S. Gordon, I. Jacobson, R. Kauffman, L. McNair, and A. Muir.** 2007. Results of an interim analysis of a phase 2 study of telaprevir (VX 950) with peginterferon alpha 2a and ribavirin in previously untreated subjects with hepatitis C. *J. Hepatol.* **42**(Suppl. 1): S296. (Abstract.)
33. **Nevens, F., T. Roskams, H. Van Vlierberghe, Y. Horsmans, D. Sprengers, A. Elewaut, V. Desmet, G. Leroux-Roels, E. Quinaux, E. Depla, S. Dincq, C. Vander Stichele, G. Maertens, and F. Hulstaert.** 2003. A pilot study of therapeutic vaccination with envelope protein E1 in 35 patients with chronic hepatitis C. *Hepatology* **38:**1289–1296.
34. **Niederau, C., T. Heintges, S. Lange, G. Goldmann, C. M. Niederau, L. Mohr, D. Häussinger.** 1996. Long-term follow-up of HBeAg-positive patients treated with interferon alfa for chronic hepatitis B. *N. Engl. J. Med.* **334:**1422–1427.
35. **Poynard, T., V. Ratziu, F. Charlotte, Z. Goodman, J. McHutchison, and J. Albrecht.** 2001. Rates and risk factors of liver cirrhosis progression in patients with chronic hepatitis C. *J. Hepatol.* **34:**730–739.
36. Reference deleted.
37. **Roberts, S., G. Cooksley, D. Shaw, H. K. Berns, M. T. Brandl, S. H. Fettner, G. Hill, D. Ipe, K. Klumpp, M. Mannino, E. O'Mara, Y. Tuo, and C.B. Washington.** 2006. Interim results of a multiple ascending dose study of R1 626, a novel nucleoside analog targeting HCV polymerase in chronic HCV patients. *J. Hepatol.* **44**(Suppl. 2):S269. (Abstract.)

37a. **Rodriguez-Luna, H., and H. E. Vargas.** 2005. Management of hepatitis C virus infection in the setting of liver transplantation. *Liver Transpl.* **11:**479–489.

38. **Romero-Marrero, C. J., S. Fu, V. Thyagarajan, R. J. Fontana, A. S. Lok, S. Pelletier, and J. A. Marrero.** 2007. Predictors of dropout from transplant waiting list among patients listed for hepatocellular carcinoma using the UNOS/OPTN Database. *Hepatology* **46**(Suppl. 1):241A. (Abstract.)
39. **Ruiz, J. D., F. Molitor, R. K. Sun, J. Mikanda, M. Facer, J. M. Colford, Jr., G. W. Rutherford, and M. S. Ascher.** 1999. Prevalence and correlates of hepatitis C virus infection among inmates entering the California correctional system. *West. J. Med.* **170:**156–160.
40. **Sarrazin, C., R. Rouzier, F. Wagner, N. Forestier, D. Larrey, S. K. Gupta, M. Hussain, A. Shah, D. Cutler, J. Zhang, and S. Zeuzem.** 2007. SCH 503034, a novel hepatitis C virus protease inhibitor, plus pegylated interferon alpha-2b for genotype 1 nonresponders. *Gastroenterology* **132:**1270–1278.
41. **Schneider, J., W. Halota, D. Delic, Z. Nesic, D. Prokopowicz, R. Flisiak, J. Kuydowicz, M. Jablkowski, J. Cianciara, T. Mach, R. Modrzewska, M. Fabri, D. Tomic, A. Horban, W. Krycka, and M. Cripps.** 2006. A novel primboost therapeutic vaccine induces sustained seroconversion at 52 weeks in patients with HBeAg+ chronic hepatitis B: a phase IIa clinical trial. *J. Clin. Virol.* **36**(Suppl. 2):S30. (Abstract.)
42. **Sharma, P., V. Balan, J. L. Hernandez, A. M. Harper, E. B. Edwards, H. Rodriguez-Luna, T. Byrne, H. E. Vargas, D. Mulligan, J. Rakela, and R. H. Wiesner.** 2004. Liver transplantation for hepatocellular carcinoma: the MELD impact. *Liver Transpl.* **10:**36–41.
43. **Shiffman, M. L.** 1999. Improvement in liver histopathology associated with interferon therapy in patients with chronic hepatitis C. *Viral Hepatol. Rev.* **5:**27–43.
44. **Sun, C. A., D. M. Wu, C. C. Lin, S. N. Lu, S. L. You, L. Y. Wang, M. H. Wu, and C. J. Chen.** 2003. Incidence and cofactors of hepatitis C virus-related hepatocellular carcinoma: a prospective study of 12,008 men in Taiwan. *Am. J. Epidemiol.* **157:**674–682.
45. Reference deleted.
46. **Wakita, T., T. Pietschmann, T. Kato, T. Date, M. Miyamoto, Z. Zhao, K. Murthy, A. Habermann, H. G. Kräusslich, M. Mizokami, R. Bartenschlager, and T. J. Liang.** 2005. Production of infectious hepatitis C virus in tissue culture from a cloned viral genome. *Nat. Med.* **11:**791–796.
47. Wang, Z., Y. Tanaka, Y. Huang, F. Kirbanov, J. Chen, G. Zeng, B. Zhou, M. Mizokami, and J. Hou. 2007. Clinical and virological characteristics of hepatitis B virus subgenotypes Ba, C1, and C2 in China. *J. Clin. Microbiol.* **45:**1491–1496.
48. **Yang, H. I., S. N. Lu, Y. F. Liaw, S. L. You, C. A. Sun, L. Y. Wang, C. K. Hsiao, P. J. Chen, D. S. Chen, C. J. Chen, and Taiwan Community-Based Cancer Screening Project Group.** 2002. Hepatitis B e antigen and the risk of hepatocellular carcinoma. *N. Engl. J. Med.* **347:**168–174.
49. **Yang, S. H., C. G. Lee, S. H. Park, S. J. Im, Y. M. Kim, J. M.**

Son, J. S. Wang, S. K. Yoon, M. K. Song, A. Ambrozaitis, N. Kharchenko, Y. D. Yun, C. M. Kim, C. Y. Kim, S. H. Lee, B. M. Kim, W. B. Kim, and Y. C. Sung. 2006. Correlation of antiviral T-cell responses with suppression of viral rebound in chronic hepatitis B carriers: a proof-of-concept study. *Gene Ther.* **13:**1110–1117.

50. **Yano, M., H. Kumada, M. Kage, K. Ikeda, K. Shimamatsu, O. Inoue, E. Hashimoto, J. H. Lefkowitch, J. Ludwig, and K. Okuda.** 1996. The long-term pathological evolution of chronic hepatitis C. *Hepatology* **23:**1334–1340.

51. **Yuan, H. J., M. F. Yuen, D. Ka-Ho Wong, E. Sablon, and C. L. Lai.** 2005. The relationship between HBV-DNA levels and cirrhosis-related complications in Chinese with chronic hepatitis B. *J. Viral Hepat.* **12:**373–379.

Sequelae and Long-Term Consequences of Infectious Diseases
Edited by Pina M. Fratamico, James L. Smith, and Kim A. Brogden
© 2009 ASM Press, Washington, DC

Chapter 21

Slow Viral Infections

Rafik Samuel and Robert L. Bettiker

There are many viruses that are not cleared from the body after they infect an individual. Some of these include the herpes simplex viruses, hepatitis B, and the five viruses discussed in this chapter. The first four viruses discussed are similar because they are lentiviruses (viruses that carry negative-stranded RNA) that produce human infection in a similar fashion. These include human T-lymphotropic virus type 1 (HTLV-1), HTLV-2, human immunodeficiency virus type 1 (HIV-1), and HIV-2. In fact, HIV-1 was termed HTLV-3 when first discovered and quickly was renamed as more information was uncovered about it. These four viruses infect lymphocytes and lead to many chronic sequelae as a result. In addition, this chapter will cover one of the herpesviruses, human herpesvirus 8 (HHV-8), because of its close relationship with HIV-1. The viruses will be presented in chronologic fashion based on discovery, focusing on the possible sequelae that chronic infection with these viruses can cause.

HTLV-1 AND -2

HTLV-1 was first isolated from a man with a cutaneous T-cell lymphoma (mycosis fungoides) (144) and from another with a cutaneous T-cell leukemia (Sézary syndrome) (145). Called human T-lymphotropic virus, it was the first retrovirus that infects humans to be isolated (200).

In 1982, a similar but distinct virus was isolated from a man with a form of T-cell malignancy called hairy cell leukemia (87). This second virus was called HTLV-2, but the already described HTLV-1 is now believed to be the cause of hairy cell leukemia. HTLV-2 appears to be the cause of a disease similar to HTLV-1-associated myelopathy/tropical spastic paraparesis (HAM/TSP) (47, 158).

Molecular Mechanism of Infection

Once integrated into DNA, HTLV-1's and HTLV-2's Tax proteins regulate viral growth and replication and are heavily involved in disease pathogenesis. These proteins are transcriptional activators and are the main culprits in transformation of the T lymphocyte (157, 175). Interleukin (IL)-2 and the IL-2 receptor genes are activated, which stimulate T-cell proliferation. Tax also switches on the proto-oncogenes c-*fos* and c-*erg*. Increases in gamma interferon, stimulated by Tax, may trigger the inflammatory state responsible for HAM/TSP (24).

Clinical Sequelae of Infection

HTLV-1 is associated with a multitude of disorders (149). The most feared include adult T-cell lymphoma/leukemia (ATLL) and HAM/TSP (62, 136, 153), but the virus is also strongly associated with uveitis (118, 119, 141, 142, 203), infective dermatitis (24, 103), polymyositis (17, 24, 122), synovitis (131), thyroiditis (92), strongyloidiasis (126), and bronchioalveolar pneumonitis (24). In addition, HTLV-1 infection appears to cause a relative immunodeficient state (123).

In contrast, HTLV-2 has been conclusively linked only to HTLV-2-associated myelopathy/tropical spastic paresis (also abbreviated HAM/TSP) (158). Although HTLV-2-infected individuals appear to have a higher incidence of pneumonia, bronchitis, tuberculosis, and urinary tract infections, the mechanism is unknown. There are many case reports of hematologic abnormalities in persons with HTLV-2 (including the individual from whom the virus was initially isolated [87]), but systematic studies show no association.

Rafik Samuel and Robert L. Bettiker • Section of Infectious Diseases, Temple University School of Medicine, Philadelphia, PA 19140.

ATLL

ATLL, an aggressive leukemia/lymphoma, remains a difficult disease to treat. It has various clinical findings: cutaneous skin involvement, lytic bone lesions, generalized lymphadenopathy, visceral involvement, and cells in the peripheral blood with pleiotropic features, called flower cells (196). It generally presents decades after infection with HTLV-1 (24, 124), with a lifetime risk of 1 to 4% (187). Seven hundred cases of ATLL are diagnosed in Japan alone each year (202), and it is the most common lymphoid malignancy in Jamaica (70).

The Lymphoma Study Group in Japan has classified ATLL into four clinical types using clinical and cytologic criteria: smoldering (5%), chronic (19%), lymphoma/leukemia (19%), and acute (57%) (172). Transformation to the acute phase from the smoldering or chronic phase can occur at any time (24).

Smoldering ATLL is defined by 5% or more abnormal T cells in the periphery and skin involvement. The lactate dehydrogenase is normal, as is the total T-cell count. Skin lesions may resemble mycosis fungoides and present as erythema or infiltrative tumors or plaques. This stage may last for years. *Chronic ATLL* is characterized by a T-cell lymphocytosis of $>3.5 \times 10^9$/liter. The lactate dehydrogenase may be elevated, and there may be lymphadenopathy, hepatosplenomegaly, and pulmonary and skin involvement, but usually no other organ system involvement. The median survival time is 2 years. *Lymphoma/leukemia* ATLL's hallmark is lymphadenopathy without lymphocytosis with ATLL shown on biopsy. Survival time is approximately 10 months. *Acute ATLL* is diagnosed by leukemic T cells with the characteristic pleiomorphic morphology, which may include flower cells (Sézary cells) (109). Skin lesions, hepatosplenomegaly, hypercalcemia, and lymphadenopathy are common, as are lytic bone lesions and visceral involvement. The survival time is approximately 10 months. In ATLL, the ultimate cause of death is usually due to a massive proliferation of clonal tumor cells, hypercalcemia, sepsis, or opportunistic infections, as seen in HIV infection (24).

HTLV-1 may predispose a person to other types of malignancies. One case report spoke of HTLV proviral DNA found integrated in the tumor cells of small-cell cancer of the lung (24). Additionally, HTLV-1 infection may be associated with invasive cervical cancer (180), although confounding risk factors for the two diseases make interpretation of the data difficult.

HAM/TSP

Tropical spastic paraparesis, found in the Caribbean, and HTLV-associated myelopathy, first described in Japan, are now known to be the same disease (155) and are abbreviated HAM/TSP (201). HAM/TSP is a chronic progressive demyelinating disease that affects the spinal cord and white matter of the central nervous system (CNS) (24, 63, 79, 136). It affects females more than males, in a 2.3:1 ratio (127) and has a lifetime risk of approximately 5% in chronic HTLV carriers. The incubation period is unclear and originally was thought to be years to decades, but a recent survey showed that HAM/TSP developed in 50% of transfusion-associated HTLV-1 infections. Symptoms include spasticity or hyperreflexia of lower extremities in 98%, urinary bladder dysfunction in 94%, leg weakness in 88%, sensory disturbances—often in the thoracic dermatomes—in 56%, and ataxia in 5 to 20%. Cranial nerves and cognitive abilities are rarely involved (79).

A spastic bladder is often an early feature (80). Spinal cord atrophy or swelling has been reported in a few cases, as has subclinical involvement of white matter, spinal roots, and the spinothalamic tract (63). Some patients may have an amyotrophic lateral sclerosis-like picture, white matter lesions, or cerebellar symptoms (79). Microscopically, the disease is most commonly characterized by bilateral loss of axons and myelin in the lateral and anterior columns of the spinal cord, with lymphocyte and macrophage infiltration (135).

Elevated levels of neopterin in cerebrospinal fluid—a consequence of cellular immune activation—are useful to differentiate HAM/TSP from other myelopathies, such as multiple sclerosis (132). Brain MRI examination most often shows many high-intensity lesions in subcortical and deep structures on T2-weighted images (79).

HAM/TSP caused by HTLV-2 gives similar symptoms to those caused by HTLV-1, although case reports exist of different neurologic manifestations associated with the virus: spinocerebellar atrophy in two Native American sisters (75) and four cases of an ataxia and cognitive disorder (171). With HTLV-2, the disease has much lower levels of antibodies and proviral DNA in cerebrospinal fluid than those of HTLV-1 (125). HAM/TSP might also occur less frequently in HTLV-2-infected individuals.

HTLV-1-associated uveitis

Ohba et al. were the first to link HTLV-1 with ocular disease by describing three types of manifestations: (i) opportunistic infections and tumor in ATLL patients; (ii) ocular alterations in HAM/TSP patients, including Sjögren syndrome (SS), optic atrophy, cotton-wool spots, vitreous opacities, retinal pigmentary degeneration, and retinal vasculitis; and (iii) uveitis in HTLV-1 asymptomatic carriers (24, 134). The mean age of onset is approximately 46 years (range 19 to 75 years). Grave's disease may be associated with HTLV-1 uveitis—16 of 93 patients in one series had an episode of Grave's prior to their uveitis (119, 203). Symptoms include blurred vision, foggy vision, and floaters (118, 128). Nearly half of cases involved both eyes, and episodes can last from 2 weeks to 10 years. Relapses occur in half of patients, and 10% in one study of 112 patients had six or greater relapses (188).

Pathologic examination demonstrates inflammatory cells, including lymphocytes and histiocytes, infiltrating the intraocular tissues (135). HTLV-1 proviral DNA can be found in 60% of intraocular T cells, suggesting that these infected cells are the cause of inflammation in this disease (163).

HTLV-1 arthropathy and SS

HTLV-1 disrupts the immune system and may predispose infected individuals to certain autoimmune disorders, such as arthropathy, autoantibodies, hypergammaglobulinemia, and SS (81, 130). HTLV-1 arthropathy is characterized by joint destruction, massive proliferation of synovium, and occasional bone lesions. The clinical presentation and laboratory findings may be similar to that of rheumatoid arthritis with some key differences. The disease predominantly afflicts women, with an average age of onset at 49 years. The wrists, shoulders, and knees are preferentially involved. In a survey of 45 patients with HTLV-1 arthropathy, 36 were positive for rheumatoid factor, and 10 of these had other autoantibodies present. High levels of anti-HTLV-1 immunoglobulin M (IgM) antibodies were found in the synovial fluid. Histologic examination shows synovial proliferation with atypical lymphocytes with nuclear indentations similar to those found in ATLL (131). HTLV-1 can infect synovial cells directly (97, 164), and the *tax* gene product has been implicated in the synovial proliferation.

SS is thought to be an autoimmune disorder characterized by salivary and lacrimal gland insufficiency. Lymphocytes and plasma cells infiltrate and destroy the gland in a manner similar to rheumatoid arthritis. SS patients in the Nagasaki Prefecture in Japan have a high prevalence of HTLV-1 infection and salivary anti-HTLV-1 IgA secretion (52, 130), and interestingly, DNA sequences homologous to HTLV-1's *tax* gene were detected in the salivary glands of SS patients not infected with HTLV-1, but not in healthy controls (112, 185).

Other diseases associated with HTLV-1

Infective dermatitis in Jamaican children is a chronic eczema associated with HTLV-1 seropositivity, although only about 5% of infected children develop the disease. Nonvirulant *Staphylococcus aureus* and beta-hemolytic streptococcus cause a relapsing infection. HTLV-1-associated dermatitis has subsequently been reported in other areas where HTLV-1 is endemic (102, 103). HTLV-1 proviral DNA has been isolated from lymphocytes obtained from skin biopsies.

HTLV-1-associated alveolitis is often asymptomatic but can cause lymphocytic nodular infiltrates visible on chest X-ray (181). HTLV-1 has been detected from bronchoalveolar washes from patients with alveolitis (149). Histologically, one finds bronchial mucosa epithelium proliferation with a thickened basement membrane and mild fibrosis. Lymphocytes, along with some plasma cells, histiocytes, and neutrophils, infiltrate into the epithelial layer and mucosa (135).

HTLV-1 infection has been associated with endemic parasitic infections, such as trypanosomiasis (116), leishmaniasis (22), and especially *Strongyloides stercoralis* infection (126, 129). Such infections are thought to reflect relative immunodeficiency caused by the virus (166).

HIV-1

Introduction

No virus leads to as many chronic complications as does HIV-1. HIV quickly disseminates when entering the host and leads to complications in practically every organ system of the body. These sequelae may be the result of direct virus damage, such as with the immune system; indirect damage, by allowing entry of immune cells into an organ (cardiac); or the production of severe cellular immunodeficiency, leading to opportunistic infections. In this section we will briefly review the natural course of HIV in the infected individual and follow it with an in-depth review of the major sequelae, listed by organ system.

Immune System

The immune system takes the brunt of the effects of HIV since these cells are the target of the virus. As an individual becomes infected, HIV quickly decimates the immune system. Upon mucosal infection, dendritic cells are the first cells that become infected. Dendritic cells can lead to dissemination of the virus in two ways. They fuse with CD4 cells (syncytia formation) and release large amounts of virus (147). They also present HIV antigens to CD4 and CD8 cells, leading to activation and an increase in HIV production. In a short time, dendritic cells decrease in numbers, probably due to apoptosis (14).

Dendritic cells also initiate a rapid CD4 cell proliferation. Despite the activation of CD4 cells, the immune response does not adequately control the virus. In fact, there is a qualitative dysfunction in the CD4 response, which leads to decreased proliferation with reduced expression of IL-2 receptors, induction of T-cell anergy, and apoptosis of T cells (159).

The cytotoxic T-cell response plays the major role in decreasing the viral load in acute infection and maintaining the set point of circulating virus. This response includes the CD8 cells and the natural killer cells. Unfortunately, these cells do not clear the HIV. A few explanations include apoptosis of the CD8 and natural killer cells, HIV mutation to avoid the CD8 epitopes, and downregulation of the HLA expression induced by HIV (65, 189).

Unlike many other infections, the humoral immune system does not control infection with HIV. The body does mount a humoral response to HIV; however, it is not effective. Antibodies directed to the virus develop 2 to 6 weeks after acquisition, but the virus evades the antibody response because the sugars on the viral envelope make it difficult for antibodies to detect and attach to the virus (86).

Recent studies have led to a better understanding of the role of the gastrointestinal (GI) tract plays in host immunity. There are a large amount of immune cells in the lymphoid tissue of the GI tract that are rapidly lost early in HIV infection. Several mechanisms likely lead to the loss of these cells. First, a large number of these cells are $CD4^+$ cells, which HIV preferentially infects (27). Second, HIV has recently been shown to infect natural killer cells via integrin $\alpha_4\beta_7$, a different mechanism than the CD4 receptor. Activation of $\alpha_4\beta_7$ leads to release of another integrin, leukocyte function-associated antigen 1, which promotes junction formation within the cells and allows cell-to-cell transmission of HIV (9). Via these mechanisms, the virus quickly depletes the immune cells within the gut (82). As a result of this immune destruction there may be chronic bacterial entry into the blood stream, as evidenced by increased lipopolysaccharide A (endotoxin) in patients with chronic HIV (137a).

Even though the patient is usually asymptomatic, there is tremendous turnover of virus and infected immune cells. Over years, the infected person becomes symptomatic, either from the virus, opportunistic infections, or malignancies. The time to symptomatic disease varies from one individual to another, but the average person develops symptoms or severe immunosuppression in about 7 years. Many variables of the host and virus lead to different rates of progression.

Neurologic

One of the most frequent sites of end organ damage as a result of HIV infection is the nervous system. Involvement of the CNS can lead to HIV-associated dementia (HAD or AIDS dementia complex) or minor cognitive motor disorder (MCMD). Involvement of the peripheral nervous system can lead to peripheral neuropathy. In addition, infections can lead to a variety of different CNS complications (toxoplasmosis, primary CNS lymphoma, and others) or peripheral nervous system dysfunction, such as cytomegalovirus (CMV) radiculopathy. Medications used to treat HIV can lead to peripheral neuropathies (didanosine, stavudine) or cognitive/psychosocial difficulties (efavirenz). Here we will focus first on the effect of HIV itself and only briefly mention the infections that can affect the nervous system.

CNS

Prior to antiretroviral therapy, up to 30% of HIV-infected individuals developed HAD. This is a syndrome that includes short-term memory impairment, reduced concentration, leg weakness, personality changes with apathy, and social withdrawal. In its most advanced form it can lead to a vegetative state. In the highly active antiretroviral therapy (HAART) era, HIV-associated dementia is uncommon, but a different type of CNS involvement, MCMD, can occur. Patients with MCMD have well-controlled HIV infection, develop loss of memory, and develop cognitive dysfunction, but at a much slower rate than that seen with HAD. Both syndromes are identical by pathology, with evidence of neuroinvasion by the virus. The degree of viral invasion is likely associated with the amount of HIV circulating in the bloodstream (64, 162). In patients on HAART, there may be incomplete suppression of virus in the CNS and thus a slower progression of impairment (51).

HIV most likely enters the brain via circulating T cells and monocytes. Multiple crossovers into the CNS during the course of infection lead to genetically distinct viral variants. It is unclear how the virus causes CNS neuronal death. There are two hypotheses as to how HAD and MCMD develop. In the direct injury hypothesis, gp120 (an envelope glycoprotein of the virus) is thought to elicit chemokine activation, leading to neuronal injury (91). In the so-called bystander effect hypothesis, peripheral chemokines secreted due to HIV infection lead to activation of T cells and monocytes that then enter the CNS. These activated T cells and macrophages cause proliferation and apoptosis of astrocytes. As the astrocytes decrease in number, the chemokines secreted in the CNS subsequently lead to neuronal cell death (64). Both theories have been supported in the literature, and it is still not clear what is occurring.

Treatment of HAD includes initiating antiretroviral agents that enter the CNS. The use of these agents, including zidovudine, have been reported to improve HAD (106). Since neuronal death is also a result of an inflammatory response, antiretroviral agents alone may not improve HAD. Other agents that have been studied in animals for the treatment of HAD include *N*-methyl-D-aspartate receptor antagonists, such as memantine (191).

Peripheral nervous system

Peripheral neuropathies have become the most common neurologic complication in the HAART era. They have been classified as inflammatory demyelination polyradiculoneuropathy, mononeuropathy multiplex or radiculopathy, distal symmetric polyneuropathy (DSP), and toxic neuropathy from antiretroviral therapy. During early infection with HIV, an acute demyelination neuropathy can occur, which is usually an autoimmune phenomenon (similar to Guillain-Barré syndrome). A mononeuropathy can also occur as a result of an autoimmune process, from CMV (CMV radiculopathy), or due to vasculitis (96).

The most common form of neuropathy encountered is DSP. This syndrome is usually found in patients with advanced HIV infection with CD4 counts less than 200 and those with >10,000 copies/ml of HIV RNA (41). The symptoms are sensory and usually associated with hyperalgesia and allodynia. The symptoms begin gradually in the lower legs with aching, burning, or numbness, then progress proximally, and eventually can involve the upper extremities as well (96).

The symptoms are due to degeneration of the long axons, similar to the neuropathy associated with diabetes. Biopsies demonstrate macrophage activation at the site of the axonal degeneration. As seen with HAD, the neurotoxicity is likely due to immune activation and not directly due to the HIV itself (138). Treatment includes the use of antiretroviral therapy in conjunction with pain relievers. Commonly used pain medications include gabapentin, lamotrigine, and narcotics. The only agent found to be effective compared to placebo is lamotrigine (173).

Toxic neuropathy is usually due to the nucleoside reverse transcriptase inhibitors (NRTI), mainly didanosine, stavudine, zidovudine, and zalcitabine. The clinical symptoms of toxic neuropathy are similar to DSP. The NRTI likely lead to mitochondrial toxicity, which then causes neuronal death (107). The treatment of toxic neuropathy includes removal of the offending agents and the use of the pain medications similar to the treatment of DSP.

Infections

Infections of the nervous system in HIV-positive individuals are numerous. Some of the frequently encountered causes of peripheral neuropathy include varicella zoster virus, causing herpes zoster with resultant postherpetic neuralgia, and CMV, resulting in a peripheral radiculopathy. CNS involvement ranges from parenchymal infections to meningeal infections. Common parenchymal infections include toxoplasmosis, tuberculosis, JC virus, nocardiosis, opportunistic mold infections, and others. Meningitis due to *Cryptococcus*, tuberculosis, listeriosis, and the typical bacteria, such as pneumococcus and meningococcus, are also seen with these patients.

Cardiac and Metabolic

Cardiac involvement in HIV patients is not uncommon. Many different manifestations of cardiac disease have been noted, including pericarditis, myocarditis, cardiomyopathy, and coronary artery disease. The most frequent of these is pericarditis. Pericardial involvement can occur in up to 20% of patients not receiving antiretroviral therapy. Most patients have a small effusion that is asymptomatic, and the etiology of the pericarditis is usually not identified. Rarely, large effusions are detected, and an infection such as tuberculosis or a malignancy such as lymphoma may be found. Evaluation and treatment of these patients should follow the usual work-up for pericarditis, including pericardiocentesis and even pericardial biopsy. Nevertheless, outcome is poor in this population, with mortality over 60% if antiretrovirals are not started (23, 71).

Myocardial involvement is difficult to assess without biopsy. In an HIV pre-HAART autopsy series, myocarditis was found in over 9 percent of individuals. In only 20% of these cases were infectious agents, such as *Toxoplasma*, coxsackievirus, adenovirus, or CMV identified (76).

In the other 80% of patients with myocarditis, no etiology is found. Microscopically, one can see focal collections of mononuclear cells or myocardial necrosis (3). It is likely that these findings are the result of HIV infection; however, it is not clear how HIV enters the myocyte since there are no CD4 receptors on these cells. HIV may enter when other immune cells (usually monocytes) enter the myocyte for other inflammatory reasons, which then results in myocarditis (12, 168).

True cardiomyopathy occurs rarely, usually in about 4% of HIV infected individuals. The cardiomyopathy may be a result of the focal myocarditis but is more likely a result of other comorbidities such as alcohol consumption, cocaine use, or hypertension. Management of dilated cardiomyopathy should include antiretroviral therapy, which may reverse the cardiomyopathy in certain individuals. In addition, treatment with the usual medications for cardiomyopathy is indicated (12).

Metabolic changes affecting the body occur during chronic HIV infection and with the use of antiretroviral therapy. These include insulin resistance, hyperlipidemia, changes in body fat distribution with peripheral lipoatrophy and visceral obesity, and changes in circulating inflammatory markers. Triglycerides are increased and glucose intolerance can be seen with HIV infection itself and with antiretroviral therapy. One theory for glucose intolerance includes insulin resistance at the site of the muscle through changes in body composition and also through direct inhibition of GLUT4, the enzyme that allows glucose into the muscle. Decreased adipocyte differentiation by inhibition of the Ppar γ enzyme is the major theory leading to peripheral lipoatrophy and central visceral obesity (88, 165).

HIV-infected people not on antiretroviral agents have increased circulating immune mediators, such as IL-6 and tumor necrosis factor alpha. These patients were found to have increased cardiac events when compared to those who were on antiretroviral medications (101a). Multiple studies have shown an increase in cardiac events in those on antiretroviral therapy (56, 161), while others have shown an increase in those that had therapy stopped (179). At this point in time, it appears the cardiac risk of antiretroviral therapy is minimal when compared to the benefits of these medications. In addition, the risk of cardiac disease from the classic risk factors of smoking, diabetes, hypertension and hyperlipidemia still carry much more risk than HAART (56).

Pulmonary

The respiratory tract is frequently involved in HIV-infected individuals. Most of these complications are related to opportunistic infections. There are a few direct complications due to HIV itself. Pulmonary hypertension, nonspecific interstitial pneumonitis, and lymphocytic interstitial pneumonitis have been reported (77). Although pulmonary hypertension (PAH) may be associated with HHV-8 and is described elsewhere in this chapter, HIV has been associated with pulmonary hypertension when no other organisms have been identified. In HIV-associated PAH, findings on biopsy of the artery include abnormal endothelial cells, intimal disruption, thrombosis, medial hypertrophy, and luminal obliteration (111). This syndrome is rare, occurring in less than 1% of AIDS patients (174). Published mortality due to PAH is low because the majority of cases were described prior to the HAART era, when these patients died of other causes. Treatment of PAH is similar to that for those without HIV. Studies have shown conflicting results with the use of HAART (206).

The majority of respiratory diseases are due to infections. Upper respiratory infections and lower tract infections may be due to typical bacteria, atypical bacteria, mycobacteria, fungi, protozoa, and other viruses (77).

Renal

Renal involvement is relatively common in patients infected with HIV. The kidney manifestation encountered most often is a focal glomerulosclerosis called HIV-associated nephropathy (HIVAN). HIVAN occurs in 2 to 10 percent of HIV-infected patients, is usually seen with those with high amounts of replicating virus and lower CD4 counts and occurs mainly in black patients (69).

The pathogenesis of HIVAN may be related to direct replication of HIV within the renal cells (glomerular epithelial cells, mesangial cells, and tubular cells) (66). Another theory is that the virus may stimulate release of cytokines that are responsible for the renal injury. The relationship with host factors is also important because blacks are at particularly high risk for HIVAN (156). The histology of HIVAN includes collapse and sclerosis of the glomerular tuft, severe tubular injury with microcystic formation, and tubular degeneration (98). Patients with HIVAN present with nephrotic syndrome, which includes edema, heavy proteinuria, and hypoalbuminemia. Treatment with antiretroviral therapy and angiotensin-converting enzyme inhibitors is warranted; however, not all studies have demonstrated improvement with HAART (69).

Other causes of renal injury include toxicity from medications used for the treatment of HIV or opportunistic infections. Commonly used medications that can lead to renal complications include indinavir or atazanavir, which can cause nephrolithiasis; trimethoprim/sulfamethoxazole, which can lead to acute interstitial nephritis; and tenofovir, which has been linked to Fanconi syndrome (154). Some of the common infections encountered in HIV-infected individuals that can lead to renal insufficiency include hepatitis B and C, which lead to membranous glomerulonephritis or postinfectious glomerulonephritis from *Streptococcus pyogenes* pharyngitis (186).

Gastrointestinal and Hepatobiliary Disease

The whole GI tract from the oropharynx to the anus is commonly affected in HIV infection with a variety of different infections that are too numerous to review here. As mentioned earlier, HIV affects the GI tract, resulting in immune dysfunction. As a result, HIV enteropathy, a chronic diarrhea and malabsorption syndrome can occur. The virus directly causes apoptosis of gastrointestinal epithelial cells, leading to mucosal inflammation and subsequent increased susceptibility to infection and malabsorption (100).

There are many causes of hepatobiliary disease in the HIV-infected individual. Currently, complications of end-stage liver disease is a major cause of mortality in the HIV-infected patient (199). Hepatobiliary disease is usually due to chronic viral hepatitis, infiltrative disease from infection, AIDS-related cholangiopathy, and drug-related liver injury. By far, the most common cause of hepatic disease in HIV patients is viral hepatitis. Chronic coinfection with hepatitis C virus (HCV) can occur in up to 80% of individuals who acquired HIV via injection drug use. HIV has been shown to increase the progression to cirrhosis and hepatocellular carcinoma in HCV patients compared to the non-HIV-infected patient (115). In addition, treatment of HCV is more difficult in this population. Combination therapy with pegylated interferon and ribavirin may clear the HCV in only 19 to 40% of patients treated (43, 192). Hepatitis B virus (HBV) coinfection occurs in 5 to 10% of patients with HIV. Treatment of HBV in the HIV-infected patient should include a combination of tenofovir and either emtricitabine or lamivudine since these agents can treat both infections (143, 150).

Hepatotoxicity due to HAART is a major concern with the HIV patient, especially if he or she is coinfected with HBV or HCV or consumes alcohol. All protease inhibitors and nonnucleoside reverse transcriptase inhibitors and some nucleosides can cause hepatotoxicity (182, 183, 197). Two agents, indinavir and atazanavir, can cause elevated bilirubin as a result of inhibiting glucuronidation without causing hepatotoxicity (29, 207). In addition to the usual hepatic complications, initiation of antiretroviral therapy in the hepatitis coinfected patient can lead to an immune reconstitution inflammatory response to the hepatitis viruses, leading to an acute flare of hepatitis (104).

Not frequently seen anymore but worth mentioning is AIDS cholangiopathy, a syndrome of biliary obstruction due to infections of the biliary tract that result in strictures of the biliary ducts. The most commonly associated organism is *Cryptosporidium parvum*. Patients develop right upper quadrant pain and diarrhea and less frequently jaundice and fever (39). Endoscopic retrograde cholangiopancreatography with sphincterotomy is the treatment of choice. *C. parvum* treatment in addition to HAART is also recommended to prevent further strictures (38).

Other hepatic infectious agents include mycobacteria (*Mycobacterium tuberculosis* or *Mycobacterium avium* complex), fungi (*Histoplasma capsulatum*), bacteria (*Bartonella henselae*), and viruses (CMV). Liver biopsy may be required to identify the organism causing the disease, and each of these infections should be treated appropriately (94).

Hematology

HIV can lead to many different syndromes affecting the blood cell lines. Neutropenia, anemia, and thrombocytopenia can be seen in up to 70% of HIV-infected individuals (205). The incidence of these disorders increases as HIV disease progresses. Neutropenia is usually multifactorial and can be due to infection, malignancy, reactions to medications, or to HIV itself. The more common infections that can infiltrate bone marrow and lead to neutropenia are mycobacterial and fungal. Medications associated with neutropenia include zidovudine, trimethoprim/sulfamethoxazole, and ganciclovir. Malignancies including lymphoma can lead to neutropenia as well (117). Treatment of the underlying infection and malignancy or discontinuation of any bone marrow-toxic medication is warranted. When no etiology of the neutropenia is found, HAART and the use of colony-stimulating factors can be helpful (60).

Anemia is another frequent complication of HIV infection, occurring in up to 60 to 80% of AIDS patients (205). Risk factors for development of anemia include a mean corpuscular volume less than 80 fl, a CD4 count of <200, an HIV viral load of $>50{,}000$ copies, and the use of zidovudine. Anemia is associated with increased mortality, independent of the CD4 count (21). The most common finding in HIV-infected patients is an anemia of chronic disease. In most cases, however, the additive effects of other infections, medications, malignancy, or hemolysis complicate the anemia, sometimes leading to the requirement of urgent care (184).

Opportunistic infections such as mycobacteria and fungi can disseminate into the bone marrow and lead to anemia. Viral infections, in particular parvovirus B19, can lead to a chronic and severe anemia. Up to 30% of patients with parvovirus B19 have hematocrits below 20%. Those infected with parvovirus

B19 often require intravenous immune globulin therapy to help treat the anemia (40). Medications such as zidovudine or trimethoprim/sulfamethoxazole or infiltration of the bone marrow by malignancy can also lead to anemia. Hemolysis may be drug induced, antibody mediated, or due to microangiopathy. Drugs that can cause hemolysis in glucose-6-phosphate dehydrogenase-deficient individuals are used frequently in the HIV-infected patient (e.g., dapsone). In addition, antibodies directed against red cells are common, with a positive direct antiglobulin test found with up to 18% of patients (193). Treatment with HAART to decrease the inflammatory state, erythropoietin therapy to improve the anemia, removal of any toxic medications, and treatment of the infection or malignancy are the mainstays of anemia therapy (74).

Thrombocytopenia has been reported in 40% of patients with AIDS (205). The degree of thrombocytopenia varies in individuals; however, its incidence increases as the HIV infection progresses (176). The most common cause of thrombocytopenia is termed primary HIV-associated thrombocytopenia. This is very similar to idiopathic thrombocytic purpura. Treatment of primary HIV-associated thrombocytopenia is similar to the treatment of idiopathic thrombocytic purpura, except for the addition of HAART (8). Thrombotic thrombocytopenia purpura-hemolytic uremic syndrome occurs uncommonly (0.009/100 person years) but is life threatening. Its manifestations and treatment are similar to those of thrombotic thrombocytopenia purpura in non-HIV-infected patients. Treatment with HAART and plasma exchange is recommended since individuals treated with plasma exchange alone, without HAART, can develop recurrences (16, 133).

Endocrine

The endocrine systems are not spared in patients with HIV infection. HIV affects the pituitary, adrenal, thyroid, and testes. Although the anterior pituitary function is well preserved in HIV infection, the posterior pituitary can be affected. Syndrome of inappropriate anti-diuretic hormone secretion has been reported in up to 15% of hospitalized AIDS patients with hyponatremia (1). In addition, defects in growth hormone (GH) response have been demonstrated. Decreased levels of insulin-like growth factor-1 and insulin-like growth factor-1 binding protein-3 have been found in the setting of increased GH. This relative GH resistance is believed to be one of the contributing factors of AIDS wasting syndrome (101).

The thyroid is usually not involved in HIV, with the exception of the euthyroid sick state in which thyroid-stimulating hormone is low-normal with T3 and T4 levels also low due to impaired conversion of T4 to T3 (110). Rarely, an autoimmune thyroiditis can occur in the setting of immune reconstitution after initiation of HAART (85). Other manifestations of thyroid disease can occur at the same rates as in non-HIV-infected individuals and are treated in a similar fashion as in the non-HIV-infected person (18).

The adrenal axis can also be involved in HIV-infected individuals. Adrenal insufficiency can occur in those with advanced HIV infection. It is important to note that the lipo-hypertrophy syndrome (increased abdominal girth and development of a dorsal cervical fat pad) is not associated with changes in the adrenal axis. In patients with suspected adrenal insufficiency, it is important to measure the a.m. cortisol with an adrenal corticotropic hormone stimulation test because the a.m. cortisol may be normal, but the response to adrenal corticotropic hormone may be insufficient. Infections with mycobacteria, fungi, and CMV may lead to significant adrenal insufficiency; however, the cortisol levels should be decreased. Evaluation for these infections should be done when significant adrenal insufficiency is suspected (53).

Early in the HIV epidemic it was clear that men with advanced HIV had hypogonadism. Up to 50% of men with advanced disease were hypogonadal, with 75% of them hypogonadotropic (50). These hypogonadal men had a normal response to gonadotropin-releasing hormone when it was administered, suggesting that hypothalamic failure is responsible in many cases. These results may be due to many factors, including chronic illness and possibly effects of HIV itself (148). Men with HIV should have their testosterone levels evaluated and if low, corrected with exogenous testosterone given to those with hypogonadism (152).

Other Chronic Manifestations of HIV

Malignancies

Some malignancies are more common in HIV-infected individuals, while others occur at the same rate. Kaposi's sarcoma (KS), lymphoma (Hodgkin's and non-Hodgkin's), and primary CNS lymphoma are the classic malignancies described with patients with HIV. Recent studies, however, have shown that cancers of the liver, cervix, lung, oropharynx, colon, anus, and kidney, along with leukemia, and malignant melanoma occur at rates much greater than the non-HIV-infected population (140).

Musculoskeletal

Both muscle damage as well as bone abnormalities can occur in HIV-infected patients. Osteonecrosis of the hips, generalized osteopenia, and osteoporosis occur more frequently in HIV⁺ individuals (137). It is unclear whether the bone abnormalities are due only to HIV itself, immune activation leading to bone mineral density decrease, and hypogonadism, or due to antiretroviral agents. In any case, much more research in this area is needed (32).

NRTIs, opportunistic infections, and HIV itself can cause myopathy. HIV myopathy is similar to idiopathic polymyositis. As with many of the organ systems described above, it is difficult to tell if the muscle damage is due to the direct effects of HIV itself or an immune mechanism. As HIV is rarely isolated in muscle tissue, an immune mechanism is more likely. Diagnosis must be made by biopsy showing endomysial mononuclear cell infiltrates. Treatment with high-dose steroids is the standard of care (83). Other causes of muscle damage include NRTI-associated toxicity usually due to zidovudine treatment, which includes stopping AZT (46). Other causes include infections such as pyomyositis due to *S. aureus* or infections with toxoplasmosis.

Dermatology

Cutaneous disorders occur in almost all HIV-infected individuals. As one can imagine, the majority of these are due to dermatologic manifestations of systemic illness or reactions to medications. There are two disorders worth mentioning: eosinophilic folliculitis and atopic dermatitis. Eosinophilic folliculitis is a chronic disorder in patients with advanced HIV. The etiology is not yet known, but it usually occurs when CD4 cells drop below 100 cells/microliter. Eosinophilic folliculitis is manifested by small pink edematous follicular papules on the upper trunk and is extremely pruritic. Topical steroids help with the pruritus, but immune restoration with antiretroviral therapy is important. Atopic dermatitis or eczema is extremely common in HIV patients at any stage of their disease. Treatment with steroids and immune reconstitution is helpful (160).

HIV-2

HIV-2 was first described in Senegal in 1985 and continues to be seen almost exclusively in persons in or from western Africa. It is a lentivirus whose genome has about 40% overlap with the genome of HIV-1. In general, the diseases that it causes are the same as those caused by HIV-1, except it is much more difficult to acquire HIV-2, and HIV-2 leads to complications at a much slower rate than HIV-1. That said, HIV-2 does have some differences compared to HIV-1 that are worth mentioning. First, a higher proportion of individuals infected with HIV-2 develop HAD. This may be a result of longer time of circulating inflammatory markers before severe immunosuppression occurs, thus allowing patients to develop more severe neurologic disease before acquiring an opportunistic infection. Disseminated CMV infection and cholangiopathy are more common as well. These differences may be associated with less access to care and more exposure to infections than in other regions. On the other hand, KS occurs much less frequently with HIV-2. It is believed that the transactivating protein Tat in HIV-1 has angiogenic properties that interact with HHV-8 and lead to KS. It is noted that HIV-2 Tat does not have this property, while HIV-1 Tat does (25). For all the other chronic complications associated with HIV-2, please refer to the HIV-1 section above.

HHV-8

HHV-8, also known as KS herpesvirus (KSHV), was first isolated from a KS lesion in an HIV-1 infected patient in 1994 (36). It has been subsequently isolated in B cells in primary effusion lymphomas (PEL) (34) in multicentric Castleman's disease (178) and in primary pulmonary hypertension (44).

Molecular Mechanism of Disease

HHV-8 is capable of both lytic and latent infection, and thus infection is lifelong (93). Nearly all of HHV-8's genes are devoted to lytic infection, in which the infected cell dies and releases viral progeny into the environment. Only approximately five genes are active during latent infection, and the gene products tend to encourage cell survival (4, 120). Several HHV-8 genes have been incorporated from their human host genome, including IL-6 and a G protein coupled receptor (GPCR). Of great interest is this viral GPCR (vGPCR) (11, 35, 67, 68, 146, 169). Viral GPCR binds to multiple different chemokines but also appears to be constitutively active. This receptor, which appears to be homologous to the human IL-8 receptor, is both angiogenic and oncogenic. Approximately 30% of mice transgenic for vGPCR develop KS-like lesions (68), and 100% of nude mice injected with these lesions develop tumors (67). Viral GPCR is active only in the lytic phase of the viral life cycle, which results in death of the host cell. Viral GPCR thus cannot induce tumorgenicity in the classic sense since the cell dies, but it appears to induce proliferation in surrounding cells via cytokines with a paracrine effect.

Viral GPCR's tumorigenesis is enhanced by the HIV-1 Tat protein (5, 6, 67, 204). Although HIV-1 and HHV-8 tend to not infect the same cells, a CD8$^+$ response to the HHV-8 infection of endothelial cells may attract HIV-1-infected cells that are secreting Tat into the local environment. HIV-1 Tat's interaction with viral GPCR may explain why KS is far more common in HIV-1-infected persons than in HIV-2-infected ones (7).

HHV-8 differentially expresses genes when infecting either an endothelium-derived spindle cell or a B cell. Latency-associated nuclear antigen 2 is expressed in B cells, but not in spindle cells, and it inhibits apoptosis. HHV-8's genome encodes a viral IL-6 (vIL-6), which promotes B-cell growth. Alpha interferon, secreted by the infected host cell, downregulates the IL-6 receptor and arrests the cell cycle, but the HHV-8 vIL-6 promoter is activated by the alpha IFN pathway and allows it to bind to a separate receptor, allowing for infected B-cell proliferation (13).

KS

KS is a highly vascularized tumor that usually involves the skin, beginning as purplish lesions and evolving into plaques that may become brown with hemosiderin deposition (72, 93). The disease progresses differently depending upon the epidemiologic group to which the host belongs. Histologically, KS lesions initially have inflammatory cell infiltration with endothelial cell activation and angiogenesis. Early in the disease, they have more of a proliferative character than an actual malignancy (54). Endothelium-derived spindle-shaped cells then appear, surrounded by vascular slits with entrapped red cells. As the lesions progress, the spindle cells increase in number, and malignant transformation occurs (4, 54, 93). Nearly all of the spindle cells in KS lesions are latently infected with HHV-8, and very few of them are in the lytic stage.

KS has since been described as four variants, based upon the host characteristics: classic, endemic, transplant or immunosuppression associated, and epidemic or AIDS associated (4). HHV-8 DNA has been found in all KS variants (2, 36, 37, 78, 95, 121).

Classic KS affects older men of Mediterranean or Eastern European origin. It afflicts men over women at a rate of 15:1, with an average age of onset of 67 years (49). It has a relatively benign course and usually involves the feet and legs with multiple firm, reddish nodules. Lymphedema may precede the appearance of skin lesions. Approximately 10% of cases will develop mucosal or visceral involvement after a period of years, and untreated skin lesions will often expand and become confluent. Survival is measured in decades (4).

The endemic form of KS was first described in sub-Saharan Africa and was the cause of 3 to 9% of all cancers in Uganda in 1971 (190). A decade later in Uganda, Bayley described a sudden increase in a particularly aggressive KS that is now known to be AIDS-associated KS (15). Patients with endemic KS have a life expectancy of months to years (4). Endemic and epidemic KS now accounts for half of all tumors in men in some areas of Africa (198). African children are also afflicted by an aggressive and often fatal KS (72, 93), and endemic and epidemic KS is responsible for up to half of all sarcomas in this group (10).

KS is also associated with organ transplantation or other conditions requiring immunosuppression, involving perhaps 1% of transplants (84). The disease is often found in persons at risk for endemic KS, and survival is measured in months to years (151, 170).

In June 1981, the reported increased incidence of *Pneumocystis jirovecii* and KS in men who have sex with men (MSM) heralded the AIDS epidemic and also the AIDS-associated or epidemic KS (33). KS was 20,000 times more common in AIDS patients than in the general population, and it occurred in 21% of AIDS patients who were MSM but in only 1% of hemophiliac patients (20). The demographics of this variant of the disease suggested a sexually transmitted agent as the cause and eventually led to the identification of HHV-8. In the San Francisco Men's Health Study, men who were seropositive for both HIV and HHV-8 had a 50% probability of developing KS within 10 years (113). In the Multicenter AIDS Cohort study, a KS diagnosis in 21 patients was preceded by HHV-8 seroconversion by a median of 33 months (59). The disease is particularly aggressive in AIDS patients, and survival was measured in weeks to months (4). Contrary to classic KS, epidemic KS often involves the face, including the nose; genitalia; palate; and gingiva (93) and is particularly aggressive and resistant to treatment (54). The HIV Tat protein as well as its immunosuppressive effects is thought to contribute to the poor outcomes in AIDS-associated KS (67, 204).

In cases of immune suppression, KS often resolves with the restoration of the immune system, either with the use of HAART for epidemic KS (114,

167) or with a reduction of immunosuppression in transplant-associated KS (72, 93, 95). Nevertheless, KS can develop after initiation of HAART (105) and is thought to be due to the immune reconstitution inflammatory response (26).

PEL

First described with AIDS patients in 1989 (99), PEL is a rare B-cell lymphoma of the pericardial, pleural, or peritoneal cavities that accounts for only 3% of AIDS-related lymphomas and 0.4% of non-AIDS-associated large-cell non-Hodgkin's lymphomas (30, 93). The B lymphocytes responsible for PEL are often coinfected with the Epstein-Barr virus (EBV) and HHV-8 (34). EBV is known to cause B-cell lymphomas, such as Burkitt's lymphoma, but activation of the c-myc oncogenes so necessary in Burkitt's (108) does not appear to have occurred in the body cavity lymphomas. Coinfecting viruses may complement each other in transforming the cell, as evidenced by the ability of HHV-6 to activate the replicative cycle of EBV (55). Although the exact interaction between EBV and HHV-8 is unknown, HHV-8's vIL-6 is thought to improve survival in infected B cells (4, 13). Death usually occurs within months of the diagnosis. A fatal case of PEL was reported in a cardiac transplant patient who also had developed KS. He died approximately 6 months after the PEL diagnosis (84).

Multicentric Castleman's Disease

Castleman's disease is a rare B-cell lymphoproliferative disorder occurring in localized (31) and multicentric (57) forms. HHV-8 is associated with nearly all AIDS-associated multicentric Castleman's, but only about half of non-HIV-associated disease (61, 178). Patients with multicentric Castleman's often have fever, hepatosplenomegaly, and generalized lymphadenopathy. IL-6, which induces B-cell differentiation, is present at high levels in the affected lymph nodes (139). The disease is often fatal, many times due to infection or the development of lymphoma or KS. Interestingly, Castleman's disease has been reported in one patient from Cape Verde who was coinfected with HIV-2 and HHV-8 (177).

Primary Pulmonary Hypertension

Severe pulmonary hypertension is characterized by markedly elevated pulmonary artery pressures and possible right heart failure and death (42). The etiologies of primary pulmonary hypertension are currently uncertain, and cases are designated as either familial or sporadic (44, 48), and it is also associated with HIV-1 infection. Histologically, the lungs contain plexiform lesions—complex lesions that can occlude vascular structures—as well as vascular smooth muscle proliferation. Endothelial cells in these areas appear to proliferate monoclonally and are in close association with T- and B-cell infiltrates (194, 195). Similarities between the plexiform and KS lesions led Cool et al. to seek out and find HHV-8 DNA and latency-associated nuclear antigen 1 in these lesions in primary but not secondary pulmonary hypertension in a small number of patients (44). Nevertheless, multiple subsequent studies have not found this association (19, 28, 45, 58, 73, 90), and the preponderance of evidence argues against a role for HHV-8 in primary pulmonary hypertension (89).

CONCLUSION

As evidenced by the descriptions above, these five viruses lead to chronic infection, resulting in modulation of the immune system and many chronic sequelae. At this point in time, medications are available to suppress some of these viruses; however, without the ability to eradicate them, these chronic changes will continue to lead to sequelae that we must be able to recognize and treat appropriately.

REFERENCES

1. **Agarwal, A., A. Soni, M. Ciechanowsky, P. Chander, and G. Treser.** 1989. Hyponatremia in patients with the acquired immunodeficiency syndrome. *Nephron* **53:**317–321.
2. **Ambroziak, J. A., D. J. Blackbourn, B. G. Herndier, R. G. Glogau, J. H. Gullett, A. R. McDonald, E. T. Lennette, and J. A. Levy.** 1995. Herpes-like sequences in HIV-infected and uninfected Kaposi's sarcoma patients. *Science* **268:**582–583.
3. **Anderson, D. W., R. Virmani, J. M. Reilly, T. O'Leary, R. E. Cunnion, M. Robinowitz, A. M. Macher, U. Punja, S. T. Villaflor, and J. E. Parrillo.** 1988. Prevalent myocarditis at necropsy in the acquired immunodeficiency syndrome. *J. Am. Coll. Cardiol.* **11:**792–799.
4. **Antman, K., and Y. Chang.** 2000. Kaposi's sarcoma. *N. Engl. J. Med.* **342:**1027–1038.
5. **Aoki, Y., and G. Tosato.** 2004. HIV-1 Tat enhances Kaposi sarcoma-associated herpesvirus (KSHV) infectivity. *Blood* **104:**810–814.
6. **Aoki, Y., and G. Tosato.** 2007. Interactions between HIV-1 Tat and KSHV. *Curr. Top. Microbiol. Immunol.* **312:**309–326.
7. **Ariyoshi, K., Schim van der Loeff, M., P. Cook, D. Whitby, T. Corrah, S. Jaffar, F. Cham, S. Sabally, D. O'Donovan, R. A. Weiss, T. F. Schulz, and H. Whittle.** 1998. Kaposi's sarcoma in the Gambia, West Africa is less frequent in human immunodeficiency virus type 2 than in human immunodeficiency virus type 1 infection despite a high prevalence of human herpesvirus 8. *J. Hum. Virol.* **1:**193–199.

8. **Arranz Caso, J. A., C. Sanchez Mingo, and J. Garcia Tena.** 1999. Effect of highly active antiretroviral therapy on thrombocytopenia in patients with HIV infection. *N. Engl. J. Med.* **341:**1239–1240.
9. **Arthos, J., C. Cicala, E. Martinelli, K. Macleod, D. Van Ryk, D. Wei, Z. Xiao, T. D. Veenstra, T. P. Conrad, R. A. Lempicki, S. McLaughlin, M. Pascuccio, R. Gopaul, J. McNally, C. C. Cruz, N. Censoplano, E. Chung, K. N. Reitano, S. Kottilil, D. J. Goode, and A. S. Fauci.** 2008. HIV-1 envelope protein binds to and signals through integrin alpha4beta7, the gut mucosal homing receptor for peripheral T cells. *Nat. Immunol.* **9:**301–309.
10. **Athale, U. H., P. S. Patil, C. Chintu, and B. Elem.** 1995. Influence of HIV epidemic on the incidence of Kaposi's sarcoma in Zambian children. *J. Acquir. Immune Defic. Syndr. Hum. Retrovirol.* **8:**96–100.
11. **Bais, C., B. Santomasso, O. Coso, L. Arvanitakis, E. G. Raaka, J. S. Gutkind, A. S. Asch, E. Cesarman, M. C. Gershengorn, and E. A. Mesri.** 1998. G-protein-coupled receptor of Kaposi's sarcoma-associated herpesvirus is a viral oncogene and angiogenesis activator. *Nature* **391:**86–89.
12. **Barbaro, G., G. Di Lorenzo, B. Grisorio, G. Barbarini, et al.** 1998. Incidence of dilated cardiomyopathy and detection of HIV in myocardial cells of HIV-positive patients. *N. Engl. J. Med.* **339:**1093–1099.
13. **Barozzi, P., L. Potenza, G. Riva, D. Vallerini, C. Quadrelli, R. Bosco, F. Forghieri, G. Torelli, and M. Luppi.** 2007. B cells and herpesviruses: a model of lymphoproliferation. *Autoimmun. Rev.* **7:**132–136.
14. **Barron, M. A., N. Blyveis, B. E. Palmer, S. MaWhinney, and C. C. Wilson.** 2003. Influence of plasma viremia on defects in number and immunophenotype of blood dendritic cell subsets in human immunodeficiency virus 1-infected individuals. *J. Infect. Dis.* **187:**26–37.
15. **Bayley, A. C.** 1984. Aggressive Kaposi's sarcoma in Zambia, 1983. *Lancet* **i:**1318–1320.
16. **Becker, S., G. Fusco, J. Fusco, R. Balu, S. Gangjee, C. Brennan, J. Feinberg, and Collaborations in HIV Outcomes Research/US Cohort.** 2004. HIV-associated thrombotic microangiopathy in the era of highly active antiretroviral therapy: an observational study. *Clin. Infect. Dis.* **39:**S267–S275.
17. **Beilke, M. A., V. TrainaDorge, J. D. England, and J. L. Blanchard.** 1996. Polymyositis, arthritis, and uveitis in a macaque experimentally infected with human T lymphotropic virus type I. *Arthritis Rheum.* **39:**610–615.
18. **Beltran, S., F. X. Lescure, R. Desailloud, Y. Douadi, A. Smail, I. El Esper, S. Arlot, J. L. Schmit, and Thyroid and VIH Group.** 2003. Increased prevalence of hypothyroidism among human immunodeficiency virus-infected patients: a need for screening. *Clin. Infect. Dis.* **37:**579–583.
19. **Bendayan, D., R. Sarid, A. Cohen, D. Shitrit, I. Shechtman, and M. R. Kramer.** Absence of human herpesvirus 8 DNA sequences in lung biopsies from Israeli patients with pulmonary arterial hypertension. *Respiration* **75:**155–157.
20. **Beral, V., T. A. Peterman, R. L. Berkelman, and H. W. Jaffe.** 1990. Kaposi's sarcoma among persons with AIDS: a sexually transmitted infection? *Lancet* **335:**123–128.
21. **Berhane, K., R. Karim, M. H. Cohen, L. Masri-Lavine, M. Young, K. Anastos, M. Augenbraun, D. H. Watts, and A. M. Levine.** 2004. Impact of highly active antiretroviral therapy on anemia and relationship between anemia and survival in a large cohort of HIV-infected women: women's interagency HIV study. *J. Acquir. Immune Defic. Syndr.* **37:**1245–1252.
22. **Biggar, R. J., B. K. Johnson, C. Oster, P. S. Sarin, D. Ocheng, P. Tukei, H. Nsanze, S. Alexander, A. J. Bodner, and T. A. Siongok.** 1985. Regional variation in prevalence of antibody against human T-lymphotropic virus types I and III in Kenya, East Africa. *Int. J. Cancer* **35:**763–767.
23. **Blanchard, D. G., C. Hagenhoff, L. C. Chow, H. A. McCann, and H. C. Dittrich.** 1991. Reversibility of cardiac abnormalities in human immunodeficiency virus (HIV)-infected individuals: a serial echocardiographic study. *J. Am. Coll. Cardiol.* **17:**1270–1276.
24. **Blattner, W., and M. Charurat.** 2005. Human T-cell lymphotropic virus types I and II, p. 2098–2118. *In* G. L. Mandell, J. E. Bennett, and R. Dolin (ed.), *Principles and Practices of Infectious Diseases,* 6th ed. Elsevier, Philadelphia, PA.
25. **Bock, P. J., and D. M. Markovitz.** 2001. Infection with HIV-2. *AIDS* **15:**S35–S45.
26. **Bower, M., M. Nelson, A. M. Young, C. Thirlwell, T. Newsom-Davis, S. Mandalia, T. Dhillon, P. Holmes, B. G. Gazzard, and J. Stebbing.** 2005. Immune reconstitution inflammatory syndrome associated with Kaposi's sarcoma. *J. Clin. Oncol.* **23:**5224–5228.
27. **Brenchley, J. M., T. W. Schacker, L. E. Ruff, D. A. Price, J. H. Taylor, G. J. Beilman, P. L. Nguyen, A. Khoruts, M. Larson, A. T. Haase, and D. C. Douek.** 2004. CD4+ T cell depletion during all stages of HIV disease occurs predominantly in the gastrointestinal tract. *J. Exp. Med.* **200:**749–759.
28. **Bresser, P., M. I. Cornelissen, W. van der Bij, C. J. van Noesel, and W. Timens.** 2007. Idiopathic pulmonary arterial hypertension in Dutch Caucasian patients is not associated with human herpes virus-8 infection. *Respir. Med.* **101:** 854–856.
29. **Busti, A. J., R. G. Hall, and D. M. Margolis.** 2004. Atazanavir for the treatment of human immunodeficiency virus infection. *Pharmacotherapy* **24:**1732–1747.
30. **Carbone, A., A. Gloghini, E. Vaccher, V. Zagonel, C. Pastore, P. Dalla Palma, F. Branz, G. Saglio, R. Volpe, U. Tirelli, and G. Gaidano.** 1996. Kaposi's sarcoma-associated herpesvirus DNA sequences in AIDS-related and AIDS-unrelated lymphomatous effusions. *Br. J. Haematol.* **94:**533–543.
31. **Castleman, B., L. Iverson, and V. Menendez Pardo.** 1956. Localized mediastinal lymph-node hyperplasia resembling thymoma. *Cancer* **9:**822–830.
32. **Cazanave, C., M. Dupon, V. Lavignolle-Aurillac, N. Barthe, S. Lawson-Ayayi, N. Mehsen, P. Mercie, P. Morlat, R. Thiebaut, F. Dabis, and Groupe d'Epidemiologie Clinique du SIDA en, Aquitaine.** 2008. Reduced bone mineral density in HIV-infected patients: prevalence and associated factors. *AIDS* **22:**395–402.
33. **Centers for Disease Control (CDC).** 1981. Kaposi's sarcoma and pneumocystis pneumonia among homosexual men--New York City and California. *MMWR Morb. Mortal. Wkly. Rep.* **30:**305–308.
34. **Cesarman, E., Y. Chang, P. S. Moore, J. W. Said, and D. M. Knowles.** 1995. Kaposi's sarcoma-associated herpesvirus-like DNA sequences in AIDS-related body-cavity-based lymphomas. *N. Engl. J. Med.* **332:**1186–1191.
35. **Cesarman, E., R. G. Nador, F. Bai, R. A. Bohenzky, J. J. Russo, P. S. Moore, Y. Chang, and D. M. Knowles.** 1996. Kaposi's sarcoma-associated herpesvirus contains G protein-coupled receptor and cyclin D homologs which are expressed in Kaposi's sarcoma and malignant lymphoma. *J. Virol.* **70:**8218–8223.
36. **Chang, Y., E. Cesarman, M. S. Pessin, F. Lee, J. Culpepper, D. M. Knowles, and P. S. Moore.** 1994. Identification of herpesvirus-like DNA sequences in AIDS-associated Kaposi's sarcoma. *Science* **266:**1865–1869.
37. **Chang, Y., J. Ziegler, H. Wabinga, E. Katangole-Mbidde, C. Boshoff, T. Schulz, D. Whitby, D. Maddalena, H. W.**

Jaffe, R. A. Weiss, P. S. Moore, et al. 1996. Kaposi's sarcoma-associated herpesvirus and Kaposi's sarcoma in Africa. *Arch. Intern. Med.* **156:**202–204.

38. **Chen, X. M., J. S. Keithly, C. V. Paya, and N. F. LaRusso.** 2002. Cryptosporidiosis. *N. Engl. J. Med.* **346:**1723–1731.
39. **Chen, X. M., and N. F. LaRusso.** 2002. Cryptosporidiosis and the pathogenesis of AIDS-cholangiopathy. *Semin. Liver Dis.* **22:**277–289.
40. **Chernak, E., G. Dubin, D. Henry, S. J. Naides, R. L. Hodinka, R. R. MacGregor, and H. M. Friedman.** 1995. Infection due to parvovirus B19 in patients infected with human immunodeficiency virus. *Clin. Infect. Dis.* **20:**170–173.
41. **Childs, E. A., R. H. Lyles, O. A. Selnes, B. Chen, E. N. Miller, B. A. Cohen, J. T. Becker, J. Mellors, and J. C. McArthur.** 1999. Plasma viral load and CD4 lymphocytes predict HIV-associated dementia and sensory neuropathy. *Neurology* **52:**607–613.
42. **Chin, K. M., and L. J. Rubin.** 2008. Pulmonary arterial hypertension. *J. Am. Coll. Cardiol.* **51:**1527–1538.
43. **Chung, R. T., J. Andersen, P. Volberding, G. K. Robbins, T. Liu, K. E. Sherman, M. G. Peters, M. J. Koziel, A. K. Bhan, B. Alston, D. Colquhoun, T. Nevin, G. Harb, C. van der Horst, and AIDS Clinical Trials Group A5071 Study Team.** 2004. Peginterferon Alfa-2a plus ribavirin versus interferon alfa-2a plus ribavirin for chronic hepatitis C in HIV-coinfected persons. *N. Engl. J. Med.* **351:**451–459.
44. **Cool, C. D., P. R. Rai, M. E. Yeager, D. Hernandez-Saavedra, A. E. Serls, T. M. Bull, M. W. Geraci, K. K. Brown, J. M. Routes, R. M. Tuder, and N. F. Voelkel.** 2003. Expression of human herpesvirus 8 in primary pulmonary hypertension. *N. Engl. J. Med.* **349:**1113–1122.
45. **Daibata, M., I. Miyoshi, H. Taguchi, H. Matsubara, H. Date, N. Shimizu, and Y. Ohtsuki.** 2004. Absence of human herpesvirus 8 in lung tissues from Japanese patients with primary pulmonary hypertension. *Respir. Med.* **98:**1231–1232.
46. **Dalakas, M. C., I. Illa, G. H. Pezeshkpour, J. P. Laukaitis, B. Cohen, and J. L. Griffin.** 1990. Mitochondrial myopathy caused by long-term zidovudine therapy. *N. Engl. J. Med.* **322:**1098–1105.
47. **de The, G., M. Kazanji, and G. de The.** 1996. An HTLV-I/II vaccine: from animal models to clinical trials? *J. Acquir. Immune Defic. Syndr. Hum. Retrovirol.* **13**(Suppl. 1):S191–S198.
48. **Deng, Z., J. H. Morse, S. L. Slager, N. Cuervo, K. J. Moore, G. Venetos, S. Kalachikov, E. Cayanis, S. G. Fischer, R. J. Barst, S. E. Hodge, and J. A. Knowles.** 2000. Familial primary pulmonary hypertension (gene PPH1) is caused by mutations in the bone morphogenetic protein receptor-II gene. *Am. J. Hum. Genet.* **67:**737–744.
49. **DiGiovanna, J. J., and B. Safai.** 1981. Kaposi's sarcoma. Retrospective study of 90 cases with particular emphasis on the familial occurrence, ethnic background and prevalence of other diseases. *Am. J. Med.* **71:**779–783.
50. **Dobs, A. S., M. A. Dempsey, P. W. Ladenson, and B. F. Polk.** 1988. Endocrine disorders in men infected with human immunodeficiency virus. *Am. J. Med.* **84:**611–616.
51. **Dougherty, R. H., R. L. Skolasky, Jr., and J. C. McArthur.** 2002. Progression of HIV-associated dementia treated with HAART. *AIDS Read.* **12:**69–74.
52. **Eguchi, K., N. Matsuoka, H. Ida, M. Nakashima, M. Sakai, S. Sakito, A. Kawakami, K. Terada, H. Shimada, and Y. Kawabe.** 1992. Primary Sjogren's syndrome with antibodies to HTLV-I: clinical and laboratory features. *Ann. Rheum. Dis.* **51:**769–776.
53. **Eledrisi, M. S., and A. C. Verghese.** 2001. Adrenal insufficiency in HIV infection: a review and recommendations. *Am. J. Med. Sci.* **321:**137–144.
54. **Fiorelli, V., G. Barillari, E. Toschi, C. Sgadari, P. Monini, M. Sturzl, and B. Ensoli.** 1999. IFN-gamma induces endothelial cells to proliferate and to invade the extracellular matrix in response to the HIV-1 Tat protein: implications for AIDS-Kaposi's sarcoma pathogenesis. *J. Immunol.* **162:**1165–1170.
55. **Flamand, L., I. Stefanescu, D. V. Ablashi, and J. Menezes.** 1993. Activation of the Epstein-Barr virus replicative cycle by human herpesvirus 6. *J. Virol.* **67:**6768–6777.
56. **Friis-Moller, N., C. A. Sabin, R. Weber, A. d'Arminio Monforte, W. M. El-Sadr, P. Reiss, R. Thiebaut, L. Morfeldt, S. De Wit, C. Pradier, G. Calvo, M. G. Law, O. Kirk, A. N. Phillips, J. D. Lundgren, and Data Collection on Adverse Events of Anti-HIV Drugs (DAD) Study Group.** 2003. Combination antiretroviral therapy and the risk of myocardial infarction. *N. Engl. J. Med.* **349:**1993–2003.
57. **Gaba, A. R., R. S. Stein, D. L. Sweet, and D. Variakojis.** 1978. Multicentric giant lymph node hyperplasia. *Am. J. Clin. Pathol.* **69:**86–90.
58. **Galambos, C., J. Montgomery, and F. J. Jenkins.** 2006. No role for kaposi sarcoma-associated herpesvirus in pediatric idiopathic pulmonary hypertension. *Pediatr. Pulmonol.* **41:**122–125.
59. **Gao, S. J., L. Kingsley, D. R. Hoover, T. J. Spira, C. R. Rinaldo, A. Saah, J. Phair, R. Detels, P. Parry, Y. Chang, and P. S. Moore.** 1996. Seroconversion to antibodies against Kaposi's sarcoma-associated herpesvirus-related latent nuclear antigens before the development of Kaposi's sarcoma. *N. Engl. J. Med.* **335:**233–241.
60. **Garavelli, P. L., and P. Berti.** 1993. Efficacy of recombinant granulocyte colony-stimulating factor in the long-term treatment of AIDS-related neutropenia. *AIDS* **7:**589–590.
61. **Gessain, A., A. Sudaka, J. Briere, N. Fouchard, M. A. Nicola, B. Rio, M. Arborio, X. Troussard, J. Audouin, J. Diebold, and G. de The.** 1996. Kaposi sarcoma-associated herpes-like virus (human herpesvirus type 8) DNA sequences in multicentric Castleman's disease: is there any relevant association in non-human immunodeficiency virus-infected patients? *Blood* **87:**414–416.
62. **Gessain, A., J. C. Vernant, L. Maurs, F. Barin, O. Gout, A. Calender, and G. De Thé.** 1985. Antibodies to human T-lymphotropic virus type-I in patients with tropical spastic paraparesis. *Lancet* **326:**407–410.
63. **Gessain, A., and O. Gout.** 1992. Chronic myelopathy associated with human T-lymphotropic virus type I (HTLV-1). *Ann. Intern. Med.* **117:**933–946.
64. **Gonzalez-Scarano, F., and J. Martin-Garcia.** 2005. The neuropathogenesis of AIDS. *Nature Rev. Immunol.* **5:**69–81.
65. **Goulder, P. J., and B. D. Walker.** 1999. The great escape - AIDS viruses and immune control. *Nat. Med.* **5:**1233–1235.
66. **Green, D. F., L. Resnick, and J. J. Bourgoignie.** 1992. HIV infects glomerular endothelial and mesangial but not epithelial cells in vitro. *Kidney Int.* **41:**956–960.
67. **Guo, H. G., S. Pati, M. Sadowska, M. Charurat, and M. Reitz.** 2004. Tumorigenesis by human herpesvirus 8 vGPCR is accelerated by human immunodeficiency virus type 1 Tat. *J. Virol.* **78:**9336–9342.
68. **Guo, H. G., M. Sadowska, W. Reid, E. Tschachler, G. Hayward, and M. Reitz.** 2003. Kaposi's sarcoma-like tumors in a human herpesvirus 8 ORF74 transgenic mouse. *J. Virol.* **77:**2631–2639.
69. **Gupta, S. K., J. A. Eustace, J. A. Winston, I. I. Boydstun, T. S. Ahuja, R. A. Rodriguez, K. T. Tashima, M. Roland, N. Franceschini, F. J. Palella, J. L. Lennox, P. E. Klotman,**

S. A. Nachman, S. D. Hall, and L. A. Szczech. 2005. Guidelines for the management of chronic kidney disease in HIV-infected patients: recommendations of the HIV Medicine Association of the Infectious Diseases Society of America. *Clin. Infect. Dis.* **40:**1559–1585.

70. **Hanchard, B.** 1996. Adult T-cell leukemia/lymphoma in Jamaica: 1986-1995. J. Acquir. *Immune Defic. Syndr. Hum. Retrovirol.* **13:**S20–S25.

71. **Heidenreich, P. A., M. J. Eisenberg, L. L. Kee, C. A. Somelofski, H. Hollander, N. B. Schiller, and M. D. Cheitlin.** 1995. Pericardial effusion in AIDS. Incidence and survival. *Circulation* **92:**3229–3234.

72. **Hengge, U. R., T. Ruzicka, S. K. Tyring, M. Stuschke, M. Roggendorf, R. A. Schwartz, and S. Seeber.** 2002. Update on Kaposi's sarcoma and other HHV8 associated diseases. Part 1: epidemiology, environmental predispositions, clinical manifestations, and therapy. *Lancet Infect. Dis.* **2:**281–292.

73. **Henke-Gendo, C., M. Mengel, M. M. Hoeper, K. Alkharsah, and T. F. Schulz.** 2005. Absence of Kaposi's sarcoma-associated herpesvirus in patients with pulmonary arterial hypertension. *Am. J. Respir. Crit. Care Med.* **172:**1581–1585.

74. **Henry, D. H., P. A. Volberding, and G. Leitz.** 2004. Epoetin alfa for treatment of anemia in HIV-infected patients: past, present, and future. *J. Acquir. Immune Defic. Syndr.* **37:**1221–1227.

75. **Hjelle, B., N. Torrez-Martinez, R. Mills, O. Appenzeller, R. Jahnke, S. Alexander, G. Ross, and B. Hjelle.** 1992. Chronic neurodegenerative disease associated with HTLV-II infection. *Lancet* **339:**645–646.

76. **Hofman, P., M. D. Drici, P. Gibelin, J. F. Michiels, and A. Thyss.** 1993. Prevalence of toxoplasma myocarditis in patients with the acquired immunodeficiency syndrome. *Br. Heart J.* **70:**376–381.

77. **Huang, L.** 2008. Respiratory disease, p. 1225–1252. *In* R. Dolin, H. Masur, and M. Saag (ed.), *AIDS Therapy*, 3rd ed. Elsevier Inc., Philadelphia, PA.

78. **Huang, Y. Q., J. J. Li, M. H. Kaplan, B. Poiesz, E. Katabira, W. C. Zhang, D. Feiner, and A. E. Friedman-Kien.** 1995. Human herpesvirus-like nucleic acid in various forms of Kaposi's sarcoma. *Lancet* **345:**759–761.

79. **Ijichi, S., M. Nakagawa, F. Umehara, I. Higuchi, K. Arimura, S. Izumo, and M. Osame.** 1996. HAM/TSP: recent perspectives in Japan. *J. Acquir. Immune Defic. Syndr. Human Retrovirol.* **13:**S26–S32.

80. **Imamura, A., T. Kitagawa, Y. Ohi, and M. Osame.** 1991. Clinical manifestation of human T-cell lymphotropic virus type-I-associated myelopathy and vesicopathy. *Urol. Int.* **46:**149–153.

81. **Irving, W., P. White, and G. Cambridge.** 1989. Antibodies to HTLV-I in sera from patients with connective tissue diseases. *Ann. Rheum. Dis.* **48:**80.

82. **Johnson, R. P.** 2008. How HIV guts the immune system. *N. Engl. J. Med.* **358:**2287–2289.

83. **Johnson, R. W., F. M. Williams, S. Kazi, M. M. Dimachkie, and J. D. Reveille.** 2003. Human immunodeficiency virus-associated polymyositis: a longitudinal study of outcome. *Arthritis Rheum.* **49:**172–178.

84. **Jones, D., M. E. Ballestas, K. M. Kaye, J. M. Gulizia, G. L. Winters, J. Fletcher, D. T. Scadden, and J. C. Aster.** 1998. Primary-effusion lymphoma and Kaposi's sarcoma in a cardiac-transplant recipient. *N. Engl. J. Med.* **339:**444–449.

85. **Jubault, V., A. Penfornis, F. Schillo, B. Hoen, M. Izembart, J. Timsit, M. D. Kazatchkine, J. Gilquin, and J. P. Viard.** 2000. Sequential occurrence of thyroid autoantibodies and Graves' disease after immune restoration in severely immunocompromised human immunodeficiency virus-1-infected patients. *J. Clin. Endocrinol. Metab.* **85:**4254–4257.

86. **Kahn, J. O., and B. D. Walker.** 1998. Acute human immunodeficiency virus type 1 infection. *N. Engl. J. Med.* **339:** 33–39.

87. **Kalyanaraman, V. S., M. G. Sarngadharan, M. Robert-Guroff, I. Miyoshi, D. Golde, and R. C. Gallo.** 1982. A new subtype of human T-cell leukemia virus (HTLV-II) associated with a T-cell variant of hairy cell leukemia. *Science* **218:**571–573.

88. **Kamin, D. S., and S. K. Grinspoon.** 2005. Cardiovascular disease in HIV-positive patients. *AIDS* **19:**641–652.

89. **Katano, H., and C. M. Hogaboam.** 2005. Herpesvirus-associated pulmonary hypertension? *Am. J. Respir. Crit. Care Med.* **172:**1485–1486.

90. **Katano, H., K. Ito, K. Shibuya, T. Saji, Y. Sato, and T. Sata.** 2005. Lack of human herpesvirus 8 infection in lungs of Japanese patients with primary pulmonary hypertension. *J. Infect. Dis.* **191:**743–745.

91. **Kaul, M., and S. A. Lipton.** 1999. Chemokines and activated macrophages in HIV gp120-induced neuronal apoptosis. *Proc. Natl. Acad. Sci. USA* **96:**8212–8216.

92. **Kawai, H., T. Mitsui, K. Yokoi, M. Akaike, K. Hirose, K. Hizawa, and S. Saito.** 1996. Evidence of HTLV-I in thyroid tissue in an HTLV-I carrier with Hashimoto's thyroiditis. *J. Mol. Med.* **74:**275–278.

93. **Kaye, K. M.** 2005. Kaposi's sarcoma-associated herpesvirus (human herpesvirus type 8), p. 1827–1832. *In* G. L. Mandell, J. E. Bennett, and R. Dolin (ed.), *Principles and Practices of Infectious Diseases*, 6th ed. Elsevier, Philadelphia, PA.

94. **Keaveny, A. P., and M. S. Karasik.** 1998. Hepatobiliary and pancreatic infections in AIDS: Part II. *AIDS Patient Care STDS* **12:**451–456.

95. **Kedda, M. A., L. Margolius, M. C. Kew, C. Swanepoel, and D. Pearson.** 1996. Kaposi's sarcoma-associated herpesvirus in Kaposi's sarcoma occurring in immunosuppressed renal transplant recipients. *Clin. Transplant.* **10:**429–431.

96. **Keswani, S. C., C. A. Pardo, C. L. Cherry, A. Hoke, and J. C. McArthur.** 2002. HIV-associated sensory neuropathies. *AIDS* **16:**2105–2117.

97. **Kitajima, I., K. Yamamoto, K. Sato, Y. Nakajima, T. Nakajima, I. Maruyama, M. Osame, and K. Nishioka.** 1991. Detection of human T cell lymphotropic virus type I proviral DNA and its gene expression in synovial cells in chronic inflammatory arthropathy. *J. Clin. Investig.* **88:** 1315–1322.

98. **Klotman, M.** 1998. Potential role for G-protein coupled receptors in HIV-associated nephropathy. *Kidney Int.* **54:** 2243–2244.

99. **Knowles, D. M., G. Inghirami, A. Ubriaco, and R. Dalla-Favera.** 1989. Molecular genetic analysis of three AIDS-associated neoplasms of uncertain lineage demonstrates their B-cell derivation and the possible pathogenetic role of the Epstein-Barr virus. *Blood* **73:**792–799.

100. **Kotler, D. P.** 2005. HIV infection and the gastrointestinal tract. *AIDS* **19:**107–117.

101. **Koutkia, P., B. Canavan, J. Breu, and S. Grinspoon.** 2005. Growth hormone (GH) responses to GH-releasing hormone-arginine testing in human immunodeficiency virus lipodystrophy. *J. Clin. Endocrinol. Metab.* **90:**32–38.

101a. **Kuller, L., and SMART Study Group**. 2008. Abstr. 15th Conf. Retrovir. Opportunistic Infect., abstr. 139.

102. **LaGrenade, L.** 1996. HTLV-I-associated infective dermatitis: past, present, and future. *J. Acquir. Immune Defic. Syndr. Human Retrovirol.* **13:**S46–S49.

103. **LaGrenade, L., B. Hanchard, V. Fletcher, B. Cranston, and W. Blattner.** 1990. Infective dermatitis of Jamaican children: a marker for HTLV-I infection. *Lancet* **336:**1345–1347.

104. **Lascar, R. M., R. J. Gilson, A. R. Lopes, A. Bertoletti, and M. K. Maini.** 2003. Reconstitution of hepatitis B virus (HBV)-specific T cell responses with treatment of human immunodeficiency virus/HBV coinfection. *J. Infect. Dis.* **188:**1815–1819.
105. **Ledergerber, B., M. Egger, V. Erard, R. Weber, B. Hirschel, H. Furrer, M. Battegay, P. Vernazza, E. Bernasconi, M. Opravil, D. Kaufmann, P. Sudre, P. Francioli, and A. Telenti.** 1999. AIDS-related opportunistic illnesses occurring after initiation of potent antiretroviral therapy: the Swiss HIV Cohort Study. *JAMA* **282:**2220–2226.
106. **Letendre, S. L., J. A. McCutchan, M. E. Childers, S. P. Woods, D. Lazzaretto, R. K. Heaton, I. Grant, R. J. Ellis, and HNRC group.** 2004. Enhancing antiretroviral therapy for human immunodeficiency virus cognitive disorders. *Ann. Neurol.* **56:**416–423.
107. **Lewis, W., and M. C. Dalakas.** 1995. Mitochondrial toxicity of antiviral drugs. *Nat. Med.* **1:**417–422.
108. **Lombardi, L., E. W. Newcomb, and R. Dalla-Favera.** 1987. Pathogenesis of Burkitt lymphoma: expression of an activated c-myc oncogene causes the tumorigenic conversion of EBV-infected human B lymphoblasts. *Cell* **49:**161–170.
109. **Lutzner, M., R. Edelson, P. Schein, I. Green, C. Kirkpatrick, and A. Ahmed.** 1975. Cutaneous T-cell lymphomas: the Sezary syndrome, mycosis fungoides, and related disorders. *Ann. Intern. Med.* **83:**534–552.
110. **Madeddu, G., A. Spanu, F. Chessa, G. M. Calia, C. Lovigu, P. Solinas, M. Mannazzu, A. Falchi, M. S. Mura, and G. Madeddu.** 2006. Thyroid function in human immunodeficiency virus patients treated with highly active antiretroviral therapy (HAART): a longitudinal study. *Clin. Endocrinol.* (Oxford) **64:**375–383.
111. **Marecki, J. C., C. D. Cool, J. E. Parr, V. E. Beckey, P. A. Luciw, A. F. Tarantal, A. Carville, R. P. Shannon, A. Cota-Gomez, R. M. Tuder, N. F. Voelkel, and S. C. Flores.** 2006. HIV-1 Nef is associated with complex pulmonary vascular lesions in SHIV-nef-infected macaques. *Am. J. Respir. Crit. Care Med.* **174:**437–445.
112. **Mariette, X., F. Agbalika, M. T. Daniel, M. Bisson, P. Lagrange, J. C. Brouet, and F. Morinet.** 1993. Detection of human T lymphotropic virus type I tax gene in salivary gland epithelium from two patients with Sjogren's syndrome. *Arthritis Rheum.* **36:**1423–1428.
113. **Martin, J. N., D. E. Ganem, D. H. Osmond, K. A. Page-Shafer, D. Macrae, and D. H. Kedes.** 1998. Sexual transmission and the natural history of human herpesvirus 8 infection. *N. Engl. J. Med.* **338:**948–954.
114. **Martinez, V., E. Caumes, L. Gambotti, H. Ittah, J. P. Morini, J. Deleuze, I. Gorin, C. Katlama, F. Bricaire, and N. Dupin.** 2006. Remission from Kaposi's sarcoma on HAART is associated with suppression of HIV replication and is independent of protease inhibitor therapy. *Br. J. Cancer* **94:**1000–1006.
115. **McGovern, B. H.** 2007. Hepatitis C in the HIV-infected patient. *J. Acquir. Immune Defic. Syndr.* **45:**S47–S56.
116. **Merino, F., M. Robert-Guroff, J. Clark, M. Biondo-Bracho, W. A. Blattner, and R. C. Gallo.** 1984. Natural antibodies to human T-cell leukemia/lymphoma virus in healthy Venezuelan populations. *Int. J. Cancer* **34:**501–506.
117. **Meynard, J. L., M. Guiguet, S. Arsac, J. Frottier, and M. C. Meyohas.** 1997. Frequency and risk factors of infectious complications in neutropenic patients infected with HIV. *AIDS* **11:**995–998.
118. **Mochizuki, M., K. Tajima, T. Watanabe, and K. Yamaguchi.** 1994. Human T lymphotropic virus type 1 uveitis. *Br. J. Ophthalmol.* **78:**149–154.
119. **Mochizuki, M., A. Ono, E. Ikeda, N. Hikita, T. Watanabe, K. Yamaguchi, K. Sagawa, and K. Ito.** 1996. HTLV-I uveitis. *J. Acquir. Immune Defic. Syndr. Hum. Retrovirol.* **13:**S50–S56.
120. **Moore, P. S., C. Boshoff, R. A. Weiss, and Y. Chang.** 1996. Molecular mimicry of human cytokine and cytokine response pathway genes by KSHV. *Science* **274:**1739–1744.
121. **Moore, P. S., and Y. Chang.** 1995. Detection of herpesvirus-like DNA sequences in Kaposi's sarcoma in patients with and without HIV infection. *N. Engl. J. Med.* **332:**1181–1185.
122. **Morgan, O. S., C. Mora, P. Rodgers-Johnson, and G. Char.** 1989. HTLV-1 and polymyositis in Jamaica. *Lancet* **334:**1184–1187.
123. **Mueller, N., A. Okayama, S. Stuver, and N. Tachibana.** 1996. Findings from the Miyazaki Cohort Study. *J. Acquir. Immune Defic. Syndr. Hum. Retrovirol.* **13:**S2–S7.
124. **Murphy, E. L., B. Hanchard, J. P. Figueroa, W. N. Gibbs, W. S. Lofters, M. Campbell, J. J. Goedert, and W. A. Blattner.** 1989. Modelling the risk of adult T-cell leukemia/lymphoma in persons infected with human T-lymphotropic virus type I. *Int. J. Cancer* **43:**250–253.
125. **Murphy, E. L.** 1996. The clinical epidemiology of human T-lymphotropic virus type II (HTLV-II). *J. Acquir. Immune Defic. Syndr. Human Retrovirol.* **13:**S215–S219.
126. **Nakada, K., M. Kohakura, H. Komoda, and Y. Hinuma.** 1984. High incidence of HTLV antibody in carriers of *Strongyloides stercoralis*. *Lancet* **323:**633–633.
127. **Nakagawa, M., S. Izumo, S. Ijichi, H. Kubota, K. Arimura, M. Kawabata, and M. Osame.** 1995. HTLV-I-associated myelopathy: analysis of 213 patients based on clinical features and laboratory findings. *J. Neurovirol.* **1:**50–61.
128. **Nakao, K., M. Matsumoto, and N. Ohba.** 1991. Seroprevalence of antibodies to HTLV-I in patients with ocular disorders. *Br. J. Ophthalmol.* **75:**76–78.
129. **Nera, F. A., E. L. Murphy, A. Gam, B. Hanchard, J. P. Figueroa, and W. A. Blattner.** 1989. Antibodies to *Strongyloides stercoralis* in healthy Jamaican carriers of HTLV-1. *N. Engl. J. Med.* **320:**252–253.
130. **Nishioka, K.** 1996. HTLV-I arthropathy and Sjogren syndrome. *J. Acquir. Immune Defic. Syndr. Hum. Retrovirol.* **13:**S57–S62.
131. **Nishioka, K., I. Maruyama, K. Sato, I. Kitajima, Y. Nakajima, and M. Osame.** 1989. Chronic inflammatory arthropathy associated with HTLV-I. *Lancet* **333:**441–441.
132. **Nomoto, M., Y. Utatsu, Y. Soejima, and M. Osame.** 1991. Neopterin in cerebrospinal fluid: a useful marker for diagnosis of HTLV-I-associated myelopathy/tropical spastic paraparesis. *Neurology* **41:**457.
133. **Novitzky, N., J. Thomson, L. Abrahams, C. du Toit, and A. McDonald.** 2005. Thrombotic thrombocytopenic purpura in patients with retroviral infection is highly responsive to plasma infusion therapy. *Br. J. Haematol.* **128:**373–379.
134. **Ohba, N., M. Matsumoto, M. Sameshima, Y. Kabayama, K. Nakao, K. Unoki, F. Uehara, K. Kawano, I. Maruyama, and M. Osame.** 1989. Ocular manifestations in patients infected with human T-lymphotropic virus type I. *Jpn. J. Ophthalmol.* **33:**1–12.
135. **Ohshima, K.** 2007. Pathological features of diseases associated with human T-cell leukemia virus type I. *Cancer Sci.* **98:**772–778.
136. **Osame, M., K. Usuku, S. Izumo, N. Ijichi, H. Amitani, A. Igata, M. Matsumoto, and M. Tara.** 1986. HTLV-I associated myelopathy, a new clinical entity. *Lancet* **327:**1031–1032.
137. **Pan, G., Z. Yang, S. W. Ballinger, and J. M. McDonald.** 2006. Pathogenesis of osteopenia/osteoporosis induced by

highly active anti-retroviral therapy for AIDS. *Ann. N. Y. Acad. Sci.* **1068:**297–308.

137a. **Papasavvas, E., M. Pistilli, A. Hancock, G. Reynolds, A. Mackiewicz, C. Gallo, J. Kostman, K. Mounzer, J. Shull, and L. Montaner.** 2008. Abstr. 15th Conf. Retrovir. Opportunistic Infect., abstr. 299.

138. **Pardo, C. A., J. C. McArthur, and J. W. Griffin.** 2001. HIV neuropathy: insights in the pathology of HIV peripheral nerve disease. *J. Peripher. Nerv. Syst.* **6:**21–27.

139. **Parravicini, C., M. Corbellino, M. Paulli, U. Magrini, M. Lazzarino, P. S. Moore, and Y. Chang.** 1997. Expression of a virus-derived cytokine, KSHV vIL-6, in HIV-seronegative Castleman's disease. *Am. J. Pathol.* **151:**1517–1522.

140. **Patel, P., D. L. Hanson, P. S. Sullivan, R. M. Novak, A. C. Moorman, T. C. Tong, S. D. Holmberg, J. T. Brooks, and Adult and Adolescent Spectrum of Disease Project and HIV Outpatient Study,Investigators.** 2008. Incidence of types of cancer among HIV-infected persons compared with the general population in the United States, 1992–2003. *Ann. Intern. Med.* **148:**728–736.

141. **Pinheiro, S. R., A. B. Carneiro-Proietti, M. V. Lima-Martins, F. A. Proietti, A. A. Pereira, and F. Orefice.** 1996. HTLV-I/II seroprevalence in 55 Brazilian patients with idiopathic uveitis. *Rev. Soc. Bras. Med. Trop.* **29:**383–384.

142. **Pinheiro, S. R., M. A. Lana-Peixoto, A. B. Proietti, F. Orefice, M. V. Lima-Martins, and F. A. Proietti.** 1995. HTLV-I associated uveitis, myelopathy, rheumatoid arthritis and Sjogren's syndrome. *Arq. Neuropsiquiatr.* **53:**777–781.

143. **Piroth, L., D. Sene, S. Pol, I. Goderel, K. Lacombe, B. Martha, D. Rey, V. Loustau-Ratti, J. F. Bergmann, G. Pialoux, A. Gervais, C. Lascoux-Combe, F. Carrat, and P. Cacoub.** 2007. Epidemiology, diagnosis and treatment of chronic hepatitis B in HIV-infected patients (EPIB 2005 study). *AIDS* **21:**1323–1331.

144. **Poiesz, B. J., F. W. Ruscetti, A. F. Gazdar, P. A. Bunn, J. D. Minna, and R. C. Gallo.** 1980. Detection and isolation of type C retrovirus particles from fresh and cultured lymphocytes of a patient with cutaneous T-cell lymphoma. *Proc. Natl. Acad. Sci. USA* **77:**7415–7419.

145. **Poiesz, B. J., F. W. Ruscetti, M. S. Reitz, V. S. Kalyanaraman, and R. C. Gallo.** 1981. Isolation of a new type C retrovirus (HTLV) in primary uncultured cells of a patient with Sezary T-cell leukaemia. *Nature* **294:**268–271.

146. **Polson, A. G., D. Wang, J. DeRisi, and D. Ganem.** 2002. Modulation of host gene expression by the constitutively active G protein-coupled receptor of Kaposi's sarcoma-associated herpesvirus. *Cancer Res.* **62:**4525–4530.

147. **Pope, M.** 1999. Mucosal dendritic cells and immunodeficiency viruses. *J. Infect. Dis.* **179:**S427–S430.

148. **Poretsky, L., S. Can, and B. Zumoff.** 1995. Testicular dysfunction in human immunodeficiency virus-infected men. *Metabolism* **44:**946–953.

149. **Proietti, F. A., A. B. Carneiro-Proietti, B. C. Catalan-Soares, and E. L. Murphy.** 2005. Global epidemiology of HTLV-I infection and associated diseases. *Oncogene* **24:**6058–6068.

150. **Puoti, M., C. Torti, R. Bruno, G. Filice, and G. Carosi.** 2006. Natural history of chronic hepatitis B in co-infected patients. *J. Hepatol.* **44:**S65–70.

151. **Qunibi, W., M. Akhtar, K. Sheth, H. E. Ginn, O. Al-Furayh, E. B. DeVol, and S. Taher.** 1988. Kaposi's sarcoma: the most common tumor after renal transplantation in Saudi Arabia. *Am. J. Med.* **84:**225–232.

152. **Rietschel, P., C. Corcoran, T. Stanley, N. Basgoz, A. Klibanski, and S. Grinspoon.** 2000. Prevalence of hypogonadism among men with weight loss related to human immunodeficiency virus infection who were receiving highly active antiretroviral therapy. *Clin. Infect. Dis.* **31:**1240–1244.

153. **Rodgers-Johnson, P., D. Carleton Gajdusek, O. Morgan, V. Zaninovic, P. Sarin, and D. Graham.** 1985. HTLV-I and HTLV-III antibodies and tropical spastic paraparesis. *Lancet* **326:**1247–1248.

154. **Roling, J., H. Schmid, M. Fischereder, R. Draenert, and F. D. Goebel. 2006.** HIV-associated renal diseases and highly active antiretroviral therapy-induced nephropathy. *Clin. Infect. Dis.* **42:**1488–1495.

155. **Román, G., and M. Osame.** 1988. Identity of HTLV-I-associated tropical spastic paraparesis and HTLV-I-associated myelopathy. *Lancet* **331:**651–651.

156. **Ross, M. J., and P. E. Klotman.** 2004. HIV-associated nephropathy. *AIDS* **18:**1089–1099.

157. **Ross, T. M., S. M. Pettiford, and P. L. Green.** 1996. The *tax* gene of human T-cell leukemia virus type 2 is essential for transformation of human T lymphocytes. *J. Virol.* **70:**5194–5202.

158. **Roucoux, D. F., and E. L. Murphy.** 2004. The epidemiology and disease outcomes of human T-lymphotropic virus type II. *AIDS Rev.* **6:**144–154.

159. **Rychert, J., S. Saindon, S. Placek, D. Daskalakis, and E. Rosenberg.** 2007. Sequence variation occurs in CD4 epitopes during early HIV infection. *J. Acquir. Immune Defic. Syndr.* **46:**261–267.

160. **Saavedra-Lauzon, A., and R. A. Johnson.** 2008. Dermatologic disease, p. 1121–1156. *In* R. Dolin, H. Masur, and M. Saag (ed.), *AIDS Therapy*, 3rd ed. Elsevier, Inc., Philadelphia, PA.

161. **Sabin, C. A., S. W. Worm, R. Weber, P. Reiss, W. El-Sadr, F. Dabis, S. De Wit, M. Law, A. D'Arminio Monforte, N. Friis-Moller, O. Kirk, C. Pradier, I. Weller, A. N. Phillips, and J. D. Lundgren.** 2008. Use of nucleoside reverse transcriptase inhibitors and risk of myocardial infarction in HIV-infected patients enrolled in the DAD study: a multicohort collaboration. *Lancet* **371:**1417–1426.

162. **Sacktor, N.** 2002. The epidemiology of human immunodeficiency virus-associated neurological disease in the era of highly active antiretroviral therapy. *J. Neurovirol.* **8:**115–121.

163. **Sagawa, K., M. Mochizuki, K. Masuoka, K. Katagiri, T. Katayama, T. Maeda, A. Tanimoto, S. Sugita, T. Watanabe, and K. Itoh.** 1995. Immunopathological mechanisms of human T cell lymphotropic virus type 1 (HTLV-I) uveitis. Detection of HTLV-I-infected T cells in the eye and their constitutive cytokine production. *J. Clin. Investig.* **95:**852–858.

164. **Sakai, M., K. Eguchi, K. Terada, M. Nakashima, I. Yamashita, H. Ida, Y. Kawabe, T. Aoyagi, H. Takino, and T. Nakamura.** 1993. Infection of human synovial cells by human T cell lymphotropic virus type I. Proliferation and granulocyte/macrophage colony-stimulating factor production by synovial cells. *J. Clin. Investig.* **92:**1957–1966.

165. **Samaras, K.** 2008. Metabolic consequences and therapeutic options in highly active antiretroviral therapy in human immunodeficiency virus-1 infection. *J. Antimicrob. Chemother.* **61:**238–245.

166. **Sato, Y., and Y. Shiroma.** 1989. Concurrent infections with Strongyloides and T-cell leukemia virus and their possible effect on immune responses of host. *Clin. Immunol. Immunopathol.* **52:**214–224.

167. **Scadden, D. T.** 2003. AIDS-related malignancies. *Annu. Rev. Med.* **54:**285–303.

168. **Shannon, R. P., M. A. Simon, M. A. Mathier, Y. J. Geng, S. Mankad, and A. A. Lackner.** 2000. Dilated cardiomyopathy

associated with simian AIDS in nonhuman primates. *Circulation* **101:**185–193.

169. **Shepard, L. W., M. Yang, P. Xie, D. D. Browning, T. Voyno-Yasenetskaya, T. Kozasa, and R. D. Ye.** 2001. Constitutive activation of NF-kappa B and secretion of interleukin-8 induced by the G protein-coupled receptor of Kaposi's sarcoma-associated herpesvirus involve G alpha(13) and RhoA. *J. Biol. Chem.* **276:**45979–45987.
170. **Shepherd, F. A., E. Maher, C. Cardella, E. Cole, P. Greig, J. A. Wade, and G. Levy.** 1997. Treatment of Kaposi's sarcoma after solid organ transplantation. *J. Clin. Oncol.* **15:**2371–2377.
171. **Sheremata, W. A., W. J. Harrington, P. A. Bradshaw, S. K. H. Foung, S. P. Raffanti, J. R. Berger, S. Snodgrass, L. Resnick, and B. J. Poiesz.** 1993. Association of '(tropical) ataxic neuropathy' with HTLV-II. *Virus Res.* **29:**71–77.
172. **Shimoyama, M.** 1991. Diagnostic criteria and classification of clinical subtypes of adult T-cell leukaemia-lymphoma. A report from the lymphoma study group (1984–87). *Br. J. Haematol.* **79:**428–437.
173. **Simpson, D. M., J. C. McArthur, R. Olney, D. Clifford, Y. So, D. Ross, B. J. Baird, P. Barrett, A. E. Hammer, and Lamotrigine HIV Neuropathy Study Team.** 2003. Lamotrigine for HIV-associated painful sensory neuropathies: a placebo-controlled trial. *Neurology* **60:**1508–1514.
174. **Sitbon, O., C. Lascoux-Combe, J. F. Delfraissy, P. G. Yeni, F. Raffi, D. De Zuttere, V. Gressin, P. Clerson, D. Sereni, and G. Simonneau.** 2008. Prevalence of HIV-related pulmonary arterial hypertension in the current antiretroviral therapy era. *Am. J. Respir. Crit. Care Med.* **177:**108–113.
175. **Slamon, D. J., K. Shimotohno, M. J. Cline, D. W. Golde, and I. S. Y. Chen.** 1984. Identification of the putative transforming protein of the human T-cell leukemia viruses HTLV-I and HTLV-II. *Science* **226:**61–65.
176. **Sloand, E. M., H. G. Klein, S. M. Banks, B. Vareldzis, S. Merritt, and P. Pierce.** 1992. Epidemiology of thrombocytopenia in HIV infection. *Eur. J. Haematol.* **48:**168–172.
177. **Sophie, B., M. Anne-Genevieve, F. Nathalie, R. Stephanie, D. Florence, T. Micheline, and D. Nicolas.** 2007. The first reported case and management of multicentric Castleman's disease associated with Kaposi's sarcoma in an HIV-2-infected patient. *AIDS* **21:**1492–1494.
178. **Soulier, J., L. Grollet, E. Oksenhendler, P. Cacoub, D. Cazals-Hatem, P. Babinet, M. F. d'Agay, J. P. Clauvel, M. Raphael, and L. Degos.** 1995. Kaposi's sarcoma-associated herpesvirus-like DNA sequences in multicentric Castleman's disease. *Blood* **86:**1276–1280.
179. **Strategies for Management of Antiretroviral Therapy (SMART) Study Group, W. M. El-Sadr, J. D. Lundgren, J. D. Neaton, F. Gordin, D. Abrams, R. C. Arduino, A. Babiker, W. Burman, N. Clumeck, C. J. Cohen, D. Cohn, D. Cooper, J. Darbyshire, S. Emery, G. Fatkenheuer, B. Gazzard, B. Grund, J. Hoy, K. Klingman, M. Losso, N. Markowitz, J. Neuhaus, A. Phillips, and C. Rappoport.** 2006. CD4+ count-guided interruption of antiretroviral treatment. *N. Engl. J. Med.* **355:**2283–2296.
180. **Strickler, H. D., C. Rattray, C. Escoffery, A. Manns, M. H. Schiffman, C. Brown, B. Cranston, B. Hanchard, J. M. Palefsky, and W. A. Blattner.** 1995. Human T-cell lymphotropic virus type I and severe neoplasia of the cervix in Jamaica. *Int. J. Cancer* **61:**23–26.
181. **Sugimoto, M., H. Nakashima, S. Watanabe, E. Uyama, F. Tanaka, M. Ando, S. Araki, and S. Kawasaki.** 1987. T-lymphocyte alveolitis in HTLV-I-associated myelopathy. *Lancet* **ii:**1220.
182. **Sulkowski, M. S., S. H. Mehta, R. E. Chaisson, D. L. Thomas, and R. D. Moore.** 2004. Hepatotoxicity associated with protease inhibitor-based antiretroviral regimens with or without concurrent ritonavir. *AIDS* **18:**2277–2284.
183. **Sulkowski, M. S., D. L. Thomas, S. H. Mehta, R. E. Chaisson, and R. D. Moore.** 2002. Hepatotoxicity associated with nevirapine or efavirenz-containing antiretroviral therapy: role of hepatitis C and B infections. *Hepatology* **35:**182–189.
184. **Sullivan, P. S., D. L. Hanson, S. Y. Chu, J. L. Jones, and J. W. Ward.** 1998. Epidemiology of anemia in human immunodeficiency virus (HIV)-infected persons: results from the multistate adult and adolescent spectrum of HIV disease surveillance project. *Blood* **91:**301–308.
185. **Sumida, T., F. Yonaha, T. Maeda, Y. Kita, I. Iwamoto, T. Koike, and S. Yoshida.** 1994. Expression of sequences homologous to HTLV-I tax gene in the labial salivary glands of Japanese patients with Sjogren's syndrome. *Arthritis Rheum.* **37:**545–550.
186. **Szczech, L. A., S. K. Gupta, R. Habash, A. Guasch, R. Kalayjian, R. Appel, T. A. Fields, L. P. Svetkey, K. H. Flanagan, P. E. Klotman, and J. A. Winston.** 2004. The clinical epidemiology and course of the spectrum of renal diseases associated with HIV infection. *Kidney Int.* **66:**1145–1152.
187. **Tajima, K., and T. Kuroishi.** 1985. Estimation of rate of incidence of ATL among ATLV (HTLV-I) carriers in Kyushu, Japan. *Jpn. J. Clin. Oncol.* **15:**423–430.
188. **Takahashi, T., H. Takase, T. Urano, S. Sugita, K. Miyata, N. Miyata, and M. Mochizuki.** 2000. Clinical features of human T-lymphotropic virus type 1 uveitis: a long-term follow-up. *Ocul. Immunol. Inflamm.* **8:**235–241.
189. **Tan, R., X. Xu, G. S. Ogg, P. Hansasuta, T. Dong, T. Rostron, G. Luzzi, C. P. Conlon, G. R. Screaton, A. J. McMichael, and S. Rowland-Jones.** 1999. Rapid death of adoptively transferred T cells in acquired immunodeficiency syndrome. *Blood* **93:**1506–1510.
190. **Taylor, J. F., A. C. Templeton, C. L. Vogel, J. L. Ziegler, and S. K. Kyalwazi.** 1971. Kaposi's sarcoma in Uganda: a clinico-pathological study. *Int. J. Cancer* **8:**122–135.
191. **Toggas, S. M., E. Masliah, and L. Mucke.** 1996. Prevention of HIV-1 gp120-induced neuronal damage in the central nervous system of transgenic mice by the NMDA receptor antagonist memantine. *Brain Res.* **706:**303–307.
192. **Torriani, F. J., M. Rodriguez-Torres, J. K. Rockstroh, E. Lissen, J. Gonzalez-Garcia, A. Lazzarin, G. Carosi, J. Sasadeusz, C. Katlama, J. Montaner, H. Sette, Jr., S. Passe, J. De Pamphilis, F. Duff, U. M. Schrenk, D. T. Dieterich, and G. APRICOT Study.** 2004. Peginterferon alfa-2a plus ribavirin for chronic hepatitis C virus infection in HIV-infected patients. *N. Engl. J. Med.* **351:**438–450.
193. **Toy, P. T., M. E. Reid, and M. Burns.** 1985. Positive direct antiglobulin test associated with hyperglobulinemia in acquired immunodeficiency syndrome (AIDS). *Am. J. Hematol.* **19:**145–150.
194. **Tuder, R. M., B. Groves, D. B. Badesch, and N. F. Voelkel.** 1994. Exuberant endothelial cell growth and elements of inflammation are present in plexiform lesions of pulmonary hypertension. *Am. J. Pathol.* **144:**275–285.
195. **Tuder, R. M., and N. F. Voelkel.** 1998. Pulmonary hypertension and inflammation. *J. Lab. Clin. Med.* **132:**16–24.
196. **Uchiyama, T., J. Yodoi, K. Sagawa, K. Takatsuki, and H. Uchino.** 1977. Adult T-cell leukemia: clinical and hematologic features of 16 cases. *Blood* **50:**481–492.
197. **Van Huyen, J. P., A. Landau, C. Piketty, M. F. Belair, D. Batisse, G. Gonzalez-Canali, L. Weiss, R. Jian, M. D.**

Kazatchkine, and P. Bruneval. 2003. Toxic effects of nucleoside reverse transcriptase inhibitors on the liver. Value of electron microscopy analysis for the diagnosis of mitochondrial cytopathy. *Am. J. Clin. Pathol.* **119:**546–555.

198. **Wabinga, H. R., D. M. Parkin, F. Wabwire-Mangen, and J. W. Mugerwa.** 1993. Cancer in Kampala, Uganda, in 1989–91: changes in incidence in the era of AIDS. *Int. J. Cancer* **54:**26–36.

199. **Weber, R., C. A. Sabin, N. Friis-Moller, P. Reiss, W. M. El-Sadr, O. Kirk, F. Dabis, M. G. Law, C. Pradier, S. De Wit, B. Akerlund, G. Calvo, A. Monforte, M. Rickenbach, B. Ledergerber, A. N. Phillips, and J. D. Lundgren.** 2006. Liver-related deaths in persons infected with the human immunodeficiency virus: the D:A:D study. *Arch. Intern. Med.* **166:**1632–1641.

200. **Weiss, R.** 1981. A virus associated with human adult T-cell leukaemia. *Nature* **294:**212.

201. **World Health Organization.** 1989. Virus diseases: human T-lymphotropic virus type I, HTLV-I. *WHO Wkly. Epidemiol. Rec.* **49:**382–383.

202. **Yamaguchi, K., and T. Watanabe.** 2002. Human T lymphotropic virus type-I and adult T-cell leukemia in Japan. *Int. J. Hematol.* **76:**240–245.

203. **Yamaguchi, K., M. Mochizuki, T. Watanabe, K. Yoshimura, M. Shirao, S. Araki, N. Miyata, S. Mori, T. Kiyokawa, and K. Takatsuki.** 1994. Human T lymphotropic virus type 1 uveitis after Graves' disease. *Br. J. Ophthalmol.* **78:**163–166.

204. **Zeng, Y., X. Zhang, Z. Huang, L. Cheng, S. Yao, D. Qin, X. Chen, Q. Tang, Z. Lv, L. Zhang, and C. Lu.** 2007. Intracellular Tat of human immunodeficiency virus type 1 activates lytic cycle replication of Kaposi's sarcoma-associated herpesvirus: role of JAK/STAT signaling. *J. Virol.* **81:**2401–2417.

205. **Zon, L. I., C. Arkin, and J. E. Groopman.** 1987. Haematologic manifestations of the human immune deficiency virus (HIV). *Br. J. Haematol.* **66:**251–256.

206. **Zuber, J. P., A. Calmy, J. M. Evison, B. Hasse, V. Schiffer, T. Wagels, R. Nuesch, L. Magenta, B. Ledergerber, R. Jenni, R. Speich, M. Opravil, and the Swiss HIV Cohort Study Group.** 2004. Pulmonary arterial hypertension related to HIV infection: improved hemodynamics and survival associated with antiretroviral therapy. *Clin. Infect. Dis.* **38:**1178–1185.

207. **Zucker, S. D., X. Qin, S. D. Rouster, F. Yu, R. M. Green, P. Keshavan, J. Feinberg, and K. E. Sherman.** 2001. Mechanism of indinavir-induced hyperbilirubinemia. *Proc. Natl. Acad. Sci. USA* **98:**12671–12676.

Sequelae and Long-Term Consequences of Infectious Diseases
Edited by Pina M. Fratamico, James L. Smith, and Kim A. Brogden

Chapter 22

Complications of Superficial Mycoses

ADAM REICH, ROBERT A. SCHWARTZ, AND JACEK C. SZEPIETOWSKI

Superficial fungal infections are common infections limited to the skin, mucous membranes, hair, and nails. They are caused by three different groups of pathogens: dermatophytes, yeasts, and molds. Dermatophytes are filamentous fungi with high affinity to keratin belonging to three genera: *Trichophyton* (e.g., *T. rubrum, T. mentagrophytes, T. tonsurans*), *Microsporum* (*M. canis* and *M. audouini*), and *Epidermophyton* (*E. floccosum*). Fungal skin infections caused by dermatophytes are frequently named "tinea" or "ringworm." These pathogens have a worldwide distribution and produce different skin lesions and, depending on the particular pathogen and the localization of the disease, are defined as tinea capitis, tinea faciei, tinea barbae, tinea corporis, tinea manuum, tinea cruris, tinea pedis, and onychomycosis. Some dermatophytes are found mainly in humans (antropophilic dermatophytes), while others are noted in humans only occasionally, after contact with infected animals (so called zoophilic dermatophytes) or soil (geophilic dermatophytes).

Yeasts are common commensals of the human body but are also responsible for many pathologic conditions. *Malassezia* species or *Candida* species are the major yeast pathogens, although other genera like *Trichosporon*, *Hendersonula*, and *Phaeoannellomyces* also cause skin infections, especially in immunocompromised patients (9, 31). The *Malassezia* yeasts are normal human saprophytes that sometimes switch from a yeast to a pathogenic mycelial form and cause pityriasis (tinea) versicolor and *Malassezia* folliculitis (82). They are also associated with several other skin diseases, such as seborrheic dermatitis and some forms of confluent and reticulate papillomatosis (Gougerot-Carteaud syndrome) (27). New speciation of *Malassezia* genus has subdivided this lipophilic yeast into new categories, with *M. globosa* and *M. sympodialis* now more closely linked to tinea versicolor than *M. furfur* (82). *Candida* species can cause oral thrush, atrophic glossitis, intertrigo, granuloma gluteale infantum, or chronic mucocutaneous candidiasis. The incidence of superficial candidal infections has increased substantially over the years due to an increasing population of patients who are chronically immunosuppressed (31).

Molds are saprophytic microorganisms and do not usually cause disease in immunocompetent hosts. As pathogens, they are more likely to be found as secondary invaders in previously damaged tissue (e.g., dystrophic nails). However, sometimes, especially in immunocompromised individuals, molds could also be responsible for severe, life-threatening diseases (31). Regarding the skin, the following molds can be found in skin or adnexal lesions: *Aspergillus* species, *Fusarium* species, *Penicillium* species, *Scopulariopsis brevicaulis, Scytalidium* species, and many others (9).

Superficial fungal skin infections, although usually limited to the skin or mucous membranes, may be responsible for significant complications, some of which can be life threatening. Therefore, every patient with dermatomycosis should be treated with antifungals. Many topical and systemic formulations are currently available for therapy of fungal skin infections, and nowadays it is possible to control the disease effectively.

COMPLICATIONS OF SUPERFICIAL DERMATOMYCOSES

Cellulitis

Tinea pedis, usually interdigital type, and toenail onychomycosis are significant risk factors for bacterial cellulitis of the lower legs (76, 91). The odds ratio for patients having tinea pedis to develop cellulitis was estimated to be between 1.7 to 3.9 (8, 76). Importantly, in the study by Björnsdóttir et al.

Adam Reich and Jacek C. Szepietowski • Department of Dermatology, Venereology, and Allergology, Wroclaw Medical University, 50-368 Wroclaw, Poland. **Robert A. Schwartz** • Department of Dermatology, New Jersey Medical School, Newark, NJ 07103.

(8), tinea pedis interdigitalis was found to be significantly associated with cellulitis only when the presence of bacteria in the toe web was excluded from the analysis. Other independent risk factors of lower-limb cellulitis included previous history of bacterial cellulitis, the presence of *Staphylococcus aureus* and/or β-hemolytic streptococci in the toe webs, diabetes mellitus, chronic venous insufficiency, the presence of leg erosions or ulcers, leg edema, and prior saphenectomy (6, 8, 50, 76).

A wet occlusive environment in the infected area leads to cutaneous maceration and fissuring (2, 42). This weakens the natural barriers of the skin and may serve as an entry point for pathogenic bacteria, mainly β-hemolytic streptococci, *S. aureus, Streptococcus pneumoniae,* and gram-negative bacilli, all of which have been shown to cause cellulitis (2, 15). It is important to underscore that toe-web intertrigo, irrespective of the causative agent, is a strong risk factor for erysipelas and cellulitis of the leg (21). It was also demonstrated that thorough examination of the patient's feet and interdigital spaces will often reveal active tinea pedis (2). Treatment of this condition could significantly reduce the number of cellulitis episodes. Sometimes, identification of fungal pathogens could be difficult, as some gram-negative bacteria may inhibit fungal growth and make it harder to detect fungal hyphae by direct microscopic examination. However, aggressive treatment of the underlying tinea as well as the gram-negative bacterial infection can lead to amelioration of cellulitis in these patients (2, 3).

Recently, it was reported that dermatophytoses could be complicated by preseptal cellulitis (51, 92). Preseptal cellulitis is a common infection of the eyelid and periorbital soft tissues, characterized by acute eyelid erythema and edema. Velazquez et al. (92) documented a 10-year-old boy having a 15-day history of worsening right-sided preseptal cellulitis. The patient presented with pruritic vesicular lesions on the eyelids, with photophobia and pain in the eyelid region. Empiric therapy with oral antibacterial and antiviral medications failed to resolve the disease. Lid cultures revealed saprophytic bacteria and *Trichophyton* species. Subsequently, the infection was successfully cured with two courses of oral itraconazole (92) A similar case was also described by Kulkarni and Aggarwal (51).

Alopecia

Tinea capitis may be complicated by patchy alopecia. Usually a transient hair loss is noted, which improves after the successful antimycotic treatment. However, in some patients a persistent, scarring alopecia could be observed. Persistent hair loss is found mainly in patient having favus, characterized by the presence of yellowish, cup-shaped crusts called "scutula" on the scalp and glabrous skin. This chronic tinea is due to *T. schoenleinii* or *T. mentagrophytes* var. *quinckeanum* infection (7, 22, 34, 47, 61). The mechanism of alopecia in favus is unknown; however, it was suggested that scutulae may exert a local pressure provoking blood vessel occlusion and impaired microcirculation, which leads to scarring and persistent hair loss. Fortunately, improvements in living conditions and hygiene in developing countries in the 20th century led to the almost complete disappearance of dermatophytes responsible for favus. This infection, apart from regions where it is endemic in Africa and other tropical regions, is diagnosed only occasionally (47).

Another reason for scarring alopecia could be a severe inflammatory fungal infection called a kerion, an entity sometimes misdiagnosed as a bacterial abscess. Severe scarring and permanent hair loss may occur even if appropriate therapy has been introduced (11, 31, 37, 75).

id Reactions (Autoeczematization) to Fungal Allergens

A fungal id reaction is defined as a distant skin eruption in patients with established fungal infection, most probably due to an allergic response to the fungal antigens (9). To document an id reaction, the pathogen of superficial fungal infection has to be isolated by culture and the patient must have a positive delayed skin test to fungal antigens (45). In most patients, zoophilic fungi were found (45). Distant id lesions are free from fungal pathogens and most commonly associated with tinea pedis. Typically, when tinea pedis is flaring, the patient will simultaneously develop a dyshidrotic reaction with pruritic vesicles and/or blisters on both hands and feet (9, 10). This form of mycotic id reaction has to be differentiated from pyoderma, pompholyx, and contact eczema. A generalized id-type skin eruption was also described in a patient with tinea pedis (40).

Other Cutaneous Reactions to Fungal Allergens

Noneczematous forms of cutaneous reactions include erythema nodosum (see below), psoriasiform lesions (35), annular erythema (85), erythema multiforme (36, 72, 77), or erysipelas-like dermatophytid (64). In some patients with follicular invasion, a residual, sterile granuloma (Majocchi's granuloma) may develop which resolves with time (2). Sometimes an id reaction may be evident at the moment when systemic antifungal therapy is initiated and should not be interpreted as an adverse drug reaction (30, 75). Rarely, id reactions may be the only sign of an asymptomatic tinea pedis infection (2).

Occasionally, these reactions manifest as erythema nodosum, mainly in patients with a kerion. This was noted in patients having kerion due to *E. floccosum* (71), *T. rubrum* (30), or different zoophilic dermatophytes (e.g., *T. mentagrophytes, Trichophyton verrucosum, T. gypseum,* and *T. sulfureum*) infection (11, 16, 18, 55, 75). Erythema nodosum was also documented in patients with tinea pedis and onychomycosis (39). The causative role of fungal allergens was confirmed by the observation that subcutaneous injection of *Trichophyton* antigens in these patients resulted in the development of lesions imitating erythema nodosum (39).

The rarest fungal id reaction is lichen trichophyticus, evident as disseminated, small pale red grouped or diffuse follicular papules on the trunk. This eruption is symmetrical, usually pronounced on the trunk, but in severe cases extending down to the lower limbs, and sometimes involving the face (64). It should be differentiated from lichen planus, lichen syphiliticus, and lichen scrofulosorum (9).

Allergic Diseases

Fungal antigens in patients with superficial fungal infections may be responsible for aggravation of preexisting allergic diseases. *Candida* species and *Malassezia* species are the most important pathogens in the induction of fungal allergy and may be responsible for allergic rhinitis, allergic sinusitis, atopic asthma, urticaria, or allergic eczema (49, 58, 67, 78, 79, 84). The importance of hypersensitivity to fungal allergens was underscored in patients suffering from atopic dermatitis, in whom fungal allergens could provoke severe exacerbations (28, 54, 56, 62, 78–81). In Nordvall and Johansson's study (63), *M. furfur*-specific immunoglobulin E (IgE) antibodies were detected in about 20% of children suffering from atopic dermatitis. A significantly higher percentage of patients with *M. furfur* antibodies had eczema at the time of examination than those without detectable IgE antibodies to *M. furfur* ($p < 0.0001$) (63). In addition, bronchial asthma and IgE-mediated food allergy were both significantly more prevalent among children with IgE against *M. furfur* than among those without ($P < 0.05$) (63). In another study (78), all atopic dermatitis patients with severe eczema and a majority (77%) of those having moderate eczema had positive *Candida albicans* skin-prick tests in comparison to 39% with mild and 33% with no eczema. Antifungal therapy in atopic dermatitis patients with proven hypersensitivity to *C. albicans* and *M. furfur* resulted in significant reduction of the total serum level of IgE, as well as the level of specific IgE fractions to these allergens (5). In addition, improvement of eczema cruris was found with patients with onychomycosis having positive prick tests with some fungal allergens after an oral antifungal therapy (74). Besides *C. albicans* and *M. furfur*, other fungi responsible for dermatomycoses, including dermatophytes, could also play an important role in induction of allergic diseases (49, 54, 59, 60, 97). For instance, *T. rubrum* has been implicated as a potential trigger of atopic dermatitis flares (49). In another report (97), it was observed that an atopic dermatitis patient with onychomycosis had recalcitrant hand and foot eczema. This patient showed immediate hypersensitivity to *Trichophyton*, as well as elevated IgE antibody directed against *Trichophyton*. Remarkably, allergic skin lesions resolved after systemic antifungal therapy for onychomycosis (97). Based on this case presentation, the authors concluded that atopic dermatitis may be exacerbated by chronic dermatophyte infection due to *Trichophyton* hypersensitivity. Interestingly, the contact hypersensitivity to trichophytin (a filtrate from *Trichophyton* culture) was dependent on the localization and type of tinea (90). The highest proportion of positive patch tests was found in vesiculobullous tinea pedis (83%), and the lowest one in tinea corporis (37%) and hyperkeratotic tinea pedis (36%) (90). It was also suggested that positive trichophytin tests for some patients with atopic dermatitis may be due to a cross-reactivity to mold allergens (44, 73).

Fungal allergens should also be considered as important inducers of asthma and allergic rhinitis. Skin reactivity to fungal allergens such as *Alternaria* species has been reported to be especially common in patients with life-threatening asthma (66). Mold sensitization was shown to be associated with severe asthma attacks requiring hospital admission (65). Akiyama et al. (1) described two patients having atopic asthma due to *C. albicans* allergens. Both patients had high levels of serum IgE antibodies against the fungal acid protease and showed positive conjunctival and immediate bronchial responses when challenged with the protease. Significant histamine release was detected in both patients when their peripheral leukocytes were challenged with the protease antigen (1). Many asthmatic patients demonstrated bronchospasm following inhalation challenge with different fungal antigens (1, 38, 93). Gumowski et al. (38) observed an immediate response following inhalation challenge in 50% of asthma patients and 68% of patients having allergic rhinitis. Of note, after 2 years of hyposensitization treatment against fungal allergy, almost 60% of studied subjects demonstrated a good to excellent response (38). Some patients with asthma could also be hypersensitive to *Trichophyton* antigens (93). Moreover, a higher percentage of patients with hypersensitivity to *Trichophyton* was found among patients suffering from intrinsic asthma (63%) in comparison to patients with atopic asthma (47%) (59). Kivity et al. (48) reported coexistence of perennial rhinitis and fungal skin or toenail infection. All these patients demonstrated type I hypersensitivity to *Trichophyton,* and oral fungicidal therapy resulted in significant improvement of both their skin and nasal symptoms (48).

Superficial fungal infections were also described to induce allergic diseases de novo (24, 74). Elewski and Schwartz (24) described a patient who developed bronchial asthma subsequent to an infection of tinea pedis and toenail onychomycosis. Interestingly, antifungal management resulted in full resolution of his tinea pedis, onychomycosis, and asthma, supporting the idea, that fungal allergens were causative agents of asthma in this subject (24).

Some data indicated that fungi could be related occasionally to chronic or acute urticaria (23, 26, 32, 41, 57, 83, 95). Mostly *Candida* species were reported (23, 32, 83), but *E. floccosum* (57), *T. rubrum* (26, 41, 95), and *T. tonsurans* (17) were also described to induce urticarial lesions. However, it is still not fully clear whether these two processes are actually related to each other, occur simultaneously, or are influenced by medications taken by the patients (57).

The mechanism of fungal allergy is still not fully known. Many possible allergens have been identified (64). Most fungi may induce delayed hypersensitivity or immediate hypersensitivity responses. Savolainen et al. (79) demonstrated that *Candida* induced a strong TH1-associated response, activating the releasing of interleukin (IL)-2, specific IgG, and gamma interferon. Opposite observations were made after exposure to *Malassezia* allergens, which were responsible for a stronger TH2-like response (42, 43, 46, 79). Stimulation with *T. rubrum* antigens led to release of IL-4 from peripheral blood mononuclear cells in atopic dermatitis patients (45). It was also observed that *C. albicans* could activate $CD69^+$ as well as $CD25^+$ lymphocytes (13). Exposure to *C. albicans* allergens led to significant upregulation of IL-5 expression and release in peripheral blood mononuclear cells derived from patients having asthma and atopic dermatitis (58, 79). As IL-5 is a cytokine required for the differentiation, activation, and survival of eosinophils, fungal allergens may also be important for activation of eosinophils.

COMPLICATIONS IN IMMUNOSUPPRESSED PATIENTS

Superficial skin infections may disseminate in patients who are immunosuppressed or that have an immature immune system, such as neonates. Several authors documented that *Malassezia* species, normal human saprophytes, may be responsible for fungemia, especially in neonates having a central venous catheter and being fed with intravenous fat emulsions (14, 33, 70, 86, 96). It is difficult to characterize specific manifestations of *Malassezia* fungemia; however, neonates often had thrombocytopenia and the signs and symptoms of sepsis (apnea and bradycardia, low-grade fever in spite of broad-spectrum antibiotics, interstitial pneumonia, leukocytosis with elevated neutrophil band counts), whereas fever may be the only manifestation in adults (14, 70, 86). Some patients may be asymptomatic (14). *Malassezia* fungemia seems to be an underreported problem for patients with central venous catheters and receiving lipid emulsions, because the organism requires selective enrichment media for growth (e.g., Sabouraud's dextrose agar) with a source of fatty acids (e.g., sterile olive oil overlay) (14, 33, 96). Therefore, *Malassezia* species have to be considered in the differential diagnosis of opportunistic infections in patients receiving central hyperalimentation, and the laboratory should be informed of this possibility since routine blood culture techniques are not appropriate for the isolation of this lipid-dependent organism (33, 86). Treatment of this condition consists of catheter removal and discontinuation of lipid administration (14, 70, 86). A case of *Malassezia* fungemia in a neonate who recovered on discontinuation of the lipid emulsion, without removal of the central venous catheter, was also described (96). The role of antifungal therapy has not yet been well established.

Similarly, other fungi may disseminate in immunocompromised subjects. Arrese et al. (4) described a patient who developed a *Fusarium* big toenail infection following bone marrow transplantation due to B-lymphoblastic lymphoma. Nine months later, during the lymphoma relapse, a septicemic dissemination of *Fusarium* species occurred, and the patient died due to fungal sepsis, despite amphotericin B therapy (4). Also other molds, like *Aspergillus terreus*, have been reported to disseminate from cutaneous inoculation following immunosuppression (12). Another interesting report documented that *C. tropicalis*-infected fingernails of the medical staff were a reservoir of the pathogen responsible for sepsis in premature neonates (29). The risk factors for developing *C. tropicalis* fungemia were receiving a large number of antibiotics and a prolonged period of total parental nutrition (29). *Trichosporon* infections, which may rarely be evident as white piedra and onychomycosis in the same patient (25), may disseminate, primarily in those with neutropenia and rarely, with AIDS, with widespread cutaneous papules or purpuric nodules (68, 82). Remarkably, dermatophytes have also occasionally been reported to be responsible for widespread and invasive infections in immunosuppressed patients (52).

QUALITY OF LIFE IMPAIRMENT

Several studies demonstrated that chronic dermatomycoses, mainly onychomycosis, significantly reduced patients' quality of life (19, 20, 53, 69, 84, 87, 88, 94). Affected persons experienced reduced self-confidence and were less willing to participate in social and leisure activities (84). Patients with onychomycosis have decreased overall mental health, social functioning, and physical appearance as well as low body image and self-esteem and increased feelings of inadequacy and depression (19, 20). Patients with onychomycosis also felt stigmatized and reported concerns about nail appearance and embarrassment, as well as fear of injury or spreading the infection to others (69, 88, 89). More than half of patients with toenail onychomycosis experienced a variable degree of pain, 86% had problems when cutting their nails, and 82% could not wear the shoes they wanted (88). The majority of patients believed that the nail condition would last for the rest of their lives and claimed that other people found it unpleasant to look at their nails (88).

REFERENCES

1. **Akiyama, K., T. Shida, H. Yasueda, H. Mita, T. Yamamoto, and H. Yamaguchi.** 1994. Atopic asthma caused by *Candida albicans* acid protease: case reports. *Allergy* **49:**778–781.
2. **Al Hasan, M., S. M. Fitzgerald, M. Saoudian, and G. Krishnaswamy.** 2004. Dermatology for the practicing allergist: Tinea pedis and its complications. *Clin. Mol. Allergy* **2:**5.
3. **Anarella, J. J., C. Toth, and J. A. DeBello.** 2001. Preventing complications in the diabetic patient with toenail onychomycosis. *J. Am. Podiatr. Med. Assoc.* **91:**325–328.
4. **Arrese, J. E., C. Piérard-Franchimont, and G. E. Piérard.** 1996. Fatal hyalohyphomycosis following Fusarium onychomycosis in an immunocompromised patient. *Am. J. Dermatopathol.* **18:**196–198.
5. **Bäck, O., and J. Bartosik.** 2001. Systemic ketoconazole for yeast allergic patients with atopic dermatitis. *J. Eur. Acad. Dermatol. Venereol.* **15:**34–38.
6. **Baddour, L. M. , and Bisno A. L.** 1984. Recurrent cellulitis after coronary bypass surgery. Association with superficial fungal infection in saphenous venectomy limbs. *JAMA* **251:** 1049–1052.
7. **Besbes, M., F. Cheikhrouhou, H. Sellami, F. Makni, S. Bouassida, and A. Ayadi.** 2003. Favus due to Trichophyton mentagrophytes var. quinckeanum. *Mycoses* **46:**358–360.
8. **Björnsdóttir, S., M. Gottfredsson, A. S. Thórisdóttir, G. B. Gunnarsson, H. Ríkardsdóttir, M. Kristjánsson, and I. Hilmarsdóttir.** 2005. Risk factors for acute cellulitis of the lower limb: a prospective case-control study. *Clin. Infect. Dis.* **41:** 1416–1422.
9. **Braun-Falco, O., G. Plewig, H. H. Wolff, and W. H. C. Burgdorf.** 2000. Fungal diseases, p. 313–358. *In* O. Braun-Falco, G. Plewig, H. H. Wolff, and W. H. C. Burgdorf (ed.), *Dermatology,* 2nd ed. Springer-Verlag, Berlin, Germany.
10. **Bryld, L. E., T. Agner, and T. Menné.** 2003. Relation between vesicular eruptions on the hands and tinea pedis, atopic dermatitis and nickel allergy. *Acta Derm. Venereol.* **83:**186–188.
11. **Calista, D., S. Schianchi, and M. Morri.** 2001. Erythema nodosum induced by kerion celsi of the scalp. *Pediatr. Dermatol.* **18:**114–116.
12. **Cooke, F. J., E. Terpos, J. Boyle, A. Rahemtulla, and T. R. Rogers.** 2003. Disseminated *Aspergillus terreus* infection arising from cutaneous inoculation treated with caspofungin. *Clin. Microbiol. Infect.* **9:**1238–1241.
13. **Cozon, G. N. J., J. L. Bunet, and D. Peyramond.** 2000. Detection of specific T lymphocytes in systemic abnormal delayed type hypersensitivity to *Candida albicans. Inflamm. Res.* **49**(Suppl. 1):S39–S40.
14. **Dankner, W. M., S. A. Spector, J. Fierer, and C. E. Davis.** 1987. Malassezia fungemia in neonates and adults: complication of hyperalimentation. *Rev. Infect. Dis.* **9:**743–753.
15. **Day, M. R., R. D. Day, and L. B. Harkless.** 1996. Cellulitis secondary to web space dermatophytosis. *Clin. Podiatr. Med. Surg.* **13:**759–766.
16. **de las Heras, C., J. Borbujo, A. Pizarro, and M. Casado.** 1990. Erythema nodosum caused by kerion of the scalp. *Clin. Exp. Dermatol.* **15:**317–318.
17. **Deuell, B., L. K. Arruda, M. L. Hayden, M. D. Chapman, and T. A. Platts-Mills.** 1991. *Trichophyton tonsurans* allergen. I. Characterization of a protein that causes immediate but not delayed hypersensitivity. *J. Immunol.* **147:**96–101.
18. **Dickey, R. F.** 1972. Erythema nodosum caused by *Trichophyton mentagrophytes* granuloma (kerion). *Cutis* **9:**679–682.
19. **Drake, L. A., R. K. Scher, E. B. Smith, G. A. Faich, S. L. Smith, J. J. Hong, and M. J. Stiller.** 1998. Effect of onychomycosis on quality of life. *J. Am. Acad. Dermatol.* **38:** 702–704.
20. **Drake, L. A., D. L. Patrick, P. Fleckman, J. Andre, R. Baran, E. Haneke, C. Sapede, and A. Tosti.** 1999. The impact of onychomycosis on quality of life: development of an international onychomycosis-specific questionnaire to measure patient quality of life. *J. Am. Acad. Dermatol.* **41:**189–196.
21. **Dupuy, A., H. Benchikhi, J. C. Roujeau, P. Bernard, L. Vaillant, O. Chosidow, B. Sassolas, J. C. Guillaume, J. J. Grob, and S. Bastuji-Garin.** 1999. Risk factors for erysipelas of the leg (cellulitis): case-control study. *Br. Med. J.* **318:** 1591–1594.
22. **Eggert, A. O., S. Grunewald, I. Müller, S. Lempert, E. B. Bröcker, and M. Goebeler.** 2004. Chronic favus caused by infection with *Trichophyton schönleinii. J. Dtsch. Dermatol. Ges.* **2:**855–857.
23. **Eidelman, D., I. Neuman I, E. S. Kuttin, M. Pinto, and A. M. Beemer.** 1978. Dental sepsis due to *Candida albicans* causing urticaria: Case report. *Ann. Allergy* **41:**179–181.
24. **Elewski, B. E., and H. J. Schwartz.** 1999. Asthma induced by allergy to *Trichophyton rubrum. J. Eur. Acad. Dermatol. Venereol.* **12:**250–253.

25. **Elmer, K. B., D. M. Elston, and L. F. Libow.** 2002. *Trichosporon beigelii* infection presenting as white piedra and onychomycosis in the same patient. *Cutis* **70:**209–211.
26. **Espiritu, B. R., A. Szpindor-Watson, H. J. Zeitz, and L. L. Thomas.** 1988. IgE-mediated sensitivity to *Tricophyton rubrum* in a patient with chronic dermatophytosis and Cushing's syndrome. *J. Allergy Clin. Immunol.* **81:**847–851.
27. **Faergemann, J.** 1999. *Pityrosporum* species as a cause of allergy and infection. *Allergy* **54:**413–419.
28. **Faergemann, J.** 2002. Atopic dermatitis and fungi. *Clin. Microbiol. Rev.* **15:**545–563.
29. **Finkelstein, R., G. Reinhertz, N. Hashman, and D. Merzbach.** 1993. Outbreak of *Candida tropicalis* fungemia in a neonatal intensive care unit. *Infect. Control Hosp. Epidemiol.* **14:**587–590.
30. **Foti, C., A. Diaferio, M. Daddabbo, and G. Angelini.** 2001. Tinea barbae associated with erythema nodosum in an immunocompetent man. *J. Eur. Acad. Dermatol. Venereol.* **15:**250–251.
31. **Friedlander, S. E., M. Rueda, B. K. Chan, and H. Caceres-Rios.** 2003. Fungal, protozoal, and helmintic infections. p. 1093–1140. *In* L. A. Schachner and R. C. Hansen (ed.), *Pediatric Dermatology*, 3rd ed. Mosby Elsevier Limited, Edinburgh, United Kingdom.
32. **Gallenkemper, G., and D. Reinel.** 1992. Urticaria in the presence of intestinal yeasts-exacerbatic by chance of persorption? *Mycoses* **35:**181–184.
33. **Garcia, C. R., B. L. Johnston, G. Corvi, L. J. Walker, and W. L. George.** 1987. Intravenous catheter-associated Malassezia furfur fungemia. *Am. J. Med.* **83:**790–792.
34. **García-Sánchez, M. S., M. Pereiro, Jr., M. M. Pereiro, and J. Toribio.** 1997. Favus due to *Trichophyton mentagrophytes* var. quinckeanum. *Dermatology* **194:**177–179.
35. **Gianni, C., R. Betti, and C. Crosti.** 1996. Psoriasiform id reaction in tinea corporis. *Mycoses* **39:**307–308.
36. **Gilaberte, Y., C. Coscojuela, M. D. García-Prats, and M. P. Mairal.** 2003 Erythema multiforme associated with inflammatory ringworm on the hand. *Br. J. Dermatol.* **149:**1078–1079.
37. **Grunewald, S., U. Paasch, Y. Gräser, H. J. Glander, J. C. Simon, and P. Nenoff.** 2006. Scarring tinea profunda in the pubic area due to *Trichophyton verrucosum*. *Hautarzt* **57:**811–813.
38. **Gumowski, P., B. Lech, I. Chaves, and J. P. Girard.** 1987. Chronic asthma and rhinitis due to *Candida albicans*, Epidermophyton, and Trichophyton. *Ann. Allergy* **59:**48–51.
39. **Hicks, J. H.** 1977. Erythema nodosum in patients with tinea pedis and onychomycosis. *South. Med J.* **70:**27–28.
40. **Iglesias, M. E., A. España, M. A. Idoate, and E. Quintanilla.** 1994. Generalized skin reaction following tinea pedis (dermatophytids). *J. Dermatol.* **21:**31–34.
41. **Jang, K. A., D. H. Chi, J. H. Choi, K. J. Sung, K. C. Moon, and J. K. Koh.** 2000. Tinea pedis in Korean children. *Int. J. Dermatol.* **39:**25–27.
42. **Janniger, C. K., J. C. Szepietowski, R. A. Schwartz, and A. Reich.** 2005. Intertrigo and common secondary skin infections. *Am. Fam. Phys.* **72:**833–838.
43. **Johansson, C., H. Eshaghi, M. T. Linder, E. Jakobson, and A. Scheynius.** 2002. Positive atopy patch test reaction to *Malassezia furfur* in atopic dermatitis correlates with a T helper 2-like peripheral blood mononuclear cells response. *J. Invest. Dermatol.* **118:**1044–1051.
44. **Kaaman, T.** 1978. The clinical significance of cutaneous reactions to trichophytin in dermatophytosis. *Acta Derm. Venereol.* **58:**139–143.
45. **Kaaman, T., and J. Torssander.** 1983. Dermatophytid—a misdiagnosed entity? *Acta Derm. Venereol.* **63:**404–408.
46. **Kanda, N., K. Tani, U. Enomoto, K. Nakai, and S. Watanabe.** 2002. The skin fungus-induced Th1- and Th2-related cytokine, chemokine and prostaglandin E2 production in peripheral blood mononuclear cells from patients with atopic dermatitis and psoriasis vulgaris. *Clin. Exp. Allergy* **32:**1243–1250.
47. **Khaled, A., L. Ben Mbarek, M. Kharfi, F. Zeglaoui, A. Bouratbine, B. Fazaa, and M. R. Kamoun Barek.** 2007. Tinea capitis favosa due to *Trichophyton schoenleinii*. *Acta Dermatovenerol. Alp. Panonica Adriat.* **16:**34–36.
48. **Kivity, S., Y. Schwarz, and E. Fireman.** 1992. The association of perennial rhinitis with Trichophyton infection. *Clin. Exp. Allergy* **22:**498–500.
49. **Klein, P.A., R. A. Clark, and N. H. Nicol.** 1999. Acute infection with *Trichophyton rubrum* associated with flares of atopic dermatitis. *Cutis* **63:**171–172.
50. **Koutkia, P., E. Mylonakis, and J. Boyce.** 1999. Cellulitis: evaluation of possible predisposing factors in hospitalized patients. *Diagn. Microbiol. Infect. Dis.* **34:**325–327.
51. **Kulkarni, A. R., and S. P. Aggarwal.** 2006. Preseptal cellulitis: an unusual presentation of *Trichophyton interdigitale* in an adult. *Eye* **20:**381–382.
52. **Kwon, K. S., H. S. Jang, H. S. Son, C. K. Oh, Y. W. Kwon, K. H. Kim, and S. B. Suh.** 2004. Widespread and invasive *Trichophyton rubrum* infection mimicking Kaposi's sarcoma in a patient with AIDS. *J. Dermatol.* **31:**839–843.
53. **Lubeck, D. P., D. L. Patrick, P. McNulty, S. K. Fifer, and J. Birnbaum.** 1993. Quality of life of persons with onychomycosis. *Qual. Life Res.* **2:**341–348.
54. **Mari, A., P. Schneider, V. Wally, M. Breitenbach, and B. Simon-Nobbe.** 2003. Sensitization to fungi: epidemiology, comparative skin tests, and IgE reactivity of fungal extracts. *Clin. Exp. Allergy* **33:**1429–1438.
55. **Martinez-Roig, A., J. Llorens-Terol, and J. M. Torres.** 1982. Erythema nodosum and kerion of the scalp. *Am. J. Dis. Child.* **136:**440–442.
56. **Mayser, P., and A. Gross.** 2000. IgE antibodies to *Malassezia furfur, M. sympodialis* and *Pityrosporum orbiculare* in patients with atopic dermatitis, seborrheic eczema or pityriasis versicolor, and identification of respective allergens. *Acta Derm. Venereol.* **80:**357–361.
57. **Méndez, J., A. Sánchez, and J. C. Martínez.** 2002. Urticaria associated with dermatophytosis. *Allergol. Immunopathol.* (Madrid) **30:**344–345.
58. **Mori, A., Y. Ikeda, M. Taniguchi, C. Aoyama, Y. Maeda, M. Hasegawa, N. Kobayashi, and K. Akiyama.** 2001. IL-5 production by peripheral blood Th cells of adult asthma patients in response to *Candida albicans* allergens. *Int. Arch. Allergy Immunol.* **125**(Suppl. 1):48–50.
59. **Mungan, D., S. Bavbek, V. Peksari, G. Çelik, E. Gürgey, and Z. Misirligil.** 2001. *Trichophyton* sensitivity in allergic and nonallergic asthma. *Allergy* **56:**558–562.
60. **Nenoff, P., B. Muller, U. Sander, G. Kunze, M. Broker, and U. F. Haustein.** 2001. IgG and IgE immune response against the surface glycoprotein gp200 of *Saccharomyces cerevisiae* in patients with atopic dermatitis. *Mycopathologia* **152:**15–21.
61. **Niczyporuk, W., E. Krajewska-Kułak, and C. Łukaszuk.** 2004. Tinea capitis favosa in Poland. *Mycoses* **47:**257–260.
62. **Nissen, D., L. J. Petersen, R. Esch, E. Svejgaard, P. S. Skov, L. K. Poulsen, and H. Nolte.** 1998. IgE-sensitization to cellular and culture filtrates of fungal extracts in patients with atopic dermatitis. *Ann. Allergy Asthma Immunol.* **81:**247–255.
63. **Nordvall, S. L., and S. Johansson.** 1990. IgE antibodies to *Pityrosporum orbiculare* in children with atopic diseases. *Acta Paediatr. Scand.* **79:**343–348.

64. **Nowicki, R.** 2003. Allergic phenomena in the course of dermatomycoses. *Pol. Merkur. Lekarski* **14:**532–534.
65. **O'Driscoll, B. R., L. C. Hopkinson, and D. W. Denning.** 2005. Mold sensitization is common amongst patients with severe asthma requiring multiple hospital admissions. *BMC Pulm. Med.* 5:4.
66. **O'Hollaren, M. T., J. W. Yunginger, K. P. Offord, M. J. Somers, E. J. O'Connell, D. J. Ballard, and M. I. Sachs.** 1991. Exposure to an aeroallergen as a possible precipitating factor in respiratory arrest in young patients with asthma. *N. Engl. J. Med.* **324:**359–363.
67. **Palma-Carlos, A. G., M. L. Palma-Carlos, and A. C. Costa.** 2002. *Candida* and allergy. *Allergie Immunol.* (Paris) **34:**322–324.
68. **Panagopoulou, P., J. Evdoridou, E. Bibashi, J. Filioti, D. Sofianou, G. Kremenopoulos, and E. Roilides.** 2002. *Trichosporon asahii*: an unusual cause of invasive infection in neonates. *Pediatr. Infect. Dis. J.* **21:**169–170.
69. **Potter, L.P., S. D. Mathias, M. Raut, F. Kianifard, and A. Tavakkol.** 2006. The OnyCOE-t™ questionnaire: responsiveness and clinical meaningfulness of patient-reported outcomes questionnaire for toenail onychomycosis. *Health Qual. Life Outcomes* **4:**50.
70. **Powell, D.A., J. Aungst, S. Snedden, N. Hansen, and M. Brady M.** 1984. Broviac catheter-related *Malassezia furfur* sepsis in five infants receiving intravenous fat emulsions. *J. Pediatr.* **105:**987–990.
71. **Provini, A., M. G. Cacciaguerra, C. Angelo, C. Pedicelli, and M. Paradisi.** 2003. Erythema nodosum induced by kerion celsi in a child with hypomelanosis of Ito. *Minerva Pediatr.* **55:**621–624.
72. **Rahman, S. A., M. Setoyama, M. Kawahira, and M. Tashiro.** 1995 Erythema multiforme associated with superficial fungal disease. *Cutis* **55:**249–251.
73. **Rajka, G., and C. Barlinn.** 1979. On the significance of the trichophytin reactivity in atopic dermatitis. *Acta Derm. Venereol.* **59:**45–47.
74. **Reich, A., J. Szepietowski, and J. Gawlik.** 2004. Eczema as a hypersensitivity to fungal allergens in the patients with onychomycosis. *Mikol. Lek.* **11:**337–341.
75. **Reich, A., J. Szepietowski, L. Hirschberg, and E. Baran.** 2005. Zoophilic tinea cutis – therapeutic aspects. *Mikol. Lek.* **12:**211–215.
76. **Roujeau, J. C., B. Sigurgeirsson, and H. C. Korting.** 2004. Chronic dermatomycoses of the foot as risk factors for acute bacterial cellulitis of the leg: a case-control study. *Dermatology* **209:**301–307.
77. **Salim, A., and E. Young.** 2002 Erythema multiforme associated with *Trichophyton mentagrophytes* infection. *J. Eur. Acad. Dermatol. Venereol.* **16:**645–646.
78. **Savolainen, J., K. Lammintausta, K. Kalimo, and M. Viander.** 1993. *Candida albicans* and atopic dermatitis. *Clin. Exp. Allergy* **23:**332–339.
79. **Savolainen, J., P. Lintu, J. Kosonen, O. Kortekangas-Savolainen, M. Vianders, J. Pène, K. Kalimo, E. O. Terho, and J. Bousquet.** 2001. *Pityrosporum* and *Candida* specific and non-specific humoral, cellular and cytokine responses in atopic dermatitis patients. *Clin. Exp. Allergy* **31:**125–134.
80. **Scalabrin, D. M. F., S. Bavbeck, M. S. Perzanowski, B. B. Wilson, T. A. E. Platts-Mills, and L. M. Wheatley.** 1999. Use of specific IgE in assessing the relevance of fungal and dust mite allergens to atopic dermatitis: a comparison with asthmatic and nonasthmatic control subjects. *J. Allergy Clin. Immunol.* **104:**1273–1279.
81. **Scheynius, A., C. Johansson, E. Buentke, A. Zargari, and M. T. Linder.** 2002. Atopic eczema/dermatitis syndrome and *Malassezia*. *Int. Arch. Allergy Immunol.* **127:**161–169.
82. **Schwartz, R. A.** 2004. Superficial fungal infections. *Lancet* **364:**1173–1182.
83. **Serrano, H.** 1975. Hypersensitivity to *Candida albicans* and other fungi in patients with chronic uticaria. *Allergol. Immunopathol.* **3:**289–298.
84. **Shaw, J. W., V. N. Joish, and S. J. Coons.** 2002. Onychomycosis: health-related quality of life considerations. *Pharmacoeconomics* **20:**23–36.
85. **Stachowitz, S., D. Abeck, T. Schmidt, and J. Ring.** 2000. Persistent annular erythema of infancy associated with intestinal Candida colonization. *Clin. Exp. Dermatol.* **25:**404–405.
86. **Surmont, I., A. Gavilanes, J. Vandepitte, H. Devlieger, and E. Eggermont.** 1989. *Malassezia furfur* fungaemia in infants receiving intravenous lipid emulsions. A rarity or just underestimated? *Eur. J. Pediatr.* **148:**435–438.
87. **Szepietowski, J. C., A. Reich, M. Woźniak, and E. Baran.** 2006. Evaluation of quality of life in patients with onychomycosis using the Polish version of Dermatology Life Quality Index. *Mikol. Lek.* **13:**193–198.
88. **Szepietowski, J. C., A. Reich, P. Pacan, E. Garlowska, and E. Baran.** 2007. Evaluation of quality of life in patients with toenail onychomycosis by Polish version of an international onychomycosis-specific questionnaire. *J. Eur. Acad. Dermatol. Venereol.* **21:**491–496.
89. **Szepietowski, J. C., and A. Reich.** 2008. Stigmatisation in onychomycosis patients: a population-based study. *In Mycoses*, in press. [Epub ahead of print.]
90. **Tagami, H., S. Watanabe, S. Ofuji, and K. Minami.** 1977. Trichophytin contact sensitivity in patients with dermatophytosis. *Arch. Dermatol.* **113:**1409–1414.
91. **Torres-Rodríguez, J. M., and M. Sellart-Altisent.** 2006. Bilateral proximal cellulitis and onychomycosis in both big toes due to *Fusarium solani*. *Rev. Iberoam. Micol.* **23:**241–244.
92. **Velazquez, A. J., M. H. Goldstein, and W. T. Driebe.** 2002. Preseptal cellulitis caused by trichophyton (ringworm). *Cornea* **21:**312–314.
93. **Ward, G. W. Jr., G. Karlsson, G. Rose, and T. A. Platts-Mills.** 1989. Trichophyton asthma: sensitisation of bronchi and upper airways to dermatophyte antigen. *Lancet* **i:**859–862.
94. **Warshaw, E. M., J. K. Foster, P. M. Cham, J. P. Grill, and S. C. Chen.** 2007. NailQoL: a quality-of-life instrument for onychomycosis. *Int. J. Dermatol.* **46:**1279–1286.
95. **Weary, P. A., and J. L. Guerrant.** 1967. Chronic urticaria in association with dermatophytosis. *Arch. Dermatol.* **95:** 400–401.
96. **Weiss, S. J., P. E. Schoch, and B. A. Cunha.** 1991. Malassezia furfur fungemia associated with central venous catheter lipid emulsion infusion. *Heart Lung* **20:**87–90.
97. **Wilson, B. B., B. Deuell, and T. A. Mills.** 1993. Atopic dermatitis associated with dermatophyte infection and Trichophyton hypersensitivity. *Cutis* **51:**191–192.

Sequelae and Long-Term Consequences of Infectious Diseases
Edited by Pina M. Fratamico, James L. Smith, and Kim A. Brogden

Chapter 23

Sequelae and Long-Term Consequences of Systemic and Subcutaneous Mycoses

Elsa Vásquez-del-Mercado, Gabriela Moreno, and Roberto Arenas

In this chapter we will review the complications of the most common systemic and subcutaneous mycoses, including histoplasmosis, coccidioidomycosis, paracoccidioidomycosis, blastomycosis, mycetoma, sporotrichosis, and chromoblastomycosis. Systemic mycoses almost always begin as pulmonary diseases after inhalation of the causal agent. Subcutaneous mycoses are chronic diseases of tropical and subtropical areas in which the etiologic agent is acquired after traumatic infection.

SYSTEMIC MYCOSES

Histoplasmosis

Histoplasmosis, also known as Darling's disease or American histoplasmosis, is a systemic disease of the reticuloendothelial system caused by the dimorphic fungus *Histoplasma capsulatum* var. *capsulatum*. It is found in bat or bird feces and is acquired through inhalation of the spores. In 95% of the cases, the disease is self limited; however, progressive pulmonary, disseminated, or chronic cutaneous forms may be seen and can be lethal in patients with preexisting conditions. Immunocompromised patients may develop the disease after the first contact with the fungal spores or by endogenous reactivation. For this reason, a high index of suspicion is required to make the diagnosis, and patients must always be interrogated about recent travels or former residence in areas where it is endemic (4). The clinical symptoms and the radiological evidence found in patients with pulmonary histoplasmosis are variable, and it may mimic a lung neoplasm, requiring more-invasive studies, such as thoracoscopy or open lung biopsy to establish a definitive diagnosis (48).

In the progressive disseminated disease, after the fungus enters the individual through the respiratory tract, pneumonitis may be seen, especially in the inferior lobes of the lungs. Before cell-mediated immunity is activated, the organism gains access to the circulation through the lymphatics and disseminates widely through the body. After the activation of macrophages, the ingested fungi are killed, leading to the production of granulomas, which eventually heal with fibrosis. After the acute phase of the infection, the organisms are suppressed by the immune system, as in tuberculosis, and thus, reactivation of the infection is possible, particularly if the individual is immunosuppressed. In children and human immunodeficiency virus (HIV)-positive patients, there is meager granuloma formation. Progressive disseminated disease was reported in HIV-infected patients in 1981 and 1987; therefore, with the increasing number of cases in this population, it was accepted as an AIDS-defining illness (34, 50).

In adults, the chronic form is characterized by the presence of polymorphous cutaneous lesions. Up to 75% of the patients have mucosal involvement, mainly in the tongue, gingiva, and larynx; half of them have hepatic enlargement; and 3% have splenomegaly. Ocular involvement can manifest as uveitis or panophtalmitis, with the formation of granulomas in the uvea during the active phase of the infection. More frequently, it presents as the ocular histoplasmosis syndrome, first described in 1959 by Woods and Wahlen, where posterior uveitis or choroiditis are the key manifestations. The disease is unilateral in most of the cases (90%) (18).

H. capsulatum var. *duboisii* has been reported to cause orbital disease (6, 55). Uncommon clinical pictures include gastrointestinal and skin ulcers, intracerebral lesions and meningitis, endocarditis,

Elsa Vásquez-del-Mercado, Gabriela Moreno, and Roberto Arenas • Mycology Section, Dr. Manuel Gea González General Hospital, Tlalpan 4800, México DF 14000, Mexico.

Addison's disease, or disseminated intravascular coagulation, all of which carry a poor prognosis. In the fulminant form, the clinical presentation is accompanied by fever, malaise, hepatosplenomegaly, and pancytopenia.

African histoplasmosis is caused by the fungus *H. capsulatum* var. *duboisii*, which causes granulomatous or suppurative lesions, mainly on the skin, subcutaneous tissue, or bones. The course may be benign when the disease is limited to the skin, subcutaneous tissue, lymphatics, and bones but may be severe when lungs, bone marrow, liver, or spleen are involved.

Complications

Immunocompromised patients are very susceptible to the complications and sequelae of histoplasmosis. Gastrointestinal involvement in patients with AIDS is rare but has been reported; symptoms vary from diarrhea and abdominal pain to intestinal perforation (10, 30). Granulomatous mediastinitis or mediastinal granuloma is secondary to the infection of the mediastinal lymph nodes. The nodes enlarge and undergo caseation necrosis, instead of calcification following the initial pulmonary infection. The disease is usually asymptomatic, but there may be compression of the superior vena cava, bronchi, or the esophagus, leading to symptoms related to the affected organ. It can also spontaneously drain into soft tissues of the neck, airway, or even the pericardium. However, fibrosing mediastinitis does not occur. A mediastinal mass with granuloma formation, chest pain, and enlargement of regional lymph nodes, requires adequate antifungal therapy to avoid mediastinal fibrosis (39).

Fibrosing mediastinitis is a rare but lethal complication of the infection in which the mediastinal structures become trapped in the excessive fibrotic tissue caused by the disease of the regional lymph nodes. When there is unilateral involvement, patients may survive and a stable condition results. It appears to occur in a specific group of patients who, for unknown reasons, respond to the infection by *H. capsulatum* with the production of exuberant fibrous tissue. The disease progresses slowly over the years, gradually encroaching upon the superior vena cava, the pulmonary arteries and veins, or the bronchi. Less often, the thoracic duct, recurrent laryngeal nerve, and right atrium become involved. Symptoms include increasing dyspnea, cough, hemoptysis, and chest pain. Signs of superior vena cava syndrome or right heart failure may be seen.

The acute phase of a pulmonary infection is self-limited, but recurrences are common, presenting with the typical symptoms of pericarditis, pleural effusion, mediastinal lymphadenopathy, and pneumonia. Pericarditis may be a complication, particularly in younger patients. Disseminated disease can also manifest as endovascular infection causing embolic ischemia, requiring surgical revascularization along with antifungal therapy. Although cardiovascular complications are rare, histoplasmosis is also known to cause infection in cardiac valves and aortic aneurysms (9). Pericardial and pleural effusions can be hemorrhagic and may be a consequence of the host's reaction to the infection.

Among the rare complications of the disease are bronchopleuralcutaneous fistula, culture-positive effusions, and massive pleural effusions with fibrosis associated with a trapped lung. Broncholithiasis, lithoptysis, hemoptysis, and wheezing can sometimes be seen. Partial pericardial calcification may occur, but constrictive pericarditis rarely develops (34).

Liver disease secondary to the formation of granulomas is a rare complication, for which a high index of suspicion is needed to make an early diagnosis in order to avoid the potentially lethal consequences of disseminated disease. The infection may spread to other organs, including the suprarenal glands (manifesting as Addison's disease), kidneys (renal disease), and heart (congestive heart failure) (56, 60). Some cases of thrombocytopenic purpura with a fatal outcome have been reported, and histoplasmosis has occasionally been associated with pancytopenia (31).

Even in histoplasmosis-endemic areas, thyroid involvement in the setting of disseminated disease is rare but has been reported for immunosuppressed patients (28). The most frequent complication seen with ocular involvement is macular hemorrhage, which develops late in the course of the disease, usually 10 to 20 years after the appearance of scars. Neovascularization and scarring can lead to the loss of vision (18).

Coccidioidomycosis

Coccidioidomycosis is also known as San Joaquin's Valley disease or California Valley fever. The mycosis is caused by the dimorphic fungus *Coccidioides immitis* in the California area and by *Coccidioides posadasii* elsewhere. The microorganism acts as the primary pathogen agent in immunocompetent patients and as an opportunistic one in those who are immunosuppressed. The infection is acquired through inhalation of the fungal spores, and its primary target is the lung. It may be asymptomatic, benign, severe, or lethal. The dissemination of spherules and endospores through lymphatic or blood vessels can occur months or years after the primary infection and affect any organ (4, 51). Primary cutaneous infection after traumatic inoculation of arthroconidia rarely occurs and mimics sporotrichosis or cutaneous nocardiosis. Secondary infection may be caused by local dissemination and can generate pulmonary cavitation or a coccidioidoma, or it can evolve to a progressive pulmonary form.

Coccidioidomycosis is the third most frequently reported opportunistic infection in AIDS patients living in areas where it is endemic. Deficient cellular immunity leads to severe progressive forms, and most patients (80%) have pulmonary disease (diffuse or focal), and 15% present with extrapulmonary involvement. During pregnancy, the disease has a more aggressive behavior, with an increased risk of miscarriage or stillbirth, particularly if the infection is contracted in the third trimester (57). The disseminated form may involve the meninges, bones, joints, skin, and subcutaneous tissue; other sites include lymph nodes, liver, skin, peritoneum, kidneys, thyroid, adrenal glands, heart, pituitary, esophagus, and pancreas.

Chronic and extrapulmonary disease occurs in 5% of the patients and is more common in elderly males. Of those patients with disseminated disease, about half suffer from subacute meningitis (17). The disseminated disease is twice as frequent in males, and the incidence is higher among blacks, Indians, Filipinos, and Chinese (29). It is the most dangerous manifestation, with an incidence of 0.15 to 0.75%, requires lifelong treatment, and may coexist with tuberculosis in areas where it is endemic. Meningitis, meningoencephalitis, or meningomielitis can lead to extensive brain tissue destruction and may be accompanied by hydrocephalia, quadriplegia, or paraplegia. These cases have a high mortality rate of up to 50%, mainly in diabetic or HIV-positive patients (59). Usually patients complain of headache and present with an altered mental state, neck stiffness, and chest pain. Loss of memory, disorientation, comatose stages, paraphasia, and other signs or symptoms can be seen, particularly in advanced stages of the meningitis (12). Finding eosinophilic pleocytosis in the cerebrospinal fluid is rare (less than 3% of spinal fluid samples) and of diagnostic value for coccidioidal meningitis, particularly outside areas where it is endemic (32). A study of skin lesions and the development of meningeal infection indicated that patients with facial lesions were 11 times more likely to develop meningitis (53% compared to 9% of patients with lesions in other body parts) (5). The authors concluded that this subset of patients should, as a prophylactic measure, be treated for a longer period of time with drugs that cross the blood-brain barrier (5).

Musculoskeletal manifestations can also be seen during the disseminated form of the disease in up to half of the patients. These include a chronic granulomatous process in bones, joints, and periarticular structures. Acute arthritis develops in a third of the patients, and it is characterized as being polyarticular, usually migratory, without effusions, and the joints are painful to pressure and motion. Any joint can be involved, but those most frequently affected are the weight-bearing joints, such as ankles and knees. Generally the recovery is complete after a few weeks. There are no sequelae; however, cutaneous fistulae can develop.

Osteomyelitis of the spine and tenosynovitis, mainly of the hands, may be present. Some of the chronic sequelae caused by the disease can be evidenced by radiological changes, such as osteopenia, joint space narrowing, bony destruction, and in some instances, ankylosis (15). Osteomyelitis has been reported, too, in patients with disseminated disease. Surgery may be required in addition to antifungal treatment to control the infection (27).

A few reports mention the involvement of genitalia, including testes and epididymus late in the course of the disease. These cases required orchiectomy; however, the treatment is curative in only a few patients (2, 58).

Malnutrition, secondary to intestinal bypass procedures, has been associated with the development of tuberculosis, histoplasmosis, and coccidioidomycosis, suggesting that these infections may be a complication of the surgical technique (33). In organ transplant recipients, coccidioidomycosis may be life threatening. It can result from a reactivation of the infection, which is favored by the immunosuppressive drugs or by transmission through the transplanted organ (37).

Paracoccidioidomycosis

The systemic mycosis paracoccidioidomycosis is caused by the dimorphic fungus *Paracoccidioides brasiliensis*. The disease is acquired by inhalation of the fungal spores with initial location in the respiratory tract, which may disseminate to the oro-naso-pharyngeal mucosa, lymphatic nodes, skin, bones, or other internal organs. The disease varies from subclinical to acute, subacute, chronic, and even fatal cases.

Two major clinical pictures are recognized: the acute or juvenile and the chronic or adult form. The former is a more serious disease with a fast development. Both presentations have a high mortality rate in the absence of adequate treatment (4, 11).

The oro-naso-pharyngeal mucosa is involved in 51 to 82% of the patients, evident as nodules and/or ulcerations in the palate veil, gingiva, oral mucosa, floor of the mouth, tongue, and lips (moriform stomatitis). The teeth may loosen and detach secondary to the mucosal affection. Patients mention pain during chewing and swallowing and may limit their food ingestion, leading to cachexia.

Other organs that can be affected during the course of the disease are the cervical, axillary, and inguinal lymphatic nodes, esophagus, stomach, pancreas, suprarenal glands, bones, joints, and nervous system. Laryngeal involvement is characterized by the presence of verrucous lesions accompanied by dysphonia, dyspnea, dysphagia, and cough. In children, the disseminated form predominates, whereas with AIDS patients, the clinical picture includes prolonged fever, weight loss, generalized lymphadenopathy, spleen and/or liver enlargement, and skin lesions. During immunosuppressive maintenance therapy, the possibility of reactivation of a latent *P. brasiliensis* should be considered, particularly in the setting of AIDS or cancer chemotherapy, since acute pulmonary disease with a fatal outcome may occur (11).

Complications

Adequate treatment usually improves the patient condition, but in almost every case, the sequelae of the infection contribute to the morbidity of the disease. If the sequelae lesions harbor viable *P. brasiliensis*, relapses may occur. Remission of the disease is often accompanied by significant pulmonary fibrosis. In the chronic multifocal form, symptoms are variable, depending on specific organ involvement. The oral and nasal mucosa, skin, lymph nodes, and adrenal glands are frequently affected.

All patients with the juvenile and some patients with the chronic form of the disease suffer from lymph node hypertrophy, which may impair organ function by compression (47). Ocular or central nervous system disease, bone destruction, vascular pathology, and even genital lesions have been reported. Thyroid involvement is an infrequent finding at autopsy. Regardless of the involved tissue, all lesions heal with secondary fibrosis, which may permanently interfere with organ function. The lungs are always affected by residual lesions, manifesting later as cor pulmonale, disnea, or important cardiopulmonary restriction. Microstomy and stenosis of the glottis and trachea accompanied by dysphonia can be seen. The infection of the adrenal glands may compromise their function, leading to adrenal insufficiency or Addisonian crisis (11).

Blastomycosis

The systemic mycosis, blastomycosis, described by Walker and Montgomery in 1902, is caused by the dimorphic fungus *Blastomyces dermatitidis*. The mycosis, also known as North American blastomycosis, is commonly divided into cutaneous and systemic forms. The systemic form generally involves lungs, bones, and less frequently, the genitourinary organs, central nervous system, and gastrointestinal tract, but has been reported in other organs as well (24).

The disease is acquired by inhalation of the fungal spores, causing a primary pulmonary infection that frequently runs a subclinical course. When the disease spreads, it affects skin and bones and may produce chronic granulomatous lesions on the face or other parts of the body in immunosuppressed patients. While blastomycotic osteomyelitis is infrequent, it is one of the most frequent fungal invaders of the bones. Skeletal involvement is present in 60% of the generalized infections, commonly seen in vertebrae, ribs, skull, and also the short and long bones. It may be accompanied by mono-articular arthritis or occult osteolithic areas (13).

A series studying the frequency of the number of organs involved in blastomycosis reported that 82.8% of patients had single organ infections (predominately lungs, skin, and bones) (40). Other organs that may be involved include epididymus, testicles, and prostate as well as the central nervous system. Ocular disease manifested as keratitis, uveitis or panophthalmitis is rarely seen.

Myocardial infection may be the result of direct involvement, from extension of pericardial blastomycosis or possibly by retrograde lymphatic extension from mediastinal lymph nodes. In some of the cases of myocardial involvement, the outcome is fatal (7).

Few cases of blastomycosis have been described in pregnant women. Children are generally healthy at birth, despite the presence of disseminated disease or absence of maternal treatment during pregnancy. Nonetheless, infant death has been reported secondary to pulmonary blastomycosis (16). In immunosuppressed patients, i.e., those with an hematological malignancy or those receiving steroids, the disease becomes disseminated and involves the central nervous system. In AIDS patients, blastomycosis is rapidly progressive and fatal.

SUBCUTANEOUS MYCOSES

Mycetoma

Mycetoma is also known as Madura's foot; the syndrome is characterized by chronic inflammation of the subcutaneous tissue with multiple fistula formation which drain seropurulent exudate containing grains (aggregations of the causative organism). Some cases show ulcerated areas that resolve with retractile scars. In rare cases the infection disseminates to bones and other internal organs. The lower limbs are the most affected (64%), but any part of the body can be involved. The clinician must distinguish this disease from the incorrectly termed mycetoma that refers to a fungus ball found in a preexisting cavity in the lung or the paranasal sinuses, generally caused by *Aspergillus* species (4).

The etiological agent of mycetomas may be fungal (eumycetoma) or an actinomycete (actinomycetoma) acquired after traumatic inoculation. The geographical distribution of the infectious agents depends on the climate, pluvial precipitation, and other ecologic factors. The worldwide proportion of mycetomas is 60% actinomycetomas and 40% eumycetomas. Most of the mycetoma cases are located in Africa (Sudan has the highest incidence). The eumycetomas are slightly less inflammatory than the actinomycetomas, but otherwise, the clinical pictures are identical. Actinomycetomas are caused by aerobic actimomycetes that form microscopic grains. The most common agents are *Nocardia brasiliensis, Nocardia asteroides, Nocardia caviae, Streptomyces somaliensis, Actinomadura madurae*, and *Actinomadura pelletieri*. Eumycetomas form macroscopic grains that are white or black, depending on the fungal species. The most frequently isolated agents are *Madurella mycetomatis, Madurella grisea, Pyrenochaeta romeroi, Leptosphaeria senegalensis, Exophiala jeanselmei, Phialophora verrucosa, Pseudoallescheria boydii, Acremonium falciforme*, and *Fusarium* species. In both eumycetoma and actinomycetoma, the microorganisms live as saprophytes in the soil and are introduced by fomites or vectors such as thorns, splinters, stones, agricultural tools through traumatism of the skin, or animal bites. It is considered to be an occupational disease (4).

The incubation period varies from weeks to months or even years. In general terms, the mycetomas are asymptomatic unless bacterial infection occurs. If bacterial infection occurs, the patients present with pain, fever, and weight loss. In most cases, morbidity and disability are high, but the mortality rate is low. Diagnosis is confirmed by direct examination of the exudate with Lugol's iodine stain or saline solution. In these preparations, one can observe the characteristics of the grains that vary according to the etiological agent, such as the color and size. The causative agent can be isolated utilizing Sabouraud dextrose agar. In some cases, biopsies are useful to confirm or support the diagnosis of eumycetoma or actinomycetoma. MRI and CT scans are helpful in evaluating internal organ involvement and treatment response, particularly in cases of mycetoma of the thorax (52). Secondary bacterial infection is a complication of mycetoma, particularly those of fungal etiology. *Staphylococcus aureus* is the most frequently isolated pathogen, and patients complain of pain and increased disability (1). Bone involvement is the most important complication and is a late manifestation in actino- and eumycetomas (14). Mycetoma extends by contiguity; joints can be affected, causing arthritis and or bursitis, manifested by pain, swelling, and decreased range of motion. The knee is the most common site, although several articulations may be involved. Systemic symptoms are absent. Leukocytosis and an increased erythrocyte sedimentation rate may be found. Radiographic findings consist of osteopenia, soft tissue swelling, and lytic lesions of the articular surfaces (15). In advanced cases, it may reach tendons and nerves. Immense morbidity is caused by functional disability secondary to the fibrosis of the soft tissue, with increased volume and pain. All of these factors vary upon the localization of the infection and are greatest when an articulation is involved, leading to permanent ankylosis and claudication. Invasion of blood and lymphatic vessels may lead to dissemination of the pathogens to other areas of the body.

Granulomatous infections, such as tuberculosis and mycetoma, are still a frequent cause of infective spondylitis. In these cases, prompt treatment is essential to prevent a neurologic deficit (paraplegia) and/or spinal deformity, since the infection can affect the vertebrae, intervertebral disks, paraspinal soft tissues, the epidural space, the meninges, and/or the spinal cord (3, 52, 53).

Lesions located more laterally in the thorax can penetrate and even go through the entire thoracic cage to the other side, affecting lungs and pleura. It presents radiographically as a mass that must be distinguished from common mediastinal tumors, including thymoma or Hodgkin's disease, and thyroid goiter, parathyroid cyst, and germ cell tumors (36). Similar to tuberculosis and lung cancer, mycetomas are an important cause of hemoptysis. Patients require management in the intensive care unit for this life-threatening complication (25).

Visceral complications are directly related to the infected organ. Abdominal mycetoma rarely disseminates through blood or lymphatic vessels to other organs, like the liver and spleen. The dissemination through vessels is poorly understood, because it is thought that the grains have a larger diameter than the vessels; nevertheless, it can happen and is mainly seen in patients with some type of immunosuppression or those with prior surgical manipulation of actinomycetoma (21, 49).

Another infrequent complication is the formation of internal fistulae from skin to urethra, pleura or bronchi, with urine extravasation or expectoration of mycetoma grains (23).

Few cases of eumycetoma in the periocular area compromising the vision have been reported (46). Amputation of the affected limb is an absolutely contraindicated procedure in actinomycetoma. Unfortunately, it is still performed in settings where physicians are not familiar with the diagnosis and management of this disease. The operation permanently disables the patient and allows the dissemination of the disease through lymphatic and blood vessels to the stump as well as to other organs. In patients with eumycetoma, amputation may be curative, although there are serious socio-economic and psychological implications.

Chromoblastomycosis

Chromoblastomycosis is caused by dematiaceous (black) fungi, mostly species of *Fonsecaea, Phialophora,* and *Cladophialophora.* A common characteristic is that they form fumagoid cells (Medlar's sclerotic bodies) in their parasitic state. The disease runs a chronic course, affecting skin and subcutaneous tissues, mainly of the lower limbs. Clinically the presence of nodules, verrucous plaques, and atrophic and hypopigmented scars are classic signs. *Fonsecaea pedrosoi* is the most frequently isolated etiological agent in the Americas, especially in areas with temperatures between 20 and 25°C and a pluvial precipitation around 800 to 1600 millimeters. In this climate type, *Phialophora verrucosa* can be isolated too, but *Cladosporium carrionii* is more frequent in arid areas (4). These fungi are saprophytes of soil and plants and are inoculated into the skin through a trauma where the parasitic forms of the fungi develop. These fumagoid cells are oval shaped with thick-walled cells and reproduce by binary fission.

Chromoblastomycosis is considered an occupational disease affecting mostly male adults, living in rural areas, with ages ranging between 30 and 60 years. The incubation period is unknown. The lesions are usually unilateral and asymptomatic. Initially a papule or nodule with erythema and scales is present; after slow and gradual growth, the lesion may acquire a verrucous or tumoral appearance. Sometimes the lesions ulcerate, or satellite lesions develop. The most commonly reported form is the verrucous (53%), although the appearance may vary during the course of the disease. Up to 25% of the cases show atypical clinical forms, including the cicatricial or cerebral form (4).

When the disease resolves, it leaves extensive areas of scarring, discoloration, and lymphostasis. In general terms, the disease spares osteal structures, as well as internal organs. Nails have been reported to be affected by contiguity. Lymphatic or hematogenous dissemination is rare. Although the mucosa is said to be spared in this disease, there is a report of a patient with a lesion in the nasal mucosa that was diagnosed as chromoblastomycosis by histopathology, and the patient responded successfully to surgical treatment (54). If secondary bacterial infection occurs, then lymphangitis and recurrent celullitis result, leaving elephantiasis as an end result, which aggravates the chronic granulomatous process.

Diagnosis is made by direct examination of scales scraped from the lesions. Fumagoid cells are evident without special stains because of their dark pigmentation. The confirmation of the diagnosis can be made with a biopsy by which these cells can also be seen, and culture in Sabouraud agar can help classify the fungal species. Histopathological findings include a chronic suppurative and granulomatous reaction. Fumagoid cells appear thick walled and dark brown and measure 4 to 8 micrometers in diameter. They can be found inside the giant cells, in the dermis, or in the middle of micro-abscesses. They are easily visualized without special stains.

As with other fungal infections that predominate in tropical climates, there is confusion about the terminology used to name these diseases. Chromoblastomycosis is a term applied to infections limited to skin and subcutaneous tissues, caused by dematiaceous fungi with the characteristic formation of fumagoid cells in the infected tissues. Nonetheless, in the literature, there are reports of fungal infections caused by black fungi in internal organs which are improperly referred to as chromoblastomycosis instead of phaeohyphomycosis.

The complications and long-term consequences of chromoblastomycosis generally do not involve bones or muscle; however, periostitis can be seen. The complication rate of chromoblastomycosis is low, and probably in many cases, the disease is misdiagnosed, mostly as verrucous tuberculosis or the sequelae left by the surgical removal of the affected area.

The presence of ulcers is generally limited to lesions that become secondarily infected with bacteria. Secondary infection occurs in as many as 63% of patients with chromoblastomycosis. Long-standing plaques are usually large lesions that, over time become hyperkeratotic, resulting in limb distortion. Extensive fibrosis causes compression or blockage of the lymphatic vessels with subsequent lymphedema (20). This complication usually has a direct relationship to the duration, rather than extension of the disease. Bacterial infection is facilitated by the presence of lymphedema, which in turn is aggravated by the infection. The course of lymphedema is not modified by successful local or systemic treatment (43). Although generally not common, lymphatic spread has been reported with a subsequent lymphangitic pattern of the lesions resembling sporotrichosis (42). Hematogenous spread has rarely been described, but reports of dissemination to the central nervous system are known (26).

It has been stated that a chronic inflammatory reaction and formation of fibrous cicatricial tissue offer a favorable condition for the development of malignant skin neoplasms. The malignant potential of the lesions is similar. The origin of the tumors could be explained by the sequence of reparative processes that take place. This malignant potential has also been described in chronic ulcers and burn scars, and even the histopathological pattern of the carcinomas of these conditions is similar to chromoblastomycosis (38).

Though apparently rare, at least 14 cases of malignant transformation of chromoblastomycosis lesions have been reported in the literature (22). All of these malignancies have been of the squamous cell carcinoma type and have occurred after 10 or more years of disease (45). The carcinomas are usually well differentiated and noninvasive, with a low risk of metastatization. Recently, two carcinoma cases with aggressive behavior have been reported (38). The coincidental occurrence of chromoblastomycosis and melanoma has been described; despite an advanced clinical stage (tumor thickness of 2.3 mm), the patient was followed up for 7 years without evidence of recurrence or the presence of metastatic disease. The authors proposed that spreading of the tumor was blocked by the impairment of lymphatic drainage caused by the fibrous reaction (19).

A case of a patient with a 5-year history of a single chromoblastomycosis lesion in the leg, who later developed a similar lesion in the wrist, has been reported. The diagnosis was corroborated by histology and culture, which grew *Phialophora pedrosoi* (currently referred to as *Fonseca pedrosoi*). The authors presumed the second lesion was secondary to autoinoculation, although hematogenous spread could not be ruled out (41).

Sporotrichosis

Sporotrichosis is the most prevalent subcutaneous mycosis in the world, with a higher incidence in the intertropical areas. This granulomatous disease can run an acute or subacute course and is caused by the dimporphic fungus *Sporothrix schenkii*. The most commonly affected areas are the face and limbs; only rarely does it involve bones, articulations, and other organs. *Sporothrix schenckii* is found in soil, wood debris, leaves, and flowers. Rodents and insects are passive vectors. The disease primarily affects children and young adults of any gender, although it can be seen at any age. Sporotrichosis is an occupational disease of farmers, gardeners, florists, and carpenters. The fungus is an opportunistic pathogen in immunodepressed patients.

Sporotrichosis has lymphocutaneous (70%), fixed cutaneous (25%), and systemic (5%) forms (4). The lymphocutaneous form begins as a chancre at the inoculation site, frequently in the distal parts of the upper limbs and face. Volume increase with erythema and nodular lesions or gummas that ulcerate appear, which are generally asymptomatic. After 2 weeks, similar lesions are seen following the lymphatic vessels. Lymphocutaneous sporotrichosis must be differentiated from cutaneous tuberculosis, syphilis, and mycetoma.

The fixed cutaneous form also begins as a chancre that evolves into a verrucous lesion, covered by scale and crusts and is seen in immunocompetent patients, and for this reason, spontaneous involution is frequent. The differential diagnosis is tuberculosis verrucosa cutis, chromoblastomycosis, leishmaniasis and atypical mycobaterial infection. The systemic form is rare and is generally associated with immune alterations. It is clinically similar to the previously described lesions but affects larger areas of the body, even the mucosae, and poses a higher risk for osteal, articular, or neural infection. This form of sporotrichosis has a bad prognosis. The differential diagnosis is tuberculosis, syphilitic gummas, and coccidioidomycosis.

Pulmonary sporotrichosis is infrequent, and most of the cases are primary and run a chronic and asymptomatic course. For the diagnosis, a direct examination is not useful, but culture in Sabouraud dextrose agar is the gold standard. In biopsy specimens, small yeast can been observed in only 20% of cases, and what is normally seen is a suppurative granuloma with polymorphonuclear leukocytes and plasmatic cells or lymphocytes. The diagnosis can be supported by the sporothricin skin test. A positive skin test is specific for the disease, but it is negative in anergic or immunosuppressed patients. The positive response can be seen for many years. Serologic tests are not routinely done, and their utility depends on the sensitivity and specificity. The latex agglutination test has 100% sensitivity and specificity, whereas the immunodiffusion is positive in 80% of cases. The complement fixation test is positive only 40% of the time (4).

The complications and long-term sequelae of the extracutaneous form of sporotrichosis are rare and affect principally bones and weight-bearing joints, with or without tenosynovitis, periostitis, and ostheolisis. Arthritis is usually chronic, mono- or polyarticular; the knee is affected most often, but also the wrist and small joints of the hands and feet can be involved (15). Fungemia is a rare complication generally associated with the disseminated form of the disease, although a few reports support the presence of the fungus in the bloodstream without evidence of disseminated *sporotrichosis* (35). Some reports of fatal cases have been reported in patients with pulmonary infection by *Sporothrix schenckii* var. *luriei*, which has a different morphology from *Sporothrix schenckii* var. *schenkii* and may mimic other mycoses, causing a delay in proper diagnosis and treatment (44).

Another uncommon manifestation of sporotrichosis is ocular involvement. The commonest sites infected are the upper and lower lids, cornea, and iris, posing a serious risk for vision loss and requiring prompt treatment (8). There are a few reports of central nervous system involvement, as well as involvement of the genitourinary and digestive systems, liver, spleen, pancreas, myocardium, paranasal sinuses, kidneys, testicles, and the thyroid gland. In immunosuppressed patients, the disease can be fatal.

REFERENCES

1. **Ahmed, A. O., And E. S. Abugroun.** 1998. Unexpected high prevalence of secondary bacterial infection in patients with mycetoma. J. Clin. Microbiol. **36:**850–851.
2. **Amromin, G., and C. M. Blumenfeld.** 1953. Coccidioidomycosis of the epididymis. A report of two cases. *Calif. Med.* **78:**136–138.
3. **Arbab, M. A., I. A. el Hag, A. F. Abdul Gadir, and H. el-R. Siddik.** 1997. Intraspinal mycetoma: report of two cases. *Am. J. Trop. Med. Hyg.* **56:**27–29.
4. **Arenas, R.** 2008. *Micología médica ilustrada*, p. 113–148, 3rd ed., McGraw Hill-Interamericana, México City, México.
5. **Arsura, E. L., W. B. Kilgore, J. W. Caldwell, J. C. Freeman, H. E. Einstein, and R. H. Johnson.** 1998. Association between facial cutaneous coccidioidomycosis and meningitis. *West. J. Med.* **169:**13–16.
6. **Asbury, T.** 1966. The status of presumed ocular histoplasmosis: including a report of a survey. *Tr. Anf. Ophth. Soc.* **64:**371–400.
7. **Baker, R. D., and E. W. Brian.** 1936. Blastomycosis of the heart. Report of two cases. *Am. J. Pathol.* **13:**139–147.
8. **Bedell, A. J.** 1914. Case of chronic sporotrichosis of the eye. *Trans. Am. Ophthalmol. Soc.* **13:** 720–728.
9. **Berman, S. S., G. A. Kazlow, B. T. Fields, Jr., and S. Weinberg.** 1990. Disseminated histoplasmosis with embolic endovascular complications: a case report. *J. Vasc. Surg.* **12:**577–580.
10. **Brett, M. T., J. T. C. Kwan, and M. R. Bending.** 1988. Caecal perforation in a renal transplant patient with disseminated histoplasmosis. *J. Clin. Pathol.* **41:**992–995.
11. **Brummer, E., E. Castaneda, and A. Restrepo.** 1993. Paracoccidioidomycosis: an update. *Clin. Microbiol. Rev.* **6:**89–117.
12. **Buss, W. C., T. E. Gibson, and M. A. Gifford.** 1950. Coccidioidomycosis of the meninges. *Calif. Med.* **72:**167–169.
13. **Carnesale, P. L., and K. F. Stegman.** 1956. Blastomycosis of bone. Report of four cases. *Ann. Surg.* **114:**252–257.
14. **Castro, L. G., W. Belda, Jr., A. Salebian, and L. C. Cuce.** 1993. Mycetoma: a retrospective study of 41 cases seen in Sao Paulo, Brazil, from 1978–1989. *Mycoses* **36:**89–95.
15. **Cuellar, M. L., L. H. Silveira, and L. R. Espinoza.** Fungal arthritis. *Ann. Rheum. Dis.* **51:**690–697.
16. **Daniel, L., and I. Salit.** 1984. Blastomycosis during pregnancy. *Can. Med. Assoc. J.* **131:**759–761.
17. **Danoff, D., Z. M. Munk, B. Case, M. Finlayson, and P. Gold.** 1978. Disseminated coccidioidomycosis: clinical, immunologic and therapeutic aspects. *Can. Med. Assoc. J.* **118:**390–392.
18. **Deepe, G. S.** 2005. *Histoplasma capsulatum*, p. 3012–3026. *In* G. L. Mandell, J. E. Bennet, and R. Dolin (ed.), *Principles and Practice of Infectious Diseases*, 6th ed. Elsevier, Philadelphia, PA.
19. **dos Santos Gon, A., and L. Minelli.** 2006. Melanoma in a long-standing lesion of chromoblastomycosis. *Int. J. Dermatol.* **45:**1331–1333.
20. **Duane, R.** 2005. Agents of chromoblastomycosis, p. 2988–2991. *In* Mandell, J. E. Bennet, and R. Dolin (eds.), *Principles and Practice of Infectious Diseases*, 6th ed. Elsevier, Philadelphia, PA.
21. **Elhardello, O. A., E. S. Adam, and I. Adam.** 2007. Abdominal wall mycetoma presented as obstructed incisional hernia of cesarean section in eastern Sudan. *Infect. Dis. Obstet. Gynecol.* **7:**74643.
22. **Esterre, P., J. L. Pecarrère, C. Raharisolo, and M. Huerre.** Carcinome épidermoide développé sur des lesions de chromomycose: à propos de deux observations. *Ann. Pathol.* **19:**516–520.
23. **Fahal, A. H., A. R. Sharfi, H. E. Sheik, A. M. el Hassan, and E. S. Mahgoub.** 1996. Internal fistulae formation: an unusual complication of mycetoma. *Trans. R. Soc. Trop. Med. Hyg.* **90:**550–552.
24. **Farrel, G. E.** 1961. Blastomycosis of sacro-coccygeal area. Report of a case. *Ann. Surg.* **154:**90–92.
25. **Fartoukh, M., A. Khalil, L. Louis, M. F. Carette, B. Bazelly, J. Cadranel, C. Mayaud, and A. Parrot.** 2007. An integrated approach to diagnosis and management of severe haemoptysis in patients admitted to the intensive care unit: a case series from a referral centre. *Respir. Res.* **8:**11.
26. **Fukushiro, R.** 1983. Chromomycosis in Japan. *Int. J. Dermatol.* **22:**221–229.
27. **Gillespie, R.** 1986. Treatment of cranial osteomyelitis from disseminated coccidioidomycosis. *West. J. Med.* **145:**694–697.
28. **Goldani, L. Z., C. Klock, A. Diehl, A. C. Monteiro, and A. L. Maia.** 2000. Histoplasmosis of the thyroid. *J. Clin. Microbiol.* **38:**3890–3891.
29. **Hector, R. F., and R. Laniado-Laborin.** 2005. Coccidioidomycosis: a fungal disease of the Americas. *PLoS Med.* **2:**e2.
30. **Heneghan, S. J., J. Li, E. Petrossian, and L. S. Bizer.** 1993. Intestinal perforation from gastrointestinal histoplasmosis in acquired immunodeficiency syndrome. Case report and review of the literature. *Arch. Surg.* **128:**464–466.
31. **Hood, A. B., F. G. Inglis, L. Lowenstein, J. B. Dossetor, L. D. MacLean.** 1965. Histoplasmosis and thrombocytopenic purpura: transmission by renal homotransplantation. *Can. Med. Assoc. J.* **93:**587–592.
32. **Ismail, Y., E. Ward, and L. Arsura.** 1993. Eosinophilic meningitis associated with coccidioidomycosis. *West. J. Med.* **158:**300–301.

33. **Johnson, W.** 1981. Fatal disseminated coccidioidomycosis following an intestinal bypass operation for Obesity. *West. J. Med.* **31**:324–326.
34. **Kauffman, C. A.** 2007. Histoplasmosis: a clinical and laboratory update. *Clin. Microbiol. Rev.* **20**:115–132.
35. **Kosinski, R. M., P. Axelrod, J. H. Rex, M. Butrday, R. Sivaprasad, and A. Wreiole.** 1992. *Sporothrix schenckii* fungemia without disseminated sporotrichosis. *J. Clin. Microbiol.* **30**:501–503.
36. **Kroe, D. M., N. Shulman, C. M. Kirsch, and J. H. Wehner.** 1997. An anterior mediastinal mass with draining sternal sinus tracts due to *Nocardia. West. J. Med.* **167**:47–49.
37. **Miller, M., R. Hendren, and P. H. Gilligan.** 2004. Posttransplantation disseminated coccidioidomycosis acquired from donor lungs. *J. Clin. Microbiol.* **42**:2347–2349.
38. **Minotto, R., C. D. V. Bernardi, L. F. Mallman, M. I. Edelweiss, and M. L. Scrofemeker.** 2001. Chromoblastomycosis: a review of 100 cases in the state of Río Grande do Sul, Brazil. *J. Am. Acad. Dermatol.* **44**:585–592.
39. **Moholtz, M. S., J. H. Dauber, and S. A. Yousem.** 1994. Case report: fluconazole therapy in histoplasma mediastinal granuloma. *Am. J. Med. Sci.* **307**:274–277.
40. **Mollano, A. V., H. Shamsuddin, and J. S. Suh.** 2005. Systemic blastomycosis with osseous involvement of the foot: case report. *Iowa Orthop. J.* **25**:53–56.
41. **Morison, W. L.** 1973. Chromoblastomycosis. *Proc. Roy. Soc. Med.* **66**:178–179.
42. **Muhammed, K., G. Nandakumar, K. K. Asokan, and P. Vimi.** 2006. Lymphangitic chromoblastomycosis. *Indian J. Dermatol. Venereol. Leprol.* **72**:443–445.
43. **Ogawa, M. M., M. M. A. Alchorne, A. Barbieri, M. Castiglioni, A. P. B. Penna, and J. Tomimori-Yamashita.** 2003. Lymphoscintigraphic analysis in chromoblastomycosis. *Int. J. Dermatol.* **42**:622–625.
44. **Padhye, A. A., L. Kaufman, E. Durry, C. K. Banerjee, S. K. Jindal, P. Talwar, and A. Chakrabarti.** 1992. Fatal pulmonary sporotrichosis caused by *Sporothrix schenckii* var. *luriei* in India. *J. Clin. Microbiol.* **30**:2492–2494.
45. **Paul, C., B. Dupont, G. Pialoux, M. F. Avril, and R. Pradinaud.** 1991. Chromoblastomycosis with malignant transformation and cutaneous-synovial secondary localization. The potential role of itraconazole. *J. Med. Vet. Mycol.* **29**:313–316.
46. **Persaud, V., and J. B. M. Holroyd.** 1968. Mycetoma of the palpebral conjunctiva caused by *Allescheria boydii* (*Monosporium apiospermum*). *Brit. J.Ophthal.* **52**:857.
47. **Restrepo, A., and A. M. Tobón.** 2005. *Paracoccidiodes brasilensis,* p. 3062–3068. *In* Mandell, J. E. Bennet, and R. Dolin (ed.), *Principles and Practice of Infectious Diseases,* 6th ed. Elsevier, Philadelphia, PA.
48. **Salhab, K. H., D. Baram, and T. V. Bilfinger.** 2006.Growing PET positive nodule in a patient with histoplasmosis: case report. *J. Cardiothoracic. Surg.* **1**:23.
49. **Sánchez Navarro, L. M., M. Escobar Vázquez, R. Arenas, V. Cruz Hernández, and B. Delgado Velásquez.** 2004. Micetoma por *Nocardia* sp con localización en la pared abdominal y diseminación hemolinfática, al hígado y al bazo. *Dermatologia Rev. Mex.* **48**:90–94.
50. **Sarosi, G. A., and S. F. Davies.** 1996. Endemic mycosis complicating human immunodeficiency virus infection. *West. J. Med.* **164**:335–340.
51. **Saubolle, M. A., P. P. McKellar, and D. Sussland.** 2007. Epidemiologic, clinical, and diagnostic aspects of coccidioidomycosis. *J. Clin. Microbiol.* **45**:26–30.
52. **Sharif, H. S.** 1992. Role of MR imaging in the management of spinal infections. *Am. J. Roentgenol.* **158**:1333–1345.
53. **Sharif, H. S., D. C. Clark, M. Y. Aabed, M. C. Haddad, S. M. Al Deeb, B. Yaqub, and K. R. al Moutaery.** 1990. Granulomatous spinal infections: MR imaging. *Radiology* **177**:101–107.
54. **Symmers, W.** 1960. Chromoblastomycosis simulating rhinosporidiosis in a patient from Ceylon. *J. Clin. Path.* **13**:287–290.
55. **Tomas, P. A.** 2003. Current perspectives on ophtalmic mycoses. *Clin. Microbiol. Rev.* **16**:730–797.
56. **Tseng, T. C., S. J. Liaw, C. H. Hsiao, C. Y. Wang, L. N. Lee, T. S. Huang, and P. R. Hsueh.** 2005. Molecular evidence of recurrent histoplasmosis with 9-year latency in a patient with Addison's disease. *J. Clin. Microbiol.* **43**:4911–4913.
57. **Vaughan, J. E., and H. Ramírez.** 1951. Coccidioldomycosis as a complication of pregnancy. *Calif. Med.* **74**:121–125.
58. **Weyrauch, H. M., F. W. Norman, and J. B. Basset.** 1950. Coccidioidomycosis of the genital tract. *Calif. Med.* **72**:465–468.
59. **Wheat, J.** 1995. Endemic mycoses in AIDS: a clinical review. *Clin. Microbiol. Rev.* **8**:146–159.
60. **Wong, P., S. Houston, B. Power, E. Lalor, and V. G. Bain.** 2001. A case of histoplasma causing granulomatous liver disease and Addisonian crisis. *Can. J. Gastroenterol.* **15**:687–691.

Sequelae and Long-Term Consequences of Infectious Diseases
Edited by Pina M. Fratamico, James L. Smith, and Kim A. Brogden

Chapter 24

Prion Diseases

CHRISTOPHER J. SILVA

Transmissible spongiform encephalopathies (TSEs) or prion (140) diseases are unlike any other malady. The hallmarks of these diseases are the formation of microscopic holes in the brain (spongiform encephalopathy) and the presence of a distinct amyloid. This damage is caused by the replication of a pathogen, yet the pathogen replicates without inducing an antibody or inflammation response (141). Prion diseases have long, largely asymptomatic incubation periods. The symptomatic phase of the disease is usually relatively short and rapidly progressive. TSEs are always fatal. There is no cure, nor is there an effective treatment.

Although the name would suggest all TSEs are acquired, in fact most prion diseases have no apparent cause and are called sporadic. Some prion diseases are inherited. Most of the acquired prion diseases are iatrogenic. Sporadic, iatrogenic, and inherited prion diseases are transmissible. Prions are the only disease known to be both inherited and transmissible.

Amyloid deposits in the brains of victims are a characteristic of TSEs. A number of other diseases, such as Alzheimer's disease, are associated with amyloid deposits in the brain. These neurological diseases have been tested for transmissibility, and so far, none have been shown to be transmissible (27). Amyloid deposits are also associated with systemic amyloid diseases (126). Although these diseases may be transmissible (187), prions are not associated with systemic amyloid diseases (163).

TSEs are caused by a novel contagion once referred to as a slow virus and now called a prion. A prion is capable of converting a normal cellular prion protein (PrP^C) into a prion, thereby propagating an infection. In principle the prion is the least complicated of all of the pathogens listed in this book, since it is an oligomer consisting of a single protein. Even though they consist of a single protein, prions are capable of adapting to new hosts, replicating distinct phenotypes or strains, and responding to selection pressures like other pathogens.

Prion diseases are known to afflict a number of mammals. In sheep, goats, and wild sheep, the naturally occurring TSE disease is referred to as scrapie (54). Domestic cattle can be afflicted with bovine spongiform encephalopathy (BSE), more popularly known as "mad cow" disease (79). Feline spongiform encephalopathy is found in domestic and zoo cats (135, 185). Exotic ungulates can become afflicted with exotic ungulate encephalopathy (94). Mink have been infected with transmissible mink encephalopathy (111). Chronic wasting disease (CWD) afflicts both captive and free-ranging deer, elk, and moose (178). The human forms of these diseases include Creutzfeldt-Jakob disease (CJD) (73), Gerstmann-Sträussler-Scheinker (GSS) (107), and fatal familial insomnia (FFI) (118). Variant Creutzfeldt-Jakob disease (vCJD) is the human form of BSE (177).

Prion diseases are actually among the rarest known diseases. The incidence of CJD in the human population is about 1 or 2 cases per million people per year (103). The total number of vCJD cases since it was first described in 1996 is approximately 203, and the incidence has been rapidly decreasing (122). In the United States, more people die of the flu in a typical year than have died of prion diseases in the entire 20th century. Despite their rarity, prion diseases have attracted an astonishing level of scientific and public interest. This interest is a reflection of the fascinating nature of the prion, the science behind its discovery, and the concern about a fatal foodborne neurological disease.

SCRAPIE, SLOW VIRUSES, AND PRIONS

Scrapie is the oldest known TSE; it was first described in Europe at least 250 years ago (54). It took nearly

Christopher J. Silva • Foodborne Contaminants Research Unit, Agricultural Research Service, Western Regional Research Center, USDA, Albany, CA 94710.

200 years before it was conclusively established that scrapie was transmissible. Subsequently, a large-scale outbreak caused by a scrapie-contaminated vaccine confirmed that scrapie was transmissible and had a long asymptomatic incubation followed by rapid onset of symptoms (74). The term "slow virus" was coined to describe a collection of Icelandic sheep diseases with long incubation periods.

Although referred to as a virus, the scrapie contagion has many distinctly nonviral characteristics. The diagnostic hallmarks of scrapie are the presence of severe vacuolation in the brain (spongiform encephalopathy) and the presence of amyloid (54). In scrapie-infected sheep, in spite of the obvious cellular damage, the animals showed no evidence of fever, nor were white blood cells present in the brain during the symptomatic phase of the disease. Furthermore, there was no evidence of an antibody response to any foreign agent, even in the terminal stages of the disease (141). Formalin inactivates the viruses used to make antiviral vaccines. The scrapie agent is resistant to the formalin inactivation (74, 132). Although scrapie was shown to be transmissible, it also has the characteristics of a genetic disease (130).

The discovery of kuru, in 1957, would dramatically change the nature of "slow virus" research (65). Kuru was shown to be transmissible by ritual cannibalism among the Fore tribe in New Guinea. The publication of the pathological details of kuru prompted a veterinarian to point out the similarities of scrapie and kuru and to suggest a research program (78). Contemporaneously, the similarities of CJD, a familial and sporadic human TSE, and kuru were also recognized (95). The presence of amyloid in the brains of kuru victims suggested a relationship with a much broader category of diseases. Abruptly, an obscure neurological disease restricted to New Guinea was now related to a familial and sporadic disease of humans in Europe and a widespread disease of sheep.

The ensuing research revealed that the agent that caused TSEs was very different from any known virus or amyloidognic disease. Based on irradiation experiments, the minimum size of the scrapie agent is much smaller than any known virus. It is estimated to be on the order of a large protein (3, 17). As noted previously, the TSE agent was resistant to formalin, which inactivates viruses. Attempts to transmit other slowly developing amyloidogenic degenerative diseases, such as multiple sclerosis, amylotrophic lateral sclerosis, and Alzheimer's disease, have failed (27, 75). Kuru was definitively shown to be transmissible (66). Both sporadic and familial CJD were experimentally shown to be transmissible (27, 70). CJD was also shown to be iatrogenically transmissible by incompletely sterilized instruments and tissue transplantation (20, 58, 69).

In 1982, Prusiner proposed the controversial hypothesis that the scrapie agent was a prion, which he described as "a small proteinaceous infectious particle, which is resistant to inactivation by most procedures that modify nucleic acids" (139). Unlike other proposals describing the TSE pathogen, this hypothesis was supported by a substantial body of data (140). It remains the most widely accepted model for the etiological agent of TSEs (2).

Subsequent events would add these obscure agents to the popular lexicon. The choreographer George Balanchine died of CJD in 1983. In 1985, cases of CJD began to appear in young patients treated with human growth hormone (hGH) derived from cadaveric pituitary glands (pd-hGH) (38b). The United States banned the use of pd-hGH, opting to wait until recombinant hGH (r-hGH), derived from bacteria, became available. Other countries, most notably France, continued to use this pd-hGH, in spite of the demonstrated risks (24, 93). As dura matter transplants became more common, cases of CJD also emerged among these patients (26, 28, 38d). All of these events would be overshadowed by the discovery, in 1985, of a novel TSE of cattle referred to as BSE and more commonly known as "mad cow" disease (172). A novel form of CJD, referred to as vCJD, would be identified as the human manifestation of BSE 10 years later (177). How could a single etiological agent be responsible for familial, iatrogenic, and zoonotic transmission?

PRIONS

Soon after Prusiner proposed the prion hypothesis, researchers discovered a gene (*Prnp*) encoding a normal cellular prion protein (PrP^C) (12, 41, 127). PrP^C is a highly conserved monomeric protein found in all mammals (Fig. 1) (180). The gene codes for a protein of approximately 254 amino acids, depending on the species. The leading 22 or so amino acids are a signal sequence that is cleaved when the growing peptide is directed into the lumen of the endoplasmic reticulum (ER) (80). Inside the lumen of the ER, heterogeneous sugar antennae are covalently attached to two specific asparagine (N) residues in the peptide. The last 22 or so amino acids are cleaved when the glycophosphatidylinositol (GPI) anchor is attached (80). Fully processed PrP^C is a glycolipoprotein composed of approximately 209 amino acids (depending on the species), two sugar antennae, a GPI anchor, and a single disulfide bond. Analogues of PrP^C are found in fish, amphibians, reptiles, and birds (156).

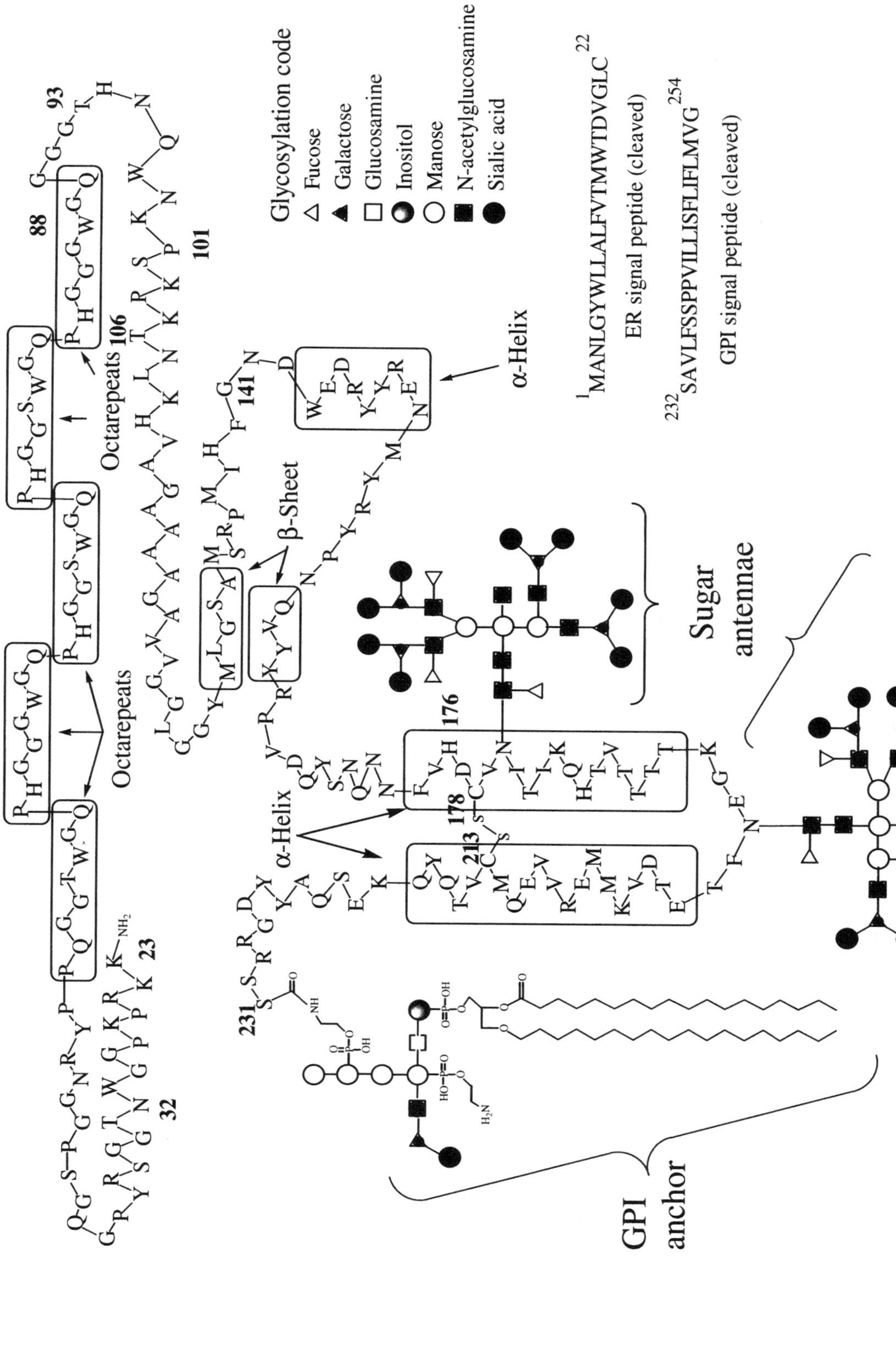

Figure 1. Version of mouse PrP^{C} (note that the sugar antennae are represented in their most complex form) (145).

The peptide portion of PrP^C contains a number of conserved structural motifs (Fig. 1). Most mammalian PrP^C sequences contain five octapeptide repeats (180). The octarepeats are thought to be involved in binding divalent cations, particularly copper (44). There are two short β-sheet sections and three α-helical elements (145). The two larger more C-terminally located α-helical elements are covalently joined by the single disulfide bond (145). Most of the PrP^C proteins the cell produces are attached to the plasma membrane by the GPI anchor. There is a highly conserved putative transmembrane domain (amino acids 112 to 134) near the middle of the protein, whose function is unclear, although it is probably involved in forming the topological isomers of PrP^C (80).

The natural function of PrP^C is not clear and is an area of active research (1, 188). It may be involved in metal chelation, protection from oxidative stress, control of circadian rhythms, sleep, and long-term memory (1, 188). Although PrP^C is highly conserved (180), it does not appear essential for normal development. Mice engineered to be devoid of PrP^C develop normally and appear to be normal (35, 108). Domestic cattle genetically engineered to be free of PrP^C appear to be normal in all respects (144). PrP^C is expressed in many tissues but is most abundant in the brain and other nervous tissue (19, 63). PrP^C is essential for the propagation of a TSE, since mice genetically engineered to be free of PrP^C are not susceptible to TSEs (34). While the function of PrP^C is unclear, prions have no known function other than to cause disease.

The structures of prions and PrP^C have been carefully analyzed by mass-spectrometric analysis (154). This analysis shows that both have identical primary amino acid sequences. In addition, they possess the same covalent posttranslational modifications: a disulfide linkage, a GPI cell membrane anchor, and two glycosylation sites. The heterogeneous sugar antennae are comparably heterogeneous in both prions and PrP^C (146). The sugar composition of the GPI anchor bound to PrP^C or to prions is similarly varied (153). PrP^C is a monomer, while prions exist as oligomers, with a minimum size estimated to be at least three monomers (3, 17). Based on nuclear magnetic resonance analysis, the secondary structure of PrP^C is composed of approximately 43% α-helix and a small amount of β-sheet (145). In contrast, prions contain less α-helix (20%) and more (34%) β-sheet secondary structure (145). PrP^C and prions thus differ only in their three-dimensional structure or conformation (154).

The information enciphered in the three-dimensional structure of a prion allows it to replicate itself and to a limited extent adapt to new hosts. More than one prion phenotype is possible for a given genetically encoded primary amino acid sequence (47). These different phenotypes are referred to as strains; prion strains have reproducible incubation times, pathologies, and physicochemical properties (30, 148). If a prion is transmitted to a host with a different PrP^C sequence, then the differences in the amino acid sequences of the prion and PrP^C (historically referred to as the species barrier) will make disease transmission less efficient than if the prion were composed entirely of the host's PrP^C sequence (92, 131). Furthermore, the species barrier is prion strain-dependent. Upon repassage in the same host species the transmission efficiency increases, since the amino acid sequence of the prion and PrP^C are now identical. In this way prion strains can adapt to new hosts and yet retain their distinct conformations (31). Mice genetically engineered to express the PrP^C of another species will readily propagate prion infections from that donor species without a species barrier (142, 149). Transgenic mice have been created that express hamster, sheep, cow, human, deer, and other forms of PrP^C (77).

Prions are more stable than their monomeric isoform, PrP^C. Prions are resistant to conventional forms of inactivation, such as formalin, UV irradiation, and autoclaving (160). BSE was spread to domestic cattle through rendered (autoclaved) meat and bone meal (175). Some cases of iatrogenically transmitted CJD occurred after appropriate conventional sterilization (20, 58, 69). Diagnosis of prion diseases often depends on the relative stability of prions to a limited proteinase K (PK) digestion. In such a limited digestion, PrP^C will be completely degraded, while a portion of the prion will be cleaved to yield a characteristic core (138). A Western blotting of this core is used to demonstrate the presence of prions and can be used to differentiate some strains (36, 89). The relative resistance of a prion to PK digestion is strain dependent (21, 67).

ROLE OF THE AMINO ACID SEQUENCE, SUGAR ANTENNAE, AND GPI IN PRIONS

The sugar antennae do not appear to be essential to propagate a prion infection but are related to strains (50, 152). Mice engineered to add only one sugar antenna or no sugar antennae to PrP^C are susceptible to prion infections, but this susceptibility is related to the prion strain (124, 167). The ratio of PrP^C glycosylation at both glycosylation sites, at only one of the two sites, or at neither site is referred to as a glycoform ratio. Differences in glycoform ratios have been observed for a number of prion strains, including CJD and vCJD (2). The observed glycoform differences in prion strains may be due to differences in the glycoform patterns of PrP^C in different regions of the brain (102). It is also possible that the structure of a given prion strain is determined by the glycoform ratio and that this is propagated as the prion replicates (46). The observed glycoform differences may be due to relative stability of the glycoform species before and after conversion to prion. Glycosylation may significantly influence the properties of a prion but does not appear to be essential for propagating a prion infection.

The GPI anchor is essential for the propagation of a prion infection (42). Mice engineered to express PrP^C devoid of the GPI anchor do not succumb to prion infections (42). When these mice are infected with prions they accumulate amyloid over time but do not develop a spongiform encephalopathy. These infected mice do suffer from other neurological problems (166). If the accumulated amyloid is inoculated into the brain of a mouse that expresses PrP^C with a GPI anchor, then the recipient mouse succumbs to a prion disease (42).

Transgenic mouse models have been used to determine the importance of the various amino acids present in PrP^C. These models have been used to show that mice expressing a form of PrP^C missing the octapeptide repeat regions (amino acids 32 to 93) are susceptible to prion infections (62). If a further 13 amino acids are removed (amino acids 32 to 106), then the mice no longer succumb to prion diseases (171). Deletion of the octapeptide repeats (amino acids 23 to 88) and amino acids 141 to 176 yield the minimum prion (mini prion 106; amino acids 89 to 140 and 177 to 231) (157). Mice expressing low levels of a protein composed of amino acids 89 to 140 and 221 to 231 in place of PrP^C die of a rapidly progressive neurological disease early in life, but this disease does not appear to be transmissible (158). The portion of mouse PrP^C believed to be responsible for the formation of prions is contained in amino acids 89 to 140.

SPORADIC PRION DISEASES

Most cases of prion disease in humans have no apparent cause and are referred to as sporadic (103, 176). Almost all of the diseases present as CJD and are referred to as sporadic CJD (sCJD). They typically occur in patients over the age of 50 and have a symptomatic phase of 6 months or less. The symptomatic phase of vCJD or iatrogenic CJD (iCJD) is typically much longer than that of sCJD. Sporadic prion diseases may result from a somatic mutation that results in the formation of prions. The resulting prions could infect surrounding cells and cause the observed disease. Sporadic prion diseases may arise from a reduction in the cells' capacity to properly process, degrade, or control the expression of PrP^C. It is even possible that they result from an unidentified rare combination of genetic factors unrelated to the human PrP^C gene (PRNP).

There is no evidence to suggest that sporadic prion diseases are the manifestation of an unrecognized epidemic. In the 1970s, there was speculation that the high rate of CJD observed in Libyan Jews resulted from the consumption of scrapie-infected sheep tissues (81, 116). Later it was shown that these patients suffered from familial CJD (fCJD) and not a human form of sheep scrapie (116). The incidence of sCJD in Australia is the same as the rest of the world and the United Kingdom (103), although Australia is one of the few countries known to be scrapie-free and BSE-free. If an unrecognized zoonotic agent caused sCJD, then Australia should have a lower rate of sCJD. CJD has been found in lifelong vegetarians (112). Epidemiological investigations have failed to associate the occurrence of sCJD with any cause except age (40, 52, 176).

FAMILIAL PRION DISEASES

Worldwide, familial prion diseases account for 10 to 15% of all prion diseases (100). All known familial prion diseases are autosomal dominant (114). In heterozygous individuals, PrP^C from the normal allele does not appear to influence the course of the disease caused by the mutant allele. Most of the cases of inherited human prion diseases are CJD (68). In humans, GSS syndrome is an exclusively heritable TSE, with an incidence rate of less than 1 person per 10,000,000 people (107). FFI occurs as rarely as GSS (100, 118). All of these diseases result from a mutation in PRNP. Even though these diseases are due to a genetic mutation, fCJD, GSS, and FFI have been transmitted to experimental animals (27, 49). Familial prion diseases are the only known examples of heritable diseases that are also transmissible.

Human PrP^C has more than 30 known polymorphisms (114). The most common variation of PrP^C occurs at position 129 (methionine [M] or valine [V]). It does not cause disease; instead, it influences the course of a prion disease. All of the known clinical cases of vCJD occur in patients who are homozygous for the amino acid M at position 129 (103). Among sCJD cases, patients homozygous for methionine

(M/M) or valine (V/V) are overrepresented compared to those patients who are heterozygous (24, 129). Among iCJD patients infected from pd-hGH, those homozygous for valine are disproportionately overrepresented (24). Among those afflicted with kuru, homozygotes had shorter incubation times than heterozygotes (39).

The 24 polymorphisms at 21 different locations in human PrP^C that are associated with inherited prion diseases are shown in Fig. 2 (114). Most of these mutations are clustered in the α-helical regions of PrP^C. The remaining polymorphisms are located in the prion portion of PrP^C. Most fCJD diseases have M at position 129. GSS phenotypes have M and V. The FFI phenotype is defined by the presence of M at 129. If V is present at position 129, the disease phenotype is fCJD.

Other mutations of human PrP^C result in fCJD or GSS prion diseases. Humans producing PrP^C with more than five or less than four octapeptide repeats will succumb to fCJD (114). Again, the polymorphism at position 129 influences the observed symptoms in these patients. Other mutations include the insertion of a stop codon at position 145 or 160, which results in the production of a truncated form of PrP^C, lacking the sugar antennae and GPI anchor. The polymorphism at position 129 is related to the length of the incubation period in these GSS patients. Mutations at positions 232 and 238 result in a familial disease, even though they occur in the GPI anchor signaling sequence, which is cleaved upon addition of the GPI anchor and is not present in fully formed PrP^C. The mutation at position 232 (M/T, methionine/threonine) results in the GSS phenotype. The mutation at position 238 results in a CJD phenotype. A recent analysis of a large group of Japanese CJD patients with a mutation at position 232 (M/R, methionine/arginine) showed that the patients had no familial history of dementia, so the relationship between the mutation at position 232 and CJD is uncertain (150).

The way that a mutation of PrP^C is turned into a prion disease is unclear (99). A number of cell-based systems have been used to show that the mutated form of PrP^C is not converted directly to a prion. The thermodynamic stability of mutated forms of PrP^C is not crucial, for many mutated forms of PrP^C appear to be as stable as normal PrP^C, while others are apparently much less stable than normal PrP^C. In engineered cell lines expressing PrP^C with the stop mutation at 145 or 160, no mutant PrP^C is produced at all. Mice engineered to express the mouse form of a mutant PrP^C (P102L) will develop a spontaneous prion disease if they overexpress the mutant form of PrP^C (87). If these mice express lower levels of mutant (P102L) PrP^C, then they do not develop a spontaneous prion disease (86). Patients producing identical mutant PrP^C (P102L) do not necessarily produce identical prion strains (137). It appears that familial prion diseases are the result of long-term misprocessing.

ACQUIRED PRION DISEASES

Kuru was the first human prion disease shown to be transmissible (65). Kuru was eliminated when local authorities intervened to persuade members of the Fore tribe to stop ritual cannibalism (106). Once the practice was halted in the late 1950s, no child born after 1959 died of the disease (65). Cases continued to be reported after 1959, but these occurred in people already infected before the halt in ritual cannibalism. It is clear that kuru is contagious, but it is not easy to become infected. Many of the people who studied the disease in the field did so under very primitive conditions, yet none of them became infected. The kuru experience showed prion diseases were not easily transmissible and that preventing exposure prevented the disease.

Iatrogenic transmission of CJD occurs through CJD-contaminated hormones, medical instruments, and transplanted tissues (26, 28). Before the advent of the biotechnology industry, hGH and gonadotrophic hormone were isolated from the pituitary glands of cadavers. Unfortunately, some of the methods used to isolate the desired hormones would also isolate infectious prions (162). In 1985, three cases of CJD appeared in young adults who had previously been treated with pd-hGH (38b). A few years later, r-hGH, produced by bacteria and CJD-free, became available. Most of the tissue transplant-associated CJD occurred from the transplantation of a particular lot of dura matter grafts (28). After 1987, a sodium hydroxide cleansing step was introduced in the processing of the dura matter. None of the dura matter grafts using this procedure have led to cases of iCJD. Other tissue transplants, such as corneas, and the use of improperly sterilized instruments have been implicated in the transmission of a few cases of CJD, but the numbers are much lower than either those of the dura matter transplants or the pd-hGH.

The emergence of BSE dramatically changed the pace of prion research. BSE was first described in 1987 (172). The incidence of BSE rose steadily until it peaked in the early 1990s (121). By the middle of the 1990s, a number of novel animal TSEs in exotic zoo animals, domestic cats, and, most disturbingly, primates had been described (94). Soon it was clear that BSE had crossed a number of species barriers

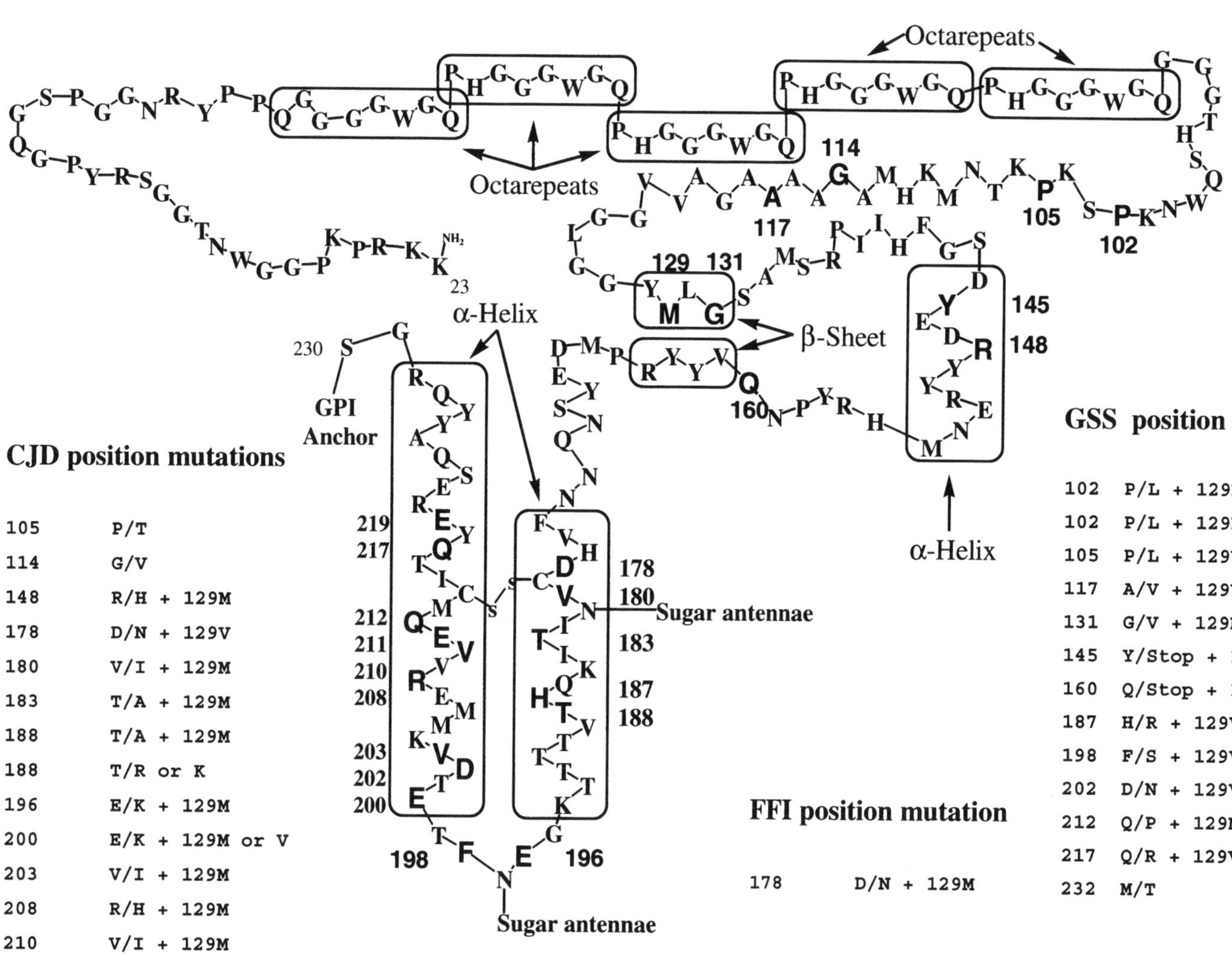

CJD position mutations

105	P/T
114	G/V
148	R/H + 129M
178	D/N + 129V
180	V/I + 129M
183	T/A + 129M
188	T/A + 129M
188	T/R or K
196	E/K + 129M
200	E/K + 129M or V
203	V/I + 129M
208	R/H + 129M
210	V/I + 129M
211	E/Q + 129M
238	P/S

FFI position mutation

178	D/N + 129M

GSS position mutations

102	P/L + 129M or V
102	P/L + 129M + 219K
105	P/L + 129V
117	A/V + 129V
131	G/V + 129M
145	Y/Stop + 129M
160	Q/Stop + 129M
187	H/R + 129V
198	F/S + 129V
202	D/N + 129V
212	Q/P + 129M
217	Q/R + 129V
232	M/T

Figure 2. Catalog of polymorphisms found in human PrP^{C}. Amino acid codes: A, alanine; D, aspartic acid; E, glutamic acid; F, phenylalanine; G, glycine; H, histidine; I, isoleucone), K, lysine; L, leucine; M, methionine; N, asparagine; P, proline; Q, glutamine; R, arginine; S, serine; T, threonine; V, valine; Y, tyrosine (114, 145).

(31, 64, 94). In the early 1990s, the health authorities in the United Kingdom established a CJD surveillance center to monitor the incidence of CJD in the United Kingdom (http://www.cjd.ed.ac.uk/). If BSE were to be transmitted to humans, then it would most likely appear as a form of CJD. CJD is typically found in adults older that 50.

By late 1995, CJD started to appear in adolescents and young adults in the United Kingdom (13, 25). These CJD cases occurred in patients with no history of fCJD, pd-hGH treatment, or dura matter grafts. The disease course was much longer than was typical of sCJD (90, 120). It became apparent that a new form of CJD, vCJD, was emerging in the United Kingdom (177). Researchers would determine that the prion causing vCJD originated from BSE (33, 50, 84, 104).

The phenotypic properties of vCJD are remarkably different from those of sCJD. vCJD is distributed throughout the body and can be detected in the appendix and the tonsil (32, 169). In cases of sCJD, it is rare for the prions to be found outside of the brain (72). sCJD has never been associated with blood transfusions, nor has it been found at higher rates among hemophiliacs (53, 59, 179). In contrast, vCJD has been linked to at least four blood transfusion-related transmissions (9).

BSE must cross a species barrier to infect humans, and the efficiency of this process appears to be very low. Between 1995 and 2008, the United Kingdom reported 165 cases of vCJD (122). In the same period, France, the only country with more than 4 indigenous cases, reported 23 cases (122). In the United Kingdom, approximately 180,000 domestic cattle have been diagnosed with BSE (184). However, it is estimated that between 1 and 3 million BSE-infected animals may have been processed for human consumption (56). In France, fewer than 2,000 animals have been diagnosed with BSE (184). Using a retrospective analysis of BSE in France, researchers estimate that more than 300,000 animals were processed for human consumption (159). This indicates that the British and French populations were exposed to significant quantities of BSE, and yet the number of vCJD cases has remained relatively low.

The prospects for the future of the BSE zoonosis are unclear. All of the known cases of vCJD have occurred in patients who were homozygous for methionine (M) at position 129 of PrP^C (103). Kuru, pd-hGH, and dura matter transplant-associated CJD cases have shorter incubation periods for patients homozygous at position 129 (either M/M or V/V) than those for heterozygous patients (4, 24, 39, 48, 129). One of the blood transfusion patients, who died of causes other than vCJD, was heterozygous (M/V) at position 129 (133). Physicians in the United Kingdom surveyed approximately 12,000 tonsils and appendices from healthy patients and discovered three prion-positive samples (85). Two of these samples were found to be homozygous for valine at position 129 (10% of the population) (88). Experiments with transgenic rodents suggest that transmission of BSE to a human homozygous for valine at position 129 would be much less efficient and would produce a disease different from vCJD (168). Recently, a patient homozygous for valine at position 129 was diagnosed with a novel type of CJD (115). It is not clear if this case is the first example of an emerging form of vCJD with a longer incubation period or if it merely represents the discovery of a previously undescribed type of CJD (115). Mathematical models suggest that a self-sustaining secondary epidemic of vCJD is unlikely (45, 55).

There have been several recent reports assessing the possibility that some U.S. cases of CJD might be caused by CWD (5, 15, 38c). One of these reports examined the association of neurological diseases and the consumption of venison (38c). Other reports examined an association between unusually young CJD patients who consumed venison and a laboratory worker who worked in a CWD testing laboratory (5, 15). These reports concluded the patients were afflicted with sCJD or fCJD or some nonprion neurodegenerative disease and not a new form of CJD (5, 15, 38c). A larger epidemiological study showed there was no enhanced risk of CJD in locations with high levels of endemic CWD (113). Experiments with transgenic mice suggest there is a substantial species barrier for the transmission of CWD to humans (98). There is no evidence to suggest that CWD is being transmitted to humans.

Although three U.S. residents have been afflicted with vCJD, all are presumed to have been infected in the United Kingdom or Saudi Arabia (11, 16). A large study of the "clustering" of cases of CJD associated with a New Jersey racetrack, showed no evidence of vCJD and no evidence of clustering (38a). Again, there is no evidence to suggest that a single case of vCJD has originated in the United States.

The emergence of acquired prion diseases has changed many aspects of medical practice. In many countries, each case of neurological pathology is closely scrutinized to determine if it is CJD and if it is a novel form of CJD. As a result, the data on the prevalence of CJD and the diagnosis of CJD are improving. Blood donations from people who have lived in the United Kingdom are restricted, as are donations from patients treated with pd-hGH or with a familial history of CJD. pd-hGH is no longer used, nor is dura matter that has not been treated with sodium hydroxide. The U.K. government acquired a number of blood banks in the United States in order to meet its needs.

DIAGNOSING PRION DISEASES

Diagnosing a prion disease is, by necessity, a diagnosis by elimination, since they are extremely rare (96, 103). The criteria for diagnosing the four existing human prion diseases are listed in Tables 1 to 3 (181, 183). Diagnosis is further complicated by the variable presentations, age of onset, and disease course of the human prion diseases (101, 186). The observed clinical symptoms of a prion disease are the result of neurological damage. Myoclonus (brief involuntary muscle twitching) is a characteristic symptom of CJD, but it is also a symptom of other, more common, diseases (23). Even diagnostic tests such as electroencephalography, magnetic resonance imaging, and the presence of cerebral spinal fluid marker proteins are insufficient to definitively diagnose a prion disease (51). In all cases, a definitive diagnosis requires a brain biopsy to confirm the pathological changes characteristic of a TSE (105, 170, 181, 183).

There are several lines of evidence to suggest that a presymptomatic diagnostic test is possible. Prions causing sCJD, iCJD, and vCJD have been found in the skeletal muscles of patients, albeit at low levels (134). The prions causing vCJD are present in the spleen, tonsil, lymph nodes, and blood (83, 189). This suggests that tissue other than brain may be tested for the presence of prions. Unfortunately, prions have not been detected in the blood of sCJD or fCJD patients (82, 189). Simple genetic testing can be used to identify patients with inherited prion diseases (170). There is some evidence that presymptomatic carriers of familial prion disease genes can be distinguished from their healthy relatives by careful observation of the patients' behaviors (71).

The BSE epizootic has led to the development of a number of tests for the presence of prions in the brain tissues of livestock. Regulators have approved tests based on Western blotting, enzyme-linked immunosorbent assay, and conformation-dependent immunoassay to detect prions in domestic cattle (76). The protein misfolding cyclic amplification assay, an in vitro means of amplifying prions (147), has been used to amplify prions from clinical cases of vCJD (91). Another approved animal diagnostic, the conformation-dependent immunoassay (148), has been used to detect prions in the tissues of patients infected with vCJD (18). Mass spectrometry has been used to detect prions at subclinical levels (128). Although it is unclear whether any of these approaches will provide a clinically useful diagnostic for human TSEs, they do show promise.

Table 1. WHO case definition for CJD (182)

Disease or type of symptom	Definition[a]
sCJD	Definite: IA *or* IB *or* IC *or* ID Probable: II *and* III (at least two symptoms) *and* IV (at least one diagnostic) Possible: II *and* III (at least two symptoms) *and* V
iCJD	Progressive cerebellar syndrome in a recipient of human cadaveric-derived pituitary hormone; or sCJD with a recognized exposure risk, e.g., antecedent neurosurgery with dura mater graft
fCJD	Definite or probable CJD plus definite or probable CJD in a first degree relative and/or neuropsychiatric disorder plus disease-specific PrP gene mutation
I	
A	Diagnosed by standard neuropathological techniques
B	Diagnosed by immunocytochemical detection
C	Diagnosed by Western blot-confirmed protease-resistant PrP
D	Diagnosed by presence of scrapie-associated fibrils
II	Progressive dementia
III	Myoclonus, visual or cerebellar disturbance, pyramidal/extrapyramidal dysfunction, or akinetic mutism
IV	Typical EEG during an illness of any duration, a positive 14-3-3 cerebrospinal fluid assay, and a clinical duration to death of <2 yr; routine investigations should not suggest an alternative diagnosis
V	No EEG or atypical EEG; and duration of <2 yr

[a]EEG, electroencephalography.

TREATMENT OF PRION DISEASES

Attempts to cure patients suffering from prion diseases have not been successful (155). The largest clinical trials have used the drugs flupirtine, quinacrine, and amantadine. A small trial using quinacrine to treat CJD victims showed some cognitive improvement, but it was transient. Amantadine showed no improvement during treatment. Treatment with flupirtine seemed to show some improvement, but in the end all patients died. Intraventricular perfusion of pentosan polysulfate was unsuccessful as well (22, 164, 173). Since all of these patients

Table 2. WHO case definition for vCJD (183)

Disease	Definition
vCJD	Definite: IA *and* neuropathological confirmation of vCJD[a]
	Probable: I *and* II (at least four symptoms) *and* III *or* I *and* IV
	Possible: I *and* II (at least four symptoms) *and* IIIA
I	
A	Progressive neuropsychiatric disorder
B.	Duration of illness >6 mo
C	Routine investigations do not suggest an alternative diagnosis
D	No history of potential iatrogenic exposure
E.	No evidence of a familial form of TSE
II	
A	Early psychiatric symptoms[b]
B.	Persistent painful sensory symptoms[c]
C	Ataxia
D	Myoclonus or chorea or dystonia
E.	Dementia
III	
A	EEG does not show the typical appearance of sporadic CJD[d] (or no EEG performed)
B.	MRI brain scan shows bilateral symmetrical pulvinar high signal[e]
IV.	Positive tonsil biopsy[f]

[a]Spongiform change and extensive PrP deposition with florid plaques, throughout the cerebrum and cerebellum.
[b]Depression, anxiety, apathy, withdrawal, and delusions.
[c]This includes both frank pain and/or dysesthesia.
[d]Generalized triphasic periodic complexes at approximately one per second. EEG, electroencephalography.
[e]Relative to the signal intensity of other deep grey matter nuclei and cortical grey matter. MRI, magnetic resonance imaging.
[f]Tonsil biopsy is not recommended routinely or in cases with EEG appearances typical of sporadic CJD but may be useful in suspect cases in which the clinical features are compatible with vCJD and where MRI does not show bilateral pulvinar high signal.

were symptomatic and their prion titers were very high, it is not, unfortunately, surprising that these drugs would have no effect.

Antibody-based approaches show promise for prophylaxis in animal models (165). Mice engineered to express antibody fragments to PrP^C are resistant to prion challenge. Mice passively immunized with anti-PrP^C antibodies also show resistance to prion diseases. This effect may be due to the antibody interfering with the PrP^C-to-prion conversion process, or it may simply be due to an enhanced degradation of PrP^C. Unfortunately, since there is no native antibody response to a prion disease, the potential for vaccines in TSE treatment is unclear (119).

The future for the treatment of prion diseases is promising. Animal models indicate that if an in vivo

Table 3. WHO neuropathological criteria for CJD and other human TSE (181, 183)

TSE	Criteria
CJD (sporadic, iatrogenic [recognized risk] or familial [same disease in first-degree relative or disease-associated PrP gene mutation])	Spongiform encephalopathy in cerebral and/or cerebellar cortex and/or subcortical grey matter; and/or encephalopathy with prion protein (PrP) immunoreactivity (plaque and/or diffuse synaptic and/or patchy/perivacuolar types)
New vCJD	Spongiform encephalopathy with abundant PrP deposition, in particular multiple fibrillary PrP plaques surrounded by a halo of spongiform vacuoles ("florid" plaques, "daisy-like" plaques) and other PrP plaques, and amorphous pericellular and perivascular PrP deposits especially prominent in the cerebellar molecular layer.
GSS disease (in family with dominantly inherited progressive ataxia and/or dementia and one of a variety of PrP gene mutations)	Encephalo(myelo)pathy with multicentric PrP plaques
FFI (in member of a family with a PrP gene mutation at codon 178 in frame with methionine at codon 129)	Thalamic degeneration, variable spongiform change in cerebrum

means of halting or substantially reducing prion replication could be developed, then it would be an effective treatment (109, 110). Researchers have developed a number of high-throughput assays that can be used to screen for anti-prion compounds (97). Once a suitable therapeutic candidate has been identified, there are a number of in vitro and in vivo methods to evaluate it (165). The European Union and the United States now have well-developed systems of identifying patients suffering from prion diseases. These patients can be enrolled in clinical trials to evaluate the efficacy of candidate therapeutics. As diagnostics improve, it may be possible to identify patients before they are symptomatic and before their prion titers are extremely high.

Historically, preventing prion diseases has been the only effective means of limiting their spread. Kuru was eradicated by preventing ritual cannibalism (65). Replacing pd-hGH with r-hGH has eliminated pd-hGH as a source of infection (26). The heightened awareness of CJD and the resulting introduction of appropriate sterilization techniques reduced the incidence of surgically acquired iCJD cases (26). Properly treating dura matter has greatly reduced its risk in transmitting CJD (26, 28). Enacting and enforcing bans on feeding ruminant tissue to ruminants has nearly eliminated BSE as a zoonotic source of vCJD (57, 184). These approaches are effective in eliminating the zoonotic sources and reducing the iatrogenic sources of prion diseases but are ineffective for sporadic or familial prion diseases, which comprise >95% of all cases.

INACTIVATING PRIONS

Prions are not indestructible, although they are resistant to many common forms of inactivation (160, 161). Prions can be completely inactivated by chlorine bleach or by combinations of sodium hydroxide and autoclaving (38, 61). Incineration at 1,000°C will completely inactivate prions (29). Complete inactivation can be accomplished by extended autoclaving at higher temperatures (38). More recent work reports that the use of acidic sodium dodecyl sulfate and autoclaving, radio-frequency gas-plasma, or phenolic cleaners will inactivate prions (14, 136, 143). The World Health Organization (WHO) and the Centers for Disease Control and Prevention (CDC) have a set of guidelines for prion decontamination (38, 182).

The biosafety guidelines for working with prions in the United States restrict work on human TSE to biosafety level 3 (BL-3) (125). The requirements for a BL-3 facility are described in the CDC guidelines (37). The same biosafety level is required for work with BSE. BSE is classified as a select agent (60). If human prions are passaged through nonhuman or primate hosts, then they are considered to be of human origin and must be treated as though they are human prions, even though they are composed of nonhuman protein. If BSE is passaged through any nonbovine, then the resulting prions must be handled as though they were BSE. If a nonhuman or nonbovine prion is passaged through transgenic mice engineered to express human or bovine PrP^C, then the resulting prion is considered as if it were of human or bovine origin, must be handled in a BL-3 facility, and may be considered to be a select agent.

PRIONS AND OTHER PROTEIN CONFORMATIONAL DISEASES

The prion hypothesis challenges a core tenet of modern molecular biology, namely that one gene encodes one protein. The existence of prion strains implies that a single gene can produce several protein isoforms with characteristic properties. Prion diseases are representatives of a much larger category of phenomena related to protein misfolding, and more than 40 nonprion diseases are associated with protein misfolding, including Alzheimer's disease and amyloid protein A (AA) amyloidosis (43).

The discovery of yeast prions demonstrated that prions can be beneficial to a host, by allowing the host organism to grow on nitrogen-poor medium (174). Protein misfolding has been invoked to explain a molecular mechanism for long-term memory (151). Prion diseases are representative of a much larger category of phenomena related to protein misfolding (43). Thus, although protein misfolding suggests a pathological process, in fact it may be a more general but relatively poorly understood biochemical process.

Prion diseases are the only known example of transmissible protein misfolding diseases. Researchers have shown that the pathological Aβ protein from Alzheimer's disease can be amplified in transgenic mice, and there seem to be different strains of Aβ (117). While these results are not evidence that Alzheimer's disease is transmissible, they do show that Aβ has prion-like properties. Captive cheetah are afflicted with a disease called amyloid protein A (AA) amyloidosis, which is associated with the accumulation of the N-terminal fragment of apolipoprotein serum amyloid A as an amyloid (187). In mouse models, the AA present in the feces of captive cheetahs will infect transgenic mice (187). The epidemiology of AA disease in cheetahs suggests that AA may be transmissible (187). However, AA disease is not associated with TSEs or prions (163). Future experimental work will determine if prion diseases will remain the only known example of a transmissible amyloidosis.

SUMMARY

TSEs comprise a set of rare fatal neurological diseases found in many mammals and include such human diseases as CJD, GSS, FFI, and kuru. TSEs are caused by prions, a novel contagion. A prion is a protein capable of converting a normal cellular protein (PrP^C) into a prion and thereby propagating an infection. PrP^C is a small, highly conserved glycoprotein with a GPI anchor. A prion and PrP^C have identical amino acid sequences and covalent posttranslational modifications. Although they differ only in their conformations, a prion is more stable to proteolysis and denaturation than is its conformer, PrP^C. There is more than one possible pathogenic conformation for a given PrP^C; these distinct and stable conformations are associated with different prion strains. The amino acid sequence, glycosylation, and GPI anchor have roles in the pathogenesis of prions and prion strains.

Prion diseases are the only diseases known to be both heritable and transmissible. Most human prion diseases are sporadic. Worldwide only 10 to 15 % of human prion diseases are inherited, and even fewer are the result of infection. Due to their rarity and variable presentation of symptoms, prion diseases are difficult to diagnose. A definitive diagnosis requires a brain biopsy. Prions are difficult to inactivate, but there are reliable methods of destroying them. Unfortunately, there is no effective treatment for prion diseases. There is promise that a treatment may be developed in the future.

The existence of prions challenges the assumption that a single gene generates a single protein with a single function. Prions are not necessarily pathological, for yeast prions facilitate the growth of the host on nitrogen-poor media. Although prions are the best known example of a protein misfolding disease, other diseases such as Alzheimer's and type II diabetes are also associated with protein misfolding. Unlike prion diseases, these are not transmissible. Recent reports suggest that AA amyloidosis may represent a new form of nonprion transmissible amyloid disease.

REFERENCES

1. **Aguzzi, A., F. Baumann, and J. Bremer.** 2008. The prion's elusive reason for being. *Annu. Rev. Neurosci.* **31:**439–477.
2. **Aguzzi, A., M. Heikenwalder, and M. Polymenidou.** 2007. Insights into prion strains and neurotoxicity. *Nat. Rev. Mol. Cell Biol.* **8:**552–561.
3. **Alper, T., D. A. Haig, and M. C. Clarke.** 1966. The exceptionally small size of the scrapie agent. *Biochem. Biophys. Res. Commun.* **22:**278–284.
4. **Alperovitch, A., I. Zerr, M. Pocchiari, E. Mitrova, J. de Pedro Cuesta, I. Hegyi, S. Collins, H. Kretzschmar, C. van Duijn, and R. G. Will.** 1999. Codon 129 prion protein genotype and sporadic Creutzfeldt-Jakob disease. *Lancet* **353:**1673–1674.
5. **Anderson, C. A., P. Bosque, C. M. Filley, D. B. Arciniegas, B. K. Kleinschmidt-Demasters, W. J. Pape, and K. L. Tyler.** 2007. Colorado surveillance program for chronic wasting disease transmission to humans: lessons from 2 highly suspicious but negative cases. *Arch. Neurol.* **64:**439–441.
6. Reference deleted.
7. Reference deleted.
8. Reference deleted.
9. **Anonymous.** 2007. Fourth case of transfusion-associated vCJD infection in the United Kingdom. *Euro. Surveill.* **12:** E070118.4.
10. Reference deleted.
11. **Anonymous.** 2006. Third case of vCJD reported in the United States. *Euro. Surveill.* **11:**E061207.2.
12. **Basler, K., B. Oesch, M. Scott, D. Westaway, M. Walchli, D. F. Groth, M. P. McKinley, S. B. Prusiner, and C. Weissmann.** 1986. Scrapie and cellular PrP isoforms are encoded by the same chromosomal gene. *Cell* **46:**417–428.
13. **Bateman, D., D. Hilton, S. Love, M. Zeidler, J. Beck, and J. Collinge.** 1995. Sporadic Creutzfeldt-Jakob disease in a 18-year-old in the UK. *Lancet* **346:**1155–1156.
14. **Baxter, H. C., G. A. Campbell, A. G. Whittaker, A. C. Jones, A. Aitken, A. H. Simpson, M. Casey, L. Bountiff, L. Gibbard, and R. L. Baxter.** 2005. Elimination of transmissible spongiform encephalopathy infectivity and decontamination of surgical instruments by using radio-frequency gas-plasma treatment. *J. Gen. Virol.* **86:**2393–2399.
15. **Belay, E. D., P. Gambetti, L. B. Schonberger, P. Parchi, D. R. Lyon, S. Capellari, J. H. McQuiston, K. Bradley, G. Dowdle, J. M. Crutcher, and C. R. Nichols.** 2001. Creutzfeldt-Jakob disease in unusually young patients who consumed venison. *Arch. Neurol.* **58:**1673–1678.
16. **Belay, E. D., J. J. Sejvar, W. J. Shieh, S. T. Wiersma, W. Q. Zou, P. Gambetti, S. Hunter, R. A. Maddox, L. Crockett, S. R. Zaki, and L. B. Schonberger.** 2005. Variant Creutzfeldt-Jakob disease death, United States. *Emerg. Infect. Dis.* **11:**1351–1354.
17. **Bellinger-Kawahara, C. G., E. Kempner, D. Groth, R. Gabizon, and S. B. Prusiner.** 1988. Scrapie prion liposomes and rods exhibit target sizes of 55,000 Da. *Virology* **164:**537–541.
18. **Bellon, A., W. Seyfert-Brandt, W. Lang, H. Baron, A. Groner, and M. Vey.** 2003. Improved conformation-dependent immunoassay: suitability for human prion detection with enhanced sensitivity. *J. Gen. Virol.* **84:**1921–1925.
19. **Bendheim, P. E., H. R. Brown, R. D. Rudelli, L. J. Scala, N. L. Goller, G. Y. Wen, R. J. Kascsak, N. R. Cashman, and D. C. Bolton.** 1992. Nearly ubiquitous tissue distribution of the scrapie agent precursor protein. *Neurology* **42:**149–156.
20. **Bernoulli, C., J. Siegfried, G. Baumgartner, F. Regli, T. Rabinowicz, D. C. Gajdusek, and C. J. Gibbs, Jr.** 1977. Danger of accidental person-to-person transmission of Creutzfeldt-Jakob disease by surgery. *Lancet* **i:**478–479.
21. **Bessen, R. A., and R. F. Marsh.** 1992. Biochemical and physical properties of the prion protein from two strains of the

transmissible mink encephalopathy agent. *J. Virol.* **66**:2096–2101.

22. **Bone, I., L. Belton, A. S. Walker, and J. Darbyshire.** 2008. Intraventricular pentosan polysulphate in human prion diseases: an observational study in the UK. *Eur. J. Neurol.* **15**:458–464.
23. **Borg, M.** 2006. Symptomatic myoclonus. *Neurophysiol. Clin.* **36**:309–318.
24. **Brandel, J. P., M. Preece, P. Brown, E. Croes, J. L. Laplanche, Y. Agid, R. Will, and A. Alperovitch.** 2003. Distribution of codon 129 genotype in human growth hormone-treated CJD patients in France and the UK. *Lancet* **362**:128–130.
25. **Britton, T. C., S. al-Sarraj, C. Shaw, T. Campbell, and J. Collinge.** 1995. Sporadic Creutzfeldt-Jakob disease in a 16-year-old in the UK. *Lancet* **346**:1155.
26. **Brown, P., J. P. Brandel, M. Preece, and T. Sato.** 2006. Iatrogenic Creutzfeldt-Jakob disease: the waning of an era. *Neurology* **67**:389–393.
27. **Brown, P., C. J. Gibbs, Jr., P. Rodgers-Johnson, D. M. Asher, M. P. Sulima, A. Bacote, L. G. Goldfarb, and D. C. Gajdusek.** 1994. Human spongiform encephalopathy: the National Institutes of Health series of 300 cases of experimentally transmitted disease. *Ann. Neurol.* **35**:513–529.
28. **Brown, P., M. Preece, J. P. Brandel, T. Sato, L. McShane, I. Zerr, A. Fletcher, R. G. Will, M. Pocchiari, N. R. Cashman, J. H. d'Aignaux, L. Cervenakova, J. Fradkin, L. B. Schonberger, and S. J. Collins.** 2000. Iatrogenic Creutzfeldt-Jakob disease at the millennium. *Neurology* **55**:1075–1081.
29. **Brown, P., E. H. Rau, P. Lemieux, B. K. Johnson, A. E. Bacote, and D. C. Gajdusek.** 2004. Infectivity studies of both ash and air emissions from simulated incineration of scrapie-contaminated tissues. *Environ. Sci. Technol.* **38**:6155–6160.
30. **Bruce, M. E.** 1993. Scrapie strain variation and mutation. *Br. Med. Bull.* **49**:822–838.
31. **Bruce, M. E., A. Chree, I. McConnell, J. Foster, G. Pearson, and H. Fraser.** 1994. Transmission of bovine spongiform encephalopathy and scrapie to mice: strain variation and the species barrier. *Philos. Trans. R. Soc. Lond. B* **343**:405–411.
32. **Bruce, M. E., I. McConnell, R. G. Will, and J. W. Ironside.** 2001. Detection of variant Creutzfeldt-Jakob disease infectivity in extraneural tissues. *Lancet* **358**:208–209.
33. **Bruce, M. E., R. G. Will, J. W. Ironside, I. McConnell, D. Drummond, A. Suttie, L. McCardle, A. Chree, J. Hope, C. Birkett, S. Cousens, H. Fraser, and C. J. Bostock.** 1997. Transmissions to mice indicate that 'new variant' CJD is caused by the BSE agent. *Nature* **389**:498–501.
34. **Bueler, H., A. Aguzzi, A. Sailer, R. A. Greiner, P. Autenried, M. Aguet, and C. Weissmann.** 1993. Mice devoid of PrP are resistant to scrapie. *Cell* **73**:1339–1347.
35. **Bueler, H., M. Fischer, Y. Lang, H. Bluethmann, H. P. Lipp, S. J. DeArmond, S. B. Prusiner, M. Aguet, and C. Weissmann.** 1992. Normal development and behaviour of mice lacking the neuronal cell-surface PrP protein. *Nature* **356**:577–582.
36. **Casalone, C., G. Zanusso, P. Acutis, S. Ferrari, L. Capucci, F. Tagliavini, S. Monaco, and M. Caramelli.** 2004. Identification of a second bovine amyloidotic spongiform encephalopathy: molecular similarities with sporadic Creutzfeldt-Jakob disease. *Proc. Natl. Acad. Sci. USA* **101**:3065–3070.
37. **Centers for Disease Control and Prevention.** 2007. Section IV, Laboratory biosafety level criteria. *In* J. Y. Richmond and R. W. McKinney (ed.), *Biosafety in Microbiological and Biomedical Laboratories (BMBL)*, 5th ed. U.S. Government Printing Office, Washington, DC. http://www.cdc.gov/od/ohs/biosfty/bmbl5/bmbl5toc.htm. Accessed 1 August 2008.
38. **Centers for Disease Control and Prevention.** 2007. Section VIII-H, Prion diseases. *In* J. Y. Richmond and R. W. McKinney (ed.), *Biosafety in Microbiological and Biomedical Laboratories (BMBL)*, 5th ed. U.S. Government Printing Office, Washington, DC. http://www.cdc.gov/od/ohs/biosfty/bmbl5/bmbl5toc.htm. Accessed 16 March 2009.

38a. **Centers for Disease Control and Prevention.** 2004. Creutzfeldt-Jakob disease not related to a common venue—New Jersey, 1995-2004. *MMWR Morb. Mortal. Wkly. Rep.* **53**:392–396.

38b. **Centers for Disease Control and Prevention.** 1985. Fatal degenerative neurologic disease in patients who received pituitary-derived human growth hormone. *MMWR Morb. Mortal. Wkly. Rep.* **34**:359–360, 365–366.

38c. **Centers for Disease Control and Prevention.** 2003. Fatal degenerative neurologic illnesses in men who participated in wild game feasts—Wisconsin, 2002. *MMWR Morb. Mortal. Wkly. Rep.* **52**:125–127.

38d. **Centers for Disease Control and Prevention.** 1987. Rapidly progressive dementia in a patient who received a cadaveric dura mater graft. *MMWR Morb. Mortal. Wkly. Rep.* **36**:49–50, 55.

39. **Cervenakova, L., L. G. Goldfarb, R. Garruto, H. S. Lee, D. C. Gajdusek, and P. Brown.** 1998. Phenotype-genotype studies in kuru: implications for new variant Creutzfeldt-Jakob disease. *Proc. Natl. Acad. Sci. USA* **95**:13239–13241.
40. **Chatelain, J., F. Cathala, P. Brown, S. Raharison, L. Court, and D. C. Gajdusek.** 1981. Epidemiologic comparisons between Creutzfeldt-Jakob disease and scrapie in France during the 12-year period 1968-1979. *J. Neurol. Sci.* **51**:329–337.
41. **Chesebro, B., R. Race, K. Wehrly, J. Nishio, M. Bloom, D. Lechner, S. Bergstrom, K. Robbins, L. Mayer, J. M. Keith, C. Garon, and A. Haase.** 1985. Identification of scrapie prion protein-specific mRNA in scrapie-infected and uninfected brain. *Nature* **315**:331–333.
42. **Chesebro, B., M. Trifilo, R. Race, K. Meade-White, C. Teng, R. LaCasse, L. Raymond, C. Favara, G. Baron, S. Priola, B. Caughey, E. Masliah, and M. Oldstone.** 2005. Anchorless prion protein results in infectious amyloid disease without clinical scrapie. *Science* **308**:1435–1439.
43. **Chiti, F., and C. M. Dobson.** 2006. Protein misfolding, functional amyloid, and human disease. *Annu. Rev. Biochem.* **75**:333–366.
44. **Choi, C. J., A. Kanthasamy, V. Anantharam, and A. G. Kanthasamy.** 2006. Interaction of metals with prion protein: possible role of divalent cations in the pathogenesis of prion diseases. *Neurotoxicology* **27**:777–787.
45. **Clarke, P., R. G. Will, and A. C. Ghani.** 2007. Is there the potential for an epidemic of variant Creutzfeldt-Jakob disease via blood transfusion in the UK? *J. R. Soc. Interface* **4**:675–684.
46. **Collinge, J.** 2005. Molecular neurology of prion disease. *J. Neurol. Neurosurg. Psychiatry* **76**:906–919.
47. **Collinge, J., and A. R. Clarke.** 2007. A general model of prion strains and their pathogenicity. *Science* **318**:930–936.
48. **Collinge, J., M. S. Palmer, and A. J. Dryden.** 1991. Genetic predisposition to iatrogenic Creutzfeldt-Jakob disease. *Lancet* **337**:1441–1442.
49. **Collinge, J., M. S. Palmer, K. C. Sidle, I. Gowland, R. Medori, J. Ironside, and P. Lantos.** 1995. Transmission of fatal familial insomnia to laboratory animals. *Lancet* **346**:569–570.
50. **Collinge, J., K. C. Sidle, J. Meads, J. Ironside, and A. F. Hill.** 1996. Molecular analysis of prion strain variation and the aetiology of 'new variant' CJD. *Nature* **383**:685–690.

51. **Collins, S. J., P. Sanchez-Juan, C. L. Masters, G. M. Klug, C. van Duijn, A. Poleggi, M. Pocchiari, S. Almonti, N. Cuadrado-Corrales, J. de Pedro-Cuesta, H. Budka, E. Gelpi, M. Glatzel, M. Tolnay, E. Hewer, I. Zerr, U. Heinemann, H. A. Kretszchmar, G. H. Jansen, E. Olsen, E. Mitrova, A. Alperovitch, J. P. Brandel, J. Mackenzie, K. Murray, and R. G. Will.** 2006. Determinants of diagnostic investigation sensitivities across the clinical spectrum of sporadic Creutzfeldt-Jakob disease. *Brain* **129:**2278–2287.
52. **D'Aignaux, J. H., S. N. Cousens, N. Delasnerie-Laupretre, J. P. Brandel, D. Salomon, J. L. Laplanche, J. J. Hauw, and A. Alperovitch.** 2002. Analysis of the geographical distribution of sporadic Creutzfeldt-Jakob disease in France between 1992 and 1998. *Int. J. Epidemiol.* **31:**490–495.
53. **Darby, S. C., S. W. Kan, R. J. Spooner, P. L. Giangrande, F. G. Hill, C. R. Hay, C. A. Lee, C. A. Ludlam, and M. Williams.** 2007. Mortality rates, life expectancy, and causes of death in people with hemophilia A or B in the United Kingdom who were not infected with HIV. *Blood* **110:**815–825.
54. **Detwiler, L. A., and M. Baylis.** 2003. The epidemiology of scrapie. *Rev. Sci. Tech.* **22:**121–143.
55. **Dietz, K., G. Raddatz, J. Wallis, N. Muller, I. Zerr, H. P. Duerr, H. Lefevre, E. Seifried, and J. Lower.** 2007. Blood transfusion and spread of variant Creutzfeldt-Jakob disease. *Emerg. Infect. Dis.* **13:**89–96.
56. **Donnelly, C. A., N. M. Ferguson, A. C. Ghani, and R. M. Anderson.** 2002. Implications of BSE infection screening data for the scale of the British BSE epidemic and current European infection levels. *Proc. Biol. Sci.* **269:**2179–2190.
57. **Donnelly, C. A., N. M. Ferguson, A. C. Ghani, M. E. Woolhouse, C. J. Watt, and R. M. Anderson.** 1997. The epidemiology of BSE in cattle herds in Great Britain. I. Epidemiological processes, demography of cattle and approaches to control by culling. *Philos. Trans. R. Soc. Lond. B* **352:**781–801.
58. **Duffy, P., J. Wolf, G. Collins, A. G. DeVoe, B. Streeten, and D. Cowen.** 1974.Possible person-to-person transmission of Creutzfeldt-Jakob disease. *N. Engl. J. Med.* **290:**692–693. (Letter.)
59. **Esmonde, T. F., R. G. Will, J. M. Slattery, R. Knight, R. Harries-Jones, R. de Silva, and W. B. Matthews.** 1993. Creutzfeldt-Jakob disease and blood transfusion. *Lancet* **341:**205–207.
60. **Federal Register.** 2005. Agricultural Bioterrorism Protection Act of 2002; possession, use, and transfer of biological agents and toxins, final rule. *Fed. Regist.* **70:**13242–13292. http://www.selectagents.gov/resources/APHISFinalRule.pdf. Accessed 16 March 2009.
61. **Fichet, G., E. Comoy, C. Duval, K. Antloga, C. Dehen, A. Charbonnier, G. McDonnell, P. Brown, C. I. Lasmezas, and J. P. Deslys.** 2004. Novel methods for disinfection of prion-contaminated medical devices. *Lancet* **364:**521–526.
62. **Flechsig, E., D. Shmerling, I. Hegyi, A. J. Raeber, M. Fischer, A. Cozzio, C. von Mering, A. Aguzzi, and C. Weissmann.** 2000. Prion protein devoid of the octapeptide repeat region restores susceptibility to scrapie in PrP knockout mice. *Neuron* **27:**399–408.
63. **Ford, M. J., L. J. Burton, R. J. Morris, and S. M. Hall.** 2002. Selective expression of prion protein in peripheral tissues of the adult mouse. *Neuroscience* **113:**177–192.
64. **Fraser, H., G. R. Pearson, I. McConnell, M. E. Bruce, J. M. Wyatt, and T. J. Gruffydd-Jones.** 1994. Transmission of feline spongiform encephalopathy to mice. *Vet. Rec.* **134:**449.
65. **Gajdusek, D. C.** 1977. Unconventional viruses and the origin and disappearance of kuru. *Science* **197:**943–960.
66. **Gajdusek, D. C., C. J. Gibbs, and M. Alpers.** 1966. Experimental transmission of a Kuru-like syndrome to chimpanzees. *Nature* **209:**794–796.
67. **Gambetti, P., Z. Dong, J. Yuan, X. Xiao, M. Zheng, A. Alshekhlee, R. Castellani, M. Cohen, M. A. Barria, D. Gonzalez-Romero, E. D. Belay, L. B. Schonberger, K. Marder, C. Harris, J. R. Burke, T. Montine, T. Wisniewski, D. W. Dickson, C. Soto, C. M. Hulette, J. A. Mastrianni, Q. Kong, and W. Q. Zou.** 2008. A novel human disease with abnormal prion protein sensitive to protease. *Ann. Neurol.* **63:**697–708.
68. **Gambetti, P., P. Parchi, and S. G. Chen.** 2003. Hereditary Creutzfeldt-Jakob disease and fatal familial insomnia. *Clin. Lab. Med.* **23:**43–64.
69. **Gibbs, C. J., Jr., D. M. Asher, A. Kobrine, H. L. Amyx, M. P. Sulima, and D. C. Gajdusek.** 1994. Transmission of Creutzfeldt-Jakob disease to a chimpanzee by electrodes contaminated during neurosurgery. *J. Neurol. Neurosurg. Psychiatry* **57:**757–758.
70. **Gibbs, C. J., Jr., D. C. Gajdusek, D. M. Asher, M. P. Alpers, E. Beck, P. M. Daniel, and W. B. Matthews.** 1968. Creutzfeldt-Jakob disease (spongiform encephalopathy): transmission to the chimpanzee. *Science* **161:**388–389.
71. **Gigi, A., E. Vakil, E. Kahana, and U. Hadar.** 2005. Presymptomatic signs in healthy CJD mutation carriers. *Dement. Geriatr. Cogn. Disord.* **19:**246–255.
72. **Glatzel, M., E. Abela, M. Maissen, and A. Aguzzi.** 2003. Extraneural pathologic prion protein in sporadic Creutzfeldt-Jakob disease. *N. Engl. J. Med.* **349:**1812–1820.
73. **Glatzel, M., K. Stoeck, H. Seeger, T. Luhrs, and A. Aguzzi.** 2005. Human prion diseases: molecular and clinical aspects. *Arch. Neurol.* **62:**545–552.
74. **Gordon, W. S.** 1946. Advances in veterinary research: Louping-ill tick-borne fever and scrapie. *Vet. Res.* **58:**516–520.
75. **Goudsmit, J., C. H. Morrow, D. M. Asher, R. T. Yanagihara, C. L. Masters, C. J. Gibbs, Jr., and D. C. Gajdusek.** 1980. Evidence for and against the transmissibility of Alzheimer disease. *Neurology* **30:**945–950.
76. **Grassi, J., S. Maillet, S. Simon, and N. Morel.** 2008. Progress and limits of TSE diagnostic tools. *Vet. Res.* **39:**33.
77. **Groschup, M. H., and A. Buschmann.** 2008. Rodent models for prion diseases. *Vet. Res.* **39:**32.
78. **Hadlow, W. J.** 1959. Scrapie and kuru. *Lancet* **274:**289–290.
79. **Harman, J. L., and C. J. Silva.** 2009. Bovine spongiform encephalopathy. *J. Am. Vet. Med. Assoc.* **234:**59–72.
80. **Harris, D. A.** 2003. Trafficking, turnover and membrane topology of PrP. *Br. Med. Bull.* **66:**71–85.
81. **Herzberg, L., B. N. Herzberg, C. J. Gibbs, Jr., W. Sullivan, H. Amyx, and D. C. Gajdusek.** 1974. Creutzfeldt-Jakob disease: hypothesis for high incidence in Libyan Jews in Israel. *Science* **186:**848. (Letter.)
82. **Hewitt, P. E., C. A. Llewelyn, J. Mackenzie, and R. G. Will.** 2006. Creutzfeldt-Jakob disease and blood transfusion: results of the UK Transfusion Medicine Epidemiological Review study. *Vox Sang.* **91:**221–230.
83. **Hill, A. F., R. J. Butterworth, S. Joiner, G. Jackson, M. N. Rossor, D. J. Thomas, A. Frosh, N. Tolley, J. E. Bell, M. Spencer, A. King, S. Al-Sarraj, J. W. Ironside, P. L. Lantos, and J. Collinge.** 1999. Investigation of variant Creutzfeldt-Jakob disease and other human prion diseases with tonsil biopsy samples. *Lancet* **353:**183–189.
84. **Hill, A. F., M. Desbruslais, S. Joiner, K. C. Sidle, I. Gowland, J. Collinge, L. J. Doey, and P. Lantos.** 1997. The same prion strain causes vCJD and BSE. *Nature* **389:**448–450, 526.
85. **Hilton, D. A., A. C. Ghani, L. Conyers, P. Edwards, L. McCardle, D. Ritchie, M. Penney, D. Hegazy, and J. W. Ironside.** 2004. Prevalence of lymphoreticular prion protein accumulation in UK tissue samples. *J. Pathol.* **203:**733–739.

86. **Hsiao, K. K., D. Groth, M. Scott, S. L. Yang, H. Serban, D. Rapp, D. Foster, M. Torchia, S. J. Dearmond, and S. B. Prusiner.** 1994. Serial transmission in rodents of neurodegeneration from transgenic mice expressing mutant prion protein. *Proc. Natl. Acad. Sci. USA* **91**:9126–9130.
87. **Hsiao, K. K., M. Scott, D. Foster, D. F. Groth, S. J. DeArmond, and S. B. Prusiner.** 1990. Spontaneous neurodegeneration in transgenic mice with mutant prion protein. *Science* **250**:1587–1590.
88. **Ironside, J. W., M. T. Bishop, K. Connolly, D. Hegazy, S. Lowrie, M. Le Grice, D. L. Ritchie, L. M. McCardle, and D. A. Hilton.** 2006. Variant Creutzfeldt-Jakob disease: prion protein genotype analysis of positive appendix tissue samples from a retrospective prevalence study. *BMJ* **332**:1186–1188.
89. **Ironside, J. W., D. A. Hilton, A. Ghani, N. J. Johnston, L. Conyers, L. M. McCardle, and D. Best.** 2000. Retrospective study of prion-protein accumulation in tonsil and appendix tissues. *Lancet* **355**:1693–1694.
90. **Ironside, J. W., K. Sutherland, J. E. Bell, L. McCardle, C. Barrie, K. Estebeiro, M. Zeidler, and R. G. Will.** 1996. A new variant of Creutzfeldt-Jakob disease: neuropathological and clinical features. *Cold Spring Harb. Symp. Quant. Biol.* **61**:523–530.
91. **Jones, M., A. Peden, C. Prowse, A. Groner, J. Manson, M. Turner, J. Ironside, I. Macgregor, and M. Head.** 2007. In vitro amplification and detection of variant Creutzfeldt-Jakob disease PrP(Sc). *J. Pathol.* **213**:21–26.
92. **Kimberlin, R. H., S. Cole, and C. A. Walker.** 1987. Temporary and permanent modifications to a single strain of mouse scrapie on transmission to rats and hamsters. *J. Gen. Virol.* **68**:1875–1881.
93. **King, S.** 2008. French doctors on trial for manslaughter. *Lancet* **371**:637.
94. **Kirkwood, J. K., and A. A. Cunningham.** 1994. Epidemiological observations on spongiform encephalopathies in captive wild animals in the British Isles. *Vet. Rec.* **135**:296–303.
95. **Klatzo, I., D. C. Gajdusek, and V. Zigas.** 1959. Pathology of Kuru. *Lab. Invest.* **8**:799–847.
96. **Knight, R.** 1998. The diagnosis of prion diseases. *Parasitology* **117**(Suppl):S3–S11.
97. **Kocisko, D. A., and B. Caughey.** 2006. Searching for anti-prion compounds: cell-based high-throughput in vitro assays and animal testing strategies. *Methods Enzymol.* **412**:223–234.
98. **Kong, Q., S. Huang, W. Zou, D. Vanegas, M. Wang, D. Wu, J. Yuan, M. Zheng, H. Bai, H. Deng, K. Chen, A. L. Jenny, K. O'Rourke, E. D. Belay, L. B. Schonberger, R. B. Petersen, M. S. Sy, S. G. Chen, and P. Gambetti.** 2005. Chronic wasting disease of elk: transmissibility to humans examined by transgenic mouse models. *J. Neurosci.* **25**:7944–7949.
99. **Kong, Q., W. K. Surewicz, R. B. Petersen, W. Q. Zou, S. G. Chen, P. Gambetti, P. Parchi, S. Capellari, L. G. Goldfarb, P. Montagna, E. Lugaresi, P. Picardo, and B. Ghetti.** 2004. Inherited prion diseases, p. 673–775. *In* S. B. Prusiner (ed.), *Prion Biology and Diseases,* 2nd ed. Cold Spring Harbor Laboratory Press, New York, NY.
100. **Kovacs, G. G., M. Puopolo, A. Ladogana, M. Pocchiari, H. Budka, C. van Duijn, S. J. Collins, A. Boyd, A. Giulivi, M. Coulthart, N. Delasnerie-Laupretre, J. P. Brandel, I. Zerr, H. A. Kretzschmar, J. de Pedro-Cuesta, M. Calero-Lara, M. Glatzel, A. Aguzzi, M. Bishop, R. Knight, G. Belay, R. Will, and E. Mitrova.** 2005. Genetic prion disease: the EUROCJD experience. *Hum. Genet.* **118**:166–174.
101. **Krasnianski, A., B. Meissner, U. Heinemann, and I. Zerr.** 2004. Clinical findings and diagnostic tests in Creutzfeldt-Jakob disease and variant Creutzfeldt-Jakob disease. *Folia Neuropathol.* **42**(Suppl. B):24–38.
102. **Kuczius, T., R. Koch, K. Keyvani, H. Karch, J. Grassi, and M. H. Groschup.** 2007. Regional and phenotype heterogeneity of cellular prion proteins in the human brain. *Eur. J. Neurosci.* **25**:2649–2655.
103. **Ladogana, A., M. Puopolo, E. A. Croes, H. Budka, C. Jarius, S. Collins, G. M. Klug, T. Sutcliffe, A. Giulivi, A. Alperovitch, N. Delasnerie-Laupretre, J. P. Brandel, S. Poser, H. Kretzschmar, I. Rietveld, E. Mitrova, P. Cuesta Jde, P. Martinez-Martin, M. Glatzel, A. Aguzzi, R. Knight, H. Ward, M. Pocchiari, C. M. van Duijn, R. G. Will, and I. Zerr.** 2005. Mortality from Creutzfeldt-Jakob disease and related disorders in Europe, Australia, and Canada. *Neurology* **64**:1586–1591.
104. **Lasmezas, C. I., J. P. Deslys, R. Demaimay, K. T. Adjou, F. Lamoury, D. Dormont, O. Robain, J. Ironside, and J. J. Hauw.** 1996. BSE transmission to macaques. *Nature* **381**:743–744.
105. **Lewis, V., G. M. Klug, A. F. Hill, and S. J. Collins.** 2008. Molecular typing of PrP(res) in human sporadic CJD brain tissue. *Methods Mol. Biol.* **459**:241–247.
106. **Liberski, P. P., and P. Brown.** 2007. Kuru—fifty years later. *Neurol. Neurochir. Pol.* **41**:548–556.
107. **Liberski, P. P., and H. Budka.** 2004. Gerstmann-Straussler-Scheinker disease. I. Human diseases. *Folia Neuropathol.* **42**(Suppl. B):120–140.
108. **Lipp, H. P., M. Stagliar-Bozicevic, M. Fischer, and D. P. Wolfer.** 1998. A 2-year longitudinal study of swimming navigation in mice devoid of the prion protein: no evidence for neurological anomalies or spatial learning impairments. *Behav. Brain Res.* **95**:47–54.
109. **Mallucci, G., A. Dickinson, J. Linehan, P. C. Klohn, S. Brandner, and J. Collinge.** 2003. Depleting neuronal PrP in prion infection prevents disease and reverses spongiosis. *Science* **302**:871–874.
110. **Mallucci, G. R., M. D. White, M. Farmer, A. Dickinson, H. Khatun, A. D. Powell, S. Brandner, J. G. Jefferys, and J. Collinge.** 2007. Targeting cellular prion protein reverses early cognitive deficits and neurophysiological dysfunction in prion-infected mice. *Neuron* **53**:325–335.
111. **Marsh, R. F., and W. J. Hadlow.** 1992. Transmissible mink encephalopathy. *Rev. Sci. Tech.* **11**:539–550.
112. **Matthews, W. B., and R. G. Will.** 1981. Creutzfeldt-Jakob disease in a lifelong vegetarian. *Lancet* **ii**:937.
113. **Mawhinney, S., W. J. Pape, J. E. Forster, C. A. Anderson, P. Bosque, and M. W. Miller.** 2006. Human prion disease and relative risk associated with chronic wasting disease. *Emerg. Infect. Dis.* **12**:1527–1535.
114. **Mead, S.** 2006. Prion disease genetics. *Eur. J. Hum. Genet.* **14**:273–281.
115. **Mead, S., S. Joiner, M. Desbruslais, J. A. Beck, M. O'Donoghue, P. Lantos, J. D. Wadsworth, and J. Collinge.** 2007. Creutzfeldt-Jakob disease, prion protein gene codon 129VV, and a novel PrPSc type in a young British woman. *Arch. Neurol.* **64**:1780–1784.
116. **Meiner, Z., R. Gabizon, and S. B. Prusiner.** 1997. Familial Creutzfeldt-Jakob disease. Codon 200 prion disease in Libyan Jews. *Medicine* (Baltimore) **76**:227–237.
117. **Meyer-Luehmann, M., J. Coomaraswamy, T. Bolmont, S. Kaeser, C. Schaefer, E. Kilger, A. Neuenschwander, D. Abramowski, P. Frey, A. L. Jaton, J. M. Vigouret, P. Paganetti, D. M. Walsh, P. M. Mathews, J. Ghiso, M. Staufenbiel, L. C. Walker, and M. Jucker.** 2006. Exogenous

induction of cerebral beta-amyloidogenesis is governed by agent and host. *Science* **313:**1781–1784.

118. **Montagna, P., P. Gambetti, P. Cortelli, and E. Lugaresi.** 2003. Familial and sporadic fatal insomnia. *Lancet Neurol.* **2:**167–176.
119. **Muller-Schiffmann, A., and C. Korth.** 2008. Vaccine approaches to prevent and treat prion infection: progress and challenges. *BioDrugs* **22:**45–52.
120. **Murray, K., D. L. Ritchie, M. Bruce, C. A. Young, M. Doran, J. W. Ironside, and R. G. Will.** 2008. Sporadic creutzfeldt-jakob disease in two adolescents. *J. Neurol. Neurosurg. Psychiatry* **79:**14–18.
121. **Nathanson, N., J. Wilesmith, and C. Griot.** 1997. Bovine spongiform encephalopathy (BSE): causes and consequences of a common source epidemic. *Am. J. Epidemiol.* **145:**959–969.
122. **National Creutzfeldt-Jakob Disease Surveillance Unit.** 2008. Variant Creuzfeldt-Jakob disease current data (February 2009). National CJD Surveillance Unit, Edinburgh, Scotland. http://www.cjd.ed.ac.uk/vcjdworld.htm. Accessed 16 March 2009.
123. Reference deleted.
124. **Neuendorf, E., A. Weber, A. Saalmueller, H. Schatzl, K. Reifenberg, E. Pfaff, and M. H. Groschup.** 2004. Glycosylation deficiency at either one of the two glycan attachment sites of cellular prion protein preserves susceptibility to bovine spongiform encephalopathy and scrapie infections. *J. Biol. Chem.* **279:**53306–53316.
125. **NIH.** Appendix B-III-D, Risk group 3 (RG3) - viruses and prions. *In NIH Guidelines for Research Involving Recombinant DNA Molecules.* National Institutes of Health, Bethesda, MD. http://www4.od.nih.gov/oba/rac/guidelines_02/NIH_Guidelines_Apr_02.htm. Accessed 16 March 2009.
126. **Obici, L., V. Perfetti, G. Palladini, R. Moratti, and G. Merlini.** 2005. Clinical aspects of systemic amyloid diseases. *Biochim. Biophys. Acta* **1753:**11–22.
127. **Oesch, B., D. Westaway, M. Walchli, M. P. McKinley, S. B. Kent, R. Aebersold, R. A. Barry, P. Tempst, D. B. Teplow, L. E. Hood, S. B. Prusiner, and C. Weissmann.** 1985. A cellular gene encodes scrapie PrP 27-30 protein. *Cell* **40:**735–746.
128. **Onisko, B. C., C. J. Silva, I. Dynin, M. Erickson, W. H. Vensel, R. Hnasko, J. R. Requena, and J. M. Carter.** 2007. Sensitive, preclinical detection of prions in brain by nanospray liquid chromatography/tandem mass spectrometry. *Rapid Commun. Mass Spectrom.* **21:**4023–4026.
129. **Palmer, M. S., A. J. Dryden, J. T. Hughes, and J. Collinge.** 1991. Homozygous prion protein genotype predisposes to sporadic Creutzfeldt-Jakob disease. *Nature* **352:**340–342.
130. **Parry, H. B.** 1962. Scrapie: a transmissible and hereditary disease of sheep. *Heredity* **17:**75–105.
131. **Pattison, I. H.** 1965. Experiments with scrapie with special reference to the nature of the agent and the pathology of the disease, p. 249–257. *In* C. J. Gajdusek, C. J. Gibbs, and M. P. Alpers (eds.), *Slow, Latent, and Temperate Virus Infections.* U.S. Government Printing Office, Washington, DC.
132. **Pattison, I. H.** 1965. Resistance of the scrapie agent to formalin. *J. Comp. Pathol.* **75:**159–164.
133. **Peden, A. H., M. W. Head, D. L. Ritchie, J. E. Bell, and J. W. Ironside.** 2004. Preclinical vCJD after blood transfusion in a PRNP codon 129 heterozygous patient. *Lancet* **364:**527–529.
134. **Peden, A. H., D. L. Ritchie, M. W. Head, and J. W. Ironside.** 2006. Detection and localization of PrPSc in the skeletal muscle of patients with variant, iatrogenic, and sporadic forms of Creutzfeldt-Jakob disease. *Am. J. Pathol.* **168:**927–935.
135. **Peet, R. L., and J. M. Curran.** 1992. Spongiform encephalopathy in an imported cheetah (*Acinonyx jubatus*). *Aust. Vet. J.* **69:**171.
136. **Peretz, D., S. Supattapone, K. Giles, J. Vergara, Y. Freyman, P. Lessard, J. G. Safar, D. V. Glidden, C. McCulloch, H. O. Nguyen, M. Scott, S. J. Dearmond, and S. B. Prusiner.** 2006. Inactivation of prions by acidic sodium dodecyl sulfate. *J. Virol.* **80:**322–331.
137. **Piccardo, P., J. C. Manson, D. King, B. Ghetti, and R. M. Barron.** 2007. Accumulation of prion protein in the brain that is not associated with transmissible disease. *Proc. Natl. Acad. Sci. USA* **104:**4712–4717.
138. **Prusiner, S. B.** 2004. An introduction to prion biology and diseases, p. 1–87. *In* S. B. Prusiner (ed.), *Prion Biology and Diseases,* 2nd ed. Cold Spring Harbor Laboratory Press, Cold Spring Harbor, New York, NY.
139. **Prusiner, S. B.** 1982. Novel proteinaceous infectious particles cause scrapie. *Science* **216:**136–144.
140. **Prusiner, S. B.** 1998. Prions. *Proc. Natl. Acad. Sci. USA* **95:**13363–13383.
141. **Prusiner, S. B.** 1984. Prions: novel infectious pathogens. *Adv. Virus. Res.* **29:**1–56.
142. **Prusiner, S. B., M. Scott, D. Foster, K. M. Pan, D. Groth, C. Mirenda, M. Torchia, S. L. Yang, D. Serban, G. A. Carlson, P. C. Hoppe, D. Westaway, and S. J. DeArmond.** 1990. Transgenetic studies implicate interactions between homologous PrP isoforms in scrapie prion replication. *Cell* **63:**673–686.
143. **Race, R. E., and G. J. Raymond.** 2004. Inactivation of transmissible spongiform encephalopathy (prion) agents by environ LpH. *J. Virol.* **78:**2164–2165.
144. **Richt, J. A., P. Kasinathan, A. N. Hamir, J. Castilla, T. Sathiyaseelan, F. Vargas, J. Sathiyaseelan, H. Wu, H. Matsushita, J. Koster, S. Kato, I. Ishida, C. Soto, J. M. Robl, and Y. Kuroiwa.** 2007. Production of cattle lacking prion protein. *Nat. Biotechnol.* **25:**132–138.
145. **Riesner, D.** 2003. Biochemistry and structure of PrP(C) and PrP(Sc). *Br. Med. Bull.* **66:**21–33.
146. **Rudd, P. M., T. Endo, C. Colominas, D. Groth, S. F. Wheeler, D. J. Harvey, M. R. Wormald, H. Serban, S. B. Prusiner, A. Kobata, and R. A. Dwek.** 1999. Glycosylation differences between the normal and pathogenic prion protein isoforms. *Proc. Natl. Acad. Sci. USA* **96:**13044–13049.
147. **Saborio, G. P., B. Permanne, and C. Soto.** 2001. Sensitive detection of pathological prion protein by cyclic amplification of protein misfolding. *Nature* **411:**810–813.
148. **Safar, J., H. Wille, V. Itri, D. Groth, H. Serban, M. Torchia, F. E. Cohen, and S. B. Prusiner.** 1998. Eight prion strains have PrP(Sc) molecules with different conformations. *Nat. Med.* **4:**1157–1165.
149. **Scott, M., D. Foster, C. Mirenda, D. Serban, F. Coufal, M. Walchli, M. Torchia, D. Groth, G. Carlson, S. J. DeArmond, D. Westaway, and S. B. Prusiner.** 1989. Transgenic mice expressing hamster prion protein produce species-specific scrapie infectivity and amyloid plaques. *Cell* **59:**847–857.
150. **Shiga, Y., K. Satoh, T. Kitamoto, S. Kanno, I. Nakashima, S. Sato, K. Fujihara, H. Takata, K. Nobukuni, S. Kuroda, H. Takano, Y. Umeda, H. Konno, K. Nagasato, A. Satoh, Y. Matsuda, M. Hidaka, H. Takahashi, Y. Sano, K. Kim, T. Konishi, K. Doh-ura, T. Sato, K. Sasaki, Y. Nakamura, M. Yamada, H. Mizusawa, and Y. Itoyama.** 2007. Two different clinical phenotypes of Creutzfeldt-Jakob disease with a M232R substitution. *J. Neurol.* **254:**1509–1517.
151. **Si, K., S. Lindquist, and E. R. Kandel.** 2003. A neuronal isoform of the aplysia CPEB has prion-like properties. *Cell* **115:**879–891.

152. **Somerville, R. A., A. Chong, O. U. Mulqueen, C. R. Birkett, S. C. Wood, and J. Hope.** 1997. Biochemical typing of scrapie strains. *Nature* **386:**564.
153. **Stahl, N., M. A. Baldwin, R. Hecker, K. M. Pan, A. L. Burlingame, and S. B. Prusiner.** 1992. Glycosylinositol phospholipid anchors of the scrapie and cellular prion proteins contain sialic acid. *Biochemistry* **31:**5043–5053.
154. **Stahl, N., M. Baldwin, D. B. Teplow, C. E. Hood, R. Beavis, J. B. Chait, B. Bibson, A. L. Bulingame, and S. B. Prusiner.** 1992. Cataloging post-translational modifications of the scrapie prion protein by mass spectrometry, p. 361–379. *In* S. B. Prusiner, J. Collinge, J. Powell, and B. Anderton (eds), *Prion Diseases of Humans and Animals*. Ellis Horwood, New York, NY.
155. **Stewart, L. A., L. H. Rydzewska, G. F. Keogh, and R. S. Knight.** 2008. Systematic review of therapeutic interventions in human prion disease. *Neurology* **70:**1272–1281.
156. **Strumbo, B., S. Ronchi, L. C. Bolis, and T. Simonic.** 2001. Molecular cloning of the cDNA coding for *Xenopus laevis* prion protein. *FEBS Lett.* **508:**170–174.
157. **Supattapone, S., P. Bosque, T. Muramoto, H. Wille, C. Aagaard, D. Peretz, H. O. Nguyen, C. Heinrich, M. Torchia, J. Safar, F. E. Cohen, S. J. DeArmond, S. B. Prusiner, and M. Scott.** 1999. Prion protein of 106 residues creates an artifical transmission barrier for prion replication in transgenic mice. *Cell* **96:**869–878.
158. **Supattapone, S., E. Bouzamondo, H. L. Ball, H. Wille, H. O. Nguyen, F. E. Cohen, S. J. DeArmond, S. B. Prusiner, and M. Scott.** 2001. A protease-resistant 61-residue prion peptide causes neurodegeneration in transgenic mice. *Mol. Cell. Biol.* **21:**2608–2616.
159. **Supervie, V., and D. Costagliola.** 2004. The unrecognised French BSE epidemic. *Vet. Res.* **35:**349–362.
160. **Taylor, D. M.** 2000. Inactivation of transmissible degenerative encephalopathy agents: a review. *Vet. J.* **159:** 10–17.
161. **Taylor, D. M.** 2004. Resistance of transmissible spongiform encephalopathy agents to decontamination. *Contrib. Microbiol.* **11:**136–145.
162. **Taylor, D. M., A. G. Dickinson, H. Fraser, P. A. Robertson, P. R. Salacinski, and P. J. Lowry.** 1985. Preparation of growth hormone free from contamination with unconventional slow viruses. *Lancet* **ii:**260–262.
163. **Tennent, G. A., M. W. Head, M. Bishop, P. N. Hawkins, R. G. Will, R. Knight, A. H. Peden, L. M. McCardle, J. W. Ironside, and M. B. Pepys.** 2007. Disease-associated prion protein is not detectable in human systemic amyloid deposits. *J. Pathol.* **213:**376–383.
164. **Todd, N. V., J. Morrow, K. Doh-ura, S. Dealler, S. O'Hare, P. Farling, M. Duddy, and N. G. Rainov.** 2005. Cerebroventricular infusion of pentosan polysulphate in human variant Creutzfeldt-Jakob disease. *J. Infect.* **50:**394–396.
165. **Trevitt, C. R., and J. Collinge.** 2006. A systematic review of prion therapeutics in experimental models. *Brain* **129:**2241–2265.
166. **Trifilo, M. J., M. Sanchez-Alavez, L. Solforosi, J. Bernard-Trifilo, S. Kunz, D. McGavern, and M. B. Oldstone.** 2008. Scrapie-induced defects in learning and memory of transgenic mice expressing anchorless prion protein are associated with alterations in the GABAergic pathway. *J. Virol.* **82:**9890–9899.
167. **Tuzi, N. L., E. Cancellotti, H. Baybutt, L. Blackford, B. Bradford, C. Plinston, A. Coghill, P. Hart, P. Piccardo, R. M. Barron, and J. C. Manson.** 2008. Host PrP glycosylation: a major factor determining the outcome of prion infection. *PLoS Biol.* **6:**e100.
168. **Wadsworth, J. D., E. A. Asante, M. Desbruslais, J. M. Linehan, S. Joiner, I. Gowland, J. Welch, L. Stone, S. E. Lloyd, A. F. Hill, S. Brandner, and J. Collinge.** 2004. Human prion protein with valine 129 prevents expression of variant CJD phenotype. *Science* **306:**1793–1796.
169. **Wadsworth, J. D., S. Joiner, A. F. Hill, T. A. Campbell, M. Desbruslais, P. J. Luthert, and J. Collinge.** 2001. Tissue distribution of protease resistant prion protein in variant Creutzfeldt-Jakob disease using a highly sensitive immunoblotting assay. *Lancet* **358:**171–180.
170. **Wadsworth, J. D., C. Powell, J. A. Beck, S. Joiner, J. M. Linehan, S. Brandner, S. Mead, and J. Collinge.** 2008. Molecular diagnosis of human prion disease. *Methods Mol. Biol.* **459:**197–227.
171. **Weissmann, C., and E. Flechsig.** 2003. PrP knock-out and PrP transgenic mice in prion research. *Br. Med. Bull.* **66:**43–60.
172. **Wells, G. A., A. C. Scott, C. T. Johnson, R. F. Gunning, R. D. Hancock, M. Jeffrey, M. Dawson, and R. Bradley.** 1987. A novel progressive spongiform encephalopathy in cattle. *Vet. Rec.* **121:**419–420.
173. **Whittle, I. R., R. S. Knight, and R. G. Will.** 2006. Unsuccessful intraventricular pentosan polysulphate treatment of variant Creutzfeldt-Jakob disease. *Acta Neurochir. (Wien)* **148:**677–679.
174. **Wickner, R. B., H. K. Edskes, B. T. Roberts, U. Baxa, M. M. Pierce, E. D. Ross, and A. Brachmann.** 2004. Prions: proteins as genes and infectious entities. *Genes Dev.* **18:**470–485.
175. **Wilesmith, J. W., G. A. Wells, M. P. Cranwell, and J. B. Ryan.** 1988. Bovine spongiform encephalopathy: epidemiological studies. *Vet. Rec.* **123:**638–644.
176. **Will, R. G., A. Alperovitch, S. Poser, M. Pocchiari, A. Hofman, E. Mitrova, R. de Silva, M. D'Alessandro, N. Delasnerie-Laupretre, I. Zerr, and C. van Duijn.** 1998. Descriptive epidemiology of Creutzfeldt-Jakob disease in six European countries, 1993-1995. EU Collaborative Study Group for CJD. *Ann. Neurol.* **43:**763–767.
177. **Will, R. G., J. W. Ironside, M. Zeidler, S. N. Cousens, K. Estibeiro, A. Alperovitch, S. Poser, M. Pocchiari, A. Hofman, and P. G. Smith.** 1996. A new variant of Creutzfeldt-Jakob disease in the UK. *Lancet* **347:**921–925.
178. **Williams, E. S.** 2005. Chronic wasting disease. *Vet. Pathol.* **42:**530–549.
179. **Wilson, K., C. Code, and M. N. Ricketts.** 2000. Risk of acquiring Creutzfeldt-Jakob disease from blood transfusions: systematic review of case-control studies. *BMJ* **321:**17–19.
180. **Wopfner, F., G. Weidenhofer, R. Schneider, A. von Brunn, S. Gilch, T. F. Schwarz, T. Werner, and H. M. Schatzl.** 1999. Analysis of 27 mammalian and 9 avian PrPs reveals high conservation of flexible regions of the prion protein. *J. Mol. Biol.* **289:**1163–1178.
181. **World Health Organization.** 1998. Global surveillance, diagnosis and therapy of human transmissible spongiform encephalopathies: report of a WHO consultation, Geneva, Switzerland, 9–11 February 1998. Report no. WHO/EMC/ZDI/98.9 World Health Organization, Geneva, Switzerland. http://www.who.int/csr/resources/publications/bse/whoemc zdi 989.pdf. Accessed 16 March 2009.
182. **World Health Organization.** 1999. WHO infection control guidelines for transmissible spongiform encephalopathies. Report of a WHO consultation, Geneva, Switzerland, 23-26 March 1999. Report no. WHO/CDS/CSR/APH/2000/3. World Health Organization, Geneva, Switzerland. http://www.who.int/csr/resources/publications/bse/whocdscsraph 2003.pdf. Accessed 16 March 2009.

183. **World Health Organization.** 2001. The revision of the surveillance case definition for variant Creutzfeldt-Jakob Disease (vCJD). Report of a WHO consultation, Edinburgh, United Kingdom 17 May 2001. Report no. WHO/CDS/CSR/EPH/2001.5. World Health Organization, Geneva, Switzerland. http://www.who.int/csr/resources/publications/bse/whocdscsreph20015.pdf. Accessed 16 March 2009.
184. **World Organisation for Animal Health** (OIE). 2008. Number of reported cases of bovine spongiform encephalopathy (BSE) in farmed cattle worldwide. July 24, 2008. World Organisation for Animal Health, Paris, France. http://www.oie.int/eng/info/en_esbmonde.htm. Accessed 16 March 2009.
185. **Wyatt, J. M., G. R. Pearson, T. N. Smerdon, T. J. Gruffydd-Jones, G. A. Wells, and J. W. Wilesmith.** 1991. Naturally occurring scrapie-like spongiform encephalopathy in five domestic cats. *Vet. Rec.* **129:**233–236.
186. **Zerr, I., and S. Poser.** 2002. Clinical diagnosis and differential diagnosis of CJD and vCJD. With special emphasis on laboratory tests. *APMIS* **110:**88–98.
187. **Zhang, B., Y. Une, X. Fu, J. Yan, F. Ge, J. Yao, J. Sawashita, M. Mori, H. Tomozawa, F. Kametani, and K. Higuchi.** 2008. Fecal transmission of AA amyloidosis in the cheetah contributes to high incidence of disease. *Proc. Natl. Acad. Sci. USA* **105:**7263–7268.
188. **Zomosa-Signoret, V., J. D. Arnaud, P. Fontes, M. T. Alvarez-Martinez, and J. P. Liautard.** 2008. Physiological role of the cellular prion protein. *Vet. Res.* **39:**9.
189. **Zou, S., C. T. Fang, and L. B. Schonberger.** 2008. Transfusion transmission of human prion diseases. *Transfus. Med. Rev.* **22:**58–69.

Sequelae and Long-Term Consequences of Infectious Diseases
Edited by Pina M. Fratamico, James L. Smith, and Kim A. Brogden

Chapter 25

Infection with *Porphyromonas gingivalis*, a Potential Risk Factor for Chronic Systemic Disease

Sophie Joly, Myriam Bélanger, Georgia K. Johnson, Ann Progulske-Fox, and Kim A. Brogden

Polymicrobial diseases in humans result from the clinical and pathological manifestations induced by the presence of multiple microorganisms (13). These diseases are complex and caused by infections with multiple viruses, multiple bacteria, multiple fungi, or any combination of viruses, bacteria, and fungi. At times, the causative microorganisms are difficult to isolate, identify, and treat. Immunocompromised individuals are particularly susceptible (13). In some instances, polymicrobial diseases lead to chronic inflammation and tissue damage that has long-term consequences for the individual.

Periodontal disease is a polymicrobial disease involving multiple microorganisms in a well-defined biofilm environment (44) (Fig. 1). If untreated, the microorganisms in these biofilms can have a detrimental effect on both oral and systemic health. In this chapter, periodontal disease will be used as an example of a polymicrobial disease that represents a potential risk factor for chronic systemic diseases. Recent research has focused on the contribution of periodontal infection to systemic infection, placing an individual at potential risk for (i) developing coronary artery disease, cerebrovascular disease, and peripheral arterial disease; (ii) delivering preterm low-birth-weight infants; (iii) developing respiratory infections; and (iv) exacerbating preexisting chronic inflammatory conditions, like rheumatoid arthritis and diabetes (Table 1). The focus will be on *Porphyromonas gingivalis,* a predominant periodontopathogenic bacterium that can leave the oral cavity, enter the circulatory system, and invade the vascular endothelium and cardiac tissues.

PERIODONTAL DISEASE AS A POLYMICROBIAL DISEASE

The oral cavity contains extensive numbers of diverse microorganisms. Saliva contains ~10^8 total microorganisms/ml, and plaque, if present, contains ~10^{11} total microorganisms/gram (149). The latter subgingival microbial community is estimated to contain more than 700 phylotypes (1, 99, 115). Also, many microorganisms within the oral cavity have site-specific tropisms. For example, the microbiota of the tongue is different from that of the gingival crevice (147).

Periodontal disease is an inflammatory disease of the supporting tissues of the teeth caused by the host response to the presence of specific microorganisms or groups of microorganisms (76). Ultimately, periodontal infection results in progressive destruction of the periodontal ligament and alveolar bone and can result in tooth loss in adults (21, 52).

Periodontal disease has a polymicrobial etiology. An extensive combination of bacteria (68, 109, 115), fungi (108), and even viruses (71, 134, 141) have been reported to be present simultaneously within infected periodontal sites. Even the *Archaea* (*Archaeobacteria*) are present in the oral cavity, where they may be associated with chronic inflammation and disease. For example, *Methanobrevibacter oralis*, a methanogen archaeal species, may be syntropic with other bacteria in the subgingival crevice and promote colonization by secondary fermenters during periodontal disease (84). Key periodontal pathogens typically include *Aggregatibacter actinomycetemcomitans, Tannerella forsythia,* and *P. gingivalis,* although *Prevotella intermedia, Campylobacter rectus, Peptostreptococcus micros,*

Sophie Joly • Dows Institute for Dental Research, College of Dentistry, The University of Iowa, Iowa City, IA 52242. **Myriam Bélanger and Ann Progulske-Fox** • Center for Molecular Microbiology and Department of Oral Biology, College of Dentistry, University of Florida, Gainesville, FL 32610. **Georgia K. Johnson** • Department of Periodontics, College of Dentistry, The University of Iowa, Iowa City, IA 52242. **Kim A. Brogden** • Dows Institute for Dental Research and Department of Periodontics, College of Dentistry, The University of Iowa, Iowa City, IA 52242.

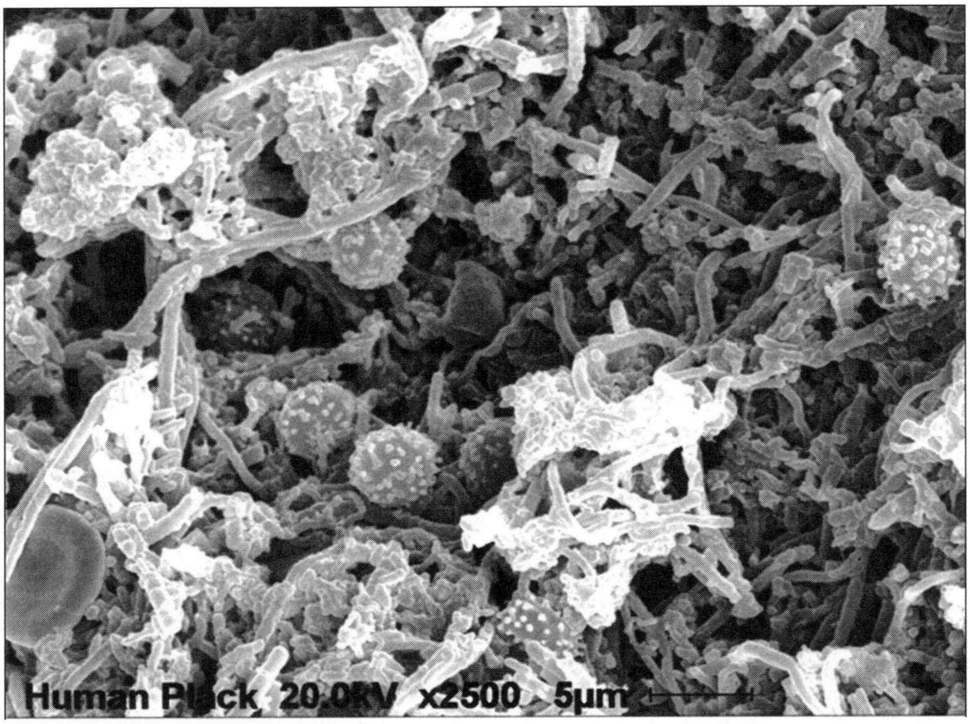

Figure 1. Polymicrobial biofilm in the oral cavity showing microorganisms, inflammatory cells, and erythrocytes in human plaque. Bar, 5 µm. (Micrograph by Janet M. Guthmiller and John Laffoon, courtesy of ASM Press.)

Fusobacterium nucleatum, Eubacterium nodatum, Streptococcus intermedius, Veillonella atypica, Actinomyces naeslundii, Treponema denticola, and others may also be involved (67, 76, 109, 126).

Three main periodontal pathogens share very similar characteristics. Indeed, *A. actinomycetemcomitans*, *T. forsythia*, and *P. gingivalis* are gram-negative anaerobes and late colonizers in the oral biofilm. They interact with the host by (i) producing toxins and proteases (75, 98, 148), which cause major tissue destruction and allow the bacteria to evade the innate immune response; (ii) producing highly toxic lipopolysaccharide, which can modulate the local inflammatory response in host cells (49, 65); and (iii) invading epithelial cells and inducing apoptosis (2, 96).

In the context of the disease progression, there are differences between the three pathogens. *A. actinomycetemcomitans* is associated with the localized aggressive form of periodontal disease (formerly called localized juvenile periodontitis) (140, 162), whereas *T. forsythia* and *P. gingivalis* are often isolated together in chronic periodontitis and are believed to lead the way to advanced periodontitis (36, 114). As mentioned above, no one pathogen is critical in the development of periodontal disease; however, recent studies have focused on early detection in order to prevent advanced disease causative of threatening systemic implication. As a result, the presence of *A. actinomycetemcomitans, P. gingivalis*, and *T. forsythia* has been proposed as a potential risk factor in periodontitis (36).

PERIODONTAL AND SYSTEMIC DISEASE INTERRELATIONSHIPS

Periodontal disease induces chronic inflammation in the oral cavity, and chronic inflammation from various sources is linked with increased cardiovascular risk (145). Therefore, individuals with periodontitis may be at an increased risk for developing cardiovascular and coronary heart diseases (8, 29, 90, 100). Furthermore, the potential role of periodontal infection as a risk factor for preterm, low-birth-weight infants (60, 87, 109) and respiratory infections (135, 137) has been proposed. There is early evidence of periodontopathogenic microorganisms in placentas of women with preeclampsia (7). Periodontitis may also exacerbate preexisting chronic inflammatory conditions, like rheumatoid arthritis (128) or diabetes mellitus (150).

Table 1. Studies suggesting an association between periodontal disease and long-term chronic systemic disease

Sequela	Association (reference[s])
Atherosclerosis	Persistent bacterial infections, including *P. gingivalis*, are thought to cause immune responses that promote atherosclerosis (18, 40, 48, 55, 70, 89, 121, 163)
Coronary artery disease	There is a growing relationship between periodontal disease and coronary artery disease and acute coronary syndrome (42, 124, 125, 127, 159)
	Periodontal disease with elevated bacterial exposure is associated with cardiovascular disease (102)
	Periodontal disease may increase the potential risk of occurrence of coronary heart disease in which inflammation might be a common factor (107)
	An association has been noted between coronary heart disease and poor periodontal status in middle-aged males (12)
Cerebrovascular disease	Individuals with periodontal disease may be at potential risk of developing stroke (30, 43, 109, 122, 123, 136)
Peripheral arterial disease	Individuals with periodontal disease may have a fivefold potential risk of developing peripheral arterial disease (16)
	Specimens from individuals with peripheral arterial disease contained *P. gingivalis* (56)
Preterm, low-birth-weight infants	Women with periodontal disease may be at potential risk of delivering preterm, low-birth-weight infants (58–60, 87, 97, 109–111)
Exacerbation of preexisting chronic conditions	An association between periodontal disease and several respiratory conditions has been reported (135, 137)
	Patients with rheumatoid arthritis may be at potential risk to get periodontal disease (41, 61)
	Patients with periodontal disease may be at potential risk to get rheumatoid arthritis (92–94)
	Patients with rheumatoid arthritis and periodontal disease have differences in inflammatory markers in gingival crevicular fluid (10)
	Periodontitis may exacerbate preexisting chronic inflammatory conditions, like diabetes mellitus (150)
	The presence of periodontal disease may have significant effects on the medical management of patients with end-stage renal disease (22, 23)

Periodontal disease may have systemic effects via different mechanisms. One mechanism involves the systemic effect of cytokines produced locally in response to periodontal infections. Here, chronic systemic exposure to inflammatory mediators of periodontal origin are thought to contribute to atheroma development and thromboembolic phenomena in cardiovascular disease (109) or adversely affect the developing fetus and trigger premature birth in pregnant females (20).

Another mechanism involves the systemic effect of microorganisms (e.g., *P. gingivalis*) migrating from periodontal infections. The underlying connective tissues of the periodontium are highly vascularized, which may serve as the primary portal allowing local organisms to enter the circulatory system (28). Once in circulation, *P. gingivalis* can attach and invade endothelial cells. This constant exposure to *P. gingivalis* may subsequently induce and contribute to atheroma development.

SEQUELAE OF PERIODONTAL INFECTION

Cardiovascular Diseases

Cardiovascular diseases are those that affect the heart or blood vessels. They include atherosclerosis, coronary artery disease, cerebrovascular disease, and peripheral arterial disease. The morbidity and mortality of cardiovascular diseases are staggering. In 2005, an estimated 80,700,000 people in the United States had one or more forms of cardiovascular disease and an estimated 16,000,000 people had a history of coronary heart disease (American Heart Association statistics).

Atherosclerosis

Atherosclerosis is a common underlying cause of cardiovascular diseases (88). Atherosclerosis is the formation and buildup of material (atheroma) within the intima and inner media of large- and medium-sized arteries. Atheromas contain cholesterol, lipoid material, cellular debris, and a number of proteins (45). They begin as an accumulation of intimal smooth muscle cells together with macrophages and T lymphocytes (88). Leukocytes are drawn to the vascular endothelium and enter at expression sites of vascular cell adhesion molecule (VCAM)-1, intercellular adhesion molecule (ICAM)-1, E-selectin, and P-selectin (116). Proinflammatory cytokines in the early atherosclerotic lesions attract monocytes. These monocytes enter the vessel wall and develop into macrophages that take up oxidized low-density lipoprotein and differentiate into foam cells (116). Lipids, cholesterol esters, and free cholesterol accumulate in the cells and the surrounding tissues. Over time, these lesions may become calcified. Inflammation, cellular breakdown, degradation of collagen, and expansion of the core with lipids and lipoproteins from dead macrophages and foam cells can convert a stable plaque to an unstable, ruptured plaque (69).

Major risk factors for atherosclerosis include age, dyslipidemia, smoking, diabetes, and hypertension (151). Potential triggers for the onset of atherosclerosis include dyslipidemia, hypercoagulability, oxidative stress, endothelial dysfunction, and infection and inflammation by certain pathogens (88, 89). Persistent bacterial infections are thought to cause localized immune responses (70, 89, 121), which are confirmed by the presence of T lymphocytes and macrophages. The presence of these cells also suggests that there is an immunologic component to the formation of atherosclerosis, perhaps due to the presence of specific bacterial antigens (85, 131).

P. gingivalis has been identified as a contributing pathogen in the process (40). Atherosclerotic plaques in individuals with periodontal disease often contain periodontal organisms, including *P. gingivalis* (55, 70, 163). DNA from *P. gingivalis* is found in stenotic coronary artery plaques and is correlated with its presence in subgingival plaque (55, 163). Other studies suggest that *P. intermedia* may have a role in the development of coronary artery disease (107), and *A. actinomycetemcomitans* may contribute to the acute coronary syndrome (133).

Coronary artery disease

Coronary artery disease is a highly prevalent disease with a significant morbidity and mortality rate (42). Plaque forms inside coronary arteries, which can restrict blood flow to cardiac tissues. Restricted blood flow then increases the potential risk of both blood clot formation and/or angina (91).

Recent epidemiological studies suggest that there is a growing relationship between periodontal disease and coronary artery disease and acute coronary syndrome. Gotsman reported that patients with severe coronary artery disease had significantly more periodontal destruction than patients with mild coronary artery disease (42). Patients with acute coronary syndrome had significantly higher dental plaque scores and subgingival *P. gingivalis* counts than stable patients. Periodontal destruction measures were significantly correlated with coronary artery disease severity, whereas periodontal infection measures were significantly associated with clinical cardiac status. In a systemic review and meta-analysis of 10 published studies, Mustapha et al. concluded that periodontal disease with elevated systemic markers of bacterial exposure, such as C-reactive protein and bacterial antibodies, was associated with cardiovascular disease (odds ratio of 1.75) and early atherogenesis (102).

Periodontal and systemic disease interrelationships can be determined by estimating the numbers of oral bacterial species and specific periodontopathogens. Direct estimates for total oral bacterial load were determined using a checkerboard DNA-DNA hybridization method (127). The oral bacterial load was higher in subjects with acute coronary syndrome and significant for 26 of 40 bacterial species, including *P. gingivalis* (127). The prevalence of *P. gingivalis* in coronary artery plaque ranged from 21.6% to 53.3% (48, 55, 121, 163). Although *P. gingivalis* is difficult to isolate from plaque samples, viable *P. gingivalis* can be detected within plaque using a cell culture invasion assay. Here, a carotid atherosclerotic plaque homogenate was incubated with ECV-304 cells, and *P. gingivalis* was detected with immunofluorescent microscopy (70).

Periodontal and systemic disease interrelationships can also be determined by measuring serum antibodies to select periodontopathogens. In separate studies, elevated levels of serum immunoglobulin G (IgG) to *P. gingivalis* were associated with the presence of coronary artery atherosclerosis (18) and coronary heart disease (125). A high IgA response to *P. gingivalis* was found to be correlated with an increased potential risk for myocardial infarction in men free of coronary heart disease (124). A more recent study suggested strain differences were important and the presence of periodontopathic bacteria with high virulence may affect atherogenesis (159). Antibody titers for two different strains of *P. gingivalis*, FDC381 and Su63, were different between individuals with coronary heart disease and periodontal disease. Individuals with periodontal disease had high antibody titers to both *P. gingivalis* FDC381 and Su63, but individuals with coronary heart disease had only high antibody titers to *P. gingivalis* Su63.

Cerebrovascular disease

There is also a growing relationship between periodontitis and the potential risk for stroke (109, 136). In a case-control study involving 6,950 subjects, those with a history of stroke more often had IgA titers to *P. gingivalis* than the controls: 79.7% versus 70.2% (123). In a follow-up study involving 8,911 subjects, those with systemic exposure to *P. gingivalis* had an increased potential risk of stroke compared to seronegative subjects (122). Men with IgA titers and women with IgG titers for *P. gingivalis* had a multivariate odds ratios of 1.63 (1.06 to 2.50) and 2.30 (1.39 to 3.78) for stroke, respectively. Higher odds ratios were observed with males who had never smoked. Compared to seronegative men, *P. gingivalis* IgA-seropositive men had a multivariate odds ratio of 3.31 (1.31 to 8.40, $P = 0.012$) for stroke. In a similar case-control study involving 603 subjects, periodontal disease was associated with an increased potential risk of ischemic stroke (30, 43). A strong independent association was seen between severe periodontal disease (odds ratio of 7.38) and gingivitis (odds ratio of 18.29) with stroke. Taken together, all of these studies suggest that systemic exposure to *P. gingivalis* is associated with an increased incidence of stroke.

Peripheral arterial disease

Peripheral arterial disease (PAD) is associated with atherosclerosis and results in obstruction of blood flow to the lower extremities. Stages of PAD range from intermittent claudication (Fontaine grade II) to resting pain (Fontaine grade III), to ischemic ulceration and gangrene (Fontaine grade IV). Individuals with periodontal disease may have a five-fold potential risk of developing PAD (16). In PAD patients, the presence of periodontal disease was associated with a significantly increased serum interleukin 6 (IL-6) and tumor necrosis factor alpha (TNF-α) response. Atherosclerotic specimens from individuals with PAD contained *P. gingivalis*, which was detected more frequently in severe PAD (e.g., Fontaine grade III and IV) than in less severe PAD (e.g., Fontaine grade I).

Periodontal bacteria, including *P. gingivalis*, were present in occluded arteries removed from patients with characteristic Buerger's disease, an inflammation of the vessels and nerves in the legs leading to reduced blood flow (56). Fourteen patients with Buerger's disease had moderate to severe periodontal disease, and periodontal bacteria were found in 14% to 43% of the arterial samples and 71% to 100% of the oral samples. No control arterial samples were positive for periodontal bacteria. Furthermore, elevated IgG titers against periodontal pathogens, including *P. gingivalis*, were found in the serum of patients with Buerger's disease (15).

Preterm, Low-Birth-Weight Infants

Women with periodontal disease may be at potential risk of delivering preterm, low-birth-weight infants (109). In a case-controlled study of pregnant women, periodontitis was a significant factor for preterm, low-birth-weight infants, with an adjusted odds ratio of 7.5 to 7.9 (110). Later studies by Jeffcoat et al. and Offenbacher et al. also suggested that periodontal disease precedes preterm births, and the more severe the periodontal disease, the more likely a baby will be born at earlier gestational ages (58–60, 87, 111). A meta-analysis demonstrated that the overall adjusted odds ratio of preterm, low-birth-weight infants in pregnant women with periodontitis was 5.28 (64). Underlying mechanisms have been studied in both small and large animal models using extracted cell products from *P. gingivalis*. In hamsters, *P. gingivalis* lipopolysaccharide suppressed fetal growth (19, 20). In sheep, intra-amniotic injections of *P. gingivalis* lipopolysaccharide induced fetal mortality (106). Only 6 of 22 fetuses survived doses of 0.1 to 10 mg of lipopolysaccharide, suggesting that sources of inflammation distant from the uterus may result in unexplained stillbirth and other complications of pregnancy. In a small animal model, Bélanger et al, demonstrated that *P. gingivalis* can invade both maternal and fetal tissues, resulting in chorioamnionitis and placentitis (9). Interestingly, strains of *P. gingivalis* differed in virulence, and maternal and fetal colonization was influenced by the infection dose and strain of *P. gingivalis*.

Treatment of periodontal disease in pregnant women improves their periodontal health and is safe. In a pilot trial of 366 pregnant women with periodontal disease, scaling and root planing reduced the rate of preterm births at less than 35 weeks from 6.3% in the reference group to 4.9% in the prophylaxis group (60). The rate of preterm births was 3.3% in the group receiving scaling and root planing in conjunction with a systemic antibiotic and 0.8% in the group receiving scaling and root planing in conjunction with a placebo. In a larger multicenter trial, scaling and root planing did not significantly reduce the potential risk of delivering a premature or low-birth-weight baby (97). Preterm birth occurred in 12.0% women in the treatment group and in 12.8% women in the control group. This study concluded that treatment of periodontal disease in pregnant women improves periodontal health and is safe but does not significantly alter rates of preterm birth or low birth weight (97).

Exacerbation of Preexisting Chronic Conditions

Periodontitis may exacerbate preexisting chronic conditions, like rheumatoid arthritis (128), renal disease, and diabetes mellitus (150). A potential interrelationship between periodontal disease and rheumatoid arthritis has been proposed (41, 61, 92–94). Both are inflammatory diseases and subjects with periodontal disease and rheumatoid arthritis produce inflammatory markers in their serum and gingival crevicular fluids. Higher concentrations of rheumatoid factors, prostaglandins, type I carboxy terminal peptide, C-reactive protein, plasminogen activator, plasminogen activator inhibitor-2, IL-1β, and prostaglandin E2 were produced in serum and gingival crevicular fluids (10), and lower concentrations of IL-4 were produced in gingival crevicular fluids (11).

Patients with rheumatoid arthritis are thought to be at potential risk for periodontal disease (41, 61). In a cross-sectional study, 50 patients with long-term active rheumatoid arthritis had substantially higher degrees of periodontal disease, including loss of teeth, compared with 101 healthy controls. Functional impairment of the upper extremities was thought to compromise oral hygiene procedures and thus amplify periodontal destruction. The long-term use of nonsteroidal anti-inflammatory drugs, corticosteroids, and disease-modifying antirheumatic drugs showed no connection with the severity of periodontal disease observed in these patients. Patients with periodontal disease are thought to be at potential risk for rheumatoid arthritis. Periodontal treatment has reduced select clinical markers of disease severity in rheumatoid arthritis patients (128). For example, erythrocyte sedimentation rates, a nonspecific marker of inflammation, were significantly reduced after scaling and root planing, although rheumatoid factors were not. This suggested that periodontal treatment reduced systemic inflammation.

Periodontal disease may complicate the medical management of end-stage renal disease patients (22, 23). Periodontal treatment decreased systemic markers such as C-reactive protein, which could have implications in the control of atherosclerotic complications, including myocardial infarction and stroke, the primary causes of mortality in end-stage renal disease patients.

P. GINGIVALIS, A PRIMARY PERIODONTOPATHOGEN

P. gingivalis is a dominant periodontopathogen (53, 76, 115). It produces capsular polysaccharide (74, 154), fimbriae (26, 157), hemagglutinins (34, 54, 63, 83, 113, 120), lipopolysaccharide (3, 4, 156), and a variety of proteolytic enzymes that facilitate, directly or indirectly, both local tissue damage and evasion of host defense mechanisms (5, 6, 24, 117, 152, 153). Although associated with periodontitis, increasing evidence clearly shows *P. gingivalis* has the ability to leave the oral cavity. Once in circulation, many of these virulence factors allow *P. gingivalis* to attach, invade, and activate cells and tissues of the cardiovascular system (Table 2).

Access to the Cardiovascular System

Oral microorganisms in the gingival crevice passively cross the inflamed gingival barrier and "spill over" into the circulatory system. This sometimes occurs while eating and chewing, but definitive proof of this mechanism is yet to be determined (37, 39, 101). It more likely occurs after physical manipulation of

Table 2. General virulence factors used by *P. gingivalis* to attach, infect, colonize, and activate cardiovascular tissues

Bacterial component	Activity and select examples of infection and colonization of cardiovascular tissues (reference[s])
Fimbrial adhesins	Fimbriae are required for adherence and invasion of aortic and heart endothelial cells (28)
	Expression of FimA is required for attachment but not for invasion (31)
	Fimbrillin induces IL-8 and MCP-1 responses in human umbilical vein endothelial cells (105)
Nonfimbrial adhesins	Hemagglutinins A, B, C, and D mediate adherence to coronary artery endothelial cells (118, 144)
Lipopolysaccharides (LPS)	LPS facilitates monocyte adhesion to vascular endothelium through sustained upregulation of ICAM-1 and VCAM-1 via TLR2-dependent mechanism (103)
	LPS induces IL-8 and MCP-1 responses in human umbilical vein endothelial cells (105)
Toxins	45-kDa hemolysin has partial sequence similarity to fimbrillin (27)
Enzymes	Proteases are essential for invasion of aortic and heart endothelial cells (28)
	Chemokine response of human umbilical vein endothelial cells is suppressed through a gingipain-mediated mechanism (105)
	Matrix metalloproteinase-9 protease activity degrades fibrous caps from autopsy samples (72)
	Gingipains reduce cyclin expression and cause early G(1) arrest, leading to the inhibition of cellular proliferation (62)
	HtrA is a heat shock protein, chaperone, and serine protease involved in H_2O_2 stress (161)

teeth and their supporting structures (32). Bacteremias involving *P. gingivalis* have been detected after toothbrushing (138), flossing (14), periodontal probing (25), scaling and root planing (73, 86), and other dental procedures (95).

P. gingivalis can be actively transported across inflamed gingival tissues, and this may occur during infection (51). In infected mice, for example, *P. gingivalis* left subcutaneous chambers via an activated kallikrein/kinin pathway. Underlying vascular permeability was blocked by kininase and kinin receptor antagonists and was enhanced by exogenous bradykinin and kininase inhibitors.

Attachment

Once in circulation, *P. gingivalis* uses both fimbrial and nonfimbrial adhesins to attach to vascular tissue surfaces. Ultrastructurally, there are three distinct fimbriae on *P. gingivalis*: major fimbriae (38), minor fimbriae (46), and Pg-II fimbriae (112). The major fimbrial type is 3 to 5 nm wide and 0.3 to 3.0 μm long, peritrichous on the microbial cell surface, and composed of 41- to 49-kDa monomers of fimbrillin (FimA) (77, 142, 143, 160). Minor fimbriae are composed of a 67-kDa component (46), and Pg-II fimbriae are composed of a 72-kDa protein (112).

P. gingivalis FimA fimbriae are grouped into six genotypes based on the nucleotide sequences of *fimA* (104). In subgingival plaque containing *P. gingivalis*, genotypes II (37.5%), I (28.6%), and IV (21.4%) were present. In cardiovascular specimens containing *P. gingivalis*, genotypes IV (45.0%), II (30.0%), and I (5%) were present.

The role of FimA in the attachment and invasion of *P. gingivalis* is not firmly established. Both highly invasive and noninvasive strains express FimA (31). For example, strains 381 and W50 were invasive and AJW4 was noninvasive, yet AJW4 had FimA expressed on its surface. Comparing the degrees of adherence and invasion of strains AJW4 (type IV FimA), W50 (type IV FimA), and 381, the adherence and invasion of AJW4 was 38.7% of that of strain 381; the amount of AJW4 recovered from within cells was 2.9% of that of strain 381; and AJW4 was 8.9-fold more adhesive yet was internalized 170-fold less (31).

In other strains, the role of FimA in the attachment and invasion of *P. gingivalis* is clearer. A *fimA* mutant, DPG3, which lacks the major fimbriae, did not attach and invade compared to strain 381: 0.001% of DPG3 adhered and invaded bovine aortic endothelial cells, whereas 0.11% of strain 381 adhered and invaded (28).

P. gingivalis has five hemagglutinins that facilitate microbial binding to host cells and erythrocytes. *hagA* encodes a 233.4-kDa protein that contains four repeating segments, each with hemagglutinating activity (119). *hagB* and *hagC* encode 42.0- and 39.3-kDa proteins, respectively (82, 119, 120). *hagD* encodes a 187.9-kDa protein (47, 82), and *hagE* encodes a 185.7-kDa protein (155). HagA and HagD have 73.8% homology; HagA and HagE have 93% homology; and HagB and HagC have 98% homology (82). The hemagglutinins also have significant sequence homology to protease genes of *P. gingivalis* (118).

HagB is a major virulence factor and among the more closely studied hemagglutinins of *P. gingivalis*. It induces proinflammatory cytokine responses in a variety of rodent cells. For example, HagB induced gamma interferon (IFN-γ), IL-2, IL-4, and IL-10 in rat splenic lymphoid cells (63); IL-4, IL-5, and IFN-γ by murine CD4$^+$ T cells (165); TNF-α, IL-12p40, IFN-γ, and IL-10 in mouse peritoneal macrophages (164); and proinflammatory cytokine responses in human myeloid dendritic cells and human keratinocytes. Human myeloid dendritic cells incubated with recombinant HagB (rHagB) produced proinflammatory cytokines (IL-6, GM-CSF, TNF-α, and IL-12p40), IL-10, and the chemokines IL-8 (CXCL8), IP-10 (CXCL10), monocyte chemoattractant protein 1 (MCP-1) (CCL2), macrophage inflammatory protein 1α (MIP-1α) (CCL3), and RANTES (CCL5). Human oral keratinocytes incubated with rHagB produced IL-6 and IL-8 (our unpublished data).

HagB is involved in the adherence of *P. gingivalis* to human coronary artery endothelial cells (HCAE) (144) (Fig. 2). *P. gingivalis* strain 381, a *P. gingivalis* 381 HagB mutant, *Escherichia coli* JM109 expressing HagB (*E. coli*-HagB), and *E. coli* JM109 containing pUC9 (*E. coli*-pUC9) all adhered differently to HCAE cells. No differences were seen between the attachments of 381 and the HagB mutant, possibly a result of the expression of HagC. Differences were seen between the attachments of the *E. coli*-HagB strain and the *E. coli*-pUC9. Further evidence showed that preincubation of HCAE cells with HagB decreased bacterial adhesion of *P. gingivalis* or *E. coli*-HagB to HCAE cells. Adding polyclonal or monoclonal antibodies to HagB significantly decreased attachment of *P. gingivalis* and *E. coli*-HagB to HCAE cells (144).

Invasion

The most convincing evidence of *P. gingivalis* as a potential risk factor for chronic systemic diseases is its ability to invade vascular endothelial and coronary artery cells. Interestingly, not all strains of *P. gingivalis* have similar invasive capabilities (57), and

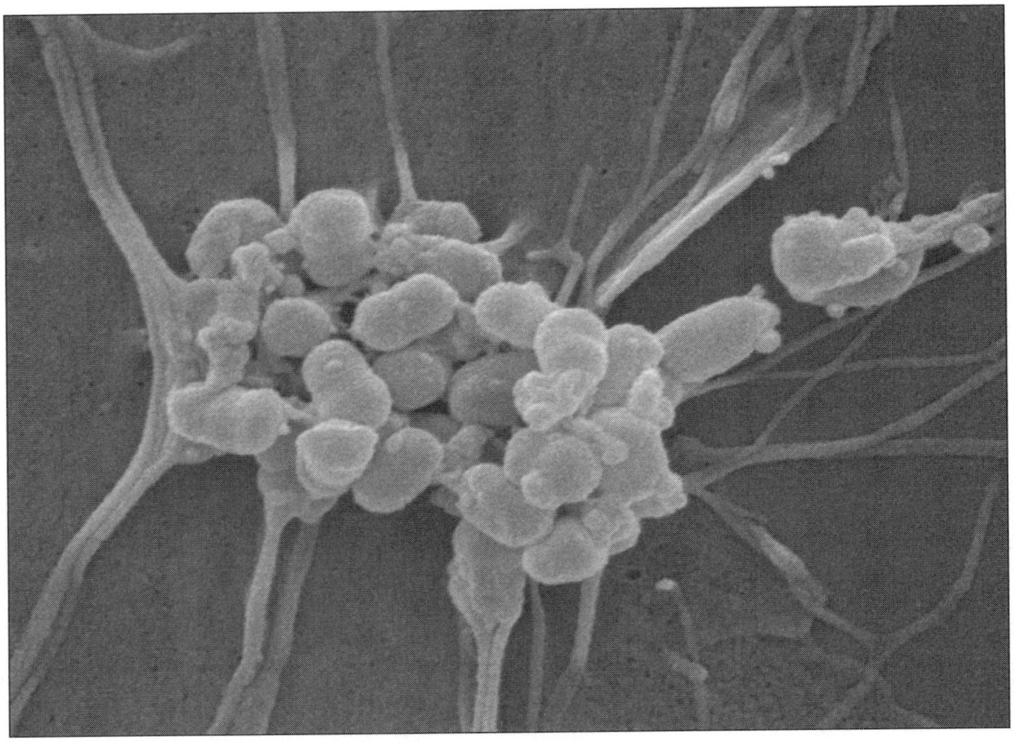

Figure 2. Scanning electron micrograph of HCAE cells infected with *P. gingivalis* 381 for 30 minutes. Bar, 2.3 μm. (Micrograph by A. Progulske-Fox.)

it likely uses different invasive mechanisms for different host cell types (31, 118). This suggests that some strains may have specialized to specific tissues. The host cell type also determines the route of *P. gingivalis* trafficking in the autophagic pathway (129).

P. gingivalis can invade fetal bovine heart endothelial cells (28), bovine aortic endothelial cells (28), HCAE cells (32, 33, 105, 118, 129, 132), heart cells (105), coronary artery smooth muscle cells (32), and human umbilical vein endothelial cells (28, 105) (Fig. 2 and 3). Invasion is initiated by the formation of microvillus-like extensions around adherent bacteria, followed by the engulfment of the pathogen within vacuoles (28, 118). Internalized bacteria were within multimembranous compartments localized with rough endoplasmic reticulum and may use components of the autophagic pathway as a means to survive intracellularly (33). After intracellular uptake, *P. gingivalis* transited from early autophagosomes to late autophagosomes and prevented the formation of autolysosomes, either by delaying the autophagosome-lysosome fusion or by redirecting the normal autophagic trafficking (129) (Fig. 3). Cytoskeletal involvement, protein phosphorylation, energy metabolism, and *P. gingivalis* proteases were all essential for this process (28, 32).

Microarray analyses show that 62 genes in *P. gingivalis* W83 are differentially expressed during invasion of primary HCAE cells (130). Upregulated genes for proteins included those involved in transport and binding; biosynthesis of cofactors, prosthetic groups, and carriers; energy metabolism; central intermediary metabolism; and the cell envelope. Downregulated genes for proteins included those involved in amino acid biosynthesis; biosynthesis of cofactors, prosthetic groups, and carriers; the cell envelope; cellular processes; energy metabolism; fate of proteins; protein synthesis; proteins for transcription; and proteins for transport and binding.

ClpB, a stress response protein, may play a role in *P. gingivalis* invasion (161). A *clpB* mutant of *P. gingivalis* W83 was more susceptible to intracellular killing than the wild-type W83 in HCAE cells. *htrA* is involved in cellular invasion and in vivo survival (161). It is a heat shock protein, chaperone, and serine protease thought to be involved in H_2O_2 stress.

Overall, these studies show that *P. gingivalis* is an extremely successful pathogen. It can leave the oral environment, enter the circulatory system, evade systemic immune defenses, and invade host endothelial cells.

Activation

P. gingivalis and its extracellular products induce the production of proinflammatory cytokines in epithe-

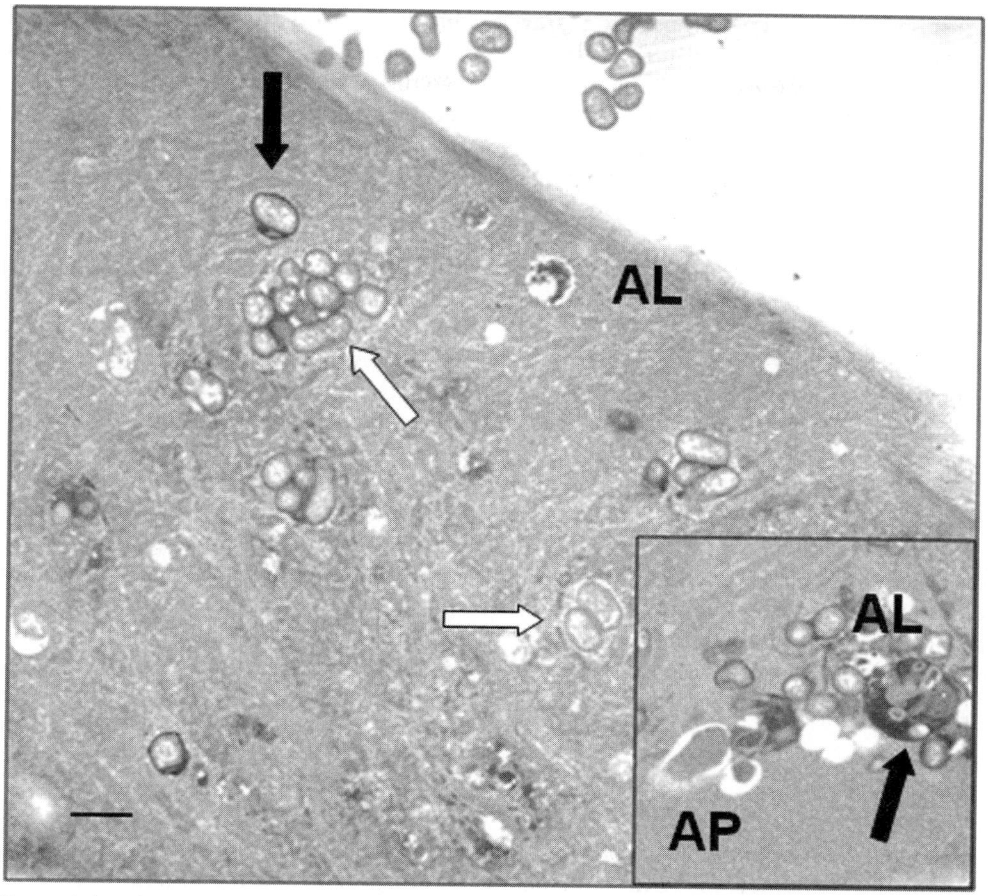

Figure 3. Transmission electron micrograph of HCAE cells infected with *P. gingivalis* W83. After 3 hours of infection, *P. gingivalis* W83 was found in vacuoles that either contained (black arrow) or lacked (white arrow) acid phosphatase. Nascent autophagosomes (AP) that had not yet acquired acid phosphatase and mature autolysosomes (AL) that contained acid phosphatase were observed in infected cells. The presence of autophagic vacuoles and autolysosomes in the infected HCAE cells suggests that *P. gingivalis* is capable of promoting autophagy. *P. gingivalis* W83 is localized predominantly in vacuoles which contained multiple bacteria but lacked lysosomal acid phosphatase. Bar, 1 μm. (Micrograph by M. Bélanger, W.A. Dunn, Jr., and A. Progulske-Fox.)

lial cells (66, 164) and induce the production of proinflammatory cytokines, cell adhesion molecules, and inflammatory genes in endothelial cells. Human aortic endothelial cells exposed to invasive *P. gingivalis* strain 381 produced increased mRNA levels for cytokine genes, cytokine receptor genes, adhesion molecule genes, enzyme genes, angiogenesis growth factor genes, genes involved in apoptosis and cell death, and genes involved in signal transduction, many playing essential roles in the pathobiology of atherosclerosis (17). Human aortic endothelial cells exposed to invasive *P. gingivalis* strains 381 and 381MF1 (expressing major fimbriae) produced GRO2 (17), GRO3 (17), IL-1β (146), IL-6 (17, 132), IL-8 (17, 132, 146), MCP-1 (132, 146), ICAM-1 (17, 132, 146), VCAM-1 (17, 132, 146), E-selectin (17, 132, 146), and Cox-2 (17). Interestingly, human aortic endothelial cells exposed to nonfimbrial *P. gingivalis* mutants DPG3 or DPGMFB did not produce MCP-1, IL-8, IL-1β, or cell adhesion molecule mRNA (146).

Under some circumstances, human umbilical vein endothelial cells exposed to live *P. gingivalis* do not produce IL-8 and MCP-1 (105). The lack of a cytokine response was likely due to the presence of proteases, because treatment with protease inhibitors prior to the addition of *P. gingivalis* to human umbilical vein endothelial cells restored the production of IL-8 and MCP-1. Bovine coronary artery endothelial cells and human microvascular endothelial cells treated with gingipains lost cell adhesion properties as well as lost N- and VE-cadherin and integrin. Apoptotic cell death followed (139). These effects were inhibited by preincubation of gingipains with protease inhibitor.

Human aortic endothelial cells exposed to major or minor fimbriae from *P. gingivalis* produce MCP-1 and IL-8, but not IL-1β. These cells exposed to major or minor fimbriae also have increased mRNA levels for ICAM-1, VCAM-1, and E-selectin, but not increased levels of P-selectin (146). The human aortic endothelial cell response to major or minor fimbriae was highly dependent upon maintenance and rearrangement of an intact endothelial actin cytoskeleton (146).

Endothelial cells exposed to *P. gingivalis* lipopolysaccharide or heat-killed whole cell preparations also produce modest IL-8 and MCP-1 responses (105). Coronary artery endothelial cells exposed to *P. gingivalis* lipopolysaccharide produced ICAM-1, but not VCAM-1 (50). Coronary artery endothelial cells or human umbilical vein endothelial cells exposed to *P. gingivalis* lipopolysaccharide stimulated Toll-like receptor 2 (TLR2), but not TLR4-dependent cell signaling (35). Extended exposure of human umbilical vein endothelial cells to *P. gingivalis* lipopolysaccharide facilitated mononuclear cell adhesion to vascular endothelium via a TLR2-dependent mechanism (103). *P. gingivalis* lipopolysaccharide significantly upregulated ICAM-1 and VCAM-1 in these cells.

Apoptosis

P. gingivalis and its extracellular products induce apoptosis-associated events in bovine coronary artery endothelial cells and human microvascular endothelial cells, like annexin V, caspase-3 activation, and cleavage of caspase substrates poly(ADP-ribose) polymerase and topoisomerase I (139). In cardiac cells, infection with *P. gingivalis* increased DNA fragmentation, nuclear condensation, and activated apoptotic caspase-3, -8, and -9 proteins (81). Use of inhibitors in multiple studies suggested that cellular hypertrophy and apoptosis by *P. gingivalis* and its extracellular products in cardiomyoblast cells were mediated via different signaling pathways (78, 80), including the calcineurin signaling pathway (79, 81) and the P38 mitogen-activated protein kinase pathway (158).

CONCLUSIONS

Individuals with periodontal disease may be at increased potential risk of developing various chronic systemic diseases and complications, although a cause-and-effect relationship has not been proven. The association between periodontitis and systemic diseases, such as cardiovascular disease, may be due to a common inflammatory phenotype and exacerbation of preexisting systemic conditions due to increased levels of circulation cytokines as a result of chronic periodontal infection. On the other hand, infiltration of periodontal bacteria and their products into the systemic circulation may have a direct effect. Because of its many virulence factors, *P. gingivalis* has received considerable attention in periodontal-systemic connections. *P. gingivalis* may passively or actively migrate from the oral cavity and enter the cardiovascular system. The presence of *P. gingivalis* or DNA from *P. gingivalis* in subgingival plaque correlates with the presence of *P. gingivalis* or DNA from *P. gingivalis* in atherosclerotic plaque. Likewise, antibodies to *P. gingivalis* may be used as a marker of increased exposure. Inflammatory mediators or bacterial products from *P. gingivalis* may place pregnant women at potential risk for delivering preterm, low-birth-weight infants. Finally, work from Ann Progulske-Fox and colleagues clearly shows that not all strains of *P. gingivalis* are similar (57). Some strains are invasive and may have a more important role in the potential risk and onset of chronic systemic diseases.

Further studies are needed to explore the relationship between *P. gingivalis* and systemic diseases in order to identify the active mechanism by which *P. gingivalis* successfully leaves the oral cavity and colonizes and invades various other niches. The variability of virulent properties among strains may reflect the extreme adaptability of *P. gingivalis* and the ability to specialize in the function of the tissue, thereby becoming a catalyst to the development of chronic systemic diseases.

Acknowledgments. This work was supported by funds from grant number R01 DE014390 from the National Institute of Dental and Craniofacial Research, National Institutes of Health. We are grateful to Elizabeth A. Schmitt (Cairn Communications, Mahtomedi, MN) for critically reading the manuscript.

REFERENCES

1. **Aas, J. A., B. J. Paster, L. N. Stokes, I. Olsen, and F. E. Dewhirst.** 2005. Defining the normal bacterial flora of the oral cavity. *J. Clin. Microbiol.* **43:**5721–5732.
2. **Arakawa, S., T. Nakajima, H. Ishikura, S. Ichinose, I. Ishikawa, and N. Tsuchida.** 2000. Novel apoptosis-inducing activity in *Bacteroides forsythus*: a comparative study with three serotypes of *Actinobacillus actinomycetemcomitans*. *Infect. Immun.* **68:**4611–4615.
3. **Bainbridge, B. W., and R. P. Darveau.** 1999. Lipopolysaccharide from oral bacteria: role in innate host defense and chronic inflammatory disease, p. 899–913. *In* H. Brade, S. M. Opal, S. N. Vogel, and D. C. Morrison (ed.), *Endotoxin in Health and Disease*. Marcel Dekker, Inc., New York, NY.
4. **Bainbridge, B. W., and R. P. Darveau.** 2001. *Porphyromonas gingivalis* lipopolysaccharide: an unusual pattern recognition receptor ligand for the innate host defense system. *Acta Odontol. Scand.* **59:**131–138.
5. **Banbula, A., M. Bugno, J. Goldstein, J. Yen, D. Nelson, J. Travis, and J. Potempa.** 2000. Emerging family of proline-specific

peptidases of *Porphyromonas gingivalis*: purification and characterization of serine dipeptidyl peptidase, a structural and functional homologue of mammalian prolyl dipeptidyl peptidase IV. *Infect. Immun.* **68:**1176–1182.

6. **Banbula, A., P. Mak, M. Bugno, J. Silberring, A. Dubin, D. Nelson, J. Travis, and J. Potempa.** 1999. Prolyl tripeptidyl peptidase from *Porphyromonas gingivalis*. A novel enzyme with possible pathological implications for the development of periodontitis. *J. Biol. Chem.* **274:**9246–9252.
7. **Barak, S., O. Oettinger-Barak, E. E. Machtei, H. Sprecher, and G. Ohel.** 2007. Evidence of periopathogenic microorganisms in placentas of women with preeclampsia. *J. Periodontol.* **78:**670–676.
8. **Beck, J., R. Garcia, G. Heiss, P. S. Vokonas, and S. Offenbacher.** 1996. Periodontal disease and cardiovascular disease. *J. Periodontol.* **67:**1123–1137.
9. **Belanger, M., L. Reyes, K. Von Deneen, M. K. Reinhard, A. Progulske-Fox, and M. B. Brown.** 2008. Colonization of maternal and fetal tissues by *Porphyromonas gingivalis* is strain-dependent in a rodent animal model. *Am. J. Obstet. Gynecol.* **199:**86.e1–86.e7.
10. **Biyikoglu, B., N. Buduneli, L. Kardesler, K. Aksu, G. Oder, and N. Kutukculer.** 2006. Evaluation of t-PA, PAI-2, IL-1beta and PGE(2) in gingival crevicular fluid of rheumatoid arthritis patients with periodontal disease. *J. Clin. Periodontol.* **33:**605–611.
11. **Bozkurt, F. Y., Z. Yetkin Ay, E. Berker, E. Tepe, and S. Akkus.** 2006. Anti-inflammatory cytokines in gingival crevicular fluid in patients with periodontitis and rheumatoid arthritis: a preliminary report. *Cytokine* **35:**180–185.
12. **Briggs, J. E., P. P. McKeown, V. L. Crawford, J. V. Woodside, R. W. Stout, A. Evans, and G. J. Linden.** 2006. Angiographically confirmed coronary heart disease and periodontal disease in middle-aged males. *J. Periodontol.* **77:**95–102.
13. **Brogden, K. A.** 2002. Polymicrobial diseases of animals and humans, p. 3–20. *In* K. A. Brogden and J. M. Guthmiller (ed.), *Polymicrobial Diseases*. ASM Press, Washington, DC.
14. **Carroll, G. C., and R. J. Sebor.** 1980. Dental flossing and its relationship to transient bacteremia. *J. Periodontol.* **51:**691–692.
15. **Chen, Y. W., T. Iwai, M. Umeda, T. Nagasawa, Y. Huang, Y. Takeuchi, and I. Ishikawa.** 2007. Elevated IgG titers to periodontal pathogens related to Buerger disease. *Int. J. Cardiol.* **122:**79–81.
16. **Chen, Y. W., M. Umeda, T. Nagasawa, Y. Takeuchi, Y. Huang, Y. Inoue, T. Iwai, Y. Izumi, and I. Ishikawa.** 2008. Periodontitis may increase the risk of peripheral arterial disease. *Eur. J. Vasc. Endovasc. Surg.* **35:**153–158.
17. **Chou, H. H., H. Yumoto, M. Davey, Y. Takahashi, T. Miyamoto, F. C. Gibson III, and C. A. Genco.** 2005. *Porphyromonas gingivalis* fimbria-dependent activation of inflammatory genes in human aortic endothelial cells. *Infect. Immun.* **73:**5367–5378.
18. **Colhoun, H. M., J. M. Slaney, M. B. Rubens, J. H. Fuller, A. Sheiham, and M. A. Curtis.** 2008. Antibodies to periodontal pathogens and coronary artery calcification in type 1 diabetic and nondiabetic subjects. *J. Periodontal. Res.* **43:**103–110.
19. **Collins, J. G., M. A. Smith, R. R. Arnold, and S. Offenbacher.** 1994. Effects of *Escherichia coli* and *Porphyromonas gingivalis* lipopolysaccharide on pregnancy outcome in the golden hamster. *Infect. Immun.* **62:**4652–4655.
20. **Collins, J. G., H. W. Windley III, R. R. Arnold, and S. Offenbacher.** 1994. Effects of a *Porphyromonas gingivalis* infection on inflammatory mediator response and pregnancy outcome in hamsters. *Infect. Immun.* **62:**4356–4361.
21. **Coventry, J., G. Griffiths, C. Scully, and M. Tonetti.** 2000. ABC of oral health: periodontal disease. *BMJ* **321:**36–39.
22. **Craig, R. G.** 2008. Interactions between chronic renal disease and periodontal disease. *Oral Dis.* **14:**1–7.
23. **Craig, R. G., M. A. Spittle, and N. W. Levin.** 2002. Importance of periodontal disease in the kidney patient. *Blood Purif.* **20:**113–119.
24. **Curtis, M. A., J. Aduse-Opoku, and M. Rangarajan.** 2001. Cysteine proteases of *Porphyromonas gingivalis*. *Crit. Rev. Oral Biol. Med.* **12:**192–216.
25. **Daly, C. G., D. H. Mitchell, J. E. Highfield, D. E. Grossberg, and D. Stewart.** 2001. Bacteremia due to periodontal probing: a clinical and microbiological investigation. *J. Periodontol.* **72:**210–214.
26. **Dashper, S. G., N. M. O'Brien-Simpson, P. S. Bhogal, A. D. Franzmann, and E. C. Reynolds.** 1998. Purification and characterization of a putative fimbrial protein/receptor of *Porphyromonas gingivalis*. *Aust. Dent. J.* **43:**99–104.
27. **Deshpande, R. G., and M. B. Khan.** 1999. Purification and characterization of hemolysin from *Porphyromonas gingivalis* A7436. *FEMS Microbiol. Lett.* **176:**387–394.
28. **Deshpande, R. G., M. B. Khan, and C. A. Genco.** 1998. Invasion of aortic and heart endothelial cells by *Porphyromonas gingivalis*. *Infect. Immun.* **66:**5337–5343.
29. **DeStefano, F., R. F. Anda, H. S. Kahn, D. F. Williamson, and C. M. Russell.** 1993. Dental disease and risk of coronary heart disease and mortality. *BMJ* **306:**688–691.
30. **Dorfer, C. E., H. Becher, C. M. Ziegler, C. Kaiser, R. Lutz, D. Jorss, C. Lichy, F. Buggle, S. Bultmann, M. Preusch, and A. J. Grau.** 2004. The association of gingivitis and periodontitis with ischemic stroke. *J. Clin. Periodontol.* **31:**396–401.
31. **Dorn, B. R., J. N. Burks, K. N. Seifert, and A. Progulske-Fox.** 2000. Invasion of endothelial and epithelial cells by strains of *Porphyromonas gingivalis*. *FEMS Microbiol. Lett.* **187:**139–144.
32. **Dorn, B. R., W. A. Dunn, Jr., and A. Progulske-Fox.** 1999. Invasion of human coronary artery cells by periodontal pathogens. *Infect. Immun.* **67:**5792–5798.
33. **Dorn, B. R., W. A. Dunn, Jr., and A. Progulske-Fox.** 2001. *Porphyromonas gingivalis* traffics to autophagosomes in human coronary artery endothelial cells. *Infect. Immun.* **69:**5698–5708.
34. **Dusek, D. M., A. Progulske-Fox, J. Whitlock, and T. A. Brown.** 1993. Isolation and characterization of a cloned *Porphyromonas gingivalis* hemagglutinin from an avirulent strain of *Salmonella typhimurium*. *Infect. Immun.* **61:**940–946.
35. **Erridge, C., C. M. Spickett, and D. J. Webb.** 2007. Non-enterobacterial endotoxins stimulate human coronary artery but not venous endothelial cell activation via Toll-like receptor 2. *Cardiovasc. Res.* **73:**181–189.
36. **Ezzo, P. J., and C. W. Cutler.** 2003. Microorganisms as risk indicators for periodontal disease. *Periodontology 2000* **32:**24–35.
37. **Forner, L., T. Larsen, M. Kilian, and P. Holmstrup.** 2006. Incidence of bacteremia after chewing, tooth brushing and scaling in individuals with periodontal inflammation. *J. Clin. Periodontol.* **33:**401–407.
38. **Fujiwara, T., S. Morishima, I. Takahashi, and S. Hamada.** 1993. Molecular cloning and sequencing of the fimbrilin gene of *Porphyromonas gingivalis* strains and characterization of recombinant proteins. *Biochem. Biophys. Res. Commun.* **197:**241–247.
39. **Geerts, S. O., M. Nys, M. P. De, J. Charpentier, A. Albert, V. Legrand, and E. H. Rompen.** 2002. Systemic release of endotoxins induced by gentle mastication: association with periodontitis severity. *J. Periodontol.* **73:**73–78.

40. **Gibson, F. C., III, T. Ukai, and C. A. Genco.** 2008. Engagement of specific innate immune signaling pathways during *Porphyromonas gingivalis* induced chronic inflammation and atherosclerosis. *Front. Biosci.* **13:**2041–2059.
41. **Gleissner, C., B. Willershausen, U. Kaesser, and W. W. Bolten.** 1998. The role of risk factors for periodontal disease in patients with rheumatoid arthritis. *Eur. J. Med. Res.* **3:**387–392.
42. **Gotsman, I., C. Lotan, W. A. Soskolne, S. Rassovsky, T. Pugatsch, L. Lapidus, Y. Novikov, S. Masrawa, and A. Stabholz.** 2007. Periodontal destruction is associated with coronary artery disease and periodontal infection with acute coronary syndrome. *J. Periodontol.* **78:**849–858.
43. **Grau, A. J., H. Becher, C. M. Ziegler, C. Lichy, F. Buggle, C. Kaiser, R. Lutz, S. Bultmann, M. Preusch, and C. E. Dorfer.** 2004. Periodontal disease as a risk factor for ischemic stroke. *Stroke* **35:**496–501.
44. **Guthmiller, J. M., and K. F. Novak.** 2002. Periodontal diseases, p. 137–152. *In* K. A. Brogden and J. M. Guthmiller (ed.), *Polymicrobial Diseases*. ASM Press, Washington, DC.
45. **Guyton, J. R., and K. F. Klemp.** 1996. Development of the lipid-rich core in human atherosclerosis. *Arterioscler. Thromb. Vasc. Biol.* **16:**4–11.
46. **Hamada, N., H. T. Sojar, M. I. Cho, and R. J. Genco.** 1996. Isolation and characterization of a minor fimbria from *Porphyromonas gingivalis*. *Infect. Immun.* **64:**4788–4794.
47. **Han, N., G. Lepine, J. Whitlock, L. Wojciechowski, and A. Progulske-Fox.** 1998. The *Porphyromonas gingivalis* prtP/kgp homologue exists as two open reading frames in strain 381. *Oral Dis.* **4:**170–179.
48. **Haraszthy, V. I., J. J. Zambon, M. Trevisan, M. Zeid, and R. J. Genco.** 2000. Identification of periodontal pathogens in atheromatous plaques. *J. Periodontol.* **71:**1554–1560.
49. **Hasebe, A., A. Yoshimura, T. Into, H. Kataoka, S. Tanaka, S. Arakawa, H. Ishikura, D. T. Golenbock, T. Sugaya, N. Tsuchida, M. Kawanami, Y. Hara, and K. Shibata.** 2004. Biological activities of *Bacteroides forsythus* lipoproteins and their possible pathological roles in periodontal disease. *Infect. Immun.* **72:**1318–1325.
50. **Honda, T., T. Oda, H. Yoshie, and K. Yamazaki.** 2005. Effects of *Porphyromonas gingivalis* antigens and proinflammatory cytokines on human coronary artery endothelial cells. *Oral Microbiol. Immunol.* **20:**82–88.
51. **Hu, S. W., C. H. Huang, H. C. Huang, Y. Y. Lai, and Y. Y. Lin.** 2006. Transvascular dissemination of *Porphyromonas gingivalis* from a sequestered site is dependent upon activation of the kallikrein/kinin pathway. *J. Periodontal. Res.* **41:**200–207.
52. **Hujoel, P. P., B. G. Leroux, H. Selipsky, and B. A. White.** 2000. Non-surgical periodontal therapy and tooth loss. A cohort study. *J. Periodontol.* **71:**736–742.
53. **Hutter, G., U. Schlagenhauf, G. Valenza, M. Horn, S. Burgemeister, H. Claus, and U. Vogel.** 2003. Molecular analysis of bacteria in periodontitis: evaluation of clone libraries, novel phylotypes and putative pathogens. *Microbiology* **149:**67–75.
54. **Inoshita, E., A. Amano, T. Hanioka, H. Tamagawa, S. Shizukuishi, and A. Tsunemitsu.** 1986. Isolation and some properties of exohemagglutinin from the culture medium of *Bacteroides gingivalis* 381. *Infect. Immun.* **52:**421–427.
55. **Ishihara, K., A. Nabuchi, R. Ito, K. Miyachi, H. K. Kuramitsu, and K. Okuda.** 2004. Correlation between detection rates of periodontopathic bacterial DNA in coronary stenotic artery plaque and in dental plaque samples. *J. Clin. Microbiol.* **42:**1313–1315. (Erratum **42:**5437)
56. **Iwai, T., Y. Inoue, M. Umeda, Y. Huang, N. Kurihara, M. Koike, and I. Ishikawa.** 2005. Oral bacteria in the occluded arteries of patients with Buerger disease. *J. Vasc. Surg.* **42:**107–115.
57. **Jandik, K. A., M. Belanger, S. L. Low, B. R. Dorn, M. C. K. Yang, and A. Progulske-Fox.** 2008. Invasive differences among *Porphyromonas gingivalis* strains from healthy and diseased periodontal sites. *J. Periodontal. Res.* **42.**
58. **Jeffcoat, M. K., N. C. Geurs, M. S. Reddy, S. P. Cliver, R. L. Goldenberg, and J. C. Hauth.** 2001. Periodontal infection and preterm birth: results of a prospective study. *J. Am. Dent. Assoc.* **132:**875–880.
59. **Jeffcoat, M. K., N. C. Geurs, M. S. Reddy, R. L. Goldenberg, and J. C. Hauth.** 2001. Current evidence regarding periodontal disease as a risk factor in preterm birth. *Ann. Periodontol.* **6:**183–188.
60. **Jeffcoat, M. K., J. C. Hauth, N. C. Geurs, M. S. Reddy, S. P. Cliver, P. M. Hodgkins, and R. L. Goldenberg.** 2003. Periodontal disease and preterm birth: results of a pilot intervention study. *J. Periodontol.* **74:**1214–1218.
61. **Kasser, U. R., C. Gleissner, F. Dehne, A. Michel, B. Willershausen-Zonnchen, and W. W. Bolten.** 1997. Risk for periodontal disease in patients with longstanding rheumatoid arthritis. *Arthritis Rheum.* **40:**2248–2251.
62. **Kato, T., T. Tsuda, H. Inaba, S. Kawai, N. Okahashi, Y. Shibata, Y. Abiko, and A. Amano.** 2008. *Porphyromonas gingivalis* gingipains cause G(1) arrest in osteoblastic/stromal cells. *Oral Microbiol. Immunol.* **23:**158–164.
63. **Katz, J., K. P. Black, and S. M. Michalek.** 1999. Host responses to recombinant hemagglutinin B of *Porphyromonas gingivalis* in an experimental rat model. *Infect. Immun.* **67:**4352–4359.
64. **Khader, Y. S., and Q. Ta'ani.** 2005. Periodontal diseases and the risk of preterm birth and low birth weight: a meta-analysis. *J. Periodontol.* **76:**161–165.
65. **Kiley, P., and S. C. Holt.** 1980. Characterization of the lipopolysaccharide from *Actinobacillus actinomycetemcomitans* Y4 and N27. *Infect. Immun.* **30:**862–873.
66. **Kinane, D. F., D. R. Demuth, S. U. Gorr, G. N. Hajishengallis, and M. H. Martin.** 2007. Human variability in innate immunity. *Periodontology 2000* **45:**14–34.
67. **Kolenbrander, P. E.** 1993. Coaggregation of human oral bacteria: potential role in the accretion of dental plaque. *J. Appl. Bacteriol.* **74:**79S–86S.
68. **Kolenbrander, P. E., R. N. Andersen, K. Kazmerzak, R. Wu, and R. J. Palmer, Jr.** 1999. Spatial organization of oral bacteria in biofilms. *Methods Enzymol.* **310:**322–332.
69. **Kolodgie, F. D., H. K. Gold, A. P. Burke, D. R. Fowler, H. S. Kruth, D. K. Weber, A. Farb, L. J. Guerrero, M. Hayase, R. Kutys, J. Narula, A. V. Finn, and R. Virmani.** 2003. Intraplaque hemorrhage and progression of coronary atheroma. *N. Engl. J. Med.* **349:**2316–2325.
70. **Kozarov, E. V., B. R. Dorn, C. E. Shelburne, W. A. Dunn, Jr., and A. Progulske-Fox.** 2005. Human atherosclerotic plaque contains viable invasive *Actinobacillus actinomycetemcomitans* and *Porphyromonas gingivalis*. *Arterioscler. Thromb. Vasc. Biol.* **25:**e17–e18.
71. **Kubar, A., I. Saygun, A. Ozdemir, M. Yapar, and J. Slots.** 2005. Real-time polymerase chain reaction quantification of human cytomegalovirus and Epstein-Barr virus in periodontal pockets and the adjacent gingiva of periodontitis lesions. *J. Periodontal. Res.* **40:**97–104.
72. **Kuramitsu, H. K., M. Qi, I. C. Kang, and W. Chen.** 2001. Role for periodontal bacteria in cardiovascular diseases. *Ann. Periodontol.* **6:**41–47.

73. **Lafaurie, G. I., I. Mayorga-Fayad, M. F. Torres, D. M. Castillo, M. R. Aya, A. Baron, and P. A. Hurtado.** 2007. Periodontopathic microorganisms in peripheric blood after scaling and root planing. *J. Clin. Periodontol.* **34:**873–879.
74. **Laine, M. L., and A. J. van Winkelhoff.** 1998. Virulence of six capsular serotypes of *Porphyromonas gingivalis* in a mouse model. *Oral Microbiol. Immunol.* **13:**322–325.
75. **Lally, E. T., E. E. Golub, I. R. Kieba, N. S. Taichman, J. Rosenbloom, J. C. Rosenbloom, C. W. Gibson, and D. R. Demuth.** 1989. Analysis of the *Actinobacillus actinomycetemcomitans* leukotoxin gene. Delineation of unique features and comparison to homologous toxins. *J. Biol. Chem.* **264:**15451–15456.
76. **Ledder, R. G., P. Gilbert, S. A. Huws, L. Aarons, M. P. Ashley, P. S. Hull, and A. J. McBain.** 2007. Molecular analysis of the subgingival microbiota in health and disease. *Appl. Environ. Microbiol.* **73:**516–523.
77. **Lee, J. Y., H. T. Sojar, G. S. Bedi, and R. J. Genco.** 1991. *Porphyromonas (Bacteroides) gingivalis* fimbrillin: size, amino-terminal sequence, and antigenic heterogeneity. *Infect. Immun.* **59:**383–389.
78. **Lee, S. D., S. H. Chang, W. H. Kuo, T. H. Ying, W. W. Kuo, P. C. Li, H. H. Hsu, M. C. Lu, H. Ting, and C. Y. Huang.** 2006. Role of mitogen-activated protein kinase kinase in *Porphyromonas gingivalis*-induced myocardial cell hypertrophy and apoptosis. *Eur. J. Oral Sci.* **114:**154–159.
79. **Lee, S. D., W. W. Kuo, D. Y. Lin, T. H. Chen, W. H. Kuo, H. H. Hsu, J. Z. Chen, J. Y. Liu, Y. L. Yeh, and C. Y. Huang.** 2006. Role of calcineurin in *Porphyromonas gingivalis*-induced myocardial cell hypertrophy and apoptosis. *J. Biomed. Sci.* **13:**251–260.
80. **Lee, S. D., C. C. Wu, Y. C. Chang, S. H. Chang, C. H. Wu, J. P. Wu, J. M. Hwang, W. W. Kuo, J. Y. Liu, and C. Y. Huang.** 2006. *Porphyromonas gingivalis*-induced cellular hypertrophy and MMP-9 activity via different signaling pathways in H9c2 cardiomyoblast cells. *J. Periodontol.* **77:**684–691.
81. **Lee, S. D., C. C. Wu, W. W. Kuo, J. A. Lin, J. M. Hwang, M. C. Lu, L. M. Chen, H. H. Hsu, C. K. Wang, S. H. Chang, and C. Y. Huang.** 2006. *Porphyromonas gingivalis*-related cardiac cell apoptosis was majorly co-activated by p38 and extracellular signal-regulated kinase pathways. *J. Periodontal. Res.* **41:**39–46.
82. **Lepine, G., R. P. Ellen, and A. Progulske-Fox.** 1996. Construction and preliminary characterization of three hemagglutinin mutants of *Porphyromonas gingivalis. Infect. Immun.* **64:**1467–1472.
83. **Lepine, G., and A. Progulske-Fox.** 1996. Duplication and differential expression of hemagglutinin genes in *Porphyromonas gingivalis. Oral Microbiol. Immunol.* **11:**65–78.
84. **Lepp, P. W., M. M. Brinig, C. C. Ouverney, K. Palm, G. C. Armitage, and D. A. Relman.** 2004. Methanogenic Archaea and human periodontal disease. *Proc. Natl. Acad. Sci. USA* **101:**6176–6181.
85. **Libby, P.** 2002. Inflammation in atherosclerosis. *Nature* **420:**868–874.
86. **Lofthus, J. E., M. Y. Waki, D. L. Jolkovsky, J. Otomo-Corgel, M. G. Newman, T. Flemmig, and S. Nachnani.** 1991. Bacteremia following subgingival irrigation and scaling and root planing. *J. Periodontol.* **62:**602–607.
87. **Madianos, P. N., S. Lieff, A. P. Murtha, K. A. Boggess, R. L. Auten, Jr., J. D. Beck, and S. Offenbacher.** 2001. Maternal periodontitis and prematurity. Part II: maternal infection and fetal exposure. *Ann. Periodontol.* **6:**175–182.
88. **Mallika, V., B. Goswami, and M. Rajappa.** 2007. Atherosclerosis pathophysiology and the role of novel risk factors: a clinicobiochemical perspective. *Angiology* **58:**513–522.
89. **Matsuura, E., K. Kobayashi, and L. R. Lopez.** 2008. Preventing autoimmune and infection triggered atherosclerosis for an enduring healthful lifestyle. *Autoimmun. Rev.* **7:**214–222.
90. **Mattila, K. J., M. S. Nieminen, V. V. Valtonen, V. P. Rasi, Y. A. Kesaniemi, S. L. Syrjala, P. S. Jungell, M. Isoluoma, K. Hietaniemi, and M. J. Jokinen.** 1989. Association between dental health and acute myocardial infarction. *BMJ* **298:**779–781.
91. **McCullough, P. A.** 2007. Coronary artery disease. *Clin. J. Am. Soc. Nephrol.* **2:**611–616.
92. **Mercado, F., R. I. Marshall, A. C. Klestov, and P. M. Bartold.** 2000. Is there a relationship between rheumatoid arthritis and periodontal disease? *J. Clin. Periodontol.* **27:**267–272.
93. **Mercado, F. B., R. I. Marshall, and P. M. Bartold.** 2003. Inter-relationships between rheumatoid arthritis and periodontal disease. A review. *J. Clin. Periodontol.* **30:**761–772.
94. **Mercado, F. B., R. I. Marshall, A. C. Klestov, and P. M. Bartold.** 2001. Relationship between rheumatoid arthritis and periodontitis. *J. Periodontol.* **72:**779–787.
95. **Messini, M., I. Skourti, E. Markopulos, C. Koutsia-Carouzou, E. Kyriakopoulou, S. Kostaki, D. Lambraki, and A. Georgopoulos.** 1999. Bacteremia after dental treatment in mentally handicapped people. *J. Clin. Periodontol.* **26:**469–473.
96. **Meyer, D. H., P. K. Sreenivasan, and P. M. Fives-Taylor.** 1991. Evidence for invasion of a human oral cell line by *Actinobacillus actinomycetemcomitans. Infect. Immun.* **59:**2719–2726.
97. **Michalowicz, B. S., J. S. Hodges, A. J. DiAngelis, V. R. Lupo, M. J. Novak, J. E. Ferguson, W. Buchanan, J. Bofill, P. N. Papapanou, D. A. Mitchell, S. Matseoane, and P. A. Tschida.** 2006. Treatment of periodontal disease and the risk of preterm birth. *N. Engl. J. Med.* **355:**1885–1894.
98. **Moncla, B. J., P. Braham, L. K. Rabe, and S. L. Hillier.** 1991. Rapid presumptive identification of black-pigmented gram-negative anaerobic bacteria by using 4-methylumbelliferone derivatives. *J. Clin. Microbiol.* **29:**1955–1958.
99. **Moore, W. E., and L. V. Moore.** 1994. The bacteria of periodontal diseases. *Periodontology 2000* **5:**66–77.
100. **Morrison, H. I., L. F. Ellison, and G. W. Taylor.** 1999. Periodontal disease and risk of fatal coronary heart and cerebrovascular diseases. *J. Cardiovasc. Risk* **6:**7–11.
101. **Murphy, A. M., C. G. Daly, D. H. Mitchell, D. Stewart, and B. H. Curtis.** 2006. Chewing fails to induce oral bacteraemia in patients with periodontal disease. *J. Clin. Periodontol.* **33:**730–736.
102. **Mustapha, I. Z., S. Debrey, M. Oladubu, and R. Ugarte.** 2007. Markers of systemic bacterial exposure in periodontal disease and cardiovascular disease risk: a systematic review and meta-analysis. *J. Periodontol.* **78:**2289–2302.
103. **Nakamura, N., M. Yoshida, M. Umeda, Y. Huang, S. Kitajima, Y. Inoue, I. Ishikawa, and T. Iwai.** 2008. Extended exposure of lipopolysaccharide fraction from *Porphyromonas gingivalis* facilitates mononuclear cell adhesion to vascular endothelium via Toll-like receptor-2 dependent mechanism. *Atherosclerosis* **196:**59–67.
104. **Nakano, K., H. Inaba, R. Nomura, H. Nemoto, H. Takeuchi, H. Yoshioka, K. Toda, K. Taniguchi, A. Amano, and T. Ooshima.** 2008. Distribution of *Porphyromonas gingivalis*

fimA genotypes in cardiovascular specimens from Japanese patients. *Oral Microbiol. Immunol.* **23:**170–172.

105. **Nassar, H., H. H. Chou, M. Khlgatian, F. C. Gibson III, T. E. Van Dyke, and C. A. Genco.** 2002. Role for fimbriae and lysine-specific cysteine proteinase gingipain K in expression of interleukin-8 and monocyte chemoattractant protein in *Porphyromonas gingivalis*-infected endothelial cells. *Infect. Immun.* **70:**268–276.
106. **Newnham, J. P., A. Shub, A. H. Jobe, P. S. Bird, M. Ikegami, I. Nitsos, and T. J. Moss.** 2005. The effects of intra-amniotic injection of periodontopathic lipopolysaccharides in sheep. *Am. J. Obstet. Gynecol.* **193:**313–321.
107. **Nonnenmacher, C., M. Stelzel, C. Susin, A. M. Sattler, J. R. Schaefer, B. Maisch, R. Mutters, and L. Flores-de-Jacoby.** 2007. Periodontal microbiota in patients with coronary artery disease measured by real-time polymerase chain reaction: a case-control study. *J. Periodontol.* **78:**1724–1730.
108. **O'Sullivan, J. M., H. F. Jenkinson, and R. D. Cannon.** 2000. Adhesion of *Candida albicans* to oral streptococci is promoted by selective adsorption of salivary proteins to the streptococcal cell surface. *Microbiology* **146:**41–48.
109. **Offenbacher, S.** 1996. Periodontal diseases: pathogenesis. *Ann. Periodontol.* **1:**821–878.
110. **Offenbacher, S., V. Katz, G. Fertik, J. Collins, D. Boyd, G. Maynor, R. McKaig, and J. Beck.** 1996. Periodontal infection as a possible risk factor for preterm low birth weight. *J. Periodontol.* **67:**1103–1113.
111. **Offenbacher, S., S. Lieff, K. A. Boggess, A. P. Murtha, P. N. Madianos, C. M. Champagne, R. G. McKaig, H. L. Jared, S. M. Mauriello, R. L. Auten, Jr., W. N. Herbert, and J. D. Beck.** 2001. Maternal periodontitis and prematurity. Part I: obstetric outcome of prematurity and growth restriction. *Ann. Periodontol.* **6:**164–174.
112. **Ogawa, T., K. Yasuda, K. Yamada, H. Mori, K. Ochiai, and M. Hasegawa.** 1995. Immunochemical characterisation and epitope mapping of a novel fimbrial protein (Pg-II fimbria) of *Porphyromonas gingivalis. FEMS Immunol. Med. Microbiol.* **11:**247–255.
113. **Okuda, K., A. Yamamoto, Y. Naito, I. Takazoe, J. Slots, and R. J. Genco.** 1986. Purification and properties of hemagglutinin from culture supernatant of *Bacteroides gingivalis. Infect. Immun.* **54:**659–665.
114. **Papapanou, P. N., V. Baelum, W. M. Luan, P. N. Madianos, X. Chen, O. Fejerskov, and G. Dahlen.** 1997. Subgingival microbiota in adult Chinese: prevalence and relation to periodontal disease progression. *J. Periodontol.* **68:**651–666.
115. **Paster, B. J., S. K. Boches, J. L. Galvin, R. E. Ericson, C. N. Lau, V. A. Levanos, A. Sahasrabudhe, and F. E. Dewhirst.** 2001. Bacterial diversity in human subgingival plaque. *J. Bacteriol.* **183:**3770–3783.
116. **Plutzky, J.** 2001. Inflammatory pathways in atherosclerosis and acute coronary syndromes. *Am. J. Cardiol.* **88:**10K–15K.
117. **Potempa, J., and J. Travis.** 1996. *Porphyromonas gingivalis* proteinases in periodontitis, a review. *Acta Biochim. Pol.* **43:**455–465.
118. **Progulske-Fox, A., E. Kozarov, B. Dorn, W. Dunn, Jr., J. Burks, and Y. Wu.** 1999. *Porphyromonas gingivalis* virulence factors and invasion of cells of the cardiovascular system. *J. Periodontal. Res.* **34:**393–399.
119. **Progulske-Fox, A., S. Tumwasorn, and S. C. Holt.** 1989. The expression and function of a *Bacteroides gingivalis* hemagglutinin gene in *Escherichia coli. Oral Microbiol. Immunol.* **4:**121–131.
120. **Progulske-Fox, A., S. Tumwasorn, G. Lepine, J. Whitlock, D. Savett, J. J. Ferretti, and J. A. Banas.** 1995. The cloning, expression and sequence analysis of a second *Porphyromonas gingivalis* gene that codes for a protein involved in hemagglutination. *Oral Microbiol. Immunol.* **10:**311–318.
121. **Pucar, A., J. Milasin, V. Lekovic, M. Vukadinovic, M. Ristic, S. Putnik, and E. B. Kenney.** 2007. Correlation between atherosclerosis and periodontal putative pathogenic bacterial infections in coronary and internal mammary arteries. *J. Periodontol.* **78:**677–682.
122. **Pussinen, P. J., G. Alfthan, P. Jousilahti, S. Paju, and J. Tuomilehto.** 2007. Systemic exposure to *Porphyromonas gingivalis* predicts incident stroke. *Atherosclerosis* **193:**222–228.
123. **Pussinen, P. J., G. Alfthan, H. Rissanen, A. Reunanen, S. Asikainen, and P. Knekt.** 2004. Antibodies to periodontal pathogens and stroke risk. *Stroke* **35:**2020–2023.
124. **Pussinen, P. J., G. Alfthan, J. Tuomilehto, S. Asikainen, and P. Jousilahti.** 2004. High serum antibody levels to *Porphyromonas gingivalis* predict myocardial infarction. *Eur. J. Cardiovasc. Prev. Rehabil.* **11:**408–411.
125. **Pussinen, P. J., P. Jousilahti, G. Alfthan, T. Palosuo, S. Asikainen, and V. Salomaa.** 2003. Antibodies to periodontal pathogens are associated with coronary heart disease. *Arterioscler. Thromb. Vasc. Biol.* **23:**1250–1254.
126. **Quirynen, M., R. Vogels, M. Pauwels, A. D. Haffajee, S. S. Socransky, N. G. Uzel, and D. van Steenberghe.** 2005. Initial subgingival colonization of 'pristine' pockets. *J. Dent. Res.* **84:**340–344.
127. **Renvert, S., T. Pettersson, O. Ohlsson, and G. R. Persson.** 2006. Bacterial profile and burden of periodontal infection in subjects with a diagnosis of acute coronary syndrome. *J. Periodontol.* **77:**1110–1119.
128. **Ribeiro, J., A. Leao, and A. B. Novaes.** 2005. Periodontal infection as a possible severity factor for rheumatoid arthritis. *J. Clin. Periodontol.* **32:**412–416.
129. **Rodrigues, P. H., M. Belanger, W. Dunn, Jr., and A. Progulske-Fox.** 2008. *Porphyromonas gingivalis* and the autophagic pathway: an innate immune interaction? *Front. Biosci.* **13:**178–187.
130. **Rodrigues, P. H., and A. Progulske-Fox.** 2005. Gene expression profile analysis of *Porphyromonas gingivalis* during invasion of human coronary artery endothelial cells. *Infect. Immun.* **73:**6169–6173.
131. **Ross, R.** 1993. The pathogenesis of atherosclerosis: a perspective for the 1990s. *Nature* **362:**801–809.
132. **Roth, G. A., B. Moser, F. Roth-Walter, M. B. Giacona, E. Harja, P. N. Papapanou, A. M. Schmidt, and E. Lalla.** 2007. Infection with a periodontal pathogen increases mononuclear cell adhesion to human aortic endothelial cells. *Atherosclerosis* **190:**271–281.
133. **Sakurai, K., D. Wang, J. Suzuki, M. Umeda, T. Nagasawa, Y. Izumi, I. Ishikawa, and M. Isobe.** 2007. High incidence of *Actinobacillus actinomycetemcomitans* infection in acute coronary syndrome. *Int. Heart J.* **48:**663–675.
134. **Saygun, I., A. Kubar, A. Ozdemir, and J. Slots.** 2005. Periodontitis lesions are a source of salivary cytomegalovirus and Epstein-Barr virus. *J. Periodontal Res.* **40:**187–191.
135. **Scannapieco, F. A.** 1999. Role of oral bacteria in respiratory infection. *J. Periodontol.* **70:**793–802.
136. **Scannapieco, F. A., R. B. Bush, and S. Paju.** 2003. Associations between periodontal disease and risk for atherosclerosis, cardiovascular disease, and stroke. A systematic review. *Ann. Periodontol.* **8:**38–53.
137. **Scannapieco, F. A., R. B. Bush, and S. Paju.** 2003. Associations between periodontal disease and risk for nosocomial bacterial pneumonia and chronic obstructive

pulmonary disease. A systematic review. *Ann. Periodontol.* **8:**54–69.

138. **Sconyers, J. R., J. J. Crawford, and J. D. Moriarty.** 1973. Relationship of bacteremia to toothbrushing in patients with periodontitis. *J. Am. Dent. Assoc.* **87:**616–622.
139. **Sheets, S. M., J. Potempa, J. Travis, C. A. Casiano, and H. M. Fletcher.** 2005. Gingipains from *Porphyromonas gingivalis* W83 induce cell adhesion molecule cleavage and apoptosis in endothelial cells. *Infect. Immun.* **73:**1543–1552.
140. **Slots, J.** 2000. *Actinobacillus actinomycetemcomitans* and *Porphyromonas gingivalis* in periodontal disease: introduction. *Periodontology* **20:**7–13.
141. **Slots, J., and A. Contreras.** 2000. Herpesviruses: a unifying causative factor in periodontitis? *Oral Microbiol. Immunol.* **15:**277–280.
142. **Slots, J., and R. J. Gibbons.** 1978. Attachment of *Bacteroides melaninogenicus* subsp. *asaccharolyticus* to oral surfaces and its possible role in colonization of the mouth and of periodontal pockets. *Infect. Immun.* **19:**254–264.
143. **Sojar, H. T., J. Y. Lee, G. S. Bedi, M. I. Cho, and R. J. Genco.** 1991. Purification, characterization and immunolocalization of fimbrial protein from *Porphyromonas (Bacteroides) gingivalis*. *Biochem. Biophys. Res. Commun.* **175:**713–719.
144. **Song, H., M. Belanger, J. Whitlock, E. Kozarov, and A. Progulske-Fox.** 2005. Hemagglutinin B is involved in the adherence of *Porphyromonas gingivalis* to human coronary artery endothelial cells. *Infect. Immun.* **73:**7267–7273.
145. **Spahr, A., E. Klein, N. Khuseyinova, C. Boeckh, R. Muche, M. Kunze, D. Rothenbacher, G. Pezeshki, A. Hoffmeister, and W. Koenig.** 2006. Periodontal infections and coronary heart disease: role of periodontal bacteria and importance of total pathogen burden in the Coronary Event and Periodontal Disease (CORODONT) study. *Arch. Intern. Med.* **166:**554–559.
146. **Takahashi, Y., M. Davey, H. Yumoto, F. C. Gibson III, and C. A. Genco.** 2006. Fimbria-dependent activation of pro-inflammatory molecules in *Porphyromonas gingivalis* infected human aortic endothelial cells. *Cell. Microbiol.* **8:** 738–757.
147. **Tanner, A. C., B. J. Paster, S. C. Lu, E. Kanasi, R. Kent, Jr., T. Van Dyke, and S. T. Sonis.** 2006. Subgingival and tongue microbiota during early periodontitis. *J. Dent. Res.* **85:**318–323.
148. **Tanner, A. C., M. N. Strzempko, C. A. Belsky, and G. A. McKinley.** 1985. API ZYM and API An-Ident reactions of fastidious oral gram-negative species. *J. Clin. Microbiol.* **22:**333–335.
149. **Tannock, G.** 1999. *Medical Importance of the Normal Microflora.* Kluwer Academic Publishers, Norwell, MA.
150. **Taylor, G. W., B. A. Burt, M. P. Becker, R. J. Genco, M. Shlossman, W. C. Knowler, and D. J. Pettitt.** 1996. Severe periodontitis and risk for poor glycemic control in patients with non-insulin-dependent diabetes mellitus. *J. Periodontol.* **67:**1085–1093.
151. **Teramoto, T., J. Sasaki, H. Ueshima, G. Egusa, M. Kinoshita, K. Shimamoto, H. Daida, S. Biro, K. Hirobe, T. Funahashi, K. Yokote, and M. Yokode.** 2007. Risk factors of atherosclerotic diseases. Executive summary of Japan Atherosclerosis Society (JAS) guideline for diagnosis and prevention of atherosclerosis cardiovascular diseases for Japanese. *J. Atheroscler. Thromb.* **14:**267–277.
152. **Travis, J., A. Banbula, and J. Potempa.** 2000. The role of bacterial and host proteinases in periodontal disease. *Adv. Exp. Med. Biol.* **477:**455–465.
153. **Travis, J., R. Pike, T. Imamura, and J. Potempa.** 1997. *Porphyromonas gingivalis* proteinases as virulence factors in the development of periodontitis. *J. Periodontal. Res.* **32:**120–125.
154. **van Winkelhoff, A. J., B. J. Appelmelk, N. Kippuw, and J. de Graaff.** 1993. K-antigens in *Porphyromonas gingivalis* are associated with virulence. *Oral Microbiol. Immunol.* **8:**259–265.
155. **Veith, P. D., G. H. Talbo, N. Slakeski, S. G. Dashper, C. Moore, R. A. Paolini, and E. C. Reynolds.** 2002. Major outer membrane proteins and proteolytic processing of RgpA and Kgp of *Porphyromonas gingivalis* W50. *Biochem. J.* **363:**105–115.
156. **Wilson, M.** 1995. Biological activities of lipopolysaccharides from oral bacteria and their relevance to the pathogenesis of chronic periodontitis. *Sci. Prog.* **78:**19–34.
157. **Wu, H., and P. M. Fives-Taylor.** 2001. Molecular strategies for fimbrial expression and assembly. *Crit. Rev. Oral Biol. Med.* **12:**101–115.
158. **Wu, H. C., Y. L. Yeh, W. W. Kuo, S. K. Huang, W. H. Kuo, D. J. Hsieh, C. L. Wu, C. H. Tsai, S. D. Lee, and C. Y. Huang.** 2008. P38 mitogen-activated protein kinase pathways are involved in the hypertrophy and apoptosis of cardiomyocytes induced by *Porphyromonas gingivalis* conditioned medium. *Cell. Biochem. Funct.* **26:**246–255.
159. **Yamazaki, K., T. Honda, H. Domon, T. Okui, K. Kajita, R. Amanuma, C. Kudoh, S. Takashiba, S. Kokeguchi, F. Nishimura, M. Kodama, Y. Aizawa, and H. Oda.** 2007. Relationship of periodontal infection to serum antibody levels to periodontopathic bacteria and inflammatory markers in periodontitis patients with coronary heart disease. *Clin. Exp. Immunol.* **149:**445–452.
160. **Yoshimura, F., K. Takahashi, Y. Nodasaka, and T. Suzuki.** 1984. Purification and characterization of a novel type of fimbriae from the oral anaerobe *Bacteroides gingivalis*. *J. Bacteriol.* **160:**949–957.
161. **Yuan, L., P. H. Rodrigues, M. Belanger, W. A. Dunn, Jr., and A. Progulske-Fox.** 2008. *Porphyromonas gingivalis* htrA is involved in cellular invasion and in vivo survival. *Microbiology* **154:**1161–1169.
162. **Zambon, J. J., L. A. Christersson, and J. Slots.** 1983. *Actinobacillus actinomycetemcomitans* in human periodontal disease. Prevalence in patient groups and distribution of biotypes and serotypes within families. *J. Periodontol.* **54:**707–711.
163. **Zaremba, M., R. Gorska, P. Suwalski, and J. Kowalski.** 2007. Evaluation of the incidence of periodontitis-associated bacteria in the atherosclerotic plaque of coronary blood vessels. *J. Periodontol.* **78:**322–327.
164. **Zhang, P., M. Martin, S. M. Michalek, and J. Katz.** 2005. Role of mitogen-activated protein kinases and NF-kappaB in the regulation of proinflammatory and anti-inflammatory cytokines by *Porphyromonas gingivalis* hemagglutinin B. *Infect. Immun.* **73:**3990–3998.
165. **Zhang, P., M. Martin, Q. B. Yang, S. M. Michalek, and J. Katz.** 2004. Role of B7 costimulatory molecules in immune responses and T-helper cell differentiation in response to recombinant HagB from *Porphyromonas gingivalis*. *Infect. Immun.* **72:**637–644.

Sequelae and Long-Term Consequences of Infectious Diseases
Edited by Pina M. Fratamico, James L. Smith, and Kim A. Brogden

Chapter 26

Diseases with Long-Term Consequences in Search of a Microbial Agent

James L. Smith and Pina M. Fratamico

The chapters presented in the current volume indicate that microorganisms can initiate diseases with long-term consequences (i.e., chronic diseases) in the infected host. A chronic disease is an illness that is prolonged, does not resolve spontaneously, is rarely cured completely, and has a duration of 3 months or longer. A listing of such chronic diseases in which infectious agents have been demonstrated is presented by Carbone et al. (22). However, there are other chronic diseases that are suspected of having an infectious origin, but proof is lacking, and among these diseases are multiple sclerosis (MS), inflammatory bowel disease (IBD), chronic fatigue syndrome (CFS), and others (22).

Host factors that may contribute to long-term consequences as a result of infections include the genetic background of the host (major histocompatibility complex status or genetic defects that increase susceptibility to disease), concomitant infections, age, gender, hormonal status, immune status, nutritional status, environmental factors, and behavioral attitudes (22, 122, 128). Important microbial factors include integration of microbial DNA into the host genome (leading to inactivation of essential genes of the host or promotion of oncogenesis), microbial latency (persistence), ability of a pathogen to bind to mucosal surfaces or tissues, high mutation rate of the microorganism, ability of the microorganism to evade the immune response (coating itself with host proteins, living within cells, or occupying immune privileged sites, such as the brain, eye, or testis), ability of a bacterial antigen to mimic a host molecule, biofilm formation (on medical implants or on tissues), malignant transformation (cells acquire the properties of cancer), and ability to induce inflammation (22, 23, 122, 128).

There are a number of reasons why it is difficult to demonstrate an infecting organism-disease connection: (i) the infecting organism is ubiquitous (many people carry the organism but few show signs of illness); (ii) the organism has a long latency period which makes it hard to connect the disease with the infecting organism; (iii) a complicated syndrome makes it problematic to associate the disease with a causative organism; (iv) if an affected tissue is relatively inaccessible (i.e., the brain), attempts to differentiate between infected and uninfected individuals are difficult; (e) current methodology may not be adequate to detect the organism; (f) a causative agent may not be identified if an illness occurs after the organism has been cleared from the host; (g) when a disease occurs at a nonsterile site, it is virtually impossible to associate a particular organism with the disease; and (h) strict adherence to Koch's postulates when studying a chronic disease may hinder the detection of the inciting pathogen (22, 46).

In the present chapter, the symptoms and long-term consequences of chronic diseases, including autism, rheumatoid arthritis (RA), IBD, CFS, and MS, are discussed. In addition, studies of potential candidates for causative pathogens for these illnesses will be presented.

CHRONIC DISEASES SUSPECTED OF HAVING A MICROBIAL TRIGGER

Autism

Autism in children is a behavior-defined syndrome and is diagnosed on the basis of clinical history. There are no known biomarkers. Autism is one of the autistic spectrum disorders (ASDs); these disorders include a diverse group of conditions which present with consistent abnormal behavior patterns (67). Therefore, ASDs are etiologically, biologically, and clinically heterogeneous neurobehavioral syndromes.

James L. Smith and Pina M. Fratamico • Microbial Food Safety Research Unit, Eastern Regional Research Center, Agricultural Research Service, United States Department of Agriculture, 600 East Mermaid Lane, Wyndmoor, PA 19038-6520.

There are three main clusters of behavior in ASD: (i) impairment of social interactions (the autistic individual has little interest in interacting with others and tends to be a "loner"); (ii) impairment in communication and language skills; and (iii) rigid, stereotyped, and repetitive patterns of behavior, interests, and activities (18, 71, 82). Aberrant brain development leads to errors in neural information processing, resulting in behavior abnormalities characteristic of autism and ASDs (12). Symptoms can vary from mild to very severe; therefore, autism symptoms are diverse, and there is a wide spectrum of autistic behavior. Most individuals with autism appear abnormal from birth (often with craniofacial defects), and most are severely retarded. Thus, early onset autism should be viewed as a birth defect (139). Twenty to 30% of children demonstrate apparently normal development until 18 to 24 months of age before they show regression in their normal behavior and display the signs of autistic behavior (regressive autism) (69, 82). Autism occurs in 1 or 2 babies/1,000 births and occurs three or four times more often in boys than girls; however, ASDs occur in 4 to 6 babies/1,000 births (18, 82, 140). The Autism and Developmental Disabilities Monitoring Network presented data from six sites in the United States for the year 2000 which indicated that ASD prevalence was 6.7/1,000 children (24).

Genetic susceptibility appears to be a necessary component of autism, and the genetic picture is quite complex. Chromosomal disarrangements, rare single gene mutations, and multiplicative effects of common gene variants are involved in autism and the ASDs and are influenced by environmental factors (56, 67, 115, 158, 166). Thus, there is a great deal of genetic heterogeneity in autism and ASDs, indicating that many genetic loci are involved. The concordance rate in monozygotic twins for developing autism is 70%, and it increases to 90% for ASDs. The concordance rate for dizygotic twins is 5 to 10%. The risk that a sibling of an autistic child will develop autism is 4.5% (12, 147). Recent work has indicated that candidate genes for ASDs may be found by studying targeted mutations in a mouse model. If the consequence of a mutation is a phenotype analogous to human ASD, then that gene may play an important role in the disorder (30, 159).

Potential triggers that may induce autism and ASDs include microbial infections, chemicals, food products, drugs, and medications, but at the present time, no inducing agent has been identified. Infections in utero or drugs and/or medications taken during pregnancy could be potential triggers for early-onset autism, whereas exposure of a child to an infection, a chemical, or toxin could trigger regressive autism.

Utilizing data from 403 children with ASDs and 2,100 controls, Rosen et al. (140) studied the association between infections and ASDs. They found that children with subsequent diagnosis of ASD did not have more infections in the first 2 years of life than children without ASD. However, it can not be ruled out that for autism-prone children any of the infections reported by Rosen et al. (140) could have induced the symptoms of autism, while such infections would not induce autism in the nonsusceptible child. In a study involving age-matched (approximately 8 years of age) ASD patients and control subjects, Nicolson et al. (119) determined that there was a higher prevalence of *Mycoplasma* species, *Chlamydia pneumoniae*, and human herpes virus 6 (HHV-6) infections in ASD patients (46/48; 95.8%) compared to control children (7/45; 15.6%). However, it is not clear whether these infections triggered autism or were opportunistic infections.

Does the immune system have a role in the induction of autism? ASD patients show signs of immune dysregulation, higher levels of autoantibodies to brain antigens, and increased incidence of familial autoimmune diseases (2). However, no definitive autoantibody pattern has been found in ASD patients. There is dysregulation or dysfunction of various components of the immune system of ASD patients (3). These immune aberrations include abnormal T cells or skewed TH1/TH2 cytokine profiles, decreased lymphocyte numbers, decreased T-cell mitogen response, and an imbalance of serum immunoglobulin levels. The dysregulation or dysfunction of the immune system during neurodevelopment may lead to neurological dysfunctions characteristic of the ASDs (3).

All children should be evaluated for ASD at their pediatric 9-, 18-, and 24- or 30-month visits (82). In the management of autism and ASDs, early intervention is a must. Better outcomes in children with regressive autism are seen if intensive and structured education is begun early. The education treatment must be combined with behavior management and family support. There must be an emphasis on functional communication (100, 117, 131). Psychotropic medication is used in extreme cases for which behavior management has failed; however, such drugs are not used as routine treatments (131). Considering the heterogeneity of autistic behaviors, treatment for ASD children must be done on an individual basis.

It is clear that the ASDs comprise several disorders with separate and specific etiologies, including genetic, environmental, immunological, and neurological factors, and that all the disorders share a common behavioral diagnosis (3). The literature indicates that genetics play a major role in autism and ASDs, and it seems logical that an infection or a chemical insult to a genetically susceptible child will induce autism. However, at the present time, the triggering mechanism, be it an infectious agent, chemical agent, or toxin, is unknown.

RA

RA is a chronic inflammatory disease involving the synovial membranes and articular structures of the joints, resulting in pain, stiffness, and swelling of the joints. Chronic RA results in progressive joint destruction, deformity, and a decline in functional status, unless the disease is treated aggressively (113). Thus, RA cripples patients by progressively destroying cartilage and bone. Extra-articular symptoms are common and include rheumatic nodules, vasculitis (inflammation of blood and lymphatic vessels), pleuropericarditis (inflammation of the pleura and pericardium), and lung involvement as well as other systemic effects. The prevalence of RA is approximately 1% among the general population worldwide, and all races are affected. The female to male ratio is approximately 3:1. Rheumatoid arthritis can occur at any age but the incidence increases with increasing age (57, 113).

Genetics play an important role in RA. Studies involving monozygotic twins indicate that up to one-third of the twins of patients with RA can expect to be eventually affected. There is only a slight increase of RA prevalence in dizygotic twins and offspring of affected parents (151). Susceptibility and severity of RA depends on the inheritance of genes in the major histocompatibility complex locus, which encodes cell surface proteins, known as the human leukocyte antigens (HLAs). Rheumatoid arthritis is closely associated with alleles of *HLA-DR* genes, in particular, alleles of the *HLA-DRB1* and *-DR4* genes. Only about 30% of the genetic risk of RA is due to HLA genes and gender (45, 53). Plenge et al. (129) tested 17 alleles of 14 genes in 2,370 RA cases and 1,757 controls (from North America and Sweden). They found that the *PTPN22* gene (encodes lymphoid protein tyrosine phosphatase, nonreceptor type 22), the *CTLA4* gene (encodes cytotoxic T-lymphocyte-associated protein 4), and the *PAD14* gene (encodes peptidylarginine deiminase citrullinating enzyme, type IV) are associated with susceptibility to RA. A genetic variant at the *TRAF1-C5* locus (*TRAF1* encodes tumor necrosis factor [TNF] receptor-associated factor 1; *C5* encodes complement component 5) on chromosome 9 has been shown to be an RA susceptibility gene in ACPA (anti-citrullinated protein/peptide antibodies)-positive individuals (130). Undoubtedly, other RA susceptibility genes are present, and Gulko (55) discusses the use of rodent models of autoimmune arthritis as a method to elucidate the genes that may be involved in susceptibility to and severity of RA.

T cells infiltrate the synovium, and most of these T cells express the CD4 phenotype and recognize antigens in restriction in the context of HLA-DR molecules. The fact that T cells infiltrate the synovium and that HLA-DR is associated with RA are strong indications that CD4 T cells play a role in RA pathogenesis (53). In addition, the efficacy of rituximab (an anti-CD20 monoclonal antibody) as a B cell-targeted therapy in the treatment of RA indicates that B cells also are involved in the pathogenesis of RA (20).

Autoantibodies are produced in RA patients. Rheumatoid factor (RF), an immunoglobulin M (IgM) antibody directed towards IgG, is found in 80 to 90% of RA patients, on examination of joint fluid. However, RF is not specific for RA, since it can be found in healthy individuals as well as patients with a number of other morbidities, and the prevalence of RF increases with age in healthy individuals (53, 112). While not present in all patients and not a requirement for developing RA, RF is a major hallmark for RA and is associated with severity and development of extra-articular symptoms. Another autoantibody found in RA patients is an antibody against peptides and proteins containing the amino acid citrulline (ACPAs). Arginine is acted on by peptidylarginine deiminases (PADs) in the presence of Ca^{++} to produce citrulline. PADs are found in monocytes and macrophages in synovial fluid (164, 170). Sixty to 70% of RA patients produce ACPAs, and these autoantibodies are specific for RA, since they are rarely detected in patients with other diseases or in healthy controls. There is a strong association between ACPAs and the presence of the *HLA-DRB1* gene and the *PAD14* gene (encodes a citrullinating enzyme) (164). A comparison of 228 RA patients with ACPAs to 226 RA patients who were negative for ACPAs indicated that patients with ACPAs develop a more severe disease course, with more evidence of joint destruction as detected by radiography (163). Thus, both RF and ACPAs are associated with radiographic severity of RA; however, they are independent markers of severity (114). Immunity against citrullinated antigens may play a critical role in RA because the citrullinated antigens are found in the inflamed joints, ACPAs are present before RA is apparent, and ACPAs are highly specific for RA (164). However, it is not clear that ACPAs incite the pathology leading to the symptoms associated with RA.

Cytokines play a key role in a broad range of inflammatory processes involved in the pathogenesis of RA (109, 151). An imbalance between proinflammatory and anti-inflammatory cytokines contributes to autoimmunity, chronic inflammation, and tissue destruction (joint damage). Extensive synovial hyperplasia and infiltration by lymphocytes, monocytes, macrophages, and fibroblasts are marked in RA. Aberrant $CD4^+$ T cells stimulate monocytes and macrophages to produce inflammatory cytokines (including interleukin-1 [IL-1], IL-6, TNF-α) and proteolytic enzymes, leading to the destruction of the synovium, cartilage, and underlying bone (109, 151). The role of cytokines in immunological processes involved in RA pathogenesis is quite complicated and somewhat confusing.

A microbiological cause for the induction of RA, while logical, has not been identified. RA patients exhibit significantly greater frequency and severity of periodontal disease compared to control individuals without RA (141). *Porphyromonas gingivalis*, an oral gram-negative, nonmotile, facultative anaerobe, is strongly correlated with adult-onset periodontitis (141). McGraw et al. (107) isolated the citrullinating enzyme, PAD, from *P. gingivalis* and Rosenstein et al. (141) and Weissmann (171) have suggested that in genetically predisposed individuals, the PAD of the oral pathogen would induce the production of citrullinated autoantigens, leading ultimately to the formation of ACPAs, an indication of impending RA and a marker of RA severity.

Latent Epstein-Barr virus ([EBV] a DNA herpes virus), cytomegalovirus ([CMV] a DNA herpes virus), and B19 virus (a DNA parvovirus) have been isolated from synovial tissue of RA patients (111). EBV is a latent virus that can be found in blood and lymphoid tissue and infects >98% of the human population by age 40 (29). Thus, EBV infection is one the most common infections found in humans. There is a wide range of clinical manifestations, and many individuals have subclinical infections (123). Baldandraud et al. (5) demonstrated a high EBV load in peripheral blood mononuclear cells from RA patients. The mean copy number (number of EBV genomes/150,000 peripheral blood mononuclear cells) of EBV was 15.64 for RA patients ($n = 84$), 1.89 for healthy controls ($n = 69$), and 5.73 for patients with rheumatic conditions other than RA ($n = 22$). The high EBV load in RA patients indicates that these patients have difficulty controlling the viral infection and suggests that EBV could be an etiologic agent of RA. If EBV is a trigger for RA in genetically predisposed individuals, then exposure to such a common virus could explain the ubiquity of RA worldwide.

EBV is present in synovial cells of the joints of some RA patients. Saal et al. (144) demonstrated EBV DNA in the synovial membranes of 34.5% of 84 RA patients, whereas only 11% of osteoarthritis patients showed the presence of EBV DNA. Individuals with EBV DNA were 5.5 times more likely to present with RA than individuals lacking EBV DNA. Patients with RA-linked HLA-DRB1 alleles and EBV were more likely to acquire RA than individuals lacking EBV DNA and the RA-linked HLA genotypes (144). EBV DNA was present in synovial tissue of 15/32 (46.9%) RA patients; no viral DNA was found in the synovial tissue from 30 patients with osteoarthritis (160). Other studies also indicate that EBV genes are present in the synovial cells of RA patients (145).

Pratesi et al. (132) demonstrated the presence of antibodies (ACPAs) specific for a citrullinated peptide of EBV in approximately 50% of Italian RA patients ($n = 170$), whereas the incidence of antibodies against the citrullinated peptide was seen in <5% of 77 healthy individuals or 161 patients with other diseases. That there are specific ACPAs for citrullinated EBV indicates that this virus is susceptible to the deiminating enzyme PAD. Therefore, ACPAs from RA patients react with an EBV-deiminated peptide, suggesting that EBV may play a role in RA induction (132).

Since there is no cure for RA, ameliorating symptoms (pain and inflammation) and improving the quality of life for RA patients have been the normal approach to therapy. Therapy that has proven useful includes nonsteroidal anti-inflammatory drugs, cyclooxygenase-2 inhibitors, disease-modifying agents (methotrexate, hydroxychloroquine, gold, D-penicillamine, sulfasalazine, cyclosporine A, minocycline, azathioprine, leflunomide, infliximab, and etanercept), glucocorticoids, and immunosuppressive agents (57, 85). Recent approaches to therapy target agents that induce tissue injury, such as the proinflammatory cytokines, and immune cells, such as T cells and B cells (7, 108, 151, 152).

The studies with EBV suggest that a viral infection may trigger the induction of RA. However, if infection is indeed a trigger for RA, it is probable that infections by a variety of agents can elicit the arthritis.

IBD

IBD refers to ulcerative colitis (UC) and Crohn's disease (CD). IBD is more common in industrialized countries than in developing countries. Both UC and CD are chronic inflammatory diseases of the GI tract, and the etiology of these diseases is unknown. UC is a chronic recurrent inflammatory disease of the mucosal surface of the rectum and extends proximately through the colon in a continuous manner. Most patients exhibit urgency to defecate, diarrhea, rectal bleeding, abdominal pain, and passage of mucus in the stool. The clinical course typically is of chronic intermittent exacerbations, followed by periods of remission. Complications of UC may include toxic megacolon (dilation of the colon) and/or perforation, anemia, and colonic adenocarcinoma (73). Any area of the GI tract may be involved in CD, but the affected areas are discontinuous, with skipped areas of unaffected tissue. Involvement of the ileocecal portion of the bowel is present in approximately 40% of CD patients; about 30% have CD involvement of the terminal ileal portion, and approximately 25% have CD restricted to the colon (73). Unlike UC, CD affects all of the layers of the bowel, not just the mucosa and submucosa. The bowel wall can be thickened, fibrotic, and narrowed, and deep fissures can develop. The mucosa may present a cobblestone appearance (73). Complications of CD include stenosis (stricture leading to partial or complete bowel obstruction), vitamin B_{12} and fat-soluble vitamin deficiency, malabsorption of bile salts and lipids, fistulae, formation of urinary calcium oxalate stones, and carcinoma (73). Extraintestinal manifestations of IBD include arthritis, liver complications (intrahepatic and biliary tract diseases), cutaneous manifestations, and ocular symptoms (32, 73).

IBD affects 0.5 to 1.0% of the population in western countries; it is second to rheumatoid arthritis as a cause of chronic inflammation. The incidence has been increasing throughout the world, possibly as a result of populations switching to a more western style of life (142). The incidence of IBD in the United States is 70 to 150 cases/100,000 population. The incidence is slightly higher in females than in males. The peak onset of IBD occurs between 15 and 30 years, but the disease can occur at any age. IBD in young children results in growth retardation in addition to the intestinal symptoms (142, 149). In the United States, IBD accounts for approximately 700,000 visits to physicians, 100,000 hospitalizations, and disability in 119,000 patients. Up to 75% of CD patients and 25 to 33% of UC patients will require surgery (60).

Approximately 10% of IBD patients have a first-degree relative (parent, sibling, child) with the disease, and first-degree relatives of IBD patients have a 10- to 15-fold increased risk of developing IBD (73). A positive family history is the largest independent risk factor for the development of IBD. Patients with CD have a first-degree relative with CD in 2.2 to 16.2% of cases, and patients with UC have a first-degree relative with UC in 5.7 to 15.5% of cases (9). The concordance rate for CD in monozygotic twins ranged from 42 to 58%, whereas concordance for UC ranges between 6 and 17%. The concordance rate for CD in dizygotic twins is 4 to 12%, and for UC it is 0 to 5%. A concordance rate of 100% would indicate that the IBDs have only genetic factors as the cause (66). A monozygotic co-twin of a CD patient has a relative risk of developing CD of 667, whereas the monozygotic co-twin of a UC patient has a relative risk of developing UC of 71. The relative risk of developing CD in the dizygotic co-twin of a CD patient was zero, but the dizygotic co-twin of a UC patient has a relative risk of 22 for developing UC (143). These data indicate that there is a strong genetic basis in the development of IBD, particularly for CD. Hugot et al. (75) mapped a susceptibility locus for CD to chromosome 16, associated with three variants of the *NOD2* gene. The gene is now labeled *CARD15* and is often written as *NOD2/CARD15* (105). NOD2 is an intracellular protein that senses bacterial products such as muramyl dipeptide, a bacterial peptidoglycan product, and activates components of the immune system. However, homozygous mutations in *NOD2/CARD15* account for only about 20% of CD cases (74). Other, less clearly characterized, genetic loci appear to be associated with susceptibility to CD (9, 48, 105, 133, 165). Since IBD is a quite complex genetic disorder, it is probable that a defect in a single gene does not account for all cases of CD and UC, and therefore, each susceptibility gene only partially contributes to the disease risk (74).

Environmental factors associated with IBD include smoking cigarettes (active smoking decreases risk for UC but increases risk for CD), appendectomy (decreases risk for UC), breast feeding (decreases risk for CD), early infection (increases risk for IBD), economic status (higher status increases risk for IBD), geographic location (IBD more common in western countries and northern regions), sanitation (lower standard of cleanliness decreases risk for IBD), occupation (increased IBD in white collar workers compared to blue collar), and gastrointestinal infections (increases risk for IBD) (6, 9).

In CD, naïve T cells (TH0) cells are transformed into TH1 cells under the influence of IL-12. These cells produce the proinflammatory cytokines, gamma interferon (IFN-γ), IL-2, and TNF-α (60, 76). However, UC does not appear to be a TH1-mediated disease but is rather an atypical TH2-mediated disease. These TH2 cells produce the cytokines IL-5 and IL-13 (60, 88). The cytokines IL-5 and IL-13 are involved in hypersensitivity immune reactions. People with CD have difficulty clearing overreactive or autoreactive T cells due to a defective apoptosis mechanism. Inappropriate control of T-cell proliferation and death leads to an accumulation of T cells and subsequent increase in inflammation (39). Intestinal tissue destruction in IBD involves reactive oxygen and nitrogen species as well as proteolytic enzymes released through degranulation by polymorphonuclear leucocytes (granulocytes) recruited to the site by cytokine action (60, 89, 90).

Intestinal inflammation does not occur in germfree mice, and there is a general opinion that in the absence of intestinal bacteria, there can be no IBD (6, 157). Therefore, there is strong evidence that intestinal commensal bacteria (or their products), rather than conventional pathogens, are the drivers of dysregulated immunity and IBD (157, 175). Normal individuals have a tolerance for their own intestinal bacteria and do not develop an immune response against those organisms; however, IBD patients lose that tolerance, and the immune response is upregulated toward the host's intestinal bacteria. In genetically susceptible individuals, there is an aggressive immune response toward the luminal bacteria or luminal bacterial constituents, with the end result of IBD (148, 157, 161). Thus, there is a malfunction of the immune system in IBD which gives an inappropriate response to the intestinal indigenous flora and/or luminal antigens. Individuals genetically disposed to IBD have an increased permeability of the intestinal barrier which allows access of commensal organisms to the underlying mucosal tissue. The antigens from the commensal bacteria trigger and maintain an inflammatory response. Intestinal dendritic cells improperly recognize the commensal bacteria as pathogens and promote differentiation of naïve T cells into TH1, TH17, TH2, and natural killer cells, leading to inflammatory responses (9, 60). It is probable that the interplay of luminal gut bacteria, a weakened intestinal barrier, genetic susceptibility, and a dysregulated immune system account for a large number of UC and CD cases.

Some students of IBD pathogenesis have postulated that a specific bacterial pathogen is the cause of IBD, particularly CD. Studies indicate that adherent invasive *Escherichia coli* (AIEC) strains are prevalent in the intestinal contents of CD patients (41). Utilizing intestinal epithelial cells (IEC), Eaves-Pyles et al. (41) demonstrated that an AIEC strain adhered and invaded IEC. In addition, the strain induced cytokine secretion and promoted the migration of immune cells through the IEC. Eaves-Pyles et al. (41) suggested that AIEC contributes to the chronic inflammation seen in CD.

Ruminants, infected by *Mycobacterium avium* subsp. *paratuberculosis* acquire Johne's disease, a chronic, wasting enteritis with clinical symptoms, gross pathology, and epidemiology reminiscent of human CD (54). A number of studies suggest *M. avium* subsp. *paratuberculosis* is associated with CD. The organism has been demonstrated in tissue and blood of CD patients by PCR and culture (25, 54, 118). In addition, serum antibodies against *M. avium* subsp. *paratuberculosis* proteins have been demonstrated in CD patients (25, 54). Mucosal biopsy specimens obtained from irritable bowel syndrome (IBS) and CD patients and a healthy control group at a university hospital in Italy were subjected to PCR for *M. avium* subsp. *paratuberculosis* (146). *M. avium* subsp. *paratuberculosis* was detected in 75.0% (15/20) of IBS patients, 87.0% (20/23) of CD patients, and 15.0% (3/20) of controls. However, it is not clear if *M. avium* subsp. *paratuberculosis* was present before the onset of IBS or CD or was a secondary invader of the inflamed tissues. Feller et al. (42) did a systemic review and meta-analysis of 28 case-control studies comparing the presence of *M. avium* subsp. *paratuberculosis* in CD patients, UC patients, and non-IBD individuals. Positive tests for *M. avium* subsp. *paratuberculosis* (PCR of tissue or enzyme-lined immunosorbent assay of serum) were substantially more common with CD patients than with UC patients or individuals without IBD; thus, there seems to be a specific association of *M. avium* subsp. *paratuberculosis* with CD (42). Feller and his coworkers (42) stated that it was not possible to confirm or exclude *M. avium* subsp. *paratuberculosis* as the causal agent in CD. Other groups also have concurred that the case against *M. avium* subsp. *paratuberculosis* as a cause of CD has not been proven (54).

Animal models have shown some usefulness in the study of IBD. Mouse models of IBD do not reproduce the human disease completely; however, these models have provided some insight into the disease process. These models include mice with targeted mutations or mice with transgenes (mice containing human genes), mice in which colitis is induced by exogenous agents, or mice in which colitis is due to a defective induction of regulatory cells (16, 66, 157). These mouse models emphasize the importance of genetics and environmental factors, the role of commensal microorganisms, and the role of immune-mediated tissue injury.

Since IBD is a chronic recurrent disease with no cure, treatment depends on controlling acute attacks, inducing remission, and maintaining remission. Kuhbacher and Fölsch (91) have published guidelines to follow in treatment of IBS. Older drugs useful for the treatment of IBD include aminosalicyclates, corticosteroids, and immunosuppressive drugs (73, 91). Increased knowledge concerning the role of the immune process in IBD has led to the concept of drugs that target various aspects of the inflammatory process.

Monoclonal antibodies have been developed that modulate key inflammatory cytokines (particularly TNF-α), block inflammatory cell migration and adhesion, and block T cells (10, 88, 91). Colectomy may be necessary in cases of IBD. For CD, the lifetime risk of surgery is 70 to 80%, whereas, for total UC, the risk is 20 to 30% (138).

An exciting area of research in the treatment of IBD is the use of probiotics. Since the gut microflora play a prominent role in the development of IBD, that microflora can be targeted as a therapeutic intervention. The administration of probiotic microorganisms to IBD patients should, in theory, restore microbial homoeostasis in the gut, downregulate intestinal inflammation, and ameliorate the disease. And unlike drugs, probiotics are generally safe and have little or no side effects (4, 49, 124). Probiotics may be defined as "live microorganisms, which when administered in adequate amounts, confer a health benefit on the host" (64). Generally, species from the genera *Lactobacillus* and *Bifidobacterium* are used as probiotics; however, species from other genera have been used (64). In animal models of IBD, the animals showed improvement of symptoms on the administration of probiotics (49, 124), but trials with human patients have been shown to be less successful than trials with animals. Limited studies indicate that probiotics may be useful in treating CD and UC patients (104); however, large, double-blind, placebo-controlled trials are needed to prove that probiotics are therapeutically useful in IBD. The function of probiotics is not completely understood. Possible mechanisms of action include (i) production of inhibitory substances, (ii) blocking of adhesion sites, (iii) stimulation of the immune system, and (iv) promotion of gut integrity (4, 161).

CFS

A common symptom of many illnesses is fatigue; typically, the fatigue is transient, self limiting, and explained by the patient's illness. However, CFS differs in that there is no known etiology; it presents as a severe debilitating long-lasting fatigue featuring impairments in concentration and short-term memory, sleep disturbances, and musculoskeletal pain (38, 47). Some investigators use the term chronic fatigue syndrome/myalgic encephalomyelitis (CFS/ME) (17, 167). The diagnosis of CFS is based on clinical criteria; currently, there is no laboratory test for the identification of CFS. In a diagnosis of CFS, the patient must have (i) an unexplained persistent chronic fatigue of 6 months duration or longer (not the result of ongoing exertion), which is not alleviated by rest and results in a substantial reduction in previous activities and (ii) the concurrent occurrence of four or more of the following: significant impairment in short-term memory or severe loss in the ability to concentrate, sore throat, tender cervical or axillary lymph nodes, muscle pain, multijoint pain without swelling or redness, headaches of a new type, unrefreshing sleep, and aggravation of symptoms after physical activity. Patients without cognitive dysfunction should not be considered to have CFS (31, 38, 162). Physical and psychiatric diseases which may cause fatigue must be excluded from the description of CFS. Bowen et al. (17) pointed out that the diagnosis of CFS/ME is difficult for the general practitioner since there are no specific disease markers or validated laboratory tests to confirm the syndrome.

The syndrome is most common in young to middle-aged adults and occurs more often in females than in males; all age groups can be affected. CFS has a worldwide distribution (31). Using a population sample from Chicago, IL, Jason et al. (81) found a prevalence rate for CFS of approximately 0.42% in a random community-based sample; the prevalence rate for females was 0.52%, and that for males was 0.29%. In addition, Jason et al. (81) found that ethnicity played no role in susceptibility to CFS. In a similar study, Reyes et al. (135), utilizing a population sample from Wichita, KS, found that the prevalence rate for CFS was 0.24%; the rate was higher for females (0.24%) than for males (0.08%). Reeves et al. (134) studied the prevalence of CFS in metropolitan, urban, and rural populations in Georgia. The overall prevalence was quite similar for adults suffering from CFS in metropolitan, urban, and rural populations, with a mean rate of 2.54%. Interestingly, Reeves et al. (134) found that in metropolitan populations, the prevalence of CFS in females was 11.2 times that of males, but there was no significant difference in the ratio of CFS in males and females from urban and rural populations. Approximately 300 million people live in the United States; thus, a 2.54% prevalence rate translates into about 7.5 million people suffering from CFS.

Cairns and Hotopf (21) did a systematic review of studies describing the prognosis of CFS and found that full recovery from CFS is rare; the median full recovery rate was approximately 7%. The median proportion of patients who showed some improvement in their CFS symptoms was 39.5%, and there was no increase in deaths due to CFS. Three of the studies reported that a return to work by CFS patients ranged from 8 to 30% (21). Thus, most CFS patients do not return to full functionality. Using the data of CFS patients from Wichita, KS, obtained by Reyes et al. (135), Reynolds et al. (136) estimated that there was a 37% decline in household productivity (including both the caretaker and CFS patient) and 54% reduction in the national labor force productivity for patients with CFS. The loss of productivity as a result of CFS represents a great economic loss both to the individual person and to the nation, since most CFS patients either cannot work or cannot work to full capacity.

The pathogenesis of CFS is not clear, but it is considered to be multifactorial and involves host and environmental factors. Devanur and Kerr (38) presented a short review of various immune responses observed with CFS patients; however, Afari and Buchwald (1), Lyall et al. (103), and Peakman et al. (125) indicate that no consistent pattern of immunological parameters (T-cell function or activation, cytokine levels, or immunoglobulins) have been associated with CFS. The cytokine levels of 22 CFS patients diagnosed with EBV, Ross Valley virus (RRV), or *Coxiella burnetii* were compared with those of 42 individuals who had the same infections but had recovered (showing no signs of CFS); the data demonstrated that serum cytokine levels did not differ between the two groups (169).

Up to 85% of CFS patients complain about impairment in concentration, decrease in attention span, and decline in short-term memory; however, neuropsychological studies have not shown consistent results that would explain these symptoms (1). Genetics does not seem to play a major role in pathogenesis of CFS. In a twin study of women, (both monozygotic and dizygotic), Buchwald et al. (19) found that the concordance rate for CFS in monozygotic twins was somewhat higher than that for dizygotic twins, but the difference was not significant. Environmental factors were more important than genetic factors.

Cases of CFS often start with a flu-like illness, which suggests that the syndrome has an infectious origin (38). It is likely that CFS is due to infection by a heterogeneous group of microbial agents. Potential pathogenic candidates for the induction of CFS include enteroviruses, EBV, CMV, HHV-6, parvovirus B19, recurrent varicella-zoster virus, hepatitis C virus, *C. pneumoniae,* and *C. burnetii* (27, 38). It is probable that infections by other microorganisms also may be able to induce CFS.

In a study involving 200 CFS patients, Chia and Chia (27) demonstrated that infections by enteroviruses (coxsackievirus and echovirus) were the probable cause of the syndrome in 109 patients (54.5%); the second leading probable cause was infection by *C. pneumoniae* (18/200; 9.0%). Nicolson et al. (120) compared 200 CFS patients to 100 matched control subjects and found that 29.0% of the CFS patients and 88.0% of the controls did not have an apparent infection. Using PCR, Nicolson et al. (120) found HHV-6 in 30.5% of the CFS patients and in 9% of the controls; PCR studies indicated that *Mycoplasma* species were present in 52.0% of the CFS patients and 7.0% of the controls; and 7.5% of the CFS patients had a positive PCR for *C. pneumoniae* in comparison to 1.0% for the controls. In addition, some patients were infected with multiple strains of *Mycoplasma* as well as with mixed infections of *Mycoplasma* and HHV-6 or *Mycoplasma* and *C. pneumoniae* (120). Thus, CFS may be induced by mixed infections. In another study, Nijs et al. (121), studying 261 CFS patients (83.5% female), found that 68.6% of the patients showed evidence of infection with *Mycoplasma* species compared to 5.5% of healthy controls. IgG antibodies against EBV were detected in 9/44 CFS patients in Japanese hospitals (77).

In a group consisting of 68 individuals with confirmed EBV infection, 60 with confirmed RRV infection, and 43 with confirmed *C. burnetii* infection, 87 individuals showed signs of postinfectious fatigue at 6 weeks, 67 at 3 months, and 28 at 6 months. The 28 individuals with postinfectious fatigue at 6 months were defined as CFS patients: 5 had been infected with EBV, 3 with *C. burnetii*, and 13 with RRV (70). Thus, CFS may be the sequel of postinfectious fatigue due to different infections.

Komaroff (87) has suggested that an infection by HHV-6 may trigger and maintain CFS in some patients. Viral sequences of HHV-6 were detected in the peripheral blood leukocytes of 3/17 CFS patients and in 2/20 blood donors; sequences of HHV-7 were found in 4/17 CFS patients and in 12/20 blood donors; and viral sequences of both HHV-6 and -7 were present in 10/17 CFS patients and 3/20 blood donors (26). A questionnaire survey of 108 individuals infected with *C. burnetii* during an outbreak in 1989 in the United Kingdom indicated that 14 individuals met the criteria for CFS; these CFS patients demonstrated the presence of antibodies against the agent (173). Iwakami et al. (79) found that 4 out of 8 CFS patients were positive for *C. burnetii* DNA or antibodies, and Ikuta et al. (77) demonstrated the presence of anti-*C. burnetii* IgG antibodies in 6 of 22 CFS patients in Japan. Three of 90 patients with *C. burnetii* infections were diagnosed with CFS in Croatia (96). These limited studies indicate that *C. burnetii*, HHV-6, and HHV-7 may be inducing pathogens for CFS.

In a study involving monozygotic twins, discordant for CFS, Koelle et al. (86) found that assays for various viruses did not differ between CFS twins and healthy twins; the viruses included HHV-6, -7, and -8, CMV, EBV, herpes simplex virus, varicella-zoster virus, JC virus, BK virus (BKV), and parvovirus.

Thus, the data presented by Koelle et al. (86) do not indicate a major contribution by viruses in the induction and perpetuation of CFS; however, their data do not exclude the possibility that bacterial infections may trigger CFS. However, only 22 sets of twins were studied, and the overall significance of this small study is not clear.

The ambiguous etiology and the diagnostic uncertainty of CFS make treatment of the disease difficult. Thus, there are no firmly established recommendations for the treatment of CFS. In general, treatment has been aimed at relieving symptoms and improving bodily and mental functions. Since CFS is considered to be associated with microbial infections, various antibacterial and antiviral therapies have been tried with various degrees of success (1, 38). Similarly, therapies directed toward alleviating the symptoms and distress induced by CFS indicate that these treatments do not always offer adequate relief to CFS sufferers (1, 38). Clinicians may find that the "trial and error" system of treatment of the CFS patient is the best way to give some measure of relief.

Thus, limited data suggest that infections by *C. pneumoniae, C. burnetii, Mycoplasma* species, enteroviruses, HHV-6, HHV-7, EBV, or RRV are associated with CFS and may act as triggers of the illness. However, it not clear if the infective agent is the inducer of the illness, if the infective agent is a consequence of suffering from CFS, or if the infection was transmitted to the CFS patient via contact with an infected individual.

MS

MS is an inflammatory, demyelinating chronic disease that affects the CNS. During the disease course, the affected individual may suffer from a variety of symptoms, including loss of sensation, muscle weakness, visual problems, speech difficulties, fatigue, depression, cognitive impairment, motor and autonomic problems, coordination and balance difficulties, and pain (33, 95). The three signs associated with MS are dysarthria (difficulty in articulating words), ataxia, and tremor (168).

In the United States, MS is the most common incapacitating disease among young adults; the disease is not common in individuals younger than 20 years or older than 50 years (33, 95). Thus, MS causes a great deal of disability in those individuals who make up the main work force in the United States. The incidence of MS is 0.5 to 1.0 cases/1,000 persons in the United States, and worldwide, the incidence is approximately one out of a million individuals. MS is more common in women than men with a ratio of about 2:1. The incidence is higher in Caucasians and higher in temperate climates (33, 95). However, Christensen (28) states that the classic paradigm in the epidemiology of MS that prevalence of the disease increases as the distance from the equator increases and that MS is a disease almost exclusively of Caucasians is changing, since the disease is being seen in the areas around the Mediterranean basin and is emerging in African nations. People with MS usually die from complications (recurrent infections) rather than from MS itself (33, 95).

There are several clinical subtypes of MS. Relapsing-remitting MS (RRMS) describes the subtype seen in most MS patients. It is characterized by short-term relapses (i.e., attacks) followed by full or partial recovery between relapses. Secondary progressive MS (SPMS) is seen in approximately 40% of RRMS patients. It starts out like RRMS, but as time progresses, patients show shorter and shorter periods of recovery between attacks. The overall trend in SPMS is increasing disability (58, 168). Approximately 10% of MS patients do not demonstrate remission after their initial MS symptoms in primary progressive MS (PPMS); thus, there is a continual decline without any apparent attacks, and the patient shows gradually worsening symptoms. This subtype is usually seen with individuals who are older (>40 years) at disease inception (58, 168). Relapses in MS are often unpredictable, but certain events may trigger relapses, including infections (respiratory or gastroenteritis) and emotional or physical stresses. However, the role of stress as a trigger for MS relapse is controversial. Relapses are more frequent during the spring and summer months (168). The relapse rate is decreased during pregnancy but increases drastically following birth of the child, with an eventual return to the baseline relapse rate (168).

The pathology of MS is due to an unrelenting assault on the CNS by the innate and adaptive immune system which results in widespread demyelination, loss of oligodendrocytes (cells that synthesize and maintain the myelin sheath of axons), and deterioration of axons leading to neurodegeneration. The peripheral nervous system is spared in MS (63, 110). In the healthy individual, the blood-brain barrier (BBB) restricts the nonspecific flux of ions, proteins, and other substances into the CNS environment, which protects neurons from harmful compounds circulating in the blood. The BBB also allows the transport of essential molecules into the CNS (52). In MS, the BBB becomes more permeable and leaky (102). The tight permeability of the BBB can be disrupted by the proinflammatory cytokines IFN-γ and TNF-α as well as by other cytokines such as IL-1, Il-4, IL-13, transforming growth factor alpha, vascular endothelial growth factor, and insulin-like growth factor I and -II. Oxidative stress and mediator compounds of oxidative injury (hydrogen peroxide, nitric oxide) also increase permeability of the BBB (52, 155, 174).

The inflammatory lesions (demyelinated plaques in white matter and gray matter) of MS are characterized by massive infiltration of both cellular and soluble immune factors, such as T cells, B cells, macrophages, microglia, cytokines, chemokines, antibodies, complement, and other toxic substances through the disrupted BBB. The appearance of the lesions is associated with relapse episodes. During remission, there is clinical improvement due to resolution of inflammation and to remyelination (myelination is generally incomplete). The immunopathology of MS is very complex, and thorough discussions of the topic are provided in the reviews of Hauser and Oksenberg (63), Lassmann et al. (93), McQualter and Bernard (110), and Sospedra and Martin (154).

While MS is not an inherited disease, genetics does have a role in susceptibility of the individual to MS. Twin studies indicate that the concordance rate for MS in monozygotic twins is 20 to 30% compared to 2 to 5% in same-sex dizygotic twins (40, 154). The rate for first-degree relatives (the affected individual's parents or children) is approximately the same for dizygotic twins. The risk of MS for offspring of two parents with MS is approximately the same as that of monozygotic twins. Adopted children in families that have an MS patient do not show an increased risk of contacting MS (40). The strongest genetic factor influencing MS susceptibility is the *HLA-DRB1* gene; it is probable, however, that the susceptibility profile of MS consists of many risk alleles, each of which contributes only a small overall risk effect (43, 126, 154). The genetic data indicate that familial aggregation of MS is genetically determined, whereas a shared environment showed no effect.

An animal model of neuroinflammatory diseases, including MS, is experimental autoimmune encephalomyelitis (EAE). The animal disease is a T cell-mediated inflammatory disease of the CNS with demyelination and axonal damage induced by immunization of the animal with myelin antigens. While EAE is not completely similar to MS, its study has given information on the basic mechanisms of neural inflammation and degeneration (11, 65, 110). However, a large number of therapies effective for EAE did not demonstrate clinical effectiveness in MS (11).

Many workers believe that MS is an immune-mediated disease that is triggered by an infection; however, there is no hard evidence to show a direct link of an infectious agent to MS. Stratton and Wheldon (156) and Giovannoni et al. (51) have suggested *C. pneumoniae* as a candidate pathogen for MS. However, a relationship between *C. pneumoniae* and MS has really not been shown (50). Individuals who have had a prior case of EBV-induced infectious mononucleosis have more than a twofold increased risk for MS compared to individuals who were infected with EBV but not showing signs of infectious mononucleosis (51, 101). Levin et al. (97) and DeLorenze et al. (36) demonstrated that anti-EBV antibody titers (using stored blood samples) were elevated in MS patients 5 to 20 years before the onset of symptoms compared to healthy controls, suggesting that EBV infection may be a trigger for MS. Utilizing blood collected 1 to 11 years before onset of MS in 245 cases, Levin et al. (97) found that the serum level of antibodies against the latency-associated EBV nuclear antigen complex was two- to threefold higher than the antibody level in 265 controls, indicating that heightened serum levels of EBV nuclear antigen complex was strongly predictive for MS. Other viruses have been suggested as triggering organisms for MS, including HHV-6, retroviuruses, coronaviruses, and polyoma JC virus, but there is little evidence that these viruses are involved with the induction of MS (50).

Targeting the immune response has been the only successful therapy for MS. While immunotherapy helps to resolve inflammation, there is no effective therapy for the complete recovery of neurological function in MS patients, since regeneration of the CNS eventually fails. In the early stages of MS, IFN-β and glatiramer acetate (an amino acid polymer which mimics a protein region of myelin) reduces the number of relapses and inflammatory activity, but these drugs are ineffective for SPMS and primary progressive MS (33, 65, 78, 154). Hafler et al. (59) stated that a neglected area of MS treatment is the use of combination therapies, such as the complex drug cocktails that prolong graft survival in transplant patients. Insufficient mobilization or loss of endogenous stem cell populations may account for the transitory regenerative myelinization seen with MS during the periods between relapses; McQualteer and Bernard (110) suggest that stem cell transplantation into the CNS may be a means of regenerating myelin in MS.

Studies strongly suggest that an EBV infection can trigger MS, but it is unlikely that a single infective agent accounts for all MS cases. It is probable that a number of microbial agents or environmental insults can trigger the disease.

Other Diseases

Systemic lupus erythematosus (SLE) is a multisystem, autoimmune disorder in which the immune system (autoantibodies) attacks various bodily cells and tissues. There is a broad range of clinical presentations. Individuals with Asian or African ancestry are at greater risk for SLE than Caucasians. The disease is more common in women than men (9:1 ratio). The incidence of SLE worldwide is approximately 5/100,000 individuals, with a death rate approximately three times that of the general population. Twin studies indicate concordance rates of 2 to 5% for dizygotic twins and a rate of 24 to 60% for monozygotic twins (8, 35, 150). The genetics of SLE is complicated, and a large number of genes may be involved in susceptibility to the disease. The strongest genetic associations reside in the HLA-DR2 and –DR3 regions of the human leukocyte antigens (150).

SLE-specific autoantibodies have been shown to arise from antibodies against EBV nuclear antigen 1, which bind to SLE-specific autoantigens (61, 106). It can be concluded that in genetically susceptible individuals, EBV infections can act as a trigger for induction of SLE. However, EBV infections are probably not the only triggering infection for SLE, and other infections or environmental insults play a role.

It is estimated that prostate cancer causes 10% of cancer deaths in males. The BKV (a polyomavirus) infects the urinary tract and encodes tumor antigens that inactivate tumor suppressors (indicating that the virus has oncogenic properties); the virus has been postulated to have a role in the induction of prostate cancers (34). Das et al. (34) demonstrated the presence of BKV DNA in 11/15 (73.3%) cancerous prostates; however, BKV DNA was found in only 3/14 (21.4%) normal prostates. The virus was not detected in advanced stages of prostate cancer progression, but only in the early stages (34). However, Lau et al. (94) were unable to show a relationship between the presence of BKV and prostate cancer.

Preeclampsia occurs at any period after the 20th week of gestation and is characterized by increased blood pressure and proteinuria or excessive edema. The disease is the third leading cause of death in pregnancy, with a frequency estimated at 750 maternal deaths/100,000 live births. The death rate is higher for African-American women than for white women. Preeclampsia occurs in approximately 5% of pregnancies, with an incidence of 23.6 cases/1,000 deliveries in the United States (83). Pregnant women younger than 20 years have a slightly increased risk of preeclampsia, whereas older women (>35 years) have a markedly increased risk. A urinary tract infection during pregnancy is associated with an increased risk of preeclampsia (68, 72). Similarly, periodontal disease during pregnancy has been linked with preeclampsia (13, 14). Boggess et al. (15) found that pregnant women were more at risk for preeclampsia if they had severe periodontal disease at the time of delivery or if the periodontal disease progressed during pregnancy. However, it is not clear if precclampsia is induced by a urinary tract infection or periodontal disease or if the infections are triggered by ecclampsia.

Parkinson's disease (PD) is an idiopathic progressive neurodegeneration disorder. Symptoms include tremors that occur at rest, shuffling gait, rigid muscles, and postural instability. The major neuropathological finding in PD is the loss of pigmented dopaminergic neurons. Sixty to 80% of the dopaminergic neurons are lost before symptoms appear (62, 80). PD is approximately 1.5 times more common in women than men, and the disease incidence and prevalence increases with age. The average age at onset of PD is 60 years. The disease affects 1 to 2% of the adult population >50 years of age. At the present time, approximately 4.1 million persons in the United States are affected by PD and the disease is expected to increase as the population grows older (62, 80). The current cost of PD to the United States economy is around $8 billion per year. Weller et al. (172) have suggested that inflammatory products induced by a *Helicobacter pylori* infection may be the triggering mechanism that leads to PD. However, Jang et al. (80) suggested that viral infections, in particular, influenza, may precipitate the development of PD. It is probable that host and environmental factors play a role in the etiology of PD. While there is little evidence to indicate that the induction of PD has an infectious origin, research to determine a potential infectious trigger for PD seems worthwhile.

It has been proposed that children who experience tics or obsessive-compulsive disorders are suffering from an autoimmune response to group A β-hemolytic streptococci (GABHS) infections. These symptoms are termed "pediatric autoimmune neuropsychiatric disorders associated with streptococcal infections" (PANDAS) (92). Tourette's syndrome probably should be classified as one of the diseases caused by PANDAS since GABHS infections have been associated with the syndrome (112, 116). A study of children with tics and obsessive-compulsive disorder showed that the frequency of these disorders was significantly higher in first-degree relatives (parents and siblings) than in the normal population, suggesting that genetics plays a role in PANDAS (37). Similarly, the concordance rate for Tourette's syndrome in monozygotic twins was 53%, whereas it was 8% for dizygotic twins. Tic symptoms in Tourette's syndrome patients were present in 77% of monozygotic twins and 23% of dizygotic twins (137). The prevalence of Tourette's syndrome is 5 to 10/10,000 population and is approximately four times higher in males than females (137). A prior infection with GABHS has been correlated with the onset of tics, obsessive-compulsive disorder, and Tourette's syndrome (44, 84, 112, 116, 153). Thus, the clinical literature indicates that genetically susceptible children who have had an antecedent GABHS infection show the symptoms of PANDAS and Tourette's syndrome; the symptoms are probably due to the activation of an autoimmune response. However, Perrin et al. (127) were not able to show an association between a streptococcal infection and PANDAS. It is not certain that infection by microorganisms other than GABHS can induce the disease symptoms.

CONCLUSIONS

Lorber (98, 99) asked the question: Are all diseases infectious? He then discussed a number of chronic diseases that might be induced by infectious agents. He advised clinicians to "maintain a healthy skepticism" but also keep an open mind and consider that chronic illnesses (with no apparent inducing pathogen) may have an infectious origin. One of the problems in identifying a pathogen as the inducing agent for such chronic diseases is that Koch's idea of "one organism, one disease" may not always be applicable to complex chronic diseases. It is more probable that many of these chronic illnesses are induced by infection per se rather than due to an infection by a particular organism. Many of the chronic diseases without an apparent inducing pathogen have a strong genetic component, and genetically susceptible individuals have a higher risk of chronic disease if they undergo an infection. Lünemann et al. (101) suggest that many chronic diseases are induced by ubiquitous pathogens, such as EBV or CMV, which are highly prevalent in the population. However, it is not always clear if the detected organism is the causative agent or if the microorganism is merely present as an opportunistic pathogen because of immunosuppression due to the disease.

REFERENCES

1. **Afari, N., and D. Buchwald.** 2003. Chronic fatigue syndrome: a review. *Am. J. Psychiatry* **160:**221–236.
2. **Ashwood, P., and J. van de Water.** 2006. Is autism an autoimmune disease? *Autoimmun. Rev.* **3:**557–562.
3. **Ashwood, P., S. Wills, and J. Van de Water.** 2006. The immune response in autism: a new frontier for autism research. *J. Leukoc. Biol.* **80:**1–15.
4. **Bai, A.-P., and Q. Ouyang.** 2006. Probiotics and inflammatory bowel disease. *Postgrad. Med. J.* **82:**376–382.
5. **Balandraud, N., J. B. Meynard, I. Auger, H. Sovran, B. Mugnier, D. Reviron, J. Roudier, and C. Roudier.** 2003. Epstein-Barr virus load in the peripheral blood of patients with rheumatoid arthritis. Accurate quantification using real-time polymerase chain reaction. *Arth. Rheum.* **48:**1223–1228.
6. **Bamias, G., M. R. Nyce, S. A. De La Rue, and F. Cominelli.** 2005. New concepts in the pathophysiology of inflammatory bowel disease. *Ann. Intern. Med.* **143:**895–904.
7. **Barksby, S. R. Lea, P. M. Preshaw, and J. J. Taylor.** 2007. The expanding family of interleukin-1 cytokines and their role in destructive inflammatory disorders. *Clin. Exp. Immunol.* **149:**217–225.
8. **Bartels, C. M., J. Hildebrand, and D. Muller.** 2007. Systemic lupus erythematosus. htttp://www.emedicine.com/med/topic 2228.htm Accessed 2 January 2008.
9. **Baumgart, D. C., and S. R. Carding.** 2007. Inflammatory bowel disease: cause and immunobiology. *Lancet* **369:**1627–1640.
10. **Baumgart, D. C., and W. J. Sandborn.** 2007. Inflammatory bowel disease: clinical aspects and established and evolving therapies. *Lancet* **369:**1641–1657.
11. **Baxter, A. G.** 2007. The origin and application of experimental autoimmune encephalomyhelitis. *Nat. Rev. Immunol.* **7:**904–912.
12. **Belmonte, M. K., E. H. Cook, G. M. Anderson, J. L. R. Rubenstein, W. T. Greenough, A. Beckel-Mitchener, E. J. Courchesne, L. M. Boulanger, S. B. Powell, P. E. Lwcirr, W. K. Pweey, Y. Y. Jiang, T. M. DeLory and E. Tierney.** 2004. Autism as a disorder of neural information processing: directions for research and targets for therapy. *Mol. Psychiatry* **9:**646–663.
13. **Boggess, K. A.** 2005. Pathogenicity of periodontal pathogens during pregnancy. *Am. J. Obstr. Gynecol.* **193:**311–312
14. **Boggess, K. A., and B. L. Edelstein.** 2006. Oral health in women during preconception and pregnancy: implications for birth outcomes and infant oral health. *Matern. Child Health J.* **10:**S169–S174.
15. **Boggess, K. A., S. Lieff, A. P. Murtha, K. Moss, J. Beck and S. Offenbacher.** 2003. Maternal periodontal disease is associated with an increased risk for preeclampsia. *Obstet. Gynecol.* **101:**227–231.
16. **Bouma, G., and W. Strober.** 2003. The immunological and genetic basis of inflammatory bowel disease. *Nat. Rev. Immunol.* **3:**521–533.
17. **Bowen, J., D. Pheby, A. Charlett, and C. McNulty.** 2005. Chronic fatigue syndrome: a survey of GPs' attitudes and knowledge. *Fam. Pract.* **22:**389–393.
18. **Brasic, J. R.** 2006. Pervasive developmental disorders: autism. http://www.emedicine.com/ped/topic180.htm. Accessed 29 May 2007.
19. **Buchwald, D., R. Herrell, S. Ashton, M. Belcourt, K. Schmaling, P. Sullivan, M. Neale, and J. Goldberg.** 2001. A twin study of chronic fatigue. *Psychosom. Med.* **63:**936–943.
20. **Bugatti, S., V. Codullo, R. Caporali, and C. Montecucco.** 2007. B cells in rheumatoid arthritis. *Autoimmun. Rev.* **7:**137–142.
21. **Cairns, R., and M. Hotopf.** 2005. A systematic review describing the prognosis of chronic fatigue syndrome. *Occup. Med.* **55:**20–31.
22. **Carbone, K. M., R. B. Luftig, and M. R. Buckley.** 2005. Microbial triggers of chronic human illness. American Society for Microbiology, Washington, DC. http://www.asm.org/ASM/files/ccLibraryFiles/FILENAME/000000001497/ASM.MicroTriggers.pdf. Accessed 3 April 2007.
23. **Casadevall, A., and L. Pirofski.** 2003. The damage-response framework of microbial pathogenesis. *Nat. Rev. Microbiol.* **1:**17–24.
24. **CDC.** 2007. Prevalence of autism spectrum disorders—Autism and Developmental Disabilities Monitoring Network,

six sites, United States, 2000. *MMWR Morb. Mortal. Wkly. Rep.* **56**:1–11.

25. **Chamberlin, W. M., and S. A. Naser.** 2006. Integrating theories of the etiology of Crohn's disease. On the etiology of Crohn's disease: questioning the hypotheses. *Med. Sci. Monit.* **12**:RA27–RA33.
26. **Chapenko, S., A. Krumina, S. Kozireva, Z. Nora, A. Sultanova, L. Viksna, and M. Murovska.** 2006. Activation of human herpesviruses 6 and 7 in patients with chronic fatigue syndrome. *J. Clin. Virol.* **37**(Suppl. 1):S47–S51.
27. **Chia, J. K. S., and A. Chia.** 2003. Diverse etiologies for chronic fatigue syndrome. *Clin. Infect. Dis.* **36**:671–672.
28. **Christensen, T.** 2007. Human herpesviruses in MS. *Int. MS J.* **14**:41–47.
29. **Costenbader, K. H., and E. W. Karson.** 2006. Epstein-Barr virus and rheumatoid arthritis: is there a link? *Arthritis Res. Ther.* **8**:204.
30. **Crawley, J. N.** 2007. Testing hypotheses about autism. *Science* **318**:56–57.
31. **Cunha, B. A.** 2006. Chronic fatigue syndrome. http://www.emedicine.com/med/topic3392.htm Accessed 7 November 2007.
32. **Danese, S., S. Semeraro, A. Papa, I. Roberto, F. Scaldaferri, G. Fedeli, G. Gasbarrini, and A. Gasbarrini.** 2005. Extraintestinal manifestations in inflammatory disease. *World J. Gastroenterol.* **11**:7227–7236.
33. **Dangond, F.** 2006. Multiple sclerosis. http://www.emedicine.com/NEURO/topic228.htm. Accessed 27 December 2007.
34. **Das, D., K. Wojno and M. J. Imperiale.** 2008. BKV as a cofactor in the etiology of prostate cancer in its early stages. *J. Virol.* **82**:2705–2714.
35. **D'Cruz, D. P., M. A. Khamashta and G. R. V. Hughes.** 2007. Systemic lupus erythematosus. *Lancet* **369**:587–596.
36. **DeLorenze, G. N., K. L. Munger, E. T. Lennette, N. Osrentreich, J. H. Vogelman, and A. Ascherio.** 2006. Epstein-Barr virus and multiple sclerosis. *Arch. Neurol.* **63**:839–844.
37. **de Oliveira, S. K.** 2007. PANDAS: a new disease? *J. Pediatr.* (Rio J) **83**:201–208.
38. **Devanur, L. D., and J. R. Kerr.** 2006. Chronic fatigue syndrome. *J. Clin. Virol.* **57**:139–150.
39. **Dignass, A. U., D. C. Baumgard, and A. Sturm.** 2004. Review article: the aetiopathogenesis of inflammatory bowel disease–immunology and repair mechanisms. *Aliment. Pharmacol. Ther.* **20**(Suppl. 4):9–17.
40. **Dyment, D. A., G. C. Ebers, and A. D. Sadovnick.** 2004. Genetics of multiple sclerosis. *Lancet Neurol.* **3**:104–110.
41. **Eaves-Pyles, T., C. A. Allen, J. Taormina, A. Swidsinski, C. B. Tutt, C. E. Jezek, M. Islas-Ilas, and A. G. Torres.** 2008. *Escherichia coli* isolated from a Crohn's patient adheres, invades, and induces inflammatory responses in polarized intestinal epithelial cells. *Int. J. Med. Microbiol.* **298**:397–409.
42. **Feller, M., K. Hujwiler, R. Stephan, E. Altpeter, A. Shang, H. Furrer, G. F. Pfyffer, T. Jemmi, A. Baumgartner, and M. Egger.** 2007. *Mycobacterium avium* subspecies *paratuberculosis* and Crohn's disease: a systematic review and meta-analysis. *Lancet Infect. Dis.* **7**:607–613.
43. **Fernald, G. H., R.-F. Yeh, S. L. Hauser, J. R. Oksenberg and S. E. Baranzini.**2005. Mapping gene activity in complex disorders: integration of expression and genomic scans for multiple sclerosis. *J. Neuroimmunol.* **167**:157–169.
44. **Fernández Ibieta, M., J. T. Ramos Amador, I. Auñón Martínc , M. A. Marin, M. I. González Tomé, and R. Simón de las Heras.** 2005. Trastornos neuropsiquiátricos asociados a estreptococo. *An Pediatr.* (Barcelona) **62**:475–478.
45. **Firestein, G. S.** 2003. Evolving concepts of rheumatoid arthritis. *Nature* **423**:356–361.
46. **Fredricks, D. N., and D. A. Relman.** 1996. Sequence-based identification of microbial pathogens: a reconsideration of Koch's postulates. *Clin. Microbiol. Rev.* **9**:18–33.
47. **Fukuda, K., S. E. Straus, I. Hickie, M. C. Sharpe, J. G. Dobbins, A. Komaroff, and the International Chronic Fatigue Syndrome Study Group.** 1994. The chronic fatigue syndrome: a comprehensive approach to its definition and study. *Ann. Intern. Med.* **121**:953–959.
48. **Gaya, D. R., R. K. Russell, E. R. Nimmo, and J. Satsangi.** 2006. New genes in inflammatory bowel disease: lessons for complex diseases? *Lancet* **367**:1271–1284.
49. **Geier, M. S., R. N. Butler, and G. S. Howarth.** 2007. Inflammatory bowel disease: current insights into pathogenesis and new therapeutic options; probiotics, prebiotics and synbiotics. *Int. J. Food Microbiol.* **115**:1–11.
50. **Gilden, D. H.** 2005. Infectious causes of multiple sclerosis. *Lancet Neurol.* **4**:195–202.
51. **Giovannoni, G., G. R. F. Cutter, J. Lunemann, R. Martin, C. Münz, S. Sriram, I. Steiner, M. R. Hammerschlag, and C. A. Gaydos.** 2006. Infectious causes of multiple sclerosis. *Lancet Neurol.* **5**:887–894.
52. **Gloor, S. M., M. Wachtel, M. F. Bolliger, H. Ishihara, R. Landmann, and K. Frei.** 2001. Molecular and cellular permeability control at the blood-brain barrier. *Brain Res. Rev.* **36**:258–264.
53. **Goronzy, J. J., and C. M. Weyand.** 1997. Rheumatoid arthritis. A. Epidemiology, pathology, and pathogenesis, p. 155–161. *In* J. H. Klippel (ed.), *Primer of the Rheumatic Diseases*, 11th ed., Arthritis Foundation, Atlanta, GA.
54. **Grant, I. R.** 2005. Zoonotic potential of *Mycobacterium avium* ssp. *paratuberculosis*: the current position. *J. Appl. Microbiol.* **98**:1282–1293.
55. **Gulko, P. S.** 2007. Contribution of genetic studies in rodent models of autoimmune arthritis to understanding and treatment of rheumatoid arthritis. *Genes Immun.* **8**:523–531.
56. **Gupta, A. R., and M. W. State.** 2007. Recent advances in the genetics of autism. *Biol. Psychiatry* **61**:429–437.
57. **Gupta, K., J. J. Nicholas, and S. M. Bhagia.** 2006. Rheumatoid arthritis. http://www.emedicine.com/PMR/topic124.htm Accessed 6 August 2007.
58. **Hafler, D. A.** 2004. Multiple sclerosis. *J. Clin. Investig.* **113**:788–794.
59. **Hafler, D. A., J. M. Slavik, D. E. Anderson, K. C. O'Conner, P. de Jager and C. B. Allan.** 2005. Multiple sclerosis. *Immunol. Rev.* **2004**:208–231.
60. **Hanauer, S. B.** 2006. Inflammatory bowel disease: epidemiology, pathogenesis, and therapeutic opportunities. *Inflamm. Bowel Dis.* **12**(Suppl. 1):S3–S9.
61. **Harley, J. B., and J. A. James.** 2006. Epstein-Barr virus infection induces lupus autoimmunity. *Bull. NYC Hosp. J. Dis.* **64**:45–50.
62. **Hauser, R. A., R. Pahwa, K. E. Lyons, and T. A. McClain.** 2007. Parkinson disease. http://www.emedicine.com/NEURO/topic 304.htm. Accessed 19 September 2008.
63. **Hauser, S. L., and J. R. Oksenberg.** 2006. The neurobiology of multiple sclerosis: genes, inflammation, and neurodegeneration. *Neuron* **52**:61–76.
64. **Heczko, P. B., M. Strus, and P. Kochan.** 2006. Critical evaluation of probiotic activity of lactic acid bacteria and their effects. *J. Physiol. Pharmacol.* **57**(Suppl. 9):5–12.
65. **Hemmer, B., S. Nessler, D. Zhou, B. Kieseier and H.-P. Hartung.** 2006. Immunopathogenesis and immunotherapy of multiple sclerosis. *Nat. Clin. Pract. Neurol.* **2**:201–211.
66. **Hendrickson, B. A., R. Gokhale, and J. H. Cho.** 2002. Clinical aspects and pathophysiology of inflammatory bowel disease. *Clin. Microbiol. Rev.* **15**:79–94.

67. **Herbert, M. R., J. P. Russo, S. Yang, J. Roohi, M. Blaxill, S. G. Kahler, L. Cremer, and E. Hatchwell.** 2006. Autism and environmental genomics. *Neurotoxicology* **27:**671–684.
68. **Herrera, J. A., G. Chaudhuri, and P. López-Jaramillo.** 2001. Is infection a major risk factor for preeclampsia? *Med. Hypotheses* **57:**393–397.
69. **Hertz-Picciotto, I., L. A. Croen, R. Hansen, C. R. Jones, J. van de Water, and I. N. Pessah.** 2006. The CHARGE Study: an epidemiologic investigation of genetics and environmental factors contributing to autism. *Environ. Health Perspect.* **114:**1119–1125.
70. **Hickie, I., T. Davenport, D. Wakefield, U. Vollmer-Conna, B. Cameron, S. D. Vernon, W. C. Reeves, A. Lloyd, and the Dubbo Infection Outcomes Study Group.** 2006. Post-infective and chronic fatigue syndromes precipitated by viral and non-viral pathogens: prospective cohort study. *Br. Med. J.* **333:**575.
71. **Hilt, R. J., and W. P. Metz.** 2006. Autistic spectrum disorders. http://www.emedicine.com/med/topic3202.htm. Accessed 29 May 2007.
72. **Hsu, C. D., and F. R. Witter.** 1995. Urogenital infection in preeclampsia. *Int. J. Gynecol. Obstet.* **49:**271–275.
73. **Huang, C. S., L. J. Saubermann, and F. A. Farraye.** 2007. Inflammatory bowel disease, p. 406–441. *In* T. E. Andreoli, C. C. J. Carpenter, R. C. Griggs and I. J. Benjamin (eds.), *Andreoli and Carpenter's Cecil Essentials of Medicine,* 7th ed., Saunders Elsevier, Philadelphia, PA.
74. **Hugot, J.-P.** 2004. Inflammatory bowel disease: a complex group of genetic disorders. *Best Pract. Res. Clin. Gastroenterol.* **18:**451–462.
75. **Hugot, J.-P., M. Chamaillard, H. Zouall, S. Lesage, J.-P. Cézard, J. Belaiche, S. Almer, C. Tysk, C. A. O'Moraln, M. Gassull, V. Binder, Y. Finkel, A. Cortot, R. Modigllani, P. Laurent-pulg, C. Gower-Rousseau, J. Macry, J.-F. Colombel, M. Sahbatou, and G. Thomas.** 2001. Association of NOD2 leucine-rich repeat variants with susceptibility to Crohn's disease. *Nature* **411:**599–603.
76. **Hyun, F. G., and L. Mayer.** 2006. Mechanisms underlying inflammatory bowel disease. *Drug Discov. Today* **3:**457–462.
77. **Ikuta, K., T. Yamada, T. Shimomura, H. Kuratsune, R. Kawahara, S. Ikawa, E. Ohnishi, Y. Sokawa, H. Fukushi, K. Hirai, Y. Watanabe, T. Kurata, T. Kitani, and T. Sairenji.** 2003. Diagnostic evaluation of 2', 5'-oligoadenylate synthetase activities and antibodies against Epstein-Barr virus and *Coxiella burnetii* in patients with chronic fatigue syndrome in Japan. *Microb. Infect.* **5:**1096–1102.
78. **Inglese, M.** 2006. Multiple sclerosis: new insights and trends. *Am. J. Neuroradiol.* **27:**954–957.
79. **Iwakami, E., Y. Arashima, K. Kato, T. Komiya, Y. Matsukawa, T. Ikeda, Y. Arakawa, and S. Oshida.** 2005. Treatment of chronic fatigue syndrome with antibiotics: pilot study assessing the involvement of *Coxiella burnetii* infection. *Intern. Med.* **44:**1258–1263.
80. **Jang, H., D. A. Boltz, R. G. Webster, and R. J. Smeyne.** 2008. Viral parkinsonism. *Biochim. Biophys. Acta* [Epub ahead of print.] doi:10.1016/j.bbadis.2008.08.001.
81. **Jason, L. A., J. A. Richman, A. W. Rademaker, K. M. Jordan, A. V. Plioplys, R. R. Taylor, W. McCready, C.-F. Huang, and S. Plioplys.** 1999. A community-based study of chronic fatigue syndrome. *Arch. Intern. Med.* **159:**2129–2137.
82. **Johnson, C. P., S. M. Myers, and the Council on Children with Disabilities.** 2007. Identification and evaluation of children with autism spectrum disorders. *Pediatrics* **120:**1183–1215.
83. **Jung, D. C.** 2007. Pregnancy, Preeclampsia. http://www.emedicine.com/EMERG/topic480.htm. Accessed 4 February 2008.
84. **Kim, S. W., J. E. Grant, S. I. Kim, T. A. Swanson, G. A. Bernstein, W. B. Jaszcz, K. A. Williams, and P. M. Schlievert.** 2004. A possible association of recurrent streptococcal infections and acute onset of obsessive-compulsive disorder. *J. Neuropsychiatry Clin. Neurosci.* **16:**252–260.
85. **King, R. W.** 2006. Arthritis, Rheumatoid. http://www.emedicine.com/emerg/topic48.htm. Accessed 6 August 2007.
86. **Koelle, D. M., S. Barcy, M.-L. Huang, R. L. Ashley, L. Corey, J. Zeh, S. Ashton, and D. Buchwald.** 2002. Markers of viral infection in monocygotic twins discordant for chronic fatigue syndrome. *Clin. Infect. Dis.* **35:**518–525.
87. **Komaroff, A. L.** 2006. Is human herpesvirus-6 a trigger for chronic fatigue syndrome? *J. Clin. Virol.* **37**(Suppl. 1)**:**S39–S46.
88. **Korzenik, J. R., and D. K. Podolsky.** 2006. Evolving knowledge and therapy of inflammatory bowel disease. *Nat. Rev. Drug Discov.* **5:**197–209.
89. **Kruidenier, L., I. Kuiper, W. van Duijn, M. A. X. Mieremet-Ooms, R. A. van Hogezand, C. B. H. W. Lamers, and H. W. Verspaget.** 2003. Imbalanced secondary mucosal antioxidant response in inflammatory bowel disease. *J. Pathol.* **201:**17–27.
90. **Kruidenier, L., and H. W. Verspaget.** 2002. Review article: oxidative stress as a pathogenic factor in inflammatory bowel disease – radicals or ridiculous? *Aliment. Pharmacol. Ther.* **16:**1997–2015.
91. **Kuhbacher, T., and U. R. Fölsch.** 2007. Practical guidelines for the treatment of inflammatory bowel disease. *World J. Gastroenterol.* **28:**1149–1155.
92. **Kurlan, R., and E. L. Kaplan.** 2004. The pediatric autoimmune neuropsychiatric disorders associated with streptococcal infection (PANDAS) etiology for tics and obsessive-compulsive symptoms: hypothesis or entity? Practical considerations for the clinician. *Pediatrics* **113:**883–886.
93. **Lassmann, H., W. Brücke and C. F. Lucchinetti.** 2007. The immunopathology of multiple sclerosis: an overview. *Brain Pathol.* **17:**210–218.
94. **Lau, S. K., S. F. Lacey, Y.-Y. Chen, W.-G. Chen and L. M. Weiss.** 2007. Low frequency of BK virus in prostatic adenocarcinomas. *APMIS* **115:**743–749.
95. **Lazoff, M.** 2007. Multiple sclerosis. http://www.emedi cine.com/EMERG/topic321.htm. Accessed 27 December 2007.
96. **Ledina, D., N. Bradarić, I. Milas, I. Ivić, N. Brnčić, and N. Kuzmičić.** 2007. Chronic fatigue syndrome after Q fever. *Med. Sci. Monit.* **13:**CS88–CS92.
97. **Levin, L. I., K. L. Munger, M. V. Rubertone, C. A. Peck, E. T. Lennette, D. Spiegelman, and A. Ascherio.** 2005. Temporal relationship between elevation of Epstein-Barr virus antibody titers and initial onset of neurological symptoms in multiple sclerosis. *JAMA* **293:**2496–2500.
98. **Lorber, B.** 1996. Are all diseases infectious? *Ann. Intern. Med.* **125:**844–851.
99. **Lorber, B.** 1999. Are all diseases infectious? Another look. *Ann. Intern. Med.* **131:**989–990.
100. **Lord, C., E. H. Cook, B. L. Leventhalm and D. G. Amaral.** 2000. Autism spectrum disorders. *Neuron* **28:**355–363.
101. **Lünemann, J. D., T. Kamradt, R. Martin and C. Münz.** 2007. Epstein-Barr virus: environmental trigger of multiple sclerosis? *J. Virol.* **81:**6777–6784.
102. **Lutton, J. D., R. Winston, and T. C. Rodman.** 2004. Multiple sclerosis: etiological mechanisms and future directions. *Exp. Biol. Med.* **229:**12–20.
103. **Lyall, M., M. Peakman, and S. Wessely.** 2003. A systematic review and critical evaluation of the immunology of chronic fatigue syndrome. *J. Psychosom. Res.* **55:**79–90.

104. **Mach, T.** 2006. Clinical usefulness of probiotics in inflammatory bowel diseases. *J. Physiol. Pharmacol.* **57**(Suppl. 9):23–33.

105. **Mathew, C. G., and C. M. Lewis.** 2004. Genetics of inflammatory bowel disease: progress and prospects. *Hum. Mol. Genet.* **13**(Suppl.):R161–R168.

106. **McClain, M. T., B. D. Poole, B. F. Bruner, K. M. D. Kaufman, J. B. Harley, and J. A. James.** 2006. An altered immune response to Epstein-Barr virus nuclear antigen 1 in pediatric systemic lupus erythematosus. *Arth. Rheum.* **54**:360–368.

107. **McGraw, W. T., J. Potempa, D. Farley, and J. Travis.** 1999. Purification, characterization, and sequence analysis of a potential virulence factor from *Porphyromonas gingivalis*, peptidylarginine deiminase. *Infect. Immun.* **67**:3248–3256.

108. **McInnes, I. B., and F. Y. Liew.** 2005. Cytokine networks–towards new therapies for rheumatoid arthritis. *Nat. Clin. Pract. Rheumatol.* **1**:31–39.

109. **McInnes, I. B., and G. Schett.** 2007. Cytokines in the pathogenesis of rheumatoid arthritis. *Nat Rev. Immunol.* **7**:429–442.

110. **McQualter, J. L., and C. C. A. Bernard.** 2007. Multiple sclerosis: a battle between destruction and repair. *J. Neurochem.* **100**:295–306.

111. **Mehraein, Y., C. Lennerz, S. Ehlhardt, K. Remberger, A. Ojak, and K. D. Zang.** 2004. Latent Epstein-Barr virus (EBV) infection and cytomegalovirus (CMV) infection in synovial tissue of autoimmune chromic arthritis determined by RNA- and DNA-in situ hybridization. *Mod. Pathol.* **17**:781–789.

112. **Mell, L. K., R. L. Davis, and D. Owens.** 2005. Association between streptococcal infection and obsessive-compulsive disorder, Torette's syndrome, and tic disorder. *Pediatrics* **116**:56–60.

113. **Merkel, P. A., and R. W. Simms.** 2007. Rheumatoid arthritis, p. 804–808. *In* C. C. J. Carpenter, R. C. Griggs, and I. J. Benjamin (ed.), *Andreoli and Carpenters's Cecil Essentials of Medicine,* 7th ed., Saunders-Elsevier, Philadelphia, PA.

114. **Mewar, D., A. Coote, D. J. Moore, I. Marinou, J. Keyworth, M. C. Dickson, D. S. Montogmery, M. H. Binks, and J. A. G. Wilson.** 2006. Independent associations of anti-cyclic citrullinated peptide antibodies and rheumatoid factor with radiographic severity of rheumatoid arthritis. *Arthritis Res. Ther.* **8**:R128.

115. **Morrow, E. M., S.-Y. Yoo, S. W. Flavell, T.-K. Kim, Y. Lin, R. S. Hill, N. M. Mukaddes, S. Balkhy, G. Gascon, A. Hashmi, S. Al-Saad, J. Ware, R. M. Joseph, R. Greenblatt, D. Gleason, J. A. Erteit, K. A. Apse, A. Bodell, J. N. Partlow, B. Barryu, H. Yao, K. Markianos, R. J. Ferland, M. E. Greenberg, and C. A. Walsh.** 2008. Identifying autism loci and genes by tracing recent shared ancestry. *Science* **321**:218–223.

116. **Müller, N., B. Kroll, M. J. Schwarz, M. Riedel, A. Straube, R. Lütticken, R. R. Reinert, T. Reineke, and O. Kühnemund.** 2001. Increased titers of antibodies against streptoccal M12 and M19 proteins in patients with Tourette's syndrome. *Psychiatry Res.* **101**:187–193.

117. **Myers, S. M., C. P. Johnson, and the Council on Children with Disabilities.** 2007. Management of children with autism spectrum disorders. *Pediatrics* **120**:1162–1182.

118. **Naser, S. A., G. Ghobrial, C. Romero, and J. F. Valentine.** 2004. Culture of *Mycobacterium avium* subspecies *paratuberculosis* from the blood of patients with Crohn's disease. *Lancet* **364**:1039–1044.

119. **Nicolson, G. L., R. Gan, N. L. Nicolson, and J. Haier.** 2007. Evidence for *Mycoplasma* spp., *Chlamydia pneumoniae* and human herpes virus-6 co-infections in the blood of patients with autistic spectrum disorders. *J. Neurosci. Res.* **85**:1143–1148.

120. **Nicolson, G. L., R. Gan, and J. Haier.** 2003. Multiple co-infections (*Mycoplasma, Chlamydia*, human herpes virus-6) in blood of chronic fatigue syndrome patients: association with signs and symptoms. *APMIS* **111**:557–566.

121. **Nijs, J., G. L. Nicolson, P. de Becker, D. Coomans, and K. de Meirleir.** 2002. High prevalence of *Mycoplasma* infections among European chronic fatigue syndrome patients. Examination of four *Mycoplasma* species in blood of chronic fatigue syndrome patients. *FEMS Immunol. Med. Micrbiol.* **34**:2009–214.

122. **O'Connor, S. M., C. E. Taylor, and J. M. Hughes.** 2006. Emerging infectious determinants of chronic diseases. *Emerg. Infect. Dis.* **12**:1051–1057.

123. **Ollier, W.** 2000. Rheumatoid arthritis and Epstein-Barr virus: a case of living with the enemy? *Ann. Rheum. Dis.* **59**:497–499.

124. **Pagnini, C., and F. Cominelli.** 2006. Probiotics in experimental and human inflammatory bowel disease: discussion points. *Dig. Liver Dis.* **38**(Suppl. 2):S270–S273.

125. **Peakman, M., A. Deale, R. Field, M. Mahalingam, and S. Wessely.** 1997. Clinical improvement in chronic fatigue syndrome is not associated with lymphocyte subsets of function or activation. *Clin. Immunol. Immunopathol.* **82**:83–91.

126. **Peltonen, L.** 2007. Old suspects found guilty – the first genome profile of multiple sclerosis. *New Engl. J. Med.* **357**:927–929.

127. **Perrin, E. M., M. L. Murphy, J. R. Casey, M. E. Pichichero, D. K. Runyan, W. C. Miller, L. A. Snider, and S. E. Swedo.** 2004. Does group A β-hemolytic streptococcal infection increase risk for behavioral and neuropsychiatric symptoms in children? *Arch. Pediatr. Adolesc. Med.* **158**:848–856.

128. **Pincus, S.** 2005. Potential role of infections in chronic inflammatory diseases. *ASM News* **71**:529–535.

129. **Plenge, R. M., L. Padyukov, E. F. Remmers, S. Purcell, A. T. Lee, E. W. Karlson, F. Wolfe, D. L. Kastner, L. Alfredsson, A. Altshuler, P. K. Gregersen, L. Klareskog, and J. D. Rioux.** 2005. Replication of putative candidate-gene associations with rheumatoid arthritis in >4,000 samples from North America and Sweden: association of susceptibility with *PTPN22, CTLA4,* and *PAD14*. *Am. J. Hum. Genet.* **77**:1044–1060.

130. **Plenge, R. M., M. Seiekstad, L. Padyukov, A. T. Lee, E. F. Remmers, B. Ding, A. Liew, H. Khalili, A. Chandrasekaran, L. R. L. Davies, W. Li, A. K. S. Tan, C. Bonnard, R. T. H. Ong, A. Thalamuthu, S. Pettersson, C. Liu, C. Tian, W. V. Chen, J. P. Carulli, E. M. Beckman, D. Altschuler, L. Alfredsson, L. A. Criswell, C. I. Amos, M. F. Seldin, D. L. Kastner, L. Klareskog, and P. K. Gregersen.** 2007. *TRAF1-C5* as a risk locus for rheumatoid arthritis–a genomewide study. *New Eng. J. Med.* **357**:1199–1209.

131. **Prater, C. D., and R. G. Zylstra.** 2002. Autism: a medical primer. *Am. Fam. Physician* **66**:1667–1674.

132. **Pratesi, F., C. Tommasi, C. Anzilotti, D. Chimenti, and P. Migliorini.** 2006. Deiminated Epstein-Barr virus nuclear antigen 1 is a target of anti-citrullinated protein antibodies in rheumatoid arthritis. *Arth. Rheum.* **54**:733–741.

133. **Raelson, J. V., R. D. Little, A. Ruether, H. Fournier, B. Paquin, P. Van Eerdewegh, W. E. C. Bradley, P. Croteau, Q. Nguyen-Huu, J. Segal, S. Debrus, R. Allard, P. Rosenstiel, A. Franke, G. Jacobs, S. Nikolaus, J-M. Vidal, P. Szego, N. Laplante, H. F. Clark, R. J. Paulussen, J. W. Hooper, T. P. Keith, A. Belouchi, and S. Schreiber.** 2007. Genome-wide association study for Crohn's disease in the Quebec founder

population identifies multiple validated disease loci. *Proc. Natl. Acad. Sci. USA* **104:**14747–14752.

134. **Reeves, W. C., J. F. Jones, E. Maloney, C. Heim, D. C. Hoaglin, R. S. Boneva, M. Morrissey, and R. Devlin.** 2007. Prevalence of chronic fatigue syndrome in metropolitan, urban, and rural Georgia. *Popul. Health Metr.* **5:**5.
135. **Reyes, M., R. Nisenbaum, D. C. Hoaglin, E. R. Unger, C. Emmons, B. Randall, J. A. Stewart, S. Abbey, J. F. Jones, N. Grantz, S. Minden, and William C. Reeves.** 2003. Prevalence and incidence of chronic fatigue syndrome in Wichita, Kansas. *Arch. Intern. Med.* **163:**1530–1536.
136. **Reynolds, K. J., S. D. Vernon, E. Bouchery, and W. C. Reeves.** 2004. The economic impact of chronic fatigue syndrome. *Cost Eff. Resour. Alloc.* **2:**4 http://www.resource.allocation.com/content/2/1/4. Accessed 10 December 2007.
137. **Riederer, F., M. Stamenkovic, S. D. Schindler, and S. Kasper.** 2002. Das Tourette-Syndrom. Eine Übersicht. *Nervenarzt.* **73:**805–819.
138. **Roberts, S. E., J. G. Williams, D. Yeates, and M. J. Goldacre.** 2007. Mortality in patients with and without colectomy admitted to hospital for ulcerative colitis and Crohn's disease: record linkage studies. *Br. Med. J.* **335:**1033.
139. **Rodier, P. M.** 2004. 2003 Warkany lecture: autism as a birth defect. *Birth Defects Res. A* **70:**1–6.
140. **Rosen, N. J., C. K. Yoshida, and L. A. Croen.** 2007. Infection in the first 2 years of life and autism spectrum disorders. *Pediatrics* **119:**e61–e69.
141. **Rosenstein, D. D., R. A. Greenwald, L. J. Kushner, and G. Weissmann.** 2004. Hypothesis: the humoral immune response to oral bacteria provides a stimulus for the development of rheumatoid arthritis. *Inflammation* **28:**311–318.
142. **Russel, M. G. V. M.** 2000. Changes in the incidence of inflammatory bowel disease: what does it mean. *Eur. J. Intern. Med.* **11:**191–196.
143. **Russell, R. K., and J. Satsangi.** 2004. IBD: a family affair. *Best Pract. Res. Clin. Gastroenterol.* **18:**525–539.
144. **Saal, J. G., M. Krimmel, M. Steidle, F. Gerneth, S. Wagner, P. Fritz, S. Koch, J. Zacher, S. Sell, H. Einsele, and C. A. Müller.** 1999. Synovial Epstein-Barr virus infection increases the risk of rheumatoid arthritis in individuals with the shared HLA-DR4 epitope. *Arth. Rheum.* **42:**1485–1496.
145. **Sawada, S., M. Takei, H. Inomata, T. Nozaki, and H. Shiraiwa.** 2007. What is after cytokine-blocking therapy, a novel therapeutic target–synovial Epstein-Barr virus for rheumatoid arthritis. *Autoimmune Rev.* **6:**126–130.
146. **Scanu, A. M., T. J. Bull, S. Cannas, J. D. Sanderson, L. A. Sechi, G. Dettori, S. Zanetti, and J. Hermon-Taylor.** 2007. *Mycobacterium avium* subspecies *paratuberculosis* infection in cases of irritable bowel syndrome and comparison with Crohn's disease and Johne's disease: common neural and immune pathogenicities. *J. Clin. Microbiol.* **45:**3883–3890.
147. **Sebat, J., B. Lakshmi, D. Malhotra, J. Troge, C. Lese-Martin, T. Walsh, B. Yamrom, S. Yoon, A. Krasnitz, J. Kendall, A. Leotta, D. Pai, R. Zhang, y-H. Lee, J. Hicks, S. J. Spence, A. T. Lee, K. Puura, T. Lehtimäki, D. Ledbetter, K. K. Gregersen, J. Bregman, J. S. Sutcliffe, V. Jobanputra, W. Chung, D. Warburton, M-C. King, D. Skuse, D. H. Geschwind, T. C. Gilliam, K. Ye, and M. Wigler.** 2007. Strong association of de novo copy number mutations with autism. *Science* **316:**445–449.
148. **Shanahan, F.** 2002. Crohn's disease. *Lancet* **359:**62–69.
149. **Shapiro, W.** 2006. Inflammatory bowel disease. http://www.emedicine.com/EMERG/topic106.htm. Accessed 28 May 2007.
150. **Simard, J. F., and K. H. Costenbader.** 2007. What can epidemiology tell us about systemic lupus erythematosus? *Int. J. Clin. Pract.* **61:**1170–1180.
151. **Smith, J. B., and M. K. Haynes.** 2002. Rheumatoid arthritis–a molecular understanding. *Ann. Intern. Med.* **136:**908–922.
152. **Smolen, J. S., D. Aletaha, M. Koeller, M. H. Weisman and P. Emery.** 2007. New therapies for treatment of rheumatoid arthritis. *Lancet* **370:**1861–1874.
153. **Snider, L. A., and S. E. Swedo.** 2003. Childhood-onset obsessive-compulsive disorder and tic disorders: case report and literature review. *J. Child. Adolesc. Psychopharmacol.* **13**(Suppl. 1)**:**S81–S88.
154. **Sospedra, M., and R. Martin.** 2005. Immunology of multiple sclerosis. *Annu. Rev. Immunol.* **23:**683–747.
155. **Stamatovic, S. M., O. B. Dimitrijevic, R. F. Keep, and A. V. Andjelkovic.** 2006. Inflammation and brain edema: new insights into the role of chemokines and their receptors. *Acta Neurochir.* **96**(Suppl.)**:**444–450.
156. **Stratton, C. W., and D. B. Wheldon.** 2006. Multiple sclerosis: an infectious syndrome involving *Chlamydophila pneumoniae. Trends Microbiol.* **14:**474–479.
157. **Strober, W., I. Fuss, and P. Mannon.** 2007. The fundamental basis of inflammatory bowel disease. *J. Clin. Investig.* **117:**514–521.
158. **Sutcliffe, J. S.** 2008. Insights into the pathogenesis of autism. *Science* **321:**208–209.
159. **Tabuchi, K., J. Blundell, M. R. Etherton, R. E. Hammer, X. Liu, C. M. Powell, and T. C. Südhof.** 2007. A neurologin-3 mutation implicated in autism increases inhibitory synaptic transmission in mice. *Science* **318:**71–76.
160. **Takeda, T., Y. Mizugaki, L. Matsubara, S. Imai, T. Koike, and K. Takada.** 2000. Lytic Epstein-Barr virus infection in the synovial tissue of patients with rheumatoid arthritis. *Arth. Rheum.* **43:**1218–1225.
161. **Thompson-Chagoyán, O. C., J. Maldonado, and A. Gil.** 2005. Aetiology of inflammatory bowel disease (IBD): role of intestinal microbiota and gut-associated lymphoid tissue immune response. *Clin. Nutr.* **24:**339–352.
162. **Tolan, R. W., J. M. Stewart, and B. Carter.** 2007. Chronic fatigue syndrome. http://www.emedicine.com/ped/topic2795.htm Accessed 7 November 2007.
163. **van der Helm-van Mil, A. H. M., K. N. Verpoort, F. C. Brfeedveld, R. E. M Toes, and T. W. J. Huizinga.** 2005. Antibodies to citrullinated proteins and differences in clinical progression of rheumatoid arthritis. *Arthritis Res. Ther.* **7:**R949–R958.
164. **van Gaalen, F., A. Ioan-Facsinay, T. W. J. Huizinga, and R. E. M. Toes.** 2005. The devil in the details: the emerging role of anticitrulline autoimmunity in rheumatoid arthritis. *J. Immunol.* **175:**5575–5580.
165. **van Heel, D. A., S. A. Fisher, A. Kirby, M. J. Daly, J. D. Rioux, C. M. Lewis, and the Genome Scan Meta-Analysis Group of the IBD International Genetics Consortium.** 2004. Inflammatory bowel disease susceptibility loci defined by genome scan meta-anlysis of 1952 affected relative pairs. *Hum. Mol. Genet.* **13:**762–770.
166. **Veenstra-VanderWeele, J., and E. H. Cook.** 2004. Molecular genetics of autism spectrum discorder. *Mol. Psychiatry* **9:**819–832.
167. **Viner, R., and M. Hotopf.** 2004. Childhood predictors of self-reported chronic fatigue syndrome/myalgic encephalomyelitis in adults: national birth cohort study. *Brit. Med. J.* **329:**941.
168. **Vollmer, T.** 2007. The natural history of relapses in multiple sclerosis. *J. Neurol. Sci.* **256:**S5–S13.

169. **Vollmer-Conna, U., B. Cameron, D. Hadzi-Pavlovic, K. Singletary, T. Davenport, S. Vernon, W. C. Reeves, I. Hickie, D. Wakefield, A. R. Lloyd, and the Dubbo Infective Outcomes Group.** 2007. Postinfective fatigue syndrome is not associated with altered cytokine production. *Clin. Infect. Dis.* **45**:732–735.

170. **Vossenaar, E. R., T. R. D. Radstake, A. van der Heijden, M. A. M. van Mansum, C. Dieteren, D.-J. de Rooij, P. Barrera, A. J. W. Zendman, and W. J. van Venrooij.** 2004. Expression and activity of citrullinating peptidylarginine deiminase enzymes in monocytes and macrophages. *Ann. Rheum. Dis.* **63**:373–381.

171. **Weissmann, G.** 2006. The pathogenesis of rheumatoid arthritis. *Bull. NYU Hosp. J. Dis.* **64**:12–15.

172. **Weller, C., N. Oxlade, S. M. Dobbs, R. J. Dobbs, A. Charlett, and I. T. Bjarnason.** 2005. Role of inflammation in gastrointestinal tract in aetiology and pathogenesis of idiopathic parkinsonism. *FEMS Immunol. Med. Microbiol.* **44**:129–135.

173. **Wildman, M. J., E. G. Smith, J. Groves, J. M. Beattie, E. O. Caul, and J. G. Ayres.** 2002. Chronic fatigue following infection by *Coxiella burnetii* (Q fever): ten-year follow-up of the 1989 UK outbreak cohort. *Q. J. Med.* **95**:527–538.

174. **Wong, D., K. Dorovini-Zia, and S. R. Vincent.** 2004. Cytokines, nitric oxide, and cGMP modulate the permeability of an in vitro model of the human blood brain barrier. *Exp. Neurol.* **190**:446–455.

175. **Xavier, R. J., and D. K. Podolsky.** 2007. Unraveling the pathogenesis of inflammatory bowel disease. *Nature* **448**:427–434.

Sequelae and Long-Term Consequences of Infectious Diseases
Edited by Pina M. Fratamico, James L. Smith, and Kim A. Brogden

Chapter 27

Epidemiological Methods To Implicate Specific Microorganisms with Long-Term Complications

Kåre Mølbak

Many chronic or recurrent conditions have over the years been accused of being late consequences of acute infections. Rigorous research has later been able to confirm, refute, or modify such "links" for which the scientific basis and evidence had varied at the time when the hypothesis was created. In this context, epidemiological studies have played— and will also in the future continue to play—an important role. Thus, epidemiological studies were important in order to associate *Campylobacter* species infection with Guillain-Barré syndrome (54, 85); staphylococcal infections and toxic shock syndrome (61, 71); *Helicobacter pylori* infection and peptic ulcer (59, 63); Epstein-Barr virus and malignant disease, including Burkitt's lymphoma (22) and Hodgkin's disease (13, 34); hepatitis B virus and liver cancer (49); human herpesvirus 8 and Kaposi's sarcoma (12, 62); and human papilloma virus (HPV) and cervical cancer (45, 64). These studies are by no means an exhaustive list of references but are examples of highlights in public health and epidemiology. They are research papers that have found important associations between acute infections and later manifestations and were able to provide a public health perspective to basic or clinical research. As discussed later, there are also examples of large-scale epidemiological studies that were equally important because they were unable to confirm hypotheses that arose from smaller case series or from basic research.

The aim of this chapter is to present the epidemiological methods to implicate microorganisms with long-term complications. The discussion will address the design of epidemiological studies, the validity of such studies, and the importance of population- and registry-based research.

EPIDEMIOLOGICAL STUDIES TO IMPLICATE SPECIFIC MICROORGANISMS WITH LONG-TERM COMPLICATIONS

A variety of observational studies have been important in raising or substantiating hypotheses or models of disease mechanisms. Such studies include case reports and case series, outbreak investigations with follow-up of exposed individuals, and large population-based studies (Table 1). Whereas basic science and studies of animal models are pivotal to understanding pathogenesis and disease mechanisms of long-term complications, analytical epidemiological studies are important to (i) confirm or refute hypotheses, (ii) quantify the magnitude of an association, and (iii) provide a public health perspective to an association, including expanding studies of the burden of illness to include long-term sequelae. For the last objective—determining the burden of illness—it should be underscored that for many infections, a careful estimation of the costs for society is dependent on an understanding of the associated complications and sequelae. Thus, the burden of illness due to *Campylobacter* is due largely to Guillain-Barré syndrome (26), prevention of hepatocellular carcinoma and liver cirrhosis are prime motivations for vaccination against hepatitis B (72), and the primary aim by introducing vaccination against HPV is the prevention of cervical cancer and other HPV-associated malignant diseases (16). On the other hand, the associations between acute bacterial infections and irritable bowel syndrome and, in particular, inflammatory bowel disease remain somehow controversial (41, 73, 74). Although epidemiological studies have indicated such associations, their causal nature is not clear. Whether or not these associations are accepted

Kåre Mølbak • Statens Serum Institut, 5 Artillerivej, 2300 Copenhagen S, Denmark.

Table 1. Infectious disease associations with long-term complications

How can an infectious disease be associated with a late outcome?
Concerns or rumors raised by affected individuals, interest groups, or clinicians
Hypotheses raised from basic science or from experimental or animal models
Observations, from ecological studies, that acute infections and outcomes follow similar temporal trends
Observations from outbreak investigations or clinical studies (case series)
Results from analytical epidemiological studies (cohort or case-control studies)

as "cause and effect" and thus included in the burden of illness estimates becomes essential for the determination of costs for society and thus for priority setting (26, 57).

Two Families of Design Options

Two types of epidemiologic designs—and variations thereof—are commonly used to study the association between acute infections and later outcomes, such as complications and sequelae. The two "families" of design options—the cohort study and the case-control study—are described in standard epidemiological textbooks (23, 68). In the present context, the term "exposure" commonly used in epidemiological textbooks refers to the acute infectious event or microbial agent under study, and the "outcome" to the chronic condition or sequelae that may or may not be linked to the infectious event. Each study type has advantages and disadvantages (Table 2). In a cohort study, infected ("exposed") and uninfected ("unexposed") individuals are followed over time to determine the rate of specified outcomes, such as complications and sequelae. The rates of outcomes in these two groups are compared, and the association between infection and outcome is expressed in terms of the relative incidence rate or a similar measure. On this basis, a number of other measures can be derived, including the attributable fraction of complications and sequelae that may be accredited to the acute infection, and the number of infections "needed" to "cause" one complication.

In a case-control study, patients with the specific complications or manifestations are identified, and the evidence of prior infections (by interview, historical clinical records, or serological evidence) is measured and compared with the evidence of prior infections in control subjects without the complications or manifestations of interest. The result of such a study usually will be expressed in terms of an odds ratio, i.e., the odds of prior infection in cases relative to the odds of prior infection in controls.

As indicated in Table 2, each study has advantages and disadvantages. The choice of a particular design depends on the scientific questions, available data sources, available resources, and research infrastructure. As will be discussed below, case-control studies may often be more prone to bias and confounding than cohort studies. But, on the other hand, carefully designed and rigorously conducted case-control studies are a very efficient way to obtain high-quality results. Indeed, most of the studies quoted above were designed as case-control studies (13, 33, 47, 54, 59, 61–64, 71, 85).

There are important modifications of the two types of study designs, including the nested case-control studies (where a well-defined cohort serve as a sampling frame for a case-control study), case-case studies, and case-cohort studies. Furthermore, both

Table 2. Advantages and disadvantages of the cohort and the case-control studies to implicate specific microorganisms with long-term complications

Advantage or disadvantage of: Cohort	Advantage or disadvantage of: Case-control
Several types of outcomes may be studied	Only one outcome (i.e., the criterion for which the cases are selected) may be studied
Usually only one type of infection can serve as "exposure" event	More than one infection may serve as an "exposure" event
Cohort studies can be very costly to establish and may require a large sample size, in particular if the outcomes are infrequent[a]	Are usually less expensive
In general, unbiased estimates are better if obtained from cohort studies	Sources of bias should be carefully addressed
Are particularly well suited to the study of a range of different complications that may occur a long time after the "exposure" event	Are particularly well suited to the study of well-defined complications that occur a short while after the "exposure" event, in particular if information bias can be reduced

[a]Costly studies may not be an issue for registry-based cohort studies taking advantage of existing registries and databases.

types of studies may be designed as prospective or retrospective and include some type of matching as a way to control confounding. It is beyond the scope of this chapter to discuss these issues in detail, and we refer the reader to standard textbooks (23, 68).

ASSOCIATION OR CAUSATION?

Epidemiological studies are able to provide a measure of the strength and the precision of a link between the infection (exposure) and the later complications (outcomes). However, in the interpretation of the findings of an epidemiological study, it is important to address the causal relevance of an observation. Causal inference is a special case of the more general process of scientific reasoning, which is a vast subject (67).

Koch's (Löffler) postulates are classical and well-known causal criteria for infectious diseases. In short, (1) the organism must always be present in the diseased tissue, (2) the organism should be isolated and grown in pure culture, and (3) this pure culture must be shown to induce the disease experimentally (23, 48). Although the postulates were an important advance in scientific reasoning, they are now inadequate for the validation of evidence vis-à-vis infections that allegedly are associated with later outcomes. Nonetheless, in 1984 Marshall managed to meet Koch's postulates using self inoculation by ingesting a culture of *Helicobacter pylori*, which resulted in gastritis, which was treated and cured with bismuth salts and metronidazole (51). However, limitations of Koch's postulates include the fact that the outcome may often be caused by more than one infectious exposure, the outcome will not occur in all exposed individuals, and for many reasons, the association may prove hard or unethical to confirm in animal models, not to mention human experiments.

A commonly used set of causal criteria was proposed by Hill (33). These nine criteria included the strength and consistency of an association, its specificity, temporality, biologic gradient, plausibility, coherence, experimental evidence, and finally analogy. It is, as discussed by Rothman and Greenland, also evident that the standards of epidemiological evidence offered by Hill are saddled with reservations and exceptions (67). Hill himself was ambivalent about the utility of these "standards" and did not use the word "criteria" in his paper. To quote Hill: "None of my nine viewpoints can bring indisputable evidence for or against the cause-and-effect hypothesis and none can be regarded as a *sine qua non.*" However, the fourth criteria, temporality, is a *sine qua non* for causality. If a putative outcome did precede its infectious cause, that indeed is indisputable evidence that the observed association is not causal. Therefore, to establish the timing of the infectious event and the later outcomes is an essential part of epidemiological studies.

Rothman and Greenland have developed a general epidemiological model of causation (67). In their model, a sufficient cause refers to a complete and often complex causal mechanism that can be defined as a set of minimal conditions and events that inevitably produce disease. Among these conditions, one or more may be "a necessary cause," i.e., a condition that always should be present to produce the outcome. It is, for example, generally agreed that infection with high risk HPV (hrHPV) is a necessary cause of cervical cancer (83). That is, persistent infection with hrHPV is always present prior to the development of cervical cancer. However, hrHPV infection is not a sufficient cause because only a small fraction of woman with hrHPV will develop cervical cancer. It is therefore obvious that other complement causes must be present before disease develops. These complement causes are often incompletely understood. Thus, tobacco smoking increases the risk of cervical cancer and may thus be regarded as a complement cause or "causal component" but is clearly not a necessary cause since many nonsmoking women develop cervical cancer. Behavioral factors, genetic and immunological factors, coinfections, and so on are often found as component causes for late outcomes of infectious diseases. Indeed, well-designed and well-conducted epidemiological studies are well suited to study how the necessary cause(s) interact with the component causes (18, 19, 44, 77).

VALIDITY OF EPIDEMIOLOGICAL STUDIES: BIAS AND CONFOUNDING

Three types of problems that affect the interpretation of epidemiological studies may be identified. These include selection bias, information bias, and confounding (68).

Selection Bias

Selection bias refers to distortions that result from procedures used to select subjects and from factors that influence study participation. The common element is that the relation between exposure and outcome is different for those who participate and those who originally formed the basis of the study. For example, if in a study of risk factors for Guillain-Barré syndrome, individuals with a history of *Campylobacter* infection were more willing to take part than individuals with no such history, the estimation of the association between *Campylobacter* infection and Guillain-Barré syndrome may be distorted. This is an example of self-selection bias. A special example of selection bias is "the healthy worker effect" that allow those who do not develop the outcome to stay in a cohort longer than those who develop the outcome. This could for instance be a problem if those individuals, who develop early signs of complications, simply drop out of an epidemiological study. This bias will usually result in the underestimation of the true association.

Another type of selection bias is diagnostic or "culture bias." This type of bias is important to consider in studies that associate infectious exposures with later outcomes. For example, individuals with underlying illness or persons who have traveled to foreign parts of the world may see their doctor more often and may be selected more often for microbiological examinations or other diagnostic procedures than individuals from the general population do. Hence, one may argue that the association between acute gastrointestinal infections and conditions such as inflammatory bowel disease or irritable bowel syndrome may be affected by the fact that patients with persistent bowel complaints get stool cultured more often than the general population (41). Also, when registry-based studies suggested that bacterial gastrointestinal infections may be associated with a long-term excess mortality, it was discussed to which extent this may be ascribed to case selection (32, 60). It is always important to think about why a sample was taken!

Information Bias

Information bias occurs when there are errors in the measurement of infectious exposure, the outcome, or both. This type of bias generally is classified as differential or nondifferential. A nondifferential bias will often result in a conservative estimation of the association between infectious exposure and later outcome. Thus, if a hypothetical cohort study of the relation between gastrointestinal infections and reactive complications include a number of subjects with undiagnosed infections in the "unexposed" group, the estimation of the relative rate of reactive symptoms among the exposed will be underestimated. It is important to critically consider the completeness and the specificity of the ascertainment of exposures and outcomes. An incomplete ascertainment of outcomes is very common in cohort studies, but this will have no effect on the relative rate of the outcome, provided that this information bias is nondifferential, i.e., independent of the infectious exposures.

Information bias can also be differential. This can be the situation in a case-control study if cases (i.e., individuals with the relevant outcome) or their physicians are more likely to report a history of an infectious exposure than healthy controls. Information bias is a serious issue if those who provide the information are aware of the study hypothesis.

Telescoping is an example of information bias in which study participants overestimate the rate of illness because they underestimate the time since an event took place. Thus, if a study measures the incidence of a disease within a given recall period, enthusiastic participants may decide to report an event although it did not take place within the defined period, simply because they felt it was important. Thus, in infectious intestinal disease in England, a retrospective estimate of reported diarrhea in the month before recruitment to the cohort was nearly three times the prospective estimate (84). A related bias is the so-called Hawthorne effect, which in a broad sense refers to the problem of people's behavior and performance possibly changing (often improving) following any new or increased attention (50).

Confounding

A confounder is often described as a factor related to both the outcome of interest and the infectious exposure that may lead to this outcome. Furthermore, a confounder is not part of the causal pathway that leads from infectious disease to the outcome. Confounding will affect the result of an epidemiological study if the distribution of the confounder is skewed, regarding both the infectious exposure and the outcome. The design of the study and the data analysis can deal with confounding. A classic way to deal with confounding is by matching. Matching can be undertaken in both cohort and case-control studies. Registry-based studies of the risk of complications following foodborne bacterial infections are examples of matched cohort studies, since the rate of outcomes was determined for individuals with infectious exposures (e.g., *Salmonella*, *Campylobacter*, and *Yersinia enterocolitica*) and matched subsets of the general population (28–30, 32). Frequently, matching is carried out in case-control studies. It is important to underscore that matching should be undertaken only if there are good reasons to do so (e.g., strong confounding). In addition, the analytical strategy should take this matching into consideration by an appropriate statistical method.

Multivariable analysis is a standard way to control for confounding. It is common to determine confounding by the evaluation of changes in the measures of association upon the inclusion of potential confounding factors ("change-in-estimate" approach or "noncollapsibility"). Confounding is a complex issue, and it is beyond the scope of this chapter to discuss this issue in more detail (24, 68).

Multivariable modeling or stratification may adjust for selection bias, provided that the necessary information is available. However, information bias is usually not possible to adjust for, since it represents unknown measurement errors of infectious exposure or outcome.

THE IMPORTANCE OF POPULATION- AND REGISTRY-BASED RESEARCH

Population- or community-based studies refer to large population studies in which cohorts are followed over several years. For chronic disease epidemiology, there are many examples of such studies. The Framingham Heart Study, initiated in 1949, is the most notable of several long-term follow-up studies of cardiovascular disease. This remarkable study is continuing to produce valuable findings more than 40 years after it was begun (43, 75). However, also within the area of infectious disease epidemiology, long-term follow-up studies have been essential. Examples from industrialized countries include human herpesvirus 8 and Kaposi's sarcoma in HIV-positive individuals (53), HPV and cervical cancer (45, 86), *H. pylori* and gastric cancer (10, 69), and population-based cohort studies of the epidemiology of gastrointestinal diseases (17, 84).

Demographic Surveillance

From developing countries, where patterns of morbidity and mortality are strikingly different from those of industrialized countries, population-based cohort studies have provided essential information about patterns of morbidity and mortality from infectious diseases (76). In recent years, many demographic sentinel sites have been organized in the INDEPTH network (http://www.indepth-network.org). This network serves as an international platform of sentinel demographic sites that provides health and demographic data and research to enable developing countries to set health priorities and policies based on longitudinal evidence. The mission is that data and research will guide the cost-effective use of tools, interventions, and systems to ensure and monitor progress towards national goals. INDEPTH has 38 demographic surveillance sites in 19 different countries. Of this number, 26 sites are found in Africa, 10 sites in Asia, 1 in Central Oceania and 1 in Central America. One of the oldest of these demographic sentinel sites is the Matlab site in Bangladesh run by the International Centre for Diarrhoeal Diseases Research. The objectives are to (i) provide a small-area registration system which is suitable for assessment of the effectiveness, safety, and acceptability of maternal and child health and family planning interventions, (ii) undertake research related to diarrheal diseases, and on the measurement and determinants of fertility and mortality, and (iii) develop a demographic field site that can be used for training of program planners, researchers, and implementors.

In Matlab, the long-term consequences of interventions such as immunizations, management of common infections, family planning, distribution of vitamin A capsules, and nutritional education are determined (3, 9, 11, 14, 27).

In Africa, the longest ongoing demographic surveillance has been carried out at the Bandim field site in Guinea-Bissau, West Africa. This site was established in 1978, and the area under surveillance has expanded since then. The central features of the research in Bandim are the attempts to follow long-term consequences of various infections, health conditions, and interventions. Main areas of research are determinants of measles mortality, evaluation of different measles vaccination schemes, long-term consequences of measles infection, crowding and health, epidemiology and control of diarrheal and respiratory diseases, management of childhood illnesses, impact of breast feeding and weaning on morbidity and survival, risk factors for hospitalization, immunological determinants of child survival, maternal mortality, epidemiology of HIV-2 and other retroviruses, and epidemiology and control of tuberculosis. For example, studies from the site have been pivotal in suggesting that mortality from measles was determined by and large by transmission factors (e.g, infectious dose) rather than host factors (1, 4). More recently, research has focused on positive as well as negative nontargeted effects of childhood vaccinations. It has been suggested that the overall impact of vaccines on public health may be ascribed to such effects beyond the control of illness (2, 5–8, 42, 46, 66, 80). Diarrheal diseases, in particular infection with *Cryptosporidium* species, have been shown to have long term consequences for child growth and survival (55, 56, 58, 78). Several studies have addressed the epidemiology and effects of HIV-1 infection in comparison with those of HIV-2 infection and the interactions between HIV infection and tuberculosis (25, 35, 70).

Registry-Based Research

As mentioned, results from smaller epidemiological studies or case reports have often raised the hypothesis that an acute infection may be associated with long-term complications. To refute or confirm such suggestions, large-scale population based studies have been of great value. In some countries, such as those in Scandinavia, national administrative and health care registries can be linked by the use of unique civil registry numbers. By such linkage, the entire national population can be analyzed as one cohort (20). This setup served as the basis for a number of studies of which a few examples will be summarized in the present chapter.

Long-term effects of foodborne bacterial infections

In Denmark, a series of registry-based studies was initiated to determine long-term effects of gastrointestinal infections that usually are foodborne. The objective of the largest of these studies was to determine the excess mortality associated with infections with *Salmonella*, *Campylobacter*, *Yersinia enterocolitica*, and *Shigella* and to examine the effect of preexisting illness. The study was designed as a registry-based, matched cohort study. A total of 48,857 people with gastrointestinal infections and 487,138 individuals from the general population were included. A total of 1,071 (2.2%) people with gastrointestinal infections died within 1 year after infection compared with 3,636 (0.7%) in the general age- and gender-matched population. This suggested that the mortality among persons who are diagnosed with gastrointestinal infections is 3.1 times higher in patients than in the general population. Furthermore, there was excess mortality 1 to 6 months after infection with *Y. enterocolitica* and from 6 months to 1 year after infection with *Campylobacter* and *Salmonella*. This observation remained significant even after underlying illness was included as an explanatory variable in the statistical model (32). Additional studies determined the effects of antimicrobial drug resistance in *Salmonella enterica* serovar Typhimurium (31), the excess risk of death or invasive illness due to quinolone resistance in *S. enterica* serovar Typhimurium (28), and the excess risk of death or invasive illness following infection with fluoroquinolone- or macrolide-resistant *Campylobacter* compared with susceptible strains (30).

Is infection with GBM associated with an increased risk of autoimmune diseases?

The capsular polysaccharide of group B meningococci (GBM) is structurally identical to a polysaccharide found on neural cell adhesion molecules in humans. This structural identity has raised concern that a vaccine based on the GBM capsular polysaccharide might induce autoimmune disease in vaccinated persons. Because systemic infection with GBM induces serum antibody in adults, the entire Danish population was studied in order to determine whether persons with a history of GBM disease are at increased risk of developing autoimmune diseases. The cohort included 7,467,001 individuals, who were observed for autoimmune diseases from 1977 through 2004. Persons with GBM disease had no increased risk of autoimmune diseases, either compared with persons with a history of group C meningococcal disease or compared with persons without a history of meningococcal disease (36). An additional study explored if women with a previous systemic GBM disease experienced pregnancy complications and if their offspring had increased risk of birth defects. Also these results did not support the hypothesis that GBM is associated with immunoreactive disease that may affect the course of pregnancy or the health of the offspring (37). Taken together, these findings suggest that invasive disease caused by GBM is not associated with autoimmune diseases in humans and should therefore lessen concerns regarding the development of a capsular-based GBM vaccine.

Postlicensure epidemiology of childhood vaccination

Although the focus of this book is on the complications and late outcomes of acute infections, controversy also exists regarding late outcomes of vaccinations in the form of adverse events that have not been recognized by routine safety assessment. For example, MMR vaccinations and vaccines with thimerosal as a preservative have been hypothesized to be linked with neurodevelopment disorders, including autism (21, 82). It has also been suggested that childhood vaccinations may be linked with the increase in type 1 diabetes seen in several countries (15). Many early childhood vaccinations have been viewed as promotors of asthma development either by decreasing the microbial pressure ("the hygiene hypothesis") or by affecting the immune system in an atopic TH2 direction; both explanations would shift the cytokine balance of TH1 and TH2 immunity (52,65).

Inherent limitations in the prelicensure assessment necessitate continued epidemiological evaluations of efficacy and safety issues after the introduction of vaccines into use. In Denmark, the opportunities available for epidemiological research are unique. In 2001, an initiative was undertaken to take advantage of these opportunities to study the postlicensure epidemiology of childhood vaccination with respect to effectiveness and safety (38). A number of postlicensure studies of effectiveness and safety have taken advantage of these opportunities. Specific studies have investigated the following relations: measles-mumps-rubella vaccine and autism (49), thimerosal-containing vaccine and autism (39), measles-mumps-rubella vaccine and febrile seizures (81), and childhood vaccination and type 1 diabetes (40). These studies, taken together, have lessened the concerns about such adverse events following routine childhood vaccinations.

These studies have been carried out as registry-based cohort studies. The use of a cohort with independent and prospective ascertainment of exposure and outcome minimizes concern over selection and information bias, particularly recall bias. However, the comparability of vaccinated and unvaccinated children, with respect to factors influencing risk of disease other than the possible effect of vaccination, must be considered rigorously. The classical type of confounding, in safety studies, is confounding by contraindication, in which certain groups of high-risk children are undervaccinated. Consequently, the estimated effect of vaccination will be biased towards a false protective effect (38). For studies in developing countries, where mortality is high, "survival bias" is a major methodological concern (42).

FUTURE PERSPECTIVES

Not so long ago, conditions like cervical cancer or peptic ulcer were not perceived as late outcomes of infections with specific microorganisms. Without doubt, we will in the coming years associate other chronic conditions, including malignant disease, etc., with infectious exposures earlier in life. Perhaps even more exciting, persistent viral infections, such as cytomegalovirus, may be important in the configuration of the immune system and thereby determine the "age" of the immune system. It is thus possible that we should consider immunosenescence as an infectious state and that this will have implications for the length of life and the effectiveness of interventions to preserve the health of senior citizens (79).

In the future, infections will be detected or described, and some of these may be linked to complications or sequelae that occur later in life. Epidemiological studies will, along with other lines of rigorous research, continue to be of importance to explore putative associations between infectious exposures and chronic conditions or illnesses. In particular, large-scale epidemiological cohort studies with long-term follow up that are able to yield results with a high degree of precision will be of continued significance. Therefore, it is essential to plan and invest for an infrastructure that allows for the undertaking of this type of research in a variety of settings.

In less developed countries, it is essential to maintain financial and scientific support to demographic sentinel surveillance sites that allow the study of both the natural history of infectious diseases and a critical assessment of the interventions that are put in place to control these problems. As a part of this activity, disease surveillance at the sentinel sites should be maintained and developed.

In industrialized countries, registry-based research offers an attractive and cost-effective methodology to investigate associations between infectious exposures and chronic conditions. In order to do so, it is important to include the same set of personal identifiers in surveillance registries, national hospital discharge registries, and clinical databases as well as demographic registries. In some countries, this may be difficult to achieve because of legal and political issues. However, given the great scientific and public health ramifications of such studies, decision makers should strive to overcome such barriers. Also, the greater complexity of vaccination programs and the challenges associated with globalization may give rise to unexpected findings. To prepare for this, investment in infrastructure to facilitate epidemiological research, including collections of biological material and strains, becomes pivotal.

REFERENCES

1. **Aaby, P.** 1995. Assumptions and contradictions in measles and measles immunization research: is measles good for something? *Soc. Sci. Med.* **41:**673–686.
2. **Aaby, P., C. S. Benn, J. Nielsen, I. M. Lisse, A. Rodrigues, and H. Jensen.** 2007. DTP vaccination and child survival in observational studies with incomplete vaccination data. *Trop. Med. Int. Health* **12:**15–24.
3. **Aaby, P., A. Bhuiya, L. Nahar, K. Knudsen, F. A. de, and M. Strong.** 2003. The survival benefit of measles immunization may not be explained entirely by the prevention of measles disease: a community study from rural Bangladesh. *Int. J. Epidemiol.* **32:**106–116.
4. **Aaby, P., J. Bukh, I. M. Lisse, and A. J. Smits.** 1984. Overcrowding and intensive exposure as determinants of measles mortality. *Am. J. Epidemiol.* **120:**49–63.
5. **Aaby, P., M. L. Garly, C. Bale, C. Martins, H. Jensen, I. Lisse, and H. Whittle.** 2003. Survival of previously measles-vaccinated and measles-unvaccinated children in an emergency situation: an unplanned study. *Pediatr. Infect. Dis. J.* **22:**798–805.
6. **Aaby, P., M. L. Garly, J. Nielsen, H. Ravn, C. Martins, C. Bale, A. Rodrigues, C. S. Benn, and I. M. Lisse.** 2007. Increased female-male mortality ratio associated with inactivated polio and diphtheria-tetanus-pertussis vaccines: Observations from vaccination trials in Guinea-Bissau. *Pediatr. Infect. Dis. J.* **26:**247–252.
7. **Aaby, P., and H. Jensen.** 2005. Do measles vaccines have non-specific effects on mortality? *Bull. W. H. O.* **83:**238.

8. **Aaby, P., A. Rodrigues, S. Biai, C. Martins, J. E. Veirum, C. S. Benn, and H. Jensen**. 2005. Vaccines and unexpected observations: flaws or cause for concern? *Vaccine* **23**:2407–2408.
9. **Alam, D. S., G. C. Marks, A. H. Baqui, M. Yunus, and G. J. Fuchs**. 2000. Association between clinical type of diarrhoea and growth of children under 5 years in rural Bangladesh. *Int. J. Epidemiol.* **29**:916–921.
10. **Anonymous**. 2001. Gastric cancer and *Helicobacter pylori*: a combined analysis of 12 case control studies nested within prospective cohorts. *Gut* **49**:347–353.
11. **Bennish, M. L., and B. J. Wojtyniak**. 1991. Mortality due to shigellosis: community and hospital data. *Rev. Infect. Dis.* **13**(Suppl. 4):S245–S251.
12. **Beral, V., T. A. Peterman, R. L. Berkelman, and H. W. Jaffe**. 1990. Kaposi's sarcoma among persons with AIDS: a sexually transmitted infection? *Lancet* **335**:123–128.
13. **Bernard, S. M., R. A. Cartwright, C. M. Darwin, I. D. Richards, B. Roberts, C. O'Brien, and C. C. Bird**. 1987. Hodgkin's disease: case control epidemiological study in Yorkshire. *Br. J. Cancer* **55**:85–90.
14. **Chowdhury, M. E., R. Botlero, M. Koblinsky, S. K. Saha, G. Dieltiens, and C. Ronsmans**. 2007. Determinants of reduction in maternal mortality in Matlab, Bangladesh: a 30-year cohort study. *Lancet* **370**:1320–1328.
15. **Classen, J. B.** 1996. The timing of immunization affects the development of diabetes in rodents. *Autoimmunity* **24**: 137–145.
16. **Cutts, F. T., S. Franceschi, S. Goldie, X. Castellsague, S. S. de, G. Garnett, W. J. Edmunds, P. Claeys, K. L. Goldenthal, D. M. Harper, and L. Markowitz**. 2007. Human papillomavirus and HPV vaccines: a review. *Bull. W. H. O.* **85**: 719–726.
17. **de Wit, M. A., M. P. Koopmans, L. M. Kortbeek, W. J. Wannet, J. Vinje, L. F. van, A. I. Bartelds, and Y. T. van Duynhoven**. 2001. Sensor, a population-based cohort study on gastroenteritis in the Netherlands: incidence and etiology. *Am. J. Epidemiol.* **154**:666–674.
18. **Franceschi, S.** 2005. The IARC commitment to cancer prevention: the example of papillomavirus and cervical cancer. *Recent Results Cancer Res.* **166**:277–297.
19. **Franco, E. L., N. F. Schlecht, and D. Saslow**. 2003. The epidemiology of cervical cancer. *Cancer J.* **9**:348–359.
20. **Frank, L.** 2003. Epidemiology. The epidemiologist's dream: Denmark. *Science* **301**:163.
21. **Geier, D. A., and M. R. Geier**. 2003. An assessment of the impact of thimerosal on childhood neurodevelopmental disorders. *Pediatr. Rehabil.* **6**:97–102.
22. **Geser, A., T. G. de, G. Lenoir, N. E. Day, and E. H. Williams**. 1982. Final case reporting from the Ugandan prospective study of the relationship between EBV and Burkitt's lymphoma. *Int. J. Cancer* **29**:397–400.
23. **Giesecke, J.** 2002. *Modern Infectious Disease Epidemiology*. Arnold, London, United Kingdom.
24. **Greenland, S., and H. Morgenstern**. 2001. Confounding in health research. *Annu. Rev. Public Health* **22**:189–212.
25. **Gustafson, P., V. F. Gomes, C. S. Vieira, B. Samb, A. Naucler, P. Aaby, and I. Lisse**. 2007. Clinical predictors for death in HIV-positive and HIV-negative tuberculosis patients in Guinea-Bissau. *Infection* **35**:69–80.
26. **Havelaar, A. H., M. A. de Wit, K. R. van, and K. E. van**. 2000. Health burden in the Netherlands due to infection with thermophilic *Campylobacter* spp. *Epidemiol. Infect.* **125**:505–522.
27. **Hawkes, S., L. Morison, S. Foster, K. Gausia, J. Chakraborty, R. W. Peeling, and D. Mabey**. 1999. Reproductive-tract infections in women in low-income, low-prevalence situations: assessment of syndromic management in Matlab, Bangladesh. *Lancet* **354**:1776–1781.
28. **Helms, M., J. Simonsen, and K. Molbak**. 2004. Quinolone resistance is associated with increased risk of invasive illness or death during infection with *Salmonella* serotype Typhimurium. *J. Infect. Dis.* **190**:1652–1654.
29. **Helms, M., J. Simonsen, and K. Molbak**. 2006. Foodborne bacterial infection and hospitalization: a registry-based study. *Clin. Infect. Dis.* **42**:498–506.
30. **Helms, M., J. Simonsen, K. E. Olsen, and K. Molbak**. 2005. Adverse health events associated with antimicrobial drug resistance in *Campylobacter* species: a registry-based cohort study. *J. Infect. Dis.* **191**:1050–1055.
31. **Helms, M., P. Vastrup, P. Gerner-Smidt, and K. Molbak**. 2002. Excess mortality associated with antimicrobial drug-resistant *Salmonella typhimurium*. *Emerg. Infect. Dis.* **8**:490–495.
32. **Helms, M., P. Vastrup, P. Gerner-Smidt, and K. Molbak**. 2003. Short and long term mortality associated with foodborne bacterial gastrointestinal infections: registry based study. *BMJ* **326**:357.
33. **Hill, A. B.** 1965. The environment and disease: association or causation? *Proc. R. Soc Med.* **58**:295–300.
34. **Hjalgrim, H., K. E. Smedby, K. Rostgaard, D. Molin, S. Hamilton-Dutoit, E. T. Chang, E. Ralfkiaer, C. Sundstrom, H. O. Adami, B. Glimelius, and M. Melbye**. 2007. Infectious mononucleosis, childhood social environment, and risk of Hodgkin lymphoma. *Cancer Res.* **67**:2382–2388.
35. **Holmgren, B., S. Z. da, P. Vastrup, O. Larsen, S. Andersson, H. Ravn, and P. Aaby**. 2007. Mortality associated with HIV-1, HIV-2, and HTLV-I single and dual infections in a middle-aged and older population in Guinea-Bissau. *Retrovirology* **4**:85.
36. **Howitz, M., T. G. Krause, J. B. Simonsen, S. Hoffmann, M. Frisch, N. M. Nielsen, J. Robbins, R. Schneerson, K. Molbak, and M. A. Miller**. 2007. Lack of association between group B meningococcal disease and autoimmune disease. *Clin. Infect. Dis.* **45**:1327–1334.
37. **Howitz, M., J. Simonsen, T. G. Krause, J. Robbins, R. Schneerson, K. Mølbak, and M. A. Miller**. 2009. Risk of adverse birth outcome after group B meningococcal disease: results from Danish National Cohort. *Pediatr. Infect. Dis.* **28**: 199–203.
38. **Hviid, A.** 2006. Postlicensure epidemiology of childhood vaccination: the Danish experience. *Expert Rev. Vaccines* **5**:641–649.
39. **Hviid, A., M. Stellfeld, J. Wohlfahrt, and M. Melbye**. 2003. Association between thimerosal-containing vaccine and autism. *JAMA* **290**:1763–1766.
40. **Hviid, A., M. Stellfeld, J. Wohlfahrt, and M. Melbye**. 2004. Childhood vaccination and type 1 diabetes. *N. Engl. J. Med.* **350**:1398–1404.
41. **Irving, P. M., and P. R. Gibson**. 2008. Infections and IBD. *Nat. Clin. Pract. Gastroenterol. Hepatol.* **5**:18–27.
42. **Jensen, H., C. S. Benn, I. M. Lisse, A. Rodrigues, P. K. Andersen, and P. Aaby**. 2007. Survival bias in observational studies of the impact of routine immunizations on childhood survival. *Trop. Med. Int. Health* **12**:5–14.
43. **Kannel, W. B., and R. D. Abbott**. 1984. Incidence and prognosis of unrecognized myocardial infarction. An update on the Framingham study. *N. Engl. J. Med.* **311**:1144–1147.
44. **Kjaer, S. K.** 1998. Risk factors for cervical neoplasia in Denmark. *APMIS Suppl.* **80**:1–41.
45. **Kjaer, S. K., A. J. van den Brule, G. Paull, E. I. Svare, M. E. Sherman, B. L. Thomsen, M. Suntum, J. E. Bock, P. A. Poll, and C. J. Meijer**. 2002. Type specific persistence of high risk

human papillomavirus (HPV) as indicator of high grade cervical squamous intraepithelial lesions in young women: population based prospective follow up study. *BMJ* **325**:572.

46. **Kristensen, I., P. Aaby, and H. Jensen**. 2000. Routine vaccinations and child survival: follow up study in Guinea-Bissau, West Africa. *BMJ* **321**:1435–1438.
47. **Larouze, B., G. Saimot, E. D. Lustbader, W. T. London, B. G. Werner, and M. Payet**. 1976. Host responses to hepatitis-B infection in patients with primary hepatic carcinoma and their families. A case/control study in Senegal, West Africa. *Lancet* **ii**:534–538.
48. **Löffler, E**. 1988. Mitteilungen aus den Kaiserliche Gesundheitsamt. Vol 11, 1884., p. 180. *In* D. T. Brock (ed.), *Robert Koch. A Life in Medicine and Bacteriology*. Science Technical Publishers, Madison, WI.
49. **Madsen, K. M., A. Hviid, M. Vestergaard, D. Schendel, J. Wohlfahrt, P. Thorsen, J. Olsen, and M. Melbye**. 2002. A population-based study of measles, mumps, and rubella vaccination and autism. *N. Engl. J. Med.* **347**:1477–1482.
50. **Mangione-Smith, R., M. N. Elliott, L. McDonald, and E. A. McGlynn**. 2002. An observational study of antibiotic prescribing behavior and the Hawthorne effect. *Health Serv. Res.* **37**:1603–1623.
51. **Marshall, B. J., J. A. Armstrong, D. B. McGechie, and R. J. Glancy**. 1985. Attempt to fulfill Koch's postulates for pyloric Campylobacter. *Med. J. Aust.* **142**:436–439.
52. **McDonald, K. L., S. I. Huq, L. M. Lix, A. B. Becker, and A. L. Kozyrskyj**. 2008. Delay in diphtheria, pertussis, tetanus vaccination is associated with a reduced risk of childhood asthma. *J. Allergy Clin. Immunol.* **121**:626–631.
53. **Melbye, M., P. M. Cook, H. Hjalgrim, K. Begtrup, G. R. Simpson, R. J. Biggar, P. Ebbesen, and T. F. Schulz**. 1998. Risk factors for Kaposi's-sarcoma-associated herpesvirus (KSHV/HHV-8) seropositivity in a cohort of homosexual men, 1981-1996. *Int. J. Cancer* **77**:543–548.
54. **Mishu, B., A. A. Ilyas, C. L. Koski, F. Vriesendorp, S. D. Cook, F. A. Mithen, and M. J. Blaser**. 1993. Serologic evidence of previous *Campylobacter jejuni* infection in patients with the Guillain-Barre syndrome. *Ann. Intern. Med.* **118**:947–953.
55. **Mølbak, K**. 2000. The epidemiology of diarrhoeal diseases in early childhood. A review of community studies in Guinea-Bissau. *Dan. Med. Bull.* **47**:340–358.
56. **Mølbak, K., M. Andersen, P. Aaby, N. Hojlyng, M. Jakobsen, M. Sodemann, and A. P. da Silva**. 1997. Cryptosporidium infection in infancy as a cause of malnutrition: a community study from Guinea-Bissau, west Africa. *Am. J. Clin. Nutr.* **65**:149–152.
57. **Mølbak, K., and A. H. Havelaar**. 2008. Burden of illness of campylobacteriosis and sequelae, p. 151–161. *In* I. Nachamkin, C. M. Szymanski, and M. J. Blaser (ed.), *Campylobacter*, 3rd ed. ASM Press, Washington, DC.
58. **Mølbak, K., N. Hojlyng, A. Gottschau, J. C. Sa, L. Ingholt, A. P. da Silva, and P. Aaby**. 1993. Cryptosporidiosis in infancy and childhood mortality in Guinea Bissau, West Africa. *BMJ* **307**:417–420.
59. **Nomura, A., G. N. Stemmermann, P. H. Chyou, G. I. Perez-Perez, and M. J. Blaser**. 1994. *Helicobacter pylori* infection and the risk for duodenal and gastric ulceration. *Ann. Intern. Med.* **120**:977–981.
60. **O'Brien, S. J., and R. A. Feldman**. 2003. Mortality associated with foodborne bacterial gastrointestinal infections: case selection and clinical data are important. *BMJ* **326**:1265.
61. **Osterholm, M. T., J. P. Davis, R. W. Gibson, J. S. Mandel, L. A. Wintermeyer, C. M. Helms, J. C. Forfang, J. Rondeau, and J. M. Vergeront**. 1982. Tri-state toxic-state syndrome study. I. Epidemiologic findings. *J. Infect. Dis.* **145**:431–440.
62. **Parravicini, C., S. J. Olsen, M. Capra, F. Poli, G. Sirchia, S. J. Gao, E. Berti, A. Nocera, E. Rossi, G. Bestetti, M. Pizzuto, M. Galli, M. Moroni, P. S. Moore, and M. Corbellino**. 1997. Risk of Kaposi's sarcoma-associated herpes virus transmission from donor allografts among Italian posttransplant Kaposi's sarcoma patients. *Blood* **90**:2826–2829.
63. **Parsonnet, J., G. D. Friedman, D. P. Vandersteen, Y. Chang, J. H. Vogelman, N. Orentreich, and R. K. Sibley**. 1991. *Helicobacter pylori* infection and the risk of gastric carcinoma. *N. Engl. J. Med.* **325**:1127–1131.
64. **Reeves, W. C., L. A. Brinton, M. Garcia, M. M. Brenes, R. Herrero, E. Gaitan, F. Tenorio, R. C. de Britton, and W. E. Rawls**. 1989. Human papillomavirus infection and cervical cancer in Latin America. *N. Engl. J. Med.* **320**:1437–1441.
65. **Rook, G. A., and L. R. Brunet**. 2002. Give us this day our daily germs. *Biologist* (London) **49**:145–149.
66. **Roth, A., M. Sodemann, H. Jensen, A. Poulsen, P. Gustafson, C. Weise, J. Gomes, Q. Djana, M. Jakobsen, M. L. Garly, A. Rodrigues, and P. Aaby**. 2006. Tuberculin reaction, BCG scar, and lower female mortality. *Epidemiology* **17**:562–568.
67. **Rothman, K. J., and S. Greenland**. 1998. Causation and causal inference, p. 7–28. *In* K. J. Rothman and S. Greenland (ed.), *Modern Epidemiology*. Lippincott-Raven, Philadelphia, PA.
68. **Rothman, K. J., and S. Greenland**. 1998. *Modern Epidemiology*. Lippincott-Raven, Philadelphia, PA.
69. **Sasazuki, S., M. Inoue, M. Iwasaki, T. Otani, S. Yamamoto, S. Ikeda, T. Hanaoka, and S. Tsugane**. 2006. Effect of *Helicobacter pylori* infection combined with CagA and pepsinogen status on gastric cancer development among Japanese men and women: a nested case-control study. *Cancer Epidemiol. Biomarkers Prev.* **15**:1341–1347.
70. **Schmidt, W. P., M. S. Van Der Loeff, P. Aaby, H. Whittle, R. Bakker, M. Buckner, F. Dias, and R. G. White**. 2008. Behaviour change and competitive exclusion can explain the diverging HIV-1 and HIV-2 prevalence trends in Guinea-Bissau. *Epidemiol. Infect.* **136**:551–561.
71. **Shands, K. N., G. P. Schmid, B. B. Dan, D. Blum, R. J. Guidotti, N. T. Hargrett, R. L. Anderson, D. L. Hill, C. V. Broome, J. D. Band, and D. W. Fraser**. 1980. Toxic-shock syndrome in menstruating women: association with tampon use and *Staphylococcus aureus* and clinical features in 52 cases. *N. Engl. J. Med.* **303**:1436–1442.
72. **Shepard, C. W., E. P. Simard, L. Finelli, A. E. Fiore, and B. P. Bell**. 2006. Hepatitis B virus infection: epidemiology and vaccination. *Epidemiol. Rev.* **28**:112–125.
73. **Smith, J. L., and D. Bayles**. 2007. Postinfectious irritable bowel syndrome: a long-term consequence of bacterial gastroenteritis. *J. Food Prot.* **70**:1762–1769.
74. **Spiller, R. C**. 2007. Role of infection in irritable bowel syndrome. *J. Gastroenterol.* **42**(Suppl. 17):41–47.
75. **Sytkowski, P. A., W. B. Kannel, and R. B. D'Agostino**. 1990. Changes in risk factors and the decline in mortality from cardiovascular disease. The Framingham Heart Study. *N. Engl. J. Med.* **322**:1635–1641.
76. **Tarimo, E**. 1991. Community-based studies in sub-Saharan Africa: an overview, p. 243–247. *In* R. G. Feachem and D. T. Jamison (ed.), *Disease and Mortality in Sub-Saharan Africa*. Oxford University Press, Oxford, United Kingdom.
77. **Trottier, H., and E. L. Franco**. 2006. The epidemiology of genital human papillomavirus infection. *Vaccine* **24**(Suppl. 1): S1–S15.
78. **Valentiner-Branth, P., H. Steinsland, T. K. Fischer, M. Perch, F. Scheutz, F. Dias, P. Aaby, K. Molbak, and H. Sommerfelt**.

2003. Cohort study of Guinean children: incidence, pathogenicity, conferred protection, and attributable risk for enteropathogens during the first 2 years of life. *J. Clin. Microbiol.* **41:**4238–4245.

79. **Vasto, S., G. Colonna-Romano, A. Larbi, A. Wikby, C. Caruso, and G. Pawelec.** 2007. Role of persistent CMV infection in configuring T cell immunity in the elderly. *Immun. Ageing* **4:**2.

80. **Veirum, J. E., M. Sodemann, S. Biai, M. Jakobsen, M. L. Garly, K. Hedegaard, H. Jensen, and P. Aaby.** 2005. Routine vaccinations associated with divergent effects on female and male mortality at the paediatric ward in Bissau, Guinea-Bissau. *Vaccine* **23:**1197–1204.

81. **Vestergaard, M., A. Hviid, K. M. Madsen, J. Wohlfahrt, P. Thorsen, D. Schendel, M. Melbye, and J. Olsen.** 2004. MMR vaccination and febrile seizures: evaluation of susceptible subgroups and long-term prognosis. *JAMA* **292:**351–357.

82. **Wakefield, A. J., S. H. Murch, A. Anthony, J. Linnell, D. M. Casson, M. Malik, M. Berelowitz, A. P. Dhillon, M. A. Thomson, P. Harvey, A. Valentine, S. E. Davies, and J. A. Walker-Smith.** 1998. Ileal-lymphoid-nodular hyperplasia, non-specific colitis, and pervasive developmental disorder in children. *Lancet* **351:**637–641.

83. **Walboomers, J. M., M. V. Jacobs, M. M. Manos, F. X. Bosch, J. A. Kummer, K. V. Shah, P. J. Snijders, J. Peto, C. J. Meijer, and N. Munoz.** 1999. Human papillomavirus is a necessary cause of invasive cervical cancer worldwide. *J. Pathol.* **189:**12–19.

84. **Wheeler, J. G., D. Sethi, J. M. Cowden, P. G. Wall, L. C. Rodrigues, D. S. Tompkins, M. J. Hudson, and P. J. Roderick.** 1999. Study of infectious intestinal disease in England: rates in the community, presenting to general practice, and reported to national surveillance. The Infectious Intestinal Disease Study Executive. *BMJ* **318:**1046–1050.

85. **Winer, J. B., R. A. Hughes, M. J. Anderson, D. M. Jones, H. Kangro, and R. P. Watkins.** 1988. A prospective study of acute idiopathic neuropathy. II. Antecedent events. *J. Neurol. Neurosurg. Psychiatry* **51:**613–618.

86. **Ylitalo, N., P. Sorensen, A. M. Josefsson, P. K. Magnusson, P. K. Andersen, J. Ponten, H. O. Adami, U. B. Gyllensten, and M. Melbye.** 2000. Consistent high viral load of human papillomavirus 16 and risk of cervical carcinoma in situ: a nested case-control study. *Lancet* **355:**2194–2198.

Sequelae and Long-Term Consequences of Infectious Diseases
Edited by Pina M. Fratamico, James L. Smith, and Kim A. Brogden

Chapter 28

Concluding Perspectives of Sequelae and Long-Term Consequences of Infectious Diseases—What's Next?

PINA M. FRATAMICO, JAMES L. SMITH, AND KIM A. BROGDEN

There are obstacles in establishing the concept that some infectious diseases may have sequelae with long-term consequences. As pointed out by Carbone in Chapter 1, these obstacles include (i) an impediment to demonstrating causal associations between an infectious agent and a chronic disease, (ii) technical barriers to identifying infectious causes of chronic disease, and (iii) psychological, sociological, and personal barriers to changing medical dogma. This book is an attempt to overcome the first obstacle and assess sequelae and long-term consequences of infectious diseases by bringing together a group of infectious disease experts who assess their own fields and identify the sequelae and consequences of acute and chronic infections caused by viruses, bacteria, fungi, and parasites. Here, we will briefly overview the sequelae of infectious agents, present the economic burdens associated with these infections, and suggest future directions to progress this concept.

Infectious diseases are the second leading cause of death worldwide and the third leading cause of death in the United States (7). They are also the leading cause of disability-adjusted life years or lost years of healthy life. In addition to the significant public health impact, infectious diseases and the associated complications and long-term consequences cause a substantial economic burden to society due to costs of medical care, decreased productivity, and days lost from work. For the most part, infections are self limiting or treatable. However, some infectious agents cause diseases that are not easily treatable or become chronic, and in a subset of patients, infections can lead to serious complications.

SEQUELAE AND LONG-TERM CONSEQUENCES OF INFECTIOUS DISEASES

Sequelae, of course, are the pathological conditions resulting from a prior disease. From the chapters in this book, it is obvious that sequelae differ, depending upon the etiologic agent (Table 1). However, they have a number of commonalities. First, sequelae often occur at a substantially later date, which is often weeks to years after the initial infection. Second, the underlying reasons for the sequelae are difficult to diagnose and very hard to link to the initial infection. Third, sequelae from a number of different infections are similar. Finally, some sequelae result from chronic inflammation and are very difficult to treat. Often the opportunity to eliminate the infectious microorganism is long past, leaving only the opportunity to treat the host's immunological and/or pathological reactions.

The consequences of long-term infectious diseases are yet to be fully realized. From the medical standpoint, Carbone in Chapter 1 points out that the initial proof of an infectious organism's causal link to a chronic disease often requires several years of research by various teams of researchers to isolate the organism, develop a reliable clinical test, and document the association of the organism with human disease through clinical studies. Thus, accurate documentation of infectious etiologies of chronic disease will help mainstream this concept. Her question is, then, how best to efficiently support high-quality, original, and creative hypothesis development and proof linking infectious pathogens to chronic diseases while first overcoming impediments and second avoiding erroneous associations as much as possible?

Pina M. Fratamico and James L. Smith • United States Department of Agriculture, Agricultural Research Service, Eastern Regional Research Center, 600 E. Mermaid Lane, Wyndmoor, PA 19038. **Kim A. Brogden** • Department of Periodontics and Dows Institute for Dental Research, College of Dentistry, N447 Dental Science Building, University of Iowa, Iowa City, IA 52242.

Table 1. Examples of sequelae induced by acute and chronic infections caused by viruses, bacteria, fungi, and parasites

Sequelae[a]	Infectious agent(s)	Chapter(s)
Aberrant pregnancy outcomes: intrauterine growth retardation, fetal demise, miscarriage	*Necator americanus, Ancylostoma duodenale*	17
Acute disseminated encephalomyelitis	Rubella, Measles virus, varicella virus, Epstein-Barr virus	18
Adrenal insufficiency	*Paracoccidioides brasiliensis*	23
Allergic diseases	*Trichophyton Microsporum Epidermophyton*	22
Alopecia	*Trichophyton Microsporum Epidermophyton*	22
Alzheimer's disease	*Chlamydia* species	3
Amyloid deposits	Prions	24
Ankylosing spondylitis	Enteric infections	4
Ankylosis of limb	*Dracunculus medinensis,* Guinea worm disease	17
Aortic aneurysms	*Treponema pallidum*	10
Arrhythmias	*Trichinella spiralis*	17
Arthritis	*Borrelia* species, *Dracunculus medinensis,* Guinea worm disease, rubella, *Coccidioides immitis*	2, 17, 18, 23
Arthritis (Reiter's syndrome)	*Neisseria* species	9
Ascending cholangitis	*Fasciola hepatica, Clonorchis sinensis, Opisthorchis* species	17
Asthma	*Chlamydia* species	3
Atherosclerosis	*Chlamydia* species	3
Autoeczematization	*Trichophyton Microsporum Epidermophyton*	22
Autoimmune hemolytic anemia	Epstein-Barr virus	18
Autoimmune thyroid disease	Enteric infections	4
Bacterial superinfections	*Dracunculus medinensis,* Guinea worm disease	17
Bile duct lithiasis	*Fasciola hepatica*	17
Biliary tract obstruction	*Ascaris lumbricoides, Trichuris trichiura*	17
Blindness	*Loa loa, Mansonella* species	17
Bronchial hyperreactivity	*Ascaris lumbricoides, Trichuris trichiura*	17
Cachexia	*Tropheryma whipplei*	11
Cardiac involvement	*Borrelia* species	2
Cellulitis	*Trichophyton Microsporum Epidermophyton*	22
Chagas heart disease	*Trypanosoma cruzi*	16
Chlorosis	*Necator americanus, Ancylostoma duodenale*	17
Cholangiocarcinoma	*Clonorchis sinensis* *Opisthorchis* species	17
Chronic acute gastritis	*Helicobacter* species	7
Chronic dermatitis	*Loa loa, Mansonella* species	17
Chronic diarrhea	Enteric infections, *Strongyloides stercoralis*	4, 5, 17
Chronic hepatobiliary disease	*Helicobacter* species	7
Chronic inflammation and disease	*Treponema pallidum, Chlamydia* species	3, 10
Chronic muscle pain	*Trichinella spiralis*	17
Chronic pyelonephritis	*Escherichia coli*	5
Chronic urticarial rashes	*Strongyloides stercoralis*	17
CNS inflammation	*Taenia solium*	13
Complicated seizures	*Plasmodium* species	15
Congenital toxoplasmosis	*Toxoplasma gondii*	12
Cor pulmonale	*Schistosoma haematobium*	17
Cranial neuritis	*Borrelia* species	2
Cranial osteoperiostitis	*Treponema pallidum*	10
Crohn's disease	*Escherichia coli, Mycobacterium* species	5, 8
CSF circulation dysfunction	*Taenia solium*	13
Cyclic fevers	*Plasmodium* species	15
Dementia and cognitive changes	*Tropheryma whipplei*	11
Digestive tract abnormalities	*Trypanosoma cruzi*	16
Disseminate gonococcal infection	*Neisseria* species	9
Electroencephalographic alterations	*Trichinella spiralis*	17
Encephalitis	*Toxoplasma gondii*	12

Continued

Table 1. *Continued*

Sequelae[a]	Infectious agent(s)	Chapter(s)
Endocarditis	*Neisseria* species, *Tropheryma whipplei*	9, 11
Endomyocardial fibrosis	*Loa loa, Mansonella* species	17
Epididymitis vasitis/infertility	*Neisseria* species	9
Epilepsy	*Taenia solium, Plasmodium* species	13, 15
Erythema migrans	*Borrelia* species	2
Ectopic pregnancy	*Neisseria* species	9
Failure to thrive	*Necator americanus, Ancylostoma duodenale*	17
Gallbladder carcinoma	Enteric infections	4
Gallbladder lithiasis	*Fasciola hepatica*	17
Gastric adenocarcinoma	*Helicobacter* species	7
Gastric MALT lymphoma	*Helicobacter* species	7
Gastroesophageal reflux disease	*Helicobacter* species	7
Glaucoma	*Onchocerca volvulus*	17
Glomerulonephritis	*Streptococcus/Staphylococcus*	6
Grand mal epilepsy	*Schistosoma japonicum*	17
Granulomatous lesions	*Histoplasma capsulatum*	23
Growth retardation in children	*Helicobacter* species	7
Guillain-Barré syndrome	Enteric infections, Epstein-Barr virus	4, 18
Gummatous osteomyelitis	*Treponema pallidum*	10
Hemolytic-uremic syndrome	*Escherichia coli*	5
Hydatid cyst	*Echinococcus* species	17
Hydroureter/hydronephrosis	*Schistosoma haematobium*	17
Idiopathic thrombocytopenic purpura	*Helicobacter* species	7
Immunosuppression	*Leishmania* species	16
Infective endocarditis	*Streptococcus/Staphylococcus*	6
Inflammatory bowel disease	*Escherichia coli, Mycobacterium* species	5, 8
Intellectual and cognitive impairment	*Necator americanus, Ancylostoma duodenale*	17
Intestinal obstruction	*Ascaris lumbricoides, Diphyllobothrium latum, Trichuris trichiura*	17
Intrahepatic pigment stones	*Clonorchis sinensis, Opisthorchis* species	17
Iron deficiency anemia	*Helicobacter* species, *Plasmodium* species, *Necator americanus, Ancylostoma duodenale, Schistosoma mansoni*	7, 15, 17
Irritable bowel disease	Enteric infections	4, 5
Ischemic heart disease	*Helicobacter* species	7
Keratitis	*Onchocerca volvulus*	17
Liver fibrosis	*Schistosoma mansoni*	17
Lymph node hypertrophy	*Paracoccidioides brasiliensis*	23
Lymphadenitis	*Loa loa, Mansonella* species	17
Lymphadenopathy	*Tropheryma whipplei*	11
Lymphedema	*Wuchereria bancrofti, Brugia malayi, Brugia timori*	17
Macular degeneration and depigmentation	*Chlamydia* species, *Treponema pallidum*	3, 10
Megaloblastic anemia	*Diphyllobothrium latum*	17
Meningitis	*Borrelia* species, *Escherichia coli, Neisseria* species, *Angiostrongylus cantonensis, Gnathostoma* species	2, 5, 9, 17
Micronutrient deficiencies	*Cryptosporidium*	14
Multiple sclerosis	*Chlamydia* species	3
Myalgias	*Tropheryma whipplei*	11
Myocardial infection	*Blastomyces dermatitidis*	23
Myocarditis	*Tropheryma whipplei*	11
Nerve paralysis (cranial, peripheral)	*Angiostrongylus cantonensis*	17
Nutritional deficiencies	*Ascaris lumbricoides, Trichuris trichiura*	17
Ocular toxoplasmosis	*Toxoplasma gondii*	12
Oligo- and polyarthralgias	*Tropheryma whipplei*	11
Osteomyelitis	*Coccidioides immitis*	23

Continued

Table 1. *Continued*

Sequelae[a]	Infectious agent(s)	Chapter(s)
PANDAS	*Streptococcus/Staphylococcus*	6
Paresthesias	*Angiostrongylus cantonensis*	17
Parkinson's disease	*Helicobacter* species	7
Pelvic inflammatory disease (endometritis, salpingitis)	*Chlamydia* species, *Neisseria* species	3, 9
Peptic ulcer disease	*Helicobacter* species	7
Periappendicitis	*Neisseria* species	9
Pericarditis	*Tropheryma whipplei*	11
Perihepatitis (Fitz-Hugh-Curtis syndrome)	*Neisseria* species	9
Periostitis of the long bones	*Treponema pallidum*	10
Peripheral neuropathy	*Diphyllobothrium latum*	17
Pneumonia	Influenza virus, measles virus	18
Portal hypertension	*Schistosoma mansoni, Schistosoma japonicum*	17
Prolonged dehydration and diarrhea	*Cryptosporidium* species	14
Psychiatric disturbances	*Loa loa, Mansonella* species	17
Pulmonary involvement (chronic cough, hemoptysis, pulmonary granulomas/calcifications, pleural thickening, and pulmonary hemorrhages)	*Paragonimus westermani, Paragonimus* species	17
Radiculitis	*Borrelia* species	2
Reactive arthritis	Enteric infections	4, 5
Recurrent urinary tract infections	*Escherichia coli*	5
Renal disease	Enteric infections	4
Renal failure	*Loa loa, Mansonella* species, *Schistosoma haematobium*	17
Respiratory disease	*Helicobacter* species	7
Retinitis	*Onchocerca volvulus*	17
Reye syndrome	Varicella	18
Rheumatic fever	*Streptococcus/Staphylococcus*	6
Rhinoscleroma and ozena	Enteric infections	4
Sacroiliitis	*Neisseria* species	9
Scarlet fever	*Streptococcus/Staphylococcus*	6
Seizures/visual disturbances	*Paragonimus westermani, Paragonimus* species	17
Severe combined degeneration	*Diphyllobothrium latum*	17
Spongiform encephalopathy	Prions	24
Squamous cell bladder carcinoma	*Schistosoma haematobium*	17
Supranuclear ophthalmoplegia	*Tropheryma whipplei*	11
Synovitis	*Dracunculus medinensis,* guinea worm disease	17
Syphilitic pseudo-rheumatism	*Treponema pallidum*	10
Tapir nose	*Leishmania* species	16
Toxic shock syndrome	*Streptococcus/Staphylococcus*	6
Transverse myelitis	*Schistosoma mansoni*	17
Tubal factor infertility	*Neisseria* species	9
Urethral stricture	*Neisseria* species	9
Vitamin B_{12} deficiency	*Helicobacter* species, *Diphyllobothrium latum*	7, 17

[a]CNS, central nervous system; CSF, cerebrospinal fluid; MALT, mucosa-associated lymphoid tissue; PANDAS, pediatric autoimmune neuropsychiatric disorders associated with streptococcal infections.

Even well-intended, well-designed scientific studies and techniques and their conclusions can be subverted by sampling and sample-processing procedures that go awry.

Etiology

There are many chronic syndromes and diseases for which there is a suspicion of an infectious etiology. For example, *Mycobacterium paratuberculosis* and possibly other pathogens could be triggers of inflammatory bowel disease or Crohn's disease (Table 1). Studies suggest that the onset of type 1 diabetes is accelerated in genetically susceptible individuals and may be triggered by rotavirus infection (11). Rotavirus may trigger pancreatic islet autoimmunity through a molecular mimicry process. Lorber points out possible links between infectious and "noninfectious" diseases and chronic illnesses (15–17). These include the association between nanobacteria and kidney stones, enteroviruses and insulin-dependent diabetes mellitus, and various types of infectious agents and mental disorders, including schizophrenia, bipolar disorder, depression, psychosis, Tourette's syndrome, obsessive compulsive disorder, and others.

It is estimated that less than one percent of microorganisms that can be observed by microscopy are culturable (26), and there are likely many organisms that may be involved in human diseases that have not yet been identified. A major stumbling block hindering the ability to associate specific microorganisms with chronic illnesses is our inability to culture the organism or to detect the presence of pathogens in affected tissues, for example, by using PCR to look for signature microbial sequences. However, although an organism may be detected in the diseased tissue, it does not necessarily prove causality; the causative organism may no longer be present in the affected site or may have initiated an infection in a location different than the diseased site. Uncovering the links between established, emerging, and hitherto unidentified microorganisms and chronic infections will require a multidisciplinary approach, involving microbiologists, geneticists, pathologists, epidemiologists, physicians, public health officials, and teams of researchers with different knowledge sets and skills. In Chapter 27, Mølbak highlights the importance of large-scale epidemiological studies and registry- or population-based research to investigate the associations between infectious exposures and chronic illnesses. Knowledge of the sequence of the human genome and of numerous microbial genomes and use of bioinformatics tools and DNA microarray technology to understand gene function and expression is leading to a greater understanding of microbial pathogenesis and host susceptibility to infectious diseases and related chronic illnesses.

Diagnosis

As pointed out by Carbone in Chapter 1, the modern medical community is getting better at identifying and linking new infectious agents to disease syndromes. Often the increase in incidence or prevalence of a syndrome is enough to trigger a medical search for the association of the symptoms with an underlying infectious agent. Recent advances include human immunodeficiency virus as the etiology of the acquired immunodeficiency syndrome; human coronavirus as the cause of severe acute respiratory syndrome: role of hepatitis B/C virus infection in liver cancer; role of human papilloma virus infection in cervical cancer; role of *Helicobacter pylori* in gastric cancer; and association of *Borrelia burgdorferi*, lymphoma, and Epstein-Barr virus infections with the formation of arthritis. It is estimated that approximately 16% of all cancers may be linked to a microbial agent (21). Continued investigation may link infection with *C. pneumoniae* to inflammation in allergic asthmatics (Hammerschlag et al. Chapter 3). Some infectious agents are eliminated easily, whereas others, like *B. burgdorferi* have been isolated sporadically by culture months to years after infection (Hovius et al., Chapter 2). As our ability to identify infectious agents, to diagnose infectious disease, and to delineate host responses improves, we will be able to more accurately determine if physiological, immunological, and pathological reactions have an underlying infectious disease etiology.

Treatment

Lyme disease is a controversial illness (Hovius et al., Chapter 2). The medical community is divided on whether the disease is easily diagnosed, treated, and cured (9, 25). Some groups, represented by the Infectious Diseases Society of America (IDSA), believe that the disease is relatively rare and easily treatable with a short course of antibiotics and that infection with *Borrelia* is rarely associated with chronic infection and long-term consequences. It has been suggested that persistent symptoms can be attributed to an autoimmune response to an eradicated infection. Other groups, represented by the International Lyme and Associated Diseases Society, argue that Lyme disease may persist after antibiotic treatment and become a chronic infection, leading to a range of medically unexplained symptoms beyond the known manifestations of late Lyme disease. These cases require long-term antibiotic treatment. However, a study by Klempner and coworkers (12) that was published in the *New England Journal of Medicine* in 2001 reported that prolonged treatment with antibiotics provided no further benefit to patients with chronic symptoms. Based on this study, the IDSA released new guidelines on the doses and durations of antimicrobial therapy recommended for treatment and prevention of Lyme disease, which limited treatment options for patients. Insurance companies denied antibiotic treatment beyond the 2- to 4-week IDSA limit. The study by Klempner and coworkers is being challenged, and several studies that were subsequently conducted showed some benefits of different antibiotic treatment regimes for chronic Lyme disease (25).

Economic Burden

From an economic standpoint, the costs associated with the short- and long-term consequences of disease can be excessive. Sexually transmitted diseases caused by agents, including *Chlamydia*, *Treponema*, *Neisseria*, hepatitis B virus, human papilloma virus, herpes simplex virus, and HIV, are excellent examples. In 2000, it was estimated that there were 9 million cases of STDs among people aged 15 to 24 years, and the cost of STDs among all age groups was estimated to be $9.3 to $15.5 billion in the United States, mainly associated with viral STDs (5). Thus, the economic burden due to STD infections is substantial. There is a need to educate people, particularly adolescents, about the risks for sexually transmitted diseases and the associated long-term sequelae.

Diarrheal diseases rank third among the leading infectious causes of death worldwide (7). Furthermore, a number of chronic sequelae may result from food- and water-borne infections. Some estimates indicate that 2 to 3% of food-borne disease cases may result in long-term consequences, and the public health impact and economic burden of these sequelae may be greater than those of the acute disease (14). Helms and coworkers (10) examined short- and long-term mortality associated with *Salmonella*, *Campylobacter*, *Yersinia*, and *Shigella* infections in 48,857 people suffering from these infections compared to 487,138 control subjects. Patients with gastrointestinal infections had 3.1 times higher mortality than controls, reflecting both acute and long-term sequelae of food-borne illness and the effect of underlying diseases. Frenzen estimated the annual direct costs related to Guillain-Barré syndrome (GBS) due to loss of productivity and premature death at about $1.7 billion ($1.6 to $1.9 billion) (8). The mean cost for a patient with GBS was $318,969 ($278,378 to $359,554). In 11 studies that examined stools of individuals (480 patients) with GBS at the onset of their neurologic symptoms, 27.5% were positive for *C. jejuni* (19). Therefore, the estimated cost of GBS due to *Campylobacter* infections would be $480 million, with a cost for each patient of $87,716.

Urinary tract infections are common and occur more frequently in women than in men. *Escherichia coli* is the cause of these infections in a high percentage of cases. Russo and Johnson (22) estimated that in the United States, the number of cases ranged from 6.5 to 8.3 million, with medical costs of approximately $1.5 billion. The annual direct costs attributed to irritable bowel syndrome (IBS) in the United States was $1.7 billion, with most of the medical costs due to hospitalization. The total indirect cost (loss in productivity due to absenteeism) was approximately $20 billion (1). Acute bacterial gastroenteritis has been linked to approximately 15% of IBS cases (23); therefore, the direct costs of postinfectious IBS would be approximately $255 million and the indirect costs, approximately $3 billion.

There is a strong genetic element associated with ankylosing spondylitis (AS); however, the illness may also have a microbial trigger. *Klebsiella pneumoniae* infection has been suggested as a triggering or perpetuating factor in the pathogenesis of AS through a molecular mimicry process. A survey by Kobelt and coworkers, examining 1,413 patients with AS in the United Kingdom, was conducted to investigate the burden of the disease in terms of cost and to estimate the cost-effectiveness of treatment with infliximab (13). The annual mean total direct cost per patient was estimated at £2,853, and the total indirect cost per patient was £3,913, giving a total cost of £6,765. For patients treated with infliximab, there was a reduction in costs of 31%, excluding treatment, and the total gain in quality of life was calculated at 0.175, equivalent to 2 months of full health.

OTHER CHALLENGES AND FUTURE DIRECTIONS

Polymicrobial Diseases

The sequelae and long-term consequences of infectious disease induced by a single etiologic infectious agent were portrayed in this book in a reductionist format. However, we realize that many infections can occur in polymicrobial formats either concurrently or sequentially. Polymicrobial diseases represent the clinical and pathological manifestations induced by the presence of multiple microorganisms (3, 4). These diseases result from multiple viral infections (e.g., multiple hepatotropic viral infections, multiple retroviral infections, viruses associated with multiple sclerosis, etc.), multiple bacterial infections (e.g., bacterial vaginosis, periodontal disease, abscesses, etc.), diseases involving viruses and bacteria (e.g., respiratory disease, otitis media, intestinal disorders, etc.), and multiple mycotic infections. Often stress, physiologic abnormalities, and metabolic disease favor the colonization of multiple organisms.

It is not known what sequelae or long-term consequences will result from these infections. It is likely that the downstream consequences will be additive across many of the infectious agents and increasingly complex in nature.

Biofilms as a Source of Continual Infection

Infections involving biofilms will likely have sequelae. Biofilms are a common cause of persistent infections (6, 20). Here, bacteria attach and aggregate in polymeric matrixes on various mucosal surfaces (2, 24,

27). Organisms in these communities are more resistant to antimicrobial agents and host defense mechanisms (18). They also are a source of continual release of microorganisms in a planktonic state and may induce continual chemokine and cytokine release.

CONCLUSIONS

Indeed, the chapters in this text have given emphasis to the transmissible agents that play important roles in diseases that were not known to be infectious in origin. Furthermore, there are a large number of putative associations between microbes and chronic illnesses that are strongly suspected and must be proved or disproved by rigorous research. Some of these links may be proved wrong; however, if they are substantiated, such as the association of *H. pylori* and ulcers, these findings will lead to new treatments and prevention strategies for various types of cancers and chronic illnesses, including the development of new vaccines. These developments are keenly awaited.

REFERENCES

1. **American Gastroenterological Association.** 2001. The burden of gastrointestinal diseases. http://www.gastro.org/clinicalRes/pdf/burden-report.pdf. Accessed 15 August 2008.
2. **Anderson, G. G., J. J. Palermo, J. D. Schilling, R. Roth, J. Heuser, and S. J. Hultgren.** 2003. Intracellular bacterial biofilm-like pods in urinary tract infections. *Science* **301:**105–107.
3. **Brogden, K. A., and J. M. Guthmiller** (ed.). 2002. *Polymicrobial Diseases.* ASM Press, Washington, DC.
4. **Brogden, K. A., and J. M. Guthmiller.** 2003. Polymicrobial diseases, a concept whose time has come. *ASM News* **69:**69–73.
5. **Chesson, H. W., J. M. Blandford, T. L. Gift, G. Tao, and K. L. Irwin.** 2004. The estimated direct medical cost of sexually transmitted diseases among American youth, 2000. *Perspect. Sex. Reprod. Health* **36:**11–19.
6. **Costerton, J. W., P. S. Stewart, and E. P. Greenberg.** 1999. Bacterial biofilms: a common cause of persistent infections. *Science* **284:**1318–1322.
7. **Fauci, A. S.** 2001. Infectious diseases: considerations for the 21st century. *Clin. Infect. Dis.* **32:**675–685.
8. **Frenzen, P. D.** 2008. Economic cost of Guillain-Barré syndrome in the United States. *Neurology* **71:**21–27.
9. **Halperin, J. J.** 2008. Prolonged Lyme disease treatment: enough is enough. *Neurology* **70:**986–987.
10. **Helms, M., P. Vastrup, P. Gerner-Smidt, and K. Molbak.** 2003. Short and long term mortality associated with foodborne bacterial gastrointestinal infections: registry based study. *Brit. Med. J.* **326:**357.
11. **Honeyman, M. C., B. S. Coulson, N. L. Stone, S. A. Gellert, P. N. Goldwater, C. E. Steele, J. J. Couper, B. D. Tait, P. G. Colman, and L. C. Harrison.** 2000. Association between rotavirus infection and pancreatic islet autoimmunity in children at risk of developing type 1 diabetes. *Diabetes* **49:**1319–1324.
12. **Klempner, M. S., L. T. Hu, J. Evans, C. H. Schmid, G. M. Johnson, R. P. Trevino, D. Norton, L. Levy, D. Wall, J. McCall, M. Kosinski, and A. Weinstein.** 2001. Two controlled trials of antibiotic treatment in patients with persistent symptoms and a history of Lyme disease. *N. Engl. J. Med.* **345:**85–92.
13. **Kobelt, G., P. Andlin-Sobocki, S. Brophy, L. Jonsson, A. Calin, and J. Braun.** 2004. The burden of ankylosing spondylitis and the cost-effectiveness of treatment with infliximab (Remicade). *Rheumatology* **43:**1158–1166.
14. **Lindsay, J. A.** 1997. Chronic sequelae of foodborne disease. *Emerg. Infect. Dis.* **3:**443–452.
15. **Lorber, B.** 1996. Are all diseases infectious? *Ann. Intern. Med.* **125:**844–851.
16. **Lorber, B.** 1999. Are all diseases infectious? Another look. *Ann. Intern. Med.* **131:**989–990.
17. **Lorber, B.** 2005. Infection and mental illness: do bugs make us batty? *Anaerobe* **11:**303–307.
18. **Mah, T. F., and G. A. O'Toole.** 2001. Mechanisms of biofilm resistance to antimicrobial agents. *Trends Microbiol.* **9:**34–39.
19. **Nachamkin, I., B. M. Allos, and T. W. Ho.** 2000. *Camypylobacter jejuni* infection and the association with Guillain-Barré syndrome, p. 155–175. *In* I. Nachamkin and M. L. Blaser (ed.), *Campylobacter*, 2nd ed. ASM Press, Washington, DC.
20. **Parsek, M. R., and P. K. Singh.** 2003. Bacterial biofilms: an emerging link to disease pathogenesis. *Annu. Rev. Microbiol.* **57:**677–701.
21. **Pisani, P., D. M. Parkin, N. Munoz, and J. Ferlay.** 1997. Cancer and infection: estimates of the attributable fraction in 1990. *Cancer Epidemiol. Biomarkers Prev.* **6:**387–400.
22. **Russo, T. A., and J. R. Johnson.** 2003. Medical and economic impact of extraintestinal infections due to *Escherichia coli:* focus on an increasingly important endemic problem. *Microbes Infect.* **5:**449–456.
23. **Smith, J. L., and D. Bayles.** 2007. Postinfectious irritable bowel syndrome: a long-term consequence of bacterial gastroenteritis. *J. Food Prot.* **70:**1762–1769.
24. **Starner, T. D., N. Zhang, G. Kim, M. A. Apicella, and P. B. McCray, Jr.** 2006. *Haemophilus influenzae* forms biofilms on airway epithelia: implications in cystic fibrosis. *Am. J. Respir. Crit. Care Med.* **174:**213–220.
25. **Stricker, R. B., and L. Johnson.** 2007. Lyme disease: a turning point. *Expert Rev. Anti Infect. Ther.* **5:**759–762.
26. **Torsvik, V., and L. Ovreas.** 2002. Microbial diversity and function in soil: from genes to ecosystems. *Curr. Opin. Microbiol.* **5:**240–245.
27. **Veeh, R. H., M. E. Shirtliff, J. R. Petik, J. A. Flood, C. C. Davis, J. L. Seymour, M. A. Hansmann, K. M. Kerr, M. E. Pasmore, and J. W. Costerton.** 2003. Detection of *Staphylococcus aureus* biofilm on tampons and menses components. *J. Infect. Dis.* **188:**519–530.

INDEX